Comprehensive Respiratory Care

Comprehensive Respiratory Care

◆

David R. Dantzker, M.D.
President and Chief Executive Officer
Long Island Jewish Medical Center
New Hyde Park, New York
Professor of Medicine
Albert Einstein College of Medicine
New York, New York

Neil R. MacIntyre, M.D.
Associate Professor of Medicine
Duke University Medical Center
Durham, North Carolina

Eric D. Bakow, M.A., R.R.T.
Director, Department of Respiratory Care and Neurodiagnostics
University of Pittsburgh Medical Center
Pittsburgh, Pennsylvania

W.B. SAUNDERS COMPANY
A Division of Harcourt Brace & Company
Philadelphia London Toronto Montreal Sydney Tokyo

W.B. SAUNDERS COMPANY
A Division of
Harcourt Brace & Company

The Curtis Center
Independence Square West
Philadelphia, Pennsylvania 19106

Library of Congress Cataloging-in-Publication Data

Comprehensive respiratory care / [edited by] David R. Dantzker, Neil R. MacIntyre, Eric D. Bakow; with 74 contributors.—1st ed.

  p.   cm.

Includes bibliographical references and index.

ISBN 0–7216–2844–3

1. Respiratory therapy.   2. Respiratory organs—Diseases.
    3. Pulmonary manifestations of general diseases.
I. Dantzker, David R.   II. MacIntyre, Neil R.
III. Bakow, Eric D.

[DNLM: 1. Respiratory Tract Diseases—therapy.
2. Respiratory Therapy.   WF 140 C737 1995]

RC735.I5C65 1995

616.2′0046—dc20
DNLM/DLC   94–34397

COMPREHENSIVE RESPIRATORY CARE   ISBN 0–7216–2844–3

Printed in the United States of America.

Last digit is the print number: 9   8   7   6   5   4   3   2   1

To my wife, Sherrye Roberta Dantzker,
whose contributions are incalculable

DD

To my wife, Suzanne, and my children

NM

To Cindy and Justin,
for the smile they bring to my life

EB

Contributors

Delorese Ambrose, Ed.D.
Adjunct Professor of Management, Carnegie Mellon University, Heinz
School of Public Policy and Management, Pittsburgh, Pennsylvania
Managing Organizational Change

Eric D. Bakow, M.A., R.R.T.
Director, Department of Respiratory Care, University of Pittsburgh
Medical Center, Pittsburgh, Pennsylvania
*Bronchial Hygiene; Atelectasis: Pathophysiology and Treatment;
Management Principles*

Arthur S. Banner, M.D.
Adjunct Associate Professor of Medicine, Dartmouth Medical School;
Lecturer, Harvard Medical School; Veterans Affairs Medical Center,
Manchester, New Hampshire
Physical Examination

James R. Bengtson, M.D., M.P.H.
Director of Research, Michigan Heart and Vascular Institute, Ann
Arbor, Michigan
Myocardial Ischemia

Morris I. Bierman, M.D.
Assistant Professor, Department of Anesthesiology/Critical Care
Medicine, University of Pittsburgh; Director, Cardiothoracic Surgical
Intensive Care Unit, Presbyterian University Hospital, Pittsburgh,
Pennsylvania
Respiratory Monitoring

Nicholas G. Bircher, M.D., F.C.C.M.
Assistant Professor of Anesthesiology and Critical Care Medicine,
University of Pittsburgh; Associate Director, Surgical Intensive Care
Unit and Staff Anesthesiologist, Montefiore University Hospital,
University of Pittsburgh Medical Center, Pittsburgh, Pennsylvania
Cardiopulmonary Resuscitation

Stephen Blumberg, M.D.
Attending Physician, Department of Cardiology, Long Island Jewish
Medical Center, New Hyde Park, New York
Electrocardiography

Charles W. Boig, Jr., R.R.T.
Home Care Educator/Discharge Planner, Children's Hospital of Pittsburgh, Pittsburgh, Pennsylvania
Pediatric Respiratory Care

Thomas H. Breedlove
DeVry Technical Institute, Electronics Engineering and Rollins College, Winter Park, Florida
Managing Quality in Health Care

Suzanne M. Burns, R.N., M.S.N., R.R.T., C.C.R.N.
Practitioner/Teacher and Assistant Professor of Nursing and Critical Care, University of Virginia School of Nursing, University of Virginia Health Sciences Center; Practitioner/Teacher-Clinician V MICU, Charlottesville, Virginia
Clinical Application of Laboratory Examinations

Paul W. Burrowes, M.D., F.R.C.P.(C.)
Clinical Assistant Professor, Faculty of Medicine, Department of Radiology, University of Calgary, Calgary, Alberta, Canada; Active Staff, Department of Radiology, Foothills Hospital, Calgary, Alberta, Canada
Conventional Chest Radiography

Robert L. Chatburn, R.R.T.
Instructor, Department of Pediatrics, Case Western Reserve University; Director, Respiratory Care Department, Rainbow Babies and Children's Hospital, University Hospitals of Cleveland, Cleveland, Ohio
Research and Statistics for the Clinician

Donald E. Craven, M.D.
Professor of Medicine and Epidemiology, Boston University Schools of Medicine and Public Health; Director, Clinical AIDS Program, Boston City Hospital, Boston, Massachusetts
Nosocomial Respiratory Tract Infection: Perspectives for Prevention and Respiratory Care

Philip B. Crosby
Member, Board of Trustees, Rollins College; Former Member, Board of Directors, Winter Park Memorial Hospital, Winter Park, Florida
Managing Quality in Health Care

Gilbert E. D'Alonzo, D.O.
Professor of Medicine, Department of Medicine, Division of Pulmonary and Critical Care Medicine, Temple University School; Attending Physician, Temple University Hospital, Philadelphia, Pennsylvania
Pulmonary Thromboembolic Disease

David R. Dantzker, M.D.
President and Chief Executive Officer, Long Island Jewish Medical Center, New Hyde Park, New York; Professor of Medicine, Albert Einstein College of Medicine, New York, New York
Lung Anatomy and Development; Respiratory Muscles; Pulmonary

Gas Exchange; Ventilatory Control; Tissue Oxygen Delivery; Obstructive Lung Disease; Respiratory Failure; Cor Pulmonale and Pulmonary Hypertension

R. Phillip Dellinger, M.D.
Professor and Chief, Division of Pulmonary and Critical Care Medicine, University Hospitals and Clinics, and Harry S. Truman Veterans Hospital, Columbia, Missouri
General Management Principles of Poisoning and Overdose

Michael A. DeVita, M.D.
Assistant Professor, Department of Anesthesiology/Critical Care Medicine and Medicine, University of Pittsburgh; Medical Director, Surgical Intensive Care Unit, Montefiore University Hospital, University of Pittsburgh Medical Center, Pittsburgh, Pennsylvania
Neuromuscular Disorders

Charles G. Durbin, Jr., M.D.
Professor of Anesthesiology and Surgery, University of Virginia Health Sciences Center; Medical Director, Respiratory Care, and Medical Director, Surgical Intensive Care Unit, University of Virginia Health Sciences Center, Charlottesville, Virginia
Hemodynamic Monitoring

Steven J. L. Evans, M.D.
Assistant Professor of Medicine, Albert Einstein College of Medicine, New York, New York; Director, Department of Cardiac Electrophysiology, Long Island Jewish Hospital, New Hyde Park, New York
Electrocardiography

John Frank, R.R.T.
Clinical Specialist, Respironics, Murryville; Formerly Supervisor, Respiratory Therapy, Children's Hospital of Pittsburgh, Pittsburgh, Pennsylvania
Pediatric Respiratory Care

David J. Frid, M.D.
Assistant Professor of Medicine, Division of Cardiology, The Ohio State University; Director, Department of Preventive and Rehabilitative Cardiology, The Ohio State University Medical Center, Columbus, Ohio
Cardiovascular Anatomy and Physiology

William K. Fulkerson, M.D.
Associate Professor of Medicine, Duke University School of Medicine, Durham, North Carolina
Barotrauma in Mechanical Ventilation

Michael S. Gorback, M.D.
Assistant Consulting Professor of Anesthesiology, Duke University Medical Center, Durham, North Carolina; Anesthesiologist, WCA Hospital, Jamestown, New York
Airway Management

Mark E. Hamer, M.D.
Fellow in Cardiology, Duke University Medical Center, Durham, North Carolina
Myocardial Ischemia

David K. Handshoe, M.D.
Director, Intensive Care Unit, Trident Regional Medical Center, Charleston, South Carolina
Barotrauma in Mechanical Ventilation

Sunil Hegde, M.D.
Medical Director for Rehabilitation, Huntington Memorial Hospital, Pasadena, California
Neuromuscular Disorders

Dean Hess, M.Ed., R.R.T.
Instructor in Anesthesia, Harvard Medical School; Assistant Director of Respiratory Care, Massachusetts General Hospital, Boston, Massachusetts
Aerosol Therapy; Research and Statistics for the Clinician

George H. Hicks, M.S., R.R.T.
Instructor and Clinical Coordinator, Allied Health Division, Mt. Hood Community College, Gresham, Oregon
Blood Gas and Acid-Base Measurement

Jay A. Johannigman, M.D., F.A.C.S.
Assistant Professor of Surgery, Uniformed Services University of the Health Sciences, Bethesda, Maryland; Director, Surgical Critical Care Services, and Staff Trauma Surgeon, Wilford Hall Medical Center, Lackland Air Force Base, San Antonio, Texas
Respiratory Care

Amal Jubran, M.D.
Assistant Professor of Medicine, Division of Pulmonary and Critical Care Medicine, Loyola University of Chicago, Stritch School of Medicine and Edward Hines, Jr., Veterans Administration Hospital, Hines, Illinois
Aspiration Pneumonia

Peter S. Kussin, M.D.
Assistant Professor of Medicine, Division of Pulmonary Critical Care Medicine, Duke University Medical Center, Durham, North Carolina
Dyspnea: Pathophysiology and Clinical Evaluation; Respiratory Tract Infections

Stephen E. Lammers, B.A., M.A., Ph.D.
Helen H.P. Manson Professor, Religion Department, Lafayette College, Easton, Pennsylvania; Ethics Consultant, Lehigh Valley Hospital, Allentown, Pennsylvania
Ethics and Patient Care

Nelson E. Leatherman, Ph.D. Bioengineering
Research Associate, Duke University Medical Center, Durham, North Carolina
Pulmonary Rehabilitation

R. Alan Leonard, R.R.T.
Assistant Director, Respiratory Care Services, Duke University
Medical Center, Durham, North Carolina
*Unconventional Support Techniques for Ventilation and Oxygenation;
Pathophysiology-Based Approach to Neonatal Respiratory Care*

Ann Parks Linn, BSJ
The Creative Factory, Winter Park, Florida
Managing Quality in Health Care

J. Peter Longabaugh, M.D.
Ward Instructor, Duke University; Attending Physician, St. Joseph
Mercy Hospital, Ypsilanti, Michigan
Myocardial Ischemia

John M. Luce, M.D.
Professor of Medicine and Anesthesia, University of California;
Associate Director, Medical-Surgical Intensive Care Unit, San
Francisco General Hospital, San Francisco, California
Neurologic Monitoring

Jane Luchsinger, M.S., R.P.F.T.
Instructor, State University of New York at Stony Brook, Stony Brook,
New York; Director, Pulmonary Function Laboratory, Long Island
Jewish Medical Center, New Hyde Park, New York
Pulmonary Function Testing

Neil R. MacIntyre, M.D.
Associate Professor of Medicine, Duke University Medical Center,
Durham, North Carolina
*Mechanical Ventilatory Support; Oxygenation Support;
Unconventional Support Techniques for Ventilation and Oxygenation;
Weaning Mechanical Ventilatory Support*

Vincent F. Maher, Esq., J.D., M.S., M.A., R.N., C.R.N.A.
Associate Professor of Health Care Programs, Iona College, New
Rochelle, New York
Legal Aspects of Critical Care

Rich Malloy, R.R.T.
Chief of Cardiopulmonary Care, Fox Chase Cancer Center,
Philadelphia, Pennsylvania
Oxygen Therapy

James R. Mault, M.D.
Chief Resident, Department of General and Thoracic Surgery, Duke
University Medical Center, Durham, North Carolina
Nutrition

Susan L. McInturff, R.C.P., R.R.T.
Clinical Director, Bay Area Home Health Care, Novato, California
Home Care

Jon N. Meliones, M.D.
Associate Professor of Pediatrics and Anesthesia, Duke University
Medical School; Director, Pediatric Intensive Care Unit and Pediatric
Respiratory Care, Duke University Medical Center, Durham, North
Carolina
Pathophysiology-Based Approach to Neonatal Respiratory Care

Richard E. Moon, M.D., F.A.C.P., F.C.C.P., F.R.C.P.(C.)
Associate Professor, Department of Anesthesiology, and Assistant
Professor, Department of Pulmonary Medicine, Duke University;
Attending Anesthesiologist and Pulmonologist Medical Director,
Hyperbaric Center, Duke University Medical Center, Durham, North
Carolina
Hyperbaric Oxygen Therapy

Rodolfo Morice, M.D.
Associate Professor and Chief, Pulmonary and Critical Care Medicine
Section, The University of Texas M.D. Anderson Cancer Center,
Houston, Texas
Pleural Effusion

Edward F. Patz, Jr., M.D.
Assistant Professor of Radiology, Duke University Medical School,
Durham, North Carolina
Newer Imaging Techniques in the Thorax

Margarete Pierce, R.R.T., C.P.F.T.
Chief Respiratory Therapist, Fox Chase Cancer Center, Philadelphia,
Pennsylvania
Oxygen Therapy

Isaac Raijman, M.D.
Assistant Professor of Medicine, University of Texas Health Science
Center; Director, Therapeutic Endoscopy, University of Texas; Clinical
Assistant Professor, M.D. Anderson Cancer Center, Houston, Texas
Gastrointestinal Emergencies in the Intensive Care Unit

Carl E. Ravin, M.D.
Professor of Radiology and Chairman, Department of Radiology, Duke
University Medical Center, Durham, North Carolina
Conventional Chest Radiography

Michael Rhodes, M.D., F.A.C.S., F.C.C.M.
Associate Professor of Clinical Surgery and Chief, Division of Trauma
and Surgical Critical Care, Hahnemann University, Philadelphia,
Pennsylvania
Trauma

David D. Rice, Ph.D., R.R.T.
Associate Professor and Assistant Dean, Health and Human Service
Division, National-Louis University Evanston, Illinois
Patient, Community, and Staff Education

Leonard J. Rossoff, M.D.
Assistant Professor of Medicine, Albert Einstein College of Medicine,
New York, New York; Section Head, Department of Pulmonary

Medicine, Long Island Jewish Medical Center, New Hyde Park, New York
Cough

Scott L. Roth, M.D., F.A.C.C.
Clinical Instructor in Medicine, Albert Einstein College of Medicine, New York, New York; Staff Cardiologist and Director, Adult Electrocardiography, Long Island Jewish Medical Center, New Hyde Park, New York
Congestive Heart Failure

Wayne M. Samuelson, M.D.
Assistant Professor, Duke University Medical Center, Durham, North Carolina
Barotrauma in Mechanical Ventilation

A. Saville, R.R.T.
Supervisor of Clinical Education and Respiratory Therapy, Children's Hospital of Pittsburgh, Pittsburgh, Pennsylvania
Pediatric Respiratory Care

E. Neil Schachter, M.D.
Professor of Medicine and Community Medicine, Mount Sinai School of Medicine; Medical Director, Department of Respiratory Therapy, Mount Sinai Medical Center, New York, New York
Respiratory Care Pharmacology

Larry D. Scott, M.D.
Professor of Medicine, University of Texas-Houston Health Science Center, Houston, Texas
Gastrointestinal Emergencies in the Intensive Care Unit

Evelyn Shearer-Poor, M.D.
Assistant Professor of Medicine, Division of Pulmonary and Critical Care Medicine, University of Texas-Houston Health Science Center, Houston, Texas
Dyspnea: Pathophysiology and Clinical Evaluation

Stuart Sheifer, B.A.
Medical Student, Duke University Medical School, Durham, North Carolina
Cardiovascular Anatomy and Physiology

Alan R. Spitzer, M.D.
Professor of Pediatrics and Vice Chairman, Department of Pediatrics, Thomas Jefferson University; Pediatrician-in-Chief and Director, Division of Neonatology, Thomas Jefferson University Hospital, Philadelphia, Pennsylvania
Pathophysiology-Based Approach to Neonatal Respiratory Care

Kathleen A. Steger, R.N., M.P.H.
Assistant Professor of Public Health, Boston University School of Public Health; Associate Director, Clinical AIDS Program, Boston City Hospital, Boston, Massachusetts
Nosocomial Respiratory Tract Infection: Perspectives for Prevention and Respiratory Care

Harry Steinberg, M.D.
Associate Professor, Albert Einstein College of Medicine, New York, New York; Attending Physician and Chief, Division of Pulmonary and Critical Care Medicine, Long Island Jewish Medical Center, New Hyde Park, New York
Pulmonary Function Testing

Victor F. Tapson, M.D.
Assistant Professor of Medicine, Division of Pulmonary and Critical Care Medicine, Duke University Medical Center; Medical Director, Duke Lung Transplant Program; Director, Duke Pulmonary Clinic, Durham, North Carolina
Respiratory Tract Infections

Catherine S. Thompson, M.D.
Attending Nephrologist, Virginia Mason Hospital, Seattle, Washington
Acid-Base Disorders and Electrolyte Imbalance

Jonathon Truwit, M.D.
Assistant Professor of Medicine, University of Virginia; Director of Medical Intensive Care Unit, University of Virginia Health Sciences Center, Charlottesville, Virginia
Lung Mechanics

Shekhar T. Venkataraman, M.D.
Assistant Professor, Departments of Anesthesiology/Critical Care Medicine and Pediatrics, School of Medicine, University of Pittsburgh; Medical Director, Respiratory Care, Children's Hospital of Pittsburgh, Pittsburgh, Pennsylvania
Pediatric Respiratory Care

Joseph E. Vincent, M.D.
Chief, Pulmonary Section, Lehigh Valley Hospital, Allentown, Pennsylvania
Ethics and Patient Care

John D. Wagner, M.D.
Assistant Professor of Medicine, Albert Einstein College of Medicine, New York, New York; Head, Section of Nephrology, Long Island Jewish Medical Center, New Hyde Park, New York
Acute Renal Failure

Barbara G. Wilson, R.R.T., M.Ed.
Research Associate, Pediatric Critical Care and Respiratory Care Services, Duke University Medical Center, Durham, North Carolina
Pathophysiology-Based Approach to Neonatal Respiratory Care

Drew Wiltsie, R.R.T.
Clinical Educator, Respiratory Therapy, Children's Hospital of Pittsburgh, Pittsburgh, Pennsylvania
Pediatric Respiratory Care

Theodore J. Witek, Jr., Dr.P.H., R.R.T.
Research Assistant and Professor of Medicine and Community Medicine, Mount Sinai School of Medicine; Associate Director, Clinical

Research, Pulmonary Group, Boehringer Ingelheim Pharmaceuticals, Inc., New York, New York
Respiratory Care Pharmacology

Karl Yang, M.D.
Assistant Professor, University of Texas Medical School at Houston; Director, Hermann Sleep Disorder Laboratory, Houston, Texas
Sleep and Sleep-Disordered Breathing

Preface

The care of the patient with acute or chronic respiratory disease has become an increasingly complex matter. Our knowledge base has dramatically increased and the technology available for support, monitoring, and diagnosis has been revolutionized. Because of this, not only is a clear understanding of the traditional disciplines such as physiology and pharmacology required, but also a familiarity with subjects as diverse as biomedical engineering and molecular biology.

Patient care is increasingly being delivered by teams of professionals. This requires that each discipline appreciate the skills brought to the effort by the other members of the team, and it requires a blending and focusing of all these individual talents toward the successful care of the patient.

Individuals with respiratory illnesses rarely have isolated lung dysfunction. Thus, a clear appreciation of how disorders of other organ systems can complicate lung dysfunction or act as a primary cause of abnormal lung function is mandatory to the correct approach to the patient.

These considerations have been the driving forces in the development of *Comprehensive Respiratory Care*. By expanding the scope beyond the traditional areas covered in textbooks devoted to respiratory care, we hope to increase the book's usefulness to practitioners from all disciplines. By drawing on the expertise of people from many specialties, we hope to make it relevant to daily practice.

DAVID R. DANTZKER, M.D.
NEIL R. MACINTYRE, M.D.
ERIC D. BAKOW, M.A., R.R.T.

Acknowledgment

The production of a new book, especially one with the scope of *Comprehensive Respiratory Care*, requires the input of many people with varied talents. Unfortunately they often labor in anonymity despite the major contributions they make. We have been fortunate in having a dedicated group of specialists at the W. B. Saunders Company without whose help this project would never have been completed. We would like to recognize Evelyn Weiman and Elizabeth Gauger for their copy editing, Bruce Franklin for his production help, and Joan Wendt and Kathleen Fisher for their artistic contributions to the design and illustrations. We would especially like to thank our editors, Lisa Biello and Les Hoeltzel, who stuck with the project through thick and thin and without whose encouragement this undertaking might never have reached fruition.

DAVID R. DANTZKER, M.D.
NEIL R. MacINTYRE, M.D.
ERIC D. BAKOW, M.A., R.R.T.

Contents

SECTION **II**

DIAGNOSTIC TECHNIQUES

52 **Respiratory Care Pharmacology** 972

E. Neil Schachter, M.D. and
Theodore J. Witek, Jr., Dr. P.H., R.R.T.

53 **Pediatric Respiratory Care** 1004

Shekhar T. Venkataraman, M.D.,
A. Saville, R.R.T.,
Drew Wiltsie, R.R.T.,
John Frank, R.R.T., and
Charles W. Boig, Jr., R.R.T.

54 **Pathophysiology-Based Approach to
Neonatal Respiratory Care** 1033

Jon N. Meliones, M.D.,
Barbara G. Wilson, R.R.T., M.Ed.,
R. Alan Leonard, R.R.T., and
Alan R. Spitzer, M.D.

58 Ethics and Patient Care 1153
Joseph E. Vincent, M.D. and
Stephen E. Lammers, B.A., M.A., Ph.D.

59 Legal Aspects of Clinical Care 1182
Vincent F. Maher, Esq., J.D., M.S., M.A., R.N., C.R.N.A.

60 Patient, Community, and Staff Education 1191
David D. Rice, Ph.D., R.R.T.

SECTION V

RESPIRATORY THERAPY DEPARTMENT MANAGEMENT

Fundamentals of Anatomy and Physiology

1

⬛⚪

Lung Anatomy and Development

David R. Dantzker, M.D.

The lung, which plays a central role in the maintenance of body homeostasis, serves as

- A filter for the bloodstream
- An active metabolic organ, producing and inactivating important biologic substances
- A storage place for chemical mediators and various circulating cells

In its most obvious and important role, that of a gas exchanger, it facilitates the transfer of carbon dioxide (CO_2) and oxygen (O_2) between the surrounding air and the body cells. The evolution of the lungs into this well-designed organ occurred in concert with dramatic changes taking place in the environment and in response to the increasing complexity of the developing animal life.

EVOLUTIONARY DEVELOPMENT

For at least half of the Earth's existence, O_2 existed in only minute quantities. The earliest forms of living matter were created in this anaerobic environment, with the absence of O_2 being a necessary requirement for the creation of the first organic molecules from the primordial soup.[1]

About 2 billion years ago, the first aerobic life is thought to have evolved. The ability to use O_2 in the metabolic process markedly improved the efficiency of energy extraction from fuel because the oxidation reaction could now be carried to completion using O_2 as the terminal electron acceptor. This depended on the evolution of the cytochrome chain and adenosine triphosphate, which provided a means of extracting and storing the energy in easily controllable, small packets[2] (see Chapter 9). The first aerobic organisms are thought to have resembled present-day bacteria, in which the enzymes of the cytochrome chain reside within the cell cytoplasm as well as in the cell membrane. In present-day eukaryotic cells (which includes all organisms more complex than bacteria and blue-green algae), the cytochrome chain is found in specialized organelles, the mitochondria. In view of similarities of structure between bacteria and mitochondria, mitochondria may have originally been free-living organisms that developed a symbiotic relationship with protoplasmic elements to form a more complex cell.

About 500 million years ago, the inspired fractional concentration of O_2 (FI_{O_2}) began to rise as a result of increased photosynthetic activity. In addition, an increase in atmospheric ozone screened out sufficient ultraviolet light to permit life to move out of the sea and onto dry land. The present FI_{O_2}, which is thought to have been reached about 300 to 400 million years ago, has been essentially unchanged since, with small variations due to major changes in the volume of photosynthetic activity.

As life forms became more complex, the machinery necessary for gas transport also required modification. Single-cell organisms were able to get a continual supply of O_2 directly from the surrounding environment and to release waste products directly into it. More complex organisms, however, needed a means of transporting O_2 to the interior cells. Some developed systems using air as a carrier, still seen today in insects.[3] Fluid-based systems required the development of a closed series of tubes and a pump. As the O_2 requirements increased, delivery needed to be more efficient. This task was achieved with O_2-binding pigments, which could carry up to five times as much O_2 as body water. These exist today in the form of hemocyanin, which is found in some species of mollusks and arthropods, and in the more commonly occurring iron-containing pigment hemoglobin, which can be found either in solution or packaged in erythrocytes.

Once a fluid carrier developed, the optimal gas exchanger needed to have a surface area sufficient to provide quick, efficient transfer of gas between the air and liquid phases. In the aquatic environment, gills provided this large gas-exchanging surface, with water either pumped or passively directed across the gills providing a constant supply of O_2.[4] When life moved onto land, however, gills were no longer practical because the capillary lamellae could not be kept apart as a result of the surface tension that developed at the air-tissue fluid interphase. Thus, the gas exchanger was drawn inside of the body and gradually changed from a simple outpocketing of the foregut to a true mammalian alveolar lung.

> The basic pattern of evolutionary development can be observed during the embryonic development of the human lung.

Embryology

A full exposition of the developmental anatomy of the lung is beyond the scope of this introductory chapter, but some understanding of the steps allows an appreciation of the relevant anatomy of the adult lung.

The lung bud, forming from the embryonic foregut and pushing out into the splanchnopleural mesenchyme,[5] can be seen in the human embryo as a separate structure by 22 to 26 days of gestation (Fig. 1–1). The mesenchyme provides for the development of the pulmonary microvessels and the supporting structure of the lung, including the smooth muscle, connective tissue fibrous sheaths, and cartilage. Although the continued growth of the lung depends on the progressive differentiation, growth, and division of the lung bud into the airway and alveolar structures, the control of growth seems to be invested in the mesenchyme. The bud continues to develop only if it is in intimate contact with the mesenchyme, presumably because of growth or regulatory factors produced by this derivative of the mesoderm. At the same time that the airways develop, the trachea begins to separate from the esophagus, and finally, the larynx forms to complete the separation between the air and food pathways.

> The common origin of the esophagus and the trachea explains the occasional congenital communications between these two passages.

The pulmonary arterial supply arises from the sixth branchial arches, which grow into the mesenchyme and connect with the developing vascular plexus. The branchial arches are the equivalent of the vessels that supply the gills of fish. The pulmonary venous bud arises from the left atrium and also connects to the splanchnopleural vascular plexus.

The airways continue to grow by an irregular dichotomous division. This means that each airway divides into two daughter branches, thus doubling the number with each new generation. It is an irregular dichot-

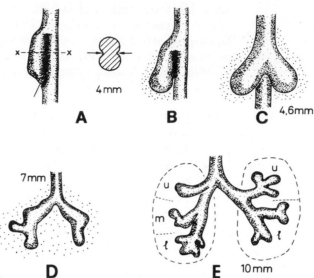

FIGURE 1–1: *A* to *E,* The embryology of the lung. The lung bud originates from the foregut *(A)* and then pushes out into the surrounding mesenchyme *B.* The combination of foregut and mesenchyme is necessary to successful lung development. The lung bud branches *(C)* and continues to grow into the mesenchyme *(D* and *E)* and develops into the embryonic lung. u, Upper lobes; m, middle lobe; l, lower lobes. (*A* to *E,* From Burri PH. Development and growth of the human lung. *In* Fishman AP, Fisher AB [eds]. Handbook of Physiology, vol 1, Bethesda, MD, American Physiological Society, 1985, p 9.)

Failure of alveolar expansion during birth results in the development of the respiratory distress syndrome in the neonate. Failure of the two vascular communications to close results in a right-to-left shunt with marked hypoxemia; this may eventually require surgical correction.

omous division because each daughter bronchus is not necessarily the same length or diameter. Between 18 and 25 weeks, when all of the cellular elements of the adult airway exist, type I and II pneumocytes begin to develop. During this time, the blood vessels acquire their smooth muscle coat and the capillary meshwork increasingly becomes a potential blood-gas interface. It will remain potential because at this stage and until the first breath of life following delivery, the airways are filled with fluid, which is continually pumped out of the lungs by fetal chest wall movement and deposited in the amniotic fluid. This conveniently allows us to sample the airway environment of the fetus by amniocentesis, providing a means of measuring the adequacy of surfactant production and therefore of dating the maturity of the lung.

At birth, if adequate surfactant is present, the lung can overcome the surface forces, allowing expansion of the terminal saccules and permitting gas exchange to take place. At the same time, the foramen ovale and ductus arteriosus close, establishing the normal separation of the systemic and pulmonary circulations.

The first 3 to 4 months of postnatal life are characterized by the conversion of the saccular lung to a true alveolar lung with alveoli developing from the walls of the saccules, markedly increasing the cross-sectional area.[6] It is estimated that in the immediate post-term period, the lung contains about 50 million alveoli. Continued growth of the lung occurs both by expansion and by addition of new units. By ages 5 to 8, the adult number of alveoli have been created, and further growth is by expansion alone.

ANATOMY OF THE LUNG AND THE AIRWAYS

The Upper Airway

The upper airway (Fig. 1–2), a complex series of passages and recesses, includes

- The external nose
- The nasal passages
- The paranasal sinuses
- The eustachian tubes
- The pharynx

Although its major role is to conduct air from the outside to the trachea, it serves a number of other important functions, including modification of the inspired air and deglutition without contamination of the lungs.[7] It also serves as an initial defense against noxious inhalants and provides for olfaction and phonation.

Although infants are obligate mouth breathers, most adults breathe through their noses until ventilatory demands become excessive (greater than 30 to 40 L/min). At the high flows required with very large ventilatory demands, such as during exercise, the use of the oral route appears to be necessary, in part to prevent nasal passage collapse due to the sharp pressure drop secondary to high resistance. The resistance to airflow through the mouth depends to a great degree on the position of the jaw and tongue; therefore, both body position and the tone of the upper airway muscles influence the resistance.

The nasal passage, which is a complex pathway built with two 90-degree bends, has a profound influence on the fate of particulate matter, with most deposited in the anterior nose. The anterior opening is wide (about 35 × 15 mm), but the passage rapidly tapers to a ribbon-like

The resistance to breathing through the nose is about twice that of the oral route and it represents almost 50% of the total respiratory airflow resistance.

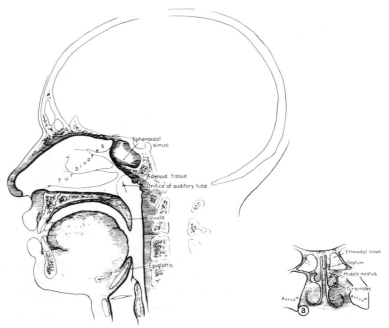

FIGURE 1–2: Sagittal view of the upper airway. (From Irwin RS, Hollingsworth HM. The upper respiratory tract. *In* Bone RC [ed]. Pulmonary and Critical Care Medicine, vol 1. St. Louis, Mosby–Year Book, 1993, p 2.)

opening with its flat side against the nasal septum. At this point, the opening may be no more than 1 to 2 mm wide. At its posterior end, it opens widely into the nasopharynx. The surface area of the nasal passages is much larger than one might expect from a simple tube of the same dimensions. Much of the increase is secondary to the bony turbinates that extend out into the nose, covering the openings to some of the paranasal sinuses. This increased cross-sectional area is important to the functioning of the nose, which serves to modify the inspired air. These modifications include an increase in the temperature and humidity of the gas and the removal of particulate matter and water-soluble gases. The nasal passages may also play a role in defense against infection, both by the entrapment of organisms in secreted mucus and possibly through the release of immunoglobulins directly into the nasal secretions. The role of the paranasal sinuses in breathing is less clear, but they are probably more important for nonrespiratory functions such as phonation and as a cushion for the brain. They require communication with the nose to allow equilibration of their internal pressure with the atmosphere in order to prevent sinus squeeze or distention.

> The total volume of the nasal passages is about 15 to 20 mL, which communicates with 40 to 60 mL in the paranasal sinuses.

At the back of the nose, the nasal septum terminates and the nasopharynx begins, continuing downward to the end of the soft palate. At this point the eustachian tubes enter. These easily collapsible structures drain the middle ear and permit equilibration of pressure in that rigid compartment. Blockage of these tubes often results in infection of the middle ear space. Below the soft palate extends the oral pharynx, which can be effectively separated by contraction of the palate to prevent soiling of the nasopharynx during swallowing and to direct expired flow through the mouth. Adequate control of the soft palate is necessary for singing and speaking. The pharynx serves mainly to conduct air and food to the correct outlets.

The larynx functions as a valve, protecting the lower respiratory tract from contamination by upper airway secretions and foodstuffs (Fig. 1–3). The importance of this can be appreciated by considering the high incidence of recurrent respiratory tract infections in patients in whom this function is compromised. The larynx also serves a number of additional important functions, including maintaining a patent airway, permitting phonation, and allowing for the increase in intrathoracic and intra-abdominal pressure required during micturition, defecation, vomiting, and parturition and before coughing.

Anatomically, the larynx is composed of a series of cartilages surrounding a lumen, which communicates with the pharynx above and the trachea below. The thyroid cartilage articulates with the cricoid cartilage posteriorly, and anteriorly they are connected by the cricothyroid membrane, which clinically allows safe access to the trachea for the creation of an emergency airway. The larynx is surrounded by a large number of muscles capable of pulling it up, pushing it down, or tilting it forward or backward, which are important during breathing, swallowing, and phonation (Fig. 1–4).

> The cricoid cartilage is the only complete cartilaginous ring in the respiratory tract.

The epiglottis arises from the posterior aspect of the anterior plate of the thyroid cartilage and expands backward along the base of the tongue. The vocal cords (the thyroarytenoid muscles), in addition to their role in phonation, protect the entrance to the trachea during swallowing through strong adduction. This is augmented by the backward and downward movement of the epiglottis, which serves mainly to protect the cords from the bolus of food and to direct the food into the esophagus. The sensory input to the larynx is from the superior laryngeal nerves,

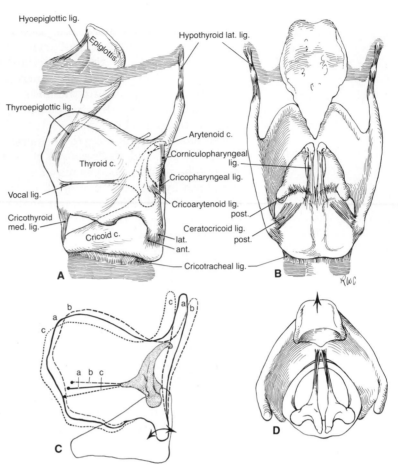

FIGURE 1–3: *A* to *D,* View of the bony structure of the larynx. As shown in *C,* the thyroid cartilage can rotate on the cricothyroid joint, with resulting lengthening of the vocal folds as demonstrated by lines a, b, and c. (*A* to *D,* From Proctor DF. Physiology of the upper airway. *In* Fenn WO, Rahn H [eds]. Handbook of Physiology. Washington, American Physiological Society, 1964, p 333.)

whereas the motor input to the upper airway and larynx comes from the fifth, seventh, ninth, tenth, and twelfth cranial nerves and the first through third cervical nerves.

The Lungs

The adult lungs are a paired organ designed to optimize the transfer of gases between the environment and the blood, and to do so with minimal energy expenditure. Because no active transport is involved, the lungs need a very large diffusion surface, which in an average adult would have to be 50 to 150 m^2 to permit sufficient reserve at all levels of metabolic demand.[8] Because a single large chamber of this size would be an inconvenient appendage, the necessary surface area has been wrapped around 300 million small sacs, or alveoli, each of which is about 0.33 mm in diameter.

Although this arrangement satisfies the requirement of a large surface area in a manageable space, it creates the problem of designing a system of tubes to deliver the gas to each alveolus with the minimal energy expenditure. The easiest way to accomplish this would be to

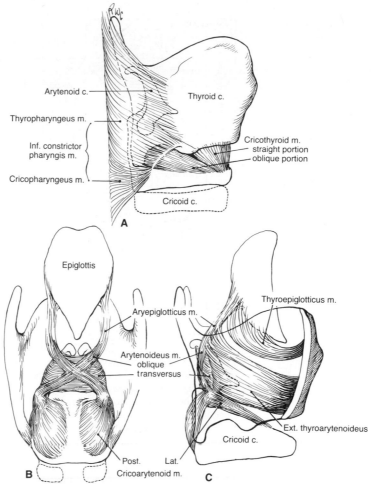

FIGURE 1–4: *A to C,* View of the laryngeal muscles. (*A to C,* From Proctor DF. Physiology of the upper airway. *In* Fenn WO, Rahn H [eds]. Handbook of Physiology. Washington, American Physiological Society, 1964, p 333.)

maximize the diameter of each airway, thus keeping airway resistance to a minimum. However, this would result in a large volume of gas (dead space) that would have to be washed out during inspiration before fresh air finally reached the diffusing surface. On the other hand, minimizing dead space by keeping the volume of the conducting airways small (i.e., decreasing airway diameter) increases the resistive work of breathing. The lung has accommodated this dilemma by developing a branching pattern of airways with gradually decreasing diameters down to the level of the respiratory bronchiole, which permits connective flow with minimal energy costs (Fig. 1–5). Beyond the respiratory bronchiole, where the predominant movement of gas is by diffusion, the diameter of the airways remains essentially unchanged, so that each subsequent division results in a doubling of the cross-sectional area, thus optimizing the conditions for diffusion.

Grossly, the lung can be divided into five lobes, three on the right and two on the left (Fig. 1–6). The lobes are separated from each other by deep fissures. The functional importance of the lobar structure is not totally clear, although the presence of the fissures tends to limit certain tumors and infections from spreading and facilitates the surgical resection of pieces of the lung. The other commonly identified subunits are

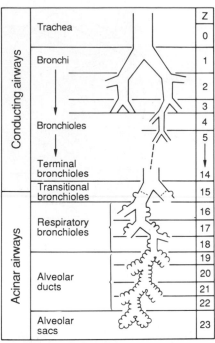

FIGURE 1–5: Branching pattern of the airways. There is a dramatic increase in the cross-sectional area of the airways as one moves from the trachea to the lung periphery. Z, generations of dichotomous branching. (From Weibel ER. Design of airways and blood vessels considered as branching trees. *In* Crystal RG, West JB [eds]. The Lung: Scientific Foundations. New York, Raven Press, 1991, pp 711–720.)

the segments, which can often be approximated well enough to permit surgical separation, although their anatomic separation is not as complete as that of the lobes. There is no obvious functional significance of the segments, and unlike the arrangement of the lobes, their distribution is often variable.

The mechanical support of the lungs consists of a continuous system of fibers that are anchored at the hilum and extend to the visceral pleura. The fibers grow out along with the airways during lung development.[9] They consist basically of two fiber types, collagen and elastin, in about a 2.5:1 ratio. The collagen fibers have a high tensile strength with almost no extensibility, whereas the elastin fibers are very extensible but have a much lower tensile strength.

Developmental or acquired abnormalities of the lung fibers will lead to rearrangement of this basic backbone of the lung, with dire consequences. For example, destruction of fibers results in emphysema, whereas overproduction leads to pulmonary fibrosis.

The Airways

The trachea, a direct continuation of the larynx, is a 10- to 12-cm tube supported by U-shaped rings that resist collapse during high intrathoracic pressures. The posterior portion consists of an unsupported muscular membrane. The trachea divides into two mainstem bronchi at the carina. The right mainstem bronchus is a more direct outgrowth of the trachea, and thus aspirated foreign bodies tend to be directed to the right

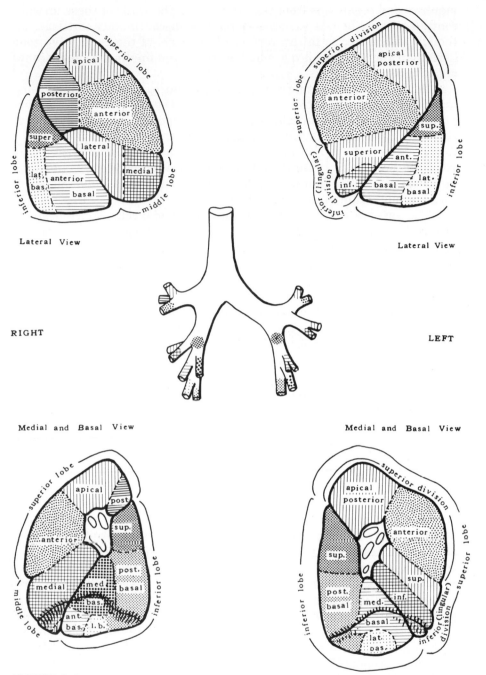

Lateral View

Lateral View

RIGHT

LEFT

Medial and Basal View

Medial and Basal View

FIGURE 1–6: The lobar and segmental anatomy of the adult lung. (From Krahl VE: Anatomy of the mammalian lung. *In* Fenn WO, Rahn H [eds]. Handbook of Physiology. Washington, American Physiological Society, 1964, p 248.)

side. Beyond the mainstem bronchi, the airways continue to divide in the already referred to irregular dichotomous branching pattern. It takes, on the average, 16 divisions of the airway to reach the terminal bronchus. The terminal bronchi mark the end of what is considered the purely conductive zone of airways, whose major function is the distribution of the inspired air toward the gas-exchanging regions of the lung (see Fig. 1–6). The conductive airways serve an additional purpose in lung defense, acting along with the upper airway to impede and remove foreign material and organisms from the air stream. The walls of these airways contain within them a variable amount of discontinuous cartilage, although as one moves to the very small airways of the conductive zone (less than 1 mm), there is a gradual decrease and finally a disappearance of the cartilage.

Beyond the conducting zone, alveoli begin to appear in increasing numbers in the walls of the airway, indicating the start of the respiratory bronchioles and the beginning of the transitional zone. These airways serve the dual role of conduction and gas exchange, gradually giving way to the alveolar ducts and finally to the alveolar space. The airways beyond the first-order respiratory bronchiole are part of the acinus, estimated to be about 5 mm in length. There are approximately 150,000 of these terminal units in the adult lung.

The airways are lined with a layer of epithelial cells, which begin as pseudostratified cells and gradually change to cuboidal and finally to squamous cells as they approach the alveoli. These cells are connected by tight junctions, suggesting that the epithelium is normally not very permeable. Fluids and molecules that pass through must do so by active transport or diffusion through the cells. Topping the airway epithelium are cilia, small hair-like projections that are covered by a layer of mucus. The cilia grip the mucus and move it gradually toward the top of the trachea, from where it is generally swallowed or expectorated. Under normal circumstances, this "ciliary escalator" is capable of clearing all of the mucus produced. Interspersed among the epithelial cells are secretory cells and rare neuroendocrine cells and Clara's cells, whose functions have yet to be clarified.

> Only when the amount of mucus produced is excessive or there is damage to the ciliary blanket is coughing necessary to clear the airway.

Beneath the basement membrane of the bronchial epithelial cells lies the smooth muscle coat. Smooth muscle, in one form or another, surrounds the airways from the trachea to the respiratory bronchioles; muscle fibers have even been identified surrounding the openings of the alveolar ducts. Contraction of these muscles can cause both a reduction in the diameter of the airways and a shortening of their length. Their major role in normal individuals may be to increase the rigidity of the airways by contracting and preventing dynamic collapse during increased respiratory demands. They may also serve to modulate the distribution of ventilation by constricting in response to a fall in airway P_{CO_2} (hypocapnic bronchoconstriction). Because a low P_{CO_2} would represent overventilation, bronchoconstriction would serve the purpose of improving the matching of ventilation to blood flow (see Chapter 6). Finally, the bronchial smooth muscle serves to protect the lungs from noxious environmental contaminants by constricting in response to stimulation of neural receptors lying beneath the epithelium. When this potentially useful reflex becomes too hyper-responsive to outside stimuli (asthma), the bronchoconstriction that is induced can cause significant problems.

The fluid that lines the airways is mainly water mixed with small amounts of mucous glycoproteins and electrolytes. It is the product of the submucosal glands as well as the goblet cells and other surface epithelial cells. Most of the fluid is from the submucosal glands, which have 40 times the capacity of the surface cells for producing it. Water moves in and out of the glands along an osmotic gradient caused by the transport of sodium and chloride in and out of the lumen through specialized channels that exist in the wall of the bronchial epithelium. Most drugs and stimuli that affect the production of mucus do so through their influence on the flux of these electrolytes. Once in the airway, the fluid forms two layers, a sol layer directly next to the epithelial lining cells

> Cystic fibrosis, a disease characterized by abnormally thick mucus, is thought to result from an abnormality in the control of electrolyte flux through the chloride channel.

and a gel layer covering this. The cilia beat in the sol layer and move the gel layer toward the mouth. The role of the fluid is almost entirely protective; all sorts of inhaled substances will cause an increase in mucus secretion. This serves to trap and dilute these substances, facilitating their removal through the ciliary escalator or by coughing.

The Blood Vessels

The lung is supplied with blood through two circulatory systems, which differ markedly in their functions and capacities. The airways are supplied by the bronchial circulation, which arises as branches directly off the aorta or from the upper intercostal arteries. The venous drainage from the large airway is through the azygous system, whereas the small airway venous blood drains directly into the pulmonary veins, accounting for a portion of the physiologic right-to-left shunt. The bronchial circulation receives between 0.5 and 1.5% of the total cardiac output and provides the nutritive circulation for all airways down to the respiratory bronchioles. These vessels, in addition, supply scar tissue and lung tumors and are probably important for lung repair.

The pulmonary circulation, which by contrast receives the entire cardiac output, has as its major role the optimal distribution of the venous blood returning from the systemic tissues to the gas-exchanging surface of the lungs. It is a very low resistance, high compliance system, which means that the pressures necessary to move blood from the arterial to the venous side are normally very low, with the walls of the vessels correspondingly thin and relatively nonmuscular. The pulmonary arteries enter the loose connective tissue sheath along with the main bronchi and travel together with the airways to the level of the respiratory bronchioles. Capillary networks originate from the arterioles intermittently along their course; thus, unlike the systemic circulation, the pulmonary arteriole is not a true terminal vessel. The pulmonary veins travel in the lobular and sublobular septum and run along the arteries only in the hilum.

The pulmonary vessels are lined with a continuous sheet of endothelial cells attached to each other by tight junctions, similar to the epithelium of the airway. However, these junctions are much leakier than those in the airway, allowing a freer exchange of fluid and solute with the perivascular interstitium. In addition to functioning as a smooth lining surface for the vessels, the endothelial cells have prodigious synthetic and degradative abilities, making the lungs an important and active metabolic organ.[10] The lungs play an endocrine role through the synthesis of various peptides, arachidonic acid products, and under abnormal conditions, classic hormones. Because the lungs filter all of the circulating blood, they are in an ideal position to act as a site of transformation and inactivation of various active compounds that are produced for local regulation but find themselves carried into the systemic circulation along with the organ's venous drainage. Many vasoactive amines, prostanoids, adenine nucleotides, and other compounds are either removed or inactivated by a single passage through the lungs. Finally, the lungs may play an important role in systemic blood pressure regulation through their ability to activate a vasoconstrictor (angiotensin) and inactivate a vasodilator (bradykinin).

A third circulatory system that plays an important role in the homeostasis of the lungs is the lymphatic drainage. The lymphatic capillaries begin in the loose connective tissue, which is in series with the connective tissue of the alveolar wall. The lymph vessels are responsible for removing water, cells, and particles from the interstitium.[11] In this role, the lymph vessels are key to both lung defense and fluid homeostasis. The lymph is directed to the hilum of the lung and through a series of lymph nodes that function as biologic filters, trapping foreign material, damaged cells, and macrophages. Within the lymph nodes are immunocompetent cells, which can be presented with antigens by the macrophages to initiate the immune response. The cleared lymph fluid is then returned to the systemic circulation.

The Alveolar-Capillary Interface

The total alveolar surface area in young adults has been estimated to range from 70 to 140 m², depending on the morphometric technique used.

At the termination of the airway lie the alveoli, the thin-walled sacs in which pulmonary gas exchange takes place. This simple structure is perfectly designed to maximize the surface area for gas diffusion in the smallest possible space. Each alveolus is a saccular outpocketing of about 0.25 mm in diameter, each wall of which is part of two alveoli, providing for increased stability and imposing an interdependency that ensures a more uniform behavior of the lungs during respiration (Fig. 1–7). Within the walls of the alveoli runs the meshwork of pulmonary capillaries, which are so densely packed that some have suggested that the meshwork actually functions as a sheet of blood rather than as individual vessels. The cross-sectional area of the capillary bed is estimated to be about 80 to 85% of the alveoli. The total volume of blood in the pulmonary capillaries at rest is approximately 70 to 80 mL, as estimated from physiologic studies. However, morphometric measurements suggest a true capillary volume of about 200 mL, a reserve that can be called on with increased gas exchange needs. The basal transit time for blood through the gas-exchanging region, about 0.75 second, shortens considerably when cardiac output increases.

The exceedingly thin alveolar-capillary membrane is made up of four layers:

- The alveolar endothelium and its basement membrane
- The capillary endothelium and its basement membrane
- The interstitial space
- The lining layer of surfactant[12] (see Fig. 1–7)

Although the thickness of this blood-gas barrier differs from one portion of the wall to another, at its thinnest it is only 0.2 μm.

The endothelial cells are typical of those already described for the arteries and veins. The epithelium is made of two important cell types. Ninety-three percent of the surface is covered by the cytoplasmic extensions of the alveolar type I cell, or squamous pneumocyte. By all standards, this is a simple, quiescent cell whose major role is to constitute the epithelial side of the gas-exchanging membrane. It is incapable of cell division and probably has no other function. The type II cell, or granular pneumocyte, is by contrast crowded with cytoplasmic organelles, suggesting very active metabolic activity. One of its most important functions is certainly the production of surfactant, which it stores in lamellated inclusion bodies and secretes onto the alveolar surface to reduce surface tension and improve alveolar stability. The type II cell, also the progenitor of the type I cell, can be seen to proliferate after lung injury. The only other cell that is typically found in the alveolus is the

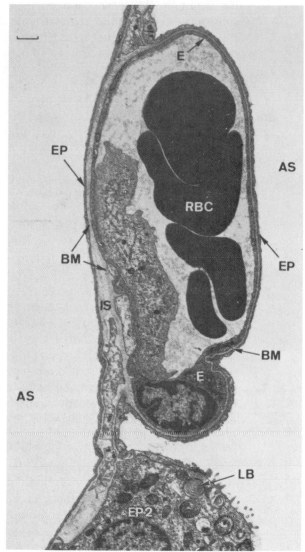

FIGURE 1–7: The gas-exchanging unit of the lung. E, endothelium; EP, type I epithelial cells; BM, basement membrane; IS, interstitial space; AS, alveolar space; EP2, type II epithelial cells; LB, lamellar body; RBC, red blood cells. (Courtesy of Ewald R. Weibel, M.D. From Murray JF. Respiration. *In* Smith LH, Thier S [eds]. Pathophysiology. Philadelphia, WB Saunders, 1985, pp 753–854.)

alveolar macrophage. This cell originates in the bone marrow and plays its role as the scavenger of the alveoli after migrating to and differentiating in the lung. In addition to its scavenger role, the alveolar macrophage may have the ability to secrete various biologically active substances. For example, it has been implicated as a possible culprit in certain forms of lung injury in which the mechanisms by which it normally kills invading microorganisms become uncontrolled, with the resultant release into the lung of toxic O_2 radicals that damage the lung itself.

Neural Innervation

Branches of the autonomic nervous system, which are found throughout the lung, play an important role in both normal function and disease. Afferent nerves from a variety of receptors in the airways and lung parenchyma monitor alterations in the lung environment. Afferent inputs influence airway and vascular tone by activating receptors, leading at times to dramatic alterations in lung function and the pattern of breathing.

The sensory inputs are grouped under three general categories.[13, 14] Stretch receptors, myelinated fibers found in the smooth muscle of the large airways, are activated by lung inflation and terminate inspiration. They mediate the Hering-Breuer reflex, which in certain animals causes apnea after a large inflation but which does not appear to be as active in normal human adults. In addition to terminating inspiration, stimulation of these receptors has also been shown to increase heart rate, decrease systemic vascular resistance, and reduce the level of normal bronchial smooth muscle tone.

Irritant receptors, another set of myelinated fibers found in the epithelial lining of the large airways, are triggered by a wide variety of chemical and mechanical stimuli to cause bronchoconstriction, tachypnea, increased mucus secretion, and cough. These stimuli may be environmental, such as noxious gases, allergens, or cold air, or they may be produced within the airway, such as histamine and other biologically active substances. Although their ostensible function appears to be the protection of the airways, when they become overactive, they are believed to contribute to the constellation of symptoms seen in asthma.

Increased activity of the C fibers causes dyspnea and often increased airway smooth muscle tone.

The final set of afferent inputs are the unmyelinated C fibers, which are found around airways and blood vessels (where they are also known as J receptors). These receptors are activated by various mediators released from mast cells and granulocytes or by increases in interstitial pressure from fluid or inflammation.

The components of the efferent autonomic system are usually classified by the neurotransmitter that is released following stimulation and that achieves its function by activating specific receptors on the cell wall.[15] In the lung, all three components of the autonomic nervous system have been demonstrated to play important physiologic roles.

Cholinergic nerves run in the vagus nerve and innervate ganglia located in the walls of the airway. From here, short postganglionic nerves travel to the airway smooth muscle and submucosal glands, where they release acetylcholine, which activates muscarinic receptors on these structures. The number of muscarinic receptors is greatest in the large airways and decreases as one moves peripherally.

Although there is a certain degree of cholinergically mediated airway tone in normal individuals, increased activation of cholinergic nerves, which is thought to play a role in asthma and chronic obstructive pulmonary disease, leads to bronchoconstriction, increased mucous gland secretion, and histamine release from the mast cells.

Adrenergic receptors, both alpha and beta, are commonly found in the lungs. They respond to both norepinephrine released from postganglionic sympathetic nerves and epinephrine released from the adrenal glands. However, because the number of sympathetic nerves actually found in the human lung is very small, direct innervation of these receptors is not likely to play a major functional role. Beta-adrenergic receptors are almost ubiquitous. They are found on airway smooth muscle at all levels of the airway, and activation results in relaxation. Unlike with cholinergic receptors, there appears to be no tonic sympathetic tone; therefore, stimulating or blocking these receptors in normal individuals has little effect. Beta-receptors have also been found on mucous glands (where they increase secretion), on epithelial cells (where they increase ion transport), on mast cells (where they inhibit degranulation and thus mediator release), and on alveolar walls (where they stimulate surfactant release). They are also found on pulmonary vessels, where they cause relaxation of the vascular smooth muscle. Alpha-adrenergic receptors are also found in airways, vessels, and mucous glands, although at much lower densities, and stimulation of these receptors leads to broncho- and vasoconstriction.

The third component of the autonomic nervous system is much less well characterized and is called, for convenience, the nonadrenergic, noncholinergic nerves. These nerves may run along with the cholinergic nerves, and there appear to be, as in the adrenergic system, two different receptors. Stimulation of an inhibitory receptor leads to bronchodilatation, whereas the stimulatory receptor causes bronchoconstriction, mucosal edema, and mediator release from inflammatory cells.

At this stage, there are as many questions as there are answers regarding the role of neural receptors in normal lung function and disease. A clear understanding of their role is complicated by the observation that these three components of the autonomic nervous system are often activated together, influencing each other in complex and often poorly characterized ways.

SUMMARY

This chapter shows that the lung is a complex yet well-designed organ, ideally suited to fulfill the many important jobs necessary to maintain the overall homeostasis of the body. The remainder of this book explores in detail how many of these functions are accomplished in normal individuals and how they are modified by disease.

References

1. Orgel LE. The Origins of Life: Molecules and Natural Selection. New York, John Wiley & Sons, 1973.
2. Broda E. The Evolution of Bio-energetic Processes. Oxford, Pergamon, 1978.
3. Wigglesworth VB. The Principles of Insect Physiology. London, Chapman & Hall, 1972.
4. Hughes GM, Morgan M. The structure of fish gills in relation to their respiratory function. Biol Rev 48:419–475, 1973.
5. Hislop A, Reid L. Growth and development of the respiratory system. In Davis JA, Dopping J (eds). Scientific Foundations of Paediatrics. London, Heineman, 1974.
6. Polgar G, Weng TR. The functional development of the respiratory system. Am Rev Respir Dis 120:625–695, 1979.
7. Proctor DF. The upper airways. Am Rev Respir Dis 115:97–129, 315–342, 1977.
8. Weibel ER. Morphometry of the Human Lung. New York, Academic Press, 1963.
9. Weibel ER. The Pathway for Oxygen. Cambridge, MA, Harvard University Press, 1963.
10. Said SI. Metabolic functions of the pulmonary circulation. Circ Res 50:325–333, 1982.
11. Leak LV. Lymphatic removal of fluids and particles in the mammalian lung. Environ Health Perspect 35:55–76, 1980.
12. Weibel ER. Morphological basis of alveolar-capillary gas exchange. Physiol Rev 53:257–312, 1973.
13. Widdicombe JG. Reflexes from the upper respiratory tract. In Cherniak NS, Widdicombe JG (eds). The Respiratory System, vol II. Control of Breathing. Bethesda, MD, American Physiological Society, 1986, pp 363–394.
14. Coleridge HM, Coleridge JCG. Reflexes evoked from tracheobronchial tree and lungs. In Cherniak NS, Widdicombe JG (eds). The Respiratory System, vol II. Control of Breathing. Bethesda, MD, American Physiological Society, 1986, pp 395–429.
15. Barnes PJ. General pharmacologic principles. In Murray JF, Nadel JA (eds). Textbook of Respiratory Medicine. Philadelphia, WB Saunders, 1988, pp 221–248.

2

Key Terms

Compliance

Elastance

Hysteresis

Resistance

Work

Pao = airway pressure

Ppl = pleural pressure

PB = barometric pressure

Lung Mechanics

Jonathon Truwit, M.D.

Ventilation occurs when a pressure gradient across the thoracic cage results in flow and volume displacement of gas. During inspiration, the respiratory muscles (spontaneously) or external positive pressure devices (a mechanical ventilator) generate this pressure gradient. The ease with which the thoracic system accepts flow and volume depends on its impedance (resistance, compliance, and inertia), whereas the quantification reflects the work performed. Measurements of respiratory mechanics permit the clinician to detect alterations in the disease process. At the bedside, these measurements may also reflect sudden changes in respiratory status, as well as subtle improvement (i.e., the patient's ability to wean from mechanical ventilation).

PRESSURE GRADIENTS

The lung, which is a relatively passive structure, expands when a pressure gradient (Pao-Ppl) occurs across it (Fig. 2–1). Gas can either be drawn into the lung by generating a negative pleural pressure (spontaneous breathing or negative pressure mechanical ventilation) or be forced in by elevating Pao above barometric pressure, PB (positive pressure mechanical ventilation).

During positive mechanical ventilation of a passive subject, expansion of the chest is governed by the Ppl-PB pressure gradient. Because a portion of the positive pressure (pressure greater than atmospheric) applied to the airway transmits to the pleural space, the Ppl-PB pressure gradient favors chest expansion. However, it appears that the chest should move inward during a spontaneous inspiration, as pleural pressure becomes more subatmospheric. This apparent paradox can be resolved by considering the activity of the chest wall muscles. The intercostals contract during inspiration and generate forces greater than pleural pressure.

RESPIRATORY MUSCLES

The dome-shaped diaphragm, the major muscle of respiration, specifically inspiration, works in concert with the intercostal muscles of the chest to distend the lungs and expand the chest cavity. The muscles reduce Ppl and create a Pao-Ppl gradient that leads to flow and volume expansion of the lung.

As the diaphragm contracts during inspiration, the zone of apposition, the portion of diaphragm that is in contact with the chest wall, decreases. As a result, the hinged ribs swing upward and outward. This movement of the ribs leads to volume expansion of the chest. Furthermore, the outward pressure of the abdomen against the zone of apposition enhances this pattern. This positive abdominal pressure that takes place during contraction occurs as a direct consequence of the descent of the central portion of the diaphragm. Additional volume expansion of the chest occurs with the contraction of the intercostals, which further serves

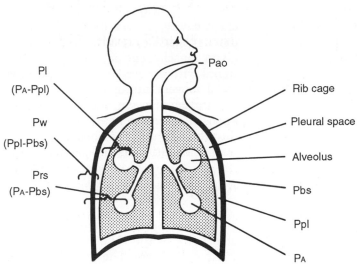

FIGURE 2–1: The respiratory system accepts flow and volume when pressure gradients favor gas movement. The difference between airway pressure (Pao) and body surface pressure (Pbs) governs the respiratory system's flow and volume expansion. The pressure difference between the alveolus and the airway opening (Palv and Pao) directs the flow within the airways. Lung expansion occurs when a pleural-alveolar pressure gradient exists (between Ppl and Palv). The chest wall is affected by the Ppl-Pbs pressure gradient. During mechanical ventilation of a passive subject, Pbs equals barometric pressure (PB). (Adapted from Murray JF. The Normal Lung, 2nd ed. Philadelphia, WB Saunders, 1986, p 85.)

to lift each rib. The scalene muscles are recruited during high minute ventilation requirements or when excessive inspiratory work is required. These muscles expand the chest cavity by directly elevating the upper chest. The elastic recoil of the chest and lungs governs the generally passive expiration. However, when the patient requires high minute ventilations or when excessive workloads exist, the abdominal muscles serve as the primary expiratory pressure generators.

The strength of the respiratory muscles can be measured by the maximal inspiratory pressure maneuver. The subject is asked to make inspiratory efforts against an occluded airway, with the most negative inspiratory pressure being termed the maximal inspiratory pressure. Respiratory muscles, like other muscles, operate best when they are at their true resting length. Maximal inspiratory pressures can be generated when the thoracic system is at residual volume. Conversely, maximal expiratory pressures are generated at total lung capacity. Hyperinflation of the chest alters the length of the diaphragmatic fibers, resulting in less ability to generate negative pleural pressures. Such is the case in chronic obstructive pulmonary disease.

In addition to lung volume, respiratory drive is also important in determining maximal inspiratory pressure. Adequate drives can be achieved in normal subjects with coaching, but they cannot necessarily be achieved in poorly cooperative patients. However, when patients must make inspiratory efforts against a one-way valve that permits only exhalation, adequate respiratory drives can be achieved. At times, the interposition of a dead space apparatus to the airway may be needed to heighten the patient's response to the maximal inspiratory pressure maneuver.

The ability to transform muscle tension into volume displacement depends on the relationship between the inspiratory muscles and the chest cavity. Severe hyperinflation, as seen in chronic obstructive pulmonary disease, results in a reduced zone of apposition; hence, for any given muscle tension, the patient inhales less gas. At the bedside, patients with severe chronic obstructive pulmonary disease may have inward movements of the lower lateral aspect of the chest wall during inspiration. Known as Hoover's sign, this results from a lost zone of apposition. As the nearly horizontal diaphragm contracts, the insertions into the ribs pull the chest inward and not upward. Patients with chest wall deformities also display reduced efficiency.

IMPEDANCES

The pressure gradient Pao-Ppl governs lung inflation. Certain characteristics of the lung determine the ease with which flow enters and volume displaces. The forces required for inspiration must overcome the lungs' resiliency to deformation (defined as elasticity) and the resistance of airways and lung tissue to expansion and flow. Inertia, an additional component of lung impedance, is considered to be minimal. The chest wall also has its impedance characteristics (resistance and elasticity). Resistance, a dynamic feature, describes the unwillingness of the thoracic system to accept flow or movement. Elasticity, a static feature, describes the unwillingness of the thoracic system to expand.

COMPLIANCE

Static measurements occur at periods of zero flow, hence the word *static*. Static measurements can be made with or without the airway interrupted, provided that at the time of measurement flow equals zero. Instead of measuring elasticity, the common practice is to measure its inverse, compliance. Compliance is determined by assessing distending pressures at two different volumes and then calculating the ratio of the change in volume divided by the change in pressure.

$$C_L = \Delta V/(\Delta Pl)$$

and

$$C_W = \Delta V/(\Delta Pw)$$

where C_L and C_W are the compliances for lung and chest wall

The distending pressures for the lung are described by the gradient $Pl = P_A - Ppl$, where Pl is transpulmonary pressure and P_A is alveolar pressure. Likewise, the distending pressure gradient for the chest wall is $Pw = Ppl - P_B$. Compliance is determined by dividing the magnitude of change in the pressure gradients after a change in volume into the magnitude of that volume. Compliance for the entire respiratory system is determined by dividing the change in volume by the change in the pressure gradient ($P_{RS} = P_A - P_B$). Elastances of two structures in series are additive.

The elastance of the respiratory system can be expressed as follows:

$$E_{RS} = E_L + E_W$$

Expressed in terms of compliance:

$$1/C_{RS} = 1/C_L + 1/C_W$$

$$C_{RS} = C_L \times C_W/(C_L + C_W)$$

Although a single value for compliance can now be determined, caution must be used. The calculated value of compliance may change with the phase of ventilation (inflation versus deflation), even when taken at the same absolute lung volume. This is known as hysteresis. Furthermore, the volume history (pattern of breathing) preceding the measurement of compliance can also alter the value, making values over time somewhat inconsistent. Lastly, compliance, as determined here, does not account for the entire lung volume because it is based on the change in volume. Compliance measurements from a patient before and after pneumonectomy differ by a factor of 2, but the unwillingness of lung tissue to distend does not change. Dividing compliance by the measured absolute lung volume (specific compliance) provides a consistent measurement permitting comparisons across patient populations and various pulmonary conditions for a given patient. The measurement of specific compliance also corrects for the seemingly great variation in compliance between lungs of infants and adults. The property of the lungs and chest wall known as elastic recoil determines the compliance. The pressure associated with the elastic recoil of the lung determines the force driving the lung to deflate to zero volume. The latter relates to the absolute lung volume. The lung remains distended because this force is offset by an equal and opposite pressure, Ppl. In the normal individual, this same pressure (Ppl) also restrains the chest wall from springing outward at functional residual capacity.

The elasticity of the lung tissue and surface forces acting on alveoli determine the elastic recoil of the lung. Elastin and collagen fibers dictate the elastic characteristics of lung tissue. In large part, surfactant determines surface tension. Surfactant, which is capable of reducing surface tension as alveolar surface area is reduced, prevents the alveolar units from collapsing at end-exhalation. If the alveolus is assumed to be spherical, alveolar pressure can be calculated from Laplace's law. If surface tension were constant, the pressure within a small alveolus would be greater than that in a larger alveolus. This would result in further emptying of the smaller alveolus into the larger, until the smaller alveolus collapsed. Surfactant prevents this collapse by reducing surface tension as alveolar size diminishes, thus keeping alveolar pressures between alveoli nearly equal.

Laplace's law:

$$P = 2T/r$$

where

T = surface tension
r = the radius of the sphere

Clinically, compliance measurements apply to the respiratory system in total (lungs and chest wall). Separating the lungs from the thorax requires a measurement of pleural pressure. Although an esophageal balloon for estimation of pleural pressure can be easily and safely placed, its use is infrequent because of patient discomfort. Because the magnitude of changes in central venous pressure parallels pleural pressure, separate chest wall and lung compliances can be determined at the bedside with central venous pressure measurements. This technique, however, has not been verified in a variety of disease states or across a range of intravascular volume states.

Clinicians determine the compliance of the respiratory system in a mechanically ventilated passive patient by estimating alveolar pressure using airway occlusions. The change in P_A can be determined by subtracting the pressure in the alveolus at end-expiration, Pex, from the alveolar pressure at end-inspiration, Ps. The change in volume between end-expiration and end-inspiration is simply tidal volume. Compliance is determined as follows: $C_{RS} = V_T/(P_S - Pex)$. In normal subjects, Pex is zero, but in patients Pex may be equivalent to preset ventilator positive end-expiratory pressure (PEEP) or the pressure associated with hyperinflation (auto-PEEP or intrinsic PEEP). Because effectively delivered tidal volume differs from machine-delivered tidal volume by the product of Ps and the tubing compressibility factor (TCF; 2 to 4 mL/cm H_2O), compliance is mathematically redefined as:

$$C_{RS} = [V_T - (P_S \times TCF)]/(P_S - Pex)$$

Compliance measurements can be obtained under "dynamic" conditions when the flow tracing crosses zero between expiration and inspiration (Pz). During mechanical ventilation of a passive patient, Pz tends to overestimate alveolar pressure. Thus, substituting Pz for Ps results in reductions of measured compliance of 10 to 15%. Greater separations in these compliance measurements occur when inhomogeneities in ventilation are more apparent, as in obstructive pulmonary disease.

Although usually reserved for ventilated patients, the practice of determining compliance from airway occlusions can be used in spontaneously breathing patients. However, tidal volumes, which are generally not constant, must be measured before each airway occlusion if reproducible data are to be expected. Analysis at zero-flow points is not possible without an esophageal balloon because airway pressure does not reflect alveolar pressure during spontaneous ventilation.

Respiratory system compliance is routinely recorded at the bedside of critically ill patients. Reductions may be noted with the onset of adult respiratory distress syndrome, cardiogenic pulmonary edema, pneumothorax, or respiratory muscle activity. Increments may follow recovery from adult respiratory distress syndrome, addition of PEEP, diuresis, pneumothorax, or paralysis resolution. Because changes in respiratory system compliance are paralleled by alterations in Ps, the clinician may choose to observe only Ps. Caution must be exercised because such analogies are appropriate only if tidal volume and Pex remain constant.

Compliance measurements need not be made solely at end-inspiration. Serial airway occlusions during inspiration and expiration provide for the construction of a static pressure-volume plot. The slope of the curve at any point defines Crs at that point of the respiratory cycle. Patients with adult respiratory distress syndrome often have very low compliances at the beginning of inspiration because great pressures are needed to open collapsed alveoli for volume expansion. These patients benefit from the addition of PEEP as alveoli are recruited for improved ventilation-perfusion matching. A simplified technique for discovering which patients might benefit from the addition of PEEP is to plot airway pressure against volume (Fig. 2–2). Patients in whom the addition of PEEP may prove beneficial can be identified by the presence of an initial horizontal portion (constant lung volume despite increasing airway pressure) followed by an inflection point. In addition, marked hysteresis will be present in the airway pressure-volume plots of these patients. As PEEP is added, the hysteresis will diminish and a leftward shift of the inflection point will be noted.

RESISTANCE

Dynamic measurements are made during gas movement (flow greater than zero). Gas movement occurs when forces overcome the frictional impedances within the airways, lung, and chest wall tissues. The complex relationship between pressure and flow depends on the type of flow present, laminar versus turbulent: $P = k1 \times \dot{V}$ for laminar flow; $P = k2 \times \dot{V}^2$ for turbulent flow. The Reynold's number permits classification of airways that are more likely to experience turbulent or laminar flows. In general, flows within the large airways and major bifurcations are turbulent, whereas flows in the more distal airways are laminar. Because the relationship between pressure and flow during laminar flow is linear (resistance = pressure/flow), clinicians have chosen to represent gas transport as being only laminar. Because Poiseuille's law applies to laminar flow, airway resistance is defined as $8\eta l/\pi r^4$, where η is gas density and l and r represent airway length and radius, respectively. The impact of radius on airway resistance is magnitudes greater than that of length. Hence, the major contributor to imposed resistance of an endotracheal

The likelihood of flow to be laminar or turbulent can be predicted by an equation:

Reynold's number = $2\dot{V}r\rho/\eta$ (values > 2000 favor turbulent flow)

where

$\dot{V}$ = airflow
r = airway radius
ρ = gas density
η = gas viscosity

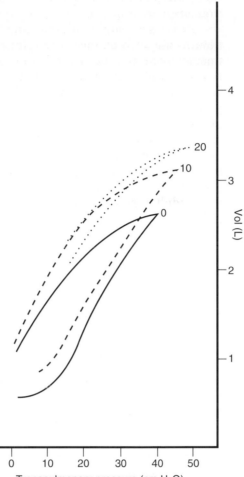

FIGURE 2–2: Pressure-volume plots of a mechanically ventilated passive patient with adult respiratory distress syndrome. As PEEP is added, the plots shift upward. Note that the pressure-volume loops become narrower (less hysteresis) and the inflection point moves toward the onset of applied inspiratory pressure. (Adapted from Benito S, Lemaire F. Pulmonary pressure-volume relationships in acute respiratory distress syndrome in adults: Role of positive end expiratory pressure. J Crit Care 5:27–34, 1990.)

tube is its radius, not its length. The effective radius of an endotracheal tube may be less in vivo than in vitro because secretions may be impacted within the lumen.

Because resistance determines the magnitude of flow when a pressure gradient is applied, resistance can be calculated more simply as $R_L = (Ppl - Pao)/\dot{V}$. Similarly, airway resistance and lung tissue resistance could be defined as $R_{AW} = (P_A - Pao)/\dot{V}$ and $R_L = (Ppl - P_A)/\dot{V}$, respectively.

As with compliance, resistance is variable over absolute lung volume. During inflation, airway resistance falls as the increasing elastic recoil exerts direct traction on small intrapleural airways and indirectly expands bronchial and extrapulmonary airways by the contribution of elastic recoil pressure to pleural pressure. The relationship between lung resistance and absolute volume is hyperbolic, with airway resistance rising markedly at absolute lung volumes less than functional residual capacity.

Pulmonary function tests provide a measurement of conductance, the inverse of resistance. The relationship between conductance and volume is linear, but the relationship between elastic recoil and conductance is not. Specific conductance, conductance divided by the absolute lung volume at which it was measured (usually functional residual capacity), permits comparisons between patients or changes in airway tone for a given patient. It is somewhat misleading to use conductance because expiratory flow reflects elastic recoil and not absolute lung volume.

In normal subjects, maximal inspiratory flow appears to be limited by respiratory muscle strength and total lung and chest resistance. Expiratory flow, however, is only limited by respiratory muscle strength during the initial phase of exhalation, after which maximal flow is limited in accordance with elastic recoil pressure or absolute lung volume (Fig. 2–3). Measurements of flow, expiratory volume, and esophageal pressure during forced exhalations provide the basis for isovolume pressure-flow plots and the flow-volume curve. Three theories have been suggested to explain flow limitation:

- Equal pressure point theory
- Starling resistance theory
- Wave-speed theory

According to the equal pressure point theory, alveolar pressure is augmented by positive pleural pressure during a forced expiration. Because this pressure is dissipated in overcoming airway resistance, intraluminal pressure along the airway is reduced from P_A. Intraluminal

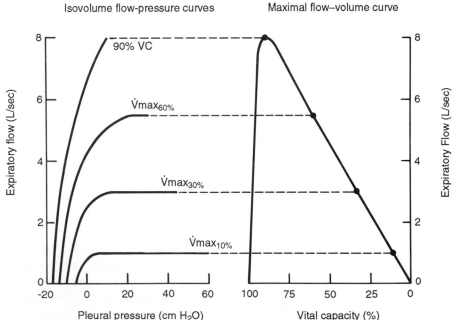

FIGURE 2–3: Measurements of expiratory flow and pleural pressure during forced expiratory maneuvers of various magnitudes provide isovolume flow-pressure curves. These curves permit generation of a maximal flow–volume curve. Note that at all lung volumes, maximal expiratory flow ($\dot{V}$max) is limited once a lung volume–specific pleural pressure is achieved. VC, vital capacity. (From Murray JF. The Normal Lung, 2nd ed. Philadelphia, WB Saunders, 1986, p 100.)

pressure may also fall along the airway to values equivalent to or below surrounding pleural pressure. Hence, the airway might be compressed and act as a chokepoint to expiration, limiting flow. The driving pressure to flow is P_A minus intraluminal pressure (Ppl). Recall that elastic recoil is defined as P_A minus Ppl.

Considering the airway as a Starling resistor provides a similar but different analysis. The airway proximal to the level of a critical transmural pressure narrows to limit flow. As a result, the driving pressure is defined as P_A minus Pcrit.

The wave-speed theory draws on principles of fluid mechanics. Flow limitation occurs when flow velocity approaches the speed of wave propagation within the wall of the airway. The speed of wave propagation is a function of cross-sectional area and the elastic properties of the airway walls. Patients with airways that have a reduced cross-sectional area are more likely to exhibit flow limitation.

In general, flow limitation in normal subjects is of consequence only during maximal expiratory efforts. However, patients with obstructive airway disease exhibit flow limitation during the respiratory cycle, without maximal effort. Characteristics of the airways in these patients provide for variable resistance values throughout the respiratory cycle.

As with compliance, determination of lung resistance during spontaneous breathing requires an esophageal balloon. The esophageal–airway pressure difference is plotted against volume, and a line connecting the pressure gradients at the zero-flow points is drawn. The difference at any volume between the curve and the newly created straight line represents the pressure responsible for driving flow. A companion flow-volume plot permits determination of flow at that volume of the breath. The convention is to determine resistance at midtidal volume because flows and driving pressures vary during spontaneous breathing.

Measurement of resistance at midtidal volume appears to be satisfactory during inspiration because the values of inspiratory resistance are generally low and are not affected by dynamic airway collapse. However, resistance values are quite variable during exhalation in patients with dynamic airway collapse, and resistance values measured at mid-exhalation will greatly underestimate those at end-exhalation.

The pressure gradient needed to overcome inspiratory resistance during a mechanically delivered constant-flow breath to a passive patient is constant. Once the pressure gradient has been established, resistance can be calculated at any point of the inspiratory cycle. As with spontaneous ventilation, the pressure gradient driving flow is defined as the difference between airway and alveolar pressure. By convention, the pressure gradient driving flow is generally determined at the end of inspiration. The pressure gradient is approximated by subtracting peak static airway pressure (end-inspiratory alveolar pressure [Ps]) from peak dynamic airway pressure (P_D). Inspiratory resistance (R_I) is then calculated as $(P_D - P_S)/\dot{V}$.

Inspiratory resistance can also be determined after defining the pressure gradient at the beginning of inspiration (Pao-P_A). Pao at time zero (P_0) is estimated by backward extrapolation of the tangent to the airway pressure tracing ramp, and P_A represents the end-expiratory alveolar pressure (Pex). Such methodology requires a linear segment in the airway pressure tracing. Overinflation of the lung at end-inspiration alters the linear ramp, resulting in inaccuracies with regard to back-extrapolation. Furthermore, P_0 may also reflect the pressure needed to

R_E = expiratory resistance

$$R_E = \frac{P_{pl} - P_{ao}}{\dot{V}}$$

Mathematically:

$$P_A(t) = P_s \times e^{-t/RC}$$

where

$P_A(t)$ = the alveolar pressure at time t into exhalation
P_s = peak static pressure (end-inspiration)
R = expiratory airway resistance
C = compliance

Solving for RC (the time constant):

$$P_A(t)/P_s = e^{-t/RC}$$

$$\ln[P_A(t)/P_s] = -t/RC$$

$$RC = -t/\ln[P_A(t)/P_s]$$

$$RC = t/\ln[P_s/P_A(t)]$$

Because the driving pressure to flow is unaltered, the product of expiratory flow and resistance before interposition ($\dot{V}b$ and Rb) equals that after ($\dot{V}a$ and Ra):

$$Rb \times \dot{V}b = (Rb + Rk) \times \dot{V}a$$

$$Rb = \dot{V}a \times Rk/(\dot{V}b - \dot{V}a)$$

recruit collapsed alveoli and thus result in overestimation of airway resistance.

Determination of expiratory resistance is traditionally performed at midtidal volume in the manner described previously. Because the esophageal balloon permits estimation of Ppl, lung resistance is calculated by dividing Ppl minus Pao by $\dot{V}$ at any time during expiration. In patients with dynamic airway collapse, magnitudes of difference may exist between R_E values during early and late exhalation. Determining R_E at midtidal volume provides a value of resistance that greatly underestimates resistance at end-exhalation in such patients.

An alternative method of determining airway resistance, the major component of R_E, during constant-volume ventilation is to examine the rate of fall in alveolar pressure during passive lung deflation. The decay in pressure is characterized by time constants that represent the product of expiratory airway resistance and compliance. If the lungs are considered as one alveolus, R_E can be determined from two estimates of alveolar pressure and the time needed for the greater value to decay to the smaller. An "average expiratory airway resistance" is obtained by dividing compliance into the time constant.

In patients with airway disease, a slightly more complicated mathematical model is needed. Two time constants, the product of compliance and airway resistance during early and late phases of exhalation, are needed to characterize the decay of alveolar pressure. These "average expiratory airway resistances" may differ greatly in magnitude.

Alternative methods for measuring resistance without the need for constant-volume ventilation include the interrupter technique and the interposition of a known resistance. Both can be performed on mechanically ventilated or spontaneously breathing patients. Because the volume at which these measurements are obtained is variable, differences in expiratory airway resistance might reflect the time during exhalation that the measurements were obtained and not changes in the clinical status of the patient.

With the interrupter technique, airway pressure is measured immediately before and shortly after airway occlusion (Pao-b and Pao-a). Simultaneous flow measurements provide for the calculation of expiratory airway resistance: $(P_{ao\text{-}a} - P_{ao\text{-}b})/\dot{V}$.

Abrupt interposition of a resistor with a known resistance (Rk) permits calculation of expiratory resistance, given the reasonable assumption of constant lung volume and elastic recoil pressure before and after interposition.

Use of an imposed resistor to caculate expiratory resistance requires an electronic or a pneumatic shutter for stepwise interposition of the resistor and simultaneous flow and pressure measurements.

Finally, airway resistance can also be calculated using plethysmographic measurements of P_A during short panting maneuvers (see Chapter 17).

WORK OF BREATHING

Work of breathing, defined as the product of the pressure needed to move gas and the volume of that gas, represents the mechanical energy expenditure for a subject to accomplish the task of ventilation. The calculation of work of breathing is generally restricted to inspiration because expiration is commonly assumed to be passive. Work does not encompass total energy expended during breathing. Ineffective energy (with regard to volume movement) is expended during isometric activity, in overcoming mechanical disadvantages, and through discoordinate contraction by opposing muscle groups. However, work is easy to calculate and serves as a measure of the impedance (resistive and elastic) to ventilation. In addition, many clinicians have used work of breathing as a guide to weaning.

The performance of work requires pressure gradients to overcome frictional and elastic impedances. Integration of the pressure gradient–flow product defines work (pressure times volume). The pressure gradient for lung and chest wall inflation has been previously defined as P_{ao}-P_B. Pressure gradients between the alveolus and the airway permit calculation of work to overcome airway resistance. The pressure gradient between the alveolus and the pleura permits definition of work performed to overcome the elastic forces of the lungs. Similarly, P_{pl}-P_B permits calculation of work expended in overcoming the elastic forces of the chest wall.

$$Pavg = (V_T/t_i) \times R + (V_T/2C) + Pex$$

Calculating work as work per liter of ventilation provides a measure of impedance defined as the average inspiratory pressure (Pavg). This can be obtained directly by dividing the integrated product of inspiratory pressure and flow by tidal volume or from the equation of motion. The latter method sums the average inspiratory pressures needed to overcome frictional and elastic forces, as well as to counterbalance the pressure associated with hyperinflation (auto-PEEP or intrinsic PEEP).

During mechanical ventilation, the inspiratory work performed can be partially or fully supplied by the ventilator. The work of ventilation of a passive subject receiving mechanical ventilation can be estimated at the bedside by multiplying the V_T by the Pavg determined by one of three techniques (Fig. 2–4):

1. Integration of the P_{AW}-time tracing or P_{AW}-volume plot
2. Measuring airway pressure at midinspiratory time or midvolume
3. $P_D - (P_S - Pex)/2$

Clinically, quantifying the ventilator work permits sequential evaluation of respiratory impedance.

Increases in the work per liter of ventilation (Pavg) during constant-flow mechanical ventilation of a passive subject parallel peak airway pressure (P_D), provided that tidal volume, flow, and end-expiratory alveo-

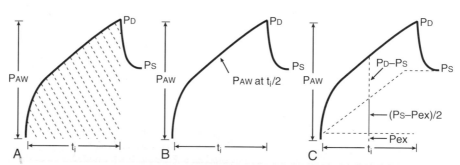

FIGURE 2–4: The airway pressure tracing permits calculation of work per liter of ventilation (Pavg) in a passive patient receiving constant-flow mechanical ventilation. Pavg is estimated by dividing the integral of the airway pressure (P_{AW}) tracing by inspiratory time (t_i) *(A)*, recording airway pressure at midinspiratory time ($t_i/2$) *(B)*, or calculating $P_D - (P_S - Pex)/2$ (the sum of the three components in *C*), where P_D is peak airway pressure and P_S and Pex are estimates of end-inspiratory and end-expiratory alveolar pressures, respectively.

lar pressure remain unchanged. Elevations of PD should alert the clinician to alterations in a patient's impedance characteristics. Simultaneous and equal elevations in Ps suggest a change in effective respiratory compliance (pulmonary edema, pneumothorax, right mainstem intubation). However, elevations in PD without changes in Ps suggest that airway resistance has changed (bronchospasm, secretions, tube biting).

The measurement of work during spontaneous breathing requires an estimate of pleural pressure (esophageal balloon pressure [Pes]), such that transpulmonary pressure can be determined throughout the respiratory cycle. As noted earlier, the work required to drive flow and expand the lungs is the integral of the product of transpulmonary pressure and flow (Fig. 2–5). However, determination of work in expanding the chest wall during spontaneous breathing is not possible. A common practice is to estimate the elastic work in expanding the chest wall from the product of tidal volume and average inflation pressure needed for chest expansion from the equation of motion ($V_T^2/2C_W$).

Bedside estimates of the work of breathing during spontaneous ventilation can be obtained from the equation of motion. Alternatively, the airway pressure tracing (PAW) from passive patients receiving constant-flow machine-delivered breaths with flows and volumes matched to the patient's spontaneous values can be integrated over time or volume. Furthermore, the work per liter of ventilation can also be estimated from the airway pressure tracing of the matched machine-delivered breaths (see Fig. 2–4):

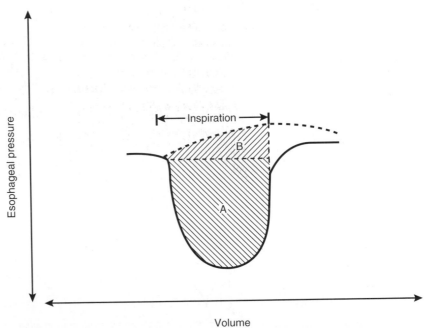

FIGURE 2–5: The work of breathing during spontaneous ventilation can be determined by planimetry of an esophageal pressure-volume plot (or integration of the product of Pes and flow). Shaded area A represents the work performed in moving gas into and expanding the lung. The work to expand the chest wall is estimated from an esophageal pressure-volume plot reproduced in the patient when the patient is passively receiving a mechanically delivered breath (B). The sum of A and B represents the total work performed by the patient. (From Truwit JD, Marini JJ. Evaluation of thoracic mechanics in the ventilated patient. Part II: Applied mechanics. J Crit Care 3:192–213, 1988.)

$$Pavg = [s\dot{V}/m\dot{V} \times (P_D - P_S)] + [(sV_T/mV_T) \times (P_S - Pex)]$$

where

s = spontaneous values
m = machine-delivered values

1. Measuring P_{AW} at midinspiratory time or volume
2. $P_D - (P_S - Pex)/2$

These estimates require a passive patient. Ventilating patients with machine-set volumes and flows that are matched to a patient's spontaneous values of tidal volume and average inspiratory flow rarely results in a passive patient. Neuromuscular blocking agents are often needed. However, patients often become passive when overventilated with large tidal volumes and average inspiratory flows. An application of the equation of motion during machine delivered breaths permits estimation of the average inspiratory pressure (Pavg) for a patient during spontaneous breathing.

The patient's respiratory muscles are usually active during machine-assisted ventilation. Determination of patient work during volume modes of mechanical ventilation (assisted-controlled or synchronized mechanical ventilation) can be established from Pes- or P_{AW}-volume plots (Fig. 2–6). The difference in area between Pes- and P_{AW}-volume plots delivered when respiratory muscles are passive (e.g., pharmacologic relaxation) and when active quantifies the work of breathing performed by the patient. P_{AW}-volume plots are more prone to errors in calculation of patient work because the technique assumes no change in airway tone and secretions between passive and active breaths.

During pressure modes of mechanical ventilation, the work of

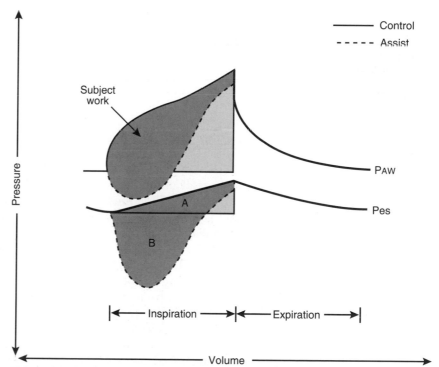

FIGURE 2–6: The work of breathing by active patients receiving mechanical ventilation can be quantified from either airway or esophageal pressure-volume plots, provided that patient-initiated breaths and machine-driven breaths are of the same flows and volumes. The difference in area between airway pressure-volume plots of a controlled, mechanically delivered breath and a patient-initiated breath represents the patient work during the latter mode. Esophageal pressure-volume plots can also be used. Region A represents the patient work in expanding the chest wall. Area B corresponds to the work performed in generating a flow and expanding the lung. (From Marini JJ. Monitoring during mechanical ventilation. Clin Chest Med 9:73–100, 1988.)

breathing can be measured from integration of the product of Pes and flow. As with spontaneous breaths, an estimation of the work performed in expanding the chest wall must be made: $(V_T)^2/(\text{chest wall compliance})$. Although more complex, PAW can be used to make estimates of the patient's muscular effort and to calculate the work of breathing during pressure modes.

PRESSURE-TIME INDEX

$$PTP = Pavg \times t_i$$

$$PTI = Pavg/MIP \times t_i/t_{tot}$$

where

Pavg = average inspiratory pressure as determined from the onset of effort and not flow

MIP = maximal inspiratory pressure that a subject can generate

t_i = the duration of inspiration

t_{tot} = the duration of a respiratory cycle

Respiratory fatigue = PTI > 0.15 to 0.18

$\dot{V}_{E_{40}}$ = (patient's Pa_{CO_2} × total minute ventilation)/(40 × body weight in kg)

WI = $(PTI \times \dot{V}_{E_{40}})/(V_T/\text{body weight in kg})$

Although work requires volume displacement, a patient may expend energy during isovolemic activity. Hence, the calculation of work may underestimate the energy utilized during ventilation. Perhaps a better method of gauging patient activity and energy consumption is to compute the pressure-time product (PTP) or the pressure-time index (PTI). Although Pavg is commonly determined from a Pes-volume plot, a Pes-time tracing would be more accurate. The PTI is useful at the bedside for spontaneously breathing patients because all components are readily available. Maximal inspiratory pressure (MIP) can be determined with a one-way valve, t_i/t_{tot} can be recorded during spontaneous ventilation, and values for Pavg during spontaneous breathing can be estimated from data obtained during mechanical ventilation.

Calculation of the PTI, or the work of breathing, provides an estimate of the impedance a subject must overcome. However, the PTI also encompasses much of the inefficient energy patients expend. In addition, the PTI references a patient's respiratory effort to respiratory strength. The PTI also relates duration of inspiration to the entire respiratory cycle and provides insight into the duration of energy expenditure in relation to the duration of respiratory muscle rest ($t_{tot} - t_i$).

The PTI has become a useful clinical tool as a marker of impending respiratory muscle fatigue. Bellemare and Grassino, while examining the human diaphragm, established a relationship between PTI and fatigue. Respiratory fatigue, as defined by the inability of a subject to perform a given respiratory task, occurred when PTI values exceeded 0.15 to 0.18. This relationship between fatigue and PTI was noted regardless of how these high PTI values were achieved (high t_i/t_{tot} and low Pavg/MIP versus low t_i/t_{tot} and high Pavg/MIP). Although their work was limited to the diaphragm, similar arguments can be made for respiratory pressures that more accurately reflect inspiratory activity (i.e., esophageal pressure). PTI can be used to predict impending respiratory fatigue for patients failing to maintain spontaneous ventilation and for those attempting to wean from mechanical ventilation.

Because dyspnea also correlates with the components of PTI, caution must be exercised when PTI is used to predict weaning. Because dyspnea is an unpleasant sensation, patients minimize their inspiratory effort to minimize dyspnea. This leads to a reduced PTI, which would favor a weaning success. However, in reducing inspiratory effort, patients also reduce tidal volume, and hence hypercapnic respiratory failure may ensue. A more complete analysis for weaning may be provided by the weaning index (WI), which accounts for patient energy expenditure (PTI), respiratory effort output (tidal volume/kg), and inefficiencies in gas exchange ($\dot{V}_{E_{40}}$). A weaning index of less than 4 suggests successful weaning from mechanical ventilation.

SUMMARY

Clinical use of lung mechanics provides the clinician with objective data on thoracic impedance and patient energy expenditure. Bedside use of the tools of lung mechanics can improve patient safety and our understanding of lung disease and the response of patients to therapy. Furthermore, combining information gained from both spontaneous and mechanical ventilation provides insight into the transition process between the two modes.

Acknowledgment

The author greatly appreciates the efforts extended by Jeanne Erickson, M.S.N., and Lee Anne Auerhan, M.D., in reviewing this chapter.

Suggested Readings

Bellemare F, Grassino A. Effect of pressure and timing of contraction on human diaphragm fatigue. J Appl Physiol 53:1190–1198, 1982.

Benito S, Lemaire F. Pulmonary pressure-volume relationships in acute respiratory distress syndrome in adults: Role of positive end expiratory pressure. J Crit Care 5:27–34, 1990.

Collett PW, Roussos C, MacHem PT. Respiratory mechanics. In Murray JF, Nadel JA (eds). Textbook of Respiratory Medicine. Philadelphia, WB Saunders, 1988, pp 85–128.

Comroe JH. Physiology of Respiration, 2nd ed. Chicago, Year Book Medical Publishers, 1974.

Fenn WO, Rahn H (eds). Respiration. Handbook of Physiology, vol 1. Washington, DC, American Physiological Society, 1964.

Hubmayr RD, Gay PC, Tayyab M. Respiratory system mechanics in ventilated patients: Techniques and indications. Mayo Clin Proc 62:358–368, 1987.

Jabour ER, Rabil DM, Truwit JD, Rochester DF. Evaluation of a new weaning index, based on gas exchange, tidal volume and effort. Am Rev Respir Dis 144:531–537, 1991.

Marini JJ, Truwit JD. Monitoring the respiratory system. In Hall JB, Schmidt GA, Wood LDH (eds). Principles of Critical Care. New York, McGraw-Hill, 1992, pp 197–219.

Marini JJ. Monitoring during mechanical ventilation. Clin Chest Med 9:73–100, 1988.

Murray JF. The Normal Lung, 2nd ed. Philadelphia, WB Saunders, 1986.

Nunn JF. Applied Respiratory Physiology, 3rd ed. London, Butterworths, 1987.

Truwit JD, Marini JJ. Evaluation of thoracic mechanics in the ventilated patient. Part I: Primary measurements. J Crit Care 3:133–150, 1988.

Truwit JD, Marini JJ. Evaluation of thoracic mechanics in the ventilated patient. Part II: Applied mechanics. J Crit Care 3:192–213, 1988.

Respiratory Muscles

David R. Dantzker, M.D.

The muscles of the thoracic cavity are responsible for expansion and contraction of the chest cavity (Fig. 3–1).[1] Abnormalities of neuromuscular function may lead to respiratory pump failure. More recently, increasing emphasis has been placed on the abnormalities of respiratory muscle function that occur secondary to abnormal pulmonary mechanics. This has led to the concept of respiratory muscle fatigue as a consequence of chronic respiratory overload, which may accompany severe obstructive or restrictive pulmonary disorders. In turn, the course of the primary pulmonary disorder may be aggravated by disordered function of the respiratory muscles. Because of its potential importance to clinical illness, increased attention has been directed to the possible role of various drugs and techniques of improving respiratory muscle function, with the ultimate goal of assisting the muscles in overcoming the increased loads imposed by various pulmonary disorders. This chapter reviews more recent concepts of the functional anatomy and physiology of the respiratory muscles, with specific emphasis on the diaphragm. In addition, various tests that can be used to assess respiratory muscle function are discussed, and therapeutic modalities aimed at improving respiratory muscle function are examined.

ANATOMY

The rib cage and the abdomen, which are separated by the diaphragm, constitute the chest wall. The abdominal contents are essentially noncompressible and therefore behave like a liquid-filled container. A rise in intra-abdominal pressure, which occurs during the descent of the diaphragm as it contracts, causes outward movement of the anterior abdomen, essentially the only mobile component of the abdominal wall. When the ribs move up and down, there are changes in both the lateral

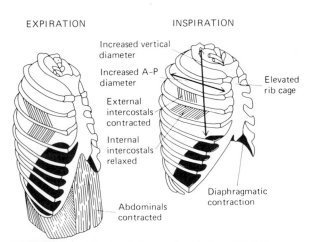

EXPIRATION   INSPIRATION

Increased vertical diameter

Increased A-P diameter

External intercostals contracted

Internal intercostals relaxed

Elevated rib cage

Diaphragmatic contraction

Abdominals contracted

FIGURE 3–1: The inspiratory and expiratory muscles. (From Luce JM, Culver BH. Critical review: Respiratory muscle function in health and disease. Chest 81:82, 1982.)

and the anteroposterior dimensions of the thorax. The necks of the upper ribs are almost parallel to the frontal plane, so that during inspiration, their predominant movement is up and forward (pump-handle motion). Because of the dorsal orientation of the necks of the lower ribs, their upward motion during inspiration results in a concomitant outward or lateral displacement, commonly described as the bucket-handle motion (Fig. 3–2).[2]

The Diaphragm

The phrenic nerves arising from the third through the fifth cervical segments innervate the diaphragm. This muscle can be thought of as an elliptical cylindroid capped by a dome. The dome is composed mainly of the central tendon, whereas the cylindrical portion is made up of the costal component, which lies in close proximity to the lower six ribs (Fig. 3–3).[2] This latter area, aptly called the zone of apposition, shortens during active diaphragmatic contraction; the resulting descent of the diaphragmatic dome is responsible for its piston-like action.[2] Diaphragmatic contraction causes a fall in pleural pressure, together with a rise in intra-abdominal pressure. With descent of the diaphragm during contraction, there is expansion of the thoracic cavity and downward displacement of the abdominal contents. This latter effect is associated with outward movement of the anterior abdominal wall.

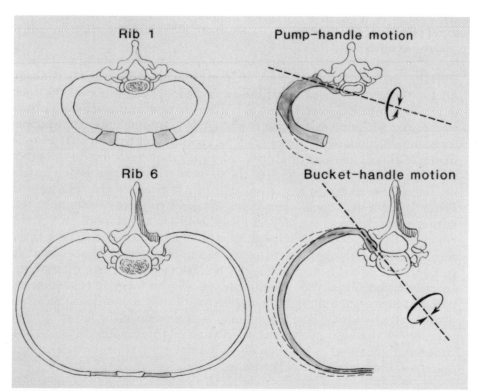

FIGURE 3–2: Functional anatomy of the human rib cage. In the upper ribs *(top)*, rotation of the rib-neck axis *(broken line)* in an inspiratory direction increases the anteroposterior diameter of the rib cage (pump-handle motion), whereas in the lower ribs *(bottom)*, rotation of the rib-neck axis causes an increase in the lateral diameter of the rib cage (bucket-handle motion). (From De Troyer A, Estenne M. Functional anatomy of the respiratory muscles. Clin Chest Med 9:177, 1988.)

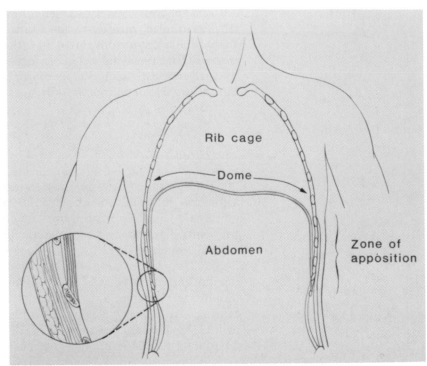

FIGURE 3–3: Frontal section of the chest wall at end-expiration illustrating the functional anatomy of the diaphragm. Note the dome of the diaphragm, which descends during inspiration. The muscle fibers in the costal portion *(inset)* run cranially and lie in close apposition to the inner aspect of the lower rib cage (zone of apposition). (From De Troyer A, Estenne M. Functional anatomy of the respiratory muscles. Clin Chest Med 9:178, 1988.)

Two factors largely account for the elevation of the lower rib cage during inspiration. The first is the craniocaudal orientation of the zone of apposition.[3–5] Reorientation of the muscle fibers in the zone of apposition occurs when hyperinflation is present. In patients with emphysema, for example, the zone of apposition is small or absent, so that muscle fibers of the diaphragm are oriented in a transverse direction rather than craniocaudal. Contraction of the diaphragm in this situation causes an indrawing of the lower costal margin (Hoover's sign). The second factor is the appositional component. The rise in intra-abdominal pressure is transmitted to the pleural recess between the diaphragm and the rib cage, thus elevating the lower rib cage during inspiration. For these mechanisms to remain operative, it is important that the abdominal contents act as a fulcrum to prevent excess descent of the diaphragm. Increased abdominal wall compliance, as seen in quadriplegic subjects, results in excess diaphragmatic descent with only a small rise in intra-abdominal pressure. Thus, the amount of expansion of the lower rib cage is small.[6] Expansion of the lower rib cage in these patients can sometimes be augmented by inflation of a pneumatic cuff (Pneumobelt), which decreases the compliance of the anterior wall.

Intercostal Muscles

The fibers of the external (superficial) and internal (deep) intercostal muscles are oriented at 90 degrees to each other, with the fibers of the external oblique muscles directed anteriorly and downward. (see Fig. 3–1). The anterior intercostal portion of the internal intercostals is referred to as the parasternal intercostals and has important inspiratory activity during quiet respiration in both humans and animals.[2] More recent animal experiments have challenged the traditional view of intercostal muscle action. Previous theory held that the orientation of the external and internal intercostal muscle fibers was responsible for inspiratory and expiratory activity, respectively. It is now believed that more important mechanisms of intercostal muscular action are related to the sequence of neuroactivation and the lung volumes at which muscle contraction occurs. The external intercostals are activated during inspiration, together with the scalenes and the parasternal intercostals, in a sequence from top to bottom that produces rib elevation. Conversely, internal intercostal activity occurs predominantly during expiration; this activity is in the reverse direction and causes descent of the ribs (Fig. 3–4).[2]

Abdominal Muscles

The abdominal muscles are primarily expiratory in action. During contraction, there is a rise in intra-abdominal and pleural pressure, with a decrease in lung volume. It is important to remember that although abdominal muscles tend to pull the ribs down and deflate the rib cage, the increase in intra-abdominal and consequently in pleural pressure in the zone of apposition causes passive diaphragmatic stretching, which raises the lower ribs in the same way as during active diaphragmatic contraction. Although the predominant action of the abdominal muscles is expiratory in nature, abdominal muscle contraction can also facilitate

Inspiratory activity
in External Intercostals

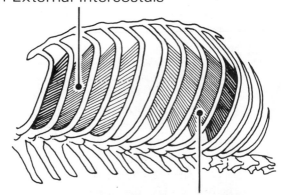

Expiratory activity
in Internal Intercostals

FIGURE 3–4: Pattern of activation of the external and internal interosseous intercostal muscles during breathing in the dog. The external intercostals in the upper portion of the rib cage are activated during inspiration along a craniocaudal gradient, whereas the internal interosseous intercostals in the lower portion of the rib cage are activated during expiration along a caudocranial gradient. A similar pattern has been observed in humans. (From De Troyer A, Ninane V. Respiratory function of intercostal muscles in supine dog: An electromyographic study. J Appl Physiol 60:1692, 1986.)

inspiration. This is seen in two circumstances. First, when a person changes from the supine to the standing position, tonic activity of the abdominal muscles becomes apparent. This acts to prevent excessive shortening of the diaphragm during inspiration and helps to optimize the length-tension characteristics of the diaphragm.[7] Second, active abdominal muscle contraction during expiration can reduce lung volume below the functional residual capacity by forcing the diaphragm further into the thoracic cavity.[2] With inspiration, there is now passive descent of the diaphragm, even before the onset of inspiratory muscle contraction. This mechanism has also been described in patients with chronic obstructive pulmonary disease, particularly during exercise, when active expiratory abdominal muscle contraction helps to counter the deleterious effects of dynamic hyperinflation.

DIAPHRAGMATIC BLOOD FLOW

An important determinant of the development of diaphragmatic fatigue is the ratio between the energy requirements of the muscle and the energy supplied. Because the resting energy stores of the diaphragm are small and are able to sustain contractions for only a few seconds, the adequacy of nutrient delivery during muscular work is critically important. This, in turn, is determined by the adequacy of diaphragmatic blood flow. Fortunately, the diaphragm is supplied by three major arteries (the internal mammary, the intercostals, and the inferior phrenic arteries), and there is a rich anastomotic network[8] among these vessels. Thus, blood supply is ensured even in the face of occlusion of a single set of vessels (Fig. 3–5). Studies have shown that over a wide range of perfu-

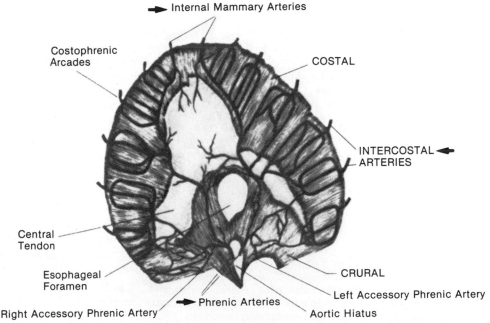

FIGURE 3–5: Abdominal view of the diaphragm illustrating the internal circle formed by the phrenic and internal mammary arteries. In addition, branches of intercostal arteries are shown communicating via costophrenic arcades with an internal circle. Arrows indicate three main arterial supplies to the diaphragm. (From Comtois A, Gorcyca W, Grassino A. Anatomy of diaphragmatic circulation. J Appl Physiol 62:242, 1987.)

sion pressures (60 to 120 mm Hg), flow is maintained relatively constant.[9]

Blood flow increases with increasing muscular activity, presumably because of the local release of vasoactive substances that cause vasodilatation. It is important to remember that there is also an opposing effect produced by the increasing tension development of the muscle, which acts to compress blood vessels.[10, 11] However, at moderate levels of diaphragmatic contraction, the net effect is an increase in diaphragmatic blood flow. Although normal individuals do not show evidence of impaired respiratory muscle performance as a result of reductions in respiratory muscle blood flow, in disease states, there may be impairment of diaphragmatic blood flow on the one hand and increased metabolic demands on the other. Together, these may result in impaired muscle performance secondary to inadequate energy delivery. This was well demonstrated in the study by Aubier and coworkers, who showed that cardiogenic shock was associated with an increase in respiratory muscle lactate production and the development of diaphragmatic fatigue, even though muscle blood flow had increased.[12] In contrast, when animals in cardiogenic shock were mechanically ventilated, diaphragmatic fatigue was prevented and blood lactate levels were lower.[12, 13] Thus, although there was impairment of blood supply, diaphragmatic energy requirements were sufficiently reduced by the mechanical ventilation so that demand did not exceed supply. Similar findings of increased diaphragmatic blood flow but increasing levels of blood lactate from the respiratory muscles have been shown in animals in which sepsis was induced by the injection of endotoxin.[13, 14]

Conditions that reduce diaphragmatic blood flow favor the development of respiratory muscle fatigue.[12, 13] Increasing diaphragmatic blood flow will reverse established diaphragmatic fatigue.[15] These studies emphasize the important relationship between diaphragmatic blood flow and diaphragmatic performance. In the absence of oxygen, adenosine triphosphate generation relies increasingly on anaerobic pathways with the generation of intracellular acids, which in turn may adversely affect muscle contractility.[16] Furthermore, Lewis and Haller have suggested that the phosphate ion concentrations, which rise in the presence of high rates of adenosine triphosphate hydrolysis, can also inhibit contractile protein adenosine triphosphatase.[17] Thus, reductions in blood flow may precipitate fatigue by increasing anaerobic glycolysis, with the accumulation of hydrogen and phosphate ions. The manipulation of respiratory muscle blood flow may have therapeutic implications in terms of the management of respiratory muscle fatigue. Measures to improve respiratory muscle blood flow (through increasing cardiac output, reducing venous pressure, or both, on the one hand and through decreasing the metabolic demands of the respiratory muscles by means of ventilatory support on the other) could be important therapeutic approaches that may prevent the development of fatigue or favor recovery in the presence of established fatigue. An improvement in diaphragmatic contractility after the administration of dopamine has been described.[18] There is no direct action of dopamine on muscle contractility, and the increase in diaphragmatic strength was ascribed to the 30% increase in blood flow to the diaphragm.

TESTS OF RESPIRATORY MUSCLE FUNCTION

Although it is common to hear that a patient required mechanical ventilation because he or she tired out, objective evidence of respiratory

At very high levels of tension development (at pressures that are at least 80% of the maximal pressure), diaphragmatic blood flow may cease entirely.

Measurements of respiratory muscle function:

- Measurements of muscle strength
- The pattern of muscle activation
- Physiologic evidence of fatigue

Stimulatory tests of ventilatory muscles in humans are feasible via transcutaneous or needle stimulation of the phrenic nerves. However, these tests are difficult to perform, require a high degree of technical competence, and at present are not ideally suited for widespread use in the critical care setting.

muscle failure or fatigue is infrequently obtained. If we are to improve our understanding of the clinical importance of this problem, more attention must be given to making the necessary measurements of respiratory muscle function.

Tests of muscle performance can be divided into measurements of static and dynamic function, and each of these can be further divided into those that are dependent on patient motivation and cooperation and those that are independent of patient performance. The latter group includes tests in which the muscles are stimulated directly or indirectly or electromyographic signals are analyzed. Obviously, patient effort influences results in tests of static and dynamic function that require patient cooperation.

Static Voluntary Tests

The contractile force of the respiratory muscles is most commonly assessed by measuring the pressure generated during voluntary contractions that are performed against obstructions at the mouth. Inspiratory pressures are generally measured from functional residual capacity or residual volume, whereas expiratory pressures are maximal at total lung capacity. The commonest measurement is mouth pressure (PI_{max}), which reflects muscle force of the total respiratory system.[19] An important variable affecting the measurement of respiratory pressures is the length of

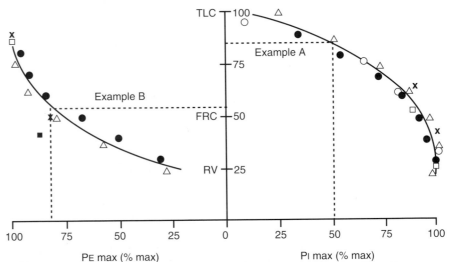

FIGURE 3–6: Relationship between maximal static respiratory pressures (PI_{max}, PE_{max}, measured at the mouth) and lung volume. Pressures are expressed as percentages of maximum, and lung volume is expressed as a percentage of total lung capacity (TLC) (Example A). A patient with emphysema has a residual volume (RV) that is 85% of predicted TLC. The expected PI_{max} at that level of hyperinflation is only 50% of the PI_{max} expected in an individual with normal lungs. Because of the lung hyperinflation, the inspiratory muscles function at a mechanical disadvantage (Example B). A patient with restrictive disease has a TLC that is only 55% of the predicted. Because the patient is unable to achieve a normal TLC, the PE_{max} expected should be reduced accordingly. For patients with abnormal lung volumes, the corrected values for PI_{max} and PE_{max} can be calculated from the product of the predicted value and the percentage adjustment. The latter value is derived from the x-axis of the graph (left side to correct PE_{max} in restrictive disease and right side to correct PI_{max} in hyperinflation). FRC, functional residual capacity. (From Rochester DF. Tests of respiratory muscle function. Clin Chest Med 9:251, 1988.)

Restrictive lung disease, which reduces total lung capacity, results in decreases in maximal expiratory pressure (PE_{max}).

the inspiratory muscles from which the contraction is initiated (Fig. 3–6).[20] The length of the muscles can be voluntarily affected, but even when this is taken into account, disease states may alter resting length so as to complicate the measurement of these pressures. The hyperinflation of chronic obstructive pulmonary disease is the prime example in which the functional residual capacity is increased, with a consequent shortening of the diaphragm and other inspiratory muscles (Fig. 3–7).[21] This shortening adversely affects the length-tension relationship, which is an important determinant of muscle contractility.

Technical factors play an important role in the measurement of these pressures. Whether a tubular or flanged mouthpiece is used affects the measurement of mouth pressure.[22] In the original description of the measurement of PI_{max}, Black and Hyatt used a tubular mouthpiece placed over pursed lips.[19] This was followed by a study that used flanged mouthpieces, making comparison with the previous data difficult.[23] As has been emphasized, the tubular mouthpiece generally gives higher values than the flanged one, except in patients with generalized muscle weakness who have difficulty in holding the pressure measuring system and the

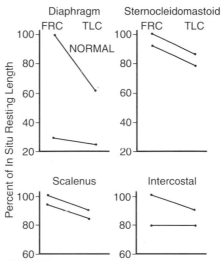

FIGURE 3–7: Lengths of inspiratory muscles, expressed as a percentage of resting in situ length at functional residual capacity (FRC) and total lung capacity (TLC) in a normal subject and a patient with chronic obstructive pulmonary disease (COPD). Muscle lengths were determined from roentgenograms. In the COPD patient, the resting lengths of the diaphragm and intercostal muscles have been so decreased by hyperinflation that they can no longer shorten during a breath from FRC to TLC. Maximal contractile tension is achieved at optimal muscle length or excessive lengthening of the muscle fiber before contraction reduces optimal tension. (From Druz WS, Danon J, Fishman HC, et al. Approaches to assessing respiratory muscle function in respiratory disease. Am Rev Respir Dis 119(2):147, 1979.)

tube firmly against the lips. In this group, use of the flanged mouthpiece produced higher values.[22] Clearly, in the critical care setting, additional complicating factors are present, in that in many cases patients may be obtunded and uncooperative. Marini and coworkers have emphasized the value of one-way expiratory valves in obtaining optimal PI_{max} values in the critical care setting.[24]

Measurement of the Transdiaphragmatic Pressure

Transdiaphragmatic pressure (Pdi) specifically reflects diaphragmatic strength (Fig. 3–8).[25, 26]

By means of the two-balloon-catheter system, with one balloon in the esophagus and the other in the stomach, pressures across the diaphragm can be measured during maximal inspiratory and expiratory maneuvers. Pdi has been measured with a variety of inspiratory techniques. These include maximal inspiratory static maneuvers against a closed shutter and maximal sniff maneuvers.[27] The latter technique has been advocated as superior to the others in that it is more easily learned, produces higher maximal Pdi values, and has a greater reproducibility.

Dynamic Voluntary Tests of Respiratory Muscle Endurance

In contrast to the static tests, there are dynamic tests of function that provide indices of respiratory muscle endurance. These tests can be performed by breathing through inspiratory resistances (loaded) or by means of sustained isocapnic hyperpnea (unloaded).

Loaded Tests of Endurance

The performance of the respiratory muscles during loaded breathing has been well described by Bellemare and Grassino.[11, 28] They measured endurance during breathing against various inspiratory pressures and combined these breathing maneuvers with variations in inspiratory time (t_i). They found that it was possible to predict endurance of the muscles during resistive breathing by means of the tension-time index of the

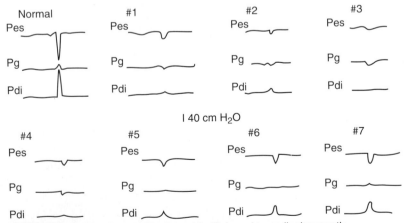

FIGURE 3–8: Esophageal (Pes), gastric (Pg), and transdiaphragmatic (Pdi) pressures during maximal sniffs in a normal subject *(top left)*, in three patients with severe diaphragm weakness (patients 1, 2, and 3; note the negative Pg during sniff), and in four patients with mild to moderate diaphragm weakness (patients 4, 5, 6, and 7; note the positive Pg during sniffs). (From Mier-Jerdrzejowicz A, Brophy C, Moxham J, Green M. Assessment of diaphragm weakness. Am Rev Respir Dis 137:880, 1988.)

diaphragm (TTIdi). This index was derived as the product of the transdiaphragmatic pressure as a percentage of the maximal transdiaphragmatic pressure (Pdi/Pdi$_{max}$) and the duty cycle during breathing (t$_i$/t$_{tot}$), where t$_{tot}$ is the total time for the breath. In their original experiments, inspiratory flow rates were kept relatively low. Additional work by McCool and colleagues has shown that inspiratory flow rate is an important additional factor that adversely affects endurance.[29] They showed that for the same tension-time index (TTI), endurance was inversely related to increasing inspiratory flow rates. This finding was corroborated in a study in which diaphragm fatigue occurred earlier in subjects who exercised with a restriction around the rib cage. In this setting, there was an increase in breathing frequency and inspiratory flow rate, which increased diaphragmatic energy expenditures to fatiguing levels even though the TTIdi was only 0.06. Thus, the critical TTIdi of 0.15 is relevant only in low-flow situations and should not be used in the setting of tachypnea or hyperpnea.[30]

Unloaded Breathing

The maximal voluntary ventilation, although dependent on airway mechanics, is affected by muscle performance and is reduced in the presence of respiratory muscle weakness.[31] A maximal voluntary ventilation less than that predicted for a certain FEV$_1$, although not specific, can be used as an indicator of possible respiratory muscle weakness. A more complicated but probably more valid test of respiratory muscle endurance is the maximal sustained ventilatory capacity. This is defined as the maximal ventilatory capacity that can be sustained for prolonged intervals; in the past, it was measured from times as short as 4 minutes to as long as 2½ hours.[32]

Static Motivation—Independent Tests of Nerve and Muscle Stimulation

Phrenic nerve stimulation can be achieved in humans by means of transcutaneous electrodes, needle electrodes, or implantation of fine wires.[33-35] The superiority of bilateral phrenic nerve stimulation over unilateral stimulation has been demonstrated. Provided that there is strict attention to detail with regard to the proximity of the stimulating electrodes to the nerve, standardization of the motor unit action potentials as recorded from surface electrodes, and maintenance of lung volume, it appears that relatively reproducible results can be obtained.[32]

After fatiguing contractions generated by means of resistive breathing, Aubier and associates showed a reduction in the twitch of the stimulated diaphragm.[33] More recently, Hubmayr and coworkers used implanted fine wires, and in some cases these were left in place for several hours, raising the possibility that this technique may be useful for repeated assessments of diaphragmatic function.[35] With transcutaneous electrodes, it has been possible to perform tetanic stimulation at increasing stimulatory frequencies from 10 through 100 Hz, although this technique generates intense pain at the sites of the electrode.[32] However, this does allow the generation of force-frequency curves of the diaphragm, which reflect the Pdi generated at increasing stimulation frequencies. This technique has been commonly used with other muscles, including the sternomastoid, as a way of measuring contractility.

Endurance—the ability to sustain a constant breathing pattern against a resistance.

No fatigue or limitation to endurance occurs when the TTIdi is approximately 15% or less, whereas there is a progressive decrease in endurance as the TTIdi increases. TTIdi values of greater than 20% are associated with ultimate failure of the muscles as a respiratory pump. When the TTIdi is only marginally elevated, fatigue occurs after approximately 1½ hours, whereas a TTIdi of 30% causes fatigue within 10 minutes.

The force-frequency curves have been used in the past to differentiate two types of fatigue, namely high-frequency fatigue and low-frequency fatigue. After the performance of repetitive muscular contraction, high-frequency fatigue is manifested in the reduced response to stimulation frequencies in the range of 50 to 100 Hz. High-frequency fatigue recovers within a short time, generally within minutes (Fig. 3–9),[36] and is believed to be related to transmission failure at the neuromuscular junction. Low-frequency fatigue, on the other hand, is demonstrated by reduced contractility to frequencies of stimulation in the 10- to 20-Hz range and is long-lasting (24 hours or more). This represents the kind of muscle fatigue seen when a muscle is overworked. Low-frequency fatigue is probably related to reduced muscular contraction in response to neural impulses (excitation contraction coupling failure)[37] and is believed by some to be the basis of the impaired muscle contractility seen in lung diseases such as obstructive airway disease, in which the respiratory muscles work continuously at high levels against high respiratory impedances. Because of the inability of the muscles to rest, it is postulated that there is persistence of low-frequency fatigue (chronic low-frequency fatigue), which in turn leads to reduced muscle contractility at the frequencies of stimulation seen during normal breathing. In such a case, therefore, respiratory drive has to be increased to compensate for the decreased muscle contractility, and this perpetuates the chronic fatigue. This hypothesis is the basis, as is discussed later, for the use of intermittent ventilatory support or rest of the respiratory muscles in order to reverse chronic fatigue.[38]

Both transmission failure (high-frequency) fatigue and excitation contraction uncoupling (low-frequency) fatigue are examples of peripheral fatigue.[37] This implies that failure of contractile strength occurs distal to the motor neuron. Central fatigue may be motivational or non-

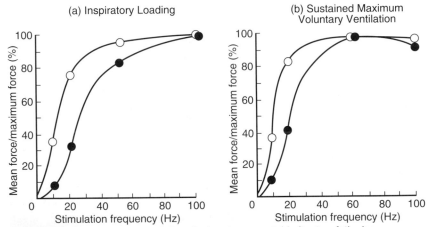

FIGURE 3–9: Low-frequency fatigue in the sternomastoid after two fatiguing respiratory maneuvers. Open circles represent the control. Closed circles show fatigue 30 minutes after inspiratory loading *(left panel)* or sustained maximal voluntary ventilation *(right panel)*. At high frequencies of stimulation (60 to 100 Hz), contractile tension recovers rapidly. Conversely, contractility at low frequencies (20 Hz) remains depressed (approximately 50% of tension in fresh muscle). This frequency fatigue requires up to 24 hours for complete recovery. The 20:50 ratio can be used to quantify the degree of low-frequency fatigue. This ratio compares the contractility at 20 Hz with the contractility at 50 Hz. The 20:50 ratio is reduced in the presence of low-frequency fatigue. (From Moxham J, Wiles CM, Newham D, Edwards HT. Sternomastoid muscle function and fatigue in man. Clin Sci 59:466, 1980.)

motivational in type. Motivational fatigue implies that with further encouragement and exhortation, the subject can improve his or her performance back to maximal levels.[37] In nonmotivational fatigue, no amount of exhortation can increase the level of respiratory effort. In this situation, the reduction in force output of the diaphragm can be partially ascribed to reduced neural output from the central nervous system. Reflex inhibition of the central nervous system from afferents originating in the diaphragm and other respiratory muscles has been suggested as the mechanism of this inhibition.[32, 39, 40] This reduced drive to the diaphragm may exist to avoid eventual contractile failure, although at the price of reduced diaphragmatic activity, decreased ventilation, and consequent hypercarbia. It has been postulated that the improved diaphragmatic function seen after rest provided by intermittent ventilation may act in part through release of these afferent inhibitory impulses from the respiratory muscles.

Central fatigue has its origins in the central nervous system along the pathway from the motor cortex to the motor neuron.

The diagnosis of central fatigue in humans can be made by the twitch interpolation method (Fig. 3–10).[34, 41] In this technique, the phrenic nerve is stimulated bilaterally and supramaximally during the performance of increasing voluntary diaphragmatic activation. If the voluntary effort activates the diaphragm maximally, superimposed stimuli cause no further twitches. Alternatively, in the presence of central fatigue, superimposed twitches are visible even when the muscle is fully activated. The severity of the central fatigue can be quantified by the ratio of the superimposed twitch during maximal activation to the size of the relaxation twitch.[34, 39]

Dynamic Motivation—Independent Tests

Breathing Pattern

Useful information can be obtained by observing a patient's pattern of breathing. Patients in the supine position use the diaphragm as the predominant muscle of respiration; thus, outward movement of the abdomen usually predominates over rib cage excursion. Two deviations from this pattern have been described.[42] The first is respiratory alternans, in which there is sequential predominance of the diaphragm and the accessory intercostal muscles as the major muscles of respiration. This may act by conserving the capabilities of the failing muscle in that the respiratory load is shifted from one muscle group to the other sequentially, thus allowing the nonworking muscle group to rest and presumably recover. The second pattern is the loss of the normal synchronous movement of the rib cage and abdomen (Fig. 3–11).[43] This can vary from asynchronous breathing, in which one compartment expands faster than another, to paradoxical motion, in which one compartment moves in a direction that opposes lung expansion. When markedly abnormal, these alterations in breathing patterns can often be evaluated by direct visualization. Quantitation, however, requires actual measurement, which is accomplished by magnetometry[44] or respiratory inductive plethysmography.[45] Some investigators have suggested that thoracoabdominal asynchrony is a hallmark of ventilatory muscle fatigue.[42] That patients who develop apparent muscle fatigue often develop these abnormal ventilatory patterns first is incontrovertible. However, Tobin and coworkers showed that thoracoabdominal asynchrony is an inevitable result of high respiratory load and does not of necessity indicate the presence of fa-

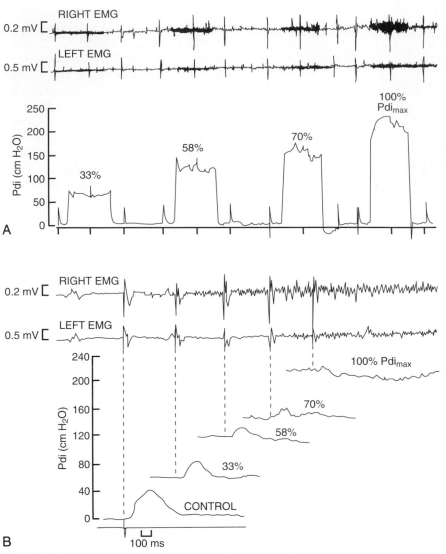

FIGURE 3–10: Typical electromyographic (EMG) *(upper)* and Pdi *(lower)* records when maximal shocks were delivered between and during combined Mueller-expulsive maneuvers of different percentages of Pdi_{max} in the sitting position. Portions of the same records displayed on a faster time base. The bottom trace in *A* and the vertical dotted lines in *B* mark the time at which the stimulus was applied. (From Bellemare F, Bigland-Ritchie B. Assessment of human diaphragm strength and activation using phrenic nerve stimulation. Respir Physiol 58:269, 1984.)

tigue.[45] In their experiments, the abnormal breathing pattern reverted to normal despite the persistence of low-frequency fatigue.

Power Spectral Analysis of the Diaphragmatic Electromyogram

Power spectral analysis of the electromyogram recorded from either esophageal or surface electrodes permits measurement of several indices, including the high-low ratio and the centroid frequency.[32, 46] The former refers to the power present in the frequency spectrum from approximately 160 to 640 Hz, as compared with the power in the lower frequencies (20 to 40 Hz). The centroid frequency is an alternative means of measuring spectral shifts because it calculates the mean power of the spectrum (Fig. 3–12).[47] When high inspiratory loads are applied to the

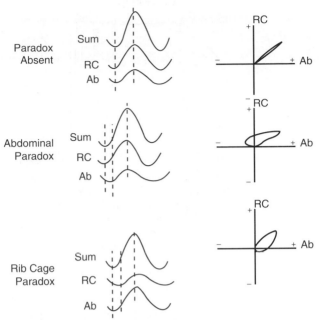

FIGURE 3–11: During normal breathing, there is neither paradoxical nor asynchronous breathing, so that an x-y plot of the rib cage (RC) against abdominal (Ab) excursion reveals a closed or slightly open loop falling between the two positive axes. During abdominal paradox, the abdomen is moving inward rather than expanding during part of inspiration. This results both in asynchrony, indicated by the clear portion of the widened RC-Ab loop, and in an area of paradox, indicated by the shaded area of the loop falling along the negative Ab axis. Similar findings are observed during rib cage paradox. (From Dantzker DR, Tobin MJ. Monitoring respiratory muscle function. Respir Care 30:427, 1985.)

The use of spectral shifts of the electromyogram as a marker of fatigue may have advantages over other techniques because it is less dependent on variability in the resting length of the muscle and on the inability of the patient to perform maximal strength maneuvers. However, it is often difficult to measure and interpret.

respiratory muscles, there is a leftward shift of the centroid frequency to a lower range. A decrease in the high-low ratio parallels a decrease in the centroid frequency. Characteristically, shifts in the power spectrum have been shown at TTIdi values of greater than 15%. Furthermore, the higher the TTIdi above 15%, the more rapidly the changes in the power spectrum occur.[28] The mechanism of the shift is not entirely understood, and it is unclear whether it actually signals the onset of fatigue or merely indicates that the muscle is working at a high percentage of its maximal output. In other words, when spectral shifts occur, the muscle is said to be in a fatiguing pattern of contraction, but it may not imply that overt fatigue has developed. In addition, the change in the electromyographic findings may have a different time course from those in fatigue. For example, the high-low ratio recovers rapidly to baseline levels after the cessation of fatiguing respiratory maneuvers, even when there is still persistence of low-frequency fatigue.[47] Additional disadvantages of this measurement are the lack of normal values and the fact that longitudinal measurements are necessary. In other words, the change in spectrum should be referenced to the power spectrum of the fresh muscle.

Inspiratory Muscle Relaxation Rate

Another manifestation of impending fatigue is a slowing of the rate at which the diaphragm and the inspiratory muscles relax.[48–50] Because

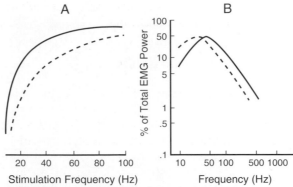

FIGURE 3–12: *A,* Frequency-force curve, and *B,* electromyographic (EMG) power spectrum during voluntary muscle contraction in fresh *(solid line)* and fatigued *(dashed line)* muscle. In the fatigued muscle, as shown by the shift in the frequency-force curve to the right, there is a shift in the power spectrum, with an increase in the power in the low (10 to 40 Hz) frequencies and a decrease in the power in the high frequencies (greater than 160 Hz). This shift can be detected by calculating the high-to-low ratio, which decreases when the muscle performs fatiguing contractions. (*A* and *B,* From Moxham J, Edwards RHT, Aubier M, et al. Changes in EMG power spectrum [high-to-low ratio] with force fatigue in humans. J Appl Physiol 53:1095, 1982.)

The maximal relaxation rate is obtained as the first derivative of pressure with respect to time (dp/dt).

this may vary with the peak inspiratory pressure or with the vigor of the contraction, it is normalized by dividing it by the peak contraction pressure. This ratio decreases with fatigue as measured by the previously described changes in centroid frequency and high-low ratios, but there is not as yet universal agreement as to the clinical utility of this index. Koulouris and colleagues demonstrated that the maximal relaxation rates of esophageal, nasopharyngeal, and mouth pressures are closely related.[49] Because nasopharyngeal and mouth pressures can be measured less invasively, these methods may have clinical utility. On the other hand, Wilcox and coworkers had technical difficulties and problems with interpretation of the data and found the maximal relaxation rate still to be of only limited value in the assessment of diaphragmatic fatigue.[51]

This discussion makes it clear that a good test of respiratory muscle fatigue is still lacking. The search for an objective, technically simple, repeatable test that does not require patient cooperation, is motivation independent, and is minimally influenced by lung volume is still ongoing.

MANAGEMENT OF RESPIRATORY MUSCLE DYSFUNCTION

The treatment of patients in whom respiratory muscle dysfunction is thought to play a central role should be directed at eliminating or correcting possible mechanisms or predisposing factors of fatigue. As a general principle, maximizing energy supplies is an important first goal. This should include nutritional replacement; correction of electrolyte abnormalities, including those of phosphorus and magnesium; elimination of hypoxemia and hypercapnia; and optimization of cardiac output. More specific treatment directed primarily at respiratory muscles includes training and conditioning, rest of the respiratory muscles, and pharmacologic manipulation.

Nutritional Repletion

The cause of weight loss in patients with chronic obstructive pulmonary disease (COPD) is not fully understood, but it may relate in part to a hypermetabolic state in which energy demand exceeds supply.[52] Donahoe and colleagues compared resting energy expenditures and the oxygen cost of augmenting ventilation in poorly nourished and well-nourished patients with COPD and in normal controls.[52] They found that both resting energy requirements and the oxygen cost of augmenting ventilation were significantly elevated in malnourished patients with COPD. This effect is probably the result of the increased mechanical load of breathing, decreased ventilatory muscle efficiency, or both. Several previous studies have indicated that caloric intake in these patients is not reduced. This suggests a greater role for the increased metabolic rate as the crucial factor.[53]

A number of factors may limit the amount of energy one can deliver to malnourished patients with COPD. These include side effects of the enteral preparations, anorexia, desaturation with meals, and ventilatory limitation in dealing with increased CO_2 production generated by the high carbohydrate load.

Several studies have documented the deleterious effects of malnutrition in both animals and humans. Animal studies have documented the characteristic atrophy of type 2 muscle fibers.[53] Type 2 fibers are responsible for most of the force exerted by the muscle. It is easy to understand, therefore, that loss of these fibers leads to muscle weakness, a feature that has been well described in underweight humans.[54] In Arora and Rochester's study, patients whose average ideal body weight was 71% of normal had marked reductions in PI_{max}, vital capacity, and maximal voluntary ventilation as compared with normally nourished individuals.[54] Although long-term nutritional repletion in underweight stable patients with COPD has shown inconsistent results, some studies have shown a positive effect of nutritional supplementation on respiratory pressures and body weight.[53, 55] The difference in outcome of these studies may be due to different periods of supplementation, greater degrees of undernutrition, and greater augmentation of caloric and protein intake in the study patients.

Weaning was more successful in a patient group receiving 2000 to 3000 calories per day than in a group receiving only 400 calories per day.[58]

After nutritional supplementation in the critical care setting, a study by Kelly and coworkers showed an increase in maximal inspiratory mouth pressures from 39.2 ± 4.8 to 52.0 ± 4.6 cm H_2O, in addition to an increase in lean body mass.[56] It has also been suggested that nutritional support is important in facilitating weaning, as demonstrated by Larca and Greenbaum.[57] They found that in patients in whom the response to hyperalimentation was favorable, weaning was successful. A study that evaluated muscle function of the adductor pollicis in malnourished patients with various gastrointestinal disorders found an improvement in contractile properties after refeeding.[59] Thus, evidence suggests that nutritional repletion improves respiratory muscle performance. Future research will focus on providing clearer guidelines regarding the timing of nutritional repletion, the optimal route and means, and whether such measures have a meaningful impact on the morbidity and mortality of these patients.

Malnutrition is clearly associated with muscle atrophy and weakness and should therefore be avoided in the critical care unit.

Conditioning and Training

Whether exercise limitation is invariably due to impaired ventilatory mechanics in COPD is unclear. Nevertheless, at peak exercise levels, patients with significant lung disease utilize a much greater percentage of their ventilatory reserve than do normal subjects. This observation supports the view that training directed specifically at the ventilatory muscles might not only improve ventilatory muscle function but also increase overall exercise capacity.[60]

Training Methods

Three main methods of ventilatory muscle training have emerged: resistive training, hyperpneic training, and threshold load training.

Resistive Method. The resistive method uses inspiratory devices with small orifices through which patients breathe, thereby loading the ventilatory muscles. During this form of training, expiration is unimpeded.

Hyperpneic Method. The patient performs voluntary hyperpnea in a rebreathing circuit, constructed so as to maintain alveolar oxygen and carbon dioxide concentrations within physiologic limits. In addition, this system provides a target ventilatory level in order to stimulate the patient's maximal performance. Sustained ventilatory levels are usually between 70 and 90% of the maximal voluntary ventilation, usually at the higher level in patients with COPD.

Threshold Load Method. The threshold load method uses an inspiratory valve that is weighted so that it opens only when a predetermined threshold inspiratory pressure is attained. Inspiration can proceed only as long as this threshold pressure is exceeded. Irrespective, therefore, of the inspiratory flow rate, the inspiratory pressure remains relatively constant.

Efficacy of Training. There is as yet no consensus on the overall efficacy of ventilatory muscle training. It is not even clear whether it is preferable to train the muscles specifically for strength or endurance, or possibly for a combination of both. Strength training is performed by means of near-maximal (high-tension, low-repetition) muscular contractions, such as may be performed by a weight lifter. This results in an increase in muscle fiber size and an obvious increase in muscle bulk. On the other hand, muscle endurance is not enhanced. Improved endurance of skeletal muscle is obtained with high-frequency (high-repetition, low-tension) activity, such as may be seen in aerobic activities (e.g., running or swimming). This training is not associated with an increase in muscle fiber size but rather with an increase in capillary number and mitochondrial density. The latter change is associated with an increase in the level of oxidative enzymes, which presumably improves the aerobic capacity of the trained muscles.

Only more recently, with the study of Harver and associates, are there data on the functional benefits of training.[61] In this study, a period of resistive training with a feedback device showed a reduction in dyspnea during activity in patients with COPD. The dyspnea was assessed by means of a questionnaire. Patients also showed an improved respiratory muscle strength. However, a Canadian study that used a threshold device showed better ventilatory muscle function but no improvement in exercise capacity.[62]

Weaning From Mechanical Ventilation

An application of particular importance to critical care is the weaning of patients from mechanical ventilators. In these patients, it is obviously important to optimize lung function and eliminate adverse metabolic factors. However, once this has been achieved, if weaning is still problematic, specific exercises aimed at improving inspiratory muscle endurance may facilitate weaning. Early case reports suggested that this may be beneficial, and more recently, a study by Aldrich and colleagues showed that almost 50% of a group of difficult-to-wean patients were ultimately weaned after a period of inspiratory resistive training. Although this study was uncontrolled, it does suggest that training may offer some benefit in difficult-to-wean patients.[63]

Some investigators have hypothesized that incorrect training may induce a state of chronic fatigue. Further muscular exercise may aggravate the fatigue rather than improve muscle function. Unfortunately, in the absence of a simple test to diagnose fatigue in patients, it has been difficult to prove this hypothesis. In this regard, however, it is interesting to speculate that the study of Brouchard and coworkers may offer a way of combining ventilatory assistance with training.[64] These investigators showed that increasing levels of pressure support ventilation progressively reduced the inspiratory work of breathing in ventilated patients. They also demonstrated that application of pressure support ventilation reduced diaphragmatic fatigue as measured by the high-low ratio of the electromyogram; interestingly, they also showed that sternomastoid muscle activity was markedly reduced when pressure support ventilation provided adequate rest to the muscles. These investigators postulated that the combination of training and graduated pressure support ventilation may be the optimal method of providing loaded breathing. In this way, it would be possible to titrate the load on the respiratory muscles without progressing to the point of fatigue. This hypothesis requires further validation, but this method offers the potential for training the muscles without the danger of precipitating or aggravating fatigue.

Resting the Ventilatory Muscles

The respiratory muscles of patients with chronic airway obstruction are required to work continuously against high loads. Several investigators have postulated that this leads to a state of chronic fatigue that further impairs respiratory muscle function.[32, 38, 65, 66] Resting the respiratory muscles by means of intermittent ventilatory support has been suggested as a way of overcoming the fatigue. Preliminary studies showed that patients with COPD and neuromuscular disease improved respiratory muscle and overall function after intermittent ventilatory support.[66] This led to a heightened interest in intermittent ventilatory support as a therapeutic modality. The early studies used negative pressure ventilation applied by means of airtight bodysuits or cuirass ventilation. Although Rochester and coworkers demonstrated that the Drinker respirator (iron lung) was capable of providing rest of the respiratory muscles, as shown by marked reductions in spontaneous diaphragmatic activity,[67] many other investigators were unable to duplicate these results with the Drinker ventilator or the bodysuit.[68-70] Success with negative pressure ventilators appears to be dependent on a cooperative, relaxed subject and considerable acclimatization and practice.[69, 70]

A potential problem with negative pressure ventilation is the development of upper airway obstruction during ventilatory support. This is associated with sleep apnea and sleep fragmentation, and it is postulated that it may result from the loss of central activation of the upper airway

Excessively high inspiratory loads can precipitate fatigue.

Simple observation of sternomastoid muscle activity may provide information about the adequacy of the ventilatory muscles in overcoming inspiratory loads during mechanical ventilation.

muscles at the onset of inspiration. Alternatively, high subglottic pressures may be generated by the negative pressure ventilator, and if these exceed the critical closing pressure of the upper airway, upper airway narrowing occurs.[71] The latter problem can be prevented by applying the negative pressure to the extrathoracic upper airway as well. Alternatively, Goldstein and coworkers showed that with nasal continuous positive airway pressure or the use of tricyclic medication, upper airway obstruction can be prevented during negative pressure ventilation.[62]

Positive Pressure Ventilation

More recently, several investigators have provided ventilatory support by means of positive pressure through a nasal mask.[40, 65, 68, 72] This has been used in patients with neuromuscular disease, such as bilateral diaphragmatic paralysis and kyphoscoliosis, and is probably superior to negative pressure ventilation in capturing the diaphragm, as shown by greater reductions in the diaphragmatic electromyogram even during wakefulness.[73, 74]

Overall, the results of intermittent ventilatory support have been most impressive with neuromuscular diseases and chest wall abnormalities such as kyphoscoliosis.[40] In these conditions, the patients' functional capacities have improved, chronic hypercapnea has been reversed, and arterial oxygen saturations have improved. Respiratory muscle strength has also increased. The results in patients with COPD have not been universally successful.[32, 69, 75, 76] Although some investigators have succeeded, even with periods of ventilatory support as short as 8 hours per day, 1 day a week, others using more frequent periods have failed to demonstrate a functional benefit. Lacking from many of these studies is the documentation that ventilatory support actually reduces spontaneous respiratory muscle activity and thus rests the muscles. This may explain some of the differences in outcome.

Although relief of muscle fatigue is one of the postulated mechanisms for the benefit of intermittent ventilatory support, it is not the only way in which this treatment may help. In the study by Ellis and coworkers in patients with kyphoscoliosis, it was believed that the chronic CO_2 retention that may develop because of nighttime hypoventilation causes resetting of the central chemoreceptors.[40] This can be reversed by nocturnal ventilation, which improves chemoreceptor sensitivity with subsequent lowering of the daytime CO_2 level.

Normalization of blood gases at night during ventilation might also counteract the direct deleterious effects of hypercapnea and hypoxemia on the respiratory muscles and may be another beneficial mechanism. Both Rochester[32] and Ellis and coworkers[40] postulated that rest of the muscles might also help to reverse the component of central fatigue, which is responsible for reduced neural drive of the respiratory muscles (see discussion on central fatigue).

Pharmacologic Manipulation

Intense interest has centered around the methylxanthines, specifically theophylline, in augmenting diaphragmatic contractility. Early observations that theophylline increased diaphragmatic contractile tension in animal experiments led to investigation of the effects of aminophylline on respiratory muscle performance in humans.[77, 78] Various techniques for measuring diaphragmatic response to theophylline have been used. They have included voluntary hyperpnea, Pdi_{max}, and muscle stimulation techniques such as twitch Pdi values and force-frequency curves of the diaphragm.

In the first of two studies by Murciano and coworkers, theophylline was reported to increase strength (as measured by the Pdi_{max}) and endurance (as measured by the high-to-low ratio during resistive breathing).[79] The former measurement is confounded by the fact that lung function improved after theophylline use (increase in FEV_1 and decrease in functional residual capacity); therefore, the increase in Pdi_{max} may have reflected improved muscle mechanics rather than increased contractility. Endurance was estimated from the rate of change in the high-low ratio and not measured directly, raising questions about the validity of the conclusion. In studies of theophylline in which endurance was measured directly, only a small effect was noted.[80] A more recent paper showed a significant reduction in dyspnea in patients with COPD.[81] Because of an improvement in the Pdi/Pdi_{max} ratio during tidal breathing, much of the improvement was ascribed to augmentation of respiratory muscle function. However, the large increases in Pdi_{max} found by Murciano and coworkers have not been substantiated by other investigators,[82] and although there may be increases in diaphragmatic strength at therapeutic concentrations of theophylline, this effect is believed to be small.

The effect of cardiac glycosides (digoxin) on diaphragmatic function has been evaluated in several animal species, but here again there is conflicting evidence and no consensus that the effect is beneficial.[83] Thus, at present there is no convincing evidence that drug therapy is likely to improve respiratory muscle function.

SUMMARY

The respiratory muscles obviously play a major role in the process of respiration. Their failure in the setting of neuromuscular disease clearly leads to respiratory failure. The significance of respiratory muscle impairment in other situations is less clear, as are the beneficial effects of strategies aimed at improving muscle strength and endurance. Clearly, more information is required before any clear-cut recommendations can be made.

References

1. Luce JM, Culver BH. Critical review: Respiratory muscle function in health and disease. Chest 81:82–90, 1982.
2. De Troyer A, Estenne M. Functional anatomy of the respiratory muscles. Clin Chest Med 9:177–193, 1988.
3. De Troyer A, Sampson M, Sigrist S, et al. Action of costal and crural parts of the diaphragm on the rib cage in dog. J Appl Physiol 53:30–39, 1982.
4. Mead J. Functional significance of the area of apposition of diaphragm to rib cage. Am Rev Respir Dis 119:31, 1979.
5. Mead J, Loring SH. Analysis of volume displacement and length changes of the diaphragm during breathing. J Appl Physiol 53:750, 1982.
6. Strohl KP, Mead J, Banzett RB, et al. Effect of posture on upper and lower rib cage motion and tidal volume during diaphragm pacing. Am Rev Respir Dis 130:320, 1984.
7. De Troyer A. Mechanical role of the abdominal muscles in relation to posture. Respir Physiol 53:341, 1983.
8. Comtois A, Gorcyca W, Grassino A. Anatomy of diaphragmatic circulation. J Appl Physiol 62:238–244, 1987.

9. Bark H, Kelsen SG, Supinski GS. The effect of changes in blood pressure on blood flow in diaphragmatic muscle strips. Am Rev Respir Dis 131:322A, 1985.
10. Bark H, Supinski GS, LaManna JC, et al. Relationship of changes in diaphragmatic muscle blood flow to muscle contractile activity. J Appl Physiol 62:291–299, 1987.
11. Bellemare F, Grassino A. Effect of pressure and timing of contraction on human diaphragm fatigue. J Appl Physiol 53:1190–1195, 1982.
12. Aubier M, Trippenbach T, Roussos C. Respiratory muscle fatigue during cardiogenic shock. J Appl Physiol 51:499–508, 1981.
13. Viires N, Sillye G, Aubier M, et al. Regional blood flow. Distribution in dog during induced hypotension and low cardiac output. J Clin Invest 72:935–947, 1983.
14. Hussain SN, Graham R, Rutledge F, et al. Respiratory muscle energetics during endotoxic shock in dogs. J Appl Physiol 60:486–493, 1986.
15. Supinski G, DiMarco AF, Ketai L, et al. Reversibility of diaphragm fatigue by mechanical hyperperfusion. Am Rev Respir Dis 138:604–609, 1988.
16. Metzger MJ, Fitts RH. Role of intracellular pH in muscle fatigue. J Appl Physiol 62:1392–1397, 1987.
17. Lewis SF, Haller RG. The pathophysiology of McArdle's disease. Clues to regulation in exercise and fatigue. J Appl Physiol 61:391–401, 1986.
18. Aubier M, Murciano D, Menir Y, et al. Dopamine effects on diaphragmatic strengths during acute respiratory failure in COPD. Ann Intern Med 110:17–23, 1989.
19. Black LF, Hyatt RE. Maximal respiratory pressures. Normal values and relationship to age and sex. Am Rev Respir Dis 99:696, 1969.
20. Rochester DF. Tests of respiratory muscle function. Clin Chest Med 9:249–261, 1988.
21. Druz WS, Danon J, Fishman HC, et al. Approaches to assessing respiratory muscle function in respiratory disease. Am Rev Respir Dis 119(2):145–149, 1979.
22. Koulouris N, Mulvey DA, Laroche CM, et al. Comparison of two different mouthpieces for the measurement of Pi_{max} and PE_{max} in normal and weak subjects. Eur Respir J 1:863–867, 1988.
23. Wilson SM, Cooke HT, Edwards RHT, Spino SG. Predicted normal values for manual respiratory pressures in caucasian adults and children. Thorax 39:535–538, 1984.
24. Marini JJ, Smith TC, Lamb V. Estimation of inspiratory muscle strength in mechanically ventilated patients. The measurement of maximal inspiratory pressure. J Crit Care 1:32–38, 1986.
25. Laporta D, Grassino A. Assessment of transdiaphragmatic pressure in humans. J Appl Physiol 58:1469, 1985.
26. Mier-Jerdrzejowicz A, Brophy C, Moxham J, Green M. Assessment of diaphragm weakness. Am Rev Respir Dis 137:877–883, 1988.
27. Miller J, Moxham J, Green M. The maximal sniff in the assessment of diaphragm function in man. Clin Sci 69:91, 1985.
28. Bellemare F, Grassino A. Evaluation of diaphragmatic fatigue. J Appl Physiol 53:1196–1206, 1982.
29. McCool FD, McCann DR, Leith DE, et al. Pressure-flow effects on endurance of inspiratory muscles. J Appl Physiol 60:299, 1986.
30. Hussain SN, Pardy RL. Inspiratory muscle function with restrictive chest wall loading during exercise in normal humans. J Appl Physiol 58:2027–2032, 1985.
31. Brown SE, Caschari RJ, Light RW. Arterial oxygen desaturation during meals in patients with severe chronic obstructive pulmonary disease. South Med J 76:194–198, 1983.
32. Rochester DF. Does respiratory muscle rest relieve fatigue or incipient fatigue? Am Rev Respir Dis 138:516–517, 1988.
33. Aubier M, Murciano D, Lercocquic Y, et al. Bilateral phrenic stimulation. A simple technique to assess diaphragmatic fatigue in humans. J Appl Physiol 58:58, 1985.
34. Bellemare F, Bigland-Ritchie B. Assessment of human diaphragm strength and activation using phrenic nerve stimulation. Respir Physiol 58:263–277, 1984.
35. Hubmayr RD, Litchy WJ, Gat PC, et al. Transdiaphragmatic twitch pressure. Am Rev Respir Dis 139:647–652, 1989.
36. Moxham J, Wiles CM, Newham D, Edwards HT. Sternomastoid muscle function and fatigue in man. Clin Sci 59:463–468, 1980.
37. Aldrich TK. Respiratory muscle fatigue. Clin Chest Med 9:225–226, 1988.
38. Macklem PT. The clinical relevance of respiratory muscle research: J. Burns Amberson lecture. Am Rev Respir Dis 134:812–815, 1986.
39. Bellemare F, Bigland-Ritchie B. Central components of diaphragmatic fatigue assessed by phrenic nerve stimulation. J Appl Physiol 62:1307–1316, 1987.
40. Ellis ER, Grunstein RR, Chan S, et al. Non invasive ventilatory support during sleep improves respiratory failure in kyphoscoliosis. Chest 94:811–815, 1988.
41. Gandevia SC, McKenzie DK. Activation of the human diaphragm during maximal static efforts. J Physiol 367:45–56, 1985.
42. Cohen CA, Zagelbaum G, Gross D, et al. Clinical manifestations of inspiratory muscle fatigue. Am J Med 73:308–316, 1982.
43. Dantzker DR, Tobin MJ. Monitoring respiratory muscle function. Respir Care 30:422–429, 1985.
44. Konno K, Mead J. Measurement of the separate volume changes of rib cage and abdomen during breathing. J Appl Physiol 22:407–422, 1967.

45. Tobin MJ, Perez W, Guenther SM, et al. Does rib cage-abdominal paradox signify respiratory muscle fatigue? J Appl Physiol 63:851, 1987.
46. Schweitzer TW, Fitzgerald JW, Bowden JA, et al. Spectral analysis of human inspiratory diaphragmatic electromyogram. J Appl Physiol 46:152, 1979.
47. Moxham J, Edwards RHT, Aubier M, et al. Changes in EMG power spectrum (high-to-low ratio) with force fatigue in humans. J Appl Physiol 53:1094–1099, 1982.
48. Esau SA, Bye PTP, Pardy RL. Changes in rate of relaxation of sniffs with diaphragmatic fatigue in humans. J Appl Physiol 55:731, 1983.
49. Koulouris N, Vianna LG, Mulvey DA, et al. Maximal relaxation rate of esophageal, nasal and mouth pressures during a sniff reflect inspiratory muscle fatigue. Am Rev Respir Dis 139:1213–1217, 1989.
50. Levy RD, Esau SA, Bye PTP, et al. Relaxation rate of mouth pressure with sniffs at rest and with inspiratory muscle fatigue. Am Rev Respir Dis 130:38, 1984.
51. Wilcox PG, Eisen A, Wiggs BJ, Pardy RL. Diaphragmatic relaxation rate after voluntary contractions and uni and bilateral phrenic stimulation. J Appl Physiol 65:675–682, 1988.
52. Donahoe M, Rogers R, Wilson D, Pennock B. Oxygen consumption of the respiratory muscles in normal and in malnourished patients with chronic obstructive pulmonary disease. Am Rev Respir Dis 140:385–391, 1989.
53. Lewis MI, Belman MJ. Nutrition and the respiratory muscles. Clin Chest Med 9:337–348, 1988.
54. Arora NS, Rochester DF. Effect of body weight and muscularity on human diaphragm muscle mass, thickness, and area. J Appl Physiol 52:64–70, 1982.
55. Efthimiou J, Fleming J, Gomes C, et al. The effect of supplemental nutrition in poorly nourished patients with chronic obstructive pulmonary disease. Am Rev Respir Dis 137:1075–1082, 1988.
56. Kelly SM, Allan R, Field S, et al. Inspiratory muscle strength and body composition in patients receiving total parenteral nutrition therapy. Am Rev Respir Dis 130:33–37, 1984.
57. Larca L, Greenbaum DM. Effectiveness of intensive nutritional regimes in patients who fail to wean from mechanical ventilators. Crit Care Med 10:297–300, 1982.
58. Laroche CM, Mier AK, Moxham J, Green M. The value of sniff esophageal pressures in the assessment of global inspiratory muscle strength. Am Rev Respir Dis 138:598–603, 1988.
59. Russell DM, Pendergast PJ, Darby PL, et al. The effect of refeeding: A comparison between muscle function and body composition in anorexia nervosa. Am J Clin Nutr 38:229–237, 1983.
60. Leith ED, Bradley M. Ventilatory muscle strength and endurance training. J Appl Physiol 41:508–516, 1976.
61. Harver A, Mahler DA, Daubenspeck JA. Targeted inspiratory muscle training improves respiratory muscle function and reduces dyspnea in patients with chronic obstructive pulmonary disease. Ann Intern Med 111:117–124, 1989.
62. Goldstein RS, Molotiu N, Skrastins R, et al. Reversal of sleep-induced hypoventilation and chronic respiratory failure by nocturnal negative pressure ventilation in patients with restrictive ventilatory impairment. Am Rev Respir Dis 135:1049–1055, 1989.
63. Aldrich TK, Karpel JP, Uhrlass RM, et al. Weaning from mechanical ventilation. Adjunctive use of inspiratory muscle training. Crit Care Med 17:143–167, 1989.
64. Brouchard L, Harf A, Lorino H, Lemaire F. Inspiratory pressure support prevents diaphragmatic fatigue during weaning from mechanical ventilation. Am Rev Respir Dis 139:513–521, 1989.
65. Braun NMT. Nocturnal ventilation—A new method [Editorial]. Am Rev Respir Dis 135:523–524, 1987.
66. Braun NMT, Marino WD. Effect of daily intermittent rest of respiratory muscles in patients with severe chronic airflow limitation (CAL). Chest 85:59S, 1984.
67. Rochester DF, Braun NMT, Lane S. Diaphragmatic energy expenditure in chronic respiratory failure: The effect of assisted ventilation with body respirators. Am J Med 63:223–232, 1977.
68. Henke KG, Arias A, Skatrud JB, et al. Inhibition of inspiratory muscle activity during sleep. Am Rev Respir Dis 138:8–15, 1988.
69. Rodenstein DO, Stanescu DC, Cuttitta G, et al. Ventilatory and diaphragmatic EMG responses to negative-pressure ventilation in airflow obstruction. J Appl Physiol 65:1621–1626, 1988.
70. Rodenstein DO, Cuttitta G, Stanescu DC. Ventilatory and diaphragmatic EMG changes during negative pressure ventilation in healthy subjects. J Appl Physiol 64:2272–2278, 1988.
71. Levy RD, Bradley TD, Newman SL, et al. Negative pressure ventilation. Effects on ventilation during sleep in normal subjects. Chest 95:95–99, 1989.
72. Celli BR, Rassulo J, Corral R. Ventilatory muscle dysfunction in patients with bilateral idiopathic diaphragmatic paralysis. Am Rev Respir Dis 136:1276–1278, 1987.
73. Belman MJ, SooHoo G, Kuei J, et al. Effectiveness of ventilatory muscle rest with positive versus negative pressure ventilation in normals and COPD patients. Am Rev Respir Dis 139:A13, 1989.
74. Carrey Z, Gottfried S, Levy R. Ventilatory muscle support in respiratory failure with nasal positive pressure ventilation. Chest 97:150–158, 1990.

75. Zibrak JD, Hill NS, Federman EC, et al. Evaluation of intermittent long-term negative-pressure ventilation in patients with severe chronic obstructive pulmonary disease. Am Rev Respir Dis 138:1515–1518, 1988.
76. Shapiro SH, Ernst P, Gray-Donald K, et al. Effect of negative pressure ventilation in severe chronic obstructive pulmonary disease. Lancet 340:1425–1429, 1992.
77. Aubier M. Pharmacotherapy of respiratory muscles. Clin Chest Med 9:311–324, 1988.
78. Rice KL, Leatherman JW, Duane PG, et al. Aminophylline for acute exacerbations of chronic obstructive pulmonary disease. Ann Intern Med 107:305–309, 1987.
79. Murciano D, Aubier M, Lecocquie Y, et al. Effects of theophylline on diaphragmatic strength and fatigue in patients with COPD. N Engl J Med 311:349–353, 1984.
80. Belman MJ, Sieck GC, Mazar A. Aminophylline and its influence on ventilatory endurance in humans. Am Rev Respir Dis 131:226–229, 1985.
81. Murciano D, Aubier M, Pariente R, et al. A randomized controlled trial of theophylline in patients with severe chronic obstructive pulmonary disease. N Engl J Med 320:1521–1525, 1989.
82. Moxham J. Aminophylline and the respiratory muscles: An alternative view. Clin Chest Med 9:325–336, 1988.
83. Sherman MS, Aldrich TK, Chaudhry I, et al. The effect of digoxin on contractility and fatigue of isolated guinea pig and rat hemidiaphragms. Am Rev Respir Dis 138:1180–1184, 1988.

4.

Key Terms

Dyspnea

Dyssynchrony

Gastroesophageal Reflux

Muscle Load

Sensory Receptors

Stridor

Transdiaphragmatic
Pressure (Pdi)

Learned responses, as well as
physiologic adaptation over time,
influence the perception of
dyspnea in any one individual.

Dyspnea: Pathophysiology and Clinical Evaluation

Evelyn Shearer-Poor, M.D., and
Peter S. Kussin, M.D.

DEFINITION OF DYSPNEA

The sensation of breathlessness, or dyspnea, is associated with a heightened awareness of the automatic and cyclic nature of respiration. In the physiologic sense, dyspnea arises from a complex interplay of neuromuscular signals, which are driven by coaxial neural mechanisms to ensure adequate ventilation and expedient motor responses. As is true with other sensory experiences, dyspneic sensations are interpreted along a continuum of severity reflecting the degree of effort required to meet physiologic demands. Dyspnea, an uncomfortable, labored sensation, can occur during normal physiologic stress such as exercise, as well as in pathophysiologic conditions. Dyspnea develops when demands to increase ventilation exceed the physiologic capacity of the neuromuscular machinery or when dyssynchrony develops. The clinician is faced with the problem of first defining the etiology of the symptom of dyspnea and then assessing the severity of the impairment or disability causing dyspnea.

No unifying hypothesis fully explains the genesis of dyspnea. Mechanisms contributing to this sensation include stimulation of the central nervous system; output from intrapulmonary, diaphragmatic, and chest wall receptors; abnormalities in respiratory muscle function; and nonpulmonary neural reflex generation. The components of this integrated system are depicted in Figure 4–1.

CENTRAL NERVOUS SYSTEM CONTROL OF RESPIRATION

The central nervous system performs an obligatory role in the control of respiration, although the relationship of these responses to the sensation of dyspnea remains obscure. Efferent signals descend from the cerebral cortex to influence brain stem respiratory control centers, spinal cord peripheral muscles, joints, and skin. Afferent signals from peripheral mechanoreceptors, chemoreceptors, and stretch receptors located in central blood vessels, lung parenchyma, muscles, joints, and skin modify output from the brain stem and the cerebral cortex. The cerebral cortex can consciously influence the depth and rate of respiration to perform functions such as speaking and can consciously alter mechanical effort by overriding autonomic stimuli. Pain, anxiety, and physical trauma can increase ventilatory demand and result in dyspnea, although the pathways for the generation of the response are not understood. The perception of dyspnea arises when there is discordance between afferent signals

55

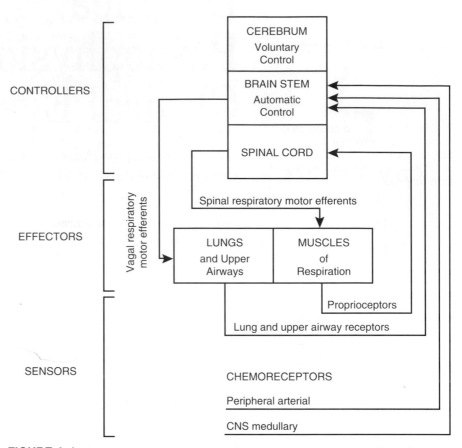

FIGURE 4–1: The respiratory control system. CNS, central nervous system. (From Berger AJ, Mitchell RA, Severinghaus JW, et al. Regulation of respiration. Reprinted, by permission, from the New England Journal of Medicine 297:92–97, 138–143, 194–201, 1977.)

from any peripheral sensory receptors and the output of the respiratory control centers. The complex pathways leading to the sensation of dyspnea are best approached by considering the various anatomic categories.

Cortical Influences

It is well appreciated that the cerebral cortex is able to override the autonomic function of the nervous system, including demands to increase minute ventilation in response to exercise, hypercarbia, or hypoxemia. Speaking, breath holding, singing, and wind instrument playing are excellent examples of the ability of the human brain to overcome the homeostatic rhythmic cycling of respiration. Interrupting vagal input and paralyzing muscular contraction may significantly prolong breath holding and mask the sensation of dyspnea. Dyspnea is not solely dependent on sensory input from muscle fibers. Eloquent studies of the relationship of anatomic lesions to changes in respiratory patterns have been performed, although the mechanisms by which these lesions influence the sensation of dyspnea are not understood.

Chemical Control of Respiration as Related to Dyspnea

Dyspnea was originally thought to occur as a result of hypoxemia, hypercarbia, and acidemia. Chemoreceptors present in the aortic arch, the carotid bifurcation, and the medulla respond to local changes in arterial oxygen, carbon dioxide, and hydrogen ion concentrations. Under normal circumstances, ventilation increases hyperbolically as the Pa_{O_2} is lowered from 100 to 40 mm Hg. Elevated Pa_{CO_2} or $[H^+]$ concentrations can also act to amplify ventilation. It is suggested that chemoreceptor response to changes in O_2 and CO_2 tensions, and regional $[H^+]$ concentration influence activation of chest wall muscle tendon organs and spindle fibers, augmenting ventilatory effort and dyspnea. Dyspnea may develop in patients with chronic obstructive pulmonary disease (COPD) in the absence of desaturation because of inefficient ventilatory effort, cardiac dysfunction, deconditioning, and chemoreceptor activation caused by hypercarbia and early exercise-induced acidosis. In contrast, patients with interstitial lung disease demonstrate an inverse correlation between gas exchange and dyspnea scores. The belief that chemoreceptor activation played an important role in dyspnea generation led to attempts to relieve dyspnea by performing bilateral carotid body resection in patients with chronic obstructive disease. These efforts succeeded in reducing the work of breathing by attenuating resting and exercise minute ventilation responses to hypoxia and hypercarbia. Unfortunately, this surgical denervation of peripheral chemoreceptors led to respiratory failure because the driving force for respiratory muscle activity had been compromised. Additional support for the concept that the carotid bodies act as a driving force in stimulating dyspnea through motor neuron activation has been demonstrated in studies in normal individuals. Exercise in the presence of high inspired fractions of CO_2 while the chest is constrained or ventilation is voluntarily inhibited exacerbates exercise-induced dyspnea. Normal individuals exposed to experimental hypercapnic ventilation do not alter their perceptions of externally applied resistive loads. Patients with chronic hypercapnia demonstrate a more complex array of responses to changes in muscle load, including much more variable and nonlinear responses than normal individuals, which suggests complicated adaptation responses from mechanoreceptors and chemoreceptors.

Brain Stem

The medulla is the central integrating center where neural afferent signals converge and are processed, resulting in rhythmic generation of the impulses responsible for cyclic breathing. The glossopharyngeal, vagal, and recurrent laryngeal nerves provide the vital connections for afferent sensory information to reach the brain stem. Higher cortical centers modulate activity in the brain stem. In the medulla, neuronal groups are activated in an oscillating pattern, influencing motor neurons in the upper airway, facial muscles, diaphragm, and thoracic and abdominal walls.

Sensory Receptors

Sensory input from the chest wall, airways, perialveolar regions, pleura, vasculature, and viscera continuously inform the brain stem of the status of muscle activation, load, volume, pressure, chemical balance, effort, and demand. Details of function and location of receptors and neural pathways in animals provide data that can be extrapolated to the clinical setting. The genesis of dyspnea due to activation of various recep-

---

Patients with chronic obstructive disease and restrictive lung disease may have a minute ventilation as much as 50% higher than normal.

Some of the exercise-induced dyspnea in patients with COPD can be alleviated with supplemental oxygen, although resting arterial oxygen tension has not been found to correlate with dyspnea on several rating scales.

tors can only be inferred from human studies. Several types of receptors are thought to be involved in the generation of dyspnea. Nonmyelinated fibers stimulated by parenchymal lung disease induce tachypnea, airway secretion, and bronchoconstriction. *Stretch receptors* distributed throughout the tracheobronchial tree relax smooth muscle and respond to changes in lung volume. Afferent pathways also exist in the upper airways as prolongation of breath holding occurs with airflow through the nose. *Irritant receptors,* rapidly adapting receptors distributed from the nasal submucosa to the alveoli, respond to chemical stimulation. It is possible to alleviate dyspnea in normal individuals with topical anesthesia of these receptors, although load sensation does not change. J receptors are present in the capillaries or the juxtacapillary regions of the interstitium of the lung parenchyma. Their stimulation, resulting from pulmonary congestion, edema, or vascular occlusion, can result in dyspnea.

Aerosolized lidocaine improves ventilatory responses to hypercapnia and inspiratory resistive loading in patients with COPD.

Chest Wall Muscle Apparatus and Dyspnea

Within the muscles of the thoracic wall are muscle spindle endings and tendon organs, which are associated with sensation of length and force, respectively. Phasic excitation and inhibition of contraction of inspiratory and expiratory muscles are accomplished through a motor loop driven by the medulla. Intrafusal sensory fibers called muscle spindles, as well as tendon organs, are sensitive to changes in muscle length. Stimulation of intercostal muscles, which inhibits inspiratory effort and duration of phrenic nerve activity, is associated with prolonged expiration. Similar responses are seen in asthma and emphysema, in which hyperinflation leads to inappropriate length-tension relationships in chest wall musculature: the external intercostal muscles are shortened and the internal intercostal muscles are stretched. Altered length-tension relationships play an important role in the generation of the sensation of dyspnea.

Stretch or mechanoreceptor stimulation in muscles, joints, or tendons of the chest wall can induce increases in respiratory rate, prolongation of expiration, and interruption of inspiration.

MEASUREMENT OF DYSPNEA

Dyspnea can arise from a multitude of stimuli. Table 4–1 lists the clinical conditions and stimuli that can provoke dyspnea. The symptom of breathlessness is modified by cognitive perception, which integrates a host of reflexive neuromechanicoreceptive properties. Historically, symptoms of dyspnea were primarily ascribed to the magnitude of respiratory effort. This construct was derived from experiments in which external loads were applied to subjects who were asked to report the first detectable change in applied load and then to note additional changes once that threshold had been determined. Although useful in defining "load detection," studies that manipulate external loads do not address the important differences between perception of dyspnea and detection of load. The advent of psychophysical measurement has since allowed investigators to reproduce and grade dyspnea reliably and to describe functional correlates of dyspnea. Improvements in dyspnea measurement have allowed physiologists to evaluate fully the influence of physiologic parameters, such as the inspired fraction of carbon dioxide or oxygen, tidal volume, applied pressure, ventilation, and resistive and elastic loads on the sensation of dyspnea.

TABLE **4-1:**   Causes of Acute and Chronic Dyspnea

Psychiatric	Cardiac disease
Hyperventilation syndrome	Myocardial infarction or ischemia
Upper airway obstruction	Tamponade
Foreign body aspiration	Dissection
Retropharyngeal abscess	Pericarditis
Epiglottitis	Intracardiac shunts
Angioedema	Valvular disease
Anaphylaxis	Arrhythmias
Vocal cord dysfunction	Chest wall deformities
Trauma, inhalation injury	Skeletal deformities
Lower airway obstruction	Ankylosing spondylitis
Acute asthma exacerbation	Kyphosis
Chronic or acute bronchitis	Scoliosis
Emphysema	Rib fracture
Cystic fibrosis	Obesity
Foreign body aspiration	Ascites
Endobronchial tumor	Pregnancy
Pulmonary parenchymal disease	Neuromuscular disease
Pneumonia	Muscular dystrophy
Cardiogenic pulmonary edema	Amyotrophic lateral sclerosis
Noncardiogenic edema	Myasthenia gravis
Adult respiratory distress syndrome	Poliomyelitis
Intrapulmonary hemorrhage	Guillain-Barré syndrome
Lymphangitic spread of malignancy	Respiratory muscle dysfunction
Pulmonary vascular disease	Thyrotoxicosis
Fat embolism	Hypothyroidism
Venous thromboemboli	Malnutrition
Tumor microemboli	Mitochondrial myopathies
Intravascular leukostasis	Acid maltase deficiency
Intrapulmonary shunts	Hematologic
Arteriovenous malformation	Anemia
Pulmonary hypertension (primary or secondary)	Hemoglobinopathies
Veno-occlusive disease	Sickle cell disease
Vasculitis	Leukoagglutinin reactions
Pleural disease	Intravascular leukostasis
Pneumothorax: spontaneous, tension	Deconditioning
Effusions	Gastroesophageal disease
Inflammation	Reflux
Fibrosis	
Malignancy or mesothelioma	

Psychophysical Parameters

Psychophysics is the study of the perception of stimulus intensity and magnitude and the characterization of sensory experiences. A way to describe this is to express the change in sensory responses as a function of baseline status, given as the relationship of ΔS/reference $S = k$ (constant). This provides a means of experimentally comparing respiratory sensation between individuals as well as between different stimuli. Threshold discrimination has been used to assess respiratory sensations resulting from the application of externally applied loads. The magnitude of threshold discrimination varies considerably between individuals. The theory of "length-tension inappropriateness" uses the application of external loads to suggest that muscle afferents in the chest wall are responsible for the sensation of dyspnea. Although magnitude scaling of externally applied loads provides clues about the genesis of dyspnea, the testing methods are cumbersome and the results do not correlate with dyspnea in the clinical sense. Scaling measurements assess the subject's perception of some magnitude related to *supra*threshold stimuli. The time-consuming methods used in scaling techniques require technical expertise, thereby limiting their use to the experimental setting. These techniques include magnitude estimation, magnitude production, Ste-

The equation $y = K\Omega^n$

where

y = the sensation magnitude
Ω = the stimulus intensity
K = an arbitrary constant of the scale unit
n = the power exponent that depends on the perceived stimulus conditions, sensory modality, and intensity

Physiologic parameters that are measured in association with dyspnea using scaling measurements include

- Minute ventilation
- Ratio of minute ventilation to maximal voluntary ventilation
- Oxygen consumption
- Ratio of pleural pressure to maximal inspiratory pressure
- Peak inspiratory flow
- Ratio of tidal volume to forced vital capacity
- Respiratory frequency
- Ratio of inspiratory time to total time
- Peak mouth pressure

vens' power law, and cross-modality matching. Magnitude estimation requires that the subject grade the magnitude of a series of suprathreshold stimuli. Two primary techniques are employed:

With *open scaling methods,* subjects assign numerical values to the perceived stimulus intensities, plotting average magnitude response as a function of the intensity of the stimulus.

With *closed scaling techniques,* numerical values are assigned by the experimenter, and subjects grade their perceptual responses within predetermined scales.

Magnitude estimation as a function of a power law serves to couple sensation of magnitude with performance under similar and dissimilar physical conditions. Linear visual analog scales provide a visual range of choices to ascertain the perceptual magnitude of dyspnea. An example of the utility of this scaling technique is seen in McGavein's Oxygen-Cost Diagram, which is a visual analog scale relating oxygen requirements to given levels of activity. Category scales, first used to grade the impact of dyspnea on activities, were adopted by the Medical Research Council and later modified by the American Thoracic Society. The linear analog and category scales are designed to measure the influence of task magnitude on provoking dyspnea. Magnitude production tasks require that subjects attempt to match their effort or response to a displayed sensory scale, and relate perceptual changes to particular work demands. Cross-modality matching requires subjects to compare sensory modalities and task intensities as a function of stimulus intensity. Stimulus values are plotted against each other. Scales have been designed to discriminate between the sensations of dyspnea and the perception of magnitude of effort during exercise, voluntary hyperventilation, with modifications in fractional inspired oxygen and carbon dioxide levels.

Functional studies of respiratory and exercise capacity correlate moderately well with dyspnea scores. The scales most widely used to measure dyspnea are the Borg Scale, the Baseline Dyspnea Index, and the Transitional Dyspnea Index. The Visual Analog Scale, the Baseline Dyspnea Index, and the Transitional Dyspnea Index have been compared favorably with physiologic assessment as tools to demonstrate changes in respiratory and exercise capacity in longitudinal studies and after clinical interventions. With exercise testing, including the 6- and 12-minute walk tests and bicycle ergometer testing, r values of .5 to .6 have been reported between exercise, oxygen uptake, power functions, and dyspnea scaling. In patients with underlying COPD, dyspnea ratings correlate modestly with FEV_1, forced vital capacity, maximal inspiratory pressure, and transdiaphragmatic pressure (Pdi). Cross-validation and reliability studies have demonstrated the clinical utility of these scales, so they are commonly used as outcome measures in clinical studies.

PHYSIOLOGIC CORRELATES OF DYSPNEA

The expression of dyspnea requires a conscious association of effort with the process of breathing. In the clinical setting, significant differences exist in the way individuals perceive dyspnea, based on learned behavior, expectations, and the underlying pathophysiology of the causative process. Variations in the rating of dyspnea with similar degrees of pulmonary impairment occur. This could be due to differences in chest wall or pulmonary compliance, variations in the functional activity of the respiratory muscles, and cardiovascular limitations. In general, individuals modify their physical responses in response to dyspnea in a relatively graduated fashion depending on the degree of impairment of the pulmonary system. Although predictable patterns of respiratory adaptation occur in patients with obstructive and restrictive disease, correlations between measures of respiratory muscle strength, spirometric values, and measures of dyspnea are only moderate and are not reproducible on all scales. For example, the DL_{CO} has been correlated with dyspnea in patients with pulmonary fibrosis, although other parameters show an extremely weak correlation. Exertional dyspnea has a weak correlation with vital capacity and the extent of parenchymal involvement (profusion index).

Contribution of the Upper Airway

The upper airway is endowed with the ability to detect flow through nasal mucosal receptors, vagally mediated muscle tone, and reflex arcs. Increased dyspnea is reported after nasal mucosal anesthesia, although this has been attributed to flow resistance secondary to mucosal edema. Intranasal receptors decrease ventilatory responses to hypercapnia and prolong breath holding. The contribution of the upper airway to the sensation of dyspnea is not well understood.

Chest Wall Mechanics

Afferent sensations from the chest wall are important in the perception of lung volume and pressure. In normal subjects, the threshold discrimination range for resistive loads is 0.5 to 1.0 cm $H_2O/L/sec$ (about 15 to 20% greater than baseline). Since their description of elastic and resistive load devices to assess threshold values for the sensation of effort, a number of investigators have assessed the change in perception of external threshold loads in patients with airway obstruction and interstitial lung diseases. With the use of magnitude scaling techniques, the relative perceived importance or magnitude of a given stimulus can be compared with the magnitudes of other stimuli. This has been used to assess discriminatory function between subjects using tidal volume, ventilation, applied pressure, and resistive and elastic loads. Perceptual scaling measures have also been used to study sensation in respiratory physiology. With the use of magnitude estimation, magnitude production, and Stevens' power law, perception of pressure change appears to be independent of lung inflation volume.

The perceived magnitudes of volume, pressure, and ventilation were similar, although that of ventilation was highest. Because patients with lung disease have greater thresholds for load detection, the sensation of dyspnea is not correlated with load detection. Adaptation to increased airway resistance reduces the dyspnea associated with chronic airflow obstruction in asthma. When imposed expiratory loads are assessed experimentally in this population, the sensation of dyspnea is reduced compared with that in controls. Pulmonary function testing results correlate best with psychophysical measurements of dyspnea and functional impairment. In patients with pulmonary fibrosis, a positive correlation was found between the sensation of dyspnea and the ratio of minute ventilation to maximal voluntary ventilation. In contrast, scores on dysp-

Patients with interstitial lung disease have greater thresholds for detection of elastic loads and do not detect increases in loads as readily as normal subjects.

nea rating scales were not correlated with load discrimination. In a study of subjects with "chronic lung disease," no correlation was noted between exertional dyspnea and detection of resistive loads. These experimental findings are confirmed in the clinical setting, in which assessment of dyspnea using detection of threshold values is much less precise than pulmonary function measurements such as flow-volume relationships, lung volume, or diffusion capacity.

In COPD, the mechanics of the chest wall and the functional state of the respiratory muscles appear to be the most important factors responsible for the genesis of dyspnea. The pressures produced by muscles of the chest wall are a function of the contractile state, resting length, and shortening velocity of the muscles. Hyperinflation and the increased work of breathing place the patient with COPD at a disadvantage. To meet ventilatory requirements, a more powerful afferent signal than normal is required to generate a given muscle tension. This is partially due to muscle fiber shortening in both the diaphragm and the chest wall, resulting in reduced maximal inspiratory pressure generation by patients with COPD. In addition, hyperinflation flattens the diaphragm and increases the elastic recoil of the thoracic cage. Despite these alterations in diaphragm structure and function, measures of dyspnea could not be correlated with diaphragmatic strength as measured by transdiaphragmatic pressure. Increases in basal airway resistance and age are additional factors that affect the perceived magnitude of a given resistive load.

Dyspnea and Exercise Testing

In the clinical evaluation of dyspnea, exercise testing may provide an objective measure of an individual patient's response to therapy or identify a primary pulmonary or cardiac etiology of dyspnea. Breathlessness is often the limiting factor to exercise in patients with pulmonary disease, although fatigue can also occur with severe deconditioning or gas-exchange abnormalities. A modest correlation between dyspnea ratings and peak oxygen consumption exists in patients with interstitial lung disease and COPD. Supplemental oxygen therapy can reduce dyspnea in this subset of patients, presumably through an increase in oxygen delivery and a reduction in resting pulmonary arterial pressure that occurs with relief of alveolar hypoxia. Exercise ability measured by walking distance but not exercise time correlated with dyspnea. Minute ventilation in patients with obstructive lung disease at rest can be as much as 50% higher than minute ventilation in normal individuals at rest. Minimal changes in exertion or physiologic stress force the muscles to operate at a disadvantage, with resulting increased expenditure of energy, increased oxygen consumption, and dyspnea.

Baroreceptor-driven mechanisms of dyspnea come into play during exercise in both restrictive and obstructive pulmonary disease, although the triggering events are different in the two processes. In the fibrotic lung, replacement of functional alveoli and loss of the vascular bed leads to reductions in lung volume. At low work rates, the pulmonary vascular bed is unable to dilate, resulting in a high ratio of dead space to tidal volume. Right atrial and pulmonary arterial pressures rise, stimulating chemoreceptors, stretch receptors, and baroreceptors. In the emphysematous lung, loss of functional lung parenchyma results in loss of vascular supply.

CLINICAL CAUSES OF DYSPNEA

Table 4–1 lists causes of dyspnea grouped by pathophysiology. In most cases, dyspnea is cardiopulmonary in origin, with the most common causes being COPD, asthma, and coronary artery disease.

Psychiatric

Hyperventilation—a syndrome manifested by induction of an acute respiratory alkalosis.

Psychogenic dyspnea remains a diagnosis of exclusion. It should be evaluated and treated by a physician specializing in psychological manifestations of the disorder. Hyperventilation, which usually arises from emotional factors, presents most commonly in women in the third to fourth decades of life. More than half of the patients complain of recurrent, nonexertional dyspnea. Common occurrences such as perioral and distal extremity paresthesias may be accompanied by dizziness, faintness, visual disturbances, and impaired psychomotor behavior. Chest radiographic, physical examination, and alveolar-arterial gradient findings will be normal; a decreased Pa_{CO_2} may be present. The work-up must exclude other etiologies of dyspnea. This syndrome may be confused with Leeuwenhoek's disease, or diaphragmatic flutter, resulting from clonic contractions of the diaphragm.

Upper Airway

Subacute and chronic forms of upper airway obstruction include thyromegaly, enlarged lymphoid tissue of the pharynx and retropharynx, tracheal malignancy, and tracheal stenosis.

In acute dyspnea accompanied by stridor, structural and functional lesions above the level of the thoracic inlet must be considered. Stridor may not always be present in these cases. Diagnoses to consider include epiglottitis, foreign body aspiration, edema, anaphylaxis, angioedema, trauma, strictures, vocal cord dysfunction, and abscesses of the pharynx, hypopharynx, or larynx. Dyspnea can occur with upper airway obstruction at any point from the oropharynx to the carina. Obstructive lesions in the upper airway result in dyspnea once the diameter of the airway has decreased to approximately 8 mm or less. The glottis is subject to vagally mediated reflexes in a fashion similar to that in the lower airways. Under normal conditions, inspiration should result in abduction of the vocal cords to allow less restricted airflow. The area of the glottal opening is relatively constant, although inspiratory widening has been noted. In histamine-induced bronchospasm, a marked expiratory narrowing of the glottis may contribute to the inspiratory wheezes seen in some patients with asthma. Epiglottitis is not common in the adult. Food may become lodged in the hypopharynx and upper larynx, causing complete airway obstruction with aphonia; the person may grasp the neck in a "universal distress signal." The middle-aged or older individual who consumes alcohol with a meal is at greatest risk for this form of airway obstruction. Anaphylactic reactions are characterized by life-threatening upper airway edema and vasodepression, which can occur within minutes of exposure. The most common precipitating events include Hymenoptera stings, shellfish ingestion, and reactions to medications. Hereditary angioneurotic edema, a derangement of function in the complement system due to a deficiency in C1 esterase activity, may present fulminantly. Facial and upper airway edema may be more prominent in this condition.

The act of inspiration requires coordinated contraction of the poste-

Other pathologic entities of the upper airway that can present as dyspnea, with or without hoarseness, wheezing, or stridor, include laryngeal or vocal cord polyps, nodules, cysts, tumors, and vocal cord dysfunction.

rior cricoarytenoid muscle, resulting in vocal cord abduction and a reduction in airflow resistance. Paradoxical inspiratory vocal cord adduction has been reported following upper respiratory infection and may accompany stress and exercise. Some patients appear to have a volitional control over this disorder. Vocal cord dysfunction is typically accompanied by wheezing (heard loudest over the larynx), normal arterial blood gas values, negative methacholine challenge results, and variable extrathoracic obstruction on pulmonary function testing. This disorder is most often described in young women; an association with the health care profession is common. Lack of response to conventional therapy for asthma, frequent emergency room visits, and normal airway function between episodes should prompt consideration of this syndrome. Patients with vocal cord dysfunction may report that dyspnea worsens with conventional treatment of the upper airways with racemic epinephrine and steroids. Inappropriate adduction of the anterior two thirds of the vocal cords during a wheezing episode is noted on direct examination, although inappropriate vocal cord adduction has also been reported during expiration and throughout the respiratory cycle. Treatment is directed toward relaxation of the laryngeal musculature and psychiatric counseling. Once a functional etiology has been ascribed to vocal cord dysfunction, associated psychological disorders should be addressed. The psychological disorders associated with laryngeal dysfunction may alter laryngeal function, although the underlying mechanism is not understood.

Vocal cord paralysis may result from antecedent surgery and may present as nocturnal or ambulatory wheezing and dyspnea. Classically, these patients have variable extrathoracic obstruction on flow-volume loops and can be diagnosed laryngoscopically. Laryngeal dyskinetic syndromes include Meige's syndrome, which is characterized by bilateral blepharospasm, and spasm of the facial, oropharyngeal, and laryngeal musculature. Women are more often affected, usually in the sixth decade of life. The etiology is unknown.

Lower Airway

Acute bronchoconstriction may develop in patients with underlying disease or after an acute toxic exposure to gases, smoke, heat, or fumes. Precipitants of bronchospasm in patients with underlying reactive airway disease include respiratory infections, aeroallergen exposure, environmental irritants, cold air, exercise, emotion, gastroesophageal reflux, and sinusitis. Progressive or acute breathlessness, orthopnea, and wheezing may be accompanied by tachypnea, tachycardia, pulsus paradoxus, and arterial desaturation. The severity of asthma cannot be ascertained by the history of breathlessness. Patients who have more frequent exacerbations of asthma have been shown to have lower dyspnea ratings than those with fewer exacerbations.

Patients suffering from chronic airflow obstruction generally complain of dyspnea on exertion and have a history of a relatively prolonged adaptation to exercise by reducing the extent or the rapidity of activities performed. Airway hyper-reactivity may coexist. The work of breathing is greater in emphysema because of airway obstruction and a reduction in the elastic recoil of the lung.

Parenchymal Disease

Any pulmonary infiltrate may induce dyspnea, either acutely or progressively, depending on the physiologic reserve and the expectations of the individual patient. Causes include infection, bleeding, and pulmonary edema of any etiology. Dyspnea in interstitial edema arises from afferent signals of perialveolar or juxtacapillary receptors, which in response to either hypoxemia, hypercapnia, or metabolic acidosis increase ventilatory drive. The diagnosis is usually suspected from the clinical scenario, although the diagnosis of infection with superimposed pulmonary edema is more problematic. The diagnosis of pneumonia is most readily made by the clinical constellation of fever, leukocytosis, radiographic infiltrate, and purulent secretions. Examination of expectorated sputum, nasotracheal suction, and bronchoscopy with a protected brush and bronchoalveolar lavage may assist in discerning the presence of infection and in identifying the pathogen, although there is considerable controversy about the best approach. The differentiation of hydrostatic pulmonary edema from permeability edema may require pulmonary artery catheterization. The patient with pulmonary hemorrhage classically presents with hemoptysis and rapid clearing of airspace disease within 24 to 48 hours. Respiratory failure can occur if hemorrhage is diffuse. This may result from perforation by intravascular catheters or erosion from tuberculoma, broncholithiasis, or granuloma. Other causes of airspace-filling diseases that may present with unexplained dyspnea include pulmonary alveolar proteinosis, hypersensitivity pneumonitis, sarcoidosis, and eosinophilic pneumonia.

Causes of pulmonary hemorrhage include vasculitis, bronchogenic carcinoma, bronchial adenoma, bronchiectasis, lung abscess, tuberculosis, mycetoma, and pulmonary vascular rupture.

Pulmonary Vascular Disease

Dyspnea, a common symptom accompanying acute pulmonary embolism, is usually associated with chest pain of a pleuritic type. The appearance of dyspnea in acute thromboembolism is due to a number of factors, including

- Hypoxemia
- Stimulation of intravascular mechanoreceptors in the pulmonary circulation or the right atrium
- Tachypnea due to increased ventilatory requirements in the setting of increased dead space

As with other lung diseases, breathlessness does not correlate with the extent of vascular occlusion in either acute or chronic thromboembolic disease.

Fat embolism occurs in the setting of trauma or surgery to long bones. It classically occurs within 48 hours of the initiating event and is associated with neurologic dysfunction, petechiae, and permeability pulmonary edema, which are believed to result from the effects of released fatty acids and endogenous mediators on cell membranes.

The dyspnea of pulmonary hypertension from primary or secondary etiologies is more insidious, although the astute practitioner can elicit the symptom of dyspnea with detailed questioning about exercise tolerance. Receptors in the pulmonary artery, the right atrium, and the right ventricle are reputed to be the source of the dyspnea. The physical examination may reveal evidence of elevated right-sided heart pressures, including a right ventricular heave, a loud pulmonic sound, regurgitant murmurs transmitted from the tricuspid and pulmonic valves, and peripheral edema. Pulmonary function testing may reveal normal or mildly restrictive lung volumes, a reduced DL_{CO}, an elevated alveolar-arterial gradient, and an exaggerated ventilatory response to exercise due to

Keys to the prompt diagnosis of pulmonary thromboembolism include

- Maintaining a high level of suspicion in the appropriate clinical setting
- Proper use of screening modalities, such as ventilation-perfusion lung scanning
- Serial noninvasive testing for the presence of deep venous thrombosis

increased demands in the face of an increased alveolar dead space ventilation. Chest radiography will reveal markedly enlarged pulmonary arteries with normal lung fields, perhaps some areas of oligemia, and right ventricular enlargement. Similarly, electrocardiography may reveal signs of right ventricular failure, strain, right atrial enlargement, or the $S_{1,2,3}$ pattern identified in cor pulmonale.

Microthromboemboli from tumor can result in dyspnea, with occlusion of small arterioles. Other potential causes of dyspnea include aggregation of leukocytes in leukemia, occlusive disease secondary to thrombocythemia, sickle cell hemoglobinopathy, obliterative diseases of scleroderma, and collagen vascular diseases.

Pleural Disease

Spontaneous pneumothoraces cause acute dyspnea and chest pain; the severity of dyspnea depends on the extent of the collapse and the degree of underlying lung disease. Only 25% are associated with strenuous activities or coughing, sneezing, and wheezing. Pleural effusions appear to induce dyspnea based on the size of the effusion and the severity of underlying parenchymal abnormalities.

Cardiac Disease

Several types of cardiac disease may present with dyspnea. The most easily diagnosed is congestive cardiomyopathy, with an enlarged cardiac silhouette on chest radiography, rales on lung examination, a diffuse or misplaced point of maximal impulse (PMI) with an S_3 or S_4 on cardiac examination, and peripheral edema. However, cardiac ischemia, acute myocardial infarction, cardiac tamponade, restrictive cardiomyopathy, aortic dissection, pericarditis, intracardiac shunts, myxomas, cardiac carcinoid, and valvular disease, especially mitral stenosis, may also present in a similar fashion. The dyspnea of the cardiac patient may be the result of metabolic acidosis at a low work rate, stimulation of right atrial stretch receptors, airway obstruction due to edema, or hypoxemia and hypercarbia due to either pulmonary edema or diaphragm fatigue. During exercise, dyspnea may occur as a result of several factors, including an increased ventilatory requirement after attainment of the anaerobic threshold and hence stimulation of chest wall receptors, increased activity of intracardiac pressure receptors, stimulation of airway irritant receptors, and enhanced activity of pulmonary vascular and J receptors. In low cardiac output states, blood flow to the diaphragm, the main inspiratory pump, may be insufficient to meet metabolic demands.

Neuromuscular Disease

Individuals with amyotrophic lateral sclerosis, muscular dystrophy, myasthenia gravis, polio, hyper- and hypothyroidism, myositis, maltase deficiency, and mitochondrial myopathy may present with dyspnea or exercise intolerance as a prominent complaint.

A restrictive pattern on pulmonary function tests with a decreased minute ventilatory volume can occur as a consequence of any disease affecting the cervical or thoracic nerve supply to the thorax and any muscular disease of primary or secondary nature. Not uncommonly, the diagnosis of a neuromuscular disorder is made in a patient presenting with exertional dyspnea as the only complaint. Acute upper respiratory tract infections have been reported to result in respiratory muscle weakness. A reduction in maximal inspiratory and expiratory pressures, which may precede changes in spirometric values and lung volumes, may be associated with uncoordinated respiratory muscle function, hypercarbia, and full-blown respiratory failure.

Chest Wall–Associated Disorders

Dyspnea occurs in disorders of the chest wall, including obesity, pregnancy, ascites, and thoracic vertebral deformities such as kyphosis and scoliosis. Chest wall receptors are primarily responsible for the sensation of breathlessness. Obesity results in deposition of fat within and around all viscera, reducing chest wall compliance, impairing diaphragmatic excursion, and requiring a greater effort to ventilate because of the added load. Hypoxemia, common in obesity, results from $\dot{V}/\dot{Q}$ inequalities, with most of the ventilation occuring in upper lung zones. Mechanical factors are of greatest importance in the dyspnea of ascites, although comorbid conditions such as malnutrition and acidosis undoubtedly play an important role as well. Pregnancy frequently elicits a sensation of dyspnea, usually in the first or second trimester. The stimulation of ventilation by elevated progesterone levels seems to be responsible, as evidenced by the mild respiratory alkalosis often noted in pregnancy. No mechanical impairment of the respiratory system has been identified to account for the symptom of dyspnea. Skeletal deformities of the chest wall or vertebrae reduce chest wall compliance, which can result in alveolar hypoventilation. These deformities also cause atelectasis, $\dot{V}/\dot{Q}$ mismatch, hypoxemia, and ultimately pulmonary hypertension.

Other Disorders

Gastroesophageal reflux may be a significant cause of dyspnea once cardiovascular diseases and deconditioning have been excluded. Although it is now well recognized that gastroesophageal reflux induces bronchoconstriction, the actual mechanism is not known. Microaspiration may lead to direct irritant bronchospasm in gastroesophageal reflux. An alternative hypothesis implicates vagally mediated neurogenic reflexes. Hematologic causes of dyspnea include anemia, resulting from decreased oxygen-carrying capacity, and vascular obstruction due to sickle cell hemoglobinopathy. When these conditions are combined with reduced cardiac output, oxygen delivery is severely impaired, which results in muscle weakness and reduced ventilatory and exercise capacity. Leukostasis within the pulmonary vasculature in leukemia can result in dyspnea, as can thrombocythemia.

CLINICAL EVALUATION OF THE PATIENT WITH DYSPNEA

A complete history taking and physical examination, a review of systems, a listing of medications, and a preliminary compilation of clinical tests are part of the initial evaluation of the patient with dyspnea. Frequently, a diagnosis can be established on the basis of the initial evaluation. The history obtained by the clinician may lead to methacholine challenge testing when the suspicion of reactive airway disease arises. Other potentially useful tests include thyroid function testing,

Because the majority of symptoms arise from the pulmonary and cardiovascular systems, initial laboratory screening should include

- Posteroanterior and lateral chest radiography
- Electrocardiography
- Complete blood count and electrolyte panel
- Pulmonary function testing and assessment of resting arterial blood gas

when hypo- or hyperthyroidism is suggested by the clinical evaluation; exercise testing, when the etiology and degree of disability are uncertain; and oral bronchoprovocation (with sulfite, tartrazine, or aspirin) or allergy testing, when suspicion of allergy is present. Ambulatory esophageal pH testing is the most sensitive method of diagnosing gastroesophageal reflux when any symptoms compatible with reflux appear. An alternative (and less expensive) strategy is empiric therapy with either antacids or H_2 antagonists. Laryngoscopy, bronchoscopy, or both are indicated in suspected laryngeal or tracheal disease, possibly preceded by tomography or computed tomography. Echocardiography may be used to evaluate ventricular function and valvular disease and to estimate right pulmonary artery pressures. Microcavitation studies performed with the echocardiogram can identify intracardiac shunts. High-resolution chest computed tomography can assist in the evaluation of radiographically inapparent interstitial lung disease, bronchiectasis, or lymphangitic metastases.

SUMMARY

The experience of dyspnea can be described as the response of the respiratory system to a change in the drive, effort, or power to ventilate; it may be acute and fulminant or insidious and chronic. Any change in the intrinsic properties of the lung may affect the work of breathing. Although the mechanisms leading to dyspnea are not completely understood, clinical success in identifying a cause of dyspnea is on the order of 80 to 95%. Most complaints of acute and chronic dyspnea can be explained on the basis of the cardiorespiratory system. The patient may require bronchial provocation or exercise studies to identify the primary organ system involved. However, in the emergency room setting, the causes of dyspnea may be life threatening and may need to be identified expeditiously so that appropriate life-supporting therapy may be administered. The number of people admitted through an emergency department for acute dyspnea is in the range of 16 to 25%, of which patients with asthma and COPD comprised 40%. The clinician should be able to match the symptoms with the possible cause and set forth a logical plan to evaluate the etiology. It is best to think of the etiologies in a systems fashion during the elicitation of the history and the physical examination, then follow with the work-up that will assist in supporting the clinical impressions.

Suggested Readings

Physiology of Dyspnea

Campbell EJM, Howell JBL. The sensation of breathlessness. Br Med Bull 19:36–40, 1963.
Killian KJ, Campbell EJM. Dyspnea and exercise. Annu Rev Physiol 45:465–479, 1983.
Wasserman K. The physiology of gas exchange and dyspnea. Clin Sci 61:7–13, 1981.

Scaling and Rating Dyspnea

Helsing KJ, Comstock GW, Speizer FE, et al. Comparison of three standardized questionnaires on respiratory symptoms. Am Rev Respir Dis 120:1221–1231, 1979.
Mahler DA, Rosiello RA, Harver A, et al. Comparison of clinical dyspnea ratings and psychophysical measurements of respiratory sensation in obstructive airway disease. Am Rev Respir Dis 135:1229–1233, 1987.

Mahler DA, Weinberg DH, Wells CK, Feinstein AR. The measurement of dyspnea: Contents, interobserver agreement, and physiologic correlates of two new clinical indexes. Chest 85/6:751–758, 1984.

Stoller JK, Ferranti R, Feinstein AR. Further specification and evaluation of a new clinical index for dyspnea. Am Rev Respir Dis 134:1129–1134, 1986.

5

Acid-Base Disorders and Electrolyte Imbalance

Catherine S. Thompson, M.D.

Volatile acids in the form of carbon dioxide (CO_2) derive from the aerobic oxidation of glucose and fatty acids and are excreted by the lung. Fixed acids, generated during the metabolism of protein, are removed by the kidney.

$$CO_2 + H_2O \leftrightarrow H_2CO_3 \leftrightarrow H^+ + HCO_3^-$$

Acid-base disorders, electrolyte disorders, or both are present in the majority of ill, hospitalized individuals. Many of these disorders exist at the time of admission; others develop in the hospital or are worsened by underlying illness, medications, or treatments. Acid-base and electrolyte disturbances often occur simultaneously. The clinical manifestations can be severe, resulting in multi–organ system dysfunction. Prompt recognition and evaluation of these conditions are important so that therapy can restore homeostasis. The reversal of acid-base and electrolyte disorders, which is essential to the overall management of the patient, has a direct impact on prognosis. This chapter reviews acid-base disorders, with an emphasis on differential diagnosis and management, and the common electrolyte disorders, including derangements of serum sodium, potassium, calcium, magnesium, and phosphorus.

ACID-BASE PHYSIOLOGY

The normal pH of arterial blood is tightly controlled between 7.38 and 7.42. The maintenance of blood pH within this narrow range is remarkable in view of the daily input of acid equivalents. The average 70-kg adult produces 15,000 mEq of volatile acids and an additional 70 to 100 mEq of fixed acids daily. The maintenance of a normal blood pH in the face of continuous input of acid depends on the complex interactions between

- The pulmonary excretion of volatile acids
- The renal excretion of fixed acids
- The effect of intracellular and extracellular buffers, which prevent wide fluctuations in blood pH

The process of alveolar ventilation facilitates the excretion of volatile acids from the lung in the form of CO_2. CO_2 is considered a "potential" form of acid because in the red blood cell, CO_2 combines with water (H_2O) in a reversible reaction to produce carbonic acid (H_2CO_3), which dissociates into hydrogen ion (H^+) and bicarbonate anion (HCO_3^-). The hydrogen ions generated by this reaction are buffered within red blood cells by hemoglobin molecules and transported to the lung, where the reaction runs in reverse, with release of CO_2 into the alveoli. CO_2 can also be transported in the blood as dissolved CO_2 or complexed with hemoglobin.

The kidney plays an important role in the regulation of acid-base balance by

- Reabsorbing the filtered load of bicarbonate from the urine
- Excreting the daily burden of fixed acids

The reabsorption of filtered bicarbonate is accomplished primarily in the proximal renal tubule (Fig. 5–1). The excretion of fixed acids occurs in the distal renal tubule, where secreted hydrogen ions either complex with ammonia (NH_3) to form ammonium ion (NH_4^+) or are eliminated as titratable acid in the form of NaH_2PO_4 (Fig. 5–2). The excretion of one hydrogen ion as ammonium or titratable acid accomplishes the net return of one bicarbonate anion to the blood. This replenishment of bicarbonate stores is critical to the preservation of extracellular buffering capacity, the third line of defense in acid-base homeostasis.

The major extracellular buffer is the carbonic acid–bicarbonate system, which serves as the first line of defense against sudden changes in blood pH. This buffer pair consists of a weak acid, carbonic acid (a proton donor), and its conjugate base, bicarbonate (a proton acceptor). The effectiveness of the carbonic acid–bicarbonate buffer system is enhanced by the independent control of the bicarbonate concentration by the kidney and of the CO_2 content by alveolar ventilation.

The relationship between carbonic acid, bicarbonate, and blood pH can be expressed according to the Henderson-Hasselbalch equation:

$$pH = pK + \log\ [HCO_3^-]/[\text{carbonic acid}]$$
$$\text{or}$$
$$pH = 6.1 + \log\ [HCO_3^-]/Pa_{CO_2}$$

where pK is the carbonic acid dissociation constant (6.1) and the carbonic acid content is expressed as a function of the CO_2 tension (Pa_{CO_2}).

In addition to the extracellular carbonic acid–bicarbonate buffer system, intracellular buffers are important in the defense of cell pH. Hemoglobin molecules, proteins, organic phosphates, and bone cartilage all serve as buffers of acid equivalents. In states of chronic metabolic acidosis, bone serves as the major intracellular buffer.

The buffer pairs are in equilibrium according to the reaction

$$CO_2 + H_2O \leftrightarrow H_2CO_3 \leftrightarrow H^+ + HCO_3^-$$

In the steady state, blood pH is a function of the ratio of [HCO_3^-] to [Pa_{CO_2}], rather than their absolute values.

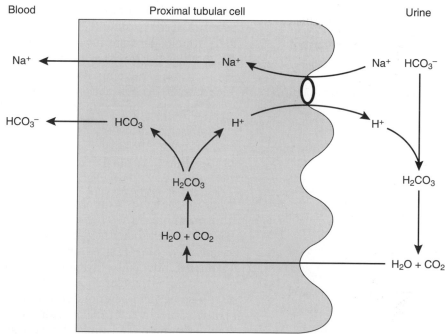

FIGURE 5–1: Bicarbonate reabsorption by the proximal renal tubular cell. The intracellular production of bicarbonate coupled with luminal Na^+-H^+ exchange results in reclamation of filtered bicarbonate. Note that the filtered bicarbonate is *not* the bicarbonate that is reclaimed but rather the bicarbonate generated within the cell.

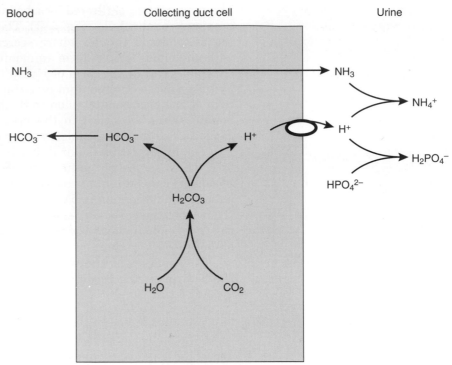

FIGURE 5–2: Bicarbonate regeneration and net H$^+$ excretion in the renal collecting duct. The hydrogen ion is secreted at the luminal surface and combines with ammonia (NH$_3$) to form ammonium (NH$_4^+$) or with HPO$_4^{2-}$ to form "titratable acid."

ACID-BASE DISORDERS

If an acidosis results in a fall in arterial blood pH below 7.35, an acidemia exists. An alkalemia is caused by an alkalosis and is manifested by an increase in arterial blood pH above 7.45.

Acid-base disorders are divided into two major categories, depending on whether the primary abnormality is metabolic or respiratory in origin. A metabolic acid-base disorder results from a primary change in the serum concentration of bicarbonate (HCO$_3^-$). A primary change in the Pa$_{CO_2}$ in blood causes a respiratory acid-base disorder. An acidosis results from either a decrease in bicarbonate concentration or an increase in Pa$_{CO_2}$. Conversely, an alkalosis is generated by either an increase in bicarbonate concentration or a decrease in Pa$_{CO_2}$.

There are four primary acid-base disorders:

- Metabolic acidosis
- Metabolic alkalosis
- Respiratory acidosis
- Respiratory alkalosis

Compensatory responses for any acid-base derangement tend to restore blood pH toward, but not actually into, the normal range.

Each of these disorders results in a physiologic compensatory response that minimizes the change in blood pH caused by the primary acid-base disorder. Metabolic acid-base disorders are compensated by ventilatory responses, and respiratory disorders are compensated by renal responses. Table 5–1 outlines the expected degree of compensation for any given acid-base disorder.

Simple acid-base disorders are defined by the presence of a single process, such as metabolic acidosis with respiratory compensation. Mixed acid-base disorders imply the coexistence of at least two, and sometimes three, independent disorders. The presence of multiple acid-base disorders may result in normal blood pH, Pa$_{CO_2}$, and bicarbonate concentrations. In these cases, calculation of the anion gap provides the clue that a mixed disorder exists.

TABLE **5–1:** Compensatory Responses in Acid-Base Disorders

Primary Disorder	Primary Abnormality	Compensatory Response	Expected Compensation
Metabolic acidosis	↓ HCO_3^- ↓ pH	↓ Pa_{CO_2}	$\Delta Pa_{CO_2} = 1.2 \times \Delta HCO_3^-$
Metabolic alkalosis	↑ HCO_3^- ↑ pH	↑ Pa_{CO_2}	$\Delta Pa_{CO_2} = 0.7 \times \Delta HCO_3^-$
Respiratory acidosis			
Acute	↑ Pa_{CO_2} ↓ pH	↑ HCO_3^-	$\Delta HCO_3^- = 0.1 \times \Delta Pa_{CO_2}$
Chronic	↑ Pa_{CO_2} ↓ pH	↑↑ HCO_3^-	$\Delta HCO_3^- = 0.35 \times \Delta Pa_{CO_2}$
Respiratory alkalosis			
Acute	↓ Pa_{CO_2} ↑ pH	↓ HCO_3^-	$\Delta HCO_3^- = 0.2 \times \Delta Pa_{CO_2}$
Chronic	↓ Pa_{CO_2} Normal to ↑ pH	↓↓ HCO_3^-	$\Delta HCO_3^- = 0.5 \times \Delta Pa_{CO_2}$

Note: ΔPa_{CO_2} and ΔHCO_3^- are the changes in concentration from normal. Pa_{CO_2} is 38–42 mm Hg. HCO_3^- is 24–28 mEq/L. Double arrows indicate more profound change.

Anion gap = Na^+ −
[Cl^- + HCO_3^-]

The anion gap is defined as the difference between serum sodium and the sum of the chloride and bicarbonate concentrations. The normal anion gap, 10 to 14 mEq/L, is an estimate of the unmeasured anions in blood. These anions include albumin molecules, other anionic serum proteins, phosphate, sulfate, and lactate. Abnormalities in the anion gap, either increases or decreases, can provide clues to the underlying acid-base disorders or other pathologic conditions (Table 5–2).

Metabolic Acidosis

Metabolic acidosis is defined as a primary decrease in the plasma concentration of bicarbonate (hypobicarbonatemia). The disorder is generated by one of three mechanisms:

- An increase in the production of fixed acids
- A decrease in the renal excretion of hydrogen ion
- An increase in bicarbonate loss from the body

TABLE **5–2:** Interpretation of the Anion Gap

Increased Anion Gap
Metabolic acidosis
  Lactic acidosis
  Ketoacidosis
  Uremic acidosis
  Intoxications
    Salicylates
    Methanol
    Ethylene glycol
Alkalemia (increased lactate production)
Administration of sodium salts
  Sodium lactate
  Sodium acetate (hemodialysis)
  Sodium citrate (blood transfusion)
  Sodium carbenicillin or ticarcillin
Hyperalbuminemia (volume contraction)

Decreased Anion Gap
Hypoalbuminemia
Multiple myeloma (cationic paraproteinemia)
Intoxications
  Bromide poisoning
  Lithium overdose
Hypercalcemia or hypermagnesemia

The cardiac effects of acidemia include hypotension, vasodilatation, and cardiac arrhythmias.

Most individuals with a metabolic acidosis are also acidemic, but in some circumstances, blood pH may be normal or alkaline if other acid-base disorders occur simultaneously. The respiratory compensation for acute metabolic acidosis is hyperventilation, which results in a fall in Pa_{CO_2} (see Table 5–1). This compensation can reduce the Pa_{CO_2} no lower than 10 to 15 mm Hg. For this reason, metabolic acidoses with serum bicarbonate concentrations of less than 10 mEq/L can be associated with severe acidemia.

The metabolic acidoses are classified into two major categories: the elevated anion gap acidoses and the normal anion gap acidoses (Table 5–3). Metabolic acidoses associated with an elevated anion gap are caused by the retention of an unmeasured anion such as lactate or ketone. Normal anion gap acidoses are generated by an excessive loss of bicarbonate, an inability of the kidney to excrete hydrogen ion, or the addition of exogenous acid equivalents.

Elevated Anion Gap Metabolic Acidosis

The reversible reaction catalyzed by the enzyme lactate dehydrogenase shown in the following equation represents the only metabolic pathway for the production of lactic acid:

$$\text{Pyruvate} + \text{NADH} + \text{H}^+ \leftrightarrow \text{lactate} + \text{NAD}^+$$

Lactic Acidosis. The development of lactic acidosis implies an imbalance between the rates of production and utilization of lactic acid. Overproduction of lactate by cells occurs most commonly as a result of tissue hypoxia, hypoperfusion, or both. Under these anaerobic conditions, the mitochondrial production of oxidized nicotinamide-adenine dinucleotide (NAD^+), an essential cofactor in the conversion of lactate into CO_2 and water, is limited and leads to excessive production of lactate.

Clinically, lactic acidosis is an acute disorder associated with a high mortality rate despite treatment. The serum lactate level typically is in excess of 5 to 10 mM but in severe cases can be greater than 30 mM. A severe acidemia (pH less than 7.20) is common.

Two categories of lactic acidosis are recognized. Type A, the most

TABLE **5–3:** Classification of Metabolic Acidosis

Elevated Anion Gap
Accumulation of endogenous acids
  Lactic acidosis
  Ketoacidosis
  Uremic acidosis
Intoxications
  Salicylates
  Methanol
  Ethylene glycol

Normal Anion Gap (Hyperchloremic Acidosis)
Bicarbonate loss
  Gastrointestinal
    Diarrhea
    Small bowel drainage
    Urinary diverting procedures
  Renal loss
    Proximal RTA
Disorders of distal tubular acidification
  Classic distal RTA
  Hyperkalemic distal RTA
    Hyporeninemic hypoaldosteronism
    Adrenal insufficiency
    Aldosterone resistance
Acid loads
  Acidifying salts
    Ammonium chloride
  Parenteral nutrition
  Dilutional ("expansion acidosis")

RTA, renal tubular acidosis.

TABLE **5–4:** Calculation of the Bicarbonate Deficit in Metabolic Acidosis

Bicarbonate space = $0.6 \times$ body weight (kg)
Bicarbonate deficit = (desired HCO_3^- − actual HCO_3^-) $\times$ bicarbonate space

Example: 70-kg man with HCO_3^- = 10 mEq/L
Desired HCO_3^- = 25 mEq/L
Bicarbonate deficit = $(25 - 10) \times 0.6$ (70 kg)
$= (15) \times (42)$
$= 630$ mEq of HCO_3^- required

Correction of the acidosis with bicarbonate infusions is a controversial issue.

common, is caused by tissue hypoxia or hypoperfusion. Cardiogenic or septic shock, severe anemia, hemorrhage, and carbon monoxide poisoning are the leading causes of this form of lactic acidosis. In type B lactic acidosis, overt tissue hypoxia or hypoperfusion is absent; therefore, the pathophysiology is unknown. A variety of disease states, including diabetes mellitus, malignancies, liver failure, and certain drugs or toxins, have been associated with the spontaneous development of type B lactic acidosis.

The management of the patient with lactic acidosis focuses on treatment of the underlying disorder with attempts to restore normal tissue perfusion, particularly in type A lactic acidosis. Most clinicians agree that bicarbonate supplements should be given to correct the arterial blood pH to 7.20. The bicarbonate deficit for any degree of acidosis can be estimated according to the formula outlined in Table 5–4.

Ketoacidosis. Metabolic acidosis caused by the accumulation of keto acids occurs most commonly in diabetic ketoacidosis, but it can develop in individuals with starvation or alcoholism. Impaired carbohydrate and fatty acid metabolism develops in these disorders as a result of increased lipolysis, insulin deficiency, or both. The keto acids, acetoacetate and beta-hydroxybutyrate, accumulate and lead to an increased anion gap metabolic acidosis.

Patients with diabetic ketoacidosis present with variable degrees of acidosis. Most are also volume depleted from an osmotic diuresis induced by hyperglycemia. Hypotension and coma may complicate the acidosis. These patients are best managed with combined intravenous hydration and insulin administration. The insulin inhibits further ketogenesis and allows for the metabolic conversion of keto acid into bicarbonate equivalents, with restoration of the acid-base balance. Administration of supplemental bicarbonate is not necessary, but correction of associated potassium and phosphorus depletion is important.

Uremic Acidosis. Advanced acute or chronic renal failure is often associated with a metabolic acidosis caused by the retention of inorganic acids such as phosphate and sulfate. These acids are usually excreted by the kidney but are retained when the glomerular filtration rate drops below 10 to 15 mL/min. The acidosis is typically mild, with bicarbonate levels rarely below 15 mEq/L. Supplemental oral bicarbonate in the form of sodium citrate can be administered before initiation of dialytic support in patients who remain acidotic.

Intoxications. Salicylate overdose leads to an accumulation of lactic and keto acids by the uncoupling of oxidative phosphorylation within mitochondria. The treatment includes induction of an alkaline diuresis; bicarbonate supplementation; and in severe intoxications, hemodialysis for removal of the drug.

The osmolar gap is defined as the difference between the measured serum osmolarity and the calculated osmolarity, as shown:

Serum osmolarity = 2 (Na$^+$) + glucose/18 + blood urea nitrogen/2.8

A positive osmolar gap indicates the presence of an unmeasured osmole in the blood, usually a drug or toxin.

Methanol or ethylene glycol poisoning can result in severe metabolic acidosis with significant morbidity and mortality. The acidosis results from the accumulation of various organic acids, such as formic and lactic acids in the case of methanol intoxication and glycolic, oxalic, and lactic acids in patients with ethylene glycol ingestion. Hemodialysis for removal of these toxins and correction of the metabolic acidosis is the preferred treatment. These intoxications can be recognized by the presence of an osmolar gap (which is defined as the difference between the measured serum osmolarity and the estimated serum osmolarity [2 (Na$^+$) + (urea/2.8) + (glucose/18)]).

Normal Anion Gap Acidosis (Hyperchloremic Acidosis)

Bicarbonate Loss. A common cause of a normal anion gap metabolic acidosis is loss of bicarbonate-rich fluid from the gastrointestinal tract in severe diarrhea or with small bowel drainage. Coexistent volume depletion is common. The kidney responds to extrarenal loss of volume and bicarbonate by excreting a concentrated, acidified urine. The urine pH is usually less than 5.5, with an osmolarity of greater than 500 mOsm/kg and a urinary sodium level of less than 10 mEq/L. Gastrointestinal bicarbonate wasting is usually self-limited and requires no specific treatment unless the acidosis is severe. Volume repletion with saline-containing fluids is advised, but supplemental bicarbonate intravenously or orally is rarely necessary unless the bicarbonate level is less than 15 mEq/L.

A less common cause of bicarbonate wasting occurs in proximal renal tubular acidosis (type II RTA). In this disorder, there is incomplete reabsorption of filtered bicarbonate from the tubular fluid, resulting in an alkaline diuresis. The metabolic acidosis is usually mild to moderate, with bicarbonate levels rarely less than 15 mEq/L. Proximal RTA can be associated with other defects of proximal renal tubular function, such as aminoaciduria, uricosuria, phosphaturia, and glycosuria (Fanconi's syndrome). Acquired proximal RTA can occur in diseases such as multiple myeloma, amyloidosis, heavy metal nephrotoxicity, and primary hyperparathyroidism. Treatment with bicarbonate supplements is not effective because the administered bicarbonate is excreted rapidly. Restriction of dietary sodium intake can help by inducing mild volume contraction and stimulating the proximal tubular reabsorption of bicarbonate.

Disorders of Distal Tubular Acidification. Disorders of distal tubular acidification, which are caused by an inability of the distal nephron to excrete adequate amounts of hydrogen ion (H$^+$) into the tubular fluid, include classic distal RTA and hyperkalemic distal RTA.

Classic distal RTA (type I RTA) is characterized by metabolic acidosis, an inappropriately alkaline urine pH (greater than 5.5), and hypokalemia. Hypercalciuria and a tendency to nephrolithiasis are associated features. Hereditary forms of the disease have been described, but most forms of classic distal RTA are acquired in association with diseases such as Sjögren's syndrome, multiple myeloma, or amyloidosis or with the administration of amphotericin B. The electrolyte disorder can be treated with supplemental potassium and bicarbonate, with the latter at a dose of 1 to 2 mEq/kg/day.

The hyperkalemic forms of distal RTA (type IV RTA) are a group of disorders caused by generalized dysfunction of the distal nephron. Hyporeninemic hypoaldosteronism, aldosterone resistance, and decreased renal ammonia genesis are all factors that have been implicated in the generation of these acidoses. A hyperkalemic, hyperchloremic metabolic acidosis and an intact ability to lower urine pH (to less than 5.5) are the hallmarks of these disorders. Clinically, chronic tubulointerstitial diseases caused by diabetes mellitus, systemic lupus erythematosus, hypertension, or analgesic abuse are the major causes of the hyperkalemic forms of distal RTA. Treatment of the hyperkalemia with dietary restriction of potassium, diuretics, or binding resins (sodium polystyrene sulfonate [Kayexalate]) is helpful in the long-term management of these patients. Oral administration of bicarbonate is indicated in refractory cases.

Other Conditions. The administration of acidifying agents such as ammonium chloride or, more commonly, the use of parenteral nutrition solutions containing acidic amino acid preparations such as lysine and arginine can induce a mild hyperchloremic acidosis. Finally, the rapid infusion of large volumes of isotonic saline can lead to a mild "expansion acidosis" with dilution of bicarbonate stores.

Metabolic Alkalosis

Metabolic alkalosis is defined as a primary increase in the plasma concentration of bicarbonate. An increase in blood pH, or alkalemia, is the hallmark of metabolic alkalosis, although the magnitude of the pH change is a function of the severity of the alkalosis, the effect of other acid-base disorders, and the degree of respiratory compensation (see Table 5–1). The systemic effects of alkalemia include lethargy, muscle weakness, seizures, and cardiac arrhythmias. In general, the clinical effects of alkalemia are more severe than those of an equivalent degree of acidemia.

Metabolic alkalosis, regardless of the underlying cause, occurs in two distinct phases: the generation phase and the maintenance phase. The alkalosis can be generated either by an excessive loss of acid through the gastrointestinal tract or the kidney or by the net gain of bicarbonate equivalents. The maintenance of metabolic alkalosis, however, is governed by the kidney, which sustains the elevated concentration of bicarbonate in blood. The renal factors that maintain metabolic alkalosis include an increased capacity of the proximal tubule to reabsorb bicarbonate and an augmented hydrogen secretory ability in the distal nephron, both of which act to perpetuate the existing alkalosis.

The causes of metabolic alkalosis are divided into two categories on the basis of the response to the infusion of chloride-containing solutions such as isotonic saline (Table 5–5). The "chloride-responsive" alkaloses,

> Respiratory compensation in metabolic alkalosis is limited, a fact that explains the presence of severe alkalemia (blood pH > 7.6) in some patients.

TABLE **5–5:** Classification of Metabolic Alkalosis

Chloride Responsive (Urine Cl⁻ < 10 mEq/L)
Gastric fluid loss (vomiting or nasogastric suction)
Diuretic use
Posthypercapneic
Villous adenoma or chloride diarrhea
Chloride Unresponsive (Urine Cl⁻ > 20 mEq/L)
Primary aldosteronism
Hypercortisolism (Cushing's syndrome)
Renin-secreting tumor
Renal artery stenosis
Licorice ingestion
Liddle's syndrome
Bartter's syndrome
Potassium depletion
Milk-alkali syndrome

disorders associated with a decrease in effective circulating volume, are typically generated by the excessive loss of fluid, acid, or both from the gastrointestinal tract or kidney. Renal factors that increase the proximal tubular reabsorption of bicarbonate or the distal nephron excretion of acid maintain these alkaloses.

The most common form of chloride-responsive alkalosis is caused by persistent vomiting or nasogastric suction. Affected patients are typically volume depleted and hypokalemic. Excessive renal loss of potassium is stimulated by high levels of aldosterone. The urine chloride content is low (less than 10 mEq/L), and the urine may be acidic (pH of less than 5.5). Other causes of gastrointestinal metabolic alkalosis include villous adenoma and congenital chloride diarrhea.

A second major cause of chloride-responsive metabolic alkalosis is the use of loop or thiazide diuretics. These drugs induce urinary losses of chloride, potassium, and extracellular fluid volume, thereby generating the alkalosis. The disorder is maintained by the effects of secondary hyperaldosteronism on the distal nephron, which promote hydrogen ion secretion.

Posthypercapneic metabolic alkalosis occurs when a patient with chronic, compensated alveolar hypoventilation experiences a sudden improvement in alveolar ventilation. The disorder is most often seen as a complication of over-aggressive mechanical ventilation. As the Pa_{CO_2} is abruptly reduced, the chronically elevated bicarbonate concentration leads to a metabolic alkalosis. The maintenance of the alkalosis is fostered by coexistent volume contraction, which stimulates bicarbonate reabsorption by the proximal tubule.

The management of chloride-responsive alkaloses includes volume repletion with isotonic saline and correction of associated potassium deficiency. Diuretic drugs should be withheld in severe cases. H_2-blocking drugs can help to reduce gastric hydrogen ion loss in patients requiring continued nasogastric suction. Refractory, severe alkaloses may on occasion require the infusion of dilute hydrochloric acid solutions (0.15 N HCl).

In contrast, the "chloride-resistant" metabolic alkaloses are characterized by a normal or an expanded extracellular fluid volume and an elevated urinary chloride concentration, and they are not corrected by the administration of isotonic saline. These alkaloses are mediated by the excessive activity of aldosterone on hydrogen ion secretion in the distal tubule. The resultant hypokalemia helps to maintain the alkalosis by further stimulating the tubular secretion of hydrogen ion.

Primary aldosteronism is an important cause of chloride-resistant metabolic alkalosis. The hypersecretion of aldosterone in this disorder is usually caused by a benign adenoma of the adrenal gland. Malignant tumors or bilateral hyperplasia of the adrenal glands can also cause this syndrome, which is characterized by hypertension, volume expansion, metabolic alkalosis, and elevated levels of aldosterone. A related disorder is hypercortisolism, or Cushing's syndrome, which can cause similar electrolyte imbalance owing to the mineralocorticoid effects of excess circulation cortisol.

RESPIRATORY ACID-BASE DISORDERS

Primary changes in Pa_{CO_2} are responsible for the generation of respiratory acid-base disorders. The change in blood pH induced by respi-

TABLE **5–6:** Causes of Acute Respiratory Acidosis

Obstructive defects
  Large airway obstruction
  Aspiration
  Obstructive sleep apnea syndrome
  Reactive airway disease (asthma)
Restrictive defects
  Pneumothorax
  Flail chest
  Acute pulmonary edema
Neuromuscular defects
  Toxins: curare, succinylcholine, organophosphates
  Myasthenia gravis
  Guillain-Barré syndrome
  Metabolic myopathy: hypokalemia, hypophosphatemia
Central nervous system depression
  Drugs: opiates
  Anesthesia
  Central sleep apnea
  Cerebral trauma or infection

The key factor in the regulation of Pa_{CO_2} is alveolar ventilation because the rates of CO_2 production and diffusion across the pulmonary capillaries are not rate-limiting functions under most conditions. Primary alveolar hypoventilation, therefore, leads to hypercapnea (increased Pa_{CO_2}) and respiratory acidosis. Conversely, alveolar hyperventilation causes hypocapnea (decreased Pa_{CO_2}) and respiratory alkalosis.

In acute compensation, the serum concentration of bicarbonate rises about 1 mEq/L for each 10-mm Hg increment rise in the Pa_{CO_2} above 40 to 45 mm Hg.

In chronic compensation, the serum concentration of bicarbonate will have increased by 3 to 4 mEq/L for each 10-mm Hg increment rise in the Pa_{CO_2} above 40 to 45 mm Hg.

ratory acid-base disorders is a function of the magnitude of change in alveolar ventilation and the effect of compensatory responses. Compensation for respiratory acid-base disorders is separated into acute and chronic phases. The acute phase occurs within minutes to hours and involves hydrogen ion shifts between the intracellular and extracellular spaces. Chronic compensation is mediated by changes in the renal handling of bicarbonate and occurs over hours to days. The expected degree of compensation for respiratory acid-base disorders is outlined in Table 5–1.

Respiratory Acidosis

A primary decrease in alveolar ventilation is responsible for the development of respiratory acidosis. Alveolar ventilation can be impaired acutely or more slowly (Tables 5–6 and 5–7). Compensatory responses to respiratory acidosis begin immediately, with buffering of hydrogen ion within cells. Chronic compensation occurs more slowly, as the kidney increases its reabsorptive capacity for bicarbonate. An increase in the renal production of ammonia, an important urinary buffer, allows for augmented excretion of hydrogen ion by the kidney. After several days of respiratory acidosis, renal compensation is at a maximum.

Patients with acute respiratory acidosis secondary to large airway obstruction or restrictive defects such as acute pulmonary edema appear

TABLE **5–7:** Causes of Chronic Respiratory Acidosis

Obstructive defects
  Chronic obstructive pulmonary disease
  Obstructive sleep apnea syndrome
  Tracheal stenosis
Restrictive defects
  Chronic pneumonitis
  Pulmonary fibrosis
  Kyphoscoliosis, pectus deformities
Neuromuscular defects
  Multiple sclerosis
  Amyotrophic lateral sclerosis
  Muscular dystrophy
Central nervous system defects
  Central sleep apnea
  Bulbar poliomyelitis

anxious and possibly disoriented. Those with central nervous system depression from drugs, trauma, or infection are typically somnolent. In contrast, individuals with chronic compensated respiratory acidosis may be relatively asymptomatic. Some complain of headache, which is a result of cerebral vasodilatation induced by the hypercapnea. In severe cases, papilledema will be observed.

The treatment of respiratory acidosis should be directed to the underlying cause of alveolar hypoventilation. Intubation and mechanical ventilation may be required in some patients with hypoventilation that is not easily reversed. Attempts to improve alveolar ventilation with bronchodilators or chest physiotherapy may be of benefit. Bicarbonate-containing solutions should not be administered because of the risk of alkalemia and volume overload. Individuals with chronic compensated respiratory acidosis are at particular risk for acute, severe alkalemia (posthypercapneic alkalosis) if they are intubated and hyperventilated.

> Chronic respiratory acidosis is usually well compensated and is associated with an arterial blood pH greater than 7.30.

Respiratory Alkalosis

Primary respiratory alkalosis, which is caused by alveolar hyperventilation, is associated with an acute fall in Pa_{CO_2} and alkalemia. The disorder is most commonly observed in its acute form in association with anxiety states ("hyperventilation syndrome"). Other conditions, such as hypoxemia, pulmonary embolism, salicylate intoxication, and cerebrovascular accidents, can also result in acute respiratory alkalosis (Table 5–8). The symptoms include dizziness, chest tightness, dyspnea, circumoral paresthesias, and in severe cases, carpopedal spasm. The neuromuscular effects of the hyperventilation syndrome are caused by a fall in the extracellular concentration of ionized calcium, an effect of increased binding of calcium to serum proteins in alkalemia. The compensatory response to acute respiratory alkalosis is a flux of hydrogen ions out of the intracellular compartment and a fall in the serum concentration of bicarbonate of 2 mEq/L for each 10-mm Hg drop in the Pa_{CO_2}.

> During pregnancy, a mild respiratory alkalosis is a normal finding.

Chronic respiratory alkalosis, a less common disorder, can be caused by chronic anxiety states, neurologic disease, or hepatic dysfunction, or it may be induced in mechanically ventilated patients (Table 5–9). Renal compensation for chronic respiratory alkalosis begins within hours and manifests as a bicarbonate diuresis with diminished net acid excretion from the kidney. These compensatory responses often result in a normal blood pH within several days of sustained hyperventilation. This contrasts with compensatory responses in other acid-base disorders, which bring blood pH toward, but not actually into, the normal range.

> In renal compensation for respiratory alkalosis, the serum bicarbonate concentration falls by 5 mEq/L for each 10-mm Hg reduction in the Pa_{CO_2}.

TABLE **5–8:** Causes of Acute Respiratory Alkalosis

Anxiety hyperventilation syndrome
Neurologic disorders
CNS trauma
CNS infection
CNS infarction or hemorrhage
Salicylate overdose
Sepsis
Tissue hypoxia
Carbon monoxide poisoning
Arterial hypoxemia: pulmonary emboli
Severe anemia
Ventilator induced

CNS, central nervous system.

TABLE **5–9:** Causes of Chronic Respiratory Alkalosis

> Chronic anxiety hyperventilation syndrome
> Neurologic diseases
>> CNS infarction
>> CNS tumor
>> CNS infections
> Hepatic failure
> Pregnancy
> Ventilator induced

CNS, central nervous system.

The treatment of the respiratory alkaloses depends on the underlying cause of hyperventilation. In the acute hyperventilation syndrome, reassurance, mild sedation, and rebreathing into a paper bag are effective maneuvers that break the attack. Acute respiratory alkalosis induced by central nervous system lesions, sepsis, or tissue hypoxia requires specific intervention directed at the underlying disease. Ventilator-induced acute respiratory alkalosis should be managed with a reduction in minute ventilation.

Chronic hyperventilation typically requires no specific treatment because the compensatory responses correct the blood pH in most cases. Patients with chronic ventilator-induced respiratory alkalosis respond to a gradual reduction in minute ventilation.

DISTURBANCES OF OSMOLARITY: HYPONATREMIA AND HYPERNATREMIA

The osmolarity of body fluid is regulated between 285 and 295 mOsm/kg water. Sodium, the major solute in extracellular fluid, and its serum concentration can be used as a gauge of total body fluid tonicity because both the intracellular and the extracellular fluid compartments exist in osmotic equilibrium. Disorders of serum sodium, both hyponatremia and hypernatremia, represent derangements in body fluid tonicity, specifically in the ratio of solute to water.

Hyponatremia

Hyponatremia may be mild (125 to 134 mEq/L), moderate (115 to 124 mEq/L), or severe (less than 115 mEq/L).

Hyponatremia is defined as a serum sodium concentration of less than 135 mEq/L. Hyponatremia does not imply a reduced total body sodium content but rather a decrease in the ratio of sodium to water in extracellular fluid. Total body sodium content may be normal, increased, or decreased depending on the underlying disorder. The disorder can develop gradually over days or acutely over hours.

Hyponatremic disorders are separated on the basis of the plasma osmolarity (Table 5–10). Isotonic hyponatremia, also termed pseudohyponatremia, is a laboratory artifact caused by an elevated lipid or protein

TABLE **5–10:** Hyponatremia: Relation of Serum Osmolarity

	Serum Na⁺	Serum Osmolarity
Isotonic hyponatremia	Low	Normal (285–295 mOsm/kg)
Hypertonic hyponatremia	Low	High (> 300 mOsm/kg)
Hypotonic hypernatremia	Low	Low (< 280 mOsm/kg)

TABLE **5–11:** Classification of Hypotonic Hyponatremia

Hypovolemic hyponatremia
  Renal losses: diuretics, salt-losing nephropathy
  Nonrenal losses: gastrointestinal, third-space losses
    (burns, muscle, retroperitoneum)
  Starvation
Hypervolemic hyponatremia
  Congestive heart failure
  Liver disease with ascites
  Nephrotic syndrome
  Acute or chronic renal failure
Normovolemic hyponatremia
  Syndrome of inappropriate antidiuretic hormone secretion
  Psychogenic polydipsia

level in the serum. This form of hyponatremia is characterized by a normal serum osmolarity, and no treatment is necessary. Hypertonic hyponatremia is observed with severe hyperglycemia (greater than 500 mg/dL) or the infusion of mannitol. Glucose and mannitol trapped in the extracellular space drive the movement of water out of cells as osmotic equilibrium across body fluid compartments is maintained. Hypotonic hyponatremia is the most significant form of hyponatremia because of its clinical sequelae. Cell swelling, the pathologic hallmark of the hypotonic state, results from the movement of water into cells. Clinically, central nervous system findings are observed, including confusion, lethargy, seizures, and coma. The most severe symptoms are seen in hyponatremias that develop acutely or are severe (Na^+ less than 115 mEq/L).

Hypotonic hyponatremias are divided into three categories on the basis of the history, physical examination, and a few simple laboratory tests (Tables 5–11 and 5–12). Hypovolemic disorders are caused by both sodium and volume depletion, with a larger deficit of sodium relative to that of water. The losses may be renal or extrarenal in origin. Hypervolemic disorders include edematous states such as congestive heart failure, advanced liver disease with ascites, and the nephrotic syndrome. The kidney is salt acquisitive and unable to excrete a water load. Normovolemic hyponatremias occur in individuals with the syndrome of inappropriate antidiuretic hormone secretion or psychogenic polydipsia. These patients are modestly volume expanded but not edematous. The common causes of the syndrome of inappropriate antidiuretic hormone secretion are outlined in Table 5–13.

TABLE **5–12:** Laboratory Features of Hypotonic Hyponatremia

	Urine Na$^+$ (mEq/L)	FeNa^{+*} (%)	Urine Osmolarity (mOsm/kg)	Uric Acid/Blood Urea Nitrogen Level
Hypovolemic hyponatremia (extrarenal)	< 20†	< 1†	Higher than serum osmolarity	Usually high
Hypovolemic hyponatremia (renal)	> 20	> 1	Usually isotonic	Usually high
Hypervolemic hyponatremia	< 20† (often < 10)	< 1†	Higher than serum osmolarity	Normal to high
Normovolemic hyponatremia (SIADH)	> 20 (usually > 50)	> 1	Inappropriately high‡	Usually low

SIADH, syndrome of inappropriate antidiuretic hormone secretion.

*FeNa$^+$ is the fractional excretion of sodium (fraction of filtered Na$^+$ that is excreted in urine). It is calculated as urine Na$^+$ × serum creatinine/serum Na$^+$ × urine creatinine × 100.

†Diuretic use may lead to a urine Na$^+$ > 20 mEq/L and an FeNa$^+$ > 1%.

‡In SIADH, urine osmolarity usually exceeds serum osmolarity but may be less. Urine osmolarity exceeds maximal diluting capacity (60–80 mOsm/kg).

TABLE **5–13:** Causes of Nonosmotic Antidiuretic Hormone Release

Syndrome of inappropriate antidiuretic hormone release
    Malignancies: lung, gastric, pancreas, prostate
    Pulmonary disorders: pneumonia, lung abscess, tuberculosis
    Cerebral disorders: head trauma, meningitis or encephalitis, tumor, cerebral
       hemorrhage
    Other: myxedema, hypokalemia, Guillain-Barré syndrome
Drugs
    Cyclophosphamide
    Vincristine
    Clofibrate
    Chlorpropamide
    Morphine sulfate
    Barbiturates

The institution of appropriate therapy for the hypotonic hyponatremic disorders depends on

- Establishing the etiology of the condition
- Determining the rapidity of its development
- Assessing the severity of the associated symptoms and signs

The clinical severity of hyponatremia is referable not only to the absolute level of serum sodium but also to its rate of decline. The most severe symptoms are observed in patients with an acute hyponatremia, defined as a serum sodium level that falls faster than 0.5 mEq/L/hr. Chronic hyponatremia develops more slowly, usually over days to weeks, and may present with few or no symptoms. The slow development of hyponatremia triggers adaptive responses, which preserve brain cell volume at near-normal levels. The extrusion of intracellular solute prevents excessive cell swelling and minimizes the symptoms and signs of hypotonicity in forms of chronic hyponatremia.

The treatment of hyponatremia depends on the disorder's underlying cause, its magnitude, and whether it is acute or chronic. Acute hyponatremia, particularly when associated with severe neurologic symptoms or signs, should be corrected rapidly (at a rate of 2 mEq/L/hr), with the target serum sodium level equal to 125 mEq/L. Chronic hyponatremia should be corrected more slowly, at a rate of 0.5 mEq/L/hr, with a target serum sodium level of 125 mEq/L. Rapid correction of hyponatremia should be avoided in the setting of chronic hyponatremia because it can lead to the development of a central pontine myelinolysis, a demyelinating lesion of the pons associated with a high mortality rate. In both acute and chronic hyponatremias, when the target sodium level of 125 mEq/L is achieved, the complete correction can be accomplished over the next 24 to 48 hours.

Table 5–14 outlines the specific approach to the treatment of hyponatremia depending on the underlying disorder and demonstrates the formula used for calculating the amount of sodium necessary for partial correction. Patients with hypovolemic hyponatremia should receive isotonic or hypertonic saline. Individuals with hypervolemic, edematous hyponatremia may require intravenous isotonic saline combined with a potent loop diuretic such as furosemide to avoid worsening of the volume overload. The syndrome of inappropriate antidiuretic hormone secretion, if severe, may necessitate the use of isotonic saline combined with furosemide to induce a water diuresis. If chronic, this syndrome can be managed with a high-sodium diet coupled with the use of a loop diuretic. The addition of oral demeclocycline, an antagonist of antidiuretic hormone action, may be of benefit.

TABLE **5–14:**   Treatment of Hyponatremia*

Hypovolemic hyponatremia
   Isotonic 0.9% saline *or*
   Hypertonic 3% saline
Hypervolemic hyponatremia
   Sodium and water restriction with loop diuretic *or*
   Isotonic 0.9% saline with loop diuretic *or*
   Hemodialysis
Normovolemic hyponatremia (SIADH)
   Water restriction *or*
   Isotonic 0.9% saline with loop diuretic

*The selection of treatment modality depends on the severity of the hyponatremia. The formula for calculating the amount of Na^+ needed for treatment is $125 - \text{measured } Na^+ \times 0.6 + \text{body weight (kg)} = \text{mEq } Na^+$ required to increase Na^+ to the target of 125 mEq/L.

SIADH, syndrome of inappropriate antidiuretic hormone secretion.

Hypernatremia

Hypernatremia is a hypertonic syndrome defined as an elevation in the serum sodium level above 145 mEq/L. The disorder represents an increase in the solute-water ratio in body fluids, although total body sodium content may be normal, increased, or decreased. The increase in body fluid tonicity in hypernatremic states obligates the movement of free water from within cells into the extracellular space. The resultant cell shrinkage results in central nervous system findings such as lethargy, confusion, coma, or intracerebral bleeding. The severity of the syndrome is a function of both the magnitude of hypernatremia and the rate of its development. As in hypotonic disorders, compensatory mechanisms are invoked, which preserve cell volume in hypernatremic states that develop slowly over days. This compensation involves the accumulation of intracellular solutes, termed idiogenic osmoles, which maintain cell volume near normal.

The causes of hypernatremia are separated into disorders resulting from losses of both sodium and water, predominately free water, and those resulting from a gain in solute (Table 5–15). Ancillary laboratory tests, including urine sodium, urine osmolarity, and urea nitrogen measurements, are helpful in distinguishing these possibilities (Table 5–16). The most common cause of hypernatremia is a combined sodium and water deficit, as seen in a debilitated patient with limited access to free water.

The goal of treatment in hypernatremic states is to restore normal tonicity of body fluids. Rapid correction of chronic hypernatremia should be avoided because of the potential for inducing cerebral edema. A fall in the serum sodium level at a rate of no greater than 1 mEq/L/hr is

TABLE **5–15:**   Classification of Hypernatremia*

Hypovolemic hypernatremia: combined Na^+ and water loss
   Extrarenal: mucocutaneous, gastrointestinal
   Renal: osmotic diuresis (hyperglycemia, mannitol, postobstructive states)
Isovolemic hypernatremia: pure free water loss
   Extrarenal: mucocutaneous (febrile states, hyperventilation, catabolic states)
   Renal: central diabetes insipidus, nephrogenic diabetes insipidus
Hypervolemic hypernatremia: excess Na^+ gain
   Intravenous: sodium bicarbonate infusions
   Oral salt poisoning: improperly mixed infant formula, overuse of sodium
     polystyrene sulfonate (Kayexalate)

*All hypernatremic states imply an inability to ingest adequate amounts of free water.

TABLE **5–16:** Laboratory Features of Hypernatremia

	Urine Na+ (nEq/L)	Urine Osmolarity (mOsm/kg)	Blood Urea Nitrogen Level
Hypovolemic hypernatremia (extrarenal)	< 20	Hypertonic	High
Hypovolemic hypernatremia (renal)	> 20	Isotonic	High
Isovolemic hypernatremia (diabetes insipidus)	< 20	Hypotonic (usually < 150)	Variable
Hypervolemic hypernatremia (salt poisoning)	> 20	Hypertonic	Variable

recommended, especially in chronic hypernatremic states. The free water deficit can be estimated according to the following formula:

$$\text{Deficit} = 0.6 \times \text{body weight (kg)} - 140/\text{actual Na}^+ \times 0.6 \times \text{body weight (kg)}$$

Ongoing losses of free water should be considered when the rate of fluid resuscitation is being determined.

Patients with a combined sodium and water deficit are volume depleted. The infusion of isotonic saline (0.9%) is advised until hemodynamic stability has been achieved. This should be followed by the administration of hypotonic saline solutions such as half-normal saline (0.45%). Dilute fluids such as 5% dextrose in water can be used if the patient is monitored and treated for the development of hyperglycemia and glycosuria.

Individuals with central or nephrogenic diabetes insipidus have an inability to concentrate the urine. Free water losses can be significant, but these persons rarely become hypernatremic unless their ability to ingest an adequate amount of water is compromised by the development of intercurrent illness. The hypernatremia in this setting is typically a free water depletion syndrome. The management includes administration of hypotonic fluids. The patient with central diabetes insipidus should also receive synthetic vasopressin, either aqueous vasopressin, 5 to 10 U intramuscularly every 3 to 4 hours, or intranasal desmopressin every 12 to 24 hours.

Salt-poisoned individuals have an excess of total body sodium and are volume overloaded. This form of hypernatremia is usually iatrogenic, most often occurring with the administration of hypertonic sodium bicarbonate ampules in patients with metabolic acidosis or cardiac arrest. Treatment includes intravenous free water replacement coupled with loop diuretics, or hemodialysis if this is not successful.

DISORDERS OF SERUM POTASSIUM

Potassium (K^+) is the major intracellular cation in body fluid. Total body potassium content amounts to 3500 mEq, 98% of which is located within cells. This is in contrast to sodium, the major extracellular cation in body fluid. The separation of sodium and potassium in distinct body fluid compartments is accomplished by the membrane-bound sodium-potassium adenosine triphosphatase pumps. These pumps maintain an intracellular K^+ concentration of 140 mEq/L, with an extracellular concentration of only 3.5 to 5.0 mEq/L. This gradient in K^+ balance is essential to the generation of the normal resting membrane potential of all cells. Interpretation of the serum potassium level can be difficult because only a small fraction of total body potassium is located in the vascular space. Small decrements in serum potassium (0.5 to 1 mEq/L) may indicate a major deficit of total body potassium. Conversely, redistribution of even a minute fraction of intracellular potassium stores into the extracellular space may cause lethal hyperkalemia.

The regulation of the serum potassium concentration within the narrow range of 3.5 to 5.0 mEq/L is a function of the balance between dietary intake, transcellular shifts, and renal excretion. The usual daily intake of potassium is 50 to 100 mEq. Ninety percent of dietary intake is excreted by the kidney, with the remainder eliminated in stool and sweat. The transcellular shifts of potassium are critical to the maintenance of a normal serum concentration, particularly when there are sudden influxes of dietary potassium. Transcellular shifts of potassium are regulated by a variety of factors, including blood pH, osmolarity, insulin, catecholamines, and aldosterone.

Hypokalemia

Hypokalemia is defined as a serum potassium concentration of less than 3.5 mEq/L. The clinical manifestations of potassium depletion include muscle weakness or paralysis, ventricular arrhythmias, rhabdomyolysis, and polyuria from impaired renal concentrating ability. The electrocardiographic changes of hypokalemia are depicted in Figure 5–3A. Mild hypokalemia (greater than 3.0 mEq/L) is often asymptomatic.

Hypokalemia may result from

- A decreased intake of potassium
- Excessive extrarenal losses

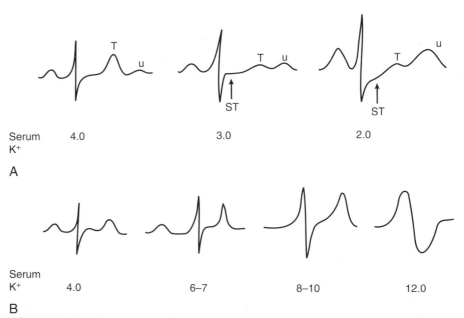

FIGURE 5–3: *A,* The electrocardiographic changes of hypokalemia. The early changes include ST segment depression and decreased amplitude of the T wave. More severe hypokalemia induces a prominent u wave, increases the amplitude of the P wave, and leads to QRS widening. *B,* The electrocardiographic changes of hyperkalemia. The initial change is a narrowing of the T wave. Widening of the QRS complex, loss of the P wave, and eventually a sine wave pattern can evolve as the hyperkalemia worsens.

TABLE **5–17:** Differential Diagnosis of Hypokalemia

Decreased intake of K^+
  Dietary
  Geophagia
Increased gastrointestinal losses*
  Diarrhea
  Enteric fistulas
  Laxative abuse
Increased or urinary losses
  Loop or thiazide diuretics*
  Primary mineralocorticoid excess
    Primary hyperaldosteronism
    Cushing's disease
    Hyper-reninism
    Bartter's syndrome
  Secondary hyperaldosteronism*
    Vomiting
    Nasogastric suction
  Hypomagnesemia*
  Drugs
    Amphotericin B
    Penicillin derivatives
Transcellular shifts of K^+
  Alkalemia
  Hyperinsulinemia
  Beta-adrenergic excess
  Periodic paralysis

*Most common causes.

- Renal potassium wasting
- An intracellular shift of potassium (Table 5–17)

Depletion of body potassium stores occurs in all of these states except for those associated with transcellular shifts of potassium. The cause of the hypokalemia can usually be determined from the patient's history. Extrarenal causes of potassium depletion are associated with a low urinary potassium excretion, less than 25 to 30 mEq/day or less than 15 mEq on a spot urine sample. The presence of coexistent acid-base disorders also aids in the differential diagnosis of hypokalemic states (Table 5–18).

Hypokalemia that results from total body potassium depletion requires treatment with either oral or intravenous potassium supplements. Factors such as volume depletion or diarrhea should be corrected, and diuretics or other drugs that aggravate the hypokalemia should be discontinued. The potassium deficit can be estimated to be 200 to 400 mEq for each 1 mEq/L fall in the serum potassium concentration. Oral repletion of potassium in mild hypokalemia (greater than 3.0 mEq/L), with 50 to 100 mEq/day in divided doses, is usually effective. For more severe hypokalemia, particularly if it is associated with cardiac arrhythmias, intravenous repletion with KCl is indicated. The rate of administration should be limited to 10 to 20 mEq/hr, with frequent monitoring of the serum potassium concentration and electrocardiography.

TABLE **5–18:** Acid-Base Disorders in Hypokalemia

Metabolic acidosis
  Diarrhea, laxative abuse
  Diabetic ketoacidosis
  Renal tubular acidosis
Metabolic alkalosis
  Diuretic therapy
  Vomiting, nasogastric suction
  Mineralocorticoid excess
  Intravenous penicillins

Hyperkalemia

Hyperkalemia is defined as a serum concentration of potassium in excess of 5.0 mEq/L. The major clinical sequelae of hyperkalemia include paresthesias, muscle weakness, and cardiac conduction defects. The electrocardiographic changes of hyperkalemia begin with peaking of the T waves and can progress to prolongation of the PR interval, widening of the QRS complex, and eventually a sine-wave pattern with cardiac arrest in severe cases (see Fig. 5–3B). These electrocardiographic changes can be unpredictable, occurring in some patients with modest elevations in the serum potassium concentration (6 to 6.5 mEq/L).

The causes of hyperkalemia can be separated by mechanism, as outlined in Table 5–19. Pseudohyperkalemia represents a laboratory artifact generated by hemolysis of the blood sample after collection. Leakage of potassium from white blood cells or platelets may also cause spurious hyperkalemia in patients with marked leukocytosis or thrombocytosis. True hyperkalemia is caused by

- Excessive dietary intake of potassium salts
- Decreased urinary excretion
- Transcellular shifts of potassium

The patient with hyperkalemia should be questioned about the dietary intake of potassium, including the use of salt substitutes (KCl). Various drugs, including the potassium-sparing diuretics, nonsteroidal anti-inflammatory agents, angiotensin-converting enzyme inhibitors, and beta-adrenergic blockers, can aggravate a hyperkalemic tendency in some patients. A history of renal disease suggests an impairment in renal excretion of potassium. The laboratory evaluation includes assessment of electrolyte, creatinine, and blood urea nitrogen levels. Renin and aldosterone levels may provide information about renal tubular disease

> As a rule, hyperkalemia does not occur with excess dietary intake of potassium unless there is impairment of renal excretory capacity.

TABLE **5–19:** Differential Diagnosis of Hyperkalemia

Pseudohyperkalemia*
  Hemolysis
  Leukocytosis
  Thrombocytosis
Increased intake†
  Dietary
  Potassium supplements*
Decreased urinary excretion
  Renal failure*
  Hypoaldosteronism
    Hyporeninemic hypoaldosteronism*
    Aldosterone resistance
    Adrenal insufficiency (Addison's disease)
    Drug induced: nonsteroidal anti-inflammatory agents, angiotensin-converting enzyme inhibitors
  Hyperkalemic distal renal tubular acidosis
  Effective circulating volume depletion*
Transcellular shifts
  Metabolic acidosis
  Insulin deficiency: uncontrolled diabetes*
  Rhabdomyolysis or tissue necrosis*
  Hyperkalemic periodic paralysis
  Drug toxicity
    Digitalis overdose
    Succinylcholine
    Beta-adrenergic blockade

*Most common causes.
†Most often combined with decreased urinary excretion of K+.

causing hyperkalemia. Pseudohyperkalemia can be excluded with a plasma potassium level rather than a serum potassium level, which can be falsely elevated.

Hyperkalemia, particularly if greater than 6.5 mEq/L or if associated with electrocardiographic changes, should be treated vigorously. The emergent management of hyperkalemia with electrocardiographic changes includes intravenous administration of calcium chloride or calcium gluconate, agents that antagonize the myocardial toxicity of hyperkalemia. Insulin, combined with glucose infusions (50% dextrose ampules), can be given to promote cellular uptake of potassium via stimulation of the sodium-potassium adenosine triphosphatase pump. Sodium bicarbonate infusions accomplish similar transcellular potassium shifts. These measures should be combined with maneuvers that remove excess potassium from the body. Loop diuretics can promote potassium loss from the kidney in patients with acceptable residual renal function. The administration of binding resins (sodium polystyrene sulfonate), either orally or by retention enema, effectively lowers the serum potassium level. Finally, hemodialysis may be necessary in patients with severe, refractory hyperkalemia or in those who have poor or no renal function.

DISORDERS OF SERUM CALCIUM

The serum concentration of calcium is regulated tightly by the interplay of hormonal and physiologic factors. Disturbances in these homeostatic mechanisms may result in either hypocalcemia or hypercalcemia, both of which have important clinical implications. The maintenance of a normal serum calcium concentration plays a critical role in cell membrane excitability and integrity, in blood coagulation, and in the intracellular function of various hormones. As depicted in Figure 5–4, mainte-

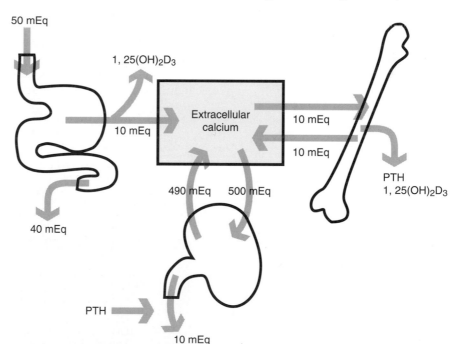

FIGURE 5–4: Calcium homeostasis as a function of gastrointestinal absorption, renal excretion, and transfer into and out of bone. Parathyroid hormone (PTH) and 1,25-dihydroxyvitamin D (1,25[OH]$_2$D$_3$) modulate the balance of calcium between body fluid and tissue compartments.

nance of the serum calcium level between 8.5 and 10 mg/dL in extracellular fluid is accomplished by the balance of gastrointestinal absorption, renal excretion, and transfer into bone. Parathyroid hormone (PTH), 1,25-dihydroxyvitamin D, and calcitonin are the hormones that modulate the movement of calcium among these organ systems.

Calcium circulates in plasma as both ionized calcium (Ca^{2+}) and protein-bound fractions. The ionized portion is available for biologic activity and constitutes about 45% of the total calcium concentration. The ionized calcium level is maintained near 4.5 mg/dL. Alterations in the protein content of blood, especially albumin, affect the total serum calcium concentration but not the ionized fraction. In general, for each 1-mg/dL decline in the serum albumin concentration, the serum calcium level falls by 0.8 mg/dL.

Hypocalcemia

The major causes of hypocalcemia are outlined in Table 5–20. Hypoparathyroidism is most often caused by true PTH deficiency resulting from disease of the parathyroid glands or as a sequela of prior thyroid or parathyroid surgery. Vitamin D deficiency is a common problem and may result from deranged metabolism at any step in the pathway of 1,25-dihydroxyvitamin D synthesis. Individuals with renal failure have at least two reasons for hypocalcemia. Decreased production of 1,25-dihydroxyvitamin D by the diseased kidney and bone resistance to the biologic effects of PTH are predictable features of advanced renal dysfunction. Hypomagnesemia can cause hypocalcemia by inhibiting PTH secretion and by impairing bone responsiveness to the effects of PTH.

Hypocalcemia is most often manifested by neuromuscular excitability. Patients complain of paresthesias in the hands, feet, and perioral region. Carpopedal spasm, Chvostek's sign (facial contraction after percussion of the facial nerve), Trousseau's sign (carpal spasm induced by inflation of a blood pressure cuff around the arm), and prolongation of the QT interval on electrocardiography can be observed. In severe cases, laryngeal stridor or seizures develop.

Symptomatic hypocalcemia requires rapid treatment with intravenous calcium supplements such as calcium chloride or calcium gluconate,

TABLE **5–20:**   Causes of Hypocalcemia

Hypoparathyroidism
  PTH deficiency
  PTH resistance (pseudohypoparathyroidism)
Vitamin D deficiency
  Malabsorption syndromes: vitamin D deficiency
  Liver disease: 25-hydroxyvitamin D deficiency
  Renal failure: 1,25-dihydroxyvitamin D deficiency
  Vitamin D–dependent rickets
  Vitamin D resistance
Chronic renal failure
Hypomagnesemia
Other
  Mithramycin
  Calcitonin
  Osteoblastic metastases
  Pancreatitis
  Rhabdomyolysis

PTH, parathyroid hormone.

TABLE **5–21:** Causes of Hypercalcemia

Increased PTH
Primary hyperparathyroidism
Tertiary hyperparathyroidism
Neoplastic production of PTH
Normal or suppressed PTH
Increased bone resorption
Malignant disorders
Osteoclast-activating factor
Prostaglandins
PTH-like factors
Vitamin A toxicity
Hyperthyroidism
Immobilization
Increased calcium absorption
Vitamin D toxicity
Milk-alkali syndrome
Sarcoidosis
Decreased calcium excretion
Thiazide diuretics
Volume contraction
Familial hypercalcemia

PTH, parathyroid hormone.

with frequent assessment of serum calcium levels. Oral calcium supplements, often combined with vitamin D, can be used for long-term management of hypocalcemic states. Magnesium repletion may be required in conjunction with calcium supplementation.

Hypercalcemia

The differential diagnosis of hypercalcemia can be divided into disorders caused by an increase in PTH activity and those in which PTH levels are suppressed (Table 5–21). Primary hyperparathyroidism is usually caused by a solitary, benign parathyroid adenoma. Tertiary hyperparathyroidism is seen in individuals with chronic renal failure whose hypertrophied, autonomous parathyroid glands continue to secrete PTH even in the presence of hypercalcemia. Malignant tumors of the lung or kidney may occasionally secrete PTH. Other causes of hypercalcemia include disorders that do not involve excessive production of PTH. Increased bone resorption of calcium occurs with a variety of malignant tumors that produce factors such as prostaglandins or osteoclast-activating factor. Increased gastrointestinal calcium absorption can occur in states of vitamin D intoxication or with sarcoidosis, a disease associated with increased endogenous production of vitamin D. Diminished excretion of calcium is commonly observed in patients receiving thiazide diuretics, although hypercalcemia is rare. Thiazide diuretics may also stimulate PTH-mediated bone resorption.

The clinical manifestations of hypercalcemia include anorexia, nausea, vomiting, and constipation. Generalized muscle weakness, lethargy, confusion, and coma can occur in severe cases. The QT interval on the electrocardiogram is shortened, and cardiac arrhythmias may develop. Hypercalcemia causes polyuria and polydipsia as a result of impaired urinary concentration and may also lead to renal insufficiency. Prolonged hypercalcemia is associated with soft tissue calcification in the skin, eyes, and viscera.

The management of severe symptomatic hypercalcemia includes intravenous administration of saline to restore extracellular fluid volume. The use of furosemide in conjunction with saline results in a calcium diuresis that is often effective in reducing the serum calcium level. Refractory hypercalcemia, particularly if associated with malignancy, can be managed with intravenous mithramycin, a chemotherapeutic agent that inhibits osteoclast resorption. Similarly, calcitonin injections may be beneficial in reducing bone resorption. Other maneuvers include the use of corticosteroids, the administration of prostaglandin synthesis inhibitors, and hemodialysis.

DISORDERS OF SERUM MAGNESIUM

The serum concentration of magnesium is maintained between 1.4 and 2.0 mEq/L (equivalent to 1.7 to 2.4 mg/dL).

Magnesium is largely an intracellular cation, with 99% of body stores located within cells or bone. Magnesium plays a critical role in the activation of cellular enzymes involved in adenosine triphosphate metabolism. Deficiency of this cation, therefore, can affect many critical cellular functions. The serum concentration of magnesium represents the balance between gastrointestinal absorption, transcellular movement, and renal excretion of magnesium. The urinary excretion of magnesium can be increased by volume expansion, sodium loading, calcium loading, diuretic use, and hypermagnesemia. Volume depletion and hypomagnesemia reduce magnesium excretion by stimulating renal tubular reabsorption.

Hypomagnesemia

Because magnesium is primarily an intracellular cation, the serum level does not always reflect body stores of magnesium. Profound magnesium depletion can occur with relatively normal serum levels. Magnesium deficiency should be suspected in patients with suggestive signs and symptoms, particularly if they occur with the conditions outlined in Table 5–22. The patient with hypomagnesemia and a urinary magnesium excretion of greater than 1 mEq/day has renal magnesium wasting. Values of less than 1 mEq/day indicate diminished intake of magnesium, either a dietary deficiency or an absorptive defect. The alcoholic individual has a multifactorial problem characterized by decreased intake as well as increased magnesium losses from the kidney.

Magnesium depletion can cause neuromuscular excitability manifesting as Chvostek's and Trousseau's signs, as well as fasciculations,

TABLE **5–22:**   Causes of Magnesium Deficiency

Gastrointestinal disorders
  Malabsorption syndromes
  Diarrhea
  Laxative abuse
  Pancreatitis
  Parenteral alimentation
Endocrine disorders
  Diabetes mellitus
  Hyperthyroidism
  Hyperparathyroidism
Alcoholism
Renal wasting of magnesium
  Diuretics
  Drug toxicity: cisplatin, aminoglycosides
  Alcohol

hyporeflexia, seizures, and cardiac arrhythmias. Symptoms include generalized weakness, nausea, and vomiting. The patient with mild magnesium depletion can be treated with an enriched magnesium diet consisting of meat, seafood, green vegetables, and dairy products. In severe or symptomatic hypomagnesemia, parenteral supplements in the form of magnesium sulfate (8 to 12 g/day) can be used, with careful attention given to the serum magnesium concentration. Oral preparations such as magnesium oxide may be necessary long term for individuals with persistent hypomagnesemia.

Hypermagnesemia

An excess of total body magnesium is usually caused by the overly vigorous administration of oral or parenteral magnesium salts, particularly in the individual with diminished renal function. Because magnesium is excreted by the kidney, patients with advanced renal failure are at risk for becoming severely hypermagnesemic if they ingest magnesium-containing antacids or cathartics. The symptoms and signs of hypermagnesemia depend on the severity of the serum elevation. Nausea, vomiting, muscle weakness, and depressed deep tendon reflexes occur with magnesium levels of 4 to 7 mEq/L. Bradycardia, vascular collapse, respiratory paralysis, and cardiac arrest can occur with levels in excess of 10 mEq/L. The management of the severely hypermagnesemic patient includes intravenous administration of calcium, which acutely reduces the magnesium level. Forced diuresis with saline and furosemide is beneficial in patients with residual renal function. Hemodialysis is another option, particularly for patients with advanced renal failure.

DISORDERS OF SERUM PHOSPHORUS

Phosphorus is a key element responsible for the maintenance of normal cell structure and function. The phospholipid bilayers of cell membranes are critical to their structural integrity. Phosphorus, an important regulator of intracellular enzymes, is involved in fuel storage and energy transformation as a constituent of adenosine triphosphate. Furthermore, phosphorus, as a component of erythrocyte diphosphoglycerate (2,3-diphosphoglycerate), plays a role in the delivery of oxygen to tissues. In the skeleton, phosphorus is a major constituent of hydroxyapatite.

The serum level of phosphorus is maintained between 2.5 and 4.5 mg/dL in healthy adults.

The serum level of phosphorus is a function of the balance between gastrointestinal absorption, transcellular flux, and renal excretion of phosphorus. Multiple factors affect this balance, including PTH, vitamin D, calcium, blood pH, insulin, and other hormones. Because 99% of body phosphorus is located within bone or soft tissue, the extracellular concentration may not always reflect total body phosphorus content. An acute rise or fall in the serum concentration of phosphorus can occur with relatively minor transcellular shifts. Similarly, a severe depletion of total body phosphorus that develops slowly may manifest with little or no change in the serum concentration.

Hypophosphatemia

Although phosphate depletion is one of the most common metabolic derangements in hospitalized patients, it is often unrecognized. The

TABLE **5–23:** Causes of Hypophosphatemia

Redistribution: transcellular shifts
    Respiratory alkalosis*
    Parenteral nutrition*
    Nutritional recovery syndrome ("refeeding hypophosphatemia")*
Gastrointestinal losses
    Decreased dietary intake
    Malabsorption
    Vitamin D deficiency
    Phosphate-binding antacids*
Renal losses: impaired tubular reabsorption
    Hyperparathyroidism
    Glycosuria
    Acid-base disorders
        Metabolic alkalosis
        Metabolic acidosis
        Respiratory acidosis
    Hypokalemia
    Hypomagnesemia
    Fanconi's syndrome
    After recovery from acute tubular necrosis

*Causes of severe hypophosphatemia.

serum phosphorus concentration in phosphate depletion is usually low (less than 2.5 mg/dL), but in some cases, particularly in diabetic ketoacidosis, it may be in the normal range. The causes of hypophosphatemia can be divided into disorders caused by a transcellular flux of phosphorus, those caused by decreased gastrointestinal absorption, and those resulting from increased renal excretion (Table 5–23). Severe hypophosphatemia, arbitrarily defined as a level of less than 1 mg/dL, is observed in a limited number of conditions, including

- Chronic alcoholism and alcohol withdrawal
- Dietary deficiency combined with the use of phosphate-binding antacids
- The recovery phase of diabetic ketoacidosis
- Respiratory alkalosis
- As a complication of parenteral nutrition or the nutritional recovery syndrome

The alcoholic patient with hypophosphatemia has a multifactorial problem. A reduced dietary intake of phosphorus coupled with increased movement of phosphorus into cells as a result of coexistent respiratory alkalosis is common. In addition, alcohol is postulated to exert a direct toxic effect on muscle, which leads to phosphate depletion. Patients with diabetic ketoacidosis lose excessive amounts of phosphorus in the urine with hyperglycemic osmotic diuresis, and when treated they may develop worsening hypophosphatemia because of insulin-stimulated intracellular flux of phosphorus. Respiratory alkalosis, a common disorder in patients with sepsis, alcohol withdrawal, and liver disease, may result in profound hypophosphatemia owing to transcellular shifts of phosphorus.

TABLE **5–24:** Clinical Effects of Hypophosphatemia

Central nervous system	Respiratory paralysis
Confusion	Congestive cardiomyopathy
Agitation	Hematologic
Seizures	Hemolysis
Coma	Impaired red blood cell oxygen delivery
Musculoskeletal	White blood cell dysfunction
Weakness	Platelet dysfunction
Rhabdomyolysis	

Hypophosphatemia is a predictable complication of parenteral nutrition that does not include adequate phosphate supplementation. This phenomenon also occurs during nutritional recovery in severely malnourished patients and is the result of transcellular shifts of potassium induced by glucose loading.

The clinical manifestations of hypophosphatemia can be life threatening, particularly when the serum level is less than 1.0 mg/dL (Table 5–24). Deaths are most often the result of respiratory muscle paralysis or heart failure. The cause of hypophosphatemia is usually apparent by the clinical setting in which it occurs. Measurement of the urinary phosphorus level can be helpful in determining if hypophosphatemia is caused by renal wasting. A 24-hour urinary phosphorus excretion of less than 150 mg or a spot urine value of less than 15 mg/dL is suggestive of extrarenal phosphorus depletion or intracellular shifts.

The treatment of hypophosphatemia depends on the magnitude of the depletion and the severity of associated symptoms. Severe hypophosphatemia (less than 1 mg/dL) should be treated with intravenous repletion, using either sodium phosphate or potassium phosphate salts. The usual dose is 2.5 to 5 mg/kg (0.08 to 0.16 mmol/kg) over 6 hours, with frequent assessment of serum phosphorus levels. For less severe depletion, oral phosphorus supplements in the form of potassium phosphate or a diet high in phosphorus can be prescribed. The risks of treatment include the development of diarrhea, hyperphosphatemia, hypocalcemia, and metastatic calcifications.

Hyperphosphatemia

As in hypophosphatemia, an elevated level of serum phosphorus can be caused by disorders of redistribution, absorption, or renal excretion (Table 5–25). Renal insufficiency resulting in reduced excretion is the most common cause of a chronically elevated serum phosphorus level. Some degree of renal dysfunction often complicates other hyperphosphatemic states caused by rhabdomyolysis, tumor cell lysis, or increased gastrointestinal absorption. A modest increase (5 to 8 mg/dL) in serum phosphorus is usually asymptomatic. Higher elevations, generally greater than 10 mg/dL, can result in acute hypocalcemia, ectopic calcification of calcium phosphorus salts in extraosseous sites, or both.

Severe hyperphosphatemia that develops in the setting of rhabdomyolysis or the tumor lysis syndrome can lead to acute oliguric renal

TABLE **5–25:** Causes of Hyperphosphatemia

Redistribution: cell destruction
Hemolytic anemia
Rhabdomyolysis*
Tumor lysis
Phosphate retention
Decreased renal excretion
Renal failure*
Hypoparathyroidism
Acromegaly
Phosphate poisoning†
Phosphate-containing enemas (Fleet's)
Phosphate-containing laxatives
Intravenous phosphate

*Most common causes.
†Usually, but not always, associated with renal insufficiency.

failure. Dialytic support may be necessary in these patients. The hyperphosphatemia of chronic renal failure is managed with oral phosphate binders such as calcium carbonate or aluminum hydroxide, which bind dietary phosphorus and prevent absorption.

SUMMARY

The kidney complements the lung as a controller of the acid-base status of the body. If the lung is the coarse control, removing about 17,000 mEq of acid per day, the kidney is the fine control, regulating both acid and base as well as fluid volume and electrolyte concentrations. Although the physiology of the kidney is complex, a thorough understanding of its many distinct parts and their functions is important in the clinical care of patients with acute and chronic illnesses.

Suggested Readings

Acid-Base Disorders

Foster DW, McGarry JD. The metabolic derangements and treatment of diabetic ketoacidosis. N Engl J Med 309:159, 1983.

Gabow PA. Disorders associated with an altered anion gap. Kidney Int 27:472, 1985.

Galla JH, Luke RG. Pathophysiology of metabolic acidosis. Hosp Pract 22:123, 1987.

Goodkin DA, Krishna GG, Narins RG. Role of the anion gap in detecting and managing mixed metabolic acid-base disorders. Clin Endocrinol Metab 13:333, 1984.

Kales A, Vela-Bueno A, Kales JD. Sleep disorders: Sleep apnea and narcolepsy. Ann Intern Med 106:434, 1987.

Kurtzman NA. Renal tubular acidosis: A constellation of syndromes. Hosp Pract 22:131, 1987.

Madias NE. Lactic acidosis. Kidney Int 29:752, 1986.

Magarian GJ. Hyperventilation syndromes: Infrequently recognized common expression of anxiety and stress. Medicine 61:219, 1982.

Morganroth ML. An analytic approach to diagnosing acid-base disorders. J Crit Ill 5:138, 1990.

Rosen RA, Julian BA, Dubovsky EV, et al. On the mechanism by which chloride corrects metabolic alkalosis in man. Am J Med 84:449, 1988.

Warnock DG. Uremic acidosis. Kidney Int 34:278, 1988.

Weinberger SE, Schwartzstein RM, Weiss JW. Hypercapnia. N Engl J Med 321:1223, 1989.

Hyponatremia and Hypernatremia

Arieff AI. Osmotic failure: Physiology and strategies for treatment. Hosp Pract 23:173, 1988.

Cluitmans FHM, Meinders AE. Management of severe hyponatremia: Rapid or slow correction? Am J Med 88:161, 1990.

Robertson GL. Abnormalities of thirst regulation. Kidney Int 25:460, 1984.

Robertson GL. Syndrome of inappropriate antidiuresis. N Engl J Med 321:538, 1989.

Snyder NA, Feigal DW, Arieff AI. Hypernatremia in elderly patients: A heterogeneous, morbid, and iatrogenic entity. Ann Intern Med 107:309, 1987.

Weisberg LS. Pseudohyponatremia: A reappraisal. Am J Med 86:315, 1989.

Disorders of Potassium Balance

Brown RS. Extrarenal potassium homeostasis. Kidney Int 30:116, 1986.

Knochel JP. Etiologies and management of potassium deficiency. Hosp Pract 22:153, 1987.

Rimmer JM, Horn JF, Gennari FJ. Hyperkalemia as a complication of drug therapy. Arch Intern Med 147:867, 1987.

Disorders of Calcium Balance

Garrick R, Goldfarb S. Differential diagnosis and pathophysiologic effects of hypercalcemia. Am J Kidney Dis 13:160, 1989.

Mundy GR, Yates AJP. Recent advances in pathophysiology and treatment of hypercalcemia of malignancy. Am J Kidney Dis 14:2, 1989.

Disorders of Magnesium Balance

Dirks JH. The kidney and magnesium regulation. Kidney Int 23:771, 1983.
Oster JR, Epstein M. Management of magnesium depletion. Am J Nephrol 8:349, 1988.
Sutton RAL, Dirks JH. Calcium and magnesium: Renal handling and disorders of metabolism. *In* Brenner BM, Rector FC Jr (eds). The Kidney, 3rd ed. Philadelphia, WB Saunders, 1986, pp 841–887.

Disorders of Phosphorus Balance

Gravelyn TR, Brophy N, Siegert C, Peters-Golden M. Hypophosphatemia associated respiratory muscle weakness in a general population. Am J Med 84:870, 1988.
Knochel JP. Hypophosphatemia in the alcoholic. Arch Intern Med 140:613, 1980.
Knochel JP. Hypophosphatemia. West J Med 134:14, 1981.

6

Key Terms

Alveolar-Arterial P_{O_2}
Difference ($P(A - a)_{O_2}$)

Anatomic Dead Space

Diffusing Capacity

O_2 Capacity

O_2 Content

O_2 Saturation

Oxyhemoglobin Dissociation
Curve

P_{50}

Respiratory Quotient (R)

Shunt

Venous Admixture

Ventilation-Perfusion Ratio
($\dot{V}/\dot{Q}$)

Pulmonary Gas Exchange

David R. Dantzker, M.D.

The tissues of the body require adequate amounts of energy in order to maintain cellular integrity and to provide for synthetic processes. Oxygen is a necessary participant in this process (see Chapter 9). In resting humans, the oxygen (O_2) requirement is about 4 to 5 mL/min/kg, and it may increase by a factor of 10 or more during periods of increased metabolic demand, such as exercise. An important byproduct of metabolism is carbon dioxide (CO_2). The amount of CO_2 produced is determined not only by the metabolic rate but also by the kind of fuel that is utilized for energy production. For example, if carbohydrate is the predominant fuel source, then the CO_2 production ($\dot{V}_{CO_2}$) is equal to the O_2 consumption ($\dot{V}_{O_2}$), and the respiratory quotient (R = $\dot{V}_{CO_2}/\dot{V}_{O_2}$) is 1.0. The R for protein is 0.8, and for fat it is 0.7.

The body's ability to store O_2 and CO_2 is minimal; thus, continuous exchange of these two gases with the environment is necessary to maintain normal cellular function and to prevent the development of respiratory acidosis (see Chapter 38). This is the major responsibility of the lungs, and the efficacy with which they carry out their task can be measured by assessing the adequacy of pulmonary gas exchange.

THE GAS-EXCHANGING UNIT OF THE LUNG

To understand how the lung functions as a gas exchanger, it is useful to consider, at the onset, a rudimentary model of the basic gas-exchanging unit (Fig. 6–1A). In this simple visualization, the lung can be viewed as a tonometer, a vessel in which blood and gas are mixed and come into equilibrium, such that the number of molecules of a gas leaving the blood phase equals the number entering the blood from the gas phase. At this point, the partial pressures of the gas in the blood and alveolar gas are equal. The total pressure in the alveolar gas equals ambient atmospheric pressure, which is 760 mm Hg at sea level but is lower at higher altitudes and higher under the unusual conditions of high pressure found in a hyperbaric chamber or when scuba diving (Table 6–1).

Ambient air contains significant amounts of three gases: O_2, nitrogen N_2, and water vapor. The remaining gases (CO_2 and the rare gases) are present in such small amounts that they are not important to consider from the standpoint of pulmonary gas exchange. Water vapor partial pressure (P_{H_2O}) depends on the ambient humidity but not on the barometric pressure (P_B). For example, P_{H_2O} is 47 mm Hg when air is fully saturated with water at body temperature at sea level (P_B of 760 mm Hg), as well as at an elevation of 18,000 feet, where the P_B is only 389 mm Hg. O_2 and N_2, in contrast, are present as a fixed percentage of the remaining pressure, approximately 0.21 and 0.79, respectively. Thus, the P_{H_2O}, which dilutes the inspired partial pressures of O_2 and N_2, will have a relatively greater impact the lower the P_B. At an altitude of 63,000 feet, where the P_B is 47 mm Hg, the other gases would not be present in

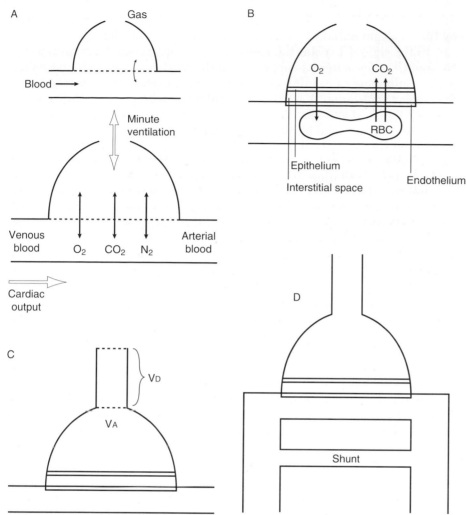

FIGURE 6–1: Models of pulmonary gas exchange. *A,* The lung modeled as a simple tonometer. There is complete equilibrium of the respiratory gases between alveolar gas and capillary blood during the time they are in contact. *B,* The addition of an alveolar-capillary membrane adds a diffusion resistance and sets up the potential for a diffusion block (an alveolar-arterial nonequilibration) to occur. *C,* The airways are a nonperfused compartment and thus add dead space to the system. This leads to a reduction in the effective component of a tidal breath (the alveolar ventilation). *D,* The presence of an unventilated compartment (shunt) provides for venous admixture. RBC, red blood cell.

TABLE **6–1:** Effect of Altitude on Barometric Pressure and Inspired P_{O_2}

Elevation (feet)	Barometric Pressure (mm Hg)	Inspired P_{O_2} (mm Hg)
63,000	47	0
29,028 (Mt. Everest)	253	43
18,000	389	72
6500 (pressurized airplane)	596	115
Sea Level	760	150
−33	1520	310
−99	3040	629

Fick's law of diffusion:

Gas flow = $D_L (P_1 - P_2)$

where

D_L = the diffusing capacity for the gas in the lung
$P_1 - P_2$ = the pressure gradient for the gas (from alveolus to blood for O_2 and in the other direction for CO_2)

The V_D, commonly referred to as the anatomic dead space, is approximately 1 mL/lb body weight at functional residual capacity. At higher lung volumes, the V_D increases as the volume of the airways increases secondary to the increase in elastic recoil pressure.

humidified inspired air. In the alveolus, the O_2 and N_2 are further diluted by the CO_2 that enters the mixture from the venous blood.

In the simple alveolar tonometer model, venous blood, containing O_2, N_2, and CO_2, flows in at a rate equal to the cardiac output ($\dot{Q}$) and mixes with inspired air containing O_2 and N_2, which exchanges at a rate equal to alveolar ventilation ($\dot{V}A$). The blood fully equilibrates with the alveolar gas and the final gas partial pressures in the blood and gas leaving the tonometer (the arterial blood and expired gas) would be equal and would depend on the partial pressures of the gases in the incoming (inspired) gas and (venous) blood, as well as on the relative rate of gas delivery and removal, the ventilation-perfusion ratio ($\dot{V}/\dot{Q}$).[1]

Unfortunately, from the standpoint of understanding pulmonary gas exchange, the actual gas-exchanging unit is not as simple as this model. Certain modifications must be made in order to approximate more closely what actually occurs in the lung. In the lung, unlike the tonometer, the blood and gas are separated by the alveolar-capillary membrane (see Fig. 6–1B). This consists of the cytoplasmic extensions of the type I pneumocyte and the pulmonary capillary endothelial cell, separated by a basement membrane and interstitial space. Gases diffuse across the membrane according to Fick's law of diffusion.

A second modification to the simple model is the addition of conducting airways within which no gas exchange takes place (see Fig. 6–1C). At the end of expiration, the conducting airways are filled with alveolar gas, which has already undergone equilibration with the blood. On inspiration, the amount of fresh gas available to raise the alveolar P_{O_2} and lower the alveolar P_{CO_2} (i.e., the alveolar volume [V_A]) is less than the volume of the breath, the tidal volume (V_T), by the volume of the conducting airways (V_D):

$$V_A = V_T - V_D$$

The final necessary addition to the model arises from the presence of venous blood, which bypasses the gas-exchanging surface and subsequently mixes with blood coming from the alveoli (see Fig. 6–1D). In normal lungs, this consists of blood from the bronchial and thebesian beds, which flows directly into the left side of the heart after nourishing the airways and heart muscle. Although this "physiologic shunt" constitutes only 1 to 3% of $\dot{Q}$, it is still capable of slightly decreasing the P_{O_2} in the arterial blood from that found in the blood exiting from the alveoli.

OXYGEN AND CARBON DIOXIDE TRANSPORT IN BLOOD

The O_2 in the blood is present in two forms:

- Dissolved in the plasma
- Combined with hemoglobin

According to Henry's law, the amount of a gas dissolved in a fluid at a specific temperature is linearly dependent on the partial pressure of the gas and its solubility. The amount of O_2 that can dissolve in plasma at body temperature is 0.003 mL/mm Hg/dL blood, or 0.3 mL/dL O_2 in normal subjects at sea level. Clearly, this is not sufficient to maintain the O_2 demands of the tissues because on average, between 3 and 5 mL of O_2 are removed from each deciliter of blood during its passage through the body. This O_2 need requires the presence of an O_2 carrier system. In humans, this is accomplished by hemoglobin, which is made up of two

Each gram of hemoglobin is theoretically capable of binding 1.39 mL of O_2, although when hemoglobin is actually exposed to a Po_2 high enough to saturate it completely, the actual binding capacity is 1.34 mL of O_2. It is this latter value that is most often used clinically.

pairs of identical polypeptide chains (two alpha-chains and two beta-chains), each encompassing an iron-porphyrin ring, the heme group.

Unlike certain primitive species, in which the O_2-carrying pigment circulates freely in the vascular space, most higher species have it packaged into erythrocytes. In humans, hemoglobin takes up almost 25% of the volume of the red blood cell, leaving little room for other organelles. For this reason, the mature erythrocyte, which depends on anaerobic metabolism for energy production, is unable to synthesize protein, making it vulnerable to injury. The biconcave shape of the red blood cell is beneficial to its function because it provides about a 70% increase in surface area over a sphere of similar volume, expediting gas exchange. The shape also increases the deformability of the cell, which facilitates its ability to squeeze through the systemic and pulmonary capillaries.

Unlike dissolved O_2, the relationship between Po_2 and the O_2 bound

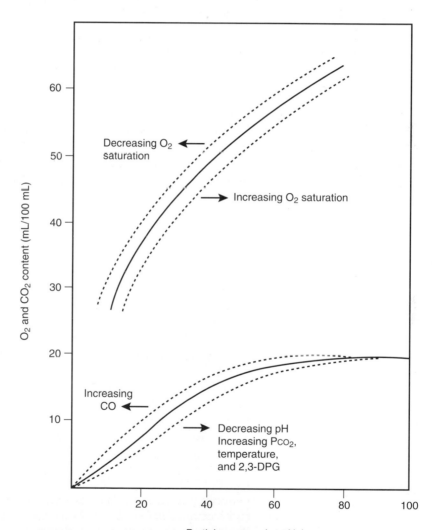

FIGURE 6–2: The oxyhemoglobin and carboxyhemoglobin dissociation curves. The carboxyhemoglobin dissociation curve is more linear than the oxyhemoglobin curve, which explains the common finding of hypoxemia without hypercapnia in many patients with lung disease (see text). Factors that may shift the position of the curves are shown. 2,3-DPG, 2,3-diphosphoglycerate. (From Dantzker DR. Pulmonary gas exchange. *In* Cardiopulmonary Critical Care, 2nd ed. Philadelphia, WB Saunders, 1991, p 29.)

to hemoglobin is described by a nonlinear, sigmoid shape (Fig. 6–2).[2] There are four separate binding sites for O_2 on the heme molecule. The avidity for binding O_2 decreases as each of the four binding sites is occupied, accounting for the peculiar shape of the oxyhemoglobin relationship. This shape has many physiologic advantages over a linear relationship. The flat upper end of the curve ensures that hemoglobin will be fully saturated with O_2, even when there is significant lung disease or the individual is exposed to a relatively hypoxic environment, such as at high altitude. The steep portion of the curve, on the other hand, allows for the extraction of large amounts of O_2 by the tissues without a large drop in the Po_2, which is necessary to ensure an adequate driving pressure for the diffusion of O_2 into the tissues.

Three definitions are important in dealing with the oxyhemoglobin relationship.

- The O_2 capacity is the total amount of O_2 an individual is able to carry combined with hemoglobin and is calculated as

$$O_2 \text{ capacity (mL/dL)} = \text{hemoglobin (g/dL)} \times 1.34$$

- The O_2 saturation is preferably measured with a cooximeter and is defined as

$$Sa_{O_2}(\%) = \text{actual } O_2 \text{ bound to hemoglobin}/O_2 \text{ capacity}$$

- The O_2 content, the total of the bound and the dissolved O_2, is then calculated as

$$O_2 \text{ content (mL/dL)} = (O_2 \text{ capacity} \times Sa_{O_2}) + (0.003 \times Pa_{O_2})$$

Of the CO_2 that is removed from the lungs, 60% comes from HCO_3, 30% from carbamino compounds, and 10% from dissolved CO_2.

CO_2 is carried in the blood in three forms. Ninety percent is carried in the form of bicarbonate (HCO_3^-) after hydration of the CO_2:

$$CO_2 + H_2O \leftrightarrow H_2CO_3 \leftrightarrow HCO_3^- + H^+$$

This reaction occurs predominantly in the red blood cell, where the presence of the enzyme carbonic anhydrase markedly increases the speed of the first reaction. The H^+ is buffered by the hemoglobin, and the HCO_3^- diffuses out into the plasma in exchange for a Cl^- to maintain electrical neutrality. Five percent of the CO_2 combines with hemoglobin to form carbamino compounds, and the remaining 5% is carried dissolved in the plasma. The relationship between the Pco_2 and the CO_2 content of the blood is described by the CO_2 dissociation curve, which is steeper and more linear than the oxyhemoglobin curve (see Fig. 6–2).

Although the shapes of the oxyhemoglobin and CO_2 dissociation curves are relatively constant, many factors can shift the position of these curves relative to the partial pressure axis. These are usually described as rightward or leftward shifts. In the case of the oxyhemoglobin dissociation curve, the position of the curve is quantified by the P_{50}, the Po_2 at which the hemoglobin is 50% saturated. The P_{50} of certain genetic variant hemoglobins may be located either to the left or to the right of normal. Occasionally, when these shifts result in a significant increase in O_2 affinity (a leftward shift), they can lead to enough of a reduction in tissue oxygenation to stimulate an increase in red blood cell production as compensation. Factors that are associated with an increased metabolic requirement for O_2 (i.e., increased Pco_2 and temperature and reduced pH) cause a rightward shift in the oxyhemoglobin curve, signaling a reduced affinity of hemoglobin for O_2. This serves to facilitate the release of O_2 at the tissue level. The Pco_2-induced shift in

The normal P_{50} in adult blood is about 27 mm Hg.

the curve is known as the Bohr effect and is mainly due to the alteration in pH rather than to the direct effect of CO_2 on oxyhemoglobin affinity. Opposite changes in these factors shift the curve to the left, which serves to increase the affinity of hemoglobin for O_2, thus assisting the onloading of O_2 in the pulmonary capillaries.

Organic phosphates can also affect the P_{50}, with increasing concentrations shifting the curve to the right. The most important of these, from a regulatory standpoint, is 2,3-diphosphoglycerate (DPG). DPG, an intermediate of glycolysis, is synthesized by the red blood cell in increasing amounts in the setting of chronic tissue hypoxia, presumably to facilitate tissue O_2 unloading.

Finally, exposure of the hemoglobin to carbon monoxide shifts the curve to the left. The clinical importance of this shift, however, is minor compared with the ability of carbon monoxide to interfere with the ability of hemoglobin to deliver O_2 to the tissues. Carbon monoxide competes with O_2 for binding sites on heme and thus effectively reduces the amount of hemoglobin available for O_2 transport.

The position of the CO_2 dissociation curve is influenced mainly by the O_2 saturation. Deoxyhemoglobin is more readily able to form carbamino compounds as well as to absorb H^+, a necessary step in the hydration of CO_2 to HCO_3^-. This shift in the CO_2 dissociation curve to the left at low O_2 saturations, the Haldane effect, increases the affinity of the blood for CO_2 in the tissues as O_2 is offloaded. Reversing this shift in the pulmonary capillaries facilitates the excretion of CO_2 in the lungs.

ABNORMAL PULMONARY GAS EXCHANGE

The normal lung, with its 300 million alveoli, is an amazingly efficient gas exchanger, responding with ease to innumerable physiologic stresses. However, there are a number of pathologic changes that can overwhelm the system and interfere with gas transfer. This section examines these problems by looking at basic underlying mechanisms rather than specific disease entities.

Reduction of the Inspired P_{O_2}

To calculate the inspired P_{O_2} (PI_{O_2}):

$$PI_{O_2} = 0.21 \times (PB - PH_2O)$$

As already discussed, O_2 constitutes 21% of the ambient air. Because barometric pressure (PB) decreases exponentially as one ascends from sea level, so does the PI_{O_2}. The PI_{O_2} is 150 mm Hg at sea level; it falls to 120 mm Hg in Denver and to 70 mm Hg in the highest continuously habitable villages in the Andes Mountains. At the highest place on Earth, the summit of Mt. Everest, the PI_{O_2} is about 43 mm Hg. Fortunately for mountain climbers, this is thought to be the lowest tolerable PI_{O_2}. At higher altitudes, such as those commonly reached by commercial airlines, supplemental oxygen is required. This is provided in airplanes by pressurizing the entire passenger compartment. The pressurization is not, however, to sea level but only to an altitude of about 6000 to 8000 feet, providing a PI_{O_2} that may be as low as 100 mm Hg. Thus, although few of us practice medicine at very high altitudes, it is quite likely that some of our patients are routinely exposed to significant reductions in PB.

The simple form of the alveolar gas equation is

$$PA_{O_2} = PI_{O_2} - (Pa_{CO_2}/R)$$

where R is the respiratory exchange ratio.

The effect that a low PB will have on the Pa_{O_2} can be estimated using the alveolar gas equation, which calculates the ideal alveolar P_{O_2} (PA_{O_2})

(assuming the lung can be modeled as a single gas-exchanging unit). With normal lung function, the difference between PA_{O_2} and Pa_{O_2}, the alveolar-arterial P_{O_2} difference ($P(A - a)O_2$), is quite small and is accounted for by a small amount of ventilation-perfusion inequality (see later discussion) and the 1 to 3% physiologic shunt. In the presence of significant lung disease, this difference progressively widens. Thus, the effect of altitude will be much more devastating on arterial oxygenation when there is concomitant lung disease (Fig. 6–3).

As the PI_{O_2} decreases, a number of physiologic compensations are invoked to maintain adequate oxygenation.[3] The most immediately available mechanism is an increase in minute ventilation, which by reducing the Pa_{CO_2} will increase the Pa_{O_2} by increasing PA_{O_2}. The PA_{O_2} will increase 1.0 to 1.25 mm Hg for each 1.0-mm Hg reduction in the Pa_{CO_2} depending on the R. In a subject with a normal $P(A - a)O_2$, this is often sufficient to raise the Pa_{O_2} to an acceptable level. The ventilatory response to the hypoxemia depends on the activity of the respiratory neurons located in the carotid body and on the ability of the ventilatory pump to respond to this stimulation. Patients with lung disease or neuromuscular problems have reduced ventilatory capacity and thus a reduced capacity to compensate. Clinicians must consider this when they advise patients about exposure to reduced barometric pressure (see Fig. 6–3). In addition, some normal subjects may have sluggish hypoxic respiratory drives, which limits their ability to function at the same altitudes as other normal subjects. The hyperventilation may also have some untoward side effects. In mountain climbers, the resultant respiratory alkalosis is thought to contribute to the development of acute mountain sickness, which is char-

During maximal hypoxic stimulation, a normal subject can decrease his or her Pa_{CO_2} to as low as 7 mm Hg.

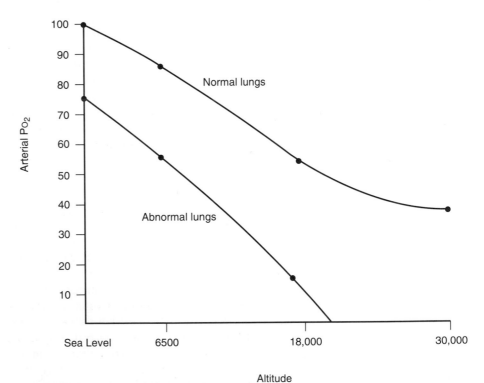

FIGURE 6–3: The effect of altitude on the arterial P_{O_2}. Patients with normal lungs can survive at high altitudes because of their narrow alveolar-arterial P_{O_2} gradient and an ability to hyperventilate. In the presence of lung disease, altitude can lead to rapidly progressive hypoxemia.

acterized by nausea, headaches, dizziness, and insomnia. The alkalosis also results in a leftward shift in the oxyhemoglobin dissociation curve. However, this effect is probably balanced in chronic altitude exposures by an increase in the DPG level. An additional compensation to chronic hypoxic exposure is an elevated red blood cell volume, which increases the amount of O_2 delivered to the tissues for any Pa_{O_2}.[4]

The most effective way to compensate for the effects of a reduction in PI_{O_2} is to provide supplemental O_2. Even in the presence of lung disease, a small increase in PO_2 is usually sufficient to ensure adequate arterial oxygenation.

Hypoventilation

CO_2 is a normal byproduct of metabolism, adding about 17,000 mEq of acid to the blood each day. To prevent the rapid development of fatal acidosis, the CO_2 must be removed at the same rate as it is produced. A complete discussion of the effects of PCO_2 on acid-base disorders is found in Chapter 5.

The alveolar and thus the arterial PCO_2 is determined by the relationship between CO_2 production ($\dot{V}CO_2$) and minute ventilation:

$$Pa_{CO_2} = \dot{V}CO_2/\dot{V}A \times K$$

where $\dot{V}A$ is the alveolar ventilation, which in any individual is a fixed percentage of minute ventilation, and K is a constant. Therefore, for a given level of metabolic activity, Pa_{CO_2} and minute ventilation are inversely proportional.

Hypoventilation is most simply defined as a minute ventilation that for a given metabolic demand is inadequate to maintain the Pa_{CO_2} in the normal range. The increase in Pa_{CO_2} that results from hypoventilation is accompanied by a fall in PA_{O_2}, as would be expected from the alveolar gas equation, and thus a fall in Pa_{O_2} (Fig. 6–4). Hyperventilation, a minute ventilation in excess of that required to keep the Pa_{CO_2} at normal levels, results in the development of respiratory alkalosis.

Although hypoventilation is usually due to a reduction in minute ventilation, $\dot{V}A$ can change with no change in $\dot{V}E$ if tidal volume (VT) and ventilatory frequency change in opposite directions. This is most easily appreciated by looking at the components of VT:

$$VT = VD + VA$$

where VD is the anatomic dead space.[5] Because VD is a fixed volume, any decrease in VT causes a fall in the proportion of the breath available for VA. Therefore, if the same $\dot{V}E$ is achieved with a smaller VT and increased frequency, the component of the $\dot{V}E$ that is VA decreases. The VA can also fall even in the face of an increase in $\dot{V}E$ in the setting of ventilation-perfusion inequality, sometimes spoken of as an increase in alveolar, as opposed to anatomic, dead space (see below).

Because $\dot{V}E$ is normally closely coupled to $\dot{V}CO_2$ by the respiratory center (see Chapter 7), an increase in Pa_{CO_2} secondary to hypoventilation usually means either a failure of the respiratory chemoreceptors in the brain or carotid body to adequately sense a change in Pa_{CO_2} or a failure of the ventilatory pump to respond to the respiratory center. As such, this mechanism of abnormal gas exchange is unique, always indicating a nonlung etiology. Hypoventilation is most commonly due to structural or pharmacologic depression of the respiratory centers, a result of neuro-

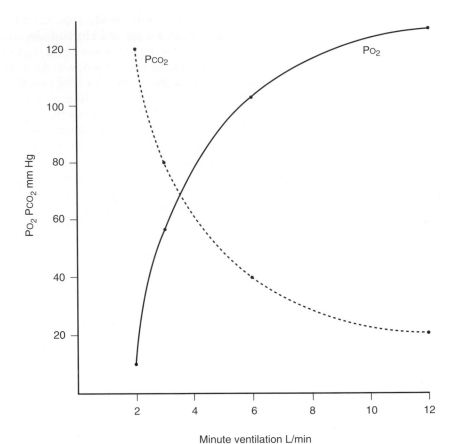

FIGURE 6–4: The effect of changes in minute ventilation on the arterial P_{O_2} and P_{CO_2} in a patient with normal lungs. Hypoventilation leads to both hypoxemia and hypercapnia.

muscular disease or secondary to a chest wall abnormality. The hypoxemia of hypoventilation is easily reversed by increasing the inspired O_2 concentration. However, the treatment must be directed at the neurologic, muscular, or chest wall abnormality in order to prevent the development of progressive acidosis. In the setting of acutely developing hypoventilation, it is often necessary to employ mechanical ventilation toward this end.

Abnormal Diffusion

The blood normally spends about 0.75 minute, on average, in the pulmonary capillaries, during which time it must equilibrate with alveolar gas. This is a passive process in which O_2 and CO_2 move across the alveolar-capillary membrane along a partial pressure gradient, with O_2 moving from the alveolus to the blood and CO_2 moving in the opposite direction. In the normal lung, complete equilibration occurs in about 0.25 second, leaving a wide margin of safety that ensures equilibration between the alveolar gas and the end-capillary blood.[6]

Because direct measurement of the diffusing capacity for the physiologic gases is impractical in humans, the diffusion pathway is usually assessed by measuring the diffusing capacity for carbon monoxide (DL_{CO}), another gas that binds with hemoglobin.

At rest, the diffusing capacity for O_2 (DL_{O_2}) is equal to about 1.23 × DL_{CO_2}. During exercise, when additional blood is recruited to the lung as a result of increasing cardiac output and pulmonary vascular pressures, the DL_{O_2} can increase by more than three times.[7]

It is often convenient to divide the diffusing capacity into two components, corresponding to the resistances the blood encounters as it moves from the alveolar gas into the blood (Fig. 6–5). The first of these is the membrane resistance, which includes the alveolar-capillary membrane, the plasma, and the red blood cell membrane. The second resistance, encountered in the combination of O_2 with hemoglobin, depends on the amount of blood present in the pulmonary capillaries as well as the kinetic rate of reaction of O_2 with hemoglobin, usually symbolized by θ. In normal lungs, these two resistances play an equal role in limiting the diffusion process.[7] In the setting of lung disease, however, the loss of pulmonary blood volume, either through vessel destruction (as in emphysema or diffuse infiltrative diseases of the lung) or through vessel occlusion (as in pulmonary vascular disease), is responsible for most of the measured decrease in the diffusing capacity.

However, just because the diffusing capacity of the lung is reduced in a given disease, it does not mean that an abnormality in the arterial blood gases can be ascribed to this mechanism. Because of the large diffusion reserve, the DL_{CO} must fall to less than 10% of normal for diffusion to be rate limiting to gas exchange at rest or to less than 25% of normal for it to interfere with the process during exercise. Usually, an abnormal diffusing capacity will lead to hypoxemia only when there is more than one significant stress on the diffusion process. These stresses might include

- A marked decrease in the inspired P_{O_2}, as is seen at high altitudes, which decreases the driving pressure for diffusion
- A reduction in the diffusing capacity of the membrane owing to an increase in the thickness of the alveolar-capillary membrane, as is seen in pulmonary fibrosis

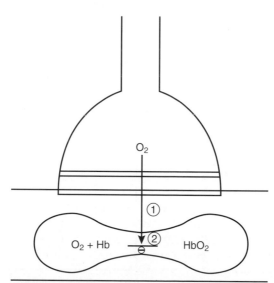

FIGURE 6–5: Components of the resistance to O_2 diffusion from the alveolus into the red blood cell. No. 1 is the resistance encountered because of the presence of the alveolar-capillary and red blood cell membranes, as well as the plasma components of blood. No. 2 involves the combination of O_2 with hemoglobin (Hb), a finite process that depends, most importantly, on the pulmonary capillary blood volume.

- A shortened residence time for blood in the pulmonary capillaries be-cause of an increase in cardiac output or a decrease in the cross-sectional area of the pulmonary capillary bed

For the most part, diffusion impairment does not play a clinically significant role in the abnormal gas exchange found in clinical practice.

Thus, in a patient with pulmonary fibrosis running on a treadmill or a mountain climber ascending to the summit of Mt. Everest, abnormal diffusion may contribute to the level of hypoxemia. However, the contribution of impaired diffusion to any observed abnormality of gas exchange, even in these settings, is small; this can easily be overcome by small increases in the $F_{I_{O_2}}$.

Ventilation-Perfusion Inequality

Although a simple model of the lung allows it to be visualized as a single gas-exchanging unit receiving all of the cardiac output and ventilation, in reality, of course, the adult lung consists of more than 300 million alveoli, each of which receives its own share of the blood flow and ventilation. All other things being equal, the ratio of ventilation to blood flow ($\dot{V}/\dot{Q}$) in each lung unit determines the alveolar and thus the end-capillary P_{O_2} and P_{CO_2}. Therefore, the arterial blood gases, a blood flow–weighted mean of the end-capillary blood from each alveolus, depends on the relative number of units with differing $\dot{V}/\dot{Q}$ that are present (i.e., the $\dot{V}/\dot{Q}$ distribution). The effect that changing the $\dot{V}/\dot{Q}$ ratio has on the end-capillary blood gases is shown in Figure 6–6. Low $\dot{V}/\dot{Q}$ units have low P_{O_2} and elevated P_{CO_2}, whereas those with a high $\dot{V}/\dot{Q}$ have the opposite values.

The $\dot{V}/\dot{Q}$ of any lung unit can vary from zero (perfused but not ventilated, or shunt) to infinity (ventilated but not perfused, or dead space).[8]

In young normal subjects, the $\dot{V}/\dot{Q}$ in the lung at rest may vary from 0.6 to 3.0, with the mean ratio being about 1.0. With increasing age, the spread in the $\dot{V}/\dot{Q}$ ratios increases (i.e., there is an increase in the degree of $\dot{V}/\dot{Q}$ mismatch or $\dot{V}/\dot{Q}$ inequality).[9] In patients with lung disease, the degree of $\dot{V}/\dot{Q}$ inequality can become quite dramatic, with lung units

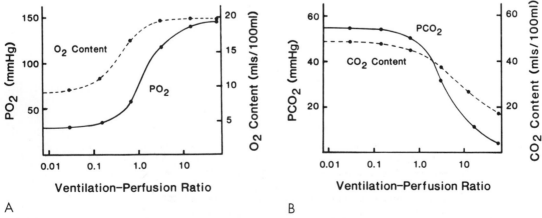

A   B

FIGURE 6–6: The effect of changing the ventilation-perfusion ratio ($\dot{V}/\dot{Q}$) in a gas-exchanging unit of the lung on the end-capillary P_{O_2}, P_{CO_2} and O_2, content. *A,* The relationship for O_2. *B,* The relationship for CO_2. (*A* and *B,* From Dantzker DR. Critical Care: A Comprehensive Approach. Park Ridge, IL, American College of Chest Physicians, 1984, p 3.)

having a very low or very high $\dot{V}/\dot{Q}$ predominating. Lung units with a low $\dot{V}/\dot{Q}$ usually develop because of a reduction in the ventilation, as seen in the setting of obstructive airway disease. However, they can also result from overperfusion, as with acute pulmonary embolism, in which blood flow is diverted from embolized to nonembolized vessels. The embolized units, from which the blood is diverted, develop an increased $\dot{V}/\dot{Q}$, whereas the overperfused, nonembolized regions have a low $\dot{V}/\dot{Q}$. The most common cause of a high $\dot{V}/\dot{Q}$ is emphysema, in which destruction of alveolar walls results in gas-exchanging units that are more poorly perfused than poorly ventilated.

The development of $\dot{V}/\dot{Q}$ inequality can have a dramatic effect on pulmonary gas exchange, interfering with the transfer of both O_2 and CO_2 (Fig. 6–7). For this reason, one might expect patients with diseases characterized by $\dot{V}/\dot{Q}$ inequality to have both hypoxemia and hypercapnia as a routine finding. However, hypercapnia is relatively uncommon because even minor increases in Pa_{CO_2} lead to a stimulation of the respiratory center, with a subsequent increase in ventilation (see Chapter 7). Because of the nature of the underlying lung pathology, most of this increased ventilation goes to already well-ventilated lung units, increasing their $\dot{V}/\dot{Q}$ above normal. Because of the shape of the oxyhemoglobin dissociation curve (see Fig. 6–2), the blood leaving these lung units is already fully saturated; therefore, the increase in the alveolar P_{O_2} is unable to load additional O_2 onto the blood. Thus, overoxygenating the already well-oxygenated blood cannot compensate for the hypoxemia due to the blood coming from lung units with low $\dot{V}/\dot{Q}$ ratios. However, the

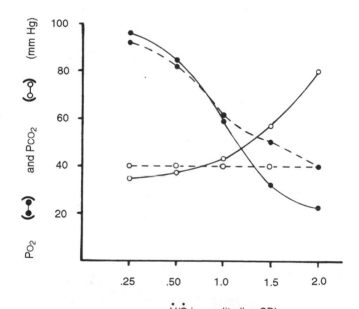

FIGURE 6–7: The effect of increasing ventilation-perfusion ($\dot{V}/\dot{Q}$) inequality on arterial P_{O_2} and P_{CO_2}. Ventilation-perfusion inequality has been increased by increasing the log SD of a log normal distribution centered on a $\dot{V}/\dot{Q}$ value of 1.0. The solid lines represent the situation when minute ventilation is held constant. The result of increasing $\dot{V}/\dot{Q}$ inequality when ventilation is allowed to increase sufficiently to keep the arterial P_{CO_2} unchanged is shown by the dotted lines. (From Dantzker DR. Gas exchange. *In* Montenegro H [ed]. Chronic Obstructive Pulmonary Disease. New York, Churchill Livingstone, 1983, p 143.)

CO_2 dissociation curve is linear throughout the physiologic range, and reductions in alveolar P_{CO_2} in the overventilated lung units remove increased amounts of CO_2 from the blood and compensate for the inefficient removal of CO_2 in the low $\dot{V}/\dot{Q}$ units.

The worse the $\dot{V}/\dot{Q}$ inequality becomes, the greater the increase in ventilation necessary to maintain a normal Pa_{CO_2} (i.e., the more CO_2 must be removed from the remaining well-ventilated units). At some point, the work of breathing and the discomfort associated with it become excessive. The respiratory muscles at this point may actually be consuming more O_2 and producing more CO_2 than are taken up or eliminated by the increased ventilation. Any further increase in minute ventilation becomes impossible or inefficient. Because the same amount of CO_2 still must be eliminated each minute to prevent death from respiratory acidosis, the Pa_{CO_2} rises. As long as ventilatory capacity can stabilize at a new, albeit reduced level, a new steady-state level is established such that each liter of ventilation is now able to eliminate more CO_2 at a higher concentration per liter. This is analogous to the manner in which the end-stage kidney eliminates the day's production of creatinine at a higher urine and serum concentration despite a reduction in the total amount of urine formed. In this setting, the rise in Pa_{CO_2} can be seen as a way of increasing the efficiency of the remaining pulmonary gas-exchanging ability. Of course, it must be accompanied by the proper changes in acid-base compensation.

The point at which this shift in strategy takes place in any given individual (i.e., a rise in Pa_{CO_2} rather than a further rise in minute ventilation) appears to depend on an interaction between the increase in mechanical work required and the set point of the respiratory center. Two patients with the same degree of $\dot{V}/\dot{Q}$ inequality may have very different levels of hypercapnia because of different sensitivities of the gain control of the respiratory center (Fig. 6–8), which may in part be genetically determined.[10] The level of hypercapnia seen in any individual may also be influenced by the strength and endurance of the respiratory muscles because they determine the level of minute ventilation that can be maintained without the development of fatigue (see Chapter 3).

Because the proper matching of ventilation and blood flow is so important to the maintenance of adequate arterial blood gases, it is not surprising that the lung has developed some intrinsic strategies for optimizing $\dot{V}/\dot{Q}$. The best studied is hypoxic vasoconstriction, by which a fall in the alveolar P_{O_2} leads to constriction of the perfusing arteriole.[11] If the cause of the alveolar hypoxia is a low $\dot{V}/\dot{Q}$, then a reduction in $\dot{Q}$ should serve to bring the ratio back toward normal. The mechanism by which the alveolar P_{O_2} is sensed and translated into vasoconstriction is unknown. It is most potent in the midranges of hypoxia (PA_{O_2} between 30 and 60 mm Hg). More severe hypoxia may actually result in vasodilatation. Hypoxic vasoconstriction should be most useful in the setting of regional lung abnormalities. Generalized hypoxia leads to a rise in pulmonary artery pressure and may cause right-sided heart failure (cor pulmonale). This etiology of cor pulmonale in severe chronic obstructive lung disease has also been implicated in the development of high-altitude pulmonary edema.

A method of minimizing lung units with a high $\dot{V}/\dot{Q}$ has also been described. The inflation of a balloon in the pulmonary artery of one lung causes a decrease in the ventilation to that lung.[12] The mechanism is thought to be a reduction in the P_{CO_2} in the airway, leading to broncho-

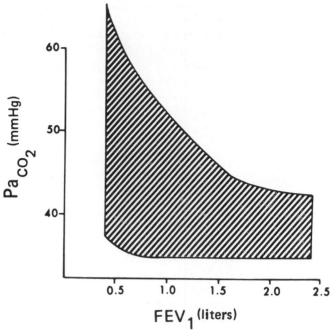

FIGURE 6–8: FEV_1 versus Pa_{CO_2} relationship in chronic obstructive lung disease. The shaded area pertains to the range of Pa_{CO_2} observed at any given level of obstruction. (From Anthonisen NR, Cherniack RM. Ventilatory control. *In* Hornbein T [ed]. Lung Disease, Regulation of Breathing, vol 2. New York, Marcel Dekker, 1981, pp 965–987.)

constriction. Hypocapnic bronchoconstriction is thus the mirror image of hypoxic vasoconstriction.

Neither of these compensatory mechanisms is very effective, as demonstrated by the altered blood gases commonly found in patients with $\dot{V}/\dot{Q}$ inequality. Moreover, each can be obviated without much difficulty. Hypoxic vasoconstriction is overcome by increases in left atrial pressure, inactivated in the presence of acute inflammation, and abolished totally or in part by the effects of many vasoactive drugs. Hypocapnic bronchoconstriction is probably eliminated by increases in tidal volume.

The treatment of abnormal gas exchange resulting from $\dot{V}/\dot{Q}$ inequality should ideally be directed at reversing the underlying cause of the mismatched ventilation and blood flow. However, acute therapy directed at the hypoxemia or hypercapnia is often necessary to prevent severe physiologic damage secondary to hypoxia or acidosis. Fortunately, the hypoxemia of $\dot{V}/\dot{Q}$ inequality responds very well to increases in the $F_{I_{O_2}}$. When the degree of $\dot{V}/\dot{Q}$ inequality is only moderately severe, the Pa_{O_2} increases almost linearly with increases in the $F_{I_{O_2}}$, and small increases ($F_{I_{O_2}}$ of 0.24 to 0.28) may be all that is necessary to provide a clinically acceptable Pa_{O_2} (Fig. 6–9). As the degree of $\dot{V}/\dot{Q}$ inequality gets worse, the resistance to a rise in Pa_{O_2} increases; under these circumstances, there may be no significant increase in Pa_{O_2} until the $F_{I_{O_2}}$ reaches 0.40 or higher.

The treatment of hypercapnia requires an increase in minute ventilation unless the underlying cause of the $\dot{V}/\dot{Q}$ inequality can be rapidly reversed. Because in most cases patients with diseases characterized by $\dot{V}/\dot{Q}$ inequality develop hypercapnia because they have exceeded their own ability to increase ventilation, the use of respiratory stimulants is of

Patients with even the worst degrees of $\dot{V}/\dot{Q}$ inequality imaginable can always be adequately oxygenated if the $F_{I_{O_2}}$ is increased sufficiently. This means that any remaining hypoxemia seen in patients breathing 100% O_2 must be a result of totally unventilated units or shunt (see later discussion).

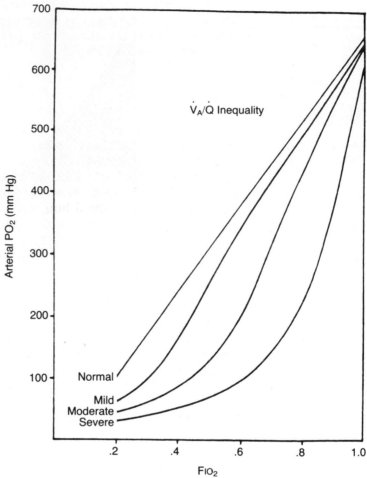

FIGURE 6–9: The effect of increasing ventilation-perfusion ($\dot{V}/\dot{Q}$) inequality on the arterial P_{O_2} at different inspired oxygen fractions ($F_{I_{O_2}}$). (From Dantzker DR. Pulmonary gas exchange. *In* Cardiopulmonary Critical Care, 2nd ed. Philadelphia, WB Saunders, 1991, p 39.)

little value. For acute and progressive hypercapnia, the only certain method of treatment is mechanical ventilation.

In the setting of chronic hypercapnia, O_2 therapy often leads to a further increase in the Pa_{CO_2}. The cause of this increase is multifactorial, with different mechanisms predominating in different individuals.[13] A further depression of respiratory drive is the usual mechanism invoked. Because these patients already have a depressed CO_2 drive, elimination of the hypoxic drive component may lead to further reductions in ventilation and worsening hypercapnia. O_2 also seems to be capable of worsening the degree of $\dot{V}/\dot{Q}$ inequality, perhaps by abolishing hypoxic vasoconstriction. Finally, in the setting of severe hypoxemia, improving the O_2 saturation also shifts the CO_2 dissociation curve to the right (the Haldane effect), decreasing the affinity of the blood for CO_2 (see Fig. 6–2). In patients unable to respond to these latter two effects by an increase in ventilation, further hypercapnia results. The clinical approach to this O_2-induced worsening of the hypercapnia depends on the magnitude of the increase and the status of the patient. Small to moderate increases in Pa_{CO_2} in a patient whose mental status is unchanged require no intervention. Progressive hypercapnia and the development of severe acidosis or central nervous system depression may require mechanical ventilation. The best treatment is to prevent O_2-induced hypercapnia, when possible, by using the smallest increases in the FI_{O_2} necessary to achieve a clinically acceptable Pa_{O_2}.

Shunt

The abnormal admixture of venous blood with the oxygenated blood returning from the alveoli is a potent mechanism of hypoxemia. This admixture may be through an anatomic channel, such as a patent ductus arteriosus, an atrial or a ventricular septal defect, or a pulmonary arteriovenous malformation. Most commonly, however, the source of the shunted blood is abnormal lung units in which perfusion is maintained but ventilation has been abolished because of the collapse of alveolar units or their filling with water or inflammatory exudate. Shunting is the mechanism of abnormal gas exchange in cardiac and noncardiac pulmonary edema, in pneumonia, and in atelectasis due to a myriad of causes. At first glance, shunt may appear to be only one extreme of $\dot{V}/\dot{Q}$ inequality, where $\dot{V}/\dot{Q}$ is zero. However, it is seen in a different spectrum of diseases and requires different therapeutic approaches; thus, it is best thought of as a separate mechanism of abnormal gas exchange.

Because the O_2 saturation of the venous blood is so low, even minor degrees of shunting cause significant reductions in the Pa_{O_2}. However, hypercapnia is never evident until the shunt gets very large (greater than 50%) (Fig. 6–10). In most clinical situations, in fact, the Pa_{CO_2} is lower than normal because ventilation increases above that required to maintain eucapnia, stimulated by the developing hypoxemia as well as

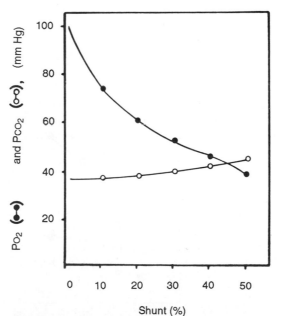

FIGURE 6–10: The effect of increasing shunt on the arterial P_{O_2} and P_{CO_2}. The P_{O_2} *(closed circles)* falls precipitously, whereas the P_{CO_2} *(open circles)* is hardly affected. (From Dantzker DR. Gas exchange. *In* Montenegro H [ed]. Chronic Obstructive Pulmonary Disease. New York, Churchill Livingstone, 1983, p 147.)

by intrapulmonary neural receptors activated by the underlying lung pathology.

The most prominent characteristic of shunt is the resistance of the resultant hypoxemia to correction by increasing the FI_{O_2}. When the shunt is small, the Pa_{O_2} can be increased by raising the FI_{O_2} and thus the O_2 content in the end-capillary blood of the ventilated alveoli. However, as the shunt approaches the levels commonly seen in pulmonary edema or pneumonia, the rise in Pa_{O_2} for a given increase in FI_{O_2} is small; even 100% O_2 is unable to correct the hypoxemia (Fig. 6–11).

Thus, unlike the other mechanisms of abnormal pulmonary gas exchange, the hypoxemia of large, clinically significant shunting is O_2 resis-

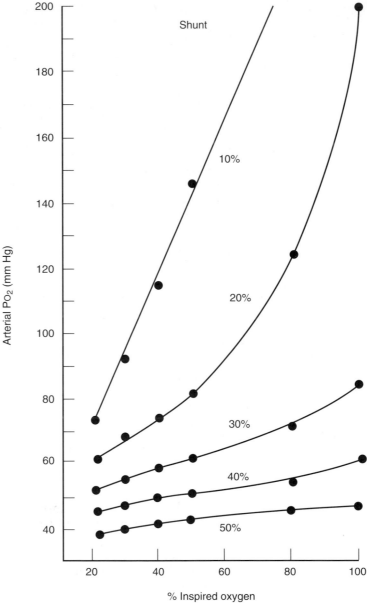

FIGURE 6–11: The effect of changing the inspired oxygen concentration on arterial Po_2 for lung shunts of 10 to 50%. The increase in Po_2 with increasing inspired oxygen concentration is small for lungs with large shunts. (From Dantzker DR. Adult respiratory distress syndrome. Clin Chest Med 3:37, 1982.)

tant. This situation must be treated by reversal of the underlying pulmonary pathology. In many conditions leading to large shunts, immediate reversal of the disease is not possible. Increases in Pa_{O_2} must be achieved without the prolonged use of a high Fi_{O_2}, which by itself may be toxic to the lung.[14] Although the exact level of Fi_{O_2} and the duration of exposure that is injurious to the lungs of humans are unknown, exposure of the lung to an Fi_{O_2} of greater than 0.60 should be kept as short as possible. For the most part, this requires the use of mechanical ventilation, which by increasing the lung volume can recruit previously unventilated units and reduce the shunt.

Nonpulmonary Factors

The earlier conceptualization of the functional unit of gas exchange in the lung stated that the steady-state alveolar gas tension was affected by changes in the partial pressure of the respiratory gases in the mixed venous blood. Because alterations in minute ventilation are so effective in compensating for any change in Pco_2, this effect is clinically significant only for changes in the mixed venous O_2 content (Ca_{O_2}) and Po_2 ($P\bar{v}_{O_2}$). The degree to which the $P\bar{v}_{O_2}$ can influence the Pa_{O_2} depends on the $\dot{V}/\dot{Q}$ of each lung unit. For shunt units, any change in the $P\bar{v}_{O_2}$ is directly translated to the end-capillary blood because there is no contact of the blood with alveolar gas. In ventilated lung units, the effect is greatest in those units with a very low $\dot{V}/\dot{Q}$ and decreases as the $\dot{V}/\dot{Q}$ increases, although even normal units ($\dot{V}/\dot{Q}$ of 1.0) are significantly affected. As the $\dot{V}/\dot{Q}$ increases above 1.0, the impact of a change in $P\bar{v}_{O_2}$ diminishes, a very useful circumstance, as will be seen subsequently. The effect on the Pa_{O_2} obviously depends on the degree of $\dot{V}/\dot{Q}$ inequality or shunting that is present (Fig. 6–12A).

The mixed venous O_2 content ($C\bar{v}_{O_2}$) is determined by the amount of O_2 extracted by the tissues, which in turn is determined by the relationship between O_2 transport and utilization. The individual factors involved can be seen by solving the Fick equation for $C\bar{v}_{O_2}$:

$$C\bar{v}_{O_2} = Ca_{O_2} - \dot{V}_{O_2}/\dot{Q}$$

Thus, a reduction in O_2 transport without a concomitant reduction in O_2 demand or an increase in O_2 requirements without a corresponding increase in O_2 transport reduces the O_2 in the mixed venous blood.

A fall in $P\bar{v}_{O_2}$ is a normal occurrence during exercise, when increased O_2 extraction is used, in addition to an increase in O_2 transfer, to meet the increased metabolic O_2 demands. A highly conditioned athlete can achieve a $P\bar{v}_{O_2}$ as low as 20 mm Hg at peak levels of exercise. What prevents this from being translated into a significant fall in Pa_{O_2} is the increase in the overall $\dot{V}/\dot{Q}$. Although cardiac output may increase four or even five times during exercise, ventilation will increase 15 times or more at peak exercise (see Fig. 6–12B).

The importance of alterations in the $P\bar{v}_{O_2}$ to the development or exaggeration of hypoxemia in disease states has been well documented.[15, 16] The coexistence of anemia or low cardiac output in the setting of chronic pulmonary disease markedly worsens the hypoxemia present for any degree of underlying lung pathology. The normal decrease in $P\bar{v}_{O_2}$ already described to occur during exercise cannot be compensated for in the setting of significant $\dot{V}/\dot{Q}$ inequality or shunting because most of the increased ventilation is distributed to the already well-ventilated

The greater the degree of $\dot{V}/\dot{Q}$ inequality or the larger the shunt, the more a change in $P\bar{v}_{O_2}$ will be translated into a change in Pa_{O_2}.

O_2 transport:

$\dot{T}o_2 = Ca_{O_2} \times \dot{Q}$

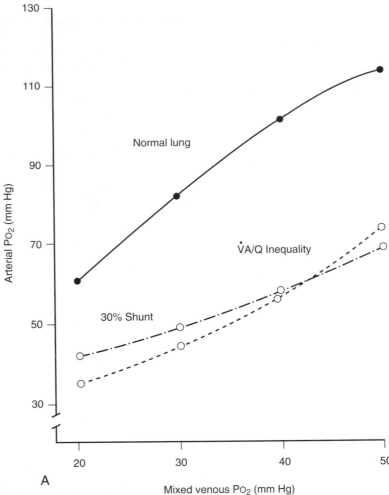

FIGURE 6–12: *A,* The effect of a change in mixed venous P_{O_2} on the arterial P_{O_2} in a theoretical lung with a normal $\dot{V}/\dot{Q}$ distribution *(solid line),* significant $\dot{V}/\dot{Q}$ inequality *(dashed line),* and a 30% shunt. The cardiac output and minute ventilation have been held constant, and the mixed venous P_{O_2} has been allowed to fall by increasing the assumed value for O_2 consumption.

lung units and thus has little or no impact on the units that are the source of the hypoxemia (see Fig. 6–12*B*). This is the major etiology of exercise-induced hypoxemia. Low cardiac output is the predominant cause of hypoxemia in pulmonary hypertension[15] and a major contributor to the low Pa_{O_2} found after acute pulmonary embolic disease.[17] In the acutely ill patient in the intensive care unit in whom the predominant abnormality of pulmonary gas exchange is shunt, it should come as no surprise that alterations in hemoglobin concentration or cardiac output may cause significant changes in Pa_{O_2}. Clearly, a change in $P\bar{v}_{O_2}$ should always be considered as a possible cause of changing Pa_{O_2}; one should not merely assume that any change seen must be the result of an alteration in the degree of lung pathology.

SUMMARY

The process of gas exchange across the alveolar-capillary membrane is a relatively simple and straightforward process of diffusion. However,

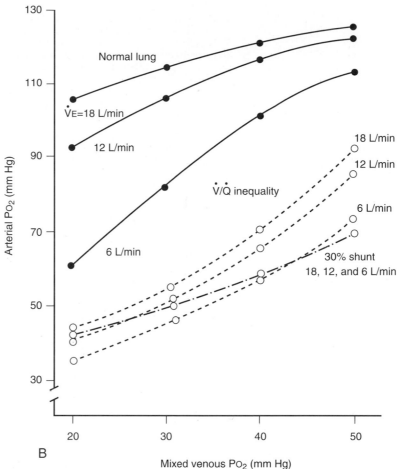

FIGURE 6–12 *Continued B,* The effect of increasing minute ventilation on the relationship between mixed venous P_{O_2} and arterial P_{O_2}. The conditions are the same as those in *A*. Increasing minute ventilation is quite effective in improving the hypoxemia in normal lungs but is much less effective when a significant ventilation-perfusion inequality or a shunt is also present. (*A* and *B,* From Dantzker DR. Cardiovascular pulmonary interaction and diseased lung. Clin Chest Med 4:149, 1983.)

the requirement for this to take place within a confined space, the thorax, and with minimal energy cost necessitated the development of a complex system for the delivery of both gas and blood to the site of interface. This opened up the potential for the inefficiencies that characterize abnormal pulmonary gas exchange and the resultant abnormalities of arterial blood gases. If the basic principles outlined in this chapter are kept in mind, one should be able to diagnose the abnormalities that are present and embark on a logical approach to treatment based on clear-cut physiologic precepts.

References

1. West JB. Ventilation-perfusion inequality and overall gas exchange in computer models of the lung. Respir Physiol 7:88–110, 1969.
2. Roughton FJW, Darling RD, Root WS. Factors affecting the determination of oxygen capacity, content and pressure in human arterial blood. Am J Physiol 142:708–720, 1944.

3. Luft U. Aviation physiology—The effects of altitude. *In* Fenn WO, Rahn H (eds). Respiration. Bethesda, MD, American Physiological Society, 1965, pp 1099–1145.
4. Hurtado A, Marino G, Delgado E. Influence of anoxemia on the hemopoietic activity. Arch Intern Med 75:284–326, 1945.
5. Krogh A, Lindhard J. The volume of the dead space in breathing and the mixing of gases in the lungs of man. J Physiol (Lond) 51:59–90, 1917.
6. Wagner PD. Diffusion and chemical reaction in pulmonary gas exchange. Physiol Rev 57:257–312, 1977.
7. Roughton FJW, Forster RE. Relative importance of diffusion and chemical reaction rates in the human lung, with special reference to true diffusing capacity of pulmonary membrane and volume of blood in the lung capillaries. J Appl Physiol 11:290–302, 1957.
8. West JB. Ventilation-perfusion relationships. Am Rev Respir Dis 116:919–943, 1977.
9. Wagner PD, Laravuso RB, Uhl RR, et al. Continuous distribution of ventilation-perfusion ratios in normal subjects breathing air and 100% O_2. J Clin Invest 54:45–68, 1974.
10. Anthonisen NR, Cherniack RM. Ventilatory control. *In* Hornbein T (ed). Lung Disease, Regulation of Breathing, vol 2. New York, Marcel Dekker, 1981, pp 965–987.
11. Fishman AP. Vasomotor regulation of the pulmonary circulation. Annu Rev Physiol 42:211–220, 1980.
12. Swensen EW, Finley TN, Guzman SV. Unilateral hypoventilation in man during temporary occlusion of one pulmonary artery. J Clin Invest 40:828–835, 1961.
13. Aubier M, Marviano D, Milic-Emili J, et al. Effects of the administration of O_2 on ventilation and blood gases in patients with chronic obstructive pulmonary disease during acute respiratory failure. Am Rev Respir Dis 122:747–754, 1980.
14. Clark JM, Lamberstsen. Pulmonary oxygen toxicity: A review. Pharmacol Rev 23:37–133, 1980.
15. Dantzker DR, D'Alonzo GE, Bower JS, et al. Pulmonary gas exchange during exercise in patients with chronic obliterative pulmonary hypertension. Am Rev Respir Dis 130:412–416, 1984.
16. Dantzker DR, D'Alonzo GE. The effect of exercise on pulmonary gas exchange in patients with severe chronic obstructive pulmonary disease. Am Rev Respir Dis 134:1135–1139, 1986.
17. Manier G, Castain Y, Guenard H. Determinants of hypoxemia during the acute phase of pulmonary embolism in humans. Am Rev Respir Dis 1985.

7 ○ Ventilatory Control

David R. Dantzker, M.D.

The amount of O_2 required ($\dot{V}O_2$) by an individual, as well as the amount of CO_2 produced ($\dot{V}CO_2$), depends on the metabolic demands of the body, which may vary widely from minute to minute. For example, the $\dot{V}O_2$ and $\dot{V}CO_2$ of a conditioned athlete may vary 10-fold or even more during the course of exercise. This feat of gas transfer must be carried out in a way that ensures that the arterial PO_2 (Pa_{O_2}) and PCO_2 (Pa_{CO_2}) levels permit adequate diffusion of O_2 from the microvessels into the tissues (see Chapter 9) and prevents significant changes in pH (see Chapter 5). This task is the major role of the ventilatory control system. In addition, the system must balance these homeostatic requirements with volitional needs for activities such as speech and breath holding. The system may also need to alter normal respiration to support other important body functions, such as the increase in abdominal pressure required for urination, defecation, and childbirth.

To oversee this wide array of functions, a complex organization of sensors, controllers, and effectors has evolved (Fig. 7–1)[1] to function as a negative feedback system with Pa_{O_2} and Pa_{CO_2} as the controlled variables. The efficacy with which any disruption is corrected depends on the adequacy of each component of the system, as well as on its correct integration. The strategy chosen by the system should result in a resolution of the abnormality in blood gases. However, it must also conform to limitations of the system caused by abnormalities of any of its constituents,

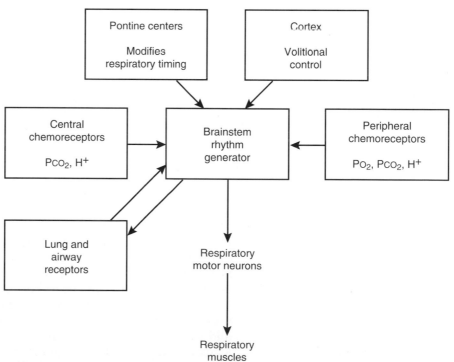

FIGURE 7–1: Model of the ventilatory control system. Multiple inputs (afferent pathways) can affect the respiratory rhythm generator in the medulla.

such as abnormal pulmonary mechanics or respiratory muscle weakness. This may force compromises in the completeness of the correction as the ventilatory control system seeks to balance the normalization of the arterial blood gases with the need to minimize the work of breathing and relieve dyspnea.

In reviewing the functions and interactions of the various elements of this important component of homeostatic control, one should keep in mind that almost all of the information about the individual portions of the ventilatory control system has been derived from experimental observations on animals. The direct transfer of these observations to humans must be undertaken with some caution. However, the integrated responses to arterial blood gas disturbances have been well studied in normal and abnormal humans, and they seem to fit the general principles derived from animal studies.

THE RESPIRATORY CONTROLLERS

Various parts of the central nervous system generate the breathing pattern. Previously, investigators thought that an autonomous rhythm generator somewhere in the brain stem acted, much as pacemaker cells in the heart, to establish some baseline rhythm, which was individualized as required by the needs of the body. Now, it seems clear that the output of the rhythm generation greatly depends on afferent input from various receptors. If the Po_2 and Pco_2 of the arterial blood are artificially maintained by some means other than breathing, such as by extracorporeal oxygenation and CO_2 removal, breathing may even cease.

The medulla is believed to play the primary role in the control of breathing.[2] Two groups of neurons have been identified. The dorsal respiratory group neurons, which are located in the ventrolateral portion of the tractus solitarius, are thought to be the initial processors of afferent information coming from peripheral sensors through cranial nerves IX and X. These neurons act predominantly during inspiration and send their message, via the bulbospinal pathway, mainly to the motor neurons of the phrenic nerve, located in the third through the sixth cervical dorsal roots. The phrenic nerve, in turn, innervates the diaphragm. The ventral respiratory group neurons act during both inspiration and expiration. Located in the nucleus ambiguus and retroambiguus, they project mainly to the motor neurons controlling the intercostal, accessory, and abdominal muscles. The exact manner by which the DRG and VRG neurons interact to determine the respiratory pattern is not well understood.

Both the DRG and VRG neurons receive input from respiratory active neurons in the pons.[3] Two areas in the pons, the apneustic center in the lower pons and the pneumotaxic center in the upper pons, have been identified. Neither of these centers appears to be necessary for rhythmic breathing, but they seem to play a role in respiratory phase switching (i.e., from inspiration to expiration). The pneumotaxic center is thought to fine tune the breathing pattern, whereas the apneustic center is responsible for the cessation of inspiration.

In animal studies, the roles of these various centers have been most graphically demonstrated by transecting the brain stem at various levels and observing the effect on respiration. Transection below the medulla leads to a cessation of breathing, indicating the importance of the medullary centers to respiration. Elimination of the respiratory neurons above the medulla, by transection at the pontomedullary junction, re-

DRG neurons—dorsal respiratory group neurons.

VRG neurons—ventral respiratory group neurons.

sults in a regular but more rapid and shallow breathing pattern than normal. The effect of transections above this level appears to depend on input from the vagus nerve. This nerve is responsible for the Hering-Breuer reflex, which normally terminates inspiration once a certain volume is reached. Bilateral vagotomy, by itself, causes a deepening and slowing of respiration. Midpontine transection, which isolates the pneumotaxic center, causes slow, deep breathing with the vagi intact but causes apneustic breathing after bilateral vagotomy. Apneustic breathing, a striking type of respiration characterized by a prolonged inspiratory phase, has been described in various brain stem disorders in humans. Transection above the pons has no discernible effect on the baseline respiratory pattern.

The stimulation of various parts of the brain above the pons, however, can have diverse effects on respiration, both excitatory and inhibitory. Although their exact role is unknown, these areas are thought to allow for override of the chemoreceptors in order to facilitate activities such as singing and speaking. They may also be involved in the coordination of breathing with locomotion and are certainly involved in the changes in respiration associated with emotion.

THE SENSORS

The ability of the ventilatory controllers to alter respiration successfully to meet the varying demands of the body depends on accurate input from receptors. These receptors sense changes in the chemical composition of both the blood and the brain interstitial fluid, as well as alterations in functions as diverse as lung volume and muscle contraction. All of these myriad afferent signals summate within the respiratory center to influence the breathing pattern. The sensors can be divided into a number of types (Table 7–1).

Central Chemoreceptors

The chemoreceptors can be divided into the central and the peripheral receptors. The central chemoreceptors, located in the medulla, are thought to lie close to its ventrolateral surface.[4] Their exact location, and the anatomic connections of the central chemoreceptors to the DRG and VRG neurons, have yet to be determined. The central chemoreceptors

TABLE **7–1:** Respiratory Sensors

Receptor	Location	Effect
Central chemoreceptor	Medulla	Stimulate breathing in response to hypercapnia and acidosis
Peripheral chemoreceptor	Carotid body	Stimulate breathing in response to hypercapnia, acidosis, and hypoxemia
Upper airway	Face and nose	"Diving reflex"
Slowly adapting stretch	Small airways	Inflation reflex and bronchodilatation
Rapidly adapting stretch	Large airways	Irritant response: cough bronchoconstriction, mucus production
Juxtacapillary (J receptors)	Airway, blood vessel, and alveolar walls	Tachypnea, hypotension, and bradycardia

increase and decrease their neural output in response to increases and decreases in the P_{CO_2} and H^+ concentration in the cerebral interstitial fluid. The interstitial fluid is in equilibrium with the cerebrospinal fluid, but not with the blood from which it is separated by the blood-brain barrier. To understand the function of these receptors fully, one must realize that CO_2 rapidly diffuses across the blood-brain barrier, but H^+ and HCO_3^- do not. Thus, the central chemoreceptors respond much more quickly to changes in ventilation than to metabolic abnormalities. The early response to alterations in metabolic acid-base disturbances is the responsibility of the peripheral chemoreceptors.

The pH of the cerebrospinal fluid is normally about 0.1 pH unit less than that of the blood. Because of a lower buffering capacity in the cerebrospinal fluid, the pH change for any alteration in P_{CO_2} or H^+ is greater than that seen in blood. However, the pH of the cerebrospinal fluid is restored more quickly than that of the blood by a system actively transporting H^+ and HCO_3^- in and out. Thus, continuing respiratory compensation for chronic alterations in metabolically induced acid-base abnormalities tends to be blunted.

Peripheral Chemoreceptors

The anatomy and physiology of the peripheral chemoreceptors, located in the carotid and aortic bodies in many animal species, are much better understood.[5] In humans, it is not clear if the aortic bodies have any role in ventilatory control. Therefore, this discussion is limited to the carotid bodies, which are located at the bifurcation of the common carotid artery. They are composed of two types of cells, the type I or glomus cell and the type II sustentacular or sheath cell. The blood flow to the carotid body, per gram of tissue, is very high. Thus, even though it is a highly metabolic organ, a very narrow arteriovenous difference exists for both O_2 and CO_2. This allows the entire organ to be exposed to arterial values for both respiratory gases. The efferent signal from the carotid body transmits via the carotid sinus nerve.

The peripheral chemoreceptors respond to changes in P_{O_2}, P_{CO_2}, and pH. The peripheral chemoreceptors do not respond to changes in O_2 content. For this reason, ventilation does not increase in carbon monoxide poisoning, methemoglobinemia, or severe anemia. The peripheral chemoreceptors are thought to contribute about 15 to 20% of the active input to the respiratory center in the medulla. This includes all of the hypoxic drive, up to 30% of the response to hypercapnia, and the entire acute response to metabolic acidosis. The carotid body can also be stimulated by a fall in blood pressure or an increase in sympathetic tone, which may account for the tachypnea associated with shock.

The carotid body, tonically active in normal healthy individuals breathing at sea level, shuts down in response to breathing 100% O_2. This may account in part for the reduction in dyspnea reported by athletes given O_2 to breathe after acute exertion, because the reduction in carotid body input leads to an abrupt decrease in minute ventilation.

Other Receptors

Various other inputs to the medullary respiratory center originate in the upper airway, trachea, lungs, and chest wall and respond to mechanical alterations as well as to a multiplicity of locally secreted chemicals. These inputs tend to modify the chemoreceptor control of ventilation and in certain pathologic states can play the dominant role in the determination of the breathing pattern.

The upper airway is known to contain a number of different receptors, although their effects on respiration have not been well defined.[6] Some appear to be designed to augment the major role of the upper airway, namely the protection of the tracheobronchial tree from noxious agents. Receptors that stimulate sneezing, cause reflex secretion of mucus glycoproteins in the lower respiratory tract, and alter bronchomotor tone would fit into this category. A more exotic response to noxious stimuli is the diving reflex. Apnea, a common response to nasal irritation, can be induced by irritants, by certain odors, and interestingly, by cold water applied to the face or into the nares. This reflex, well demonstrated in humans, presumably functions to limit the penetration of harmful substances into the lung. Along with this respiratory response, there may also be laryngeal closure, bradycardia, and peripheral vasoconstriction, which leads to a redistribution of blood to the brain and heart. Presumably, these responses protect the vital organs from the hypoxia that develops during apnea. The full manifestation of the diving reflex, namely apnea and the redistribution of blood flow, is most pronounced in diving mammals, whereas in humans, probably only infants manifest it completely.

Other upper airway receptors may help coordinate swallowing by inhibiting inspiration and stimulating glottic closure. Finally, many patients with chronic obstructive pulmonary disease describe a reduction in the sense of breathlessness when air is blown against the face and nares. The type or location of the receptor involved in this response has not been clearly defined.

RASRs—rapidly adapting stretch receptors.

SASRs—slowly adapting stretch receptors.

Three different types of receptors are found in the tracheobronchial tree:[7] the slowly adapting stretch receptors and the rapidly adapting stretch receptors (both of which are myelinated fibers in the vagus nerve), and the C fibers (unmyelinated vagal afferents). Stimulation of these receptors results in responses that probably serve as a protective reflex.

The SASRs, which are located predominantly in the small intrapulmonary airways, mediate the Hering-Breuer or inflation reflex. These mechanoreceptors respond to an increase in lung volume by inhibition of inspiratory activity, presumably through modification of the output of the DRG neurons in the medulla. Stimulation of these receptors also leads to bronchodilatation, tachycardia, and a decrease in peripheral vascular resistance. The utility of these last two responses is unclear. In contrast, the RASRs, found in highest density in the large extrapulmonary airways, respond both to an increase in lung volume and to a large number of endogenous and exogenous chemicals. The responses include hyperpnea, bronchoconstriction, cough, and increased mucus production. These "irritant receptors" and their hyper-reactivity may play an important role in certain forms of asthma. Stimulation of the RASRs probably explains the bronchospasm seen when asthmatics take a very deep inspiration. This contrasts with the reduction in airway resistance seen in normal individuals after a large breath, possibly mediated through the SASRs.

The third type of receptors, the C fibers, are found in the walls of the airways, blood vessels, and alveoli. They respond to mechanical stimuli in the form of increased interstitial pressure or congestion, as well as

The C fibers are also called the J or juxtacapillary receptors.

to a number of chemical mediators, such as histamine, bradykinin, prostaglandins, and serotonin. The response to stimulation of the C fibers is apnea, followed by rapid, shallow breathing, hypotension, and bradycardia. Activation of these fibers is thought to play an important role in the response to pulmonary edema and acute pulmonary embolism.

In addition to the lung receptors, there are also afferent inputs to the medullary ventilatory center from the respiratory muscles and other components of the chest wall. Most skeletal muscles contain muscle spindles and Golgi tendon organs, which serve to modify the response of muscles to variations in load. The spindles increase muscle recruitment and contraction in response to an increase in load, whereas the Golgi organs prevent their overloading by inhibiting the motor neuron input if the load becomes too great.

EFFECTORS

The effectors of respiration, the respiratory muscles that maintain the patency of the upper airway, alter the volume of the thoracic cage, increasing and decreasing intrathoracic pressure and moving air between the lungs and the environment (Table 7–2).[8, 9] Instructions are transmitted from the respiratory center to these muscles over various pathways. The phrenic nerves, which arise from the third to the fifth cervical roots, innervate the diaphragm. The sternocleidomastoid muscles receive their input from cranial nerve IX and C1 and C2; the scalene muscles, from C4 to C8; the intercostals, from the intercostal nerves of the thoracic roots (T1 to T12); and the abdominal muscles, from the lower thoracic and upper lumbar nerves. Interruption of any of these pathways, either at their origins in the anterior horn of the spinal column or their connections to the central nervous system via the dorsal motor tracts or through damage to the peripheral nerves, can lead to significant respiratory dysfunction. A complete discussion of the respiratory muscles is found in Chapter 3.

TESTS OF VENTILATORY FUNCTION

Because of the tightly integrated nature of the ventilatory control system, one cannot clinically assess each component individually. Instead, the tests stimulate the sensors and measure the output of the effectors. An abnormal response can thus be caused by pathology anywhere along the pathway, which makes it difficult to pinpoint clearly the

TABLE **7–2:**   Respiratory Muscles

Muscle	Neural Innervation	Action
Upper airway	Cranial nerve XII, recurrent and superior laryngeal nerves (cranial nerve X)	Maintain upper airway patency
Sternocleidomastoid	Cranial nerve IX, cervical nerves 1 and 2	Inspiration
Scalene muscles	Cervical nerves 4–8	Inspiration
Diaphragm	Phrenic nerves (cervical nerves 3–5)	Inspiration
Intercostal muscles	Thoracic nerves 1–12	Inspiration and expiration
Abdominal muscles	Lower thoracic and upper lumbar nerves	Expiration

specific site of the abnormality. In practice, clinical evaluation is limited to assessing chemoreceptor function because easily performed, specific tests for the other sensors do not exist.

Basal ventilatory drive, as well as the response to a change in P_{O_2} and P_{CO_2} can be measured. Typically, the output of the ventilatory center can be assessed by measuring minute ventilation. This can be misleading, however, when abnormal lung mechanics or neuromuscular disease makes a normal ventilatory response impossible despite normal chemoreceptor function. Under these circumstances, other output functions can be assessed.

The mouth occlusion pressure 0.1 second after the initiation of a breath against a closed airway, the $P_{0.1}$, is the most commonly used alternative to the change in minute ventilation (Fig. 7–2).[10] While the patient breathes on a test circuit, the inspiratory port is randomly occluded during expiration. The slope of the subsequent inspiratory effort, measured as the change in mouth pressure, reflects respiratory drive. Because the patient normally takes 0.3 second or longer to become aware that the airway is occluded, the slope of the line at any point before this time is considered a valid measurement of respiratory center output. In practice, the pressure at 0.1 second is measured. Because no change in lung volume and airflow occurs during the period of occlusion, abnormalities of lung mechanics play no role in the magnitude of the $P_{0.1}$. Thus, this can be a valid index of respiratory center output, even in the face of significant obstructive and restrictive lung disease. Only in the face of marked muscle weakness, or perhaps in the hyperinflated patient whose respiratory muscles are markedly shortened at functional residual capacity (see Chapter 3), will the $P_{0.1}$ be affected by factors not directly related to respiratory drive.

A more direct measurement of the output of the respiratory center can be obtained from electromyography of the diaphragm or the direct recording of the phrenic neurogram. Unfortunately, these relatively in-

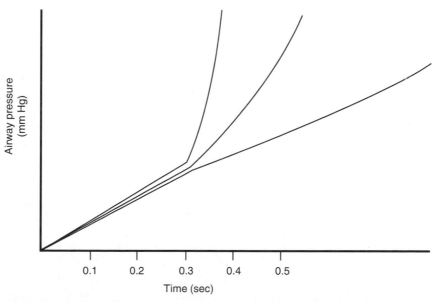

FIGURE 7–2: $P_{0.1}$ measurement. If the airway is occluded before inspiration, it will take about 0.3 second for the individual to realize it. The slope of the airway pressure–time relationship, before a conscious response, is a good measure of respiratory drive. Typically, the pressure at 0.1 second is used—the $P_{0.1}$.

vasive tests require needle electrodes or the passage of an esophageal electrode. The patient discomfort, along with the technologic difficulties in accumulating and analyzing the signal, limits their usefulness.

A final available technique, analysis of the respiratory pattern, allows the assessment of both respiratory drive and respiratory center timing.[11] This approach quantitates ventilation by assessing the tidal volume (V_T), the amount of time spent in inspiration (the inspiratory time, t_i) and the total time for the breath (t_{tot}) (Fig. 7–3). Using these variables, one can write an equation for minute ventilation ($\dot{V}_E$):

$$\dot{V}_E = (V_T/t_i) \times (t_i/t_{tot})$$

The first term, V_T/t_i, is the mean inspiratory flow rate and is a reflection of the respiratory drive. The second term, t_i/t_{tot}, is the fraction of time spent in inspiration and as such is an index of respiratory timing. In normal humans, changes in $\dot{V}_E$ are accomplished predominantly by increases in V_T rather than in t_i. The t_i also represents the duty cycle of the respiratory system and thus provides information on the time the respiratory muscles are active. The prolonged t_i seen in certain diseases is thought to predispose to respiratory muscle fatigue.

Respiratory pattern analysis has certain advantages over the other variables usually assessed in the evaluation of respiratory drive. It is typically measured using respiratory inductance plethysmography, a technique that measures the simultaneous expansion of the chest wall and abdomen via belts placed around the chest wall and abdomen. The sum of the abdominal and chest wall displacement equals V_T. Because it does not require the use of a mouthpiece or invasive techniques, the measurement is less likely to influence the output of the ventilatory center. It has been clearly demonstrated, for example, that patients breathing on mouthpieces have different breathing patterns than those performing spontaneous, unobstructed breathing, with increases in V_T and $\dot{V}_E$ and decreases in respiratory frequency.[12]

On the basis of unstimulated measurements, the normal variability of basal ventilatory control makes it difficult to draw conclusions about the status of ventilatory control. A more interpretable approach is to measure the response of any of the discussed variables in response to chemoreceptor stimulation by hypercapnia or hypoxemia. This is most efficiently accomplished with a rebreathing technique during which the patient rebreathes gas from a reservoir while O_2 and CO_2 are altered in a continually progressive fashion.

To test hypercapnic drive, the subject rebreathes from the reservoir with a starting gas concentration of 7% CO_2 and 93% O_2.[13] The high FI_{O_2} prevents any contribution from hypoxic drive. The subject's CO_2 production progressively increases the CO_2 in the inspired gas, causing the

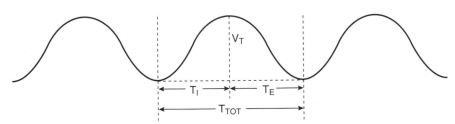

FIGURE 7–3: Recording of the respiratory cycle used to complete respiratory pattern parameters. V_T is tidal volume, t_i and t_e are inspiratory and expiratory time, and t_{tot} is the time of a whole breath. The ratio V_T/t_i is the mean inspiratory flow rate, an index of respiratory drive.

arterial and cerebral interstitial P_{CO_2} to increase at about 6 mm Hg/min. The normal response of minute ventilation to this incremental hypercapnia is a linear increase in $\dot{V}_E$ with a slope of 2 to 4 L/min/mm Hg P_{CO_2} (Fig. 7–4). However, normal CO_2 sensitivity varies, with slopes as low as 1 or as high as 8. A similar linear response is seen if $P_{0.1}$ or electromyographic measurements are the dependent variables. The slope of the CO_2 response is determined almost entirely by the central chemoreceptors, the sensitivity of which is thought to decrease somewhat with age.

The hypoxic drive is less frequently assessed because of increased technical difficulty and problems involved with quantitating the response.[14] Usually, no increase in ventilation occurs until the P_{O_2} falls below 50 to 60 mm Hg. With greater degrees of hypoxia, there is a rapid increase in $\dot{V}_E$. This response is best characterized by a hyperbolic curve (Fig. 7–5), often modeled by the equation.

$$\dot{V} = \dot{V}_0 + A/(Pa_{O_2} - 32)$$

where $\dot{V}$ is the ventilation at any given Pa_{O_2}, $\dot{V}_0$ is the initial ventilation, and A represents the sensitivity parameter and can be used to compare one individual with another. The relationship between O_2 saturation and $\dot{V}_E$ is linear, with the slope of this response sometimes used to simplify the calculation of hypoxic response. However, as already discussed, the chemoreceptor responds to P_{O_2} and not O_2 saturation.

If the Pa_{CO_2} falls during the measurement, the hypoxic response will be blunted. For this reason, CO_2 must be added to the rebreathing bag as the increased $\dot{V}_E$ associated with increasing hypoxia drives the Pa_{CO_2} down. This requirement for maintaining an isocapnic environment makes the measurement of the hypoxic response difficult. Because a sufficient clinical correlation usually exists between the hypoxic and the hypercapnic responses, the latter need not be measured. However, assessing the response to hypoxia is the only way of isolating peripheral

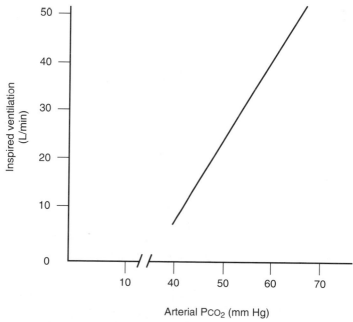

FIGURE 7–4: CO_2 response curve. There is a linear increase in minute ventilation as the arterial P_{CO_2} increases. The slope of the line defines the CO_2 response.

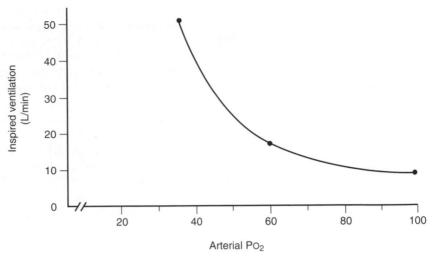

FIGURE 7–5: Hypoxic response curve. There is a nonlinear increase in minute ventilation as the arterial P_{O_2} decreases. No appreciable increase occurs until the P_{O_2} falls below 60 mm Hg.

chemoreceptor function. Table 7–3 shows situations in which the response to hypercapnia and hypoxia is abnormal.

ABNORMAL VENTILATORY PATTERNS

Apneustic breathing is sustained inspiratory pauses.

Biot's breathing is characterized by a haphazard, random fluctuation between deep and shallow breaths, with interspersed apneas.

Cheyne-Stokes respiration consists of regular cycles of tidal volume changes in a crescendo-decrescendo pattern, separated by periods of apnea or hypopnea.

For the most part, primary defects of the respiratory control system are related to neurologic disturbances. A number of characteristic breathing patterns have been described (Fig. 7–6). Apneustic breathing, sustained inspiratory pauses, is found in patients with damage in the midpons and is usually due to basilar artery infarcts. Biot's breathing, which is characterized by a haphazard, random fluctuation between deep and shallow breaths, with interspersed apneas, is usually due to disease in the medulla.

The most characteristic of the abnormal breathing patterns, Cheyne-Stokes respiration, has been described in a wide variety of diffuse neurologic disturbances but is also commonly seen in patients with heart failure.[15] In these patients, the oscillations are due to the prolongation of the circulation time, which delays the normal transmission to the brain of data concerning changes in Pa_{O_2} and Pa_{CO_2}. This leads to an instability in the feedback control such that the breathing pattern is always out of phase with the arterial blood gases. Cheyne-Stokes respiration is also seen in normal subjects, especially during light sleep. In normal individuals, it is more commonly present in older subjects and in individuals at high altitudes.

Hyperventilation, usually seen in the setting of metabolic acidosis, serves to compensate for a reduction in the HCO_3^- concentration (see Chapter 5). It can also occur as a consequence of diffuse pulmonary

TABLE **7–3:** Disorders Associated With Abnormal Ventilatory Control

Idiopathic alveolar hypoventilation	Multiple sclerosis
Cerebrovascular disease	Bacterial meningitis
Encephalitis	Hypothyroidism
Brain tumor	Obesity hypoventilation syndrome

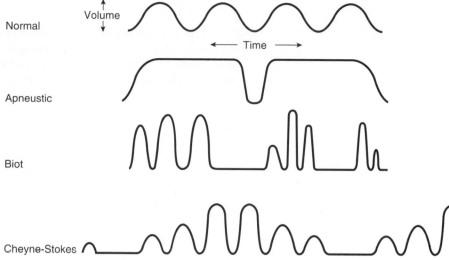

FIGURE 7–6: Examples of three abnormal breathing patterns. (See text for further discussion.)

Pain, anxiety, and other strong emotional feelings can stimulate hyperventilation. It can also be seen in the setting of hypotension, end-stage liver disease, and diffuse brain dysfunction.

parenchymal or vascular disease as the respiratory center is stimulated by mechanoreceptors within the lung. Less commonly, it is seen in the absence of clear evidence of metabolic abnormalities or lung disease. Finally, certain drugs, such as salicylates, can lead to significant respiratory alkalosis through stimulatory effects on the respiratory center. For the most part, correction of the hyperventilation can be achieved only by addressing the underlying problem.

Hypoventilation, most commonly due to the excessive use of sedating medication or to the presence of neuromuscular disease, may also be seen with severe metabolic alkalosis and complicating hypothyroidism. A small number of patients may have primary hypoventilation syndrome, sometimes referred to as Ondine's curse. Some of these rare patients suffer from a diffuse neurologic deficit occurring after brain surgery or after an episode of encephalitis. In others, there is no obvious cause. Regardless of the etiology of the hypoventilation, it characteristically worsens at night because of the predictable effect of sleep on ventilation (see Chapter 43). A number of clinical clues suggest the presence of impaired chemosensitivity leading to hypoventilation (Table 7–4). Some patients with primary hypoventilation, who have intolerable hypoxemia and hypercapnia, respond to the use of respiratory stimulants such as progesterone, although long-term success is unlikely. Nocturnal mechanical ventilation is occasionally successful, and diaphragmatic pacing has been tried. The number of reported cases is too small to draw any conclusions with regard to the efficacy of any of these therapeutic approaches.

TABLE **7–4:** Clinical Indications of Abnormal Ventilatory Control Leading to Hypoventilation

Hypoxemia with a normal alveolar-arterial P_{O_2} gradient
Disproportionally small reduction in FEV_1
Ability to achieve a normal Pa_{CO_2} with voluntary hyperventilation
Ability to generate a negative inspiration pressure of greater than 30 mm Hg (rules out respiratory muscle weakness)

SUMMARY

The ventilatory control system is a complex organization of sensors, controllers, and effectors that maintains respiration at a level necessary to provide the amount of O_2 required each minute for metabolism and to remove the amount of CO_2 produced from energy generation. Under normal circumstances, it optimizes breathing so that the work of the individual is minimal. In the setting of disease, the system is called on to make many adjustments to maintain a sufficient minute ventilation while at the same time optimizing the work of breathing. When it is unable to accomplish this adequately, dyspnea results. A clear understanding of this complex system is necessary in order to care optimally for patients with cardiorespiratory disease.

References

1. Berger AJ. Control of breathing. *In* Murray JF, Nadel JA (eds). Textbook of Respiratory Medicine. Philadelphia, WB Saunders, 1988, pp 149–166.
2. Cohen MI. Neurogenesis of respiratory rhythm in the mammal. Physiol Rev 59:1105–1173, 1979.
3. Berger AJ, Mitchell RA, Severinghaus JW. Regulation of respiration. N Engl J Med 297:92–97, 138–143, 194–201, 1977.
4. Bledsoe SW, Hornbein TF. Central chemoreceptors and the regulation of their chemical environment. *In* Hornbein TF (ed). Regulation of Breathing, part I. New York, Marcel Dekker, 1981, pp 347–428.
5. McDonald DM. Peripheral chemoreceptors: Stricture-function relationships of the carotid body. *In* Hornbein TF (ed). Regulation of Breathing, part I. New York, Marcel Dekker, 1981, pp 105–319.
6. Widdicombe JG. Reflexes from the upper respiratory tract. *In* Cherniak NS, Widdicombe JG (eds). Handbook of Physiology: The Respiratory System. Bethesda, MD, American Physiological Society, 1986, pp 363–394.
7. Coleridge HM, Coleridge JCG. Reflexes evoked from tracheobronchial tree and lungs. *In* Cherniak NS, Widdicombe JG (eds). Handbook of Physiology: The Respiratory System. Bethesda, MD, American Physiological Society, 1986, pp 395–429.
8. Lunteren EV, Strohl P. The muscles of the upper airways. Clin Chest Med 7:171–188, 1986.
9. DeTroyer A, Estenne M. Functional anatomy of the respiratory muscles. Clin Chest Med 9:175–193, 1988.
10. Whitelaw WA, Devenne JP, Milic Emili J. Occlusion pressure as a measure of respiratory center output in conscious man. Respir Physiol 23:181–199, 1975.
11. Gardner WN. The relationship between tidal volume and inspiratory and expiratory times during steady-state carbon dioxide inhalation in man. J Physiol (Lond) 272:591–611, 1977.
12. Perez W, Tobin MJ. Separation of factors responsible for change in breathing pattern induced by instrumentation. J Appl Physiol 59:1515–1526, 1985.
13. Read DJC. A clinical method for assessing the ventilatory response to carbon dioxide. Aust Ann Med 16:20–32, 1967.
14. Weil JV, Byrne-Quinn E, Sodal IE, et al. Hypoxic ventilatory drive in normal man. J Clin Invest 49:1061–1072, 1970.
15. Brown HW, Plum F. The neurological basis of Cheyne-Stokes respiration. Am J Med 30:849–861, 1961.

8

■

Cardiovascular Anatomy and Physiology

David J. Frid, M.D., and Stuart Sheifer, B.A.

Those involved in respiratory care should have a solid understanding of cardiovascular physiology because the body's cardiovascular and respiratory systems are profoundly interdependent. When functioning appropriately, these two systems work in concert to provide the body's tissues with a mechanism for oxygen delivery and waste removal. When either of these systems fails, the other suffers severe consequences.

In order to explain the physiology of the cardiovascular system and some of the ways in which it relates to the body's respiratory system, this chapter is divided into three sections. The first deals with the functional anatomy of the heart. The second focuses on how the heart works as a pump and discusses some of the basic principles of heart failure. The final section explains some of the specific mechanisms that lead to heart failure, as well as their clinical manifestations.

FUNCTIONAL ANATOMY OF THE HEART

The function of the heart is to pump blood through the body's circulatory system. In actuality, the heart is composed of two adjacent pumps: the right side of the heart, which pumps blood through the lungs, and the left side of the heart, which pumps blood through the rest of the body.

Although the specific functions and the exact structures of these two pumps differ, their anatomy is analogous. More specifically, each of these pumps contains the following components:

- Vessels to deliver blood to the pump
- A collecting chamber, known as the atrium
- A pumping chamber, known as the ventricle
- An outflow vessel
- An atrioventricular (AV) valve, separating the atrium and ventricle
- A semilunar valve, separating the ventricle and the outflow vessel

The following sections describe each of these components (Figs. 8–1 and 8–2).

Inflow Vessels

The right side of the heart is primed by deoxygenated blood from the venous system. This blood is brought to the right atrium by two large veins, the superior and inferior venae cavae. Meanwhile, the left side of the heart is primed by freshly oxygenated blood returning from the lungs. This blood is delivered to the left atrium by the pulmonary veins.

131

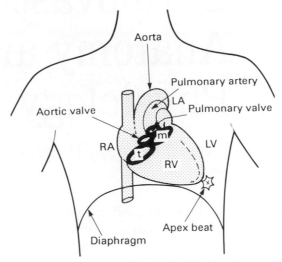

FIGURE 8–1: The heart lies obliquely across the chest. The fibrotendinous ring (*black*) forms the base of the heart. It contains the tricuspid (t), mitral (m), aortic, and pulmonary valves grouped in an oblique plane beneath the sternum. The apex of the heart is formed by the left ventricle (LV), and the anterior surface is formed by the right ventricle (RV) and the right atrium (RA). The inferior surface of the heart and the pericardium (not shown) rest on the central tendon of the diaphragm. (From Levick JR. An Introduction to Cardiovascular Physiology. Boston, Butterworths, 1991, p 14.)

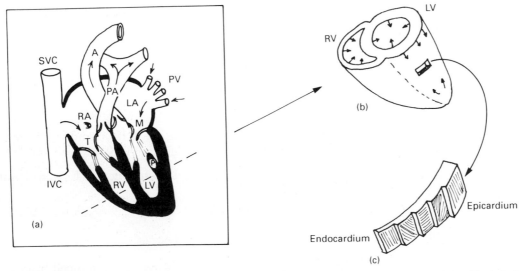

FIGURE 8–2: Sections through the heart. a, Oblique section. b, Section across the ventricles to illustrate the mode of emptying. c, Arrangement of muscle fibers in the ventricle wall. RA, LA, right and left atria. The opening just below the RA label is the coronary sinus. RV, LV, right and left ventricles; T, M, tricuspid and mitral valves; P, papillary muscle with chordae tendineae; A, aorta; PA, PV, pulmonary artery and veins; SVC, IVC, superior and inferior venae cavae. (*A* to *C*, From Levick JR. An Introduction to Cardiovascular Physiology. Boston, Butterworths, 1991, p 14.)

Diastole—the period of time when the ventricles are being filled with blood

Atria

The right and left atria lie superior to their respective ventricles. Their walls are composed of an inner epithelial layer, known as the endocardium; a middle layer of muscle, known as the myocardium; and an outer epicardial layer. Each atrium terminates in an appendage, termed an auricle, which is lined by pectinate muscle.

The atria function as primer pumps for each ventricle. During diastole, blood flows freely across the AV valve openings into the ventricles. Toward the end of this period, the atria contract to empty an additional volume of blood.

Ventricles

The ventricles are pumping chambers that contain thick muscular walls. These walls are composed of the same three layers as those of the atria, but they are typically at least five times as thick. The wall of the left ventricle is actually about 40% thicker than that of the right ventricle. The ventricles also differ in shape: whereas the left ventricle is typically globular, the right one is generally more bulging to be able to accommodate the same volume of blood with less muscle.

A muscular interventricular septum separates the two chambers and thus allows the ventricles to function independently, with the right ventricle pumping to the pulmonary circulation and the left ventricle pumping to the systemic vasculature.

Outflow Vessels

Blood flows from the right ventricle into the pulmonary artery, which subsequently branches after 4 or 5 cm into the right and left pulmonary arteries; it is these vessels that deliver deoxygenated blood to the lungs. Meanwhile, the left ventricle pumps oxygenated blood into the aorta, which subsequently delivers this blood to the entire body's arterial system.

Atrioventricular Valves

Names and Functions

The AV valve of the right side of the heart is the tricuspid valve, and the corresponding structure of the left side of the heart is the mitral valve. These valves function to allow easy entry of blood into the ventricles during diastole and to prevent backflow of blood from the ventricles into the atria during ventricular contraction, known as systole. To achieve both of these functions, the AV valves have an ingenious anatomy (Figs. 8–3 and 8–4).

Valve Framework

Each AV valve is bounded by a tough fibrous ring. Attached to this ring, and filling in the circle it creates, are fibrinous mobile cusps. The tricuspid valve contains three of these cusps, whereas the mitral valve contains two. The tip of each cusp is connected to eight to 12 fibrous

ANTERIOR

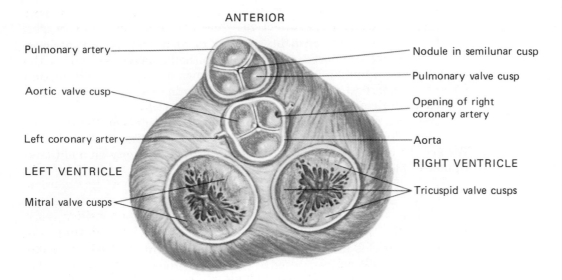

Pulmonary artery

Aortic valve cusp

Left coronary artery

LEFT VENTRICLE

Mitral valve cusps

Nodule in semilunar cusp

Pulmonary valve cusp

Opening of right coronary artery

Aorta

RIGHT VENTRICLE

Tricuspid valve cusps

POSTERIOR

FIGURE 8–3: The valves of the heart as seen from above after removal of the atria and transection of the pulmonary artery and aorta. (From Guyton AC. Anatomy and Physiology. Philadelphia, Saunders College Publishing, 1985, p 405.)

strands, known as chordae tendineae. These strands are attached inferiorly to papillary muscles, which have their origin on the inner surface of the ventricles.

Structure-Function Relationship

This anatomic framework allows the valves to achieve their two key functions. During diastole, the cusps passively protrude inferiorly, into the ventricles; the valve opening is patent; and blood passes through from the atria. Then, during ventricular contraction, the increased ventricular pressures force the AV valves superiorly, until the cusps are in

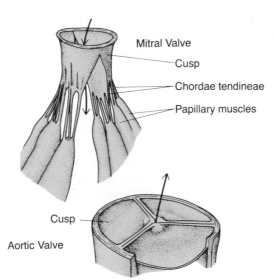

Mitral Valve

Cusp

Chordae tendineae

Papillary muscles

Cusp

Aortic Valve

FIGURE 8–4: Structure of the mitral and aortic valves. (From Guyton AC. Anatomy and Physiology. Philadelphia, Saunders College Publishing, 1985, p 405.)

apposition, and thus the valve seals off. To prevent the valves from prolapsing in the opposite direction while the ventricles contract, the papillary muscles place downward pressure on the cusps.

Semilunar Valves

The semilunar valves (see Figs. 8–3 and 8–4), which interface between the ventricles and their outflow vessels, are the pulmonic valve on the right side of the heart and the aortic valve on the left. Each of these valves contains three cusps, which are attached to the inner wall of the respective outflow vessel. These valves are not connected to any chordae tendineae or papillary muscles, as in the case of the AV valves.

During diastole, the semilunar valve cusps are in apposition, passively bulging inferiorly toward the ventricles. In contrast, during ventricular contraction, blood is forced through the valves, and the cusps are forced superiorly. The pressure generated by the blood flow causes the cusps to be pressed flat against the surface of the vessel wall, thus leaving the valve open. Once systole is over, the cusps once again passively bulge inferiorly, thereby preventing backflow from the outflow tracks back into the ventricles.

Anatomic Position of the Heart

Apex—the most distal aspect of the heart's ventricles

The heart is positioned in the chest such that its apex points inferiorly, ventrally, and to the left. Therefore, the right ventricle actually occupies the majority of the heart's ventral surface, the surface exposed as a surgeon prepares to perform coronary artery bypass grafting. Other structures visible from this angle include the pulmonary artery superiorly and portions of the left and right atria.

Protection Around the Heart

The heart is surrounded and protected by a sac known as the pericardium. This sac is composed of a membranous serous pericardium, containing inner visceral and outer parietal layers, and a fibrous pericardium.

Blood Supply to the Heart

The heart, like all other muscles, requires a mechanism to provide it with oxygen and nutrition and to remove the waste it generates. To meet these needs, the heart contains its own system of blood vessels, the coronary arteries and cardiac veins, which lie on its outer surface. Branches of these vessels penetrate inwardly to supply the myocardium (Fig. 8–5).

Coronary Arteries

The coronary arteries originate from two ostia in the proximal aorta. Oxygenated blood flows from the aorta (1) through an anterior ostium into the right coronary artery and (2) through a posterior ostium into the left coronary artery.

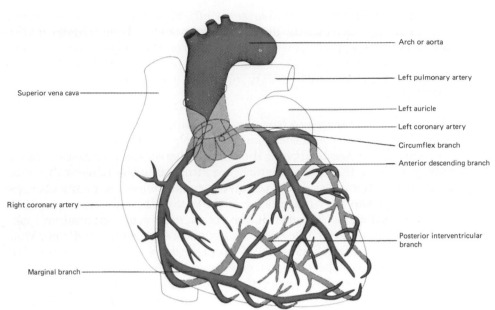

Superior vena cava

Arch or aorta

Left pulmonary artery

Left auricle

Left coronary artery

Circumflex branch

Anterior descending branch

Right coronary artery

Posterior interventricular branch

Marginal branch

FIGURE 8–5: Front view of the coronary arterial system. (From Guyton AC. Anatomy and Physiology. Philadelphia, Saunders College Publishing, 1985, p 408.)

The right coronary artery courses within the groove between the right atrium and ventricle, around the anterior surface of the right side of the heart, and subsequently over its posterior surface. In doing so, it gives off a marginal branch, which provides blood to the lateral wall of the right ventricle, and a posterior descending branch, which typically supplies blood to the posterior walls of both ventricles.

The left coronary artery initially courses posterior to the pulmonary trunk and then divides into two branches. The first of these is the left anterior descending branch, which provides blood to the anterior walls of both ventricles. The second is the circumflex branch, which supplies the posterior and lateral aspects of the left ventricle.

The left and right coronary artery systems anastomose in two locations. The circumflex branch anastomoses with the terminal portion of the right coronary artery, and the left anterior descending branch anastomoses with the posterior descending branch.

Cardiac Veins

Approximately 85% of the blood provided to the heart muscle is returned to the right atrium via the coronary sinus system. This system terminates in the coronary sinus, a large vein lying in the heart's posterior AV groove. This sinus receives deoxygenated blood from the cardiac veins and empties it directly into the right atrium.

The three major vessels that deliver blood to the coronary sinus are the great, middle, and small cardiac veins. The great cardiac vein runs first in the anterior interventricular groove and then in the left AV groove; it drains blood from both ventricles and the left atrium. The middle cardiac vein runs in the posterior interventricular groove and drains blood from the right atrium and ventricle, as well as from a portion of the left ventricle. Finally, the small cardiac vein parallels the marginal branch of the right coronary artery and drains the wall of the right ventricle.

The remaining 15% of the cardiac blood supply is returned to the right atrium directly by the anterior cardiac veins. These drain primarily the anterior walls of the right atrium and ventricle. There are also several tiny vessels, known as the thebesian veins, that lie in the walls of the atria and open individually into these chambers.

Heart's Electrical System

The contraction of the heart is driven and controlled by its electrical system (Fig. 8–6). This system originates with the sinoatrial (SA) node, which is located in the right atrium, near the entry point for the superior vena cava. Depolarization initiating from this node spreads across the atria and into the AV node, located in the interatrial septum, near the AV junction. From the AV node, messages pass into the bundle of His, a collection of large, electrically conducting cardiac muscle fibers that spread the depolarization into the ventricles. This bundle splits first into the right and left bundle branches and subsequently into individual fibers, known as Purkinje's fibers, which spread the wave of depolarization throughout the ventricular myocardium.

PRESSURE, FLOW, AND VOLUME DURING THE CARDIAC CYCLE

The pumping action of the heart is achieved in a repeated set of steps known as the cardiac cycle (Fig. 8–7 and Table 8–1). As mentioned briefly earlier, the heart's pumping action is initiated by its electrical

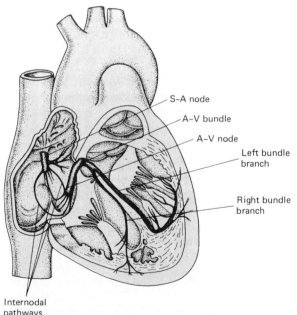

FIGURE 8–6: Transmission of the cardiac impulse from the sinoatrial (SA) node into the atria via internodal pathways, then into the atrioventricular (AV) node, and finally through the AV bundles to all parts of the ventricles. (From Guyton AC. Anatomy and Physiology. Philadelphia, Saunders College Publishing, 1985, p 417.)

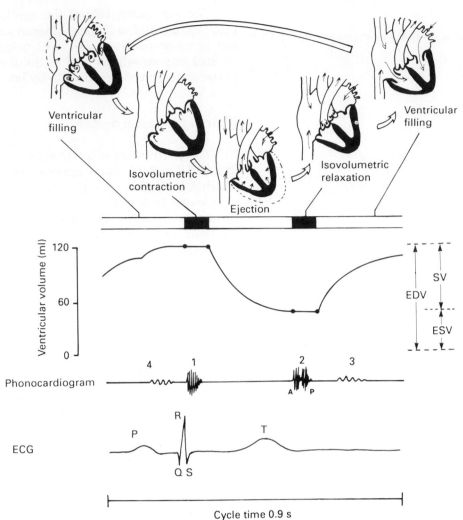

FIGURE 8–7: Changes in valve setting and ventricular volume during one cardiac cycle lasting 0.9 second. EDV, end-diastolic volume; ESV, end-systolic volume; SV, stroke volume. The ejection fraction is SV/EDV. The heart sounds on the phonocardiogram are numbered 1 to 4, and the second sound is split here into an aortic component (A) and a pulmonary component (P). (From Levick JR. An Introduction to Cardiovascular Physiology. Boston, Butterworths, 1991, p 16.)

Stroke volume—the average amount of blood expelled from the left ventricle per contraction, approximately 80 mL.

system, more specifically by the SA node. SA node depolarization leads to atrial depolarization (seen as a P wave on an electrocardiogram) and atrial contraction, which propels blood into the ventricles. The amount of blood in the ventricle after the completion of atrial contraction is known as the end-diastolic volume. The left ventricular end-diastolic volume averages approximately 120 mL.

TABLE **8–1:** Mean Pressures During the Human Cardiac Cycle*

	Right	Left
Atrium	3	8
Ventricle		
End of diastole	4	9
Peak of systole	25	120

From Levick JR. An Introduction to Cardiovascular Physiology. Boston, Butterworths, 1991.
*Pressures are of adult, resting supine.

Ventricular depolarization is seen as a T wave on an electrocardiogram.

The wave of depolarization initiated by the SA node subsequently passes through the AV node, the bundle of His, and the right and left bundle branches and across the ventricles (generating a QRS complex on an electrocardiogram). This leads to ventricular contraction, or systole. The right ventricle actually contracts slightly ahead of the left ventricle. In the first phase of ventricular contraction, known as the isovolumic period, ventricular pressures increase and the AV valves are forced shut (heard as S_1, the first heart sound). Once the AV valves close, intraventricular pressures rise rapidly. When these pressures exceed the pressures within the respective outflow tracts, systole enters the ejection period, during which the pulmonic and aortic valves open and blood flows into the pulmonary and systemic circulations.

Once depolarization and contraction of the ventricles is complete, the ventricles enter diastole, during which the myocardium begins to repolarize and relax. Decreased ventricular pressures lead to closure of the pulmonic and aortic valves (heard as S_2, the second heart sound). The initial portion of diastole is again an isovolumic period, during which the residual pressures in the ventricles are sufficient to prevent opening of the AV valves; thus, all four heart valves are closed. Subsequently, pressures fall sufficiently to allow the AV valves to open, and filling of the ventricles begins. Toward the end of this period, the SA node fires, and the cardiac cycle is reinitiated.

FACTORS IMPACTING ON THE HEART'S PUMPING FUNCTION

The most clinically important portion of the cardiac cycle is the ejection phase of ventricular systole because it is during this period that the heart is truly performing its function as a pump. Several factors intrinsic to the heart have an impact on ventricular function.

The most prominent of these factors is the length of the heart's muscle fibers during diastole. More specifically, it has been demonstrated that up to a point, as the end-diastolic length of these fibers increases, the force of their subsequent contraction during diastole also increases. This is known as the Frank-Starling mechanism.

In view of the importance of end-diastolic fiber length to ventricular function, it is necessary to identify the factors that have an impact on this key parameter. The first of these is the pressure of the blood filling the ventricle, known as the preload. The second factor is the length of time available for diastolic filling. Additional determinants of end-diastolic fiber length relate to the ability of the heart tissue to expand. These include the diastolic compliance of the ventricle and the degree of external restriction placed on the heart by the pericardium.

Cardiac output—the amount of blood pumped by the heart per minute, calculated by multiplying the heart rate by the stroke volume:

Cardiac output = heart rate × stroke volume

Two other factors intrinsic to the heart influence ventricular function. The first of these is the heart's response to a change in the resistance in the pulmonic and systemic circulations against which it must pump. This resistance is known as the ventricle's afterload. As afterload increases, the myocardium responds by generating higher intraventricular pressures. The second of these additional intrinsic factors is the heart's response, in terms of force of contraction, to a change in heart rate. Except at extreme rates, as the frequency of contraction increases, so does the force of contraction.

Several parameters can be employed to measure cardiac function. One such parameter is cardiac output. Another is the ejection fraction, the percentage of left ventricular end-diastolic volume that is ejected with each ventricular contraction. This is calculated by dividing stroke volume by left ventricular end-diastolic volume. A parameter that addresses a similar issue is the left ventricular end-diastolic pressure.

PUMP FAILURE

Heart failure—a state in which the heart muscle is incapable of pumping blood at a rate sufficient to supply the needs of the body's tissues.

Several pathophysiologic phenomena can lead the myocardium to malfunction. Each of these can result in a condition known as heart failure, or pump failure. In this condition, ventricular function decreases, which eventually leads to increased end-diastolic pressures in both ventricles. Importantly, the heart's normal response to these increased pressures may be blunted.

In certain situations, the myocardium may hypertrophy. Eventually, though, the ventricle will dilate, and left ventricular end-diastolic volume will increase. Overdistention of the ventricle leads to decreased muscular function, and thus the Frank-Starling mechanism is counteracted.

The changes seen in heart failure may be even more pronounced during exercise. These patients have an accelerated heart rate response during exercise testing; their stroke volume fails to increase. Consequently, the increase in cardiac output normally seen with exercise is markedly reduced. In addition, in order to support their blood pressures in the face of subnormal cardiac outputs, these patients maintain a high level of resistance in their peripheral blood vessels. As a result, it is even more difficult to deliver a sufficient blood flow to exercising muscle.

RELATIONSHIP OF PUMP FUNCTION TO PERIPHERAL OXYGEN DEMAND

Given that the difference between normally functioning and failing hearts is often exacerbated with exercise, a common technique for assessing cardiac pump function is to measure left ventricular end-diastolic pressure, cardiac output, and body oxygen consumption during an exercise test. Minute oxygen consumption is defined as the total amount of oxygen taken up by the body's tissues from its circulatory system each minute. It can be calculated by multiplying cardiac output by the difference in oxygen content between arterial and mixed venous blood.

In a normally functioning heart, left ventricular end-diastolic pressure is less than 12 mm Hg at rest and changes only slightly with exercise. In this same normal heart, with exercise, cardiac output increases by more than 500 mL/min for each 100-mL increase in the body's minute oxygen consumption. Thus, the heart responds to increased oxygen needs by increasing the rate of delivery of oxygenated blood to peripheral tissues.

In contrast, as mentioned previously, patients with pump failure have abnormally high left ventricular end-diastolic pressures, both at rest and during exercise. Moreover, because these patients have blunted cardiac responses to exercise, the change in their cardiac output will not be sufficient to compensate for the increase in body oxygen consumption. Thus, their hearts truly fail in their responsibility to deliver oxygen sufficient to meet the needs of the body's tissues.

CLINICAL MANIFESTATIONS OF PUMP FAILURE

Great variation exists in the clinical manifestations of pump failure, and its presentation depends on several factors, including

- The extent of and rate at which deterioration in cardiac performance occurs
- The etiology of the cardiac condition
- The age of the patient
- The precipitant of the pump failure
- Whether the right ventricle, the left ventricle, or both are involved in the process

How clinically significant the manifestations of heart failure are is also affected by how severely cardiac function is impaired and how well the patient is able to compensate. The clinical extent may range from mild (clinically manifested only with severe physical exertion) to severe (in this instance, the heart is able to maintain life only with supportive measures). This latter state is often referred to as cardiogenic shock. The remainder of this chapter reviews the various types of heart failure, their clinical findings (symptoms and physical and laboratory findings), the prognosis, the possible precipitants for their development or deterioration, and the specific clinical causes of heart failure.

Types of Heart Failure

Acute Versus Chronic Heart Failure

The clinical manifestations often depend on how quickly the heart failure develops. The ability for compensating mechanisms to occur also has an impact on the signs and symptoms present. When an acute event or decompensation suddenly develops in an otherwise normal healthy individual, a sudden reduction in the cardiac output occurs. The acute decrease in cardiac output leads to hypoperfusion of critical organs and increased pressure with rapid congestion of the vascular bed loading the affected ventricle. Associated with this are the clinical manifestations of these processes. In contrast, if the same processes developed gradually, a number of compensating mechanisms would evolve and allow the patient to adjust to and tolerate the changes with less difficulty.

Left- Versus Right-Sided Heart Failure

The initial presentation is often believed to be dependent on the ventricle that is first affected by the disease process. The prominent symptoms are the result of fluid accumulation behind the specifically failing ventricle. Left ventricular failure occurs most often because of the prevalence of disorders that affect this ventricle. Symptoms secondary to pulmonary congestion are most common as a consequence of the elevated left ventricular filling pressures. Thus, breathlessness and other respiratory symptoms are likely to be present. In the setting of right ventricular failure, systemic venous congestion and peripheral edema prevail. Although lung disease affecting the pulmonary vascular bed can produce right ventricular failure (cor pulmonale), the most common cause of right ventricular failure is prolonged left-sided failure, and in this situation many of the respiratory symptoms of left-sided failure may decrease in severity or disappear because of a decrease in the right ventricular pressures.

The process by which right ventricular failure arises from left-sided failure is not fully known. The increase in pulmonary vascular pressures alone is not enough to account for it. Ventricular interdependence is believed to play an important role. This condition arises because the ventricles share a common wall, the interventricular septum, which is affected by and contributes to the failure of the other ventricle. The precipitation of left ventricular failure by right-sided failure is uncommon, but often patients, especially elderly patients, have an independent process that affects the left ventricle to some extent. It is not unusual for patients with chronic failure, initially either right or left sided, to develop biventricular failure with the resultant symptoms related to the combined process.

Systolic Versus Diastolic Heart Failure

The failure of the ventricle to perform may be related to an abnormality in either the systolic or the diastolic function of the ventricle. One quarter to one third of patients evaluated for signs and symptoms of heart failure have normal or near-normal left ejection fractions. In these patients, an elevation in the filling pressures is required to maintain an adequate cardiac output. An abnormality in ventricular filling secondary to incomplete ventricular relaxation or poor ventricular compliance is present (diastolic dysfunction). The resultant elevated filling pressures lead to high venous pressures and pulmonary congestion.

Patients with diastolic dysfunction usually have one or more of the following three problems as the cause: left ventricular hypertrophy, myocardial ischemia that impairs ventricular relaxation and compliance, or an infiltrative disease (amyloidosis is most common). Pure systolic or diastolic dysfunction may be seen, but because of the common systolic etiologies, it is not uncommon for these conditions to occur in concert. It is important to identify the presence of systolic or diastolic dysfunction as the cause of heart failure, especially since the therapeutic approaches are significantly different. Differentiation can usually be achieved with echocardiography, radionuclide ventriculography, or cardiac catheterization.

Low- Versus High-Output Heart Failure

The separation of failure into high- and low-output failure is based primarily on differences in the clinical manifestations and the precipitants rather than the specific causes. High-output failures, described later in this chapter, are states that by their nature require an increased cardiac output, which the ventricle is not able to meet. Therefore, failure develops. Low-output failure, a much more common entity, characterizes the heart failure seen in most forms of heart disease. In low-output failure, there is evidence of impairment of the peripheral circulation, with the presence of vasoconstriction and cold, clammy, pale, and frequently cyanotic extremities. With high-output failure, the pulses are brisk and the extremities remain warm and flush. In both instances, the inability of the heart to meet the oxygen demands of the metabolic tissues is the problem. Regardless of the cause and the absolute values, the cardiac output is lower than it was and the arterial–mixed venous oxygen is higher than it was before the development of heart failure.

Clinical Findings in Heart Failure

Symptoms of Heart Failure

The symptoms of heart failure are the result of the effects of the failing heart on other systems. Thus, the clinical findings are related to the derangement of the lungs, kidneys, liver, and other organs.

Respiratory. A prominent symptom of left ventricular failure is the presence of difficulty breathing or the sensation of breathlessness. The type of circumstances under which this symptom occurs may represent an increase in the severity of the left ventricular dysfunction. Usually, the symptoms of increasing left ventricular dysfunction occur in the following order: dyspnea on exertion, orthopnea, paroxysmal nocturnal dyspnea, dyspnea at rest, and acute pulmonary edema.

Dyspnea on Exertion. Dyspnea on exertion is a common, early symptom of left-sided heart failure. The differentiation between exertional dyspnea in normal subjects and in patients with heart failure is the amount of physical activity required to manifest symptoms. Some patients may not have dyspnea on exertion even with significant left-sided heart failure. This may reflect a gradual decrease in their level of activity without their recognizing it, with patients becoming very sedentary or bedridden, or the development of a change in mental status.

Patients with other disease entities may also show dyspnea on exertion, including those with chronic lung disease, exercise-induced asthma, severe anemia, thyrotoxicosis, and physical deconditioning. The development of dyspnea on exertion over a short period is often indicative of heart failure, whereas a gradual decrease is more suggestive of the other processes. In exercise-induced asthma, wheezing is generally associated with the dyspnea on exertion.

Orthopnea. Patients with orthopnea experience dyspnea when they are in the supine position, but they have little or no dyspnea when the head is elevated or they are in the upright position. Patients usually need more pillows to obtain a comfortable night's sleep. Many patients state that they must sleep sitting in a chair or recliner in order to sleep well. Again, the degree of change is what is critical because many patients normally elevate their heads when they are in the recumbent position. The decrease in symptoms with a change in position is related to the decrease in venous return, the decrease in hydrostatic pressure in the upper lung fields, and the increase in vital capacity that occur with the head in an elevated position.

Orthopnea usually develops rapidly after the patient assumes a recumbent position and while the patient is still awake, in contrast to paroxysmal nocturnal dyspnea, which is described in the following section. Cough may also be a symptom of failure; its occurrence while the patient is lying down may be an orthopnea equivalent. In this instance, the cough is usually nonproductive in nature.

Paroxysmal Nocturnal Dyspnea. Paroxysmal nocturnal dyspnea occurs when the patient experiences a sudden awakening with dyspnea after falling asleep. The patient describes a feeling of severe anxiety and suffocation and often finds it necessary to sit on the side of the bed, to go to the window for fresh air, or to get up for a drink of water. Episodes of paroxysmal nocturnal dyspnea require a longer period than those of orthopnea to resolve. In general, the patient will be able to return to bed

Orthopnea in general is an important symptom of heart failure, but like most of the symptoms, it is not specific and may be present in other disease entities.

Of all the symptoms related to difficulty in breathing, paroxysmal nocturnal dyspnea is the one most specific to left-sided heart failure.

and sleep through the remainder of the night if the anxiety associated with the episodes is not prohibitive. If a repeated episode occurs, it is usually hours later.

Dyspnea. The patient with dyspnea complains of a feeling of breathlessness, shortness of breath, or difficulty in getting one's breath. These symptoms occur at rest and require little or no provocation. At this point, the patient has significant and severe heart failure and is often on the brink of frank pulmonary edema.

Acute Pulmonary Edema. Acute pulmonary edema is the most severe and dramatic symptom of left-sided heart failure. The patient experiences the sudden onset of the sensation of suffocation, which is usually terrifying. This is associated with an increase in heart rate and blood pressure, which further compromises left ventricular function. Extreme breathlessness develops suddenly, and patients often feel like they are drowning. Patients will usually sit upright or stand and exhibit air hunger along with anxiousness and agitation. They appear pale and sweaty, with the skin being cyanotic, cold, and clammy. The respiratory rate is rapid, and the alae nasi are often flared with use of accessory respiratory muscles and inspiratory retraction of the intercostal and supraclavicular areas. Coughing with the production of profuse pink, watery, frothy sputum occurs. Respiration is usually noisy, with expiratory gurgling and tracheal rattling sounds. Classic pulmonary edema is unambiguous. The patient is often too severely ill to talk. The lack of intervention can lead to continued deterioration, to the development of cardiogenic shock, and rapidly to death.

Patients of advanced age, with cerebrovascular disease, or with head injuries are more susceptible to Cheyne-Stokes respirations. Cheyne-Stokes respirations are exacerbated by the use of barbiturates, narcotics, and other sedative agents.

Cheyne-Stokes Respiration. A common problem in advanced left-sided heart failure is a periodic or cyclic pattern of respiration in which the patient exhibits alternating periods of hyperventilation and apnea. It is more likely to occur after the patient falls asleep; patients may awaken with dyspnea during the hyperventilatory phase but are generally unaware of the respiratory pattern. This pattern results from a decreased cardiac output, with a subsequent slowing of the circulation from the lungs to the brain. A delay develops in the normal feedback loop, and the respiratory center is not able to respond in a correct manner to changes in arterial PO_2 and PCO_2, thus leading to the episodes of apnea and hyperventilation.

Other Symptoms

Fatigue and Weakness. Fatigue and weakness are very nonspecific symptoms and may be related to a number of different causes in the patient with heart failure. They are usually secondary to low perfusion of the skeletal muscles and lactic acidosis from the low cardiac output that is common. They may also be caused by the sodium depletion, hypokalemia, and hypovolemia that may be seen with excessive diuretic use and sodium restriction. In addition, with many of the medications used to treat these patients, fatigue and weakness are common side effects.

Nocturia. Nocturia usually occurs early in the course of heart failure. Changes in the distribution of blood flow and fluid that occur at night with the assumption of a recumbent position are responsible. There is a change in the demands on cardiac output, with subsequent renal artery vasodilatation, increased renal blood flow, and increased urine formation. This increased urine formation leads to nocturia and self-induced diuresis; it may be detrimental because patients cannot obtain the rest they often require.

Oliguria. Oliguria, a late sign of heart failure, may be the result of severe hypoperfusion from a severely depressed cardiac output. In this case, urine formation is suppressed secondary to the decreased renal blood flow. Oliguria is not just a decrease in urine output: it is usually defined as a urine output of less than 20 mL/hr or 400 mL/day.

Insomnia. Left-sided heart failure may cause patients to complain of restlessness at night and the inability to sleep. The insomnia may be secondary to mild orthopnea, paroxysmal nocturnal dyspnea and the anxiety associated with it, nocturia, Cheyne-Stokes respiration, or a combination.

Cerebral Symptoms. Symptoms related to decreased cardiac output and subsequent hypoperfusion through the cerebral vasculature may occur in patients with severe heart failure, especially those with cerebrovascular disease. This may be manifested as confusion, dizziness, presyncope, somnolence, delirium, memory impairment, or even obtundation. These symptoms can often be exacerbated by the metabolic derangements and hypovolemia that occur with the use of diuretics and by the metabolic acidosis that develops from hypoperfusion. Problems with anxiety, depression, and other emotional disorders may also develop from the difficulty in accepting the severe limitations in activities and the alterations in quality of life that their disease now provokes.

Gastrointestinal Symptoms. Complaints of anorexia, nausea, vomiting, abdominal distention, constipation, diarrhea, and abdominal pain may be present. These symptoms may be due to problems with venous engorgement and congestion of the gastrointestinal tract, ascites, and hepatic congestion. Engorgement of the liver usually produces pain and tenderness of the right upper quadrant from tension on the liver capsule. Patients may also complain of easy bruising and prolonged bleeding secondary to liver congestion and subsequent hepatic dysfunction. Jaundice may occur, but this is usually the case only with the presence of cardiac cirrhosis. Most of these symptoms are found in right-sided failure or in prolonged left-sided failure with right-sided failure.

Weight Gain, Peripheral Edema, and Increased Body Girth. Weight gain, peripheral edema, and increased body girth are more likely to occur in patients with chronic heart failure and the presence of right-sided failure. These symptoms may represent

- An increase in fluid secondary to salt and water retention
- Worsening heart failure
- A change in medications or a change in responsiveness to them
- Dietary indiscretions

The patient may also report an increase in edema during the day that improves overnight, as well as a decrease in urine output during the day and an increase in nocturia. The presence of edema in left-sided failure usually indicates a more chronic and prolonged course, with the development of right-sided failure. An increase in body girth most likely indicates ascites and is more likely to occur with cirrhosis, constrictive pericarditis, restrictive cardiomyopathy, or tricuspid valve disease.

Physical Findings in Heart Failure

Cardiac

The presence of cardiomegaly is usually confirmed by a chest x-ray study, echocardiography, or cardiac catheterization.

Cardiomegaly. Enlargement of the heart is often evident from inspection, percussion, and assessment of the apical impulse by palpation. This nonspecific sign occurs in the majority of patients with chronic failure. It is less common in patients with the acute development of failure (i.e., myocardial infarction) because the heart failure may have developed before the heart had the opportunity to enlarge.

The ventricular gallop sound

- Occurs in early diastole
- Is a low-pitched sound
- Is heard best with the bell of the stethoscope

Ventricular Gallop Sound. The ventricular gallop sound, which is often referred to as the third heart sound or S_3, is considered to be the cardiac hallmark of ventricular failure. The sound results from rapid ventricular filling into a noncompliant ventricle or a ventricle that has been distended from increased preload. A left-sided gallop is heard best at the left ventricular apex, whereas a right-sided gallop is heard best over the right ventricle. Although a ventricular gallop is an abnormal sound in an adult, it may be a normal heart sound in a child or an adolescent.

When a ventricular gallop develops in a patient with heart disease, it is a fairly reliable sign of early heart failure. In certain other clinical states, a ventricular gallop can manifest without the presence of heart failure and is usually secondary to excessive ventricular volume. These instances include pregnancy, aortic regurgitation, mitral regurgitation, atrial septal defect, ventricular septal defect, patent ductus arteriosus, and anemia.

Other Heart Sounds. The development of left ventricular failure causes an elevation in pulmonary artery pressure; with this, P_2 is accentuated compared with A_2 and is more widely heard throughout the precordium. This accentuation of P_2 decreases with the resolution of heart failure. With the ventricular dilatation and the alteration in ventricular architecture that occur, systolic murmurs from mitral or tricuspid regurgitation are common. These murmurs often decrease or disappear with the treatment of the heart failure.

Pulsus alternans is characterized by a regular rhythm and the alternating of strong and weak pulses.

Pulsus Alternans. Pulsus alternans is an uncommon finding that indicates failure of the left ventricle and usually represents severe ventricular dysfunction. This may be detected by palpation of the peripheral pulses (predominantly in the femorals) or by use of the sphygmomanometer. With the sphygmomanometer, initially alternate beats are heard until the systolic pressure becomes low enough that all the beats are audible.

Pulsus alternans

- Is most common with heart failure secondary to increased constraint in left ventricular ejection, as in aortic stenosis or hypertension
- May also occur with ischemic and dilated cardiomyopathies
- Is most likely caused by an alteration in the stroke volume ejected by the left ventricle
- May be elicited by decreasing preload
- Is reduced by increasing venous return
- Also resolves with the treatment of heart failure
- Is often associated with S_3
- Tends to be more common with tachycardia

In jugular vein distention, the upper limit of normal is usually 7 cm.

Jugular Venous Distention. Distention of the deep jugular veins is a direct reflection of the right atrial pressure, the mean central venous pressure, and the right ventricular end-diastolic pressure. This is because the deep jugular veins are a direct conduit to the right atrium and are influenced by changes in the previously mentioned pressures. Jugular venous distention is usually measured with the trunk elevated 45 degrees from the supine position. In severe failure, it is often not possible to see distention at 45 degrees; in this situation, distention should be measured at 90 degrees of elevation from the supine position. The determination is made in centimeters from the horizontal line projected through the center of the right atrium to the upper level of the pulsation of the jugular venous distention.

Abnormal hepatojugular reflex test findings may also be seen in heart failure. In the hepatojugular reflex test, normal jugular venous pressure is determined. Then, after gentle liver compression, the jugular venous pressure is again measured. The reflex is considered to be abnormal if an increase in jugular venous pressure occurs with liver compression. This is secondary to the inability of the heart to compensate for the increase in venous return and central venous volume that occurs.

Lungs

Pulmonary Edema. Pulmonary edema usually results when a decrease in left ventricular output from a failing left ventricle occurs. The Frank-Starling mechanism states that the left ventricular output equals the right ventricular output. When the left ventricular output decreases, an increase in the left ventricular end-diastolic volume occurs, with an increase in the left ventricular end-diastolic pressure until left ventricular output again equals right ventricular output. With the elevation in the left ventricular end-diastolic pressure that occurs in left-sided heart failure, a compensatory rise in left atrial and pulmonary venous pressures occurs. This subsequently leads to pulmonary congestion (i.e., pulmonary edema).

Auscultatory findings with pulmonary edema include moist crackles, which are often heard at the bases of the lungs, although they may be present over the entire lung fields. Heart failure may present with pulmonary findings, especially when right-sided failure alone exists or both right- and left-sided failure coexist. Pulmonary edema may be due to causes other than heart failure, including neurogenic pulmonary edema and adult respiratory distress syndrome. Wheezing, which may also occur in the presence of pulmonary edema, has been referred to as cardiac asthma.

Pleural Effusion. When present, pleural effusion is usually bilateral. If the pleural effusion is unilateral, it is usually confined to the right side. This condition is usually secondary to a severe increase in the systemic venous pressure from such processes as tricuspid stenosis, constrictive pericarditis, or restrictive cardiomyopathy. Pleural effusions (hydrothorax) may occur in either right- or left-sided heart failure because the pleural veins drain into both of the venous systems. With the development of pleural effusions, dyspnea increases in intensity secondary to an additional reduction in vital capacity. Treatment of the deterioration in heart failure usually causes reabsorption of the fluid and lessening of dyspnea, although sometimes small interlobar effusions persist.

General

General Appearance. With mild or moderate heart failure, the patient may appear to be in no distress after a brief rest but may show significant dyspnea with activity, such as walking into the examination room or undressing. The patient with mild or moderate heart failure may become dyspneic upon lying down. With more severe failure, the patient often appears anxious and dyspneic, with signs of air hunger. Patients with acute onset of failure appear acutely ill and have marked breathlessness; however, those with chronic failure appear chronically ill, with less breathlessness even though their dyspnea may be more severe. They also often seem to be malnourished and even cachectic. This process, often referred to as cardiac cachexia, is the result of a multitude of problems that arise from prolonged low cardiac output.

- The patient may show evidence of cyanosis, pallor, and cold extremities secondary to vasoconstriction.
- Rarely, icterus and jaundice are present.
- Tachycardia with a weak and thready pulse and tachypnea are usually found.
- Systolic pressure may be reduced, especially in severe failure from decreased cardiac output, and may also represent the effects of medical therapy. Diastolic pressure may be reduced for the same reasons, but it is sometimes elevated secondary to the increased adrenergic activity that occurs as a compensatory measure. This compensatory mechanism is also responsible for the tachycardia and vasoconstriction that are observed.

Hepatomegaly. With the development of right-sided heart failure, hepatomegaly is common. The liver is usually enlarged and tender when examined. If the onset of right-sided failure is acute, severe right upper quadrant pain may also be present. Prolonged hepatic congestion may lead to cardiac cirrhosis and subsequently to liver changes consistent with cirrhosis (i.e., a shrunken, hard liver). Ascites may also develop with prolonged congestion, as described in the following section. Splenomegaly is uncommon, except in prolonged congestion. The early presence of splenomegaly should raise the suspicion of other causes (i.e., splenic infarction).

Ascites. The development of ascites is a late manifestation of right-sided heart failure and is usually associated with the presence of jugular venous distention, peripheral edema, pleural effusions, and hepatomegaly. Elevated hepatic and portal venous pressures secondary to elevated systemic venous pressures result in elevations in venous pressure in the peritoneal venous system and the development of ascites. The retention of salt and water is also an important prerequisite. The presence of ascites often leads to the abdominal symptoms described previously.

Peripheral Edema. The appearance of peripheral edema depends on whether the heart failure more severely affects the right or the left side. In significant right-sided failure, peripheral edema results. The edema is caused by a rise in the capillary pressure secondary to an increase in the venous pressure, which causes an increase in the plasma volume and a decrease in the plasma osmotic pressure. Generalized edema or anasarca, which is usually associated with severe right-sided failure, may also include the presence of ascites and pleural effusions. The genital area in particular and the abdominal and thoracic wall are involved; however, the face and arms are usually spared until the late stages of failure, when their involvement may represent a preterminal situation. Rarely does the sudden and severe development of edema lead to rupture of the skin and extravasation of the fluid. If edema is long-standing,

The location of peripheral edema is often determined by the position of the patient. The upright or erect position favors the accumulation of fluid in the feet, ankles, and lower legs. Presacral edema is more likely to be present when the patient is in the recumbent position.

chronic changes similar to those seen in venous stasis may develop, including changes in pigmentation and reddening and induration of the skin. There is also a higher propensity for the development of cellulitis.

Laboratory Findings in Heart Failure

Blood Chemistry Findings. The blood abnormalities seen in the setting of heart failure are usually a result of the effects of altered cardiac output and diminished perfusion of other organ systems or a result of therapy.

Urinalysis often shows proteinuria and an elevated specific gravity. A mildly elevated blood urea nitrogen level, as well as a mildly elevated creatinine level, may be present secondary to decreased renal blood flow and glomerular filtration rate (prerenal azotemia). The decrease in renal function, along with the extensive use of diuretic therapy and sodium restriction, may result in hyponatremia. Alterations in serum potassium levels may also occur, with the potential for hypokalemia from diuretic use and the potential for hyperkalemia from the decrease in renal function secondary to the prerenal azotemia.

Hepatic dysfunction, secondary to congestive hepatomegaly and cardiac cirrhosis, often occurs. Slight elevations in aspartate aminotransferase, alanine aminotransferase, lactic dehydrogenase, and serum bilirubin levels may be observed. The alterations may resemble viral hepatitis but usually resolve with treatment of the heart failure. Persistent changes may result from long-standing heart failure and hepatic congestion with the development of significant cardiac cirrhosis.

In addition, the erythrocyte sedimentation rate may be depressed in heart failure. This is believed to be secondary to decreased fibrinogen concentrations resulting from impaired fibrinogen synthesis.

Chest Radiography. Chest x-ray studies are very useful in evaluating patients with heart failure. Assessment of the size and shape of the cardiac silhouette may provide important information about the cause of the heart failure. An increased cardiothoracic ratio is a relatively specific indicator of an increase in the left ventricular end-diastolic volume. Further evaluation of the lung fields usually provides substantial information about the status of the patient in heart failure.

The development of elevated pulmonary venous pressures, which occur early in heart failure, may lead to early radiographic changes before clinical findings.

It is often possible to see pulmonary congestion secondary to heart failure on a chest x-ray study before it is clinically detectable. With normal pulmonary venous pressures, perfusion of the bases of the lungs is better than that of the apices when the patient is in the upright position; thus, the vessels in the lower lobes are larger. As heart failure develops, pulmonary venous hypertension occurs, with generalized dilatation of the pulmonary veins and cephalization of the pulmonary vasculature (i.e., prominence of the superior pulmonary veins) in the upright chest x-ray study. This occurs when the pulmonary capillary pressure exceeds 13 mm Hg, which is the upper limit of normal.

Interstitial edema reflects the accumulation of fluid in the tissue surrounding the pulmonary capillaries and in the interlobar connective tissue.

With further elevation of the pulmonary capillary pressure to greater than 20 to 25 mm Hg, interstitial pulmonary edema eventually occurs. Several types of findings may be present, including septal or Kerley's lines. Two types exist: B lines and A lines. B lines are horizontal peripheral markings that are seen most often in the lower lung fields and may extend to the pleural surface. A lines are similar, longer lines extending from the hilum in the upper and middle portions of the lungs to the periphery. In addition, perivascular cuffing may occur. This is exhibited as a loss of the sharpness of the central and peripheral vessels.

Kerley's lines—sharp linear densities depicting interlobular interstitial edema.

Finally, subpleural fluid may accumulate between the lung and the pleural surface and produce spindle-shaped radiographic changes.

When the pulmonary capillary pressure exceeds 25 mm Hg, alveolar edema occurs. In this instance, a cloud-like appearance develops and pulmonary edema is easily recognized. Edema usually concentrates centrally around the hilum in a "butterfly pattern." Large pleural effusions, pseudotumors, and dilatation of the azygos veins and the superior vena cava may also be evident.

Electrocardiography. Electrocardiography has no specific findings diagnostic of heart failure. Electrocardiographic findings are usually abnormal secondary to underlying severe heart disease. Electrocardiographic findings are useful in conjunction with other findings because they may point to the potential etiology of the heart failure.

Precipitants of Heart Failure

A number of factors may be responsible for the development of frank symptoms of heart failure in a patient who already has underlying heart disease and ventricular dysfunction. These factors can be divided into those that produce a high cardiac output state and those that may provoke the development of failure.

High-Output Heart Failure

Conditions that can be responsible for high-output failure include

- Anemia
- Hyperthyroidism
- Systemic arteriovenous fistulas
- Prolonged beriberi (thiamine deficiency)
- Paget's disease

A high cardiac output state, which by itself is not usually responsible for pump failure, is capable of precipitating heart failure in a patient with underlying heart disease. In these clinical conditions, the metabolic needs of the peripheral tissues can be met only by a significant increase in cardiac output. In a young, healthy heart, this increased demand for cardiac performance can often be satisfied for long periods. In the diseased heart, this is usually not the case, and some degree of heart failure develops. Its severity is governed by the extent of the underlying cardiac pathology and the severity of the high-output state.

Other Precipitants of Heart Failure

Other precipitants of heart failure include

- Systemic infection
- Pulmonary embolism
- Cardiac infection and inflammation
- Dietary changes
- Alterations in therapy or the addition of other medicines
- Development of another disease process
- Arrhythmias
- Environmental changes

These factors are often enough to push the patient over the edge, especially when the patient's condition is well regulated but on the fine line between stable and decompensated.

Clinical Manifestations in Heart Failure Secondary to Various Cardiac Diseases

Ischemic Heart Disease

Ischemia cardiomyopathy describes coronary artery disease that produces severe myocardial dysfunction with clinical manifestations often indistinguishable from those of dilated cardiomyopathy (see later discussion). Many of these patients have little or no angina; their symptoms of ischemia, related to increased left ventricular dysfunction, include dyspnea or increasing heart failure. Even in patients with a clear history of angina, this may no longer be present, and symptoms of heart failure may predominate. Patients without a history of angina or myocardial infarction may initially be diagnosed with a dilated cardiomyopathy until the presence of coronary artery disease is established. Electrocardiographic findings may not be useful in documenting coronary artery disease because they can often be misleading.

The presence of ischemic cardiomyopathy does not specifically indicate myocardial necrosis. Long-standing hypoperfusion of the myocardium may cause persistent left ventricular dysfunction. This is especially true if blood flow is sufficient to keep the myocardium viable but not enough to sustain normal function. This concept, referred to as hibernating myocardium, may play an important role in the presence of left ventricular dysfunction until adequate blood flow is restored. This then suggests that the evaluation for hibernating myocardium in left ventricular dysfunction is important because restoration of adequate blood flow may improve the situation. It is thus reasonable to evaluate these patients extensively with the potential for revascularization that may improve ventricular function and have an impact on functionality and survival. The prognosis for patients with ischemic cardiomyopathy is very poor if they are treated medically.

Valvular Heart Disease

The clinical manifestations of valvular heart disease are secondary to either valvular incompetence, stenosis, or both. Prolonged exposure to these mechanical abnormalities produces pressure or volume overload of the chamber impacted on by the defect. Compensation for these abnormalities usually involves hypertrophy and dilatation of the affected chamber. As the valvular heart disease advances, myocardial decompensation and a reduction in cardiac output occur, with the resultant development of clinical heart failure. The clinical manifestations exhibited depend on the valvular lesion present and on whether left-sided failure, right-sided failure, or both occur. Often, the development of early symptoms of heart failure is the basic indication for surgical intervention for valvular repair or replacement.

Nonischemic Cardiomyopathy

The nonischemic cardiomyopathies primarily involve the cardiac muscle, specifically the ventricular muscle. The unknown etiology is not attributable to ischemic, hypertensive, congenital, valvular, or pericardial disease. The three classifications based on functional impairment that is present are dilated, hypertrophic, and restrictive. Evaluation has been enhanced by the use of endomyocardial biopsy, although the specificity of diagnosis and the clinical utility of this technique are still uncertain.

Dilated Cardiomyopathy. Ventricular dilatation and contractile dysfunction with associated symptoms of congestive heart failure characterize dilated cardiomyopathy, which was previously known as congestive cardiomyopathy. The etiology is usually secondary to some type of insult that causes myocardial injury with resultant systolic dysfunction and dilatation of the ventricle. Some of the effects are transient, with full recovery of myocardial function, but in general this is not the case. The etiologic classification includes idiopathic, inflammatory (infectious and noninfectious), toxic, metabolic, familial, and coronary microvascular abnormalities (Table 8–2). Treatment and prognosis are related to the etiology of the dilated cardiomyopathy. In general, treatment is based on whether the process is still ongoing and is treatable, the hemodynamic state of the heart and the extent of symptoms, the risk of systemic emboli, and the risk of ventricular arrhythmias.

Hypertrophic Cardiomyopathy. In hypertrophic cardiomyopathy, inappropriate hypertrophy of the left ventricle occurs, often with asymmetrical involvement of the septum and usually with preserved or enhanced contractile function. This has been referred to by various names, including idiopathic hypertrophic subaortic stenosis, hypertrophic obstructive cardiomyopathy, and hypertrophic cardiomyopathy, the current name of choice. Both symmetrical and asymmetrical types of hypertrophic cardiomyopathy occur. The etiology is unclear, but both familial and sporadic forms exist. The genetically transmitted form of the disease is usually autosomal dominant in its inheritance. The pathogenesis of the disorder has not been firmly established, but two theories have been proposed. One is that an alteration in catecholamine function in utero affects the myocyte development, with abnormal orientation of the myofibrils. A second theory is that abnormal development is due to an excess of intracellular calcium. In addition, some have suggested that a combination of the two may be responsible. Pathologically, gross morphologic changes are seen in the septum, including hypertrophy and, histologically, cellular disarray. The basic physiologic derangement that occurs is the development of a dynamic gradient in the left ventricular outflow tract. The most common symptoms are dyspnea, fatigue, chest pain, and syncope. Dyspnea is most prevalent, worsening with exertion and mainly relating to diastolic dysfunction. Sudden death is common; patients often initially present with sudden death or syncope during strenuous exertion. Clinical deterioration is slow, except when sudden death or the development of atrial fibrillation with the loss of the "atrial kick" occurs. Many patients are only diagnosed after an immediate family member has been diagnosed. The natural history of the disease is highly variable. There is no relationship between outflow tract gradient and symptoms or prognosis. Management is based on close monitoring and the presence of symptoms. Treatment options include the use of medications and surgical interven-

TABLE **8–2:** Etiologic Classification of the Dilated Cardiomyopathies

Idiopathic	**Toxic**
Inflammatory	Ethyl alcohol
Infectious	Chemotherapeutic agents
Viral	Elemental compounds
Bacterial	Catecholamines
Mycobacterial	**Metabolic**
Parasitic	Nutritional
Rickettsial	Endocrinologic
Spirochetal	Electrolyte abnormalities
Fungal	**Familial cardiomyopathy**
Noninfectious	Neuromyopathic
Autoimmune disease	Progressive muscular dystrophy
Peripartum	Myotonic muscular dystrophy
Hypersensitivity	Friedreich's ataxia
reactions	**Abnormal coronary microvasculature**
Transplantation rejection	

tions, among them myomectomy and valve replacement and possibly heart transplantation. Genetic counseling is an important component in the treatment of these patients.

The prognosis for patients with restrictive cardiomyopathies is poor, with fewer than 10% of patients alive at 10 years.

Restrictive Cardiomyopathy. Restrictive cardiomyopathy, the least common of the three major types of cardiomyopathy, is characterized as a primary abnormality in diastolic filling with normal or near-normal systolic function. If the diastolic dysfunction is secondary to ventricular hypertrophy or the primary process is systolic dysfunction, the term *restrictive cardiomyopathy* does not apply. It has often been referred to as nonhypertrophic, nondilated cardiomyopathy because no changes in ventricular dimensions occur. The classification of restrictive cardiomyopathies is given in Table 8–3. Treatment is cause specific but is usually related to symptom relief only. Differentiation of this process from constrictive pericarditis, which has similar functional and clinical presentations, is essential because constrictive pericarditis can be surgically treated, with potential long-term relief of symptoms.

Pericardial Disease

The precipitation of symptoms similar to those seen in heart failure by diseases of the pericardium is rare and is related only to situations that affect cardiac function. Specifically, these are the development of cardiac tamponade and constrictive pericarditis.

Cardiac tamponade—a pericardial effusion of any size that compromises ventricular filling and precipitates heart failure.

Cardiac Tamponade. A multitude of etiologies exists for cardiac tamponade, with the major factor being the rapid accumulation of fluid with a rise in the intrapericardial pressure. To maintain cardiac output, diastolic filling pressure must increase. Because of the anatomy and pathophysiology of the tight pericardial space, equalization of heart pressures occurs with progressive deterioration in cardiac function. The symptoms are usually those of biventricular failure. Clinical evidence of cardiac tamponade includes elevated jugular venous pressure and a prominent x descent with a diminished y descent. Severe pulsus paradoxus is present, with a disappearance of or reduction in the arterial pulse with inspiration. Accurate quantification is done with a sphygmomanometer, with which a difference of more than 10 mm Hg is noted between the systolic blood pressure measured during inspiration and that measured during

TABLE **8–3:**   Etiologic Classification of the Restrictive Cardiomyopathies

Myocardial
 Noninfiltrative
  Idiopathic
  Scleroderma
 Infiltrative
  Amyloid
  Sarcoid
  Gaucher's disease
  Hurler's disease
 Storage diseases
  Hemochromatosis
  Fabry's disease
  Glycogen storage diseases
Endomyocardial
 Endomyocardial fibrosis
 Hypereosinophilic syndrome
 Carcinoid
 Metastatic malignancies
 Radiation
 Anthracycline toxicity

expiration. Diagnosis is by hemodynamic monitoring, with confirmation of the presence of a pericardial effusion by echocardiography. Treatment usually involves the prompt removal of pericardial fluid, either by pericardiocentesis or by the surgical creation of a pericardial window, especially if the accumulation is recurrent.

Constrictive Pericarditis. Constrictive pericarditis occurs with thickening, fibrosis, and often calcification of the pericardium, with restriction in ventricular diastolic filling. The most common causes are idiopathic, neoplasm, radiation, trauma, and connective tissue diseases. Tuberculosis and pyrogenic infections are less common causes than they were previously. The clinical findings and symptoms are those of biventricular failure. A loud third heart sound, pericardial knock, is frequently noted. Echocardiography is usually not very helpful, and the thickened pericardium is better visualized with computed tomography or magnetic resonance imaging. Differentiation from restrictive cardiomyopathy (see earlier discussion) is crucial because they mimic each other; constrictive pericarditis can be treated successfully with pericardiectomy.

SUMMARY

The function of the cardiovascular system is to provide blood flow to all organ systems of the body. The heart is composed of two pumps in a series: the right ventricle, which provides flow through the pulmonary circulation, and the left ventricle, which provides flow through the systemic circulation. These pumps have collecting chambers known as atria and pumping chambers known as ventricles. Valves exist between the atria and the ventricles and between the ventricles and the outflow vessels to maintain forward flow. The heart itself receives its blood supply through the coronary arteries. The rhythmic pumping action of the heart is controlled through the pacemaker and electrical transmission system of the heart. The volume in the heart just before contraction is known as the end-diastolic volume, and the amount of blood ejected with contraction is called the stroke volume. Stroke volume times heart rate equals cardiac output. Heart failure is pump failure, which is a state in which the heart's muscle is incapable of pumping blood at a rate sufficient to supply the needs of the body. Heart failure can be acute or chronic, is primarily left or right ventricular, and is manifest mainly as systolic or diastolic failure. Cardiac failure can occur in a number of circumstances, but the most common causes are ischemia, valvular abnormalities, and cardiomyopathies. Other causes include sepsis, pericardial disease, cardiomyopathies, and medications. The management of heart failure includes maximizing oxygen delivery to the myocardium, fluid management, weight control, the use of inotropes, and valvular surgery if the valves are the cause.

Suggested Readings

Anderson RH, Becker AE. The Heart: Structure in Health and Disease. New York, Gower Medical Publishers, 1992.

Berne RM, Levy MN. Cardiovascular Physiology. St. Louis, Mosby–Year Book, 1992.

Franciosa JA. Exercise testing in chronic congestive heart failure. Am J Cardiol 53:1447, 1984.

Garfein OB (ed). Current Concepts in Cardiovascular Physiology. San Diego, Academic Press, 1990.

Guyton AC. Anatomy and Physiology. Philadelphia, Saunders College Publishing, 1985.

Levick JR. An Introduction to Cardiovascular Physiology. Boston, Butterworths, 1991.

Mason DT (ed). Congestive Heart Failure: Mechanisms, Evaluation, and Treatment. New York, Yorke Medical Books, 1976.

Milnor WL. Cardiovascular Physiology. Oxford, Oxford University Press, 1990.

Roubin GS, Anderson SD, Shen WF, et al. Hemodynamic and metabolic basis of impaired exercise tolerance in patients with severe left ventricular dysfunction. J Am Coll Cardiol 15:986, 1990.

Sullivan MA, Higginbotham MB, Cobb FR. Exercise training in patients with severe left ventricular dysfunction. Circulation 778:506, 1988.

Zelis R, Longhurst J, Capone RJ, Mason DT. A comparison of regional blood flow and oxygen utilization during dynamic forearm testing in subjects and patients with congestive heart failure. Circulation 50:137, 1974.

9 Tissue Oxygen Delivery

David R. Dantzker, M.D.

THE METABOLIC REQUIREMENT FOR OXYGEN

The body requires a sufficient amount of energy in order to maintain the integrity of cell membranes and allow for activities such as muscular contraction, synthetic processes, and active transport. All the energy the body uses derives initially from the sun, which through photosynthesis allows green plants to make the complex sugars that form the nutrient base. A byproduct of photosynthesis is the production of oxygen, the second key ingredient in the body's ability to accumulate energy in easily usable forms. The body in turn produces the CO_2 required by green plants (in addition to sunlight) for photosynthesis (Fig. 9–1).[1]

The body extracts the energy stored in food predominantly through the process of oxidative phosphorylation via the tricarboxylic acid (TCA) or Krebs cycle (Fig. 9–2).[2] The TCA cycle is a series of oxidation-reduction

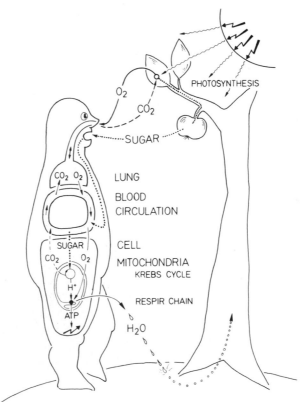

FIGURE 9–1: The oxygen cycle: the energetic needs of our body are met by solar energy. (From Weibel ER. The Pathway for Oxygen. Cambridge, MA, Harvard University Press, 1984, p 2.)

156

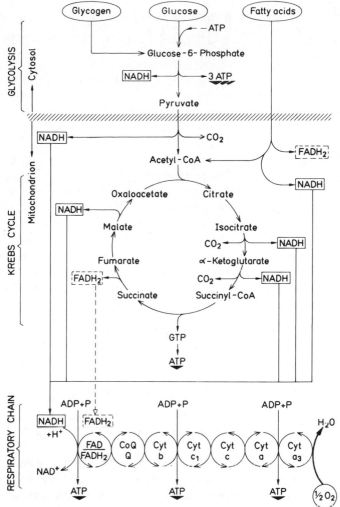

FIGURE 9–2: The three stages of oxidative metabolism: glycolysis, tricarboxylic acid cycle, and oxidative phosphorylation in the respiratory chain. ADP, adenosine diphosphate; ATP, adenosine triphosphate; CoA, coenzyme A; FAD, flavin adenine dinucleotide; $FADH_2$, reduced form of FAD; GTP, guanosine triphosphate; NAD^+, oxidized form of nicotinamide-adenine dinucleotide; NADH, reduced form of NAD. (From Wood SC, Lenfant C. Evolution of Respiratory Processes: A Comparative Approach. New York, Marcel Dekker, 1979, p 310.)

reactions during which the energy released primarily from carbohydrates and free fatty acids is captured. This involves

- The reduction of the oxidized form of nicotinamide-adenine dinucleotide (NAD^+) to the reduced form of NAD (NADH)
- A shuttling of the electrons from the NADH into the mitochondria
- The transfer of the electrons along a series of electron carrier enzymes, the cytochrome chain, located in the inner mitochondrial membrane
- The capture of the energy in the high-energy phosphate bonds of adenosine triphosphate (ATP)

In order for the TCA cycle to continue, adequate O_2 must also diffuse into the mitochondria, where it serves as the final electron acceptor reacting with cytochrome aa_3. Oxidative phosphorylation is the most efficient means of energy generation, producing 36 mol of ATP per mole of glucose metabolized. The overall equation for this reaction is

$$\text{Glucose} + 6\,O_2 + 36\,\text{ADP} + 2\,\text{Pi} \rightarrow 36\,\text{ATP} + 42\,H_2O + 6\,CO_2$$

where ADP is adenosine diphosphate and Pi is inorganic phosphate.

When O_2 is not present in sufficient amounts, ATP is produced anaerobically through glycolysis, and pyruvate becomes the terminal electron acceptor (Fig. 9–3). This much less efficient means of energy production produces only 2 mol of ATP per mole of glucose:

$$\text{Glucose} + 2\,\text{Pi} + 2\,\text{ADP} \rightarrow 2\,\text{ATP} + 2\,H_2O + 2\,\text{lactate}$$

The production of lactate as an end-product in this reaction is necessary to regenerate the NAD required for continued glycolysis. An elevated lactate level is thus a marker of anaerobic ATP production.

An alternative to glycolysis, at least in heart, skeletal muscle, and brain, is the creatine kinase reaction.[3] In this reaction, a high-energy phosphate bond transfers from the storage compound, phosphocreatine (PCr), to ADP to form ATP:

$$\text{PCr} + \text{ADP} + H^+ \rightarrow \text{ATP} + \text{creatine}$$

Although this constitutes a ready source of energy under conditions of O_2 scarcity in tissues containing PCr, its usefulness is limited by the relatively small PCr stores compared with energy requirements.

ATP diffuses out of the mitochondria to cellular sites requiring energy utilization, and the energy is released via ATP hydrolysis:

$$\text{ATP} \rightarrow \text{ADP} + \text{Pi} + H^+ + \text{energy}$$

Under conditions of sufficient O_2, the products of ATP hydrolysis are reutilized to form ATP via oxidative phosphorylation. Thus, despite the fact that as much as 150,000 mmol of H^+ is produced each day by energy utilization, there is virtually no change in pH. The H^+, however, is not

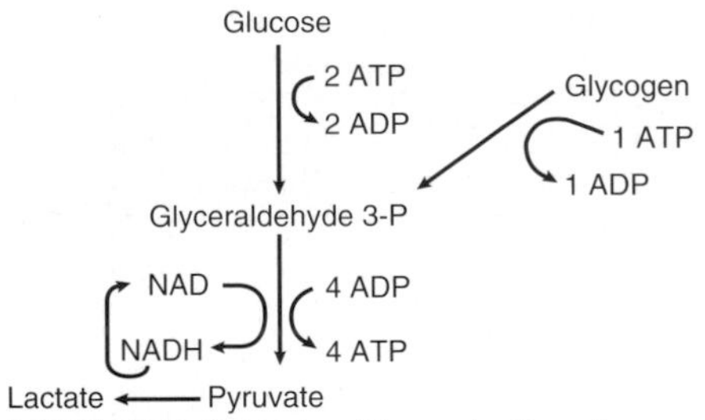

FIGURE 9–3: Anaerobic production of adenosine triphosphate (ATP) from glycolysis. When oxygen is not available, pyruvate becomes the terminal electron acceptor. In this process, 2mol of ATP is produced per mole of glucose, making this a much less efficient use of foodstuffs than aerobic phosphorylation. In addition, protons are generated, which leads to the development of metabolic acidosis. ADP, adenosine diphosphate; NAD, nicotinamide-adenine dinucleotide; NADH, reduced form of NAD. (From Dantzker DR. Interpretation of data in the hypoxic patient. *In* Bryan-Brown CW, Ayres SM [eds]. Oxygen Transport and Utilization. Fullerton, CA, Society of Critical Care Medicine, 1987, p 103.)

reutilized when ATP is produced by glycolysis, and this is the source of the acidosis associated with tissue hypoxia.[4] Thus, anaerobic metabolism leads to the production of equimolar amounts of H^+ and lactate (i.e., lactic acidosis). Note that the creatine kinase reaction utilizes H^+ in the production of ATP, therefore temporizing the development of metabolic acidosis that would otherwise occur.

The amount of O_2 required for oxidative phosphorylation is substantial. For example, it takes the O_2 found in 650 L of air to metabolize 1 mol of glucose. Yet at the level of the mitochondria, it requires a Po_2 of less than 1 mm Hg to maintain cellular respiration at maximal levels. The transport of O_2 from the environment to the cell is a complex process that is, even today, incompletely understood. This chapter reviews what is known about this transport system.

OXYGEN TRANSPORT

Oxygen is transported from the environment to the tissues by a series of diffusion and convection steps (Fig. 9–4). Convective O_2 transport to the tissues ($\dot{T}o_2$) is defined as

$$\dot{T}o_2 = \text{cardiac output} \times \text{arterial } O_2 \text{ content}$$

The determinants of Pa_{O_2} and O_2 saturation have already been covered in Chapter 5. The hemoglobin concentration is controlled predominantly through the secretion of erythropoietin, a growth factor secreted by the kidney.[5] The exact nature of the signal for erythropoietin release is un-

$\dot{T}o_2$ is determined by

- Pa_{O_2}
- O_2 saturation
- Hemoglobin concentration
- Complex factors that regulate cardiac output

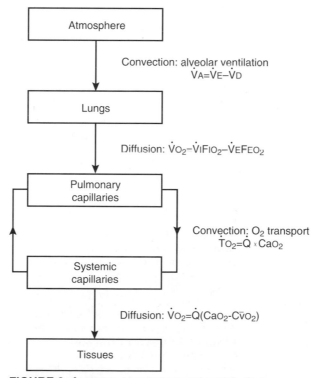

FIGURE 9–4: Model of the O_2 transport system. O_2 is transported from the atmosphere to the tissues by a series of convection and diffusion steps. The equations describing O_2 transport are shown.

known, but it must in some way relate to $\dot{T}_{O_2}$ because erythropoiesis is clearly increased in the setting of chronic reductions in tissue oxygenation.

Factors intrinsic to cardiac function, such as contractility, valvular integrity, and coronary blood flow, set limits on the cardiac output, but the moment-to-moment control of blood flow is regulated by the peripheral vasculature as it alters peripheral vascular resistance and venous return.[6] The distribution of the flow to individual organs depends on the ability of its specific vascular bed to respond to differing stresses and metabolic demands.[7]

The sympathetic adrenergic nerves innervate the heart and the systemic blood vessels, which can lead to vasodilatation and increased heart rate and contractility when beta-adrenergic receptor stimulation occurs or vasoconstriction occurs after alpha-receptor stimulation. These nerves are probably important in helping the organism respond in a coordinated fashion to environmental stresses such as change in position, hypoxia, and exercise.

Blood flow to individual organs is primarily controlled at the level of the microvasculature, which alters local vascular resistance and controls the number of open capillaries. Two mechanisms appear to be involved in maintaining the required blood flow. The first of these is myogenic control, which is responsible for keeping flow constant, in the face of varying intravascular pressures, through alterations in vascular smooth muscle tone.[8] This type of autoregulation appears to be regulated through the release of vasoactive mediators from the endothelial cells. Dilating substances such as endothelium-derived relaxing factor (EDRF) and constricting substances (endothelin) have been identified. EDRF is now known to be nitric oxide, which explains the mechanism of action of the clinically important vasodilators, sodium nitroprusside and nitroglycerine, which also release nitric oxide. Other important vasodilators, such as acetylcholine, stimulate the release of EDRF and are thus dependent on the presence of a functioning endothelium.

A second mechanism, the metabolic controller, alters local $\dot{T}_{O_2}$ to accommodate the continuously varying metabolic demands. Local blood flow is linked to local O_2 utilization, and increases in P_{O_2} constrict whereas decreases dilate the microvessels.[9] It is probably not P_{O_2} itself that is sensed but the release of some substance in response to an imbalance between O_2 requirements and supply. Possible mediators include adenosine, a potent vasodilator produced during the degradation of ATP, and inorganic phosphate, which accumulates in the setting of insufficient ATP production. The ability of any particular microvascular bed to increase flow or to recruit additional capillaries differs from organ to organ. For example, skeletal muscle can increase its capillary density by as much as three times, whereas its total flow can increase by about sevenfold. The heart, on the other hand, depends almost totally on flow. In response to various stresses, such as hypotension, hemorrhage, or hypoxemia, local vascular beds differ in their ability to respond by increasing overall $\dot{T}_{O_2}$. For example, during hypoxemia, blood flow increases to the brain, myocardium, adrenals, and skeletal muscle but declines to the kidney and most of the gastrointestinal tract.

TISSUE OXYGEN DIFFUSION

The following factors determine the diffusion of O_2 from the capillaries into the tissues:

EDRF—endothelial derived relaxing factor.

D represents the diffusing capacity of the tissues. Pc_{O_2} and $Pmito_{O_2}$ are the P_{O_2} in the capillaries and mitochondria, respectively (i.e., the driving pressure).[10]

$$O_2 \text{ transfer } = D \,(Pc_{O_2} - Pmito_{O_2})$$

D is determined, among other things, by the surface area available and the distance from the capillary to the cell. These are both functions of microvascular control, as discussed earlier. Factors that alter D, such as the presence of tissue edema or inflammation, will probably impair O_2 diffusion into the tissues.

Because the capillary P_{O_2} cannot be measured directly, it is usually calculated based on a simple model of tissue blood flow. In this model, the Pc_{O_2} falls progressively from the arterial to the venous value as it moves down the capillary (Fig. 9–5). On the basis of this concept, some have suggested that the venous value would be a good estimate of tissue P_{O_2}, but only under the condition of normal metabolic loads and when normal capillary density results in a normal diffusion distance between the capillary and the cell.[11] However, even in this simple model of the tissues, the venous P_{O_2} would be misleading as an index of tissue P_{O_2} in situations in which $\dot{T}_{O_2}$ or $\dot{V}_{O_2}$ was abnormal or in which capillary density did not change proportional to O_2 demands. Some individuals have attempted to extrapolate this theoretical study to conclude that the mixed venous P_{O_2} (i.e., the P_{O_2} of the pulmonary artery blood) can be used to reflect mean tissue P_{O_2}. They forget the cautions raised previously and that the original calculations were based on the simple model of a single core of tissue and not a value representing the blood flow–weighted mean from the entire body.

The simple tissue model described earlier also fails to take into account the time it takes for O_2 to be released from the red blood cells, which is likely to be an important determinant of Pc_{O_2}. Under conditions of reduced $\dot{T}_{O_2}$, increased $\dot{V}_{O_2}$, or reduced capillary transit time, there may be insufficient time for O_2 release from the red blood cell to keep up with its removal from the blood.[12] This would result in a lower Pc_{O_2} all the way along the capillary than might otherwise be predicted (see Fig. 9–5). In addition, the venous P_{O_2} may be higher than the end-capillary

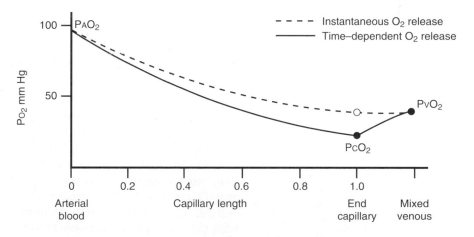

Predicted Intracapillary P_{O_2}

FIGURE 9–5: Model of the systemic capillary O_2 profile assuming time-dependent release of oxygen from hemoglobin. The capillary P_{O_2} is calculated assuming both instantaneous and time-dependent O_2 release. In the latter instance, the venous P_{O_2} overestimates the capillary, and thus certainly the mean tissue P_{O_2}. Factors that decrease O_2 delivery exaggerate this difference. (From Gutierrez G. The rate of oxygen release and its effect on capillary O_2 tension: A mathematical analysis. Respir Physiol 63:79, 1985.)

Po_2. Studies in animal models have shown that these time-related events can lead to situations in which tissue Po_2 is significantly lower than venous Po_2.

Because arteries and veins run parallel to each other as they penetrate into the tissues, O_2 may, under certain circumstances, diffuse directly from the arteries into the veins in a countercurrent system, creating an effective O_2 shunt.[13] Like the situation related to time-dependent release, this results in a venous Po_2 that is considerably higher than the capillary value. Unlike the time-dependent problem, this countercurrent shunt would be more of a problem during low-flow states because this increases the time available for diffusion.

Finally, alterations in the capillary hematocrit may affect the Po_2. As the red blood cells move through the capillaries, they orient themselves in the center of the stream and travel faster than the surrounding plasma. This serves to dilute them, producing a capillary hematocrit that may be only 75% of that found in the arterial blood.[14] The factors that alter this capillary hematocrit are not yet well defined, but if it falls low enough, the Pc_{O_2} may drop significantly. In addition, the relatively slower moving plasma layer surrounding the inside of the capillary may represent part of the barrier to O_2 diffusion. Because the value of the capillary hematocrit in any individual organ is unknown and because the effect of various stresses, such as hypoxemia, anemia, and hypotension, on this value is equally unclear, any attempt to draw conclusions about an optimal hematocrit for any given clinical problem is probably premature at this time. An additional complicating factor, which may make decisions about optimizing the hematocrit difficult, is that increasing the hematocrit alters the viscosity of the blood, increasing cardiac work and possibly altering the microvascular distribution of cardiac output. Given this complexity, it is not surprising that data can be found to support all ranges of hematocrit, from normal values to significant hemodilution. For example, the optimal hematocrit in one series of postoperative patients was found to be about 32%.[15] In the normal brain, decreasing the hematocrit to 30% increases cerebral blood flow and tissue oxygenation.[16] During experimentally induced hemorrhagic shock, whole body $\dot{V}o_2$ was maximal at a hematocrit of 45%, whereas the heart did best at a hematocrit of 25%.[17]

The normal O_2 extraction ratio =

$$\dot{V}o_2 / \dot{T}o_2 = Ca_{o_2} / Ca_{o_2} - C\bar{v}_{o_2}$$

REGULATION OF OXYGEN UTILIZATION

In normal subjects, $\dot{V}o_2$ is regulated by the body's demand for energy. During exercise, the best studied and most easily controlled alteration in metabolic demand, $\dot{T}o_2$, increases simultaneously with the onset of work (Fig. 9–6).[18] For the most part, this increase is mediated by an increase in cardiac output, although at high levels of exercise, there is some hemoconcentration, which leads to an increase in hematocrit and thus O_2 content. The increase in $\dot{T}o_2$ at maximal exercise in conditioned individuals may be as high as four to five times basal levels. However, even this prodigious increase is not sufficient to supply all of the body's requirements for increased energy because $\dot{V}o_2$ can increase 10- to 15-fold. The additional O_2 is provided by an increase in O_2 extraction. The normal O_2 extraction ratio (ER) is about 0.3, but this ratio can increase during exercise to 0.8 or higher. The ability to increase the ER results from improvements in O_2 diffusion mediated primarily by an increase in muscle capillary density.

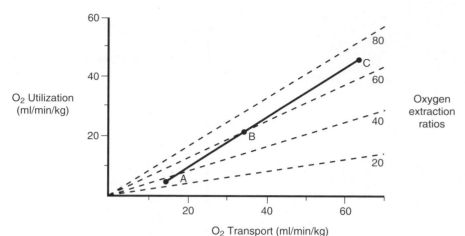

FIGURE 9–6: Relationship between O_2 transport and utilization during exercise. The increased O_2 demands are accommodated by both an increase in O_2 transport and the O_2 extraction ratio. A, basal requirements; B, anaerobic threshold; C, maximal O_2 utilization.

Even this increase in ER is usually not sufficient to supply all of the increased O_2 requirements. At some point, the body invokes glycolysis to anaerobically produce the additional ATP necessary. The level of work at which this occurs is called the AT; in sedentary individuals, this may occur at as low as 40% of maximal $\dot{V}O_2$.[19] With increased conditioning, the AT can be increased to as high as 60% or more through a combination of better cardiac performance and more effective aerobic capacity of the muscles. In patients with cardiovascular disease or those who are poorly conditioned, the AT falls. In most individuals, the ER at the AT is about 60%: that is, once the muscles need to extract more than 60% of the delivered O_2, further increases in O_2 diffusion are not sufficient to keep up with increasing demand.[20] The skeletal muscles are well designed to increase O_2 extraction because of their diffusion reserve. This ability is necessary because muscle needs to be ready to increase its workload rapidly many times over basal requirements. The visceral organs are not as well endowed with diffusion reserve.

A reduction in $\dot{T}O_2$ is an unusual occurrence in normal individuals, even under conditions of environmental reductions in FI_{O_2}. At high altitudes, an increase in cardiac output is normally sufficient to maintain a normal $\dot{T}O_2$. Even in the face of significant anemia, an increasing cardiac output is usually able to make up for the reduction in red blood cell mass, at least at rest. However, many sick patients have cardiac insufficiency, and when this is combined with hypoxemia, anemia, or both, they will be unable to match $\dot{T}O_2$ to metabolic requirements.

It is generally assumed that $\dot{T}O_2$ in normal subjects is more than sufficient to supply basal O_2 requirements (Fig. 9–7). Any reduction in $\dot{T}O_2$ should be compensated for by an increase in ER. However, experimental studies in various animals have demonstrated that if $\dot{T}O_2$ continues to fall, a point is eventually reached (the critical $\dot{T}O_2$, or $\dot{T}O_{2crit}$) at which $\dot{T}O_2$ is insufficient to sustain O_2 needs; below this point, $\dot{V}O_2$ falls.[21] The ER at which this happens (the critical ER, or ERcrit) in animal studies has varied from about 45 to 80%. The effects of a systematic reduction in $\dot{T}O_2$ cannot be studied in humans, but a similar biphasic relationship between $\dot{T}O_2$ and $\dot{V}O_2$ is believed to exist.

In patients, some studies have suggested that aerobic metabolism

AT—anaerobic threshold.

Values for the $\dot{T}O_{2crit}$ vary from 6 to 10 mL/kg/min.

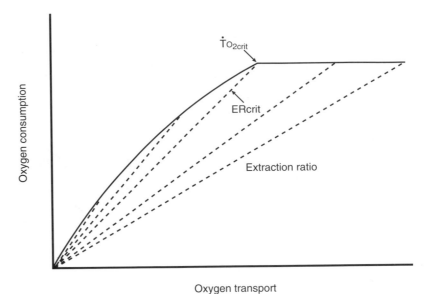

FIGURE 9–7: Relationship between oxygen consumption and oxygen transport as oxygen transport is reduced. As $\dot{T}O_2$ is reduced, a level is reached ($\dot{T}O_{2crit}$) at which transport is no longer able to sustain basal oxygen consumption despite a progressive increase in the oxygen extraction ratio (ER).

may become limited by O_2 supply at normal or even above-normal levels of $\dot{T}O_2$.[22] This so-called pathologic supply dependency has been described in acutely ill patients with sepsis, the adult respiratory distress syndrome, and hypovolemic shock. More surprisingly, patients with more chronic abnormalities of $\dot{T}O_2$, such as congestive heart failure, chronic obstructive pulmonary disease, and pulmonary hypertension, may display this dependency. In fact, it has been very difficult to demonstrate the expected biphasic relationship in individual patients, all of whom seem to have a linear relationship over the range of $\dot{T}O_2$ that has been studied.

How can the finding of an apparent "supply dependency" in such a diverse population of patients be explained? A simple explanation would be that basal $\dot{V}O_2$ increases in sick patients because of fever, hypermetabolism, inflammation, and so forth. This by itself would shift the $\dot{T}O_{2crit}$ to the right, making it more likely that a patient would be supply dependent at normal or increased $\dot{T}O_2$ (Fig. 9–8). Unfortunately, too few systematic measurements of metabolic rate in acutely ill patients have been made to allow this conclusion to be drawn.

Another explanation is that these patients have some abnormality of O_2 extraction that puts a limit on the ER (see Fig. 9–8). This might be due to an abnormality in the microcirculation or an inability of the cells to utilize available O_2 for the creation of ATP by oxidative phosphorylation. Abnormal blood flow distribution has long been postulated in patients with sepsis. Although true anatomic shunts probably do not exist, a maldistribution of blood flow with regard to actual metabolic needs is a possibility. This inability to autoregulate blood flow could occur as a result of the release of endogenous mediators such as prostaglandins. Alternatively, it could result from damage to the endothelial cells or the underlying vascular smooth muscle from hypoxia, inflammation, complement activation, or other processes thought to occur in critically ill patients. A close interaction and communication between the endothelium

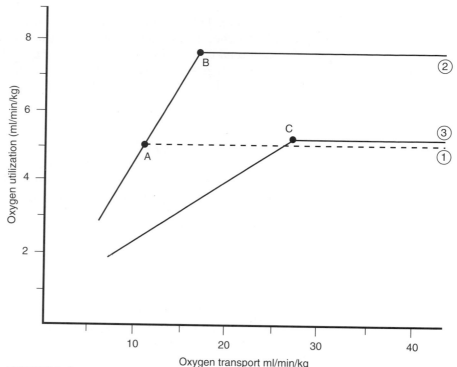

FIGURE 9–8: Proposed causes of pathologic supply dependency. No. 1 represents the hypothesized normal relationship, with the critical level of O_2 transport ($\dot{T}O_{2crit}$) at point A. In the other two situations, the $\dot{T}O_{2crit}$ is shifted to a higher level of O_2 transport. In example No. 2, the critical extraction ratio is normal, but the $\dot{T}O_{2crit}$ (point B) is shifted because of an increased metabolic rate. In example No. 3, the supply dependency is due to an abnormality of O_2 extraction ($\dot{T}O_2$ at point C).

and the vascular smooth muscle is crucial to autoregulation. All of these potential mechanisms might be accentuated by the use of the many vasoactive drugs that are given to sick patients to maintain overall blood pressure and cardiac function but that may exacerbate peripheral blood flow maldistribution.

Microvascular occlusion by inflammation with endothelial cell damage or by granulocyte or platelet aggregation or embolization could also interfere with normal O_2 extraction. A loss of capillary cross-sectional area secondary to capillary occlusion would increase diffusion distance to the tissues and interfere with capillary recruitment, the major compensation available to the organism to increase O_2 extraction. This diffusion problem may be worsened if inflammation or diffuse capillary leakage leads to the accumulation of fluid around the systemic capillaries, further increasing the distance that O_2 must diffuse to reach the cells. Finally, all of this would be exaggerated by any alteration in the time that the blood spends in the capillaries because of capillary loss or a hyperdynamic state, as seen in sepsis.

Alternatively, the problem could exist within the cell itself, with a basic metabolic abnormality leading to an inability to utilize available substrate and O_2 to form ATP. Such abnormalities have been suggested in experimental sepsis. Although this would not explain pathologic supply dependency on its own, it could play a significant augmenting role.

Another alternative has been suggested to explain the finding of supply dependency in more chronically ill individuals. Although the muscles are very good at extracting O_2 thereby achieving an ER of greater than 70% during exercise, the visceral organs are much less able to accommodate increasing extraction requirements. These organs may exceed their diffusion reserves very quickly as $\dot{T}O_2$ falls below normal. This is suggested by the findings in the only study of humans with relatively stable conditions, in whom the $\dot{T}O_{2crit}$ was seen at an ER of only 30 to 40%.[22, 23]

The finding of a linear relationship between $\dot{T}O_2$ and $\dot{V}O_2$ in many patients may, therefore, reflect a normal physiologic event. Above the $\dot{T}O_{2crit}$, $\dot{T}O_2$ follows increases and decreases in metabolic demand (i.e., is $\dot{V}O_2$ dependent). Below $\dot{T}O_{2crit}$, $\dot{V}O_2$ varies with increasing and decreasing O_2 availability (i.e., is $\dot{T}O_2$ dependent). To the degree that this hypothesis holds, graphing random $\dot{T}O_2$-$\dot{V}O_2$ points will always inscribe a straight line (Fig. 9–9).

Finally, the relationship between $\dot{T}O_2$ and $\dot{V}O_2$ that is observed may be influenced by mathematical coupling of the two measurements, making the apparent relationship really an artifact of the calculations. Because the product of cardiac output and arterial O_2 content is part of the calculation of both $\dot{T}O_2$ and $\dot{V}O_2$, variability in these measurements could force an apparent relationship where no natural one exists. This is a particular problem when the degree of change of either variable is small.

MONITORING THE ADEQUACY OF TISSUE OXYGENATION

The exact role that inadequate tissue oxygenation may play in the pathophysiology of many disease states remains unclear because of the difficulty of monitoring in the clinical setting. Available indices can be

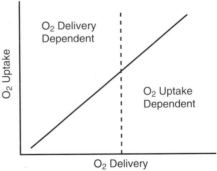

FIGURE 9–9: A possible explanation for the linearity of the relationship between O_2 delivery and O_2 transport over the very wide range seen in critically ill patients. Above a certain level of O_2 delivery, the relationship is driven by changes in O_2 uptake. This is the normal situation, in which O_2 delivery is the dependent variable. Below the critical O_2 delivery, O_2 delivery becomes the independent variable and the patient is supply dependent. (From Dantzker DR. Interpretation of data in the hypoxic patient. *In* Bryan-Brown CW, Ayres SM [eds]. Oxygen Transport and Utilization. Fullerton, CA, Society of Critical Care Medicine, 1987, p 101.)

divided, for convenience of discussion, into input, utilization, and output variables, as well as direct measurements of tissue bioenergetics (Table 9–1). Each of these parameters differs in the ease of measurement and the usefulness of the data.

The critical Pa_{O_2} is unknown in the diseased and the normal human.

The input variables are the easiest to obtain and the ones most commonly measured. The Pa_{O_2} and O_2 saturation are accurate indices of lung function but have no relationship to the peripheral tissues. Patients are rarely exposed to the levels of hypoxemia that have been shown experimentally to lead to tissue hypoxia in normal animals. $\dot{T}o_2$ monitors the bulk transport of O_2 leaving the left side of the heart. However, even though this variable is often called oxygen delivery, it does not provide any information about the actual arrival of O_2 at the tissues of any specific organ. In addition, as discussed earlier, the $\dot{T}o_{2crit}$ in humans, either normal or diseased, is unknown; like the critical Po_2, it varies, making any individual number not very useful.

Transcutaneous Po_2, which is also easily determined, may be a rough measurement of local $\dot{T}o_2$ to the skin. Unfortunately, the skin is not a good representative of the vital organs because the blood flow often changes in opposite directions to the viscera. Tissue Po_2 has been sampled in the experimental laboratory with surface or needle microelectrodes. Once again, this value is usually available only from superficial tissues, and because the minimal tissue Po_2 is unknown, even a correct value from some important organ may not prove to be useful. In addition, the critical Po_2 is likely to be so low that it will be an insensitive index to follow. In muscle, for example, a tissue Po_2 as low as 1 to 2 mm Hg is sufficient to allow high levels of work.[24]

$\dot{V}_I$ and $\dot{V}_E$ are the inspired and expired minute ventilations, $F_{I_{O_2}}$ and $F_{E_{O_2}}$ are the inspired and expired fractional concentrations of oxygen, $\dot{Q}$ is the cardiac output, and Ca_{O_2} and $C\bar{v}_{O_2}$ are the arterial and mixed venous O_2 contents.

The major utilization variable, $\dot{V}o_2$, which is a good measurement of overall aerobic metabolism, can be measured most easily using the principle of conservation of mass (Fick's equation):

$$\dot{V}o_2 = \dot{V}_I \times F_{I_{O_2}} - \dot{V}_E \times F_{E_{O_2}}$$
$$= \dot{Q}\,(Ca_{O_2} - C\bar{v}_{O_2})$$

In practice, $\dot{V}o_2$ can be measured in three different ways. It can be measured directly by rebreathing from a spirometer filled with O_2. The CO_2 is absorbed from the expired gas, and the change in the volume of the spirometer per unit time is the $\dot{V}o_2$. This technique is rarely used today because even small leaks in the spirometer circuit lead to signifi-

TABLE **9–1:**   Indices of Tissue Oxygenation

Input variables
  Arterial Po_2 and saturation
  O_2 transport
  Transcutaneous Po_2
  Tissue Po_2
Utilization variables
  O_2 consumption
  O_2 transport–O_2 consumption relationship
  O_2 extraction ratio
Output variables
  Mixed venous Po_2
  Lactate levels
  Tissue pH
  Organ function
  Adenosine triphosphate degradation
    products
Tissue bioenergetics
  Magnetic resonance spectroscopy
  Near-infrared spectroscopy

cant error. The other two techniques require that the patient is in a steady state such that metabolic demands, $\dot{V}E$, and $\dot{Q}$ are all constant. Then, the amount of oxygen taken up by the tissues is equal to the amount taken up in the lung, and $\dot{V}O_2$ can be calculated from either the blood side ($\dot{Q}[Ca_{O_2} - C\bar{v}_{O_2}]$) or the gas side ($\dot{V}I \times FI_{O_2} - \dot{V}E \times FE_{O_2}$) of the system. The method chosen in any particular clinical situation is limited by the conditions of each technique. Measurement from the gas side is noninvasive but depends on the ability to measure FI_{O_2} and FE_{O_2} accurately. In a patient breathing room air, this measurement is easy and accurate. However, in patients breathing an increased FI_{O_2}, especially those on mechanical ventilation, the accuracy reflects the consistency of the O_2 delivery system. Quantitation of $\dot{V}O_2$ from the blood side requires the measurement of cardiac output as well as the sampling of mixed venous and arterial blood. This technique bypasses the problem of consistency of inspired O_2 and thus is the method used most commonly in critically ill patients. Its major disadvantage is the large number of variables (partial pressures and saturations of arterial and mixed venous blood, hemoglobin concentration, and cardiac output) that must be measured, each of which is subject to error. When properly performed, all three methods should result in the same value for $\dot{V}O_2$.

Of the utilization variables, $\dot{V}O_2$ is a good measurement of overall aerobic metabolism, but by itself it is an unreliable measure of tissue oxygenation. In addition, the appropriate level of $\dot{V}O_2$ for any individual patient depends on metabolic demand, which varies widely both from patient to patient and from moment to moment. For this reason, monitoring the relationship between $\dot{T}O_2$ and $\dot{V}O_2$ might be useful. However, unlike the situation with laboratory experiments, patients undergo spontaneous variations in both $\dot{T}O_2$ and $\dot{V}O_2$. A primary change in $\dot{V}O_2$ would be expected to result in a concomitant change in $\dot{T}O_2$, as is seen, for example, in normal subjects during exercise. Conversely, a primary change in $\dot{T}O_2$ would likewise cause an alteration in $\dot{V}O_2$ if supply dependency is present. In the clinical setting, it may be quite difficult to tell which is the dependent and which is the independent variable without a controlled attempt to disturb one value or the other (see Fig. 9–9). In other words, it may be impossible to know if the system is behaving in a physiologic or a pathologic fashion.

If one assumes that the finding of supply dependency reflects an index of inadequate tissue oxygenation, then increasing $\dot{T}O_2$ until $\dot{V}O_2$ reaches a plateau, indicating the supply-independent region, might seem reasonable. Unfortunately, although many investigators have demonstrated that $\dot{V}O_2$ can be increased by increasing $\dot{T}O_2$, none has yet demonstrated an ability to achieve this fabled plateau.[22] However, preliminary data in a group of surgical patients show that increasing both $\dot{T}O_2$ and $\dot{V}O_2$ did improve survival.[25] Further studies may eventually show a way of using this relationship.

A low ER in the face of a low $\dot{T}O_2$ signals a poor outcome[26] and suggests an abnormality of microvascular control, perhaps a failure of autoregulation. Unfortunately, until we understand the microcirculation better and have learned how to control it, the ER may be useful only as a prognostic index.

The output variables have been the traditional measures of adequate tissue oxygenation. The $P\bar{v}_{O_2}$, or mixed venous saturation, has been commonly assumed to represent the mean tissue PO_2. Why the $P\bar{v}_{O_2}$ is not always a good approximation of the end-capillary PO_2 in the tissue, no less a helpful measure of mean PO_2, has already been discussed. The $P\bar{v}_{O_2}$

has the added disadvantage of being a blood flow—weighted mean of the venous effluent from each of the tissue beds, and it may be equal to none of them. Because the $P\bar{v}_{O_2}$ is influenced by the relative contributions from tissues with differing metabolic rates, changes in the $P\bar{v}_{O_2}$ may reflect only an alteration in blood flow distribution. For example, in sepsis, a high $P\bar{v}_{O_2}$ probably indicates inadequate tissue $\dot{V}_{O_2}$ or severe maldistribution of peripheral flow; in fact, a fall in the $P\bar{v}_{O_2}$ may actually be a good sign, indicating the return of local microvascular control. Clinical studies suggest that values of $P\bar{v}_{O_2}$ below 28 mm Hg are associated with a poor prognosis,[27] but values of $P\bar{v}_{O_2}$ that are considerably lower are found in situations in which apparently normal tissue function is present, such as during very high levels of exercise or at high altitudes. The prognostic information inherent in a low $P\bar{v}_{O_2}$ most likely stems more from its association with other physiologic abnormalities, such as low cardiac output or severe anemia, than from its ability to predict tissue P_{O_2}.

When there is insufficient O_2 to sustain oxidative phosphorylation, increased glycolysis is used to maintain tissue ATP levels, with lactate being produced. Some tissues, such as the red blood cell, the renal medulla, and portions of the eye, routinely depend on glycolysis for energy production. Their overall contribution of lactate is small, about 40 g/day. Under normal circumstances, skeletal muscle, brain, intestine, and skin may also produce small amounts of lactate; the muscle contribution can increase dramatically during exercise, especially in unconditioned individuals. The lactate may undergo further oxidation through the TCA cycle or serve as a substrate for gluconeogenesis. Both of these processes require adequate amounts of oxygen. When glycolysis is carried out under conditions of insufficient O_2, lactate accumulates.

Unfortunately, factors other than tissue hypoxia can result in increased lactate production. Lactate levels will be elevated by factors that increase the rate of glycolysis in excess of the ability of pyruvate to be utilized in the TCA cycle,[28] such as alkalosis, excess insulin or catecholamine release, as well as by factors that reduce the levels of acetyl coenzyme A, such as starvation and diabetes. During sepsis, a metabolic block may prevent substrate from entering the TCA cycle, leading to pyruvate accumulation and increased lactate production. Finally, drugs and chemicals such as ethanol, methanol, ethylene glycol, salicylates, and phenformin can elevate lactate levels by interfering with gluconeogenesis.

Other factors may limit the production of lactic acid, thus decreasing the lactate level present in the setting of significant tissue hypoxia. In malnourished patients, for example, glycogen deposits may be inadequate to supply sufficient substrate for glycolysis. More importantly, as tissue pH falls, glycolytic flux is inhibited, providing a sort of feedback control on the level of blood lactate.

On the other side of the balance sheet, the liver removes most of the lactate from the circulation. In fact, it is generally thought that the ability of the liver to remove lactate is several-fold greater than the ability of the peripheral tissues to produce it. Thus, any compromise in liver function can have a dramatic effect on the level of lactate present for any given rate of accelerated glycolysis. In addition, lactate produced by one organ can be used as substrate by another, in particular the heart and skeletal muscle. Both of these means of lactate clearance further reduce the sensitivity of lactate as an index of inadequate tissue oxygenation unless the defect is global in nature.

The normal lactate level is about 1 mEq/L; increased levels are often considered to be de facto evidence of inadequate tissue oxygenation.

Assessing the onset of individual organ hypoxia by monitoring tissue pH would provide increased sensitivity and specificity. H^+ accumulation in the tissues is an early and sensitive indication of ineffective aerobic production of ATP. Tissue pH can theoretically be measured invasively with needle electrodes or noninvasively with magnetic resonance spectroscopy (see later discussion). In the gastrointestinal tract, a good estimate of tissue pH can be obtained from tonometry using an intraluminal balloon. Preliminary studies using this technique in critically ill patients suggest that a fall in stomach mucosal pH may be a good signal of inappropriate $\dot{T}O_2$.[29] It may also prove to be a good guide to subsequent therapy.[30]

Monitoring specific organ function might seem to be the best alternative because a normally functioning organ should be an indication of adequate metabolic status and thus adequate tissue $\dot{T}O_2$. However, as with lactic acid levels, a number of factors other than inadequate tissue oxygenation can alter tissue function. More importantly, it appears that tissues will function as long as adequate ATP is present, whereas they will stop abruptly when these reserves are depleted. Because this can be a very rapid transition, a warning of impending disaster that is early enough to enable the clinician to intervene may not be available.

New monitoring techniques are on the horizon but are not yet available for routine clinical use. If ATP utilization exceeds its production, adenosine monophosphate accumulates and is then hydrolyzed through a series of steps to hypoxanthine. In tissues that contain the enzyme xanthine oxidase, predominantly the liver, the hypoxanthine can be further oxidized to xanthine and then to uric acid. This metabolic pathway generates oxygen radicals, which have been suggested to be the cause of the damage in the ischemia-reperfusion syndrome. Monitoring of these metabolic products of ATP metabolism such as hypoxanthine and adenosine has been suggested as a useful index of inadequate cellular energy production.[31] Unfortunately, the techniques that are currently available make this analysis difficult to perform accurately; their usefulness in clinical monitoring awaits clarification.

A more direct measurement of tissue bioenergetics can be obtained from the use of magnetic resonance spectroscopy. This provides a well-characterized, noninvasive means of measuring the key biologic molecules involved in the energy balance sheet.[32] When tissue is placed in a strong magnetic field and subjected to radiofrequency waves, certain isotopic species will absorb and then emit some of the energy in the form of a radiofrequency signal that can be characterized and quantitated. ^{31}P is a stable isotope that forms a part of several of the molecules playing a central role in the storage and transfer of energy in the cell: ATP, ADP, PCr, and Pi. The PCr/Pi ratio is the equivalent of the cellular phosphate potential ATP/(ADP) (Pi), the energy charge of the cell.

When $\dot{T}O_2$ is reduced, either by hypoxemia or hypoperfusion, a level is eventually reached at which PCr/Pi begins to fall. In skeletal muscle, this point has been shown to correlate with $\dot{T}O_{2crit}$.[33] In the brain, PCr/Pi falls at a PO_2 below 40 mm Hg, whereas skeletal muscle appears to be more resistant. At this point, the level of ATP is normal, supplemented in part by the creatinine kinase reaction. Whether or not glycolysis is induced at this stage as an additional source of ATP production or is invoked only when the PCr is exhausted is unclear. In the brain, the use of PCr appears to be the preferred source of anaerobically generated ATP, perhaps to decrease the generation of hydrogen ion, which is detrimental to neuronal function. In skeletal muscle, this is less clear because a fall in pH is seen to coincide with the fall in PCr/Pi, suggesting that glycolysis begins concomitantly with the use of the creatinine kinase reaction.

As tissue oxygenation becomes increasingly impaired, PCr/Pi continues to fall and the intracellular pH (also measurable by magnetic resonance spectroscopy) falls along with it. The ATP levels, however, remain normal until very severe hypoxia occurs (Pa_{O_2} of less than 18 mm Hg in the brain), when the PCr is almost entirely depleted, and only then begin to fall. In experimental preparations, decreases in ATP appear to be irreversible; thus, below this level of hypoxia, cell death may be inevitable.

Because energy levels may remain normal until the ATP-generating ability of the cell is severely taxed, organ function may remain adequate almost until cell death intervenes, which emphasizes the importance of being able to monitor the changes that take place before a fall in ATP. At the moment, unfortunately, magnetic resonance spectroscopy is impractical as a clinical tool because of the expense and complexity of the equipment and because of the logistical problems of bringing patients to the magnet on a regular basis or placing a strong magnetic field in the complicated world of the intensive care unit. However, new technology involving miniaturization and shielding may well make it practical in the near future.

Another technique for direct quantitation of cellular bioenergetics that may be closer to practical use is the optical monitoring of the oxidation-reduction status of the mitochondrial energy chain, in particular cytochrome aa_3, by near-infrared spectroscopy.[34] In the brain, the organ on which much of this work has been performed, a reduction in cytochrome aa_3 occurs with much more modest hypoxia than is necessary to result in a fall in PCr/Pi. It has been suggested that the reduction in cytochrome aa_3 could therefore be used as an early warning sign of impending tissue hypoxia. However, because of difficulty with calibrating the optical techniques, they may be useful only as a way of following trends and not as a measure of any absolute level of tissue oxygenation.

SUMMARY

The process of tissue O_2 delivery is complex, and our understanding of it is still evolving. The existing methods of evaluating the efficacy of tissue oxygenation are inadequate and do not provide a sensitive enough index on which to base therapy. Thus, we are unable at present to define clear protocols for ensuring optimal tissue oxygenation. A number of new technologies are now being tested, and it is hoped that these will overcome the shortcomings that currently exist.

References

1. Weibel ER. Oxygen and the history of life. *In* The Pathway for Oxygen. Cambridge, MA, Harvard University Press, 1984, pp 1–30.
2. Newsholme EA, Leech AR. Biochemistry for the Medical Sciences. New York, John Wiley & Sons, 1983.
3. Chance B, Leigh JS, Clark BJ, et al. Control of oxidative metabolism and oxygen delivery in human skeletal muscle: A steady state analysis of work/energy cost transfer acidosis function. Proc Natl Acad Sci USA 82:8384–8388, 1985.
4. Zilva J. The origin of the acidosis in hyperlactatemia. Ann Clin Biochem 15:40–43, 1978.

5. Spivak JL. Erythropoietin: A brief review. Nephron 52:289–294, 1989.
6. Guyton AC, Jones CE, Coleman TG. Circulatory Physiology: Cardiac Output and Its Regulation. Philadelphia, WB Saunders, 1973.
7. Heistad PD, Abboud FM. Circulatory adjustments to hypoxia. Circulation 61:463–471, 1980.
8. Johnson P. Autoregulation of blood flow. Circ Res 59:483–495, 1986.
9. Sparks HV. Effect of local metabolic factors on vascular smooth muscle. *In* Bohr DR, Somlyo AP, Sparks HV (eds). The Cardiovascular System: Vascular Smooth Muscle. Bethesda, MD, American Physiological Society, 1980, pp 475–513.
10. Krogh A. The number and distribution of capillaries in muscles with calculations of the oxygen pressure head necessary for supplying the tissue. J Physiol (Lond) 52:409–415, 1919.
11. Tenney SM. A theoretical analysis of the relationship between venous blood and mean tissue oxygen pressures. Respir Physiol 20:283–290, 1974.
12. Gutierrez G. The rate of oxygen release and its effect on capillary O_2 tension: A mathematical analysis. Respir Physiol 63:69–96, 1985.
13. Piper J, Meyer M, Scheid P. Dual role of diffusion in tissue gas exchange: Blood-tissue equilibrium and diffusion shunt. Respir Physiol 56:131–144, 1984.
14. Desjardins C, Duling BR. Micro vessel hematocrit: Measurement and implications for capillary oxygen transport. Am J Physiol 252:H494–H503, 1987.
15. Czer LSC, Shoemaker WC. Optimal hematocrit value of critically ill post operative patients. Surg Gynecol Obstet 147:363–368, 1978.
16. Brown MM, Marshall J. Regulation of cerebral blood flow in response to changes in blood viscosity. Lancet 1:604–609. 1985.
17. Jan K, Heldman J, Chen S. Coronary hemodynamics and oxygen utilization after hematocrit variations in hemorrhage. Am J Physiol 239:H326–H332, 1980.
18. Astrand P, Cuddy TE, Saltin B, Steaberg J. Cardiac output during submaximal and maximal work. J Appl Physiol 19:268–274, 1964.
19. Wasserman K, Whipp BJ, Koyal SN, Beauer WL. Anaerobic threshold and respiratory gas exchange during exercise. J Appl Physiol 35:236–243, 1973.
20. Weber K, Janicki JS. Cardiopulmonary testing for evaluation of chronic cardiac failure. Am J Cardiol 55:22A–31A, 1985.
21. Cain SM. Oxygen delivery in dogs during anemic and hypoxic hypoxia. J Appl Physiol 42:228–234, 1977.
22. Dantzker DR, Foresman B, Gutierrez G. Oxygen supply and utilization relationships: A reevaluation. Am Rev Respir Dis 143:675–679, 1991.
23. Shibutani K, Komatsu T, Kubal K, et al. Critical level of oxygen delivery in anesthetized man. Crit Care Med 11:640–643, 1983.
24. Gayeski TEJ, Honig CR. O_2 gradients from sarcolemma to cell interior in red muscle at maximal VO_2. Am J Physiol 251:H789–H799, 1986.
25. Shoemaker W, Appel P, Kram H. Prospective trial of supranormal values of survivors as therapeutic goals in high risk surgical patients. Chest 94:1176–1186, 1988.
26. Gutierrez G, Pohil RJ. Oxygen consumption is linearly related to O_2 supply in critically ill patients. J Crit Care 1:45–53, 1986.
27. Kasnitz P, Druger DL, Yorra, et al. Mixed venous oxygen tension and hyperlactatemia. JAMA 236:570–574, 1976.
28. Kreisberg RA. Lactate homeostasis and lactic acidosis. Ann Intern Med 92:227–237, 1980.
29. Gutierrez G, Bismar H, Dantzker DR, et al. Comparison of gastric intramucosal pH to measures of oxygen transport and consumption in critically ill patients. Crit Care Med 20:451–457, 1992.
30. Gutierrez G, Palizas F, Dolio G, et al. Gastric intramucosal pH as a therapeutic index of tissue oxygenation in critically ill patients. Lancet 339:195–199, 1992.
31. Grum CM, Simon RH, Dantzker DR, et al. Evidence for adenosine triphosphate degradation in critically ill patients. Chest 88:763–767, 1985.
32. Gadian DG. Nuclear Magnetic Resonance and Its Application to Living Systems. New York, Oxford University Press, 1982.
33. Gutierrez G, Pohil RJ, Strong R, et al. Bioenergetics of rabbit skeletal muscle during hypoxemia and ischemia. J Appl Physiol 65:608–616, 1988.
34. LaManna JC, Sick TJ, Pikarsky SM, et al. Detection of oxidizable function of cytochrome oxidase in intact rat brain. Am J Physiol 253:C477–C483, 1987.

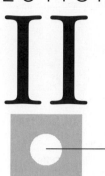

Diagnostic Techniques

Physical Examination

Arthur S. Banner, M.D.

The use of physical examination to diagnose disorders of the chest dates back to antiquity. The scientific basis for the physical examination of the chest can be attributed to Laennec, who categorized lung sounds and systematically related these findings to known underlying pathology.[1] With the advent of chest radiography and the availability of tests to measure lung and cardiac function, the physical examination has assumed a distinctly secondary role as a diagnostic modality. At present, a generational gap exists between the older physicians, who tend to retain the methods of physical examination they worked so assiduously to perfect, and the newer generation of doctors, who distrust the physical examination and rely almost exclusively on modern technology.

The following remarks take a middle ground between these opposing points of view and in so doing adopt a physiologic rather than a phenomenologic approach to physical signs. This chapter includes the classic components of the physical examination: inspection, palpation, percussion, and auscultation. It devotes little attention to the mechanics of the examination, which has been well described by others.[2] Instead, this chapter attempts to show how the physical examination can be used to generate data to support a physiologic hypothesis.

INSPECTION

Respiratory Pattern

Observation of the respiratory pattern provides important clues concerning

- The stability of the respiratory pattern generator
- The response of the respiratory system to afferent stimuli
- The response to increased loads

Classic experiments localized the respiratory generator to the medulla.[3] The respiratory pattern generator was modeled on two groups of neurons, one concerned with inspiration and the other with expiration, with activity in one group of neurons inhibiting activity in the other.[4] On the basis of this model, the respiratory pattern was analyzed in terms of tidal volume and rate. However, this model failed to explain fully the effects of altered drive and afferent feedback on the observed respiratory pattern.

More recently, the respiratory generator has been modeled on three groups of neurons, one of which provides for drive and the others of which provide for timing.[5] The group concerned with drive responds to metabolic stimuli and determines the inspiratory flow rate. The groups of neurons responsible for timing incorporate information provided by afferent nerves and serve to limit inspiratory duration, thereby determining respiratory rate and indirectly determining tidal volume. Figure 10–1 shows the manner in which afferent information interacts with drive to determine inspiratory duration and tidal volume. The observed respiratory pattern results from interaction between these neural mech-

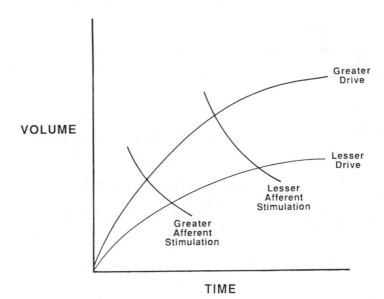

FIGURE 10–1: Two tidal volumes are shown. The larger tidal volume represents the response to increased drive and is characterized by a greater inspiratory flow rate. The effects of two levels of afferent stimulation on the tidal volume are illustrated. The effect of afferent stimulation is to decrease inspiratory time and thereby to decrease tidal volume and increase rate. The resultant effect on the inspiratory pattern is dependent on the level of drive and on the magnitude of afferent stimulation.

anisms and the mechanical function of the lungs. Looking at the generation of respiratory pattern in this way can provide insight into the underlying pathophysiology.

Stability and Adequacy of the Rhythm Generator

When confronted with a critically ill patient, the physician must immediately assess the stability and adequacy of respiration and the potential requirement for assisted ventilation. Figure 10–2 describes several stable and unstable respiratory patterns. Often, the physician must act on such information before the results of arterial blood gas measurements are known.

Several breathing patterns suggest unreliability of the brain stem rhythm generator:

- A slow respiratory rate in conjunction with small tidal volumes often results from decreased drive consequent to overall cerebral depression. Individuals exhibiting such a breathing pattern are generally obtunded and require intubation to protect the airway and assisted ventilation to ensure adequate ventilation.
- Gasping respirations are a sign of poor oxygen delivery consequent to inadequate cardiac output. Assisted ventilation will maintain ventilation while measures are taken to improve cardiac performance.
- Ataxic breathing, a pattern of breathing with unpredictable respiratory intervals and volumes on a breath-to-breath basis, generally indicates brain stem dysfunction.
- Cluster breathing, which consists of alternating apneic periods and periods of rapid, deep breathing, has the same significance as ataxic breathing.

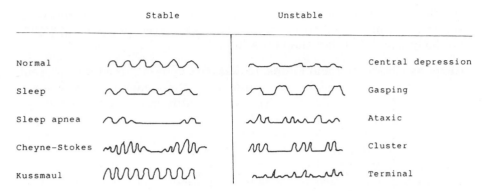

FIGURE 10–2: Stable and unstable respiratory patterns are shown. Identification of an unstable respiratory pattern is generally an indication for assisted ventilation.

- A breathing pattern consisting of irregular small breaths with an occasional gasp is a terminal breathing pattern. Although this pattern may be a consequence of multiple etiologies, it always indicates a need for assisted ventilation.
- Some breathing patterns appear irregular but are stable and require no immediate intervention. Cheyne-Stokes respiration consists of alteration between hyperpnea and hypopnea. In normal sleeping individuals, occasional short apneic periods occur in an unpredictable manner, interspersed within a regular breathing pattern. The sleep apnea syndrome is characterized by apneic periods of more prolonged duration. Some of these apneic periods are of central origin, whereas others occur secondary to intermittent upper airway obstruction. Although they are sometimes alarming to witness, immediate intervention is normally not required. However, the resulting hypoxia may have long-term detrimental effects; therefore, the patient requires some nonemergent intervention.[6]

Response to Afferent Stimuli

A rapid, shallow breathing pattern may result from heightened feedback from afferent nerves. Any process that alters lung elastic recoil, such as pulmonary interstitial or alveolar filling disease, can increase the discharge from airway stretch receptors. Irritant receptors and C fibers are located within the airways and respond to a variety of stimuli, both inhaled and endogenously produced. The discharge of these receptors could account for the rapid breathing associated with asthma, chronic obstructive pulmonary disease, pulmonary embolism, and inhalation of noxious agents. J receptors, a subclass of C fibers located within alveoli, are responsible for the rapid, shallow breathing seen in pulmonary congestion.

Response to Altered Loads

The respiratory system responds to

Elevated CO_2
Lowered Po_2
Acidosis

Response to Metabolic Loads. The respiratory system responds to an elevated CO_2, a lowered Po_2, and acidosis with an increase in drive, which leads to an increase in inspiratory flow rate. Interaction with vagal proprioceptive receptors limits an increase in tidal volume and increases rate (see Fig. 10–1). This type of breathing, termed Kussmaul's breathing, generally does not require intervention, other than for the underlying condition. However, respiratory support may be necessary when the respiratory system cannot cope with the increased demands or when the circulatory system shows impairment. In such a situation, respiratory support may preserve limited cardiac reserve, thereby supporting essential body functions other than breathing.

Response to Mechanical Loads. In disease conditions, the lungs present an increased mechanical load to the respiratory muscles. These loads may be either elastic, due to increased lung stiffness, or resistive, due to airway obstruction. In either case, the respiratory muscles must generate increased pleural pressures to overcome the load. In adults, excessive changes in pleural pressure appear as retraction of the intercostal and supraclavicular spaces. In obstructed patients, the pleural pressures may actually become positive during expiration, as evidenced by ballooning of the supraclavicular spaces and elevation of neck veins. Large changes in pleural pressure may also result in a paradoxical pulse (pulsus paradoxus). Blood pressure is thought to fall as a result of increased afterload on the left ventricle due to the large negative pleural pressure.[7]

One way that the respiratory system compensates for mechanical loading is by an increase in drive.[8] An increase in drive in the presence of altered mechanics, generally perceived as dyspnea, appears as respiratory distress.[9] This increased respiratory drive leads to augmentation of the strength of contraction of the respiratory muscles and the pattern of muscular recruitment. The following paragraphs describe the functioning of the muscles of respiration in normal circumstances and with increased mechanical loads.

The inspiratory muscles of the respiratory system are the diaphragm, the muscles of the chest wall, and the accessory muscles. A coordinated interaction of the diaphragm and the chest wall muscles allows the chest to enlarge and the pleural pressure to fall.[10] Expiration, a passive process for the most part, may involve use of the respiratory as well as the abdominal musculature during forced maneuvers or when increased resistive loads exist.

With mechanical loading, an increase in the strength of contraction of the diaphragm and the intercostal muscles occurs, as does the recruitment of additional muscle groups, such as the accessory muscles and the muscles of the abdomen. Roussos and colleagues showed that under extreme loads, there may be alternating use of the diaphragm and the chest wall muscles, presumably allowing short periods of muscular rest as each set of muscles alternately assumes the burden of breathing.[11] Konno and Mead showed that the use of particular respiratory muscles can be inferred by inspecting chest and abdominal movements.[12] Figure 10-3 illustrates the relative movements of the abdomen and chest during normal breathing, breathing with a paralyzed diaphragm, and breathing with preferential use of the diaphragm. In normal breathing, the chest and abdomen move outward as the lungs expand. The chest wall expands because of the influence of the inspiratory intercostal muscles and the positive intra-abdominal pressure asserted on the rib cage where the diaphragm is in apposition to the chest wall. With preferential use of the chest wall muscles and disuse of the diaphragm, the chest wall moves outward and the abdomen sucks inward as the diaphragm moves passively into the chest in response to the negative pleural pressure. With preferential use of the diaphragm, greater outward movement of the abdomen compared with the chest takes place. The latter situation occurs in quadriplegic patients and in normal patients during rapid eye movement sleep. For clinical purposes, it is important to recognize paradoxical breathing because such a pattern indicates diaphragmatic muscle

Paradoxical pulse—an abnormally large fall in blood pressure during inspiration

Respiratory alternans—alternating use of the diaphragm and the chest wall muscles

Paradoxical breathing—the diaphragm ascends instead of descends during inspiration

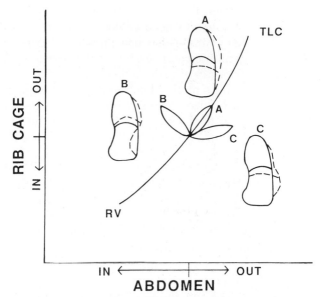

FIGURE 10–3: Konno-Mead diagram showing rib cage and abdominal movements in normal breathing (A), diaphragmatic paralysis (B), and preferential use of the diaphragm (C). The curved line from total lung capacity (TLC) to residual volume (RV) represents rib cage and abdominal movements during normal expiration. Normal breathing is situated along this line. Deviation from this line represents preferential use of the chest wall or the diaphragm. (Adapted from Fitting JW, Grassino A. Diagnosis of diaphragmatic dysfunction. Clin Chest Med 8[1]:91, 1987.)

weakness. To exclude paradoxical breathing, the breathing pattern is observed and the abdomen is palpated to detect abdominal muscle contraction during expiration. With diaphragmatic weakness, some patients aid inspiration by contracting the abdominal muscles during expiration, causing the diaphragm to move upward. During the subsequent inspiration, the abdominal wall relaxes, the diaphragm descends passively, and the abdominal wall moves outward. Thus, contraction of the abdominal muscles during expiration results in the appearance of a normal pattern of chest and abdominal movement, despite the absence of active diaphragmatic contraction.

Some investigators regard paradoxical breathing and respiratory alternans as signs of respiratory muscle fatigue and thus impending respiratory arrest.[13] However, Tobin and colleagues argue that these signs may represent a response to a high respiratory load and may not signal progressive respiratory deterioration.[14] All would agree, however, that these patterns of muscular recruitment represent an attempt to deal with potentially fatiguing loads. Patients using the respiratory muscles in this fashion must be observed closely for respiratory decompensation.

Other Signs of Respiratory Disease Evident on Inspection

Other physical signs of respiratory distress:

Speech difficulty
Patient leans forward
Pursed-lip breathing

Visual inspection of the patient can provide important clues about the presence and severity of underlying lung disease. Patients with severe respiratory impairment may hesitate while speaking in order to catch their breath. Those with severe chronic obstructive pulmonary disease tend to sit forward in their seat, so that the depressed diaphragm assumes a more advantageous configuration for contraction. These patients may also use pursed-lip breathing, which presumably prevents dynamic compression of the airways. Excessive CO_2 retention may produce a plethoric appearance of the skin owing to vascular dilatation, as well as papilledema and encephalopathy. Hypoxemia is difficult to diagnose with certainty on physical examination. Cyanosis depends on the color of the skin, perfusion, and the total quantity of desaturated hemoglobin. Thus, the presence or absence of peripheral cyanosis cannot prove or disprove the presence of hypoxemia.[15]

> The presence of central cyanosis indicates at least 5 g of desaturated hemoglobin.

Asymmetrical movement of the chest may be due to a bronchial obstruction, the presence of a pneumothorax, or a large pleural effusion. Although simple kyphosis or pectus deformities rarely result in respiratory insufficiency, the presence of kyphoscoliosis or a thoracoplasty should alert the physician to the possibility of respiratory failure due to restrictive lung disease. Although clubbing of the fingers may be a normal finding, this sign is frequently associated with suppurative lung disease and a variety of systemic disorders.

> Pulmonary osteoarthropathy—radiographic changes indicating subperiosteal new bone formation

When pulmonary osteoarthropathy exists, bronchogenic carcinoma is almost invariably present. Examination of the skin may reveal important underlying systemic disorders, such as sarcoidosis, metastatic disease, vasculitis, tuberculosis, or fungal disease.[16]

PALPATION

Palpation is often superior to inspection for detecting differences in expansion of the two lungs. Careful palpation of the ribs may provide the sole evidence of rib fracture because the radiographic findings may be minimal. The examiner may be able to detect subcutaneous emphysema because the compressible airspaces within the subcutaneous tissue elicit a sensation similar to that obtained by squeezing air-bubble packing material. Palpation can also be used to judge the use of accessory muscles and the use of abdominal muscles. Tenderness between ribs may be a sign of underlying empyema. Tactile fremitus is present when chest wall vibrations can be detected during vocalization. The chest wall can be made to vibrate when the frequency of transmitted sounds approximates the natural frequency of the chest wall structures. Hence, conditions that promote transmission of sound lead to tactile fremitus.

> Consolidation due to pneumonia may result in increased fremitus. Conditions that block transmission of sound, such as pleural disease or pneumothorax, prevent tactile fremitus.

PERCUSSION

Percussion can be used to detect the amount of air versus solid tissue underlying the chest wall. When the chest is percussed, it vibrates at its natural frequency, producing a low-pitched musical sound similar to that produced by striking a drum. Any solid tissue apposed to the chest wall dampens these oscillations, making the sound softer, higher pitched, and less musical.

> Percussion Sounds:
>
> Resonance is produced over normal lung.
> Hyper-resonance is produced over a hyperinflated chest.
> Tympany, the loudest and deepest sounds, occurs over large air-containing spaces such as lung abscesses and pneumothoraces.
> A dull sound occurs over consolidated lung or pleural effusions or when the chest wall is particularly muscular or adipose.
> The dullest sound, flatness, is produced over organs such as the heart and liver.

AUSCULTATION

Auscultation may provide important information about lung pathology. A variety of sounds can be heard at the mouth with the unaided ear and at the chest wall with the stethoscope. Past attempts to name these sounds have resulted in a chaotic classification, with little agreement on nomenclature and even less agreement on the physiologic mechanisms responsible for the production of these sounds. More recently, sound spectrograms have been used to classify sounds objectively, and attempts have been made to discern their physiologic significance. The following remarks describe the acoustic quality of these sounds and their presumed physiologic significance.

Sounds at the Mouth

Inspiratory sounds cannot be heard at the mouth in normal individuals. However, patients with airway obstruction produce noisy breathing. Forgacs showed that this sound is distributed over a wide range of frequencies and is characteristically white noise.[17] Because helium-oxygen mixtures attenuate this sound, turbulence within the airways seems to be the source.

In addition to harsh breath sounds, clicks can also be heard at the mouth in patients with chronic bronchitis. Forgacs attributes these sounds to the intermittent passage of air through lightly closed airways.[17] Wheezes may also be audible at the mouth, with the sound arising in the larynx or the lower airways.

Lung Sounds

Breath Sounds

Forgacs suggests that normal breath sounds originate from turbulent flow in the larger airways.[17] Sounds heard over the trachea are audible during inspiration and expiration and resemble white sound. The sounds heard over the chest using the stethoscope are of low frequency, since the lung acts as a low-pass filter, allowing only the lower-frequency sounds to be transmitted.

With normal breathing, inspiratory flow rates exceed those produced during expiration. Thus, the normal (vesicular) sound consists of a soft, low frequency inspiratory sound and little if any sound during expiration. With consolidation, the lung loses its filtering capacity and sounds of both high and low frequency transmit. A similar mechanism alters the transmission of sounds during vocalization.[19] Figure 10–4 shows the sound spectrograms of spoken sounds recorded over the chests of normal individuals and those with pneumonia. Air or fluid interposed between the lung and the chest wall blocks transmission of all sounds; no breath sounds can be heard with these conditions.

Adventitial Sounds

The confusing nomenclature of abnormal or added sounds has undergone considerable evolution in the last 10 years. Figure 10–5 describes the current nomenclature of adventitial sounds as provided by the American Thoracic Society.[20]

Crackles

Both Loudon and Murphy[21] and Forgacs[22] have reviewed the characteristics as well as the physiologic basis of crackles. Sound spectro-

White noise or sound—no constant waveforms, frequencies are random

Normal breath sound—only an inspiratory sound of low frequency can be discerned, the so-called vesicular sound

With pneumonia, breath sounds can be heard during both inspiration and expiration, with the sound distinctly higher in pitch than the normal vesicular sound. These are termed bronchial breath sounds.

Transmission of the higher frequencies causes "e" to sound like "a" (egophony).
Sounds corresponding to "9-9-9" transmit more faithfully (bronchophony and whispered pectoriloquy).

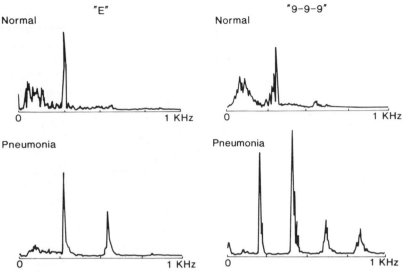

FIGURE 10–4: Sound spectrograms of spoken sounds in normal and consolidated lung. Consolidation transmits the higher frequencies, causing "e" to sound like "a" and allowing "9-9-9" to be reproduced more faithfully. (From Baughman RP, Loudon RG. Sound spectral analysis of voice-transmitted sound. Am Rev Respir Dis 134:167, 1986.)

Crackles—discontinuous sounds of short duration

grams show crackles to be discontinuous sounds of short duration. Forgacs attributes crackles to the explosive sounds produced by the sudden equalization of pressures as airways pop open.[22] Thus, crackles can be heard under any condition with lung deflation or too early airway closure. These sounds can therefore be heard in normal individuals after expiration to residual volume and in abnormal conditions such as interstitial fibrosis, atelectasis, and congestive heart failure.[23] In congestive heart failure, gravity-dependent crackles can be made to change location with positional changes. The sounds are heard during inspiration, especially at maximal lung capacity. Nath and Capel note that crackles also occur in patients with chronic obstructive lung disease.[24] However, in these patients, the crackles occur early in inspiration rather than at the end of inspiration. These authors attribute the early crackles to the opening of larger airways that remained closed after the preceding inspiration.

Wheezes

Wheezes—longer than crackles, with most of the energy contained in harmonically related frequencies

Wheezes differ from crackles by their musical quality: that is, instead of being discontinuous sounds of short duration, these sounds are longer, with most of the energy contained in harmonically related frequencies. Forgacs attributes wheezing to vibrations of airway walls that are nearly in apposition, a mechanism similar to that of a reed instrument.[22] Crackles and wheezes may occur concurrently when airway walls oscillate just before opening.

Although wheezing is often equated with diffuse airway obstruction, it can occur under any condition characterized by airway narrowing:

- Airway smooth muscle contraction
- Bronchial mucosal inflammation
- Tumors
- Foreign bodies
- External compression by lymph nodes or tumors

Acoustic Characteristics	Wave Form	Recommended Term	Associated Clinical Conditions
Discontinuous, loud explosive sound	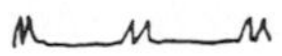 ⌇⌇⌇	Coarse Crackle	Pulmonary edema, Pneumonia
Discontinuous, softer explosive sound	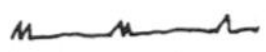 ⌇⌇⌇	Fine Crackle	Interstitial fibrosis
Continuous sound, high pitched frequency	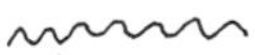 ∿∿∿	Wheeze	Airway narrowing
Continuous sound, low pitched frequency	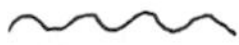 ∿∿	Rhonchus	Airway secretions

FIGURE 10–5: Nomenclature of adventitial sounds as proposed by the American Thoracic Society Ad Hoc Committee on Pulmonary Nomenclature. The acoustic characteristics represent time-expanded waveforms. (From ATS News, 16:8, 1981.)

Wheezing may also occur normally during forced expiration with dynamic compression of the airways. The significance of a wheeze can be determined by noting whether the wheeze is localized or diffuse and whether forced expiration is required to elicit the sound.

Stridor

Stridor—a loud musical sound of constant pitch

Stridor denotes upper airway obstruction. Because the upper airways tend to collapse further during inspiration, the sound is particularly loud during this phase of respiration. Confusion sometimes occurs in patients with asthma when wheezes transmit to the larynx. Similarly, stridor can transmit to the chest and simulate asthma. The distinguishing characteristics of stridor include its particular intensity during inspiration rather than during expiration and its relative localization to the upper airway. It is important to recognize stridor because upper airway obstruction may result in large increases in airway resistance and respiratory work, as well as increase the potential for respiratory muscle fatigue and arrest.

Rhonchi

Rhonchi—a continuous sound of longer duration and lower frequency than a wheeze

An American Thoracic Society panel distinguished rhonchi from wheezes by differences in sound frequency and duration.[20] The consensus was that a rhonchus, like a wheeze, has a continuous sound. However, the rhonchus had a longer duration (250 milliseconds) and a lower dominant frequency (200 versus 400 Hz). The panel described a rhonchus as a snoring sound attributable to airway secretions. Loudon and Murphy[21] and Forgacs[22] do not distinguish rhonchi from wheezes.

Pleural Friction Rubs

Pleural friction rub—a creaking or grating sound, persistant after cough

The basis of pleural friction rubs is unknown; they have been hypothesized to arise from roughened pleural surfaces rubbing against one another. The sounds, described as grating or creaking, tend to be loudest during inspiration but are frequently heard during expiration as well. To detect the rub, the examiner listens at the lower lateral and anterior chest walls. Although these sounds are sometimes confused with low-pitched, continuous sounds arising from airway secretions, pleural friction rubs can be differentiated from such sounds by their persistence after coughing.

Mediastinal crunch—a crunch heard over the heart

Mediastinal Crunch

Mediastinal crunch, a sound heard over the heart, during each heart beat, is a sign of mediastinal emphysema. This sign is more sensitive than chest radiography in detecting anterior air collections.

CARDIAC EXAMINATION

This chapter cannot give a complete description of the cardiac examination. However, attention will be paid to evaluating right ventricular function, which can be altered as a result of lung disease.

Acute right ventricular dilatation and failure may follow a sudden increase in afterload, such as after acute pulmonary embolism. Disorders affecting the pulmonary capillary bed, such as emphysema, alveolar hypoxia, or interstitial disease, lead to a chronic increase in afterload and right ventricular hypertrophy. Physical examination may aid in the diagnosis of these right ventricular disorders.

Inspection can provide information on right-sided pressures. The venous pulsations in the right internal jugular vein should be observed because this vein with no valves communicates directly with the right atrium. By noting the level of pulsations above the sternal angle, right ventricular filling pressure can be estimated. Although most books on cardiology describe several waves within this pulsation, normally all that can be discerned is a rippling appearance of the vessel. In patients with pulmonary hypertension, the A wave may appear prominent because of the subsequent rapid fall in atrial pressure due to a vigorously contracting right ventricle. A very prominent V wave results from tricuspid regurgitation due to right ventricular dilatation.

A palpable impulse in the pulmonic area suggests pulmonary arterial enlargement. A sustained thrust along the left sternal area indicates right ventricular hypertrophy. Right ventricular enlargement due to hypertrophy and dilatation results in a diffuse lift across the left precordium, with the entire left ventricle being located posteriorly.

The intensity and timing of splitting of the second heart sound provide important information related to the presence of pulmonary hypertension. The aortic and pulmonary closure sounds occur when pressures in the aortic and pulmonary arteries exceed pressures in the left and right ventricles, respectively. Normally, pulmonic closure is delayed relative to aortic closure because of the lesser pressure in the pulmonary circulation. With increasing right-sided impedance, the pulmonary valve closes sooner, the split narrows, and the intensity of the pulmonic sound increases.

Prominent pulsations caused by A waves correspond to atrial contraction.
    V waves occur at the end of systole, corresponding to the increased atrial pressure as the atrial wall stiffens and filling slows.

Conventionally, right ventricular filling pressure is taken as the vertical distance between the angle of Louis and the top of the venous pulsation. The upper normal level is considered to be 4.5 cm. If 5 cm is added, one can then estimate right atrial pressure.

DIAGNOSIS OF CONDITIONS ASSOCIATED WITH DYSPNEA

Patients frequently present to the physician acutely ill, with the sole complaint of dyspnea. Often, diagnostic pulmonary function tests cannot be performed in such individuals, and treatment is guided by a tentative diagnosis suggested by physical examination.

Obstructive Lung Disease

Patients with obstructive lung disease, particularly those with emphysema, usually appear to be struggling to breathe. The vigor of their respiratory effort belies the previously held notion that many such patients have a decreased respiratory drive. If one listens at the mouth, especially in patients with chronic bronchitis, inspiratory harsh sounds and noisy breathing due to excess turbulence of airflow in the larger airways can be discerned.[17] In such individuals, dynamic compression of airways may occur during normal breathing. Clicks can be heard at the mouth; they represent the opening of airways that were closed during the previous expiration. Auscultation may reveal a variety of sounds. In cases of emphysema, often no breath sounds can be heard because sound does not transmit through the hyperinflated lung. In patients with chronic bronchitis, early inspiratory crackles representing the opening of the larger airways can be heard. Wheezes, which are also common, reflect the fact that some airway walls are in apposition consequent to bronchoconstriction, airway inflammation, or excess secretions.

Asthma

Patients with acute asthma may have a clinical presentation similar to that of patients with exacerbations of chronic obstructive pulmonary disease. Wheezes are present to a variable extent. Baughman and Loudon showed that severe asthma is associated with wheezes of higher pitch and longer duration.[25, 26] Signs of severe asthma also include

- Decreased breath sounds
- The presence of pulsus paradoxus
- A pulse rate of greater than 130 beats per minute
- Hyperinflation
- The use of accessory muscles
- Diaphoresis
- Preference by the patient for the upright position[27]

Acute Pulmonary Edema

Patients with acute pulmonary edema may also appear to be struggling to breathe. However, unlike the patient with obstructive airway disease, who is warm and flushed, the patient with pulmonary edema is frequently cool because of a low cardiac output and peripheral vasoconstriction. Auscultation reveals wet gurgling sounds rather than the explosive crackles more characteristic of obstructive and restrictive disorders. Wheezing may also occur, obscuring other sounds. If heart sounds can be discerned above the background lung sounds, a gallop rhythm is frequently heard.

Pulmonary Vascular Disease

The hallmark of pulmonary vascular disease is the disparity between symptoms and physical signs of lung disease. Patients with pulmonary embolism may present with severe dyspnea and normal chest findings. The dyspnea in such patients has been attributed to the discharge of rapidly adapting receptors.[28] Such stimulation may give rise to a rapid respiratory rate with low tidal volumes. A cardiac examination may reveal evidence of right ventricular dilatation. Occasionally, a pleural rub can be heard despite the nearly normal chest radiographic findings.

Neuromuscular Disease

Some patients with neuromuscular disease complain of dyspnea, but the findings on physical examination of the chest appear normal. The only clue to the underlying diagnosis may be generalized weakness, in particular weakness of the respiratory muscles. Measurements of maximal respiratory pressures may be difficult to obtain because of weakness of the facial muscles and the consequent inability to maintain a seal around the mouthpiece. In such situations, testing of the accessory muscles of respiration may provide the best evidence of respiratory muscle weakness. Typically, the patient cannot raise his or her head off the pillow, and testing of the neck muscles reveals obvious weakness.

Unilateral diaphragmatic paralysis may occur from cardiac surgery, particularly after coronary bypass surgery. This can occur when the left phrenic nerve comes in contact with ice used during cardioplegia. Loh and colleagues have described the physical signs associated with diaphragmatic dysfunction.[29] Patients with unilateral diaphragmatic paralysis may exhibit excessive utilization of intercostal or accessory muscles and the use of abdominal muscles during expiration. Fluoroscopy may reveal paradoxical movements of the diaphragms, with the paretic diaphragm rising as the noninvolved diaphragm descends during inspiration and sniffing. The patient is instructed to sniff because this maneuver results in maximal diaphragmatic contraction. Bilateral diaphragmatic paralysis may be more difficult to diagnose radiographically because both diaphragms move synchronously. The radiologist will have difficulty timing diaphragmatic movement with the phase of respiration.

Physical examination may be particularly helpful under these circumstances. Such patients may be totally intolerant of the supine position; patients may also have obvious paradoxical breathing.

SUMMARY

With the advent of modern technology, the nature of abnormal structure and function can be fully delineated. In such a technologically advanced environment, the persistence of the physical examination as a phenomenologically based exercise is untenable. The physical examination retains its usefulness only to the extent that it helps us to understand and clarify the nature of disease processes. Because the pace of the research efforts in this area is encouraging, the physical examination will have an even greater impact on the care of patients as it becomes more firmly based on physiologic understanding.

References

1. Laennec RTH. De l'Auscultation Mediate au Traite du Diagnostic des Maladies des Pneumnons et du Coeur, Fonde Principalement sur ce Nouveau Moyen d'Exploration. Paris, JR Broussou et JS Chaudri, 1819.
2. Wilkins RL, Sheldon RL, Krider SJ. Clinical Assessment in Respiratory Care. St. Louis, CV Mosby, 1985, p 43.
3. Hoff HE, Breckenridge CG. The medullary origin of respiratory periodicity in the dog. Am J Physiol 158:157, 1949.

4. Wang SC, Ngai SH, Frumin MJ. Organization of central respiratory mechanisms in the brain stem of the cat: Genesis of normal respiratory rhythmicity. Am J Physiol 190:333, 1957.
5. Bradley GW, Von Euler C, Martilla I, Roos B. A model of the central and reflex inhibition of respiration in the cat. Biol Cybern 19:106, 1975.
6. Millman RP, Fishman AP. Sleep apnea syndrome. *In* Fishman AP (ed). Pulmonary Diseases and Disorders, 2nd ed. New York, McGraw-Hill Book Company, 1988, p 1347.
7. Knowles GK, Clark TJH. Pulsus paradoxus as a valuable sign indicating severity of asthma. Lancet 2:1356, 1973.
8. Cherniak NS, Milic-Emili J. Mechanical aspects of loaded breathing. *In* Roussos C, Macklem PT (eds). Thorax, Part B. New York, Marcel Dekker, 1985, p 751.
9. Campbell EJM, Howell JBL. Sensation of breathlessness. Br Med Bull 19:36, 1963.
10. De Troyer A. The mechanism of the inspiratory expansion of the rib cage. J Lab Clin Med 2:97, 1989.
11. Roussos C, Fixley M, Gross D, Macklem PT. Fatigue of inspiratory muscles and their synergic behavior. J Appl Physiol Respir Environ Exercise Physiol 46:897, 1979.
12. Konno K, Mead J. Measurement of the separate volume changes of rib cage and abdomen during breathing. J Appl Physiol 22:407, 1967.
13. Cohen CA, Zagelbaum G, Gross MD, et al. Clinical manifestations of inspiratory muscle fatigue. Am J Med 73:308, 1982.
14. Tobin MJ, Perez W, Guenther SM, et al. The pattern of breathing during successful and unsuccessful trials of weaning from mechanical ventilation. Am Rev Respir Dis 134:1111, 1986.
15. Martin L, Khalil H. How much reduced hemoglobin is necessary to generate central cyanosis? Chest 97:182, 1990.
16. Jegasothy BY, Sherertz EF. Pulmonary cutaneous disorders. *In* Fishman AP (ed). Pulmonary Diseases and Disorders, 2nd ed. New York, McGraw-Hill Book Company, 1988, p 367.
17. Forgacs P. The functional significance of clinical signs in diffuse airway obstruction. Br J Dis Chest 65:170, 1971.
18. Banaszak EF, Kory RC, Snider GL. Phonopneumography. Am Rev Respir Dis 107:449, 1973.
19. Baughman RP, Loudon RG. Sound spectral analysis of voice-transmitted sound. Am Rev Respir Dis 134:167, 1986.
20. American Thoracic Society Ad Hoc Committee on Pulmonary Nomenclature. Updated nomenclature for membership reaction. ATS News, 16:8, 1981.
21. Loudon R, Murphy RIIL Jr. Lung sounds. Am Rev Respir Dis 130:663, 1984.
22. Forgacs P. The functional basis of pulmonary sounds. Chest 73:399, 1978.
23. Workum P, Holford SK, Murphy RLH. The prevalence and character of crackles (rales) in young women without significant lung disease. Am Rev Respir Dis 126:921, 1982.
24. Nath AR, Capel LH. Inspiratory crackles—Early and late. Thorax 29:223, 1974.
25. Baughman RP, Loudon RG. Quantitation of wheezing in acute asthma. Chest 86:718, 1984.
26. Baughman RP, Loudon RG. Lung sound analysis for continuous evaluation of airflow obstruction in asthma. Chest 88:364, 1985.
27. Brenner BE. Bronchial asthma in adults: Presentation in the emergency department. Part 1: Pathogenesis, clinical manifestations, diagnostic evaluation, and differential diagnosis. Am J Emerg Med 1:50, 1983.
28. Mills J, Sellick H, Widdicombe JG. The role of lung irritant receptors in respiratory responses to multiple pulmonary embolism, anaphylaxis and histamine-induced bronchoconstriction. J Physiol (Lond) 203:337, 1969.
29. Loh L, Goldman M, Newsom Davis J. The assessment of diaphragm function. Medicine 56:165, 1977.

11

Conventional Chest Radiography

Paul W. Burrowes, M.D., and Carl E. Ravin, M.D.

Conventional chest radiography is a powerful and essential tool for accurate evaluation of the thorax. The information provided by this readily available, relatively inexpensive, low-risk procedure is almost unparalleled. The chest radiograph provides critical insight into intrathoracic pathology; when applied in appropriate situations and the findings are interpreted correctly, it is often diagnostically specific. In situations in which specificity is not possible, it is very often possible to construct a limited differential that will guide subsequent evaluation in an efficient manner. The contributions of conventional chest radiography to the assessment of the thorax are so consistent that this examination has clearly become the cornerstone for evaluation of the chest.

AIRSPACE DISEASES

The airspaces of the lung parenchyma are normally radiolucent structures; however, when they are filled with edema, pus, blood, or tumor cells, they become opacified. When gas is removed from the alveolar airspaces, as in atelectasis, a parenchymal opacity may also be created.

The first step in radiographic interpretation of an airspace opacity is to confirm that it lies in the lung parenchyma and not in the pleura, the extrapleural soft tissues, or the bones. Two radiologic signs, the "silhouette sign" and the "air bronchogram," may help to localize a radiographic opacity. The mediastinum, the heart, the diaphragm, and vascular shadows in the lung are all rendered radiographically visible owing to contrast with contiguous aerated lung. If the contiguous lung becomes opacified from any cause, the normal contrast between these structures is lost and the border between them is obliterated—the silhouette sign.[1] Perhaps the best known example of this phenomenon is loss of demarcation of the right heart border by an adjacent middle lobe pneumonia (Fig. 11–1). If vascular shadows within the lung are silhouetted, this localizes an opacity to the lung parenchyma. An air bronchogram occurs when the alveolar airspaces become filled with fluid, causing increased contrast between the air-filled bronchi and adjacent fluid-filled lung parenchyma. This renders the bronchi lucent, projecting them as branching tubular air-filled structures (Fig. 11–2). An airspace abnormality not causing an air bronchogram or not obscuring vascular structures may be pleural or extrapleural in origin.

Once the opacity has been localized to the lung parenchyma, further differentiation between the various potential causes requires careful evaluation of the entire radiograph, with attention given to the distribution of the disease, the evolution of the abnormality over time, and correlation with available clinical information. In a postoperative patient, for example, an abnormality localized only to the dependent portions of the lung may suggest a diagnosis of aspiration pneumonia. How-

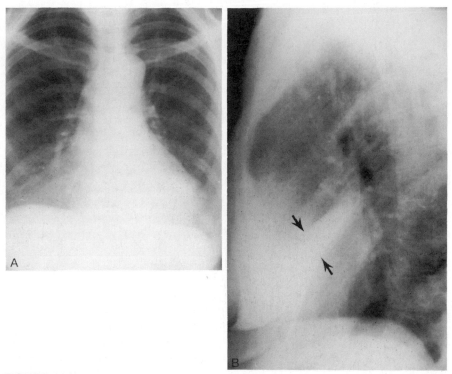

FIGURE 11–1: Silhouette sign. *A,* Posteroanterior radiograph demonstrates obliteration of the border of the right side of the heart and preservation of the silhouette of the right hemidiaphragm. Slightly increased opacity is noted adjacent to the border of the right side of the heart, but this is not nearly as prominent an observation as the obliteration of the heart border itself. This constellation of findings indicates consolidation in the right middle lobe. *B,* Lateral view of the chest demonstrates a characteristic wedge-shaped opacity projected over the heart. The sharp inferior margin *(arrow)* reflects the anteriorly displaced major fissure, whereas the sharp superior border *(arrow)* represents the inferiorly displaced minor fissure. These findings are characteristic of right middle lobe collapse.

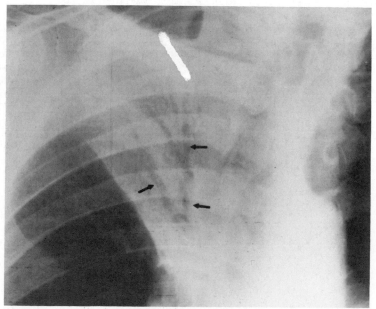

FIGURE 11–2: Air bronchogram. Branching lucencies *(arrows)* representing air-filled bronchi within an otherwise airless collapsed right upper lobe are known as "air bronchograms."

ever, a peripheral wedge-shaped opacity in the lower lobes would be more suggestive of a pulmonary infarct. In differentiating atelectasis from pneumonia, examination of serial radiographs is often invaluable because atelectasis may appear and disappear rapidly, whereas pneumonias generally take days or weeks to resolve.

Atelectasis

Atelectasis most commonly occurs secondary to interruption of the normal communication between the alveoli and the trachea. This frequently follows mucous plugging, but other causes, such as an obstructing tumor, should always be considered if atelectasis persists. If small airways obstruct, subsegmental opacities result that are often described as "discoid" or "plate-like" in appearance. Frequently seen in postsurgical patients at the lung bases, they appear as thin linear horizontal or obliquely oriented opacities (Fig. 11–3). Obstruction of large airways, on the other hand, may result in lobar atelectasis, most commonly involving the left lower lobe (66%) or the right lower lobe (22%).[2] Involvement of the left lower lobe is particularly common after cardiac surgery due to paresis of the phrenic nerve from stretching or cold cardioplegia.[3]

Although commonly a cause of a focal parenchymal opacity, the displacement of an interlobar fissure is the only direct roentgenographic sign of atelectasis that truly confirms loss of lung volume (Fig. 11–4).

Distinguishing atelectasis from pneumonia may be difficult and at times impossible, often requiring corroborative clinical information and follow-up radiographs. In comparison to pneumonia, atelectasis may appear and clear very rapidly. Air bronchograms can be seen with pneumonia or atelectasis, although they are classically absent in atelectasis secondary to obstruction. Absence of an air bronchogram in an area of persistent atelectasis may therefore be helpful because therapeutic bronchoscopy may relieve the obstruction if it is due to mucous plugging.

Atelectasis—loss of lung volume

Causes of atelectasis:

- Mucous plugging
- Obstructing tumor
- Loss of surfactant
- Compression of the lung by an adjacent space-occupying lesion
- Scarring

Indirect signs of atelectasis include hemidiaphragmatic elevation, displacement of the mediastinum or hilum, and compensatory overinflation of the remainder of the ipsilateral lung.

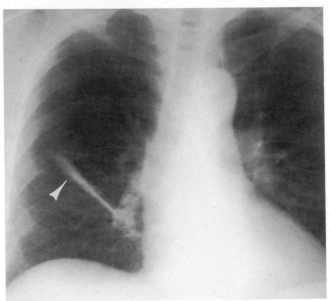

FIGURE 11–3: Discoid atelectasis. Characteristic obliquely oriented linear opacity *(arrowhead)* represents subsegmental discoid atelectasis.

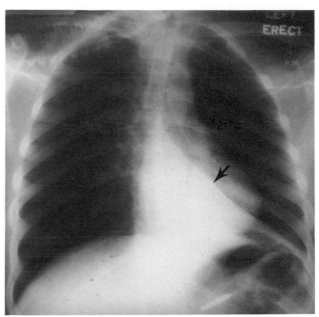

FIGURE 11–4: Left lower lobe collapse. Characteristic triangular opacity projected through the heart. The sharp lateral border *(arrow)* represents the displaced left major fissure. Note also the mild elevation of the left hemidiaphragm and the downward displacement of the left hilum, consistent with left lower lobe collapse.

Pneumonia

Pneumonia can cause a wide variety of abnormalities on the chest radiograph, resulting in segmental or lobar homogeneous opacities or scattered nonsegmental "fluffy" opacities. At times, an extensive and diffuse airspace process results. Importantly, in pneumonia, as opposed to in atelectasis, lung volume is generally preserved, and findings persist for days to weeks. Air bronchograms may or may not be present (Fig. 11–5). Associated pleural effusions may occur.

Pneumonia proves to be particularly difficult to diagnose in the intensive care unit because superimposed cardiopulmonary processes are frequently involved, such as chronic obstructive pulmonary disease, heart failure, and the adult respiratory distress syndrome. A new focal parenchymal opacity in these patients may be secondary to atelectasis, pulmonary infarct, hemorrhage, or pneumonia. Correlation with additional clinical and laboratory information is important, along with evaluation on serial radiographs.

Aspiration pneumonia is a major cause of pneumonia in hospitalized patients, especially in the intensive care unit. Factors predisposing to aspiration include

- Reduced level of consciousness
- Esophageal disorders
- Tracheostomy
- Endotracheal tube intubation
- Interference with function of the cardiac sphincter by a nasogastric tube[4–6]

Another factor to consider in aspiration is the common use of antacids

The distribution of aspiration pneumonia often helps to arrive at the diagnosis: supine patients have a predilection for the posterior segments of the upper lobes and the superior segments of the lower lobes—the dependent regions of the lung.

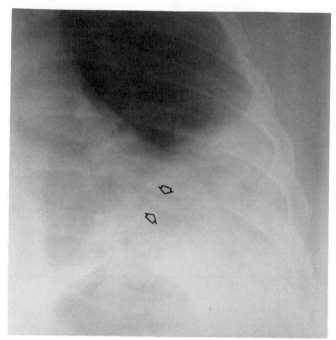

FIGURE 11–5: Left lower lobe pneumonia. Note the patchy consolidation obliterating the silhouette of the left hemidiaphragm while preserving the silhouette of the border of the left side of the heart and thus confirming the left lower lobe location. Faint air bronchograms *(open arrows)* are seen within the area of consolidation.

and drugs to reduce gastric acid production in order to prevent stress ulcers in intensive care patients, which is known to increase the bacterial colonization of the stomach because of increasing pH.[7, 8]

Occasionally, a necrotizing pneumonia, a lung abscess, or empyema may result after aspiration.[5] On plain chest radiographs, it may be difficult to differentiate a cavitated lung abscess from empyema with bronchopleural fistula. Evaluation of an air-fluid level, if present, may help to distinguish between the two: the length of the air-fluid level in a lung abscess is equal on frontal and lateral projections (Fig. 11–6), whereas in empyema, the pleural space air-fluid level usually is much longer in one projection than in the other (Fig. 11–7). At times, evaluation with computed tomography may be necessary to differentiate these two entities.[9, 10]

Pulmonary Edema

Pulmonary edema, the most common diffuse process seen on chest radiographs in the intensive care unit, is classically divided into cardiogenic and noncardiogenic causes (Fig. 11–8). Distinguishing the various causes of edema from a chest radiograph may be impossible because frequently more than one mechanism is involved.

Milne and coworkers, however, have outlined several helpful discriminating criteria.[11] In capillary permeability edema, edema is often peripherally, not gravitationally, distributed. Furthermore, the heart size is often normal, and there is usually an absence of peribronchial cuffing and septal lines. In contrast, edema due to increased hydrostatic

Noncardiogenic causes of pulmonary edema:

- Neurogenic
- Near drowning
- Overhydration
- Capillary permeability

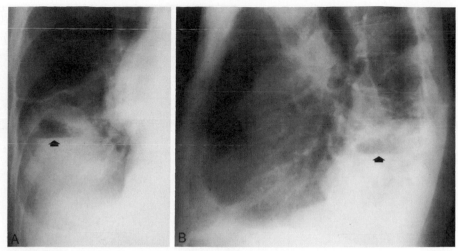

FIGURE 11–6: Lung abscess. Note the air-fluid levels *(arrows)* within an area of consolidation in the right lower lobe on both frontal *(A)* and lateral *(B)* projections. The lengths of the air-fluid levels on both projections are approximately equal, strongly suggesting an intraparenchymal location consistent with lung abscess.

pressure is often visible in connective tissue around the vessels and airways, presenting as peribronchial cuffing and blurring of vascular margins, and in the interlobar septa, presenting as septal lines. The distribution in an upright patient, unlike that seen in capillary permeability edema, is gravitationally affected, involving the lower lobes first. Other than in the acute setting, the heart size generally enlarges in hydrostatic edema. In renal failure or fluid overload, the heart size may be enlarged, with the distribution of pulmonary blood flow equalized between the upper and lower lobes but without the upper lobe redistribution seen in hydrostatic edema. Pleural fluid commonly appears in hydrostatic edema and in fluid overload, but it is uncommon in capillary permeability edema.

Several factors, however, complicate the diagnosis of pulmonary edema. Findings on low-volume films may mimic pulmonary edema (Fig. 11–9). The differences between supine and upright positioning must also

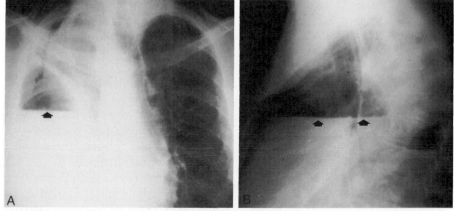

FIGURE 11–7: Empyema. Note the air-fluid levels *(arrows)* on the frontal *(A)* and lateral *(B)* projections. In this situation, the air-fluid level is much longer in one dimension than in the other, reflecting the configuration of the pleural space and strongly suggesting empyema.

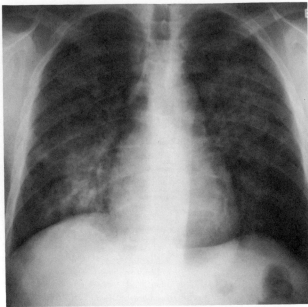

FIGURE 11–8: Noncardiogenic pulmonary edema. Note the patchy opacities on the lungs that are symmetrically distributed bilaterally, consistent with pulmonary edema. The heart size is normal. The patient was a victim of near drowning.

be recognized. Pulmonary vascular redistribution to the upper lobes, a useful sign of left ventricular failure in the upright position, becomes a normal finding in the recumbent position. Moreover, if the patient has been supine, because of the loss of gravitational effect, edema may not first present in the lower lobes. In patients with emphysema or pulmonary emboli, edema is often asymmetrical, occurring only where relatively normal perfusion exists.

The adult respiratory distress syndrome (ARDS) is a specific clinical syndrome caused by diffuse lung injury from a variety of pulmonary and nonpulmonary conditions. Pleural effusions and septal lines may occur but are uncommon.[11] The pulmonary abnormality often persists for weeks or months, with 20% of survivors showing permanent radiographic abnormalities.[12]

Because of the high ventilatory pressures often required in patients with ARDS, close monitoring is particularly important for detecting complications of barotrauma, such as pulmonary interstitial emphysema, pneumomediastinum, and pneumothorax.[13–15]

ARDS:

- Capillary permeability edema
- Decreased lung compliance
- Severe hypoxemia
- Widespread pulmonary parenchymal opacities[12]

Pulmonary Embolism

Patients in the intensive care unit are particularly prone to deep venous thrombosis and pulmonary embolism because of increased age, congestive heart failure, and other causes of low-flow states, as well as prolonged immobilization.

In most patients with pulmonary embolism, chest radiographic findings will be abnormal.[16] However, the findings are generally nonspecific and may be difficult to appreciate in a pre-existent abnormal chest radiograph. The most common findings are plate-like or discoid atelectasis, peripheral airspace consolidation, and pleural effusion. Other, less com-

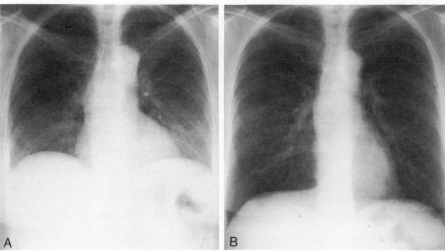

FIGURE 11–9: Expiration film mimicking pulmonary edema. *A,* A film exposed at a low lung volume demonstrates apparently increased opacity of the lung bases and indistinctness of the vessel markings in this area, suggesting mild pulmonary edema. Some redistribution of pulmonary blood flow to the upper lung zones is also noted. *B,* In the same patient, a film exposed at total lung capacity shows entirely normal findings. This comparison illustrates that films exposed at low lung volumes may mimic the radiographic findings of pulmonary edema.

Hampton's hump is characterized by a well-defined wedge-shaped opacity abutting the pleura, with the convex medial margin directed toward the hilum.

mon abnormalities are enlargement of one or both pulmonary arteries secondary to large emboli, signs of right-sided heart failure, hemidiaphragm elevation, and focal oligemia (Westermark's sign) (Fig. 11–10).[17] The so-called Hampton's hump described in association with pulmonary infarction is seen infrequently. Emboli in the ambulatory patient are more frequent in the lower lobes owing to increased blood flow in this region. However, this does not apply to patients in the intensive care unit, in whom emboli more characteristically involve the posterior segments of both upper and lower lobes because of supine positioning.[18]

Radionuclide ventilation-perfusion scanning is currently the only noninvasive modality with documented sensitivity and specificity in the diagnosis of pulmonary embolism. This test not only establishes the relative probability of pulmonary embolism but also may serve as a guide if pulmonary angiography is considered. The most common indication for pulmonary angiography is a "moderate" or "indeterminate" interpretation of a ventilation-perfusion scan.[19] However, an increasing number of angiographic studies are being performed to confirm pulmonary embolism before invasive therapeutic measures, such as embolectomy or thrombolytic infusion therapy, are undertaken. Computed tomography and magnetic resonance imaging have been performed in selected patients with pulmonary emboli, but more work is required to establish the appropriate use of these modalities.[18]

Radiographic resolution of pulmonary emboli varies and depends on the presence and size of actual lung necrosis. With complete infarction, the parenchymal opacity may resolve in weeks to months, with residual linear scarring or focal pleural thickening.[20] Without infarction, resolution usually occurs within several weeks, often without residual abnormality. With pulmonary embolism, unlike with pneumonia, resolution tends to occur from the periphery: this has been likened to the melting of an ice cube. Occasionally, cavitation from either ischemic necrosis or infection may occur during the course of resolution.

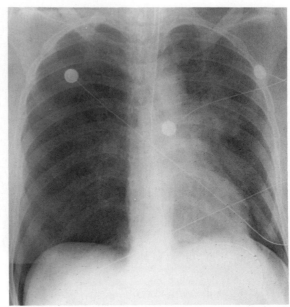

FIGURE 11–10: Westermark's sign of pulmonary embolism. There is pulmonary edema involving the left lung. The right lung is relatively clear, and the right-sided vascular markings are decreased in overall size, reflecting oligemia. The lucency of the right lung is increased.

EXTRA-ALVEOLAR AIR

Recognition of extra-alveolar air is of critical importance in thoracic imaging. "Extra-alveolar" air includes pneumothorax, pneumomediastinum, and interstitial emphysema. Each is characterized by a distinctive radiographic appearance.

Pneumothorax

The radiographic diagnosis of pneumothorax is established by identification of the "visceral pleural line" (Fig. 11–11). This thin white line represents the visceral pleura visualized between air in the pleural space laterally and air in the aerated lung medially. Although other radiographic features, including the absence of vascular markings and increased lucency in the hemithorax, are occasionally suggestive of pneumothorax, they are often misleading. Thus, the specific diagnosis of pneumothorax generally requires identification of the visceral pleural line. Visualization of the visceral pleura can be enhanced by exposing the film in expiration. With expiration, the volume of the pneumothorax remains constant, whereas the volume of the hemithorax in which it is contained is reduced; therefore, the pneumothorax occupies proportionately more of the hemithorax, facilitating visualization. Perhaps of more importance is that the orientation of the visceral pleural line relative to the overlying ribs is often changed by exposure in expiration, again facilitating visualization. A skinfold (Fig. 11–12) may mimic the visceral pleural line, but whereas the visceral pleural line is a thin line with air on both sides, a skinfold is represented as an interface in which one edge is sharp but the medial edge gradually fades away.[21]

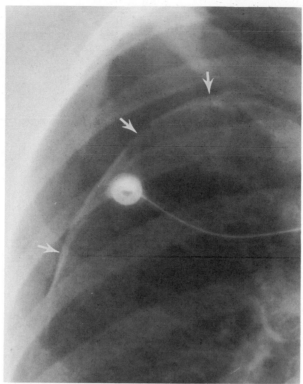

FIGURE 11–11: Pneumothorax. The visceral pleural line *(arrows)* is clearly identified between air in the pleural space laterally and air in the lung medially. (From Chiles C, Ravin CE. Radiographic recognition of pneumothorax in the intensive care unit. Crit Care Med 14(8):677–680, 1986.)

In patients radiographed in the supine position, pneumothorax will have quite a different radiographic appearance.

In patients radiographed in the upright position, free air in the pleural space generally collects over the apex of the lung. Most clinicians have been trained to look for air in this location when they suspect pneumothorax. In patients in the supine position, the highest portion of the thorax is generally the anterior costophrenic sulcus. Air free within the pleural space rises to this position, projecting over the upper abdomen and diaphragm. This results in a distinctive radiographic appearance that has been referred to as the "deep sulcus sign"[22] of pneumothorax in the supine position (Fig. 11–13). If the pneumothorax is on the left side, the apex of the heart and the pericardial fat pad will often be sharply outlined. In addition, the edge of the lung and the visceral pleural line may also be identified. In the supine projection, however, it is critically important to recognize the deep sulcus and increased lucency over the upper abdomen because direct visualization of the visceral pleura in this projection is often difficult.

In patients in the supine position, fluid free in the pleural space will layer posteriorly. Significant amounts of fluid create a generalized increased opacity over the affected hemithorax. When there is associated free air (i.e., hydropneumothorax) in a supine projection, the ability to visualize the pneumothorax depends on the relative amounts of air and fluid.[23] If sufficient air is present within the pleural space to outline the pleura laterally, a sharp pleural line can be visualized (Fig. 11–14). If the quantity of air is relatively small and the quantity of fluid is relatively large, the lateral portion of the lung may not be visualized and no pleural line will be identified. The presence of an associated pneumo-

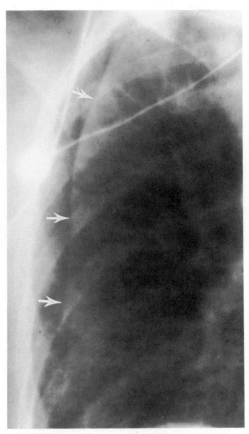

FIGURE 11–12: Skinfold mimicking pneumothorax. With a skinfold, an interface *(arrows)* is created rather than an actual line. There is a gradual fading from a sharp lateral margin medially. No distinct line is identified. The appearance may strongly mimic pneumothorax. (From Chiles C, Ravin CE. Radiographic recognition of pneumothorax in the intensive care unit. Crit Care Med 14(8):677–680, 1986.)

thorax in this setting would be evident only on an upright or a decubitus film.

Although it is often difficult to have critically ill patients radiographed in the upright position, decubitus films can be obtained in this population. Appropriate decubitus projects allow confirmation of the presence of either air or fluid free in the pleural space if their presence is suspected from conventional views.

Interstitial Emphysema

The pathophysiology of extra-alveolar air generally begins with the rupture of distal alveoli into the interstitial space and the subsequent dissection of air back toward the mediastinum or occasionally directly into the pleural space.

Radiographic recognition of this early stage of extra-alveolar air, pulmonary interstitial emphysema, is possible.[24] In general, air dissects along bronchovascular bundles, producing a very characteristic appear-

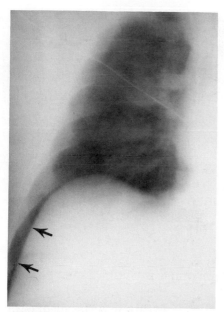

FIGURE 11–13: Deep sulcus sign of a pneumothorax. With the patient in the supine position, air will selectively collect in the anterior costophrenic sulcus, creating a "deep sulcus sign" *(arrows)*. This is characterized by increased lucency over the upper abdomen and the appearance of a deep costophrenic sulcus on the affected side.

ance of a pulmonary vessel surrounded by air (Fig. 11–15). The radiographic recognition of this frequently portends impending pneumothorax, pneumomediastinum, or both. The radiographic appearance may suggest improvement because of increased lucency in the lungs, but the characteristic configuration of air surrounding an intrapulmonary vessel should indicate the correct diagnosis.

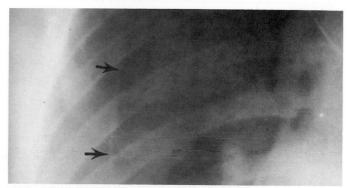

FIGURE 11–14: Hydropneumothorax. Generalized increased opacity over the right hemithorax reflects freely layering fluid in the posterior portion of the thorax. The sharply defined visceral pleural line *(arrows)* indicates an associated pneumothorax.

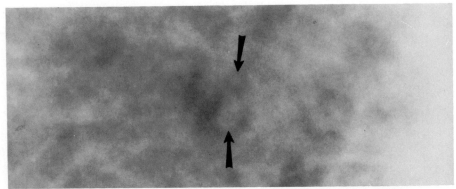

FIGURE 11–15: Pulmonary interstitial emphysema. Close-up view of the right lung demonstrates air dissecting through the interstitium and sharply outlining intrapulmonary vessels *(arrows)*.

Pneumomediastinum

Air dissecting into the mediastinum creates a characteristic radiographic appearance. The air dissects through the mediastinal tissues, creating vertical linear streaks (Fig. 11–16). Air can dissect superiorly into the neck, the muscles overlying the thorax, or both, and inferiorly into the abdomen, both intra- and extra-peritoneally. Air dissecting through the mediastinum may outline the pulmonary artery in characteristic fashion on both frontal and lateral projections.

EVALUATION OF SUPPORT AND MONITORING EQUIPMENT

Complications of tube or catheter placement are a significant cause of morbidity in hospitalized patients, and chest radiography should be routinely performed after the insertion of endotracheal tubes, chest drainage tubes, nasogastric tubes, and central venous catheters.

Endotracheal and Tracheostomy Tubes

Studies show as high as a 10% incidence of inappropriate positioning of endotracheal tubes.

If the diameter of the cuff is more than 1.5 times the tracheal diameter, severe ulceration or tracheostenosis may result.[26]

Endotracheal tubes should have a radiopaque marker for radiographic assessment. Optimal positioning requires the top of the endotracheal tube to be approximately 4 to 6 cm above the carina with the neck in the neutral position. This limits accidental extubation with neck extension and inadvertent intubation of the right mainstem bronchus (Fig. 11–17) with neck flexion.[25] The tube diameter should be one half to two thirds that of the trachea lumen, and the inflated cuff should not cause bulging of the tracheal wall.

Esophageal intubation occasionally occurs. Clues to this on the chest radiograph include projection of the endotracheal tube beyond the carina and excessive distention of the esophagus and stomach.

A tracheostomy tube should be midline, and again the cuff should not cause the tracheal wall to bulge. Optimal positioning of the tip is one half to two thirds of the distance between the stoma and the carina. A malpositioned tube may produce ulceration and hemorrhage as well as scarring. Prolonged hyperinflation of the cuff may lead to tracheomalacia, as with endotracheal cuff hyperinflation.

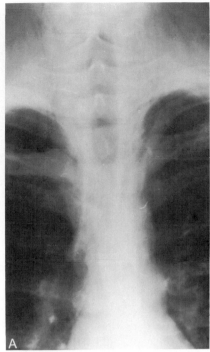
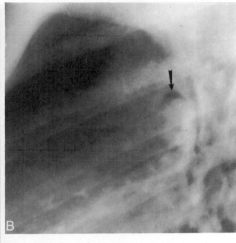

FIGURE 11–16: Pneumomediastinum. *A,* Frontal projection demonstrates multiple vertical lucencies throughout the mediastinum and lower neck, reflecting air dissecting throughout fascial planes and muscle bundles. *B,* Lateral view demonstrates air *(arrow)* dissecting over the top of the right pulmonary artery in characteristic fashion.

Chest Tubes

Chest radiographs should routinely be obtained after tube placement to detect malpositioning (Fig. 11–18) and potential complications such as pneumothorax and hemothorax.

Chest tubes are often inserted for the removal of intrapleural air or fluid. Tubes are supplied with a radiopaque marker that is interrupted by a side hole proximal to the tip. This should always be seen medial to the inner margin of the ribs. Inadvertent insertion of the tube into the soft tissues may be suspected by silhouetting of the nonopaque wall of the tube by the adjacent soft tissue density. Normally, the nonopaque wall is rendered visible by surrounding lucent lung.[26]

Optimal positioning of the tube depends on whether the air or fluid collection is free or loculated within the pleural space. Computed tomog-

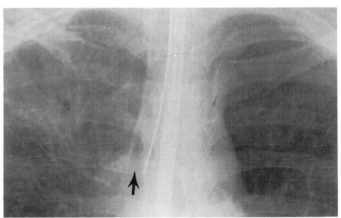

FIGURE 11–17: Right mainstem bronchus intubation. Note the distal tip of the endotracheal tube *(arrow)* extending into the proximal right mainstem bronchus.

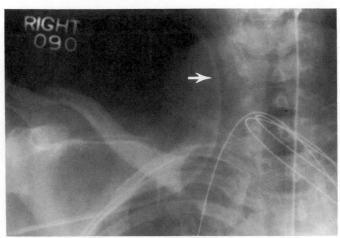

FIGURE 11-18: Malpositioned central venous catheter. A right subclavian catheter is inadvertently positioned in the right internal jugular vein *(arrow),* as opposed to the desired position in the superior vena cava.

raphy can be very helpful in directing tube placement if pleural fluid is loculated. Intraparenchymal placement may be complicated by bronchopleural fistula, pulmonary laceration, and hematoma. Placement into a fissure is associated with a 29% rate of unsatisfactory drainage.[27]

Central Venous Catheters

Common malpositions of a central venous catheter:

- Insertion into the internal mammary and azygos veins
- Insertion into the internal jugular vein in the case of subclavian line placement.

Central venous catheters are usually inserted via the subclavian or the internal jugular vein. To be able to monitor central venous pressure, the tip of the catheter must be intrathoracic and central to all venous valves. The location of the most proximal venous valve is approximated by the medial margin of the first rib.[28] The optimal position for the distal tip of central lines is at the junction of the branciocephalic vein and the superior vena cava or in the superior vena cava just proximal to the right atrium. Both the placement of catheter tips adjacent to the tricuspid valve and hypertonic instillation into the right atrium may produce arrhythmias.[4]

Swan-Ganz Catheter

Pulmonary artery catheters are commonly used to monitor pulmonary artery wedge pressures. The optimal tip position is in the right or left pulmonary artery approximately 5 cm distal to the bifurcation of the main pulmonary artery. Placement of the tip into the right ventricle predisposes to arrhythmias as well as to myocardial perforation. Too distal placement in the pulmonary artery may result in pulmonary infarction, hemorrhage, or rupture of the pulmonary artery.[29, 30] The inflated cuff should never be seen on a radiographic study.

Intra-aortic Balloon Pump

A complication of the use of the intra-aortic balloon pump is aortic dissection.

Intra-aortic balloon pumps are increasingly being used to maximize coronary artery perfusion by decreasing cardiac afterload, usually in patients with cardiogenic shock or poor left ventricular function. The catheter tip is optimally placed just distal to the left subclavian artery.[26] The balloon inflates during diastole and deflates during systole.

Nasogastric Tube

The use of a nasogastric tube is also associated with complications, the commonest of which is malpositioning. The tip and the side hole of the tube should be below the level of the gastroesophageal junction in order to avoid gastroesophageal reflux. With known gastroesophageal reflux before tube placement, more distal placement of an enteric tube is usually necessary. Misplacement of the nasogastric tube into the bronchial airway may occur, with consequent administration of fluids into the lung. Tracheal or bronchial perforation may also take place with resultant pneumomediastinum or pneumothorax.

Transvenous Pacemakers

Transvenous pacemakers are frequently used either temporarily or permanently to treat arrhythmias. The pacing leads are placed most commonly in the right ventricle in unipolar systems and in the right atrium and the right ventricle in bipolar systems. Electrode malpositioning is not an infrequent occurrence. The electrode may also migrate over time, passing into the pulmonary artery or the coronary sinus. Perforation of the myocardium is an unusual complication and should be suspected when radiographs demonstrate the electrode tip projecting beyond the right ventricle apex. Breakage of a pacing wire is an infrequent but important complication.

SUMMARY

Conventional radiography remains a fundamental component of the evaluation of the thorax. A wide variety of diseases may be diagnosed on the basis of this examination, and numerous other processes may be suspected. Correlation of radiographic imaging data with laboratory and historical data often leads to specific diagnoses. In cases in which a diagnosis is not forthcoming, the judicious application of newer imaging technology may provide additional specificity or insight.

References

1. Felson G, Felson H. Localization of intrathoracic lesions by means of the postero-anterior roentgenogram: The silhouette sign. Radiology 55:363, 1950.
2. Shevland JE, Hirleman MT, Hoang KA, Kealey GP. Lobar collapse in the surgical intensive care unit. Br J Radiol 56:531–534, 1983.
3. Wilcox P, Baile EM, Hards J, et al. Phrenic nerve function and its relationship to atelectasis after coronary artery bypass surgery. Chest 93:693–698, 1988.
4. Swensen SJ, Peters SG, LeRoy AJ, et al. Radiology in the intensive care unit. Mayo Clin Proc 66:396–410, 1991.
5. Finegold SM. Aspiration pneumonia. Rev Infect Dis 13(Suppl 9):S737–S742, 1991.
6. Torres A, Serra-Batlles J, Ros E, et al. Pulmonary aspiration of gastric contents in patients receiving mechanical ventilation: The effect of body position. Ann Intern Med 116:540–543, 1992.

7. Scheld WM, Mandell GL. Nosocomial pneumonia: Pathogenesis and recent advances in diagnosis and therapy. Rev Infect Dis 13(Suppl 9):S743–S751, 1991.
8. Goodman LR, Putman CE. Critical Care Imaging, 3rd ed. Philadelphia, WB Saunders, 1992.
9. Williford ME, Godwin JD. Computed tomography of lung abscess and empyema. Radiol Clin North Am 21:575–583, 1983.
10. Snow N, Bergin KT, Horrigan TP. Thoracic CT scanning in critically ill patients. Information obtained frequently alters management. Chest 97:1467–1470, 1990.
11. Milne ENC, Pistolesi M, Miniati M, Giuntini C. The radiologic distinction of cardiogenic and noncardiogenic edema. Am J Roentgenol 144:879–894, 1985.
12. Aberle DR, Brown K. Radiologic considerations in the adult respiratory distress syndrome. Clin Chest Med 11:737–754, 1990.
13. Suchyta MR, Clemmer TP, Elliott CG, et al. The adult respiratory distress syndrome. A report of survival and modifying factors. Chest 101:1074–1079, 1992.
14. Shale D. The adult respiratory distress syndrome—20 years on [Editorial]. Thorax 42:641–645, 1987.
15. Montgomery AB, Stager MA, Carrico CJ, Hudson LD. Causes of mortality in patients with the adult respiratory distress syndrome. Am Rev Respir Dis 132:485–489, 1985.
16. Buckner CB, Walker CW, Purnell GL. Pulmonary embolism. J Thorac Imaging 4(4):23–27, 1989.
17. Westermark N. On the roentgen diagnosis of lung embolism. Acta Radiol 19:357, 1938.
18. Dunnick NR, Newman GE, Perlmutt LM, Braun SD. Pulmonary embolism. Curr Probl Diagn Radiol 17:203–229, 1988.
19. Sostman HD, Ravin CE, Sullivan DC, et al. Use of pulmonary angiography for suspected pulmonary embolism: Influence of scintigraphic diagnosis. Am J Roentgenol 139:673–677, 1982.
20. McGoldrick PJ, Rudd TG, Figley MM, Wilhelm JP. What becomes of pulmonary infarcts? Am J Roentgenol 133:1039–1045, 1979.
21. Chiles C, Ravin CE. Radiographic recognition of pneumothorax in the intensive care unit. Crit Care Med 14(8):677–680, 1986.
22. Gordon R. The deep sulcus sign. Radiology 136:25, 1980.
23. Onik G, Goodman PC, Webb WR, Brasch RC. Hydropneumothorax: Detection on supine radiographs. Radiology 152:31–34, 1984.
24. Unger JM, England DM, Bogust GA. Interstitial emphysema in adults: Recognition and prognostic implications. J Thorac Imaging 4(1):86–94, 1989.
25. Conrady PA, Goodman LR, Lainge F, Singer MM. Alteration of endotracheal tube position: Flexion and extension of the neck. Crit Care Med 4:8–12, 1976.
26. Webb WR, Godwin JD. The obscured outer edge: A sign of improperly placed pleural drainage tubes. Am J Roentgenol 131:1062–1064, 1980.
27. Mauser JR, Friedman PJ, Wing VW. Thoracostomy tube in an interlobar fissure: Radiologic recognition of a potential problem. Am J Roentgenol 139:1155–1161, 1982.
28. Ravin CE, Putman CE, McLoud TC. Hazards of the intensive care unit. Am J Roentgenol 126:423–431, 1976.
29. Ovenfors CO. Iatrogenic trauma to the thorax. J Thorac Imaging 2(3):18–31, 1987.
30. Landay MJ, Moot AR, Estrera AS. Apparatus seen on chest radiographs after cardiac surgery in adults. Radiology 174:477–482, 1990.

12

□

Newer Imaging Techniques in the Thorax

Edward F. Patz, Jr., M.D.

Although conventional chest radiography remains the fundamental imaging procedure for the chest, several newer imaging modalities can provide significant additional information in appropriate clinical settings. These newer technologies include computed tomography, magnetic resonance imaging, and more recently, positron emission tomography. Each of these modalities has certain advantages and disadvantages (Table 12–1); therefore, their indications depend on the clinical situation.

Patients with an abnormality related to the thorax should always have plain chest radiography as the initial study. Plain chest radiography is readily available, inexpensive, and often diagnostic. If this examination does not sufficiently solve the particular problem, several questions must be addressed before further studies are performed in order to take full advantage of current imaging techniques.

- What type of abnormality is expected?
- Can the suggested study provide the necessary information?
- What will be done with the information?

If all of these questions can be appropriately answered, the additional study should be performed.

COMPUTED TOMOGRAPHY

Computed tomography (CT), the most common and readily available of the newer imaging technologies, has evolved significantly over the last decade, and the cost of performing the study and the time needed for it have decreased. With advances including high-resolution imaging for the evaluation of interstitial lung disease (Fig. 12–1) and the spiral technique, which produces multiple fast sequential images (approximately

TABLE **12–1:** Indications for CT and MRI

	Advantages	Disadvantages
Computed tomography	Readily available Easy patient monitoring Short study times Intravenous contrast is not always necessary	Axial images only Intravenous contrast may be needed for vascular abnormalities Ionizing radiation
Magnetic resonance imaging	Multiplanar capabilities Tissue characterization Evaluation of vascular and intracardiac abnormalities without intravenous contrast	Limited patient monitoring Cardiac and respiratory motion artifact Multiple sequences may be needed, causing longer study times

one image per second) (Fig. 12–2), the applications for CT have increased, and there has been continuous refinement in its diagnostic capabilities.

Because CT provides exquisite anatomic detail of the thorax, it can be used for a number of different problems, including

- Soft tissue or bony abnormalities
- Pleural abnormalities
- Lung parenchyma and interstitial disease
- Hilar or mediastinal pathology including the heart and great vessels

These general categories obviously include an entire spectrum of disease entities; depending on the clinical situation, studies should be tailored to answer specific questions. The field of view of an image can be changed in order to magnify or target regions of interest, different reconstruction algorithms can be employed for the evaluation of specific structures of different densities (Fig. 12–3), and thin sections (1 to 2 mm) can be used to produce finer detail. In addition, intravenous contrast, which can be useful for delineating vascular structures, is required in certain situations, such as aortic dissection (Fig. 12–4). Approximately 100 to 120 mL of intravenous contrast is usually sufficient for most examinations. Because most CT studies of the thorax, however, do not require the use of intravenous contrast, the additional information does not justify the low but potential risk, the cost, the additional time, or the patient discomfort.

CT can scan only in the axial plane. Because not all abnormalities are fully appreciated in this projection, some of the newer-generation CT scanners provide the software to perform multiplanar reconstructions. CT also uses ionizing radiation; although no study to date has shown a significant risk with the present doses, exposure in some patient groups, including pregnant women and children, should be limited.

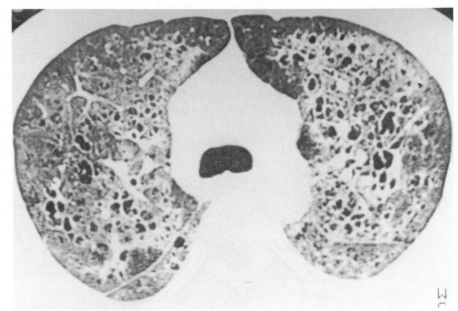

FIGURE 12–1: High-resolution CT image of the lung parenchyma in a 36-year-old with human immunodeficiency virus infection. Computed tomography demonstrates multiple thick-walled, irregular cystic lesions throughout both lungs in this patient with cystic *Pneumocystis carinii* pneumonia.

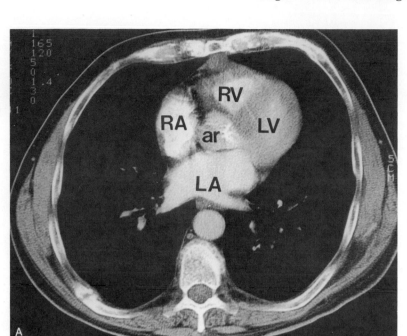

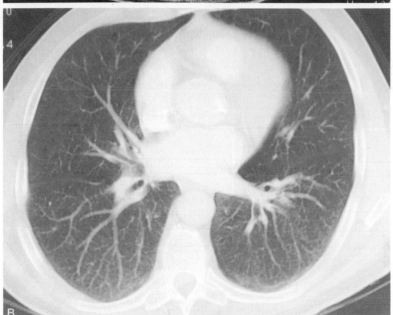

FIGURE 12–2: *A,* Spiral CT image with soft tissue windows demonstrates normal mediastinal and soft tissue structures. Intravenous contrast has been administered and is seen within each of the cardiac chambers. *B,* Lung window of the same image demonstrates normal lung parenchyma. The bronchial anatomy is also well seen on these images. RA, LA, right and left atria; RV, LV, right and left ventricles; ar, aortic root.

CT is currently the most powerful additional imaging tool available to the radiologist. Current applications are numerous, although its clinical utility with the continuously improving technology has yet to be fully defined.

MAGNETIC RESONANCE IMAGING

Magnetic resonance imaging (MRI) has become more accessible and useful as an imaging tool in the thorax. With MRI, more than with CT,

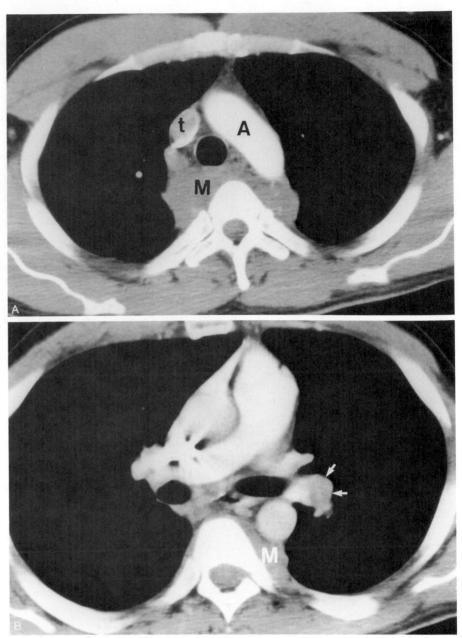

FIGURE 12–3: *A,* CT image of a 37-year-old man with Hodgkin's disease and a large posterior mediastinal mass (M). Intravenous contrast has been administered, and a soft tissue mass consistent with thrombus (t) is seen within the superior vena cava. The aorta (A) appears normal. *B,* At a more caudal level, a soft tissue mass within the left descending pulmonary artery is consistent with clot and pulmonary emboli *(arrows).* Note is again made of the extension of the posterior mediastinal mass.

the clinical questions must be answered because this study has a number of different technical parameters that need to be determined in order to tailor each study. MRI takes advantage of a well-described phenomenon, nuclear magnetic resonance, in which nuclei with odd numbers of protons and a magnetic moment become aligned when they are placed in a strong magnetic field. These protons can then be excited to a more energetic state with the addition of a radiofrequency pulse. Once allowed to relax, excited protons emit a resonance signal that is a reflection of the

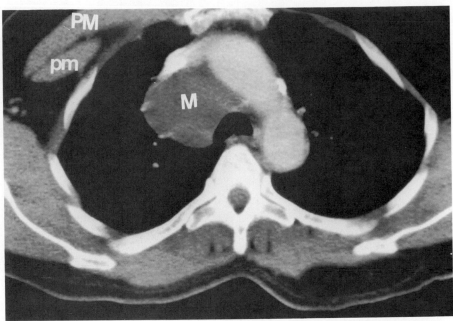

FIGURE 12–4: Soft tissue CT windows in a patient with a right paratracheal, precarinal mass (M). The mass has a low attenuation and is consistent with cystic structure. This was a surgically confirmed bronchogenic cyst. Note is made of the absence of the left pectoralis muscles from prior mastectomy. PM, right pectoralis major; pm, pectoralis minor.

number of protons and their nuclear environment. Different relaxation signals are generated depending on the pulse sequence, the way in which the protons within the nuclei are excited.

In the body, the greatest source of odd-number protons, the hydrogen nuclei, are used to create a resonance signal. Although some signals have features suggestive of a particular disease process, signal characteristics are often nonspecific.

Once a resonance signal has been generated, the information can be mathematically transformed to produce an image. MRI also provides accurate anatomic detail of the thorax. Its current indications include

- Soft tissue and bone marrow pathology
- Complicated pleural and diaphragmatic diseases
- Hilar and mediastinal abnormalities, including congenital heart disease, cardiac abnormalities, and vascular pathology

The applications of MRI are numerous, and although MRI is often complementary to CT, it has several advantages. Unlike CT, which generates images in an axial plane, MRI can produce images in any scanning plane, for greater anatomic definition. The use of intravenous contrast for thoracic MRI is almost always unnecessary. On conventional (spin-echo) images, the vessels are seen as a signal void because the protons excited do not remain in the same plane being imaged (the blood is moving). This flow phenomenon thus creates the body's own internal vascular contrast; vascular abnormalities, including dissection, require no intravenous contrast for assessment (Fig. 12–5). Additional pulse sequences (gradient-refocused images) that use different excitation patterns to produce bright signals within the vessels can be performed to demonstrate flowing blood (Fig. 12–6). MRI also has the ability to look at intracardiac pathology as the flowing blood creates a signal void (Fig.

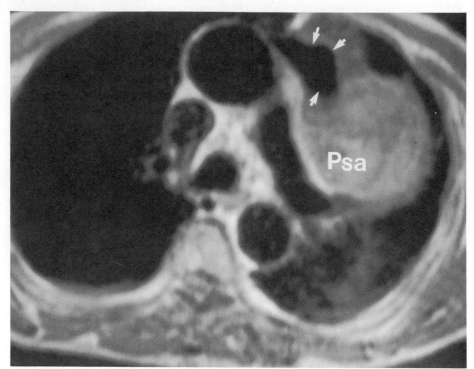

FIGURE 12–5: T_2-weighted magnetic resonance image just below the level of the transverse aortic arch demonstrates a large aortic pseudoaneurysm (Psa). Flow, seen as a signal void *(arrows)*, is entering the aneurysm from the ascending aorta.

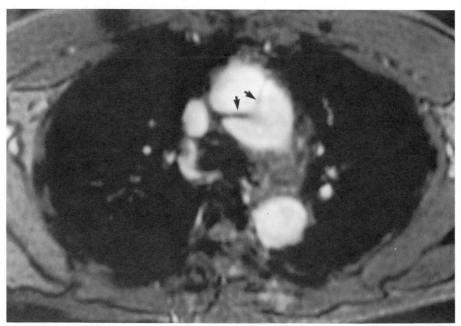

FIGURE 12–6: Gradient-refocused magnetic resonance image without intravenous contrast demonstrates a luminal flap *(arrows)* within the ascending aorta, diagnostic of a type A aortic dissection.

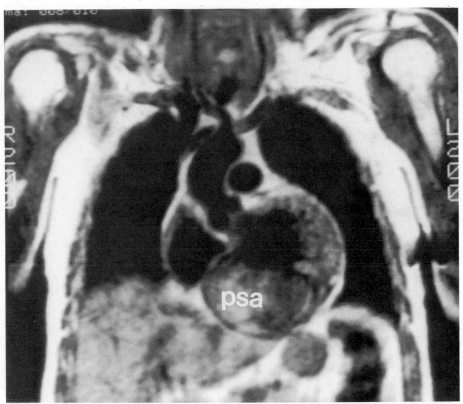

FIGURE 12–7: Coronal magnetic resonance image demonstrates regularity of the posteroinferior left ventricular wall with a heterogeneous soft tissue mass. There is no normal myocardium surrounding this collection, which is consistent with a pseudoaneurysm (psa) following myocardial infarction.

12–7). Patients with renal dysfunction are often better served by MRI because there is no need for intravenous contrast, which can be nephrotoxic. MRI, unlike CT, uses no ionizing radiation.

Some structures, however, lack sufficient free hydrogen nuclei for excitation, and thus a low signal is created. Cortical bone and lung parenchyma are the most notable areas in the chest. MRI has several other disadvantages, including limited patient monitoring capabilities and motion artifacts caused by cardiac and respiratory motion, which can obscure the images. Despite these limitations, MRI offers information not available from other modalities. The full potential of MRI in the chest, including pulmonary angiography and the evaluation of parenchymal lung disease, continues to be actively pursued. Another application of MRI in lung disease is detection of pelvic and lower extremity venous thrombosis in patients at risk for pulmonary embolism.

POSITRON EMISSION TOMOGRAPHY

The newest modality, positron emission tomography (PET), has become a recognized tool for assessing thoracic pathology. Prior PET investigations were performed almost exclusively on the brain, but now some of the same principles have been applied to thoracic abnormalities. PET, unlike the other two modalities, provides physiologic information. This test, which focuses on the biochemical properties of cells, has the ability

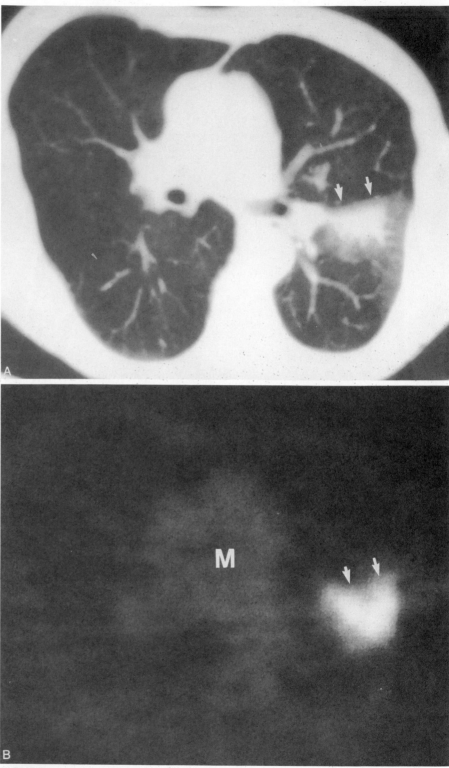

FIGURE 12–8: *A,* A 59-year-old woman has an irregular opacity within the left lower lobe *(arrows)* on computed tomography. This mass was indeterminate. *B,* Axial positron emission tomography–[18]F-fluorodeoxyglucose scan of this lesion at the same level as the computed tomography demonstrates significantly increased uptake within the lesion *(arrows)*. There is only minimal activity within the normal mediastinal vascular structures (M). This lesion proved to be an adenocarcinoma of the lung.

to analyze abnormalities quantitatively. Currently, the positron-emitting agent most commonly used in the thorax is ^{18}F-fluorodeoxyglucose (FDG). Metabolically active cells take up and trap this D-glucose analogue. The activity can then be measured and mapped out to a specific region within the thorax.

The main indication for PET is to distinguish between benign and malignant lesions in patients with pulmonary abnormalities. Preliminary data suggest that the more metabolically active transformed tumor cells will show a statistically increased amount of FDG uptake over normal tissues or a benign process. This has tremendous implications in evaluating patients with focal pulmonary abnormalities, staging bronchogenic carcinoma, and assessing tumor viability versus fibrosis after treatment. PET appears to be extremely useful in these situations for definitely separating benign from malignant lesions rather than proceding to biopsy or simply following up the patient (Fig. 12–8).

This modality has just begun to be clinically useful. As newer agents develop, this imaging technique should prove to be invaluable in patients with indeterminate abnormalities by other studies and in the management of cancer patients.

SUMMARY

The evaluation of thoracic abnormalities can be a complicated issue. Radiologic procedures should not be performed simply for further evaluation: they should instead be used judiciously, with an understanding of their capabilities. These modalities can generate a significant amount of information, some of which is complementary and some of which may be redundant. As the technology continues to improve, radiology studies will, it is hoped, become more sensitive and specific in the diagnosis of thoracic diseases.

Suggested Readings

Abe Y, Matsuzaw Y, Fujiwara T, et al. Clinical assessment of therapeutic effects on cancer using ^{18}F-2-fluoro-2-deoxy-D-glucose and positron emission tomography: Preliminary study of lung cancer. Int J Radiat Oncol Biol Phys 19:1005–1010, 1990.

Gupta NC, Frank AR, Dewan NA. Solitary pulmonary nodules: Detection of malignancy with PET with 2-[F-18]-fluoro-2-deoxy-D-glucose. Radiology 184:441–444, 1992.

Hawkins RA, Hoh CK, Glaspy J, et al. PET-FDG imaging in cancer. Appl Radiol 21(5):51–57, 1992.

Higgins CB, Hricak H. Magnetic Resonance Imaging of the Body. New York, Raven Press, 1987.

Kubota K, Matsuzawa T, Fujiwara T, et al. Differential diagnosis of lung tumor with positron emission tomography: A prospective study. J Nucl Med 31:1927–1933, 1990.

Kubota K, Yamada S, Ishiwata K, et al. Positron emission tomography for treatment evaluation and recurrence detection compared with CT in long-term follow-up cases of lung cancer. Clin Nucl Med 17:877–881, 1992.

Lee JKT, Sagel SS, Stanley RJ. Computed Body Tomography With MRI Correlation, 2nd ed. New York, Raven Press, 1989.

Naidich DP, Zerhouni EA, Siegelman SS. Computed Tomography and Magnetic Resonance of the Thorax, 2nd ed. New York, Raven Press, 1991.

13

Hemodynamic Monitoring

Charles G. Durbin, Jr., M.D.

Acrocyanosis is a sign of poor peripheral perfusion. After compression of the nail bed and subsequent release of pressure, color should return in 2 to 3 seconds if blood flow is normal. A delay of more than 5 seconds indicates circulatory insufficiency.

Supplying oxygen to peripheral tissues is the most important function of the cardiovascular system. Mitochondria use oxygen to produce energy in order to maintain intracellular processes. Oxygen permits more efficient nutrient utilization through complete oxidation of food substances. Decreased oxygen at the cellular level leads rapidly to anaerobic metabolism and lactic acidosis. Persistence of an oxygen-deficient state may lead to cell dysfunction or death. The heart and the cardiovascular system deliver blood containing oxygen to these tissues.

Assessment and support of the cardiovascular system are essential in critical illness. This chapter describes basic and advanced techniques for monitoring the cardiovascular system. Monitors can be simple or complicated, invasive or noninvasive, expensive or inexpensive. Each device or technique has advantages and disadvantages. "Routine monitoring" is a misnomer. The type and the frequency of cardiovascular assessment should be individualized to each patient and clinical situation. The stability of the patient and the understanding of the disease process dictate the appropriate monitoring methods. The risks of a particular monitor must be weighed against the "risk" of not using the device. The increased and widespread use of appropriate hemodynamic monitoring has contributed to improved patient outcome in critical illness. This chapter discusses the options for cardiovascular monitoring in detail. The application of these methods in specific diseases and critical illness is mentioned here but is more completely discussed in other chapters.

CLINICAL ASSESSMENT OF THE CIRCULATORY SYSTEM

The patient's history and the physical examination results can give important clues to the state of the cardiovascular system. Alterations in mental status frequently occur in patients with inadequate tissue perfusion. Anxiety, progressing through confusion to loss of consciousness, may indicate circulatory inadequacy. A history of recent blood loss or the recognition of ongoing bleeding would be consistent with hypovolemia as the cause of hemodynamic instability. Other organs besides the brain can provide helpful information about peripheral tissue perfusion. Skin color and capillary refill are useful signs of tissue perfusion. In septic shock, skin color and capillary refill time may be normal (if volume is maintained), but skin temperature is often elevated, and other signs of organ dysfunction (low urine output and mental status changes) are frequently present. Inadequate tissue oxygen utilization caused by toxins can present with clinical characteristics related to the agent involved (e.g., a smell of almonds in cyanide poisoning). Repeated clinical examination adds information about the process leading to illness and the need for intervention. The decision to use mechanical devices to monitor organ function is based on thorough clinical assessment.

214

Changes in urinary output lag significantly behind acute hemodynamic changes.

Pressure injury to nerves has been reported with frequent automated blood pressure determinations; this may pose an increased risk in unresponsive patients or those in shock.

Risks associated with direct arterial blood pressure monitoring:

- Local and systemic infection
- Arterial thrombosis
- Proximal and distal embolism
- Bleeding
- Pain
- Arterial spasm
- Distal ischemia

Safe use of this monitoring technique requires

- Sterile insertion technique
- Appropriate local management (frequent sterile dressing and connecting tubing changes)
- Daily visual assessment for signs of infection or thrombosis
- Prompt catheter removal when monitoring is no longer needed

The presence of a vasculitis such as Buerger's disease or Raynaud's disease is a relative contraindication to small artery cannulation. A larger artery, such as the femoral artery, should be used in these patients if cannulation is required.

Sustained mean arterial blood pressures in excess of 140 mm Hg should be treated.

Urinary output may be a useful monitor of hemodynamics. An acute decrease in urine formation accompanies decreased intravascular volume (filling pressure) or decreased cardiac output. If circulatory compromise persists, severe renal failure may occur and urinary output no longer reflects acute changes in hemodynamics. If diuretics are used or chronic renal failure is present, the reliability of urinary output as a sign of adequate hemodynamics diminishes.

ARTERIAL BLOOD PRESSURE MEASUREMENT

The most commonly used monitor of hemodynamic status is the arterial blood pressure measurement. Noninvasive auditory methods (Riva-Rocci method) and the oscillometric method (automated blood pressure measurement) are frequently used to determine this vital sign. Rapid and repeated measurements can be made with little risk to the patient.

In patients with unstable (rapidly changing) conditions, arterial blood pressure is often monitored continuously and directly. Indwelling arterial catheters are frequently used in intensive care units for several purposes. In addition to permitting continuous monitoring of blood pressure, this catheter allows frequent blood sampling for laboratory testing without patient discomfort. Despite the potential for problems, serious complications are extremely rare, and this monitoring technique is frequently employed. Continuous electronic monitoring of the indwelling line and availability of appropriately trained personnel are necessary because an accidental, unnoticed disconnection can result in exsanguination in less than 15 minutes.

Most commonly, the radial artery is used for arterial catheter insertion. Other sites include the dorsal pedal, anterior tibial, femoral, axillary, and brachial arteries. A small catheter (20 or 22 gauge) is inserted after skin preparation and local anesthetic injection. Sterile technique is maintained. The use of Allen's test for determining the adequacy of ulnar collateral circulation has been called into question and is no longer commonly used. Arterial thrombosis is common, occurring in 5 to 30% of arteries in 5 to 7 days. This is of little clinical significance because all of these vessels will become recannulated over time. Continuous, noninvasive techniques have been developed and are finding a place in the treatment of the critically ill.

In more recent years, the value of using blood pressure measurement alone to identify the shock state has been questioned. Organ blood flow is a more important oxygen delivery variable. Most tissues regulate blood flow with local vascular mechanisms to maintain appropriate perfusion. Systemic blood pressure reflects the balance between total cardiac output and tissue flow demands. Organ flow is maintained over a wide range of blood pressure (autoregulation). If blood pressure falls below a certain point (autoregulation point), organ perfusion falls and dysfunction occurs. Some tissue beds are better able to regulate their own flow than others (wider range of autoregulation).

The heart, in a unique position in the circulatory system, must supply blood flow to all other organs and tissues as well as provide its own perfusion. If the heart does not receive enough coronary perfusion, which predominantly occurs during diastole, it will fail rapidly. Autoregulation in the heart occurs between mean pressures of 40 and 150 mm Hg. When significant stenoses from coronary artery disease are present, this range shifts upward and higher pressures are necessary for perfusion. A fall below this pressure range may precipitate cardiac arrest. Brain function will fail at systolic pressures below 60 mm Hg; however, irreversible damage requires prolonged hypotension (but only brief periods of anoxia or total ischemia: i.e., 6 to 10 minutes). To prevent vital organ failure (and thus death) during periods of decreased cardiac output, hypotension, or increased (unmet) oxygen demand, hormonal-mediated systemic vasoconstriction occurs. This will deprive nonvital organs of required oxygen, and a shock state (hypoperfusion) results. Hypoperfused tissues will begin using anaerobic energy pathways to maintain basal cell function and produce lactic acid. Blood pressure may be normal despite ongoing tissue hypoperfusion. For this reason, blood pressure monitoring alone is inadequate in patients who may be in or recovering from shock. Blood flow and organ perfusion are important factors in assessing and treating the circulatory system. Blood pressure is an inadequate monitor and may be misleading in shock states.

Arterial pressure monitoring is also useful in hypertensive situations. Hypertension may cause vessel damage, may augment bleeding, and, if severe, may cause rupture of intracranial or other vascular aneurysms. Hypertension in the intensive care unit is usually a marker of excessive catecholamine release or drug effect. Pain, disorientation, and anxiety are frequent causes of hypertension in the critically ill. Systolic hypertension is less of an issue, especially if it is identified from monitoring an indwelling arterial catheter. Systolic pressures are generally 20% higher when they are measured from arterial catheters because of resonance; mean pressures maintain good correlation with those obtained from noninvasive techniques. Measured diastolic pressures are decreased by a similar percentage. The further peripherally the catheter is placed, the larger the amplification factor: that is, the dorsal pedal artery exhibits a higher systolic pressure than the radial or the femoral artery. Technical factors that influence the resonance are discussed further in the section on central venous monitoring.

Malignant hypertension, a marked, sustained increase in blood pressure that results in increased intracranial pressure, is a medical emergency that should be treated aggressively in an intensive care setting to prevent intracranial hemorrhage, cerebral edema, and other organ (renal or cardiac) failure.

OXYGEN DELIVERY: ROLE OF THE HEART

The oxygen delivery system includes the lungs (oxygenation of the blood), hemoglobin and plasma (carrying and storing oxygen), and the cardiovascular system (delivering the blood to the lungs and the peripheral tissues). An important measure of the cardiovascular system's contribution is cardiac output (CO). Often, this value is reported corrected for (divided by) body surface area as cardiac index. The smallest component of CO, that amount of blood ejected during each heartbeat, is referred to as stroke volume. Occasionally, this is also corrected for body size and reported as stroke index. Stroke volume is affected by several factors:

Cardiac output (CO)—the volume of blood ejected per minute by the heart

Cardiac index = CO/body surface area

Stroke volume—the volume of blood ejected per beat

- Preload, the initial length of the cardiac fibers
- Afterload, the resistance to the ejection of blood
- Contractility of the myocardium

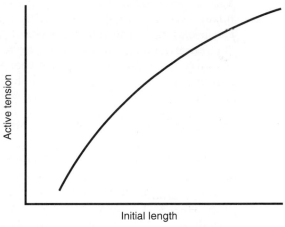

FIGURE 13–1: This figure demonstrates the increasing tension developed as a cardiac muscle fiber is progressively lengthened. This is often referred to as the Frank-Starling law of the heart.

Although this classification is simplified, it is useful because it allows a rational approach to monitoring and treatment of the cardiovascular components of oxygen delivery.

Preload in Cardiac Performance

Increasing the initial length (or stretch) of cardiac fibers before active contraction will increase the tension produced. The Frank-Starling law of the heart describes this relationship (Fig. 13–1).

Preload is the term used to describe this initial fiber condition (length). Although the Frank-Starling model is based on an isolated piece of myocardium stretched linearly, this mechanism is accepted unquestioningly in the clinical situation (Fig. 13–2). Preload is usually estimated by central venous pressure or wedge pressure, and tension is replaced by CO, cardiac index, stroke volume, or stroke index. A direct

Preload should be "optimized" in patients in all forms of shock.

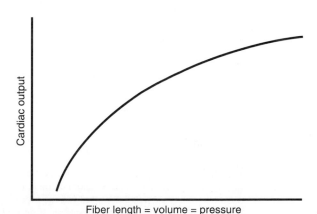

FIGURE 13–2: The Frank-Starling relationship is often translated into clinically useful terms. These assumptions are illustrated in this figure. (See Fig. 13–3 and the text for concerns about the assumptions implied in this interpretation.)

application of the Frank-Starling mechanism to the clinical situation is hazardous. The implied assumption, illustrated in Figure 13–3A, is that the pressure in the left ventricle at the end of diastole is the same as that in the other chambers, in vessels, and across valves. Even if this were true, it is further assumed that this *pressure* directly relates to the *volume* and thus the length of fibers in the left ventricular wall. This is usually not true. Any change in compliance of the ventricle, such as occurs with ischemia or vasoactive drug infusion, alters this relationship; thus, at the same pressure, there will be a different fiber length (volume).

Another equally important concern with direct application of the Frank-Starling model is ventricular geometry. A predictable (although not linear) mathematical relationship exists between the circumference of a circle and the volume of a sphere (or another regular solid object) (Fig. 13–3B). Changes in ventricular shape alter this predictable relationship. This is particularly important in conditions with increased afterload of the right ventricle. This occurs with positive airway pressure and positive end-expiratory pressure or with pathologically increased

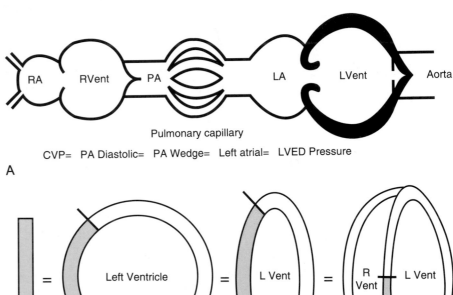

FIGURE 13–3: *A,* Assumptions implied when the Frank-Starling law is applied to the intact heart are pictured here. The pressure in the left ventricle (LV) just before contraction is assumed to be equal to the central venous pressure (CVP) or the pulmonary artery (PA) wedge pressure. This assumes that there is no pressure gradient across any cardiac valve or the pulmonary circuit. (See the text for further discussion of these factors.) *B,* Even if the pressures were equal in the left ventricle and the central venous compartment (or pulmonary capillary wedge), the relationship between a linear piece of myocardium and the intact heart is influenced by cardiac geometry, as suggested in this illustration. RA, right atrium; RV, right ventricle; LA, left atrium; LVED, left ventricular end-diastolic.

pulmonary vascular resistance, as in the adult respiratory distress syndrome. Because the nondistensible pericardium contains the heart and the two ventricles share a common wall, right ventricular overload can cause the interventricular septum to shift and distort the shape of the left ventricle. This alters the pressure–fiber length relationship by changing the cavity from a sphere-like to a half-moon–shaped structure. Changes in cardiac function due to changes in geometry are not identifiable from pressure measurement.

With these concerns, no precise information about the Frank-Starling condition of the myocardium can be obtained with indirect (pressure measurement) means alone. Although the absolute position on the Frank-Starling curve cannot be assessed with certainty, the relative position can be judged by changes seen in CO with changes in preload pressures. This is assessed by observing the changes occurring during a controlled volume infusion test. A sample protocol for such a test is illustrated in Table 13–1. When circulatory insufficiency (shock) is suspected, a fluid challenge is performed. A bolus of balanced salt solution is rapidly administered, and the effect on the preload monitor is assessed. If minimal change in this variable occurs, more fluid is rapidly given. The top of the effective Frank-Starling curve is reached when the preload monitor rises significantly with a small volume infusion. With this method, the absolute value from the monitor is not as important as the change seen with the infusion. The initial value of the preload monitor determines the size of the initial bolus for infusion, and the response identifies the relative position on the curve. As the clinical status changes, repeated infusions may be needed to optimize preload.

Afterload

Afterload is the resistance to blood being ejected from the heart.

Afterload is influenced by

- The compliance of the muscle
- Aortic pressure
- Systemic vascular resistance (SVR)
- Intracavitary pressure before contraction

A useful clinical correlate of afterload is the mean aortic pressure. In the presence of significant aortic stenosis, the afterload will be much greater

TABLE **13–1:** Suggested Plan for a Fluid Challenge*

Initial Pressure: Central Venous or Wedge (mm Hg)	Rapid Infusion Over 10 Minutes (mL)	Pressure Change (mm Hg)	Action
0–10	250	<5	Repeat bolus infusion
0–10	250	5–10	Infuse smaller bolus
0–10	250	>10	Wait 10 minutes and repeat measurement
10–20	150	<5	Repeat bolus infusion
10–20	150	5–10	Infuse smaller bolus
10–20	150	>10	Wait 10 minutes and repeat measurement
>20	75–100	<5	Repeat bolus infusion
>20	75–100	>5	Wait 10 minutes and repeat measurement

*The size of the bolus of fluid is dependent on the initial measurement of filling pressure. The change in the monitor is more important than the absolute measurement. Repeated challenges are often necessary as clinical status often changes.

$$SVR = (BP - CVP)/CO$$

where

BP = mean aortic blood pressure
CVP = central venous pressure
CO = cardiac output

SVR should not be interpreted as the size of the blood vessels.

than indicated from aortic pressure. SVR, often used to quantitate changes in afterload, is occasionally interpreted as the state of vessel smooth muscle constriction, reflecting vessel physical size. However, peripheral vessel resistance is only one of the determinants of SVR. SVR, in fact, is simply the mathematical relationship between CO and arterial blood pressure. Analogous with direct current electrical circuitry, SVR reflects the pressure drop (voltage) divided by the CO (current). It is often expressed in standard units, dynes·sec·cm^{-5}, by multiplying the number obtained previously by 80. Because SVR is only partially related to the physical state of vessels (i.e., constricted or dilated), it only partially reflects the afterload on the heart. Calculating SVR and following trends in it can help monitor therapy directed at these variables, but overinterpretation of its significance as a physical characteristic must be avoided.

Contractility

Contractility refers to the intrinsic contractile state or the potential strength of the muscle fibers. It relates on a cellular basis to the concentration of contractile elements, the available energy supplies, and the efficiency of contraction. External influences include extracellular Ca^{2+} concentration and catecholamine levels. Changes in contractility alter the shape and height of the Frank-Starling curve. There is no way to measure contractility directly. Estimates of contractility include the peak and maximal rate of rise of pressure (dp/dt) and the rate of fiber shortening or wall thickening during the ejection phase. Many of the drugs used to treat cardiovascular insufficiency affect contractility and shift the Frank-Starling curve upward, as illustrated in Figure 13–4.

Myocardial ischemia may depress the curve, indicating decreased contractility. A change in contractility is presumed if CO changes without a change in preload or afterload. This apparent change could also occur with a change in compliance or geometry. Contractility remains more of a theoretical concept than a factor to be measured in evaluating cardiac performance. After preload has been optimized, the next therapeutic intervention to improve oxygen delivery is usually to increase contractility pharmacologically (see Fig. 13–4).

Although contractility cannot be directly measured, drugs that alter it are frequently used.

Estimating Preload in Shock

Shock—inadequate tissue perfusion

Blood pressure is usually normal early in the development of shock. The pulse rate rises and the pulse pressure (the difference between systolic pressure and diastolic pressure) drops. Treatment of shock begins with the assessment and optimization of preload. The neck veins, which reflect blood return to the heart, are examined with the patient in the supine position. If there is no jugular vein distention (the external jugular veins are not visible), filling pressure is probably low. Fluid should be administered if clinical signs indicate that organ perfusion is inadequate. A primary compensatory mechanism for (relative or absolute) hypovolemia (reduced preload), an increased heart rate, serves to increase CO (smaller stroke volume × increased heart rate = maintained CO) and maintain oxygen delivery.

If the patient's neck veins are visible in the supine position, a tilt test should be performed. The patient's head and thorax are gradually raised to 45 degrees upright, and visibility of the jugular veins, pulse rate, and blood pressure are noted. If the pulse rate rises more than 15 beats or systolic blood pressure falls more than 10 mm Hg, hypovolemia is presumed to be present. If clinically appropriate fluid administration fails to restore circulatory stability and end-organ perfusion, if cardiac failure is suspected (e.g., signs of shock and distended neck veins), or if the initial shock state is severe, invasive monitoring of preload pressures is indicated.

CVP—central venous pressure

The usefulness of CVP in assessing preload and hemodynamic performance is debated. CVP reflects the filling pressure in the right side of the circulation. In normal hearts without failure, this is a reasonable reflection of the left-sided pressures as well. Most critical illnesses have major effects on cardiac and pulmonary function; therefore, the use of the CVP to monitor left ventricular preload is unreliable. A more accurate assessment of left ventricular preload is obtained from a pulmonary artery catheter (PAC). The interpretation of values obtained from either monitor is complicated by the concerns about preload described earlier with regard to the Frank-Starling model. A change in a measurement after an intervention has been made is more significant than the absolute value obtained. Trends are very useful and must be followed for appropriate therapy. A fluid challenge protocol used to optimize preload is shown in Table 13–1.

Treatment of the shock state involves optimization of preload, improvement of contractility, and reduction of afterload. The weight placed on each of these therapeutic concerns depends on the individual patient's circumstances.

CANNULATION OF A CENTRAL VEIN FOR PRESSURE MONITORING

A cutdown may be necessary

- In children
- In some adults with abnormal vascular anatomy
- After percutaneous attempts have failed

Regardless of the invasive monitor chosen (CVP or PAC), the percutaneous route is simple and is preferred to cutdown. The usual sites for catheter insertion are the subclavian, internal jugular, external jugular, brachial, and femoral veins. Equipment availability and the presence of skilled personnel are essential. The patient should be informed of the reasons for the procedure and its risks; consent should be obtained. A transducer and sterile flush solution are assembled and attached to a monitor system; the waveform is identified. In addition, the system is referenced to zero pressure at the appropriate level while calibration is confirmed.

Insertion of an intravascular monitoring device requires sterile technique. Full sterile skin preparation; field draping; and the use of mask, gown, and gloves should be employed if patient stability allows. For the conscious patient, a local anesthetic should be used to reduce discomfort, with epinephrine (1:100,000 or less) to reduce cutaneous bleeding. The right internal jugular vein is the most direct route to the central circulation and the right atrium. The left internal jugular vein is usually avoided because of possible injury to the thoracic duct, which usually enters the left subclavian vein. In addition, the path to the right atrium is longer and more circuitous from the left side, making successful cannulation less frequent. Some clinicians prefer the subclavian approach for longer-term cannulation because of the ease of securing the catheters and maintaining stability (and sterility) in this position. Brachial veins are far from the central circulation, require special-length catheters, and

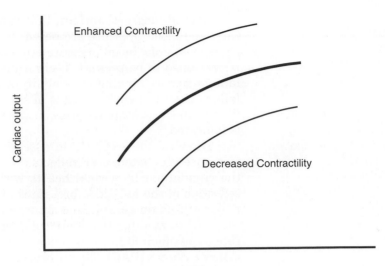

FIGURE 13–4: Contractility defines the position of the cardiac function curve. Agents or conditions that increase contractility move the curve upward and to the left. Decreased contractility depresses the curve. At any degree of contractility, the cardiac function is still determined by the initial fiber length or, in intact hearts, the filling pressure. Changes in cardiac function due to increases in filling pressure diminishes at the plateau of the curve in either case.

frequently develop venous thrombosis. The femoral route is easy and free of significant immediate complications, but it may have a higher infection rate and may be more difficult to stabilize in long-term catheterizations.

Venous Cannulation Complications

The catheter colonization rate increases with

- Duration of catheterization
- Frequency of line usage
- Number of injection ports
- Number of individuals using the line

Complications from invasive hemodynamic monitoring can be classified as early or late. Complications are listed in Table 13–2. The early complications, which are mechanical and related to the device insertion, are specific to the type of monitor chosen and the route of insertion. Pneumothorax presents as an important complication during subclavian or internal jugular vein catheterization. Another complication is line-related infection. Meticulous line maintenance and appropriate catheter changes, either with a new percutaneous needle stick or over a guide-wire, reduce the rate of catheter-related infections. Bloodstream infections caused by these monitors are less frequent than colonization but also increase with time.

Some complications are specific to the device chosen. The most lethal complication of PAC placement is pulmonary artery rupture, which occurs in 0.01 to 0.2% of PAC placements and is fatal 20 to 50% of the time. The likelihood of this occurring is increased in patients with pulmonary hypertension. Using careful balloon inflation technique, choosing safer catheters, and limiting the number of PAC wedge measurements lower the risk of this dreaded complication. Proper location of the PAC tip in the main pulmonary artery rather than in a peripheral arterial branch may help prevent this complication as well as decrease the incidence of pulmonary infarction. The tip should be within 1.5 to 2 cm of

TABLE **13–2:** Complications From Preload Monitors*

Early Complications
CVP or PAC
  Pain at insertion site
  Hematoma formation
  Arterial puncture
  Venous air embolism
  Catheter embolism
  Pneumothorax
  Hemothorax
  Pleural effusion due to infusion fluid
  Chylothorax
  Cardiac arrhythmias
  Cardiac perforation or tamponade
  Mediastinal injury (air, blood, or fluid)
  Cervical plexus injury
  Phrenic nerve injury
  Endotracheal cuff perforation
PAC
  Heart block
  Pulmonary artery rupture
  Dislocation of other catheters or pacing wires

Late Complications
Infection
Thrombosis of veins
Thrombocytopenia
Arrhythmias on removal
Pulmonary valve damage
Cardiac perforation
Catheter knotting

*Complications from preload monitors occur either at the time of venous cannulation or later. Some are specific to the device or route chosen.
CVP, central venous pressure cannula; PAC, pulmonary artery catheter.

the mediastinal shadow on chest radiography, as illustrated later in Figure 13–7.

Insertion of the PAC is often associated with benign arrhythmias. Frequent premature ventricular contractions, short runs of premature ventricular contractions, and infrequently, sustained ventricular tachycardia have been reported. These arrhythmias need not be treated; however, it is occasionally necessary to remove the catheter to terminate a malignant arrhythmia. Similar arrhythmias may occur on removal of the PAC; therefore, electrocardiographic monitoring should be used at this time. A significant problem may occur in the patient with pre-existing heart (or His bundle) block. Bifascicular block may become complete heart block as the catheter passes through the right ventricle and into the pulmonary outflow tract. This is especially likely if the patient has experienced a myocardial infarction recently.

Three types of devices are used in central venous cannulation (Fig. 13–5). For CVP cannula insertion, an over-the-needle technique is often selected. Once identification of the vein has been made by aspirating blood through the needle-and-catheter combination, the catheter is advanced over the needle into the vein. Through-the-needle devices involve threading the catheter through the needle after it has been placed in the desired vein. Movement of the catheter back and forth through the needle must be avoided because it may result in severing of the catheter tip. This will result in a catheter embolism. Strict adherence to proper technique is essential to prevent this complication.

A very useful method of catheter placement is the guidewire technique. A vein is first identified with a small-gauge needle or a catheter over a needle, through it into the vein. The needle is removed, leaving

CVP cannulas:

• Catheter through the needle
• Catheter over the needle
• Catheter over a guidewire, the Seldinger technique

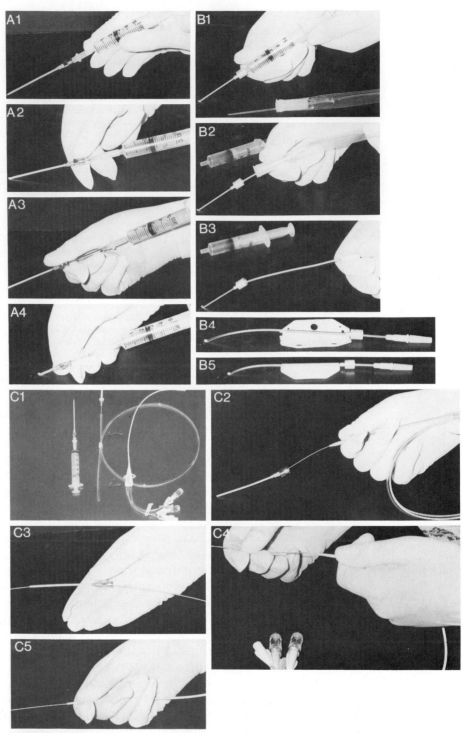

FIGURE 13–5: Devices and techniques for venous cannulation are illustrated. They are the over-the-needle cannula (A), the through-the-needle catheter (B), and a guidewire-directed technique (C). Details about and concerns with these methods are described in the text.

the guidewire in the vein. A larger catheter (and sometimes a dilator) is passed over the wire into the vein. The dilator and wire are removed, leaving the catheter in place. This technique is frequently used for placing large introducers for PACs and for changing catheter types when a vascular device is already in place.

Pressure Measurement

After a catheter has been placed in the vascular system, continuous or intermittent pressure measurements are recorded. An unbroken column of fluid connects the cannula to a transducer or strain gauge. This device converts mechanical energy to an electrical signal, which can be displayed on an oscilloscope or a paper recorder. Two aspects of this system must be ensured before accurate measurements can be obtained: the zero-pressure reference level and the system calibration. The zero-pressure reference level is arbitrarily defined as the midpoint of the left atrium; for convenience, this is set at the midpoint of the anteroposterior axillary line in the supine position. Calibration techniques are now performed during the manufacture of solid-state disposable transducers. Most monitoring systems automatically test and adjust for this factor. To set the system zero level, the monitoring line is opened to air through a stopcock. This opening should be at the midaxillary line. Internal circuitry registers this as the zero-pressure level. If the transducer fails internal calibration testing, an error message indicating a transducer failure appears on the monitor screen. A new disposable transducer should be used if this occurs.

Monitoring artifacts alter waveforms and pressure measurements. The mean pressures are most accurate.

Monitoring artifacts frequently occur with mechanical transducer systems. The fluid-filled system is capable of vibrating and producing standing waves around its natural and harmonic frequencies. This means that systolic pressure will be systematically overestimated and diastolic pressure will be underestimated. The patient's own vascular tree is also capable of producing resonance waves. The most important factors in the connecting system that increase this artifact are tubing length and stiffness. Patient factors increasing this amplification of pressure waves are stiffness of the vessels, peripheral placement of the catheters, tachycardia, and hypertension. These artifacts are more important in monitoring systemic arterial blood pressure than venous or pulmonary artery pressure. *Catheter whip* is the term used to describe the vibration artifact generated in the pulmonary artery pressure trace by the catheter movement during each heartbeat.

Resonance is not the only problem with transducer systems. A damped waveform can be caused by soft, compliant connecting tubing, air in the system, or an overdamped electrical system. In an attempt to remove the resonance artifact, some systems add a mechanical or an electronic damping system. This practice is unacceptable because it adds a new artifact to "correct" another artifact. It is better to recognize the presence of artifacts and their cause and to apply a correction mentally to interpret the values. The "mean" or average pressures are unaffected by these artifacts and should be followed to determine trends. The dynamic response of the system can be tested by snapping the fluid flush controller and observing the tracing. As illustrated in Figure 13–6, a crisp response with return to baseline in 2 to 3 cycles indicates an appropriately damped system.

Radiologic Assessment of Catheters

After hemodynamically correct placement is complete, a bedside portable anteroposterior chest radiograph is obtained and the catheter path and tip location are identified. Correct placement is confirmed, and the catheter is moved or replaced if abnormalities are seen. Pneumo-

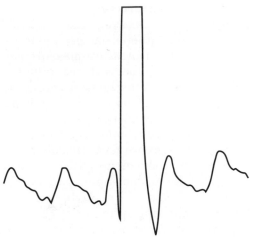

FIGURE 13–6: The dynamic response of the monitoring system should be assessed by examining how quickly the pressure trace returns to baseline. As illustrated, after a rapid flush, the system promptly returns to the patient's waveform. This indicates an appropriately damped system.

thorax is searched for in the initial image and in subsequent radiographs. In difficult situations (abnormal anatomy or very low CO), fluoroscopy may be needed to position the PAC.

In Figure 13–7, the appropriate radiographic locations of CVP and PAC tips are illustrated. The CVP tip should be above (or below, if inserted from the femoral vein) the atrium to avoid atrial perforation or arrhythmias. The catheter should be straight, and the tip should point parallel to the vein wall rather than at an acute angle to it. If this is not the case, the line should be manipulated and the radiograph repeated. The PAC should have no extra loops or knots on the chest film, and the tip should lie within 1.5 cm of the mediastinal shadow. If it lies further away from the mediastinal shadow in the periphery, the risk of permanent wedge and pulmonary infarction increases. Continuous pressure monitoring is used to identify migration of the tip into an abnormal position.

Catheter Management

Periodic flushes may be necessary to maintain catheter patency.

A continuous flush solution of 0.2 to 3.0 mL/hr of normal saline or heparin-containing (0.5 to 2 U/mL) fluid prevents the catheter lumen from clotting and becoming unusable. Dextrose-containing fluids are not used because they contribute to rouleaux formation, sluggish vessel flow, and clot formation. Some catheters are impregnated or bonded with heparin to help prevent this complication, but their effectiveness is questioned. PAC placement is associated with a slight fall in platelet count. Low-dose heparin from the infusion system and other drugs may cause thrombocytopenia.

As mentioned previously, the most serious complication of PAC placement, pulmonary artery rupture, should be suspected if massive hemoptysis or sudden shock follows balloon inflation. Patients often cough when this event occurs. Treatment of this catastrophe may require pulmonary resection. The catheter must remain in place to guide surgical

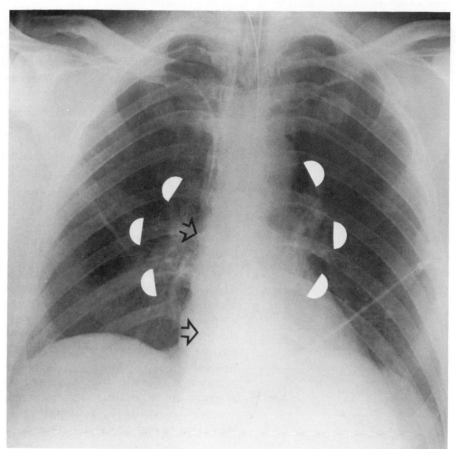

FIGURE 13–7: The pulmonary artery catheter tip should lie within 1 to 2 cm of the mediastinum. Central line tips should be located as indicated by arrows.

resection. Anecdotally, success at stopping the bleeding by balloon inflation has been reported. Separation of the lungs with a double-lumen endotracheal tube has been suggested, but this is unlikely to be accomplished because of the confusion that ensues during the resuscitation. Attempting to inflate a balloon when the PAC has drifted distally into a small vessel is a predisposing cause of this catastrophe. Careful, slow inflation techniques allow the "feel" of resistance to inflation of a wedged catheter to be identified. Some brands of PAC have noncompliant balloons that make detection of this altered resistance impossible. Daily chest radiography to identify the position of the catheter tip is essential in any patient with a PAC in place. This also helps to identify when a pulmonary infarction from dislodged clot occurs; then, the catheter should be withdrawn or replaced.

Infection rates for venous catheters are affected by the cleanliness of insertion, catheter location, dressing technique, use of the line, and duration of catheterization. With sterile technique, daily nonocclusive antibiotic dressing changes, and no inline stopcocks, a colonization rate of about 5% will be reached by 6 days. Bloodstream infections caused by indwelling catheters are less frequent, occurring one tenth as often as colonization. Controversy exists about "routine" catheter change policies. Many clinicians argue that catheters should be changed only if local or systemic signs of infection occur. There is an acceptable reduction in the

A new insertion site must be used if the colony count is greater than 15 colony-forming units.

infection rate if they are changed over a guidewire (in the absence of local infection) and the catheter tip is quantitatively cultured.

To culture a catheter tip, the skin entry site is sterilized with iodine-containing preparation solution. This is allowed to dry. The preparation is removed with alcohol and the catheter is withdrawn. The iodine will stain the catheter and mark the skin level. With sterile scissors, the last 1 to 2 cm of the catheter is cut into a dry, sterile vial. This must be immediately transported to the bacteriologic laboratory for culture by rolling the catheter on an agar plate. Broth culture of the catheter is also performed for anaerobic, aerobic, and fungal pathogens.

Pressure Waveforms

Normally, PAC placement can be accomplished by pressure transduction of the distal lumen. As the PAC passes through veins and the chambers of the heart, characteristic pressure wave patterns appear. These allow accurate bedside placement without the use of fluoroscopy. The PAC is inserted through an introducer; once the tip has been inserted past the introducer sheath and into the thoracic vessels, the balloon is inflated with 1.5 cm³ of air. PAC manufacturers recommend inflating with sterile CO_2 to minimize the effect of gas embolism if the balloon ruptures; however, this is rarely practical. Figure 13–8 illustrates the waveforms seen as the catheter passes through the cardiac structures.

A triphasic venous pressure wave should be seen first. As the catheter is slowly advanced, a right ventricular trace with higher systolic and lower diastolic pressure is seen. It is at this time that arrhythmias are frequent. Entry into the pulmonary artery is marked by an abrupt rise in diastolic pressure (and mean pressure) and an unchanged systolic pressure. Advancing the PAC further produces a fall in the pressure and a wedge tracing, similar to the previous triphasic venous tracing.

Table 13–3 lists the expected distance from the skin to the various cardiac structures from several insertion sites. If a catheter is inserted farther than the distances listed, it is probably looped on itself. Normal cardiac chamber pressures are listed in Table 13–4.

The presence of tricuspid stenosis or insufficiency often makes entry into the right ventricle difficult or impossible. With left ventricular dysfunction, mitral insufficiency, or a ventricular paced rhythm, a regurgitant V wave may distort the wedge pressure tracing, making a wedged catheter difficult to identify. A prominent V wave from mitral valvular regurgitation can obscure the normal configuration of a wedge tracing. The change from pulmonary artery tracing to wedge can be identified by noticing that the peak pressure occurs later in the cardiac cycle, as seen by timing with a simultaneous recording of the electrocardiogram.

If a wedge tracing is not seen after the catheter is inserted past 70 cm, the balloon should be allowed to deflate, the catheter should be withdrawn to 20 cm, and reinsertion should be attempted.

Inserting the PAC more than 50 cm without obtaining a ventricular trace should be avoided:

- A coil may have occurred.
- Catheter knotting is likely.

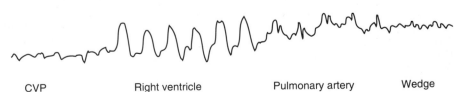

| CVP | Right ventricle | Pulmonary artery | Wedge |

FIGURE 13–8: As the pulmonary artery catheter is advanced through the chambers of the heart, this series of waveforms is seen. CVP, central venous pressure.

TABLE **13–3:** Approximate Guide for Pulmonary Artery Catheter Placement*

Insertion Site	Right Atrium	Right Ventricle	Pulmonary Artery	Wedge Position
Right internal jugular vein	22–30	25–35	30–45	40–55
Left internal jugular vein	25–30	28–38	34–48	44–58
Right external jugular vein	30–40	35–45	40–55	45–60
Left external jugular vein	35–45	40–50	45–60	50–65
Right subclavian vein	22–35	30–40	35–50	45–55
Left subclavian vein	30–40	35–45	40–55	45–60
Either femoral vein	30–40	35–45	40–55	45–60
Either brachial vein	70–90	75–95	80–110	90–120

*All values are in centimeters. Distances greater than these usually mean that the catheter has formed a coil or a knot in the right ventricle.

PACs may float past the heart into other peripheral vessels. In this case, no cardiac (ventricular) waveforms will be seen. Occasionally, a PAC will pass into the right ventricle and then loop back into the atrium. A venous waveform similar to a wedge tracing will be seen without identification first of the pulmonary artery tracing. The chest radiograph will identify this inappropriate position if clinical suspicions are not present. Occasionally, it is necessary to use fluoroscopy to ensure placement of difficult catheters. The radiation risk of this technique has been reduced, but it is not insignificant, especially to the operator.

Spontaneous breathing and mechanical ventilators alter intrathoracic pressure. These respiratory-induced pressure changes are transmitted to the vascular structures. In extreme cases, respiratory pressure variations may obscure identification of the wedge pressure. A simultaneous recording of airway pressure may help to identify the wedged catheter (as well as identification of the appropriate measurement point). Occasionally, measurement of PAC blood oxygen saturation can identify a wedged catheter when one of the previously mentioned conditions obscures the characteristic waveform. A blood sample aspirated from the distal (pulmonary artery) port will have a mixture of pulmonary capillary (fully saturated) and mixed venous blood, with a saturation higher than blood from a nonwedged catheter tip. This may even be higher than arterial oxygen saturation. A wedged continuous-reading fiberoptic mixed venous oxygen saturation monitoring PAC shows this increased O_2 saturation immediately and identifies the presence of intracardiac shunts.

Respiratory-Induced Pulmonary Artery Wedge Pressure Changes

As mentioned earlier, respiratory-induced intrathoracic pressures are transmitted to intravascular structures. In the case in which the

Patients should not be removed from mechanical ventilation or positive end-expiratory pressure for more than 1 to 3 heartbeats to measure vascular pressures because this alters hemodynamics acutely (and therefore does not represent the true clinical situation) and may cause worsening of respiratory function.

TABLE **13–4:** Normal Pressures in the Heart

Structure	Systolic Pressure (mm Hg)	Diastolic Pressure (mm Hg)	Mean Pressure (mm Hg)
Central venous pressure			0–12
Right atrium	8–15	2–4	4–12
Right ventricle	18–30	0–5	10–15
Pulmonary artery	18–30	10–15	15–25
Pulmonary artery wedge			5–15

catheter is in a segment of lung where there is no blood flow during all or part of the respiratory cycle (West's zone 1 or 2), the measured pressure may reflect only airway pressure. Even in zone 3 areas, respiratory pressures alter vascular pressures significantly. *To minimize* the effect of airway pressure on vascular pressure measurements, the end-exhalation point should be used for monitoring. A simultaneous airway (or intrathoracic) pressure tracing is helpful in identifying this point in the respiratory cycle. Automated systems for obtaining wedge pressures function poorly in patients with mixed forms of ventilation (i.e., those in whom both spontaneous and mechanical breaths are present).

DETERMINATION OF CARDIAC OUTPUT

The following equation relates O_2 consumption to CO:

$$CO = \dot{V}_{O_2}/[Ca_{O_2} - C\bar{v}_{O_2}]$$

where

Ca_{O_2} = arterial content of O_2
$C\bar{v}_{O_2}$ = mixed venous content of O_2
$\dot{V}_{O_2}$ = oxygen uptake determined from inhaled and exhaled gas analysis

Noninvasive methods have been used to determine CO. These include changes in thoracic electrical impedance, aortic Doppler flow methods, and carbon dioxide rebreathing (Fick method).

In addition to being needed for measuring preload, evaluation of CO is necessary to characterize ventricular performance. There are several ways to determine CO. The Fick principle, which uses the uptake of oxygen and the arteriovenous concentration difference to calculate CO, is often called the gold standard with which other methods are compared. Although the Fick method is considered to be the best one, there are inherent problems with it. In the presence of intracardiac shunts, this method is inaccurate in estimating forward CO. Steady-state conditions are necessary and are seldom obtained. Inaccuracies of gas analysis are compounded as the inspired O_2 percentage exceeds 40% and the inhaled-exhaled oxygen difference decreases. The Fick equation can also be used to provide a rough check on other methods of determining CO. By assuming a value for $\dot{V}_{O_2}$ (rather than measuring it directly), an estimate of CO can be made by measuring the arteriovenous O_2 content difference.

Impedance techniques use an alternating current applied to the thorax. Changes in impedance depend on the location and distribution of blood. Because the distribution of blood in the chest is changed primarily by the amount of blood in the heart (the path of lowest electrical resistance) and because this varies with systole and diastole, thoracic impedance changes should be directly related to cardiac stroke volume. Several complicated formulas have been used to calculate stroke volume with this technique. Included in the formula are the distance between cutaneous electrodes, hematocrit, left ventricular ejection time, and body temperature. This calculated stroke volume is multiplied by the heart rate to calculate CO.

The correlation between the value derived from the impedance cardiograph and other methods varies. In healthy volunteers, normal animals, and stable patients with cardiac disease, this method reflects the direction and magnitude changes in CO identified by other methods. In a critically ill population, less useful results were obtained. In one study of 27 critically ill patients, the correlation between thermodilution determinations and impedance methods was only 0.63. Both over- and underestimation of CO occurred. Technical difficulties, including maintenance of electrode placement and carotid upstroke recording (to determine left ventricular ejection time), were frequently a problem in these patients. No correlation between impedance measurements and wedge pressure could be demonstrated. No other hemodynamic variables (e.g., stroke work, resistance, CVP, or mixed venous oxygen saturation) can be derived by using this method. The authors concluded that electrical impedance CO was unsatisfactory for monitoring critically ill patients. In exercise physiology laboratories and in stable patients, this method has some value.

Doppler methods can be used to determine CO noninvasively. These depend on determining aortic cross-sectional area and average flow. These are measured by Doppler signals, and stroke volume is calculated. CO is stroke volume times heart rate. The accuracy of the velocity vector depends on maintaining a precise, optimal angle to aortic flow. As illustrated in Figure 13–9, Doppler probe placement can be extrathoracic (transthoracic), transesophageal, or transtracheal.

All of the Doppler techniques are very dependent on the location, signal direction, and acoustic contact of the Doppler ultrasound probe. User skill and experience are the keys to reproducible results. Movement of the probe is responsible for many of the changes seen clinically; artifacts are not easy to differentiate from actual cardiac functional changes. Comparison with other methods has shown variable correlation even in stable, healthy patients. These devices are large, delicate, and expensive.

A final way of determining CO noninvasively is with a pseudo–steady-state carbon dioxide rebreathing technique and the Fick relationship. An automated, microprocessor-driven device to perform this measurement is available (Gould 9000 IV System, Dayton, OH). In comparison to the bioimpedance technique, the use of this system was more accurate in normal patient volunteers who were not intubated and who were cooperative. Further work is needed to establish the reliability and usefulness of this device in clinical practice.

Steady-state CO_2 rebreathing
Using the equation

$$CO = [CO_2 \text{ uptake}]/[Cv_{CO_2} - Ca_{CO_2}]$$

CO_2 uptake is measured continuously from exhaled and inhaled respiratory gases.
Ca_{CO_2} is calculated from end-tidal P_{CO_2}.
Cv_{CO_2} is estimated from a 15-second rebreathing (with 10% CO_2) period performed intermittently.

CO can be determined from the following equation:

$$CO = (60 \times \text{indicator dose [mg]})/(\text{average concentration [mg/L]} \times \text{time [sec]})$$

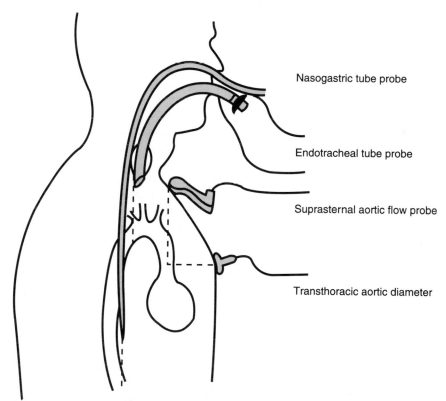

FIGURE 13–9: Determination of cardiac output from Doppler probes can be done in many ways. Illustrated here and discussed in the text are three techniques that have been reported. Optimal orientation and maintenance of the Doppler signal to aortic blood flow direction are critical for reproducible results.

Nasogastric tube probe

Endotracheal tube probe

Suprasternal aortic flow probe

Transthoracic aortic diameter

Indicator dilution (or dye dilution) methods can be used to determine CO. A bolus of colored dye (indocyanine green) is injected into a central vein, and the concentration curve of the dye in a peripheral artery is determined (Fig. 13–10). This method, widely accepted for investigations, is impractical in clinical situations because

- The dye persists for a time (until cleared by the liver), making repeated measurements less accurate.
- Blood must be withdrawn to measure the dye curve.
- Complicated mathematics (or planimetry) must be employed manually to calculate the area under the concentration curve.
- The dye stains tissues and colors urine.
- Allergic reactions to the indicator occasionally occur.

In children, smaller-volume injectates should be used to avoid excess fluid administration.

Iced fluids give a more accurate measurement of CO in most situations; however, in normal clinical situations, the accuracy with room temperature injectates is adequate.

Commonly, in critically ill patients, the thermodilution technique (with temperature difference being the indicator "dye") is used to determine CO. Most of the PACs used for pressure measurements have a thermistor for this purpose. A known quantity of cold fluid is injected proximal to the thermistor. The resultant temperature drop in pulmonary artery blood is detected. A computer integrates the temperature curve, determines an average temperature decrease for a defined period of time, and calculates the CO. Correction factors for the dead space of the PAC injection lumen and the temperature lost to surrounding structures are empirically derived and included in the calculation. This method is accurate to about 10% of the true value but has the same problems with intracardiac shunts mentioned previously for the Fick method. User factors also influence the accuracy of this method. The use of ice cold rather than room temperature fluid; an accurate volume; a rapid, constant injection speed (as with a pneumatic-powered injector); a consistent time during the respiratory cycle; and a consistent and experienced operator improve reliability. For most clinical situations, this technique is preferred, but only large changes (greater than 15%) should be considered significant. At least three measurements should be made, and the closest two (or all three) averaged. Repeated, frequent measurements are easy, with no significant accumulation of "dye." The common problems with this method are listed in Table 13–5.

If the volume or temperature is incorrectly entered into the computer, a large over- or underestimation occurs. If more indicator is injected than the computer assumes is injected (more volume or colder), an underestimation of CO will be seen. This happens if the computer thermometer is not in the ice bath but on a countertop (room temperature) when iced fluids are being used. Entering the wrong-size injectate syringe is another common mistake leading to large errors. If the distal

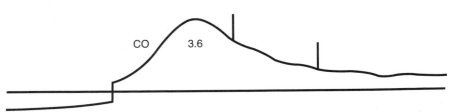

FIGURE 13–10: The injection of cold saline into the proximal lumen of a pulmonary artery catheter results in a fall in temperature at the thermistor located in the pulmonary artery. A temperature curve is illustrated here. CO, cardiac output.

TABLE **13–5:** Usual Problems Encountered With Thermodilution Cardiac Output Determination and Their Effect on the Value Obtained

Factor	Error	Effect on Cardiac Output Determination
Injectate temperature	Too warm	Overestimate
	Too cold	Underestimate
Slow injection	May warm	Overestimate
	Incomplete	Variable
Syringe size	Too small	Overestimate
	Too large	Underestimate
Injection port location	Right ventricle	Variable
	Superior vena cava	Overestimate
	Introducer	Overestimate
Pulmonary artery catheter tip location	Zone 1	Overestimate
	Zone 2	Variable
	Wedged	Overestimate

sensor is in a small vessel or wedged, the cold injectate diluted in pulmonary artery blood will not be detected and a high CO will be calculated. If the catheter is in West's zone 1, little blood or indicator may reach the catheter and a falsely elevated CO will be seen.

HEMODYNAMIC VARIABLES

BSA may be calculated from the following formula:

$$BSA = 0.202 \times weight^{0.425} (kg) \times height^{0.725} (m)$$

Once CO and filling pressures are measured, a series of useful values describing the cardiovascular system may be calculated. To adjust for variations in patient size, many are indexed to body surface area (BSA).

Table 13–6 lists the principal derived variables useful in describing hemodynamic function. These are useful for identifying abnormalities, quantitating their significance, and identifying changes over time. None of the derived variables adds information about the patient not already known from the primary, measured variables (i.e., CO, pulmonary and systemic blood pressures, right- and left-sided heart filling pressures, and heart rate).

Overinterpretation of these derived variables can lead to inappropriate therapy. For example, in hypovolemic shock with low blood pressure, systemic vascular pressure will be elevated and CO low. If SVR is believed to be a problem and a vasodilator is instituted, the patient outcome will be poor. In this case, an elevated SVR is the consequence (appropriate compensation) to prevent inadequate organ perfusion pressure when CO is profoundly decreased because of blood or fluid loss. Derived variables must not be interpreted without consideration of the measured components and the patient's clinical situation.

Stroke work, which relates the blood pressure to the stroke volume, is a measure reflecting the balance between the strength of the myocardium, filling pressure, and afterload. It is often reported corrected for BSA and in normal engineering units. Occasionally, it will be the variable representing cardiac function on a Frank-Starling curve. A list of normal values for these calculated variables is seen in Table 13–7.

OTHER MONITORS OF VENTRICULAR PERFORMANCE

An important measure of cardiac functional ability is the ejection fraction. In order to determine this fraction, ventricular systolic and

TABLE **13–6:**   Derived Values and Their Usual Units Used to Describe the Cardiovascular System

Calculated Variable	Formula	Units
Cardiac index (CI)	CI = CO/BSA	L/min/m^2
Systemic vascular resistance (SVR)	SVR = (MAP − CVP)/CO × 80	dynes•sec/cm^5
Systemic vascular resistance index (SVRI)	SVRI = (MAP − CPV) /CI × 80	dynes•sec/cm^5/m^2
Pulmonary vascular resistance (PVR)	PVR = (MPAP − PCWP)/CO × 80	dynes•sec/cm^5
Pulmonary vascular resistance index (PVRI)	PVRI = (MPAP − PCWP)/CI × 80	dynes•sec/cm^5/m^2
Stroke index (SI)	SI = CI/HR	mL/beat/m^2
Left ventricular stroke work index (LVSWI)	LVSWI = SI × (MAP − PCWP) × 0.0136	g•m/beat/m^2
Right ventricular stroke work index (RVSWI)	RVSWI = SI × (MPAP − CVP) × 0.0136	g•m/beat/m^2

BSA, body surface area; CO, cardiac output; CVP, central venous pressure; HR, heart rate; MAP, mean arterial pressure; MPAP, mean pulmonary artery pressure; PCWP, pulmonary capillary wedge pressure.

Ejection fraction is defined as the diastolic volume minus the systolic volume divided by the systolic volume (often expressed as a percentage). Normal values for this variable range from 45 to 55%.

diastolic volumes must be determined. There are several methods of measuring cardiac chamber size. Conventional radiographic techniques with ventricular injection of contrast material and biplanar views obtained in systole and diastole can be used to calculate ventricular volumes. This method requires insertion of a catheter into the left ventricle, injection of radiopaque dye, use of complicated radiographic equipment, and computer analysis of the ventriculograms obtained. It is not suitable for repeated measurements to adjust therapy or for use in unstable, critically ill patients. Other, less technically demanding techniques have been used to assess ventricular function and ejection fraction.

Gated blood pool scans have been used in stable patients with coronary artery disease, myocardial ischemia, and infarction to assess ventricular function. These techniques are replacing angiography for assessing ventricular performance and evaluating coronary blood flow. They also provide physiologic information complementary to the anatomic and structural evaluation provided by cardiac catheterization techniques. Three types of radioangiographic studies are available: radioactive isotope injection, rapidly responsive gamma radiation counters, and computer modeling techniques.

Myocardial perfusion imaging with radiolabeled ^{201}Tl is used to identify inhomogeneity of myocardial blood flow. Exercise- or vasodilator-induced normalization of hypoperfusion is the hallmark of ischemia. Persistent perfusion defects indicate myocardial infarction. Radionuclide angiocardiography is used to assess ventricular function. The first-pass method evaluates right- and left-sided heart function sequentially during a bolus administration of the tracer isotope ^{99}Tc. Rapid count images are analyzed. From these, wall motion abnormalities may be identified and the ejection fraction calculated. Differences in right- and left-sided heart

TABLE **13–7:**   Range of Normal Values for the Derived Variables

Calculated Variable	Normal Range
Cardiac output	4.6–7.5 L/min
Cardiac index	2.8–4.2 L/min
Stroke volume	60–90 mL/beat
Stroke index	30–65 mL/beat/m^2
Right ventricular stroke work	8.5–18 g•m/beat
Right ventricular stroke work index	5–10 g•m/beat/m^2
Left ventricular stroke work	80–120 g•m/beat
Left ventricular stroke work index	45–60 g•m/beat/m^2
Pulmonary vascular resistance	100–300 dynes•sec/cm^5
Pulmonary vascular resistance index	170–500 dynes•sec/cm^5/m^2
Systemic vascular resistance	1200–1600 dynes•sec/cm^5
Systemic vascular resistance index	2000–2600 dynes•sec/cm^5/m^2

function are often identified with this technique. Gated blood pool labeled angiography requires that red blood cells be radiolabeled (usually with ^{99}Tc) and that rapid repeated scans be performed during systole and diastole. In this way, the ventricular shape and size during systole and diastole can be determined and the ejection fraction calculated. This technique lends itself to repeated measurements during the half-life of the tracer. A final technique using infarct-avid labeled antibodies can be used to identify and quantitate acute infarct size.

These nuclear cardiographic techniques have added significantly to the evaluation and management of ambulatory patients with coronary artery disease. They are less invasive, less risky than angiography, and not painful. However, they require bulky, expensive gamma radiation counting equipment found only in sophisticated departments of radiology. There is some environmental risk and radiation exposure to other patients and caregivers. These techniques are not helpful for ongoing monitoring, but they can be used for diagnosis. Critically ill patients may be transported to these devices and the studies performed. Routine use of these techniques in the intensive care unit is unlikely in the near future; however, with simpler, more compact equipment, this will be possible in the future.

Ultrasound and Doppler Techniques for Evaluating Cardiac Function

The use of ultrasound and Doppler techniques for cardiac evaluation is not new. These kinds of measurements are attractive in the critically ill because they are noninvasive and indefinitely repeatable. Echocardiography uses sound waves in frequencies above the human audible range to penetrate tissues and create reflections or "echoes" that delineate cardiac chamber walls and valves. Differences in echo density create reflections at the interfaces between muscle and blood. The sound wave is produced by piezoelectrical crystals, which serve as both transmitter and receiver for the reflected waves. By sweeping the signal through an angle, a tissue plane in two dimensions can be viewed. This makes visual qualitative evaluation of cardiac chambers easy. The combination of Doppler evaluation of blood flow (a Doppler shift in frequency identifies the direction and perpendicular velocity of blood flow relative to the crystal) and echocardiography allows a complete evaluation of intracardiac shunts and valvular disorders. Septal defect sizes and valve areas can often be calculated.

Ventricular function is evaluated by qualitative assessment of wall motion. Estimates of ejection fraction can be made by examining several planes across the ventricle and calculating the systolic-diastolic change in size.

As the equipment has become smaller and more available, critically ill patients have begun to benefit from this safe form of cardiac evaluation. The usual "window" used in ambulatory patients is through the anterior chest wall between the ribs. This is less satisfactory in patients receiving mechanical ventilation because of patchy pulmonary atelectasis and hyperinflation. These lung changes adversely affect image quality and make accurate cardiac evaluation impractical. An esophageal probe, which has been used successfully to monitor patients in the operating room, is now being employed in the intensive care unit. In approaching the heart from behind, the lung is no longer an impediment to accurate visualization. The probe, mounted in the end of a gastroscope, can be rotated and flexed to obtain optimal axis views. Although this approach has been used in awake, sedated, ambulatory patients, it is ideal in patients already sedated to tolerate the typical intensive care unit interventions.

Promising results are emerging with the use of these techniques in the intensive care unit. Measuring actual ventricular size relative to filling pressure allows compliance to be calculated. Effects of airway pressures on the measured intracardiac pressures can be identified from observing heart size and contractility (as seen from wall shortening) during volume loading. The amount of data generated by this technique (about 4 million bytes per second) makes computer analysis in real time difficult. Most of the information is used in a qualitative and subjective manner; however, new algorithms for quantitative analysis are evolving.

Pressure-Volume Loops

The end-systolic pressure-volume relationship is a valuable index of ventricular function because of its independence from preload (and afterload, to some extent) and its dependence on contractility. If volume can be instantaneously measured and plotted against the intrachamber (usually the left ventricular) pressure during the cardiac cycle, a pressure-volume loop is generated (Fig. 13–11).

The components of the loop are as follows:

The interactions of preload, afterload, stroke volume, compliance, and contractility are reflected in this loop.

- A is the beginning of diastole and the opening of the mitral valve.
- B is the end of diastolic filling and the closure of the mitral valve.
- From B to C is isovolemic contraction.
- C is the opening of the aortic valve.

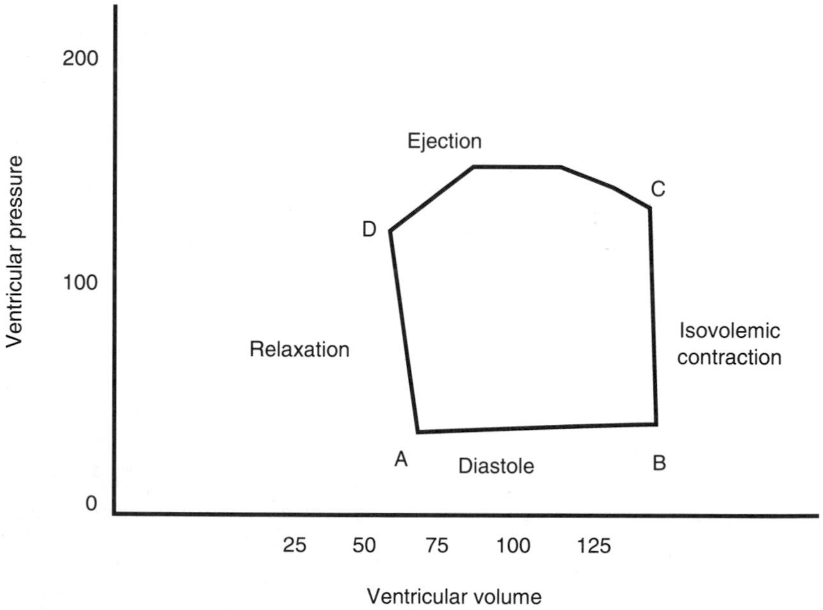

FIGURE 13–11: The complete cardiac cycle can be represented by a pressure-volume loop. Alterations in contractility, effects of various valvular lesions, and changes in heart rate, afterload, and filling pressure can be seen in alterations in this curve. Because cardiac volume is rarely known clinically, this representation is mostly applicable in theory and in experimental models.

- The period from C to D is ventricular ejection.
- D is the closure of the aortic valve and the end of ejection.

Intraventricular pressure falls between D and A when the mitral valve opens for the next cardiac cycle. In order to obtain the information needed to construct pressure-volume loops, intraventricular transducer-tipped catheters must be placed. This is rarely done in humans but is very common in experimental animal preparations. Pressure-volume loops are convenient to represent the changes seen in ventricular performance theoretically, but they are not useful in the clinical arena currently. An approximation of these curves can be obtained from echocardiographic assessment of myocardial wall segment length and pressure. This requires echodense markers to be attached to the heart and is useful in studying segmental abnormalities, such as occur with ischemia. This, as with classic pressure-volume loops, is most applicable to the experimental situation and is of little direct use in the clinical situation. The pressure-volume loop allows visual analysis of various clinical changes and the response to treatment.

Monitoring of Mixed Venous Oxygen ($S\bar{v}_{O_2}$)

PACs are available with implanted optical fibers that allow continuous measurement of hemoglobin saturation by reflectance spectrophotometry. The measurement of the saturation of venous blood may help identify pathologic states and allow titration of therapy. Changes in $S\bar{v}_{O_2}$ can be caused by changes in any (or all) of these factors: arterial saturation, hemoglobin level, cardiac output, and oxygen consumption. If several of these factors remain constant, changes in $S\bar{v}_{O_2}$ reflect changes in the other variables. Usually, the hemoglobin and oxygen consumption change only slowly. Arterial saturation can be independently assessed with pulse oximetry and is usually greater than 90%. Any acute change in $S\bar{v}_{O_2}$ is then due to a change in CO. This is a very useful monitor of CO in hemodynamically unstable patients in whom several cardiac medications are being simultaneously administered. This catheter gives immediate feedback about the direction in which the CO is changing. As a monitor of CO, this method is less helpful when more than one variable is changing. For instance, a patient who is actively shivering may have a rising CO but also a rising oxygen consumption, and the effect on $S\bar{v}_{O_2}$ depends on the balance between these opposing effects. The most important use of $S\bar{v}_{O_2}$ monitoring may be assessment of the balance between tissue oxygen delivery (primarily influenced by CO) and oxygen consumption. To this end, a new catheter capable of simultaneous continuous measurement of $S\bar{v}_{O_2}$ and CO (by thermodilution) has recently been introduced into clinical practice.

$S\bar{v}_{O_2}$ represents a flow-weighted average of all body tissues and organs. Organs vary widely in their ability to extract oxygen. The cardiac muscle extracts most of the oxygen supplied, and coronary vein P_{O_2} is between 5 and 10 mm Hg. Other tissues have some margin of reserve, with the kidney extracting very little of the delivered oxygen. Organ failure begins at an $S\bar{v}_{O_2}$ of about 50%. At values below 35% saturation (20 mm Hg), further oxygen extraction to compensate for total body inadequate delivery is not possible, and anaerobic metabolism, acidosis, and death ensue. $S\bar{v}_{O_2}$ does not identify the specific cause of the deficit but can be helpful in alerting clinicians to the presence of a problem. An

Four factors that affect $S\bar{v}_{O_2}$ are

- Arterial saturation
- Hemoglobin level
- CO
- Oxygen consumption

$S\bar{v}_{O_2}$ normally ranges between 65 and 75% ($P\bar{v}_{O_2}$ of 40 mm Hg).

$S\bar{v}_{O_2}$ can give an early warning of inadequate total body oxygen delivery.

increased serum lactate level is a marker of failure of oxygen delivery to peripheral tissues. In conditions with high CO and impairment in tissue oxygen utilization (e.g., sepsis, carbon monoxide poisoning), body oxygen consumption may be reduced and give a high value for $S\bar{v}_{O_2}$. Under these circumstances, the lactate level is useful in identifying inadequate tissue oxygenation.

HEMODYNAMIC PATTERNS IN COMMON PATHOLOGIC CONDITIONS

Table 13–8 summarizes commonly observed hemodynamic changes that occur in certain pathologic states. Additional comments relative to myocardial ischemia and pulmonary embolism are given in the following sections.

Myocardial Ischemia

The usual method for identifying an imbalance between myocardial oxygen demand and coronary artery blood flow oxygen supply is analysis of the electrocardiogram. Ischemia is suspected when the ST segments are depressed below the electrocardiographic isoelectric line or when T wave inversions or new Q waves occur. These changes are regional and occur in the distribution of the compromised circulation. Continued ischemia may progress to infarction, irreversible loss of myocardium. Detection of ischemia should lead to a modification of oxygen demand or an increase in oxygen delivery to prevent infarction. Increases in any of these may lead to or worsen the O_2 imbalance, resulting in ischemia. Heart rate is particularly important because as heart rate increases, the diastolic time when cardiac blood flow occurs decreases. Thus, increased heart rate leads to both increased O_2 demand and decreased supply. Elevation of afterload with increased blood pressure increases myocardial work and oxygen consumption, but it also raises coronary artery perfusion pressure and improves blood flow across stenotic coronary lesions. Nitroglycerine, which reduces preload and afterload, can improve the distribution of blood flow in the myocardium. Treatment of myocardial ischemia may worsen ischemia (hypoperfusion) of other organs in shock.

Myocardial ischemia may cause changes in cardiac function. As O_2 delivery begins to fail, diastolic relaxation is impaired early. Filling pressures rise acutely to high levels. Whenever a rapid rise in pulmonary artery wedge pressure is identified, myocardial ischemia must be suspected. A later change with ischemia is systolic failure. In this case, CO and blood pressure will fall along with the very high filling pressure.

Principal determinants of oxygen demand

• Heart rate
• Afterload
• Preload
• Contractility

TABLE **13–8:** Commonly Observed Hemodynamic Patterns in Disease

Disease State	Arterial Blood Pressure	Central Venous Pressure	PCWP	Pulmonary Artery Systolic Pressure	Cardiac Output
Hypovolemia	↓	↓	↓	↓	↓
Myocardial dysfunction	nl or ↓	nl or ↑	↑	nl or ↑	↓
Pulmonary embolism	nl or ↓	↑	nl or ↓	↑	nl or ↓
Sepsis	nl or ↓	nl	nl	nl	nl or ↑
Septic shock	↓	nl	nl or ↑	nl or ↑	↓

nl, normal; ↑, increased; ↓, decreased. PCWP, pulmonary capillary wedge pressure.

Earlier changes indicating ischemia are seen with echocardiography. New regional wall motion abnormalities are the hallmark of ischemia. The distribution and size of the changes identify the site of ischemia and its significance. Angiography and nuclear cardiography may also be used to confirm ischemia and infarction and to diagnose abnormal coronary artery anatomy, but they are not helpful in continuing monitoring during critical illness.

Pericardial tamponade is an infrequent complication of myocardial infarction. Tamponade may be caused by many diseases or by cardiac perforation due to line placement for monitoring. Temporary pacing catheters can penetrate an infarcted myocardium. This may be heralded by pacing of the diaphragm directly, an ominous finding. Treatment of pericardial tamponade is accomplished by pericardial fluid drainage, initially by needle and then, if needed, by surgical procedure. Chronic tamponade may present with pressures indistinguishable from those in congestive heart failure due to cardiomyopathy. Echocardiographic evaluation is necessary to make the correct diagnosis.

Acute Pulmonary Embolism

Occasionally, patients sustain acute pulmonary thromboembolism with a PAC in place. When this occurs, characteristic pressure changes follow. The magnitude of these changes depends on the size of the embolism and the amount of occluded pulmonary vasculature. The initial finding is an elevated pulmonary artery pressure. This is followed by a fall in CO and a concurrent fall in pulmonary artery wedge pressure. Right atrial pressure rises (CVP), and left atrial pressure falls. The magnitude of the pulmonary artery pressure rise correlates with the size of the embolism, except in patients with poor ventricular function.

The same acute hemodynamic pressure changes occur with venous air embolism. Larger amounts of air cause greater rises in pulmonary artery pressure. This may occur during catheter placement and can result in paradoxical arterial embolism. This is due to the increased pressure in the right atrium relative to the left atrium, with gas being pushed through a probe-patent foramen ovale. Up to 20% of the adult population is reported to have this abnormality. The treatment of air embolism is to stop the entrainment of gas by lowering the head (or cannulation site). Trapping the air in the apex of the heart by putting the patient's left side down may limit the amount in the pulmonary circulation. High inspired oxygen (100%) is helpful for improving oxygenation and absorbing the air bubbles by denitrogenating the blood. Hyperbaric chambers, which have been used to treat massive air embolism, should be considered if the clinical situation is grave and a chamber is available.

PUTTING IT TOGETHER

The question of what patients need what kind of hemodynamic monitoring is not a simple one. A rational approach to choosing methods of hemodynamic monitoring is presented in Table 13–9.

Routine clinical evaluation will identify patients unstable enough to warrant incurring the risks of invasive blood pressure monitoring. Another group of stable patients will receive aggressive monitoring because of the expectation that they may need significant interventions to pre-

---

Signs of cardiac tamponade:
- Rising CVP and wedge pressure
- Falling CO
- Eventually, equalization of pulmonary artery diastolic pressure, CVP, and wedge pressure

The combination of a rising pulmonary artery pressure and a fall in wedge pressure should alert the clinician to the possibility of pulmonary embolism. This combination is unique to pulmonary embolism and is diagnostic of this problem.

TABLE **13–9:** Summary of What Monitor to Use in What Group of Patients*

Patient Factors			Noninvasive Blood Pressure	Arterial Cannula	CVP Cannula	PAC	Fiberoptic PAC	TEE	Arteriographic Evaluation
Previous Health	Expected Course	Current Stability							
Normal	Improving	Stable	X						
Marginal	Improving	Stable		X	X?				
Poor	Improving	Stable		X		X			
Normal	Improving	Marginal		X	X				
Marginal	Improving	Marginal		X		X			
Poor	Improving	Unstable		X			X		
Normal	Declining	Stable		X		X		X	X
Poor	Declining	Marginal		X		X	X	X	X?
Poor	Declining	Unstable		X			X	X	

*The choice of the level of monitoring depends on the patient's previous health; the experience and skill of the physician; and the current stability, prognosis, and expected progress of the disease.

CVP, central venous pressure; PAC, pulmonary artery catheter; TEE, transesophageal echocardiography.

vent serious problems. This decision is based on knowledge of the disease process obtained from groups of similar patients. Most individuals will not require intervention, but the few who do will benefit significantly. In this category, those only needing monitoring cannot be separated ahead of time from those who will require treatment.

Preload assessment is necessary in all patients. In the absence of overt signs of congestive heart failure (neck vein distention, edema, and S_3 gallop), all critically ill patients are assumed initially to need more preload. The type and amount of fluid administered should be tailored to the individual patient. Urine output should be monitored at least hourly. The initial rate of fluid administration depends on the level of blood pressure and the heart rate. If blood pressure, heart rate, and urine output respond quickly, then maintenance fluids and continued noninvasive monitoring are used. If hemodynamic improvement is not rapid (rise in blood pressure, fall in heart rate, and increased urine output), placement of an invasive preload monitor should be considered. Clinicians' ability to predict filling pressures and CO correctly in critically ill patients is poor.

The added benefit of CO monitoring and the frequent discrepancy between right- and left-sided heart function and preload make the use of a PAC preferable to a CVP monitor in most situations. Often, this is for diagnosis rather than monitoring. Once the cause of shock (preload, afterload, CO, or other) has been identified, treatment is directed to this condition. Repeated fluid infusions, as described in a previous section, should be used to maintain preload in the optimal range. Patients requiring high levels of mechanical ventilation (increased airway pressure) should have aggressive monitoring of preload and cardiac function. Volume status in these patients is difficult to assess because of the effects of airway pressure on the measurement of preload, urinary perfusion, and effects on the heart chamber shape. Fluid challenges are needed to establish position on the Frank-Starling curve because pressure measurement alone is uninformative. If preload optimization is inadequate in improving the shock state, therapeutic use of agents to improve cardiac function should be considered.

CO monitoring with a thermodilution PAC will allow optimal balance between increasing contractility and afterload reduction. In very unstable patients, a PAC capable of continuous monitoring of $S\bar{v}_{O_2}$, CO, or both should be used to improve delivery of this potent therapy. If a significant discrepancy between filling pressure and myocardial performance (CO) exists, echocardiography should be used to evaluate the cardiac pressure-volume relationship and identify abnormal geometry. This is especially useful when myocardial ischemia, valvular heart disease, pericardial tamponade, or right-sided heart failure is suspected. Mechanical ventilation also alters the usual pressure-volume relationship. Management should be based on this information, and repeated measurements should be made to optimize treatment. Hemodynamic monitoring should be continued until a period of stability is established during which aggressive supportive therapy is no longer needed. Knowledge of the disease process should indicate that continued improvement is expected.

Hemodynamic and other types of monitoring in stable patients in whom catastrophic changes may occur is more controversial. This group includes many surgical patients with unrelated medical diseases. Patients with previous episodes of ischemia or recent myocardial infarction are at increased risk during the perioperative period. Invasive monitoring and optimization of cardiac function reduce the risk of myocardial failure and death in these patients. Patients who have had major vascular repairs, those who have had lung resections, those with poorly controlled hypertension, and those who have had major prolonged operations for cancer benefit from a period of intensive hemodynamic monitoring. Patients with pre-existing hepatic, lung, or kidney insufficiency and an intercurrent acute illness or operation benefit from monitoring. Elderly patients with injury or illness are often monitored, but evidence indicating improved outcome is lacking. Evidence supporting the use of specific monitors is often lacking. This is not surprising because a monitor has no direct therapeutic effect and only adds to patient risk. The use of the monitored data to make better clinical decisions adds to improved outcome but is difficult to study and prove scientifically. The value of monitoring to the patient depends on the skill and experience of the person responding to the data generated. Useful monitors help good clinicians care for critically ill patients more effectively.

SUMMARY

New tools for hemodynamic assessment are being developed. They will add less risk, deliver more and better data, integrate multiple pieces of data, and suggest therapeutic options and further studies. Artificial intelligence and decision-making techniques will be incorporated into integrated patient monitoring systems. The initial clinical assessment of patients, however, will remain paramount. The acceptance of new monitors will depend on their ease of use and on whether they provide unique information. The expected prognosis and progress of the disease process should dictate the intensity of monitoring used.

Suggested Readings

Branthwaite MA, Bradley RD. Measurement of cardiac output by thermal dilution in man. J Appl Physiol 43:434, 1968.

Bruner JMR. Handbook of Blood Pressure Monitoring. Littleton, MA, PSG Publishing, 1978.

Durbin CG. The range of pulmonary artery catheter balloon inflation pressures. J Cardiothorac Anesth 4:39, 1990.

Forrester JS, Diamond G, McHugh TJ, et al. Filling pressures in the right and left sides of the heart in acute myocardial infarction. A reappraisal of central venous pressure monitoring. N Engl J Med 285:190, 1971.

Forrester JS, Ganz W, Diamond GA, et al. Thermodilution cardiac output determination with a single flow directed catheter. Am Heart J 83:306, 1972.

Gardner RM. Direct blood pressure measurement—dynamic response requirements. Anesthesiology 54:227, 1981.

Huntsman LL, Stewart DK, Barnes SR, et al. Noninvasive Doppler determination of cardiac output in man: Clinical validation. Circulation 67:593, 1983.

Joint National Committee on Detection, Evaluation, and Treatment of High Blood Pressure. The 1984 report of the Joint National Committee. Arch Intern Med 144:1045, 1984.

Kahn JK, Sills MN, Corbett JR, Willerson JT. What is the current role of nuclear cardiology in clinical medicine? Chest 97:442, 1990.

Maki DG, Weise CE, Sarafin HW. A semiquantitative culture method for identifying intravenous-catheter-related infection. N Engl J Med 296:1305, 1977.

Michel LA, Bradpiece HA, Randour P, Pouthier F. Safety of central venous catheter change over guidewire for suspected catheter-related sepsis. A prospective randomized trial. Int Surg 73:180, 1988.

Nofleet ER, Watson CB. Continuous mixed-venous oxygen saturation measurements: A significant advance in hemodynamic monitoring. Clin Monit 1:245, 1985.

O'Quinn R, Marini J. Pulmonary artery occlusion pressure. Clinical physiology, measurement and interpretation. Am Rev Respir Dis 128:319, 1983.

Pearson D, Hudson L. Monitoring hemodynamics in the critically ill. Med Clin North Am 67:1343, 1983.

Porembka DT, Hoit BD. Transesophageal echocardiography in the intensive care patient. Crit Care Med 19:826, 1991.

Riedinger MS, Shellock FG, Swann HJC. Reading pulmonary artery and pulmonary capillary wedge pressure waveforms with respiratory variations. Heart Lung 10:675, 1981.

Seldinger SI. Catheter replacement of the needle in percutaneous arteriography. Acta Radiol 39:368, 1953.

Starling EH. The Linacre Lecture on the Law of the Heart. London, Longman's Green and Company, 1918.

Tuchschmidt J, Sharma MPO. Impact of hemodynamic monitoring in a medical intensive care unit. Crit Care Med 15:840, 1987.

Wasserman K. New concepts in assessing cardiovascular function. Circulation 78:1060, 1988.

Wiedemann HP, Matthay MA, Matthay RA. Cardiovascular-pulmonary monitoring in the intensive care unit (part I). Chest 85:537, 1984.

Wiedemann HP, Matthay MA, Matthay RA. Cardiovascular-pulmonary monitoring in the intensive care unit (part II). Chest 85:655, 1984.

14

Respiratory Monitoring

Morris I. Bierman, M.D.

The practice of respiratory monitoring has become increasingly sophisticated as technology has made possible relatively simple methods of measuring pulmonary mechanics and gas exchange. Respiratory monitoring, which is crucial to the quality of care, allows the clinician to follow the course of the disease, adjust therapy, and observe the development of complications. In addition, the ideal monitoring system enables data to be manipulated to display trends, summarize important deviations from a baseline determined by the clinician, and sound alarms to alert bedside staff to values outside predetermined boundaries. New technology has attempted to incorporate these ideal characteristics, with various degrees of success. Nevertheless, a variety of respiratory variables can be easily monitored and used in patient care.

The greatest impact of new technology has been in the monitoring of arterial blood gas parameters. Pulse oximetry, capnography, and mass spectroscopy have revolutionized our ability to observe gas exchange over time. Their clinical applications are discussed here. New technology has had less of an impact on the monitoring of respiratory mechanics. The basic measurements of flow, pressure, and volume still form the basis for assessing pulmonary mechanics. These basic measures provide a wealth of information that can be obtained with relatively simple equipment and techniques. From these basics, other measures can be derived, such as resistance, compliance, and the work of breathing.

BASIC MEASUREMENTS

Respiratory function can be characterized by observations of the respiratory rate and pattern of respiratory movements, coupled with measurement of pressure, flow, and volume.

Respiratory Motion

Observation of the patient's respiratory efforts along with measurement of the respiratory rate allows an easy assessment of overall pulmonary status. This information is most readily obtained from repeated physical examinations, although advanced techniques allow these variables to be automatically recorded and analyzed.

Respiratory Rate

Normal respiratory effort is cyclic, at a rate of 12 to 20 breaths per minute.[1]

The respiratory rate is a sensitive but nonspecific indicator of the presence or absence of respiratory pathology.[1-3] Slow rates indicate central respiratory depression, such as from drug intoxications or neurologic disease. Rapid rates may result from a wide variety of respiratory disorders and also from nonpulmonary conditions such as anxiety.

Irregular respiratory efforts can be demonstrated in normal individuals, especially with aging,[1] although they are generally regarded as nonspecific markers of dysfunction. For example, the periodic hyperpneas and apneas of Cheyne-Stokes respirations arise from a diverse etiology including severe congestive heart failure and structural lesions within the central nervous system. Other disturbances of the respiratory rhythm that have a neurologic origin include ataxic, apneustic, and cluster breathing.[4]

Pattern of Breathing

The normal motion of the thorax and abdomen is a smooth cycle of outward movement with inspiration and inward movement with expiration. Changes in this tidal motion are easily observed, with certain changes in the respiratory motion associated with the development of respiratory failure. Typically, in respiratory failure, rate increases, thoracoabdominal movements become asynchronous, and tidal volumes decrease before the patient suffers a respiratory arrest.[5] Continuous monitoring of these variables can alert the clinician to an impending respiratory catastrophe. Although discoordination and overt paradox of the normal thoracoabdominal motion are generally associated with respiratory muscle fatigue, they may be observed with increased loads on the respiratory muscles with or without fatigue.[6]

Automated methods allow respiratory rate and pattern to be monitored over time without observer bias. These methods include measurement of thoracic impedance, temperature changes at the mouth or nose, fluctuations in end-tidal carbon dioxide concentration, and airway pressure deviations in intubated patients. For monitoring respiratory movements, a number of devices can be placed around the thorax and abdomen. They include strain gauges, magnetometers, and more commonly, the respiratory inductive plethysmograph.[6]

Commercially available devices allow both breath-by-breath and trend analysis, which makes them useful in intensive care units, special care units, and sleep laboratories.

In respiratory inductance plethysmography, two electrical transducer bands are placed around the upper thorax and the abdomen, allowing accurate recording of the respiratory rate and pattern, inspiratory-expiratory timing, and the contribution of both the thoracic and the abdominal compartments to the total respiratory effort.[5, 7] Calibration of the instrument allows relative changes in respiratory volumes to be measured.[7]

Pressure

Maximal Inspiratory and Expiratory Pressures

The monitoring of airway pressure provides a wealth of information. In the spontaneously breathing patient, serial measurements of the maximal inspiratory pressure and the maximal expiratory pressure with simple aneroid pressure gauges provide an index of respiratory muscle strength.[8] These measurements are useful for observing the respiratory status over time in patients with neuromuscular disorders such as myasthenia gravis or Guillain-Barré syndrome. When the maximal inspiratory pressure decreases below 30% of its predicted value, hypercapnia can result, even in patients with no underlying lung disease.[11] In patients who are being weaned from mechanical ventilation, the maximal inspi-

Healthy men generate maximal inspiratory pressures of 106 ± 31 cm H_2O and maximal expiratory pressures of 148 ± 34 cm H_2O. These values are somewhat lower in women and also decline with age.[9, 10]

ratory pressure has been used as a predictor of weaning success, with mixed results.[12–15] As a weaning test, it is sensitive in identifying patients who can be successfully weaned, but it is not specific.[15]

These measurements are highly dependent on the patient's effort, respiratory drive,[16] understanding of the test, and coaching by the respiratory therapist. Inspiratory efforts should begin as close to residual volume as possible. Expiratory efforts should occur after full inspiration to the patient's total lung capacity. In intubated patients, the accuracy of inspiratory pressure measurements can be improved with the addition of a one-way valve[17] allowing only exhalation. This forces the patient to make serial efforts from lung volumes closer to the residual volume. Even under the best of circumstances, maximal inspiratory pressure measurements may vary widely, especially when they are taken by different personnel.[18]

Respiratory Drive

The airway pressure tracing can also be used to assess respiratory drive.[19, 20] The pressure generated in the first 0.1 second of inspiration against an airway that has been occluded without the patient's knowledge ($P_{0.1}$) reflects respiratory drive. The $P_{0.1}$ may be useful in patient assessment during weaning from mechanical ventilation.[20–22] The strength of the respiratory muscles and the lung volume at which the $P_{0.1}$ is measured can affect the test results. The special equipment required to measure $P_{0.1}$ includes an interrupter valve and a strip chart recorder, although attempts have been made to simplify the procedure.[20, 23] In patients receiving mechanical ventilation, the pressure generated in the first 100 milliseconds of an inspiratory effort, before the demand valve opens and allows airflow, is believed to be analogous to the $P_{0.1}$ measured with an occlusion valve.[20]

Positive Pressure Ventilation

Airway pressure monitoring is essential for applying and titrating positive pressure ventilation. All mechanical ventilators incorporate some type of airway pressure monitoring (peak airway pressure or positive end-expiratory pressure [PEEP]), and some include graphic displays. Ideally, these pressures should be monitored at the endotracheal tube; however, they are commonly measured within the expiratory limb or, in older machines, proximally within the inspiratory circuit.[24] Airway tracings may be obtained by inserting an adapter with a sidearm into the airway at the endotracheal tube and connecting it with pressure tubing to a standard pressure transducer generally used for intravascular monitoring. Alternatively, the pressure tubing may be connected to the port normally used for temperature monitoring. It is not necessary to use a fluid-filled system, as with intravascular pressure monitoring. To prevent artifacts, the monitoring port should be perpendicular to the direction of gas flow. On most bedside monitors, these pressure measurements can be displayed graphically as a pressure-time tracing along with a digital display of the peak and mean pressures.

Peak/Mean Airway Pressure. In intubated patients, knowledge of the peak airway pressure is crucial for the safe application of positive pressure ventilation. Peak airway pressure is influenced by both resistive and elastic elements, such as the tidal volume, lung compliance, chest wall compliance, airflow, level of PEEP, and airway resistance.[25] Exces-

Because such systems are generally designed for intravascular monitoring, they report values in millimeters of mercury. These values can be converted to the conventional units, centimeters of water, by multiplying them by 1.36.

sive peak pressures and mean airway pressures may be associated with the development of barotrauma.[26, 27] Furthermore, cyclic overpressurization and distention of the alveoli can induce injury even in otherwise normal lungs.[28–30] The peak airway pressure can also be used to assess responsiveness to bronchodilators during passive breathing if the machine settings are kept constant.[31] The mean airway pressure is also a useful variable to follow because it has been linked not only to the level of ventilation and oxygenation but also to adverse effects such as hemodynamic compromise.[32]

Positive End-Expiratory Pressure. The pressure in the thorax at end-expiration is an important but occasionally overlooked variable. PEEP is usually produced intentionally to improve oxygenation by preserving or increasing the functional residual capacity.[33] An insidious form of PEEP can develop, however, when insufficient time is allowed for exhalation such that expiratory flow persists when the next breath is initiated. For such flow to occur, PEEP must be present, generally with hyperinflation of the chest above its relaxation volume at full exhalation. This can occur in either spontaneously breathing or mechanically ventilated patients. Patients requiring a long expiratory time, such as those with airflow obstruction related to chronic obstructive pulmonary disease or asthma, are at greatest risk for the development of auto-PEEP.

Intrinsic PEEP may not be detected in mechanically ventilated patients (Fig. 14–1) unless special measurements are made.[34] With the expiratory valve open at end-expiration, the ventilator manometer reflects only the value of the applied PEEP, not the actual alveolar pressure. Occlusion of the expiratory port at end-expiration permits the manometer to equilibrate with the alveolar pressure, thereby allowing measurement of the intrinsic PEEP. Measurements can also be made from graphic tracings of pressure-volume curves[36] or pressure-flow curves.[37] Unless this occult PEEP is accounted for, significant errors in the calculation of respiratory system compliance can be made.[37]

Multiple consequences of intrinsic PEEP exist:[38]

- The end-expiratory flow created by the auto-PEEP must be terminated by the spontaneously breathing patient before the next breath can be initiated. This increases the work required to initiate a breath.[39]
- Hyperinflation of the thorax may place the respiratory muscles in an undesirable length-tension relation, which increases the work of breathing.
- Additional positive pressure in the thorax creates problems identical to those of applied PEEP, including the risks of barotrauma and hemodynamic compromise.[34]

Pressure Wave Contour. The contour of the airway pressure tracing provides additional useful information in the intubated patient (Fig. 14–2). Negative deflections in the tracing indicate patient effort and thus distinguish spontaneous breaths from mandatory breaths. The degree of the deflection indicates the adequacy of the ventilatory system relative to the patient's efforts. A delayed increase in the pressure tracing of a mechanical breath can be indicative of inadequate delivery of the breath (e.g., inadequate airflow) relative to the patient's effort (Fig. 14–3). A pressure tracing that does not return to baseline between breaths indicates an inadequate expiratory time, and one that depicts pressures lower than expected indicates a leak within the system.

Occult PEEP, also termed auto-PEEP[34] or intrinsic PEEP,[35] may be greater than the PEEP that is applied externally by the clinician.

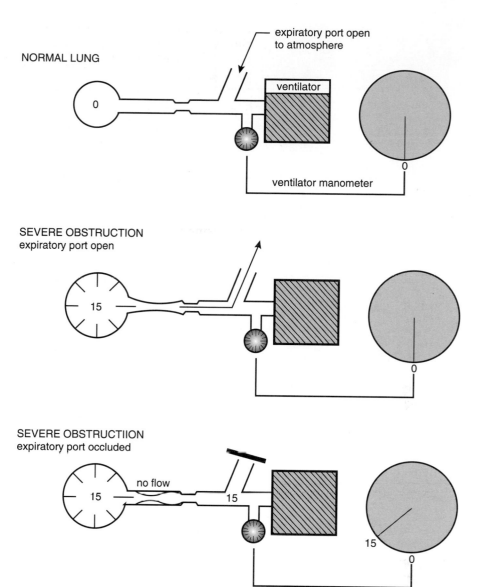

FIGURE 14–1: Measurement of auto–positive end-expiratory pressure by expiratory port occlusion. Normally *(top)*, alveolar pressure is atmospheric at the end of passive exhalation. With severe airflow obstruction *(center)*, alveolar pressure remains elevated (in this example, at 15 cm H_2O) and slow flow continues, even at the end of the set exhalation period. The ventilator manometer senses negligible pressure because it is open to the atmosphere through large-bore tubing and downstream from the site of flow limitation. With gas flow stopped by occlusion of the expiratory port at the end of the set exhalation period *(bottom)*, pressure equilibrates throughout the lung-ventilator system and is displayed on the ventilator manometer. (From Pepe PE, Marini JJ. Occult positive end-expiratory pressure in mechanically ventilated patients with airflow obstruction. Am Rev Respir Dis 126:167, 1982.)

Pleural Pressure

Monitoring the pleural pressure is of value in some circumstances. Knowledge of the pleural pressure allows differentiation of the chest wall and pulmonary components of the total respiratory system compliance. In addition, the value of the pleural pressure at end-expiration is useful for calculating the transmural pressures of the cardiac chambers to interpret hemodynamic data more accurately. Finally, negative deflections in the pleural pressure tracings can be used to measure the patient's inspiratory efforts.

Direct measurement of the pleural pressure in patients is difficult;

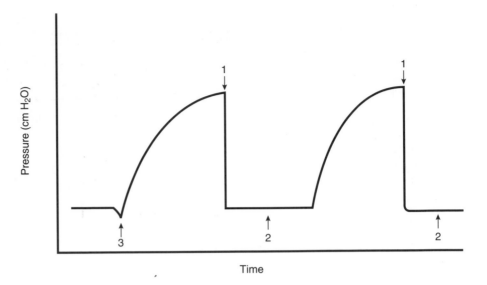

1. Peak airway pressure.
2. Positive end-expiratory pressure.
3. Negative pressure deflection due to patient effort

FIGURE 14–2: The pressure-time tracing in an intubated patient receiving mechanical ventilation. The first breath is triggered by the patient. The second represents a mandatory breath.

however, the esophageal pressure has been used to measure the pressure in the pleural space indirectly. The measurement is obtained by placing a catheter, either with or without a balloon, into the esophagus and connecting it to a pressure transducer. If a balloon-tipped catheter is used, it is placed into the stomach initially and then withdrawn into the lower third of the esophagus. The absolute value of the pleural pressure measured in this fashion is influenced by multiple factors, such as the weight of the mediastinal contents and patient position. Furthermore, the pleural pressure is not necessarily constant throughout the pleural space. Relative changes in the pleural pressure, however, can be accurately monitored.[40]

Airflow

Airflow is another important variable used to describe the mechanical properties of the respiratory system. A number of devices are available for measuring airflow in both spontaneously breathing patients and those receiving mechanical ventilation. Such devices may use rotating vanes or cogs and thermal or ultrasonic elements.[41, 42] The inertia and momentum generated by the airflow can affect the accuracy of devices that have rotating elements. The pneumotachograph, a flow measuring device, assesses the decrease in pressure across a known resistance to determine airflow.[40, 42] The resistive element may consist of screens or capillary tubes to maintain laminar flow. Routine clinical use of such a device is difficult because temperature changes, condensation, and airway secretions can all profoundly affect the measurements obtained. When flow rates outside the range of those necessary to create laminar conditions are required, a variable-orifice pneumotachograph is used. This device uses a restrictive orifice to create a pressure gradient to

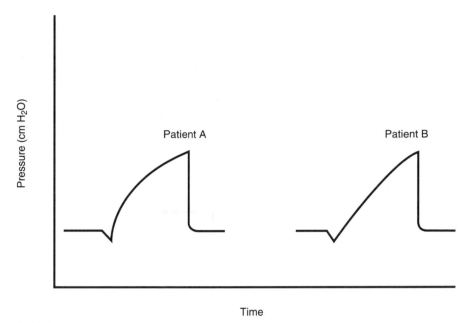

FIGURE 14–3: The pressure-time tracing in intubated patients receiving mechanical breaths. Patient A demonstrates a normal contour. Patient B is making vigorous efforts, resulting in distortion of the normally smooth rise in airway pressure during a mechanical inspiration.

measure airflow; however, the size of the orifice varies in order to accommodate moisture and condensation better. Electronic processing compensates for the turbulence in actually measuring the flow [43]

Peak Flow

In patients with asthma, peak flow has been used both to assess the severity of disease and to monitor response to treatment. Several portable devices allow patients to measure their own peak flow conveniently. Accurate measurement of the peak flow is highly dependent on patient effort, as well as on beginning the forced exhalation from a full inhalation. Repeated measurements are crucial to assess the response to therapy.

Flow-Time Curve

In the intubated patient, the flow-time curve is useful for assessing the presence or absence of intrinsic PEEP. If airflow does not decrease to zero before the next breath is initiated, then some degree of intrinsic PEEP must exist. In addition, the slope of the expiratory curve coupled with the expiratory time indirectly measures expiratory resistance (Fig. 14–4).

Lung Volume

Spirometry Testing

The final variable used to quantify respiratory mechanics is lung volume spirometry testing. Lung volumes exclusive of the functional residual capacity are easily measured with spirometry. Although the spirometer remains the preferred device for measuring lung volumes in the pulmonary function laboratory, portable devices suffice for bedside testing. Such devices must be carefully chosen to ensure that established

Normal peak flow rates vary with a patient's age and height, but they may range from 550 to 700 L/min.[44] Peak flow rates of less than 30 to 50% of the patient's predicted value (or the patient's personal best value) indicate severe airway obstruction. Peak flow rates of less than 25% of the patient's predicted value may be associated with serious hypercapnia.[44]

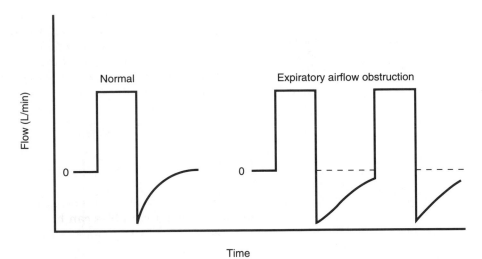

FIGURE 14–4: The flow-time curve on the left is normal; that on the right shows a delayed return to baseline in a patient with expiratory airflow obstruction. Note that if the subsequent breath follows too closely, flow will not return to zero before the next breath is initiated, which is an indirect indicator of the presence of intrinsic positive end-expiratory pressure. The inspiratory limb demonstrates a "square wave" or constant-flow pattern.

standards are met (i.e., those set by the American Thoracic Society) so that reliable data can be obtained.[45, 46] In the intubated patient, lung volume is generally quantified by integrating measurements of flow over time. Lung volumes containing the functional residual capacity are difficult to measure outside of the pulmonary function laboratory. The requirement for specialized equipment, the use of indicator gases such as helium, and manipulation of the ventilatory circuit make such measurements much too cumbersome to be used routinely.[47]

Mechanical Versus Spontaneous Ventilation

In mechanically ventilated patients, the ventilator and patient circuit may influence the measured and delivered volumes.[48] As compliance or resistance worsens, increasing amounts of gas are compressed, causing distention of the ventilator circuit as the lungs are inflated. This proportion of the tidal volume clearly does not contribute to gas exchange and thus affects the actual alveolar minute ventilation. Some ventilators compensate for this "lost" volume by adjusting the total delivered tidal volume for the compliance of the circuit, whereas others cannot.[24] Measuring the exhaled tidal volume at the endotracheal tube compensates for this wasted ventilation. Alternatively, if the compliance of the circuit is known, the proportion of the volume lost to the circuit can be calculated.

In the mechanically ventilated patient, serial monitoring of inspiratory and expiratory volumes is crucial. When these volumes are not equal, either a leak in the system exists, air trapping exists, or circuit compression volume has not been accounted for.

In spontaneously breathing patients, measurement of the vital capacity has been used to estimate respiratory muscle strength. As with pressure and flow measurements, an accurate result is highly dependent on patient cooperation and effort, as well as on the skill of the therapist in obtaining the measurement. The use of one-way valves, causing the patient to "stack" breaths, has been suggested as a means of obtaining such measurements in uncooperative patients.[50] Serial measurement of the vital capacity has been useful for monitoring the respiratory status

Graphic depictions of volume over time can also be useful. A volume curve that does not return to zero at end-exhalation indicates either air trapping or a leak within the system.

The normal vital capacity is approximately 70 mL/kg.[49]

Minimal values of approximately 10 mL/kg (vital capacity) and 5 mL/kg (tidal volume), respectively, have been reported to predict weaning success.[51]

of patients with neuromuscular disease over time. In patients receiving mechanical ventilation, the vital capacity and tidal volume have been used with limited success to predict weaning ability.[14–16] One study has demonstrated that the tidal volume is a sensitive but nonspecific indicator of weaning success.[15] Its specificity could be improved by dividing the tidal volume into the respiratory rate. This index can detect rapid breathing with small tidal volumes, which is considered a sign of impending respiratory failure.

DERIVED VARIABLES

From the basic measurements of pressure, flow, and volume, a number of additional variables can be calculated to characterize the respiratory system more fully. These variables include resistance, compliance, and the work of breathing. The following discussion of these variables relates to intubated patients. These measurements can be obtained in patients without an artificial airway, but this requires highly specialized techniques. Measurements of this type are within the capabilities of a moderately sophisticated pulmonary function laboratory but are not performed routinely.

In patients receiving mechanical ventilation, the information necessary to understand the calculations of resistance, compliance, and respiratory work can be derived from the pressure-time tracing recorded during passive inflation of the chest and lungs (Fig. 14–5). Inspiration starts either from atmospheric pressure or from the level of PEEP. Pressure in the thorax then increases to a peak as the ventilator increases positive pressure in the lungs. The rate of increase in airway pressure is determined by airway resistance, the compliance of the respiratory system (lungs and chest wall), and the flow rate and pattern. These factors, as well as the tidal volume, determine the peak pressure obtained. Inertial factors and tissue resistance also affect peak airway pressure; however, these influences are considered to be negligible.[52] If an end-inspiratory pause is imposed, the recorded pressure then decreases to a plateau pressure as the forces necessary to overcome the airway resistance dissipate and the lungs undergo stress relaxation. This pressure, which is obtained under static conditions (e.g., no airflow), is the value necessary to maintain inflation at the tidal volume given. Thus, it reflects the compliance of the respiratory system.

Airway Resistance

Resistance, which represents the pressure gradient needed to achieve a given airflow, is quantified by measuring flow and pressure. Dividing the pressure gradient needed to attain any given flow by the flow yields the resistance of the respiratory system. To obtain a meaningful number, the flow must remain constant during the time that the resistance is measured. Furthermore, the patient must not make spontaneous efforts because they distort the measured pressures.

Another confounding factor is the volume at which the resistance is measured. The diameter of the airways increases as the lungs inflate as a result of parenchymal distention as well as dilatation created by the force of the mechanical inflation. The resistance measured will thus be influenced by the volume at which it is measured and whether the measurement is taken during inspiration or expiration. When measurements

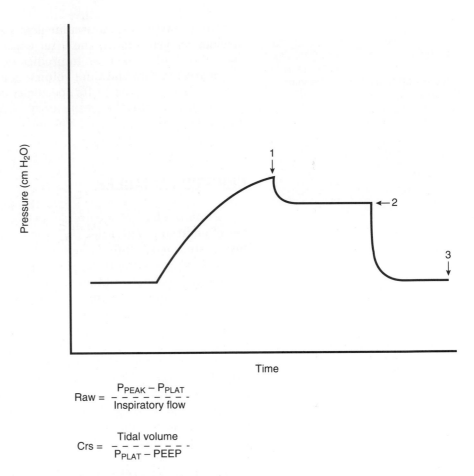

Pressure (cm H_2O)

Time

$$Raw = \frac{P_{PEAK} - P_{PLAT}}{Inspiratory\ flow}$$

$$Crs = \frac{Tidal\ volume}{P_{PLAT} - PEEP}$$

1. P_{PEAK} = Peak airway pressure
2. P_{PLAT} = Plateau pressure during inspiratory pause
3. PEEP = Positive end-expiratory pressure
4. Raw = Inspiratory airway resistance
5. Crs = Respiratory system compliance

FIGURE 14–5: The pressure-time tracing of a passive mechanical breath using constant flow in an intubated patient. An inspiratory hold allows demonstration of the plateau pressure.

are compared over time, it is crucial for them to have been taken at the same lung volume and during the same phase of respiration. In addition, in the patient with obstructive airway disease, dynamic collapse of the airway can further increase expiratory resistance and limit airflow.[35]

Inspiratory Resistance

Inspiratory resistance is calculated by dividing the pressure required to overcome the frictional resistance of the airway by the inspiratory flow. The difference between the peak airway pressure, representing the amount needed to overcome compliance and resistive factors, and the plateau pressure, representing only elastic or compliance factors, is divided by the inspiratory flow rate to obtain the inspiratory resistance (see Fig. 14–5).[52] A constant flow pattern (e.g., a "square" wave) should be used to perform the measurement to ensure constant flow rates. The resistance of the endotracheal tube will be included in the calculation unless airway pressures are measured with a catheter inserted into the trachea below it.

Expiratory Resistance

When the measurements are obtained in this fashion, the expiratory resistance of the entire system (including the lungs, endotracheal tube, expiratory circuit, and expiratory or PEEP valve) is actually being measured.

Expiratory resistance is measured by interrupting exhalation several times during deflation of the lungs.[35, 52, 53] The pressure gradient for airflow during exhalation occurs between the alveoli and the airway. Alveolar pressure is estimated by interrupting the expiratory flow, allowing equilibration between the alveolar and airway pressures. Because resistance increases as the lungs deflate, multiple interruptions during a passive exhalation are necessary to characterize the expiratory resistance fully. When dynamic airway collapse occurs, transient supranormal flows are generated that are easily recognized with the interrupter technique.[35] The creation of flow-pressure curves allows analysis of the resistive properties of the airway throughout exhalation.[31, 35]

The measurement of airway resistance is useful in assessing its contribution to the work of breathing, as opposed to that contributed by pulmonary compliance.[25] Measurements of resistance are also useful in titrating bronchodilator administration.[31, 55] A decrease in peak pressure alone is a valid measure of bronchodilator response.[31] Inspiratory resistance is easily measured using passive inflation and a square-wave flow pattern with standard monitoring equipment. The measurement of expiratory resistance, however, requires special equipment, including a shutter valve, a pneuomotachometer, and a differential transducer.

Respiratory System Compliance

The greater the compliance, the more the volume changes as pressure is applied. The reciprocal of compliance is known as elastance.

Whereas resistance is defined by the relation between airflow and pressure, compliance is defined by the relation between volume and pressure. In the lungs, the measured compliance differs between inspiration and expiration because of a number of factors, including surface tension forces and recruitment of collapsed lung units. This phenomenon is known as hysteresis. The compliance must be related to the volume against which it is measured. At full inflation, the compliance of the lung decreases as the lung pressurizes without volume change (much as the tension in a rubber band drastically increases if stretching continues once it has been pulled taut). On full exhalation, compliance also deteriorates as lung units collapse. Therefore, compliance must be measured over a range of volumes in order to produce a curve that fully characterizes the lung.

Technical Considerations

Generally, compliance refers to the compliance of the total respiratory system (lungs plus chest wall), unless otherwise specified.

Technical considerations are important in determining respiratory compliance. First, inflation of the thorax occurs as a result of expansion of both the lungs and the chest wall, so the compliance of each must be considered. If the volume change of the thorax is related to the change in airway pressure, the compliance of the total respiratory system is obtained. Relating the volume change to the pleural pressure allows one to measure actual pulmonary compliance. If the state of chest wall compliance is kept constant over time, any changes that occur can be attributed to the lungs.

The second consideration concerns the pressure measurement used to determine the compliance. As previously described, peak airway pressure is determined by both airway resistance and respiratory compliance and is therefore not appropriate for measuring the compliance. The plateau pressure, measured with an inspiratory hold, reflects the elastic forces within the lungs and chest wall. It is important that the measurement be taken from passive inflation of the lungs by the mechanical ventilator.

A third consideration relates to the presence of either externally applied PEEP or intrinsic PEEP. In measuring compliance, only the pressure change over which the lung is inflated to a given volume should be used. This means that the total PEEP (applied PEEP plus intrinsic PEEP) must be subtracted from the plateau pressure before the compliance is calculated or substantial errors may result.[37]

The final consideration concerns the tidal volume measurement. The actual exhaled tidal volume must be used after correction for the distensibility of the ventilator and circuit. Some of the newer mechanical ventilators automatically make this adjustment in reporting the tidal volume. If the compliance of the ventilator circuit is known, the applied volume can be adjusted for this distensibility. Alternatively, if the tidal volume is measured at the endotracheal tube, the need to adjust for the ventilator circuit is eliminated.

In summary, the respiratory system compliance is calculated by dividing the plateau airway pressure into the tidal volume. The tidal volume must be corrected for the distensibility of the ventilator circuit unless the measurement is taken at the endotracheal tube. The plateau pressure must also be corrected for the presence of PEEP (applied or intrinsic). If actual lung compliance is desired, pleural pressures should be used.

Static Versus Dynamic Conditions

When the plateau airway pressure is being measured, static conditions occur during the inflation hold with no airflow. This allows calculation of the "static" compliance. When the tidal volume is divided by the peak pressure, after correction for any PEEP, the "dynamic" compliance is obtained. This does not actually represent true compliance because the peak pressure is generated from both resistive and compliance elements. If the static and dynamic compliances are measured serially over a range of tidal volumes, useful clinical information can be obtained.[56] A decrease in the dynamic compliance with preservation of the static compliance indicates worsening airway resistance. Situations causing this include worsening bronchospasm and progressive occlusion of the endotracheal tube by kinking or secretions. Alternatively, when both dynamic and static compliances worsen, the site of the pathology is not likely to be in the airway. Situations causing this include pulmonary edema, diffuse lung injury (adult or infant respiratory distress syndrome), tension pneumothorax, and mainstem bronchial intubation.

Work of Breathing

Work is defined as the application of a force over a given distance. The analogy in terms of the respiratory system is the pressure applied (force) for a given volume displacement of the lungs and chest wall (distance). In the spontaneously breathing patient, the forces applied by the respiratory muscles cannot be accurately measured. In the intubated

These calculations do not account for work performed during exhalation, which can be considerable in patients with obstructive airway disease or those receiving mechanical ventilation because of the resistance of the expiratory circuit (especially the PEEP valve).[60, 61]

patient, inspiratory work performed by the ventilator can be calculated from the area beneath the pressure-volume waveform during passive inflation of the chest.[57] This calculation indicates the work performed by the ventilator to inflate the chest; however, it is difficult to relate to the patient's respiratory work during spontaneous efforts. The patient's respiratory work can be estimated by subtracting the calculations made during partial ventilatory support from those of the work of breathing made during full ventilatory support.[58, 59]

In patients with respiratory insufficiency, considerable energy can be expended in maintaining ventilation, with little work actually being performed. In these patients, measurement of the energy expenditure required for breathing allows a better estimation of respiratory effort. This can be performed with indirect calorimetry,[62] which measures the patient's baseline oxygen consumption during total respiratory support and the change in consumption during periods of decreased levels of support. If the patient's metabolic status remains constant, the differences in oxygen consumption can be attributed to change in the work of breathing.[63, 64]

Several difficulties arise with indirect calorimetry. First, the accuracy of the technique for measuring oxygen consumption is limited, especially at high levels of supplemental oxygen. The fraction of total oxygen consumption relative to the respiratory effort is quite small (1 to 4%), although in critically ill patients it may be much higher.[57] Baseline levels of oxygen consumption can vary widely. Therefore, small changes in oxygen consumption may reflect the inaccuracy of the technique rather than an actual change in the respiratory energy expenditure. Second, alterations in energy expenditure in response to changes in the level of ventilatory support may indicate the activity of muscle groups other than the respiratory muscles. For example, if the patient becomes tachycardiac during a weaning trial, the increased oxygen consumption may be due to cardiac rather than respiratory muscle demands.

NONINVASIVE MONITORING OF ARTERIAL BLOOD GAS PARAMETERS

The methods of arterial blood gas analysis and the technology of noninvasive monitoring of arterial blood gas parameters are described elsewhere in this book. This section discusses the clinical application of these techniques to estimate the arterial Po_2 (Pa_{O_2}) and Pco_2 (Pa_{CO_2}).

Measures of Arterial Oxygenation

Pulse Oximetry

Pulse oximetry permits continuous measurement of arterial saturation by measuring the pulsatile absorption of specific wavelengths of light by oxygenated and deoxygenated hemoglobin.[65] This technology has become very widely applied because it is easy to use and relatively accurate.

In using the arterial saturation as a measure of oxygenation, the shape of the oxyhemoglobin saturation curve must be considered. At its upper portion, it becomes quite flat, such that very large changes in Po_2 may be accompanied by very small changes in arterial saturation. Signif-

In patients with poor peripheral perfusion or those receiving vasoconstrictor medications, peripheral pulsatile flow may not be detectable.

icant changes in oxygenation can therefore occur that may not be reflected by the pulse oximeter. At the other end of the oxyhemoglobin saturation curve, changes in PO_2 and arterial saturation become more linear. In this range, changes in arterial saturation reflect changes in PO_2 quite well. The pulse oximeter is useful, therefore, as a monitoring device that indicates when significant desaturation occurs, but it is not helpful for following changes in Pa_{O_2} in hyperoxic patients.

The accuracy of pulse oximeter measurements (Sa_{O_2}) depends on several factors.[65, 66] First, pulsatile flow must be detected by the instrument. Second, irregular cardiac rhythms may interfere with the ability to obtain adequate pulse oximeter measurements because of the associated irregular perfusion. The pulse rate displayed by the pulse oximeter should match that determined by electrocardiographic monitoring in order to ensure accuracy. Third, the blood must be free of substances or abnormal hemoglobins that may interfere with light absorption. Methylene blue, carboxyhemoglobin, and methemoglobin all may be associated with inaccurate pulse oximeter measurements. Bilirubin has not been found to alter pulse oximeter measurements, even at high values.[67] Fourth, motion artifact can interfere with the ability of the instrument to detect pulsatile flow. Fifth, skin pigmentation can affect the quality of the measurements, with greater inaccuracy noted in dark-pigmented individuals.[68, 69] Finally, external influences such as electrocautery, certain ambient lights, or pigmented nail polish can prevent adequate pulse oximeter function.

The accuracy of the pulse oximeter is commonly cited to be $\pm 4\%$;[49] however, this defines a fairly broad range within which the true saturation may lie. The accuracy of the instruments is better assessed in terms of mean differences between pulse oximeter measurements and those obtained from blood (also known as the bias), as well as the standard deviation of this difference (the precision). One paper reviewing a series of studies cited clinically acceptable values of the bias ranging between -1.4% and $+1.9\%$, with precisions ranging between $\pm 1.6\%$ and $\pm 3.1\%$.[70] It should be noted, however, that at saturations below 90%, accuracy becomes more problematic. For example, in one study, the bias and precision increased from 1.7 ± 1.2 to 5.1 ± 2.7 when the arterial saturation dropped below 90%.[69]

Clinically, the use of pulse oximetry has become the standard of care in the operating room. It is also widely applied in the intensive care unit, although there are few studies in the adult critical care setting demonstrating its value. One study, in patients who had had cardiac surgery, showed that use of the pulse oximeter allowed a reduction in the number of blood gases utilized without compromising patient safety.[71] Furthermore, in a group in which the bedside staff were blinded to the pulse oximeter readings, clinically undetected episodes of desaturation occurred. The clinical consequence of such episodes is uncertain because they were often quite brief. Pulse oximetry has also been applied in many other locations in which patients may be at risk for significant desaturation, such as the emergency room, the endoscopy suite, and others. When used within its limitations, the pulse oximeter is an extremely useful monitoring device.

Transcutaneous Oxygen Measurement

The partial pressure of oxygen at the skin (Ptc_{O_2}) has been studied as an estimate of the Pa_{O_2}. The Ptc_{O_2} can be measured with modifications of the Clark oxygen electrode used in the laboratory to assay blood samples.[72]

The measurement of Ptc_{O_2} is affected by several factors.[73, 74] First, the skin not only provides a barrier to the diffusion of gases but also consumes oxygen. In neonates, who have very thin skin, this is less problematic; however, in others, the dermal barrier not only affects the gradient between the Ptc_{O_2} and the Pa_{O_2} but also slows the response of Ptc_{O_2} electrodes to a rapidly changing Pa_{O_2}. The dermal barrier to diffusion can be partially overcome by heating the skin with the electrode. This requires, however, that the site of the electrode be periodically changed in order to prevent thermal injuries.

The second important determinant of the Ptc_{O_2} is the perfusion status of the skin. Under conditions of low dermal perfusion, such as decreased cardiac output, the Ptc_{O_2} is greatly reduced and thus may seriously underestimate the Pa_{O_2}. The highly variable status of cutaneous perfusion in hemodynamically unstable patients makes transcutaneous monitoring extremely unreliable as a measure of the Pa_{O_2}.[75] It may be of some value, however, as an indicator of the hemodynamic or perfusion status of the patient.

Measurement of the Ptc_{O_2} for monitoring purposes has been widely applied in the management of neonates and infants, in whom arterial access can be quite limited.[73, 74, 76] Compared with pulse oximetry, however, it is technically more difficult to use and provides a slower response to rapidly changing conditions. In adults, it is unsuitable because of the large Pa_{O_2}-Ptc_{O_2} gradient. In both populations, the use of the Ptc_{O_2} as a reflection of the Pa_{O_2} becomes quite tenuous in situations of poor peripheral perfusion.[73, 77]

Measures of Arterial Carbon Dioxide

Capnography

Capnometry refers to the measurement of the concentration of CO_2 in expired gas using techniques of mass spectroscopy or infrared spectrophotometry. Mass spectroscopy has been used in the operating room because of its ability to assay multiple gases; the infrared technology has been packaged into free-standing bedside monitors for use in other locations.

The capnograph, a recording of the CO_2 concentration in expired gas over time, has a characteristic appearance (Fig. 14–6). During inspiration, the tracing is flat and shows a negligible level of CO_2. At the start of expiration, the gas expelled comes from airways not participating in gas exchange (e.g., the dead space); thus, the concentration of CO_2 remains very small. As the alveoli start to empty, the concentration of CO_2 rises quickly and then reaches a plateau as increasing amounts of alveolar gas are expired. The end-tidal CO_2 (ET_{CO_2}) is achieved just before the next inhalation, whereupon the exhaled CO_2 concentration rapidly falls once again to baseline. In order to utilize this technology safely in patient management, a thorough understanding of the physiology of the expired CO_2 concentration is mandatory. If the lungs exchanged CO_2 perfectly, the PET_{CO_2} would equal the Pa_{CO_2} exactly. In normal individuals, however, the PET_{CO_2} is less than 5 mm Hg lower than the Pa_{CO_2}.[78] As the lungs become more diseased, the gradient between the PET_{CO_2} and the Pa_{CO_2} widens, reflecting worsening ventilation-perfusion relationships.

Respiratory pattern, hemodynamic status, sampling techniques, and system leaks can all affect the PET_{CO_2} and the shape of the capnographic tracing.[79]

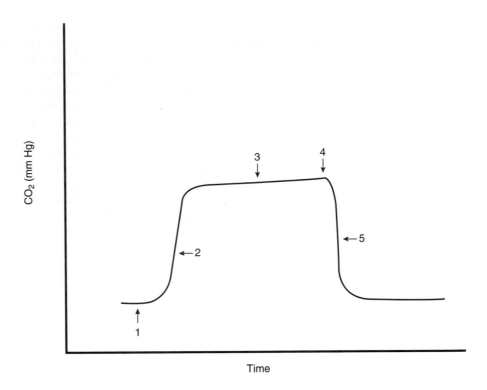

1: Exhalation of dead space gas containing no CO_2
2: Rapid rise CO_2 concentration as alveolar gas is expelled
3: Alveolar gas plateau
4: End-tidal CO_2 concentration
5: Rapid fall of the CO_2 concentration with inspiration

FIGURE 14–6: The normal capnograph.

The capnograph may provide several cues that may be useful in guiding care.[80] For example, the cyclic rising and falling of the PET_{CO_2} allows for a reliable measure of respiratory rate. Loss of these cyclic changes indicates either apnea or disconnection from the ventilator or capnometer. Failure to achieve a plateau indicates inhomogeneous alveolar emptying (e.g., small airway obstruction as in chronic obstructive pulmonary disease or asthma). Failure of the PET_{CO_2} to approximate the Pa_{CO_2} reflects ventilation-perfusion inhomogeneity. An increasing gradient between the PET_{CO_2} and the Pa_{CO_2} reflects worsening of the underlying lung disease or the imposition of additional pathology, such as pulmonary embolism. During resuscitation efforts, widening of this gradient may reflect not only ventilatory inefficiency but also failure of pulmonary perfusion. The PET_{CO_2} may be extremely low in patients receiving cardiopulmonary resuscitation because of either circulatory failure, esophageal intubation, or disconnection from the capnometer.[81, 82]

There are, however, serious technical limitations to the use of capnography. Currently, this technology can be applied only to intubated patients because no reliable means of sampling expired gas exists for patients wearing face masks or nasal cannulas. Secretions and water in the ventilatory circuits can pose problems. Leaks in the ventilatory circuit can drastically distort the capnograph and the PET_{CO_2}. Adapters placed into the ventilatory circuit for these measurements can add weight and dead space to the circuit. This is most important when such monitoring is being considered in the neonatal and infant population. Clinical studies have demonstrated a variable utility of capnography in managing patients. Some have shown advantages, such as being able to reduce the use of arterial blood gas analyses during weaning.[83] Others, however, have demonstrated serious limitations. For example, because of the tendency of the PET_{CO_2} to underestimate the Pa_{CO_2} capnographic monitoring can be quite insensitive to the presence of hypercarbia.[83] Furthermore, the Pa_{CO_2}-PET_{CO_2} gradient may not be constant: trends in the PET_{CO_2} can move opposite to those in the Pa_{CO_2} during changing ventilatory conditions.[84]

In summary, end-tidal monitoring of CO_2 has limited utility in the management of intubated patients. In those with normal ventilation-perfusion relationships and a stable hemodynamic status, capnographic estimates of the Pa_{CO_2} may be clinically useful. Unfortunately, in patients with cardiopulmonary instability, capnography may be misleading and must be used with care.

Transcutaneous P_{CO_2} Measurement

The partial pressure of carbon dioxide at the skin (Ptc_{CO_2}) has been used as an estimate of the Pa_{CO_2}, in a manner similar to the Ptc_{O_2}. Chemical and infrared electrodes have been developed for this purpose.[72, 73] Measurement of the Ptc_{CO_2} is subject to constraints similar to those encountered with the Ptc_{O_2}.[73] Because carbon dioxide is 20 times more soluble than oxygen in tissues, the dependence of the measurement on cutaneous perfusion and metabolism is decreased, although not totally eliminated. Heating the skin causes a temperature-dependent rise in the P_{CO_2}; thus, the Ptc_{CO_2} tends to overestimate the Pa_{CO_2}.[74] Several correction factors have been proposed.[77] Clinical measurement of the Ptc_{CO_2} has been most widely applied in the neonatal population, but it has applicability in other populations as well. One study noted a mean bias (Ptc_{CO_2}-Pa_{CO_2}) and precision (standard deviation of the bias) of ± 1.3 ± 3.9 mm Hg in 251 patients of all age groups. The neonatal group was not significantly different from the remainder. Hemodynamic data were not reported; however, some studies indicate that the correlation between Ptc_{CO_2} and Pa_{CO_2} is poor in hemodynamically unstable patients.[85, 86]

Widespread application of Ptc_{CO_2} monitoring has been limited by slow electrode response times,[74] the need to change the monitoring site of heated electrodes regularly in order to prevent thermal injuries, and requirements for repeated calibration.

MEASURES OF THE EFFICIENCY OF GAS EXCHANGE

Efficiency of Oxygenation

Alveolar-Arterial Oxygen Gradient

If the lungs exchanged gas perfectly, the partial pressure of oxygen in the alveolar spaces and the pulmonary venous blood would be equal. Because the gas exchange mechanisms are not perfect, the normal alveolar-arterial oxygen difference is 15 mm Hg, and it increases with age.[87] This can be accounted for by the basal level of shunting and ventilation-perfusion inequality found in normal individuals. As gas exchange be-

---

Ptc_{O_2} determinants include

- The diffusion barrier created by the skin
- Temperature
- Metabolism by the skin
- The state of cutaneous perfusion
- The Pa_{CO_2}

To use this technology effectively, knowledge of the Ptc_{O_2}-Pa_{CO_2} gradient is required; hence, the need for invasive measurement (e.g., arterial blood gas analysis) is not eliminated.

comes more inefficient in disease states, the alveolar-arterial difference for oxygen increases.

The alveolar-arterial oxygen gradient is obtained by measuring the Pa_{O_2} and then subtracting it from the calculated alveolar P_{O_2} (PA_{O_2}). The alveolar P_{O_2} is calculated from knowledge of the percentage of atmospheric or supplemental oxygen (FI_{O_2}), atmospheric pressure (PI is 760 mm Hg at sea level), and the partial pressure of water in the airways (PH_2O is 47 mm Hg at body temperature), which accounts for the humidification of the inspired gas. Knowledge of the body's metabolic efficiency, as measured by the ratio of carbon dioxide produced per oxygen consumed (e.g., the respiratory quotient [RQ]), is also needed to predict the alveolar contents. This is commonly assumed to be 0.8, although in critically ill patients it may be best to measure it with a metabolic cart.

For clinical purposes, knowledge of the $P(A - a)O_2$ is of limited usefulness for three reasons.[89] First, calculation of the PA_{O_2} is problematic, mainly because it requires that the FI_{O_2} be known precisely, which can occur only in intubated patients or those breathing room air. Second, it assumes that the alveolar and arterial PCO_2 values are equal, which may not be true in disease states. Third, in order to compare gradients at different times, the FI_{O_2} must remain constant, which is impractical in an unstable situation.[90] Finally, the hemodynamic status of the patient can influence the $P(A - a)O_2$. In patients with cardiopulmonary instability, the $P(A - a)O_2$ can be very difficult to interpret.

Arterial-Alveolar Oxygen Ratio

The arterial-alveolar oxygen ratio (Pa_{O_2}/PA_{O_2}) has a significance similar to that of the $P(A - a)O_2$. The alveolar oxygen tension is calculated as described previously and is then divided into the measured arterial oxygen tension. Like those of the $P(A - a)O_2$, the determinants of the Pa_{O_2}/PA_{O_2} include the degree of pulmonary shunting, ventilation-perfusion mismatch, FI_{O_2}, and the oxygen content of mixed venous blood. The principal advantage of this index is that it is less sensitive to the level of supplemental oxygen than the $P(A - a)O_2$.[90] This allows for the comparison of this index at varying levels of FI_{O_2}. Once calculated, the ratio can be used to predict the Pa_{O_2} at a given FI_{O_2}.[91, 92]

Arterial-Inspired Oxygen Ratio

The ratio of the Pa_{O_2} to the FI_{O_2} has been used in a fashion similar to the $P(A - a)O_2$ and the Pa_{O_2}/PA_{O_2}. The principal advantage of this index is that it does not require the calculation of the alveolar oxygen tension (PA_{O_2}). It does not account for the effect of carbon dioxide on the level of oxygenation; however, the effect is small when the FI_{O_2} is high.

Venous Admixture or Pulmonary Shunt

An additional measure of the efficiency of oxygenation results from the quantification of pulmonary shunting. A true shunt is defined as blood that is returned to the left atrium without ever having circulated through functioning alveoli. In disease states, the ratio of ventilation to perfusion may not allow full equilibration of the alveolar gas with the blood, thereby creating a shunt effect.[93] The net result of a true shunt or shunt effect is to increase the alveolar-arterial oxygen gradient. In both cases, mixed venous blood or partially oxygenated mixed venous blood is combined with that arising from normally functioning alveoli, resulting in a depression of the Pa_{O_2}.

The modified alveolar gas equation[88] is as follows:

$$PA_{O_2} = FI_{O_2}(PI - PH_2O) - PCO_2/R$$

The alveolar-arterial difference is therefore

$$P(A - a)O_2 = PA_{O_2} - Pa_{O_2}$$

In normal individuals, shunted blood accounts for less than 10% of the cardiac output.[82] This represents blood that empties into the left atrium from the bronchial circulation (originating from the aorta and supplying the large airways) and thebesian veins draining into the left ventricle (representing coronary venous blood).

Calculation of the degree of shunting requires a comparison of the arterial and mixed venous oxygen contents with the oxygen content of pulmonary end-capillary blood (Table 14–1). When the calculation is performed with the patient receiving 100% oxygen, the amount of true shunting is obtained. This is because equilibration of the blood with 100% oxygen eliminates any shunt effect (ventilation-perfusion mismatch). When the calculation is made at a lower $F_{I_{O_2}}$, the value obtained represents both true shunting and shunt effect. The hemodynamic status of the patient can have important effects on the calculated shunt.[94] Through its influence on the mixed venous oxygen content, the cardiac output can have an important effect on the amount of the calculated shunt.

Likewise, the oxygen consumption of the patient must also be considered because it affects the mixed venous oxygen content as well. In interpreting the results of repeated shunt calculations over time in following a patient's progress, it is crucial that these variables be considered.

There are three disadvantages to using the shunt calculation to follow a patient's course. First, to perform the calculation, a pulmonary artery catheter must be inserted in order to obtain mixed venous blood. Second, the calculations are cumbersome unless a programmable calculator or a computer is used. Third, multiple variables can influence the calculation, thereby making interpretation difficult. Despite these drawbacks, calculation of the shunt is required when precise measurements of the inefficiency of oxygenation are required. Other parameters, such as the $P(A - a)O_2$, the Pa_{O_2}/PA_{O_2}, and the $Pa_{O_2}/F_{I_{O_2}}$, may not correlate well with the shunt calculation in critically ill patients.[95]

Efficiency of Ventilation

Ratio of Dead Space to Tidal Volume

Dead space is defined as that portion of the respiratory system that receives ventilation but does not participate in gas exchange because of

---

TABLE 14–1: Pulmonary Shunt Equation

$$\frac{\dot{Q}s}{\dot{Q}t} = \frac{Cc'_{O_2} - Ca_{O_2}}{Cc'_{O_2} - C\bar{v}_{O_2}}$$

where

$\dot{Q}s/\dot{Q}t$ = the ratio of the shunt flow to the cardiac output

Cc'_{O_2} = the oxygen content of pulmonary end-capillary blood; this value is not measured but is calculated from the blood oxygen content equation, assuming an $F_{I_{O_2}}$ equal to the alveolar P_{O_2} (calculated from the alveolar gas equation) and 100% saturation

Ca_{O_2} = the oxygen content of arterial blood

$C\bar{v}_{O_2}$ = the oxygen content of mixed venous blood

Oxygen content is the amount of oxygen carried by hemoglobin plus that dissolved in the blood:

$$\text{Oxygen content} = (F_{I_{O_2}} \times 0.003) + (1.34 \times Hb \times SAT)$$

where

$F_{I_{O_2}}$ = the inspired oxygen concentration

0.003 = the milliliters of oxygen dissolved in 100 mL of blood per mm Hg of partial pressure

1.34 = the milliliters of oxygen carried per 100 mL of hemoglobin

Hb = the serum hemoglobin concentration (grams of hemoglobin per 100 mL of blood)

SAT = the saturation of the arterial or mixed venous blood

a lack of perfusion. There are three components to the dead space. The first is the anatomic dead space. This comprises the conducting airways, which are ventilated but do not participate in gas exchange because of a lack of alveoli. The second component is the alveolar dead space, which may be found in disease states. It consists of alveoli whose perfusion has become compromised such that gas exchange cannot occur. The combination of the anatomic and the alveolar dead space is known as the physiologic dead space. The third component is the apparatus dead space, which is found in patients using various respiratory devices, such as oxygen masks and mechanical ventilation circuits.

Minute ventilation is defined as the respiratory rate multiplied by the tidal volume. The proportion that goes to functional alveoli is known as the alveolar ventilation, whereas that going to the dead space is known as the dead space ventilation. The significance of the dead space is that ventilation going to it is wasted in that it does not participate in gas exchange. If the dead space increases, total minute ventilation must increase in order to keep the alveolar ventilation constant.

The dead space can be quantified by measuring the proportion of the tidal volume that is consumed by the physiologic dead space. This is accomplished with the Bohr equation. The $P_{E_{CO_2}}$ is obtained by collecting expired gas in a nonpermeable bag (e.g., a Douglas bag) and then withdrawing a sample for analysis. In normal individuals, V_D/V_T is less than 40%.

In following V_D/V_T over time, several factors must be considered in interpreting the values obtained. First, changes in the rate or pattern of respiration can influence this proportion independent of any process within the lung itself. Rapid, shallow breathing increases the proportion of the tidal volume occupied by the anatomic dead space. Second, changes in hemodynamic status can influence dead space measurements. Hypotensive states can increase dead space by decreasing pulmonary perfusion. Finally, changes in the metabolic rate, by influencing carbon dioxide production, can alter the respiratory rate and pattern.

The Bohr equation is as follows:

$$V_D/V_T = (Pa_{CO_2} - P_{E_{CO_2}})/Pa_{CO_2}$$

where

V_D/V_T = the ratio of the volume of dead space to tidal volume
$P_{E_{CO_2}}$ = mixed expired carbon dioxide concentration

End-Tidal–Arterial P_{CO_2} Gradient

In the ideal situation, the $P_{ET_{CO_2}}$ represents the alveolar P_{CO_2}, which in lungs with perfect gas exchange is equal to the Pa_{CO_2}. As ventilatory inefficiency increases, the gradient between the $P_{ET_{CO_2}}$ and the Pa_{CO_2} increases. This gradient is easily monitored with serial arterial blood gas analyses and measurements of the $P_{ET_{CO_2}}$ using a capnometer. The limitations of capnometry were described earlier in this chapter.

SUMMARY

Comprehensive respiratory monitoring involves techniques to assess gas exchange, respiratory mechanics, ventilator-patient interactions, and patient effort. It is useful in following the progression of disease, guiding therapy, and detecting complications. With a thorough understanding of the advantages and limitations of such techniques, the safety and efficacy of comprehensive respiratory care can be dramatically improved.

References

1. Tobin MJ, Chadha TS, Jenouri G, et al. Breathing patterns: 1. Normal subjects. Chest 84:202–205, 1983.

2. Tobin MJ, Chadha TS, Jenouri G, et al. Breathing patterns: 2. Disease states. Chest 84:286–294, 1983.
3. Gravelyn TR, Wey JC. Respiratory rate as an indicator of acute respiratory dysfunction. JAMA 244:1123–1125, 1980.
4. Plum F, Posner JB. The pathologic physiology of signs and symptoms of coma. *In* The Diagnosis of Stupor and Coma. Philadelphia, FA Davis, 1980, p 32.
5. Krieger BP. Ventilatory pattern monitoring: Instrumentation and application. Respir Care 35:697–708, 1990.
6. Tobin MJ, Perez W, Guenther SM, et al. Does rib cage-abdominal paradox signify respiratory muscle fatigue? J Appl Physiol 63:851–860, 1987.
7. Tobin MJ. Noninvasive evaluation of respiratory movement. *In* Nochomovitz ML, Cherniak NS (eds). Noninvasive Respiratory Monitoring. New York, Churchill Livingstone, 1986, pp 29–57.
8. Rochester DF. Tests of respiratory muscle function. Clin Chest Med 9:249–262, 1988.
9. Wilson SH, Cooke NT, Edwards RHT, Spiro SG. Predicted normal value for maximal respiratory pressures in Caucasian adults and children. Thorax 39:535–538, 1984.
10. Leech JA, Ghezzo H, Slevern D, Becklake MR. Respiratory pressures and function in young adults. Am Rev Respir Dis 128:17–23, 1983.
11. Braun N, Arora NS, Rochester DF. Respiratory muscle and pulmonary function in polymyositis and other proximal myopathies. Thorax 38:616–623, 1983.
12. Tahvanainen J, Salempera M, Nikki P. Extubation criteria after weaning from intermittent mandatory ventilation and continuous positive airway pressure. Crit Care Med 11:702–707, 1983.
13. DeHaven CB, Hurst JM, Branson RD. Evaluation of two different extubation criteria: Attributes contributing to success. Crit Care Med 14:92–94, 1986.
14. Krieger BP, Ershowsky PF, Becker DA, Gazeroglu HB. Evaluation of conventional criteria for predicting successful weaning from mechanical ventilatory support in elderly patients. Crit Care Med 17:858–861, 1989.
15. Yang KL, Tobin MJ. A prospective study of indexes predicting the outcome of trials of weaning from mechanical ventilation. N Engl J Med 324:1445–1450, 1991.
16. Truwit JD, Marini JJ. Validation of a technique to assess maximal inspiratory pressure in poorly cooperative patients. Chest 102:1216–1219, 1992.
17. Marini JJ, Smith TC, Lamb V. Estimation of inspiratory muscle strength in mechanically ventilated patients: The measurement of maximal inspiratory pressure. J Crit Care 1:32–36, 1986.
18. Multz AS, Aldrich TK, Prezant DJ, et al. Maximal inspiratory pressure is not a reliable test of inspiratory muscle strength in mechanically ventilated patients. Am Rev Respir Dis 142:529–532, 1990.
19. Whitelaw WA, Derenne JP, Milic-Emili J. Occlusion pressure as a measure of respiratory center output in conscious man. Respir Physiol 23:181–199, 1975.
20. Fernandez R, Blanch L, Artigas A. Respiratory center activity during mechanical ventilation. J Crit Care 6:102–111, 1991.
21. Murciano D, Bosczkowski J, Lecocguic Y, et al. Tracheal occlusion pressure: A simple index to monitor respiratory muscle fatigue during acute respiratory failure in patients with chronic obstructive pulmonary disease. Ann Intern Med 108:800–805, 1988.
22. Sassoon CS, Teresita TT, Mahutte CK, Light RW. Airway occlusion pressure: An important indicator for successful weaning in patients with chronic obstructive pulmonary disease. Am Rev Respir Dis 135:107–113, 1987.
23. Brenner M, Mukai DS, Russell JE, et al. A new method for measurement of airway occlusion pressure. Chest 98:421–427, 1990.
24. Branson RD. Enhanced capabilities of current ICU ventilators: Do they really benefit patients? Respir Care 36:362–376, 1991.
25. Hubmayr RD, Gay PC, Tayyab M. Respiratory system mechanics in ventilated patients: Techniques and indications. Mayo Clin Proc 62:358–368, 1987.
26. Haake R, Schlichtig R, Ulstad DR, Henschen RR. Barotrauma: Pathophysiology, risk factors and prevention. Chest 91:608–613, 1987.
27. Pierson DJ. Alveolar rupture during mechanical ventilation. Role of PEEP, peak airway pressure and distending volume. Respir Care 33:472–486, 1988.
28. Dreyfuss D, Soler P, Basset G, Saumon G. High inflation pressure pulmonary edema. Am Rev Respir Dis 137:1159–1164, 1988.
29. Parker JC, Hernandez LA, Longenecker GL, et al. Lung edema caused by high peak inspiratory pressures in dogs. Am Rev Respir Dis 142:321–328, 1990.
30. Tsuno K, Prato P, Lolobow T. Acute lung injury from mechanical ventilation at moderately high airway pressures. J Appl Physiol 69:956–961, 1990.
31. Gay PC, Rodarte JR, Tayyab M, Hubmayr RD. Evaluation of bronchodilator responsiveness in mechanically ventilated patients. Am Rev Respir Dis 136:880–885, 1987.
32. Marini JJ. Controlled ventilation: Targets, hazards and options. *In* Marini JJ, Roussos C (eds). Ventilatory Failure. Berlin, Springer-Verlag, 1991, pp 269–292.
33. Marini JJ, Ravenscraft SA. Mean airway pressure: Physiologic determinants and clinical importance. Crit Care Med 20:1604–1616, 1992.
34. Norwood S. Physiologic principles of conventional mechanical ventilation. *In* Kirby RR, Banner MJ, Downs JB (eds). Clinical Applications of Ventilatory Support. New York, Churchill Livingstone, 1990, pp 145–171.

35. Pepe PE, Marini JJ. Occult positive end-expiratory pressure in mechanically ventilated patients with airflow obstruction. Am Rev Respir Dis 126:166–170, 1982.
36. Gottfried SB, Rossi A, Higgs BD, et al. Noninvasive determination of respiratory system mechanics during mechanical ventilation for acute respiratory failure. Am Rev Respir Dis 131:414–420, 1985.
37. Fernandez R, Mancebo J, Blanch L, et al. Intrinsic PEEP on static pressure-volume curves. Intensive Care Med 16:233–236, 1990.
38. Rossi A, Gottfried SB, Zocchi L, et al. Measurement of static compliance of the total respiratory system in patients with acute respiratory failure during mechanical ventilation. Am Rev Respir Dis 131:672–677, 1985.
39. Rossi A, Polese G, Brandi G. Dynamic hyperinflation. In Marini JJ, Roussos C (eds). Ventilatory Failure. Berlin, Springer-Verlag, 1991, pp 199–218.
40. Marini JJ. Lung mechanics determinations at the bedside: Instrumentation and clinical application. Respir Care 35:669–696, 1990.
41. East TD. What makes monitoring tick?: A review of basic engineering principles. Respir Care 35:500–519, 1990.
42. McPherson SP. Bedside measuring and monitoring devices. In Respiratory Therapy Equipment. St. Louis, CV Mosby, 1990, pp 139–155.
43. Osborn JJ. A flow meter for respiratory monitoring. Crit Care Med 6:349–351, 1978.
44. Sheffer AL, Bailey WC, Bleeker ER, et al. Objective measures of lung function. In Guidelines for the Diagnosis and Management of Asthma. Bethesda, MD, National Asthma Education Program. National Institutes of Health Publication No. 91-3042. 1991, pp 17–25.
45. Nelson SB, Gardner RM, Crapo RO, Jensen RL. Performance evaluation of contemporary spirometers. Chest 97:288–297, 1990.
46. American Thoracic Society. Standardization of spirometry—1987 update. Am Rev Respir Dis 136:1285–1298, 1987.
47. Pierson DJ. Measuring and monitoring lung volumes outside of the pulmonary function laboratory. Respir Care 35:660–668, 1990.
48. Bartel LP, Bazik JR, Powner DJ. Compression volume during mechanical ventilation: Comparison of ventilators and tubing circuits. Crit Care Med 13:851–854, 1985.
49. Tobin MJ. Respiratory monitoring in the intensive care unit. Am Rev Respir Dis 138:1625–1642, 1988.
50. Marini JJ, Rodriguez RM, Lamb VJ. Involuntary breath stacking: An alternative method for vital capacity estimation in poorly cooperative subjects. Am Rev Respir Dis 134:694–698, 1986.
51. Irwin RS. Mechanical ventilation. Part II: Weaning. In Rippe JM, Irwin RS, Alpert JS, Fink MP (eds). Intensive Care Medicine, 2nd ed. Boston, Little, Brown and Company, 1991, pp 575–584.
52. Truwit JD, Marini JJ. Evaluation of thoracic mechanics in the ventilated patient. Part II: Applied mechanics. J Crit Care 3:199–213, 1988.
53. Bates JH, Millic-Emili J. The flow interruption technique for measuring respiratory resistance. J Crit Care 2:227–238, 1991.
54. Wright PE, Marini JJ, Bernard GR. In vitro versus in vivo comparison of endotracheal tube airflow resistance. Am Rev Respir Dis 140:10–16, 1989.
55. Gay PC, Patel HG, Nelson SB, et al. Metered dose inhalers for bronchodilator delivery in intubated, mechanically ventilated patients. Chest 99:66–71, 1991.
56. Bone RC. Diagnosis of causes for acute respiratory distress by pressure-volume curves. Chest 70:740–746, 1976.
57. Armaganidis A, Roussos C. Work of breathing in the critically ill patient. Curr Pulmonol 12:51–86, 1991.
58. Marini JJ, Capps JS, Culver BH. The inspiratory work of breathing during assisted mechanical ventilation. Chest 87:612–618, 1985.
59. Marini JJ, Rodriguez M, Lamb V. The inspiratory workload of patient-initiated mechanical ventilation. Am Rev Respir Dis 134:902–909, 1986.
60. Banner MJ, Lampotang S, Boysen PG, et al. Flow resistance of expiratory positive pressure valve systems. Chest 90:212–217, 1986.
61. Marini JJ, Culver BH, Kirk W. Flow resistance of exhalation valves and positive end-expiratory pressure devices used in mechanical ventilation. Am Rev Respir Dis 131:850–854, 1985.
62. Branson RD. The measurement of energy expenditure: Instrumentation, practical considerations and clinical application. Respir Care 35:640–659, 1990.
63. Field S, Kelly SM, Macklem PT. The oxygen cost of breathing in patients with cardiorespiratory disease. Am Rev Respir Dis 126:9–13, 1982.
64. Lewis WE, Chwals W, Benotti PN, et al. Bedside assessment of the work of breathing. Crit Care Med 16:117–122, 1988.
65. Welch JP, DeCesare R, Hess D. Pulse oximetry: Instrumentation and clinical applications. Respir Care 35:584–601, 1990.
66. Schnapp LM, Cohen NH. Pulse oximetry: Uses and abuses. Chest 98:1244–1250, 1990.
67. Veyckemans F, Baele Phillippe P, Guillaume JE, et al. Hyperbilirubinemia does not interfere with hemoglobin saturation measured by pulse oximetry. Anesthesiology 70:118–122, 1989.
68. Zeballos RJ, Weisman IM. Reliability of noninvasive oximetry in black subjects during exercise and hypoxia. Am Rev Respir Dis 144:1240–1244, 1991.

69. Jubran A, Tobin MJ. Reliability of pulse oximetry in titrating supplemental oxygen therapy in ventilator-dependent patients. Chest 97:1420–1425, 1990.
70. Technology Subcommittee of the Working Group on Critical Care, Ontario Ministry of Health. Noninvasive blood gas monitoring: A review for use in the adult critical care unit. Can Med Assoc J 146:703–712, 1992.
71. Bierman MI, Stein KL, Snyder JV. Pulse oximetry in the postoperative care of cardiac surgical patients: A randomized controlled trial. Chest 102:1367–1370, 1992.
72. Shapiro BA, Harrison RA, Cane RD, Templin R. Transcutaneous gas electrodes. *In* Clinical Application of Blood Gases, 4th ed. Chicago, Year Book Medical Publishers, 1989, pp 295–300.
73. Clark JS, Votteri B, Ariagno RL. Noninvasive assessment of blood gases. Am Rev Respir Dis 145:220–232, 1992.
74. Wiedemann HP, McCarthy K. Noninvasive monitoring of oxygen and carbon dioxide. Clin Chest Med 10:239–254, 1989.
75. Tremper KK, Shoemaker WC. Transcutaneous oxygen monitoring of critically ill adults, with and without low flow shock. Crit Care Med 9:706–709, 1981.
76. Yakaw J, Mindoff C, Levison H. The validity of the transcutaneous oxygen tension method in children with cardiorespiratory problems. Am Rev Respir Dis 124:586–587, 1981.
77. Palmisano BW, Severinghaus JW. Transcutaneous PCO_2 and PO_2: A multicenter study of accuracy. J Clin Monit 6:189–195, 1990.
78. Hess D. Capnometry and capnography: Technical aspects, physiologic aspects and clinical applications. Respir Care 35:557–576, 1990.
79. Gravenstein JS, Paulus DA, Hayes TJ. The capnogram. *In* Capnography in Clinical Practice. Boston, Butterworths, 1989, pp 11–30.
80. Carlon GC, Ray C, Miodownik S, et al. Capnography in mechanically ventilated patients. Crit Care Med 16:550–556, 1988.
81. Falk JL, Rackow EC, Weil MH. End-tidal carbon dioxide concentration during cardiopulmonary resuscitation. N Engl J Med 318:607–611, 1988.
82. Garnett AR, Ornato JP, Gonzalez ER, Johnson EB. End-tidal carbon dioxide monitoring during cardiopulmonary resuscitation. JAMA 257:512–515, 1987.
83. Niehoff J, DelCuercio C, Lamorte W, et al. Efficacy of pulse oximetry and capnometry in postoperative ventilatory weaning. Crit Care Med 16:701–705, 1988.
84. Hoffman RA, Drieger BP, Kramer MR, et al. End-tidal carbon dioxide in critically ill patients during changes in mechanical ventilation. Am Rev Respir Dis 140:1265–1268, 1989.
85. Tremper KK, Mentelos RA, Shoemaker WC. Effect of hypercarbia and shock on transcutaneous carbon dioxide at different electrode temperatures. Crit Care Med 8:608–612, 1980.
86. Tremper KK, Shoemaker WC, Slippy CR, Nolan NS. Transcutaneous PCO_2 monitoring on adult patients in the ICU and operating room. Crit Care Med 9:752–755, 1981.
87. Nunn JF. Applied Respiratory Physiology, 3rd ed. Boston, Butterworths, 1987, p 242.
88. Nunn JF. Applied Respiratory Physiology, 3rd ed. Boston, Butterworths, 1987, p 186.
89. Martin L. Abbreviating the alveolar gas equation: An argument for simplicity. Respir Care 30:964–967, 1985.
90. Hess D, Maxwell C. Which is the best index of oxygenation—$P(A - a)O_2$, PaO_2/PAO_2, or PaO_2/FiO_2? Respir Care 30:961–962, 1985.
91. Maxwell C, Hess D, Shefat D. Use of the arterial/alveolar oxygen tension ratio to predict the inspired oxygen concentration needed for a desired arterial oxygen tension. Respir Care 29:1135–1139, 1984.
92. Peris LV, Boix JH, Salom JV, et al. Clinical use of the arterial/alveolar oxygen tension ratio. Crit Care Med 11:888–891, 1983.
93. Shapiro BA, Harrison RA, Cane RD, Templin R. Applying the physiologic shunt. *In* Clinical Application of Blood Gases, 4th ed. Chicago, Year Book Medical Publishers, 1989, pp 145–163.
94. Cruz JC, Metting PJ. Understanding the meaning of the shunt fraction calculation. J Clin Monit 3:124–134, 1987.
95. Cane RD, Shapiro BA, Templin R, Walther K. The unreliability of oxygen tension based indices in reflecting intrapulmonary shunting in the critically ill. Crit Care Med 16:1243–1246, 1988.

15

Neurologic Monitoring

John M. Luce, M.D.

In a medical context, the term *monitoring* refers to the repeated or continuous assessment of patients and their physiologic function, either by direct observation or by specific procedures. Such monitoring is used most often in patients whose medical status is expected to change frequently or suddenly and has the goal of identifying abnormalities and directing appropriate therapy. The following review outlines the current neurologic monitoring techniques for serial measurements of vital signs and repeated physical examinations, assessment of central nervous system anatomy, cerebrospinal fluid analysis, electroencephalography, evoked potential recording, assessment of cerebral oxygenation, measurement of cerebral arterial flow, measurement of cerebral perfusion pressure, evaluation of arterial blood gas values, and estimation of cerebral blood flow and metabolism. Although some of the techniques are as yet experimental, they may someday be helpful in monitoring.

SERIAL MEASUREMENT OF VITAL SIGNS AND REPEATED PHYSICAL EXAMINATIONS

Initial and subsequent recording of vital signs and repeated physical examinations remain the basis of neurologic monitoring, even in technologically sophisticated institutions. Blood pressure, pulse, respiratory rate, and temperature are measured serially in most critical care units. The neurologic physical examination focuses on mental status and responsiveness, cranial nerve integrity, the optic discs, spinal reflexes, and motor, sensory, and cerebellar function. Pupillary response to light and the corneal, oculocephalic, and oculovestibular reflexes are particularly important in comatose patients. These reflexes are tested, and the complete neurologic physical examination is performed, as often as the clinical situation requires.

Several scales or diagnostic schemes based on vital signs and physical examination findings have been introduced to facilitate monitoring. One such device is the Glasgow Coma Scale of Teasdale and Jennett (1974), in which eye opening, motor responsiveness, and verbal responsiveness are measured and given a numeric score (Table 15–1). The Glasgow Coma Scale score has proved to be reliable and repeatable when used by different observers, thereby allowing comparison of the severity of coma or impaired consciousness within a single institution or among different institutions in different parts of the world.

A second approach, introduced by Plum and Posner (1980), follows the progression of neurologic signs in transtentorial herniation. This scheme focuses on five variables: level of arousal, pupillary response to light, oculocephalic or oculovestibular reflex, respiratory pattern, and motor function (Table 15–2). The level of neurologic deficit can be derived from these variables, as can a patient's deterioration or improvement. Along with corneal reflex and verbal responsiveness, three elements of this scheme—the oculocephalic reflex, the oculovestibular reflex, and motor function—have been shown to be helpful prognostic signs in patients with nontraumatic coma.

TABLE **15–1:** Glasgow Coma Scale

Patient Response	Score
Eye opening	
Spontaneous	4
To speech	3
To pain	2
Nil	1
Motor response	
Obeys commands	6
Localizes	5
Withdraws	4
Abnormal flexion	3
Extends	2
Nil	1
Verbal response	
Oriented	5
Confused conversation	4
Inappropriate words	3
Incomprehensible sounds	2
Nil	1

Although useful in the evaluation of most patients, the assessment of vital signs and the physical examination are of limited value in individuals whose neurologic status is altered by sedatives, muscle relaxants, and anesthetic agents. Neurologic signs are also unreliable in patients subjected to hypothermia and other experimental therapies. These limitations have prompted development of the monitoring procedures discussed in the following sections.

ASSESSMENT OF CENTRAL NERVOUS SYSTEM ANATOMY

Routine roentgenography of the skull, spine, and other structures may be essential in the initial evaluation of patients with neurologic disease. These radiologic studies also can be performed sequentially: for example, cervical spine films may be obtained in a patient with neck injury before and after traction is applied. In addition, cerebral angiography can evaluate and track patients with conditions such as intracranial aneurysms. Radionuclide brain scans have been used to diagnose abscesses, tumors, and other processes that disrupt the blood-brain barrier. One-dimensional ultrasonography may detect shifts in the cerebral ventricles. Two-dimensional cranial ultrasonography, in which sound

TABLE **15–2:** Progression of Neurologic Signs in Central Transtentorial Herniation

Level of Neurologic Deficit	Level of Arousal	Pupillary Response	Oculocephalic or Oculovestibular Reflex	Respiratory Pattern	Motor Function
Diencephalon	Lethargy, stupor	Small, reactive	Present	Sighs, yawns, Cheyne-Stokes respiration	Semipurposeful, decorticate
Mesencephalon (midbrain)	Coma	Midposition, fixed	Decreased or absent	Tachypneic, hyperpneic	Decerebrate
Pons	Coma	Midposition, fixed	Absent	Eupneic	Decerebrate, flaccid
Myelencephalon (medulla oblongata)	Coma	Midposition, fixed	Absent	Atactic	Flaccid

CT—computed tomography
MRI—magnetic resonance imaging

waves are directed through the anterior fontanelle to provide a dynamic view of movement of the cerebral arteries, has been employed to identify irreversible brain injury in infants and neonates. Despite their usefulness, however, these techniques are rarely performed in a serial or continuous fashion and therefore cannot be considered monitoring tools.

To date, CT and MRI provide the most precise readily available images of structures in the central nervous system. The addition of iodinated contrast medium to routine CT allows further visualization of vascular structures, whereas metrizamide can be used to delineate the anatomy of the spinal and intracranial cerebrospinal space. CT of the brain can determine which patients are at risk for intracranial hypertension, who in turn become candidates for cerebrospinal perfusion pressure monitoring. This procedure is repeated so often in the evaluation of neurologic patients that it almost constitutes a monitoring, rather than a diagnostic, technique at some centers.

CEREBROSPINAL FLUID ANALYSIS

Cerebrospinal fluid (CSF), which bathes and protects the brain, has inherent metabolic activity. Examination of CSF for cells, protein, glucose, microorganisms, and other material is important in the initial and subsequent evaluation of many patients with infectious or vascular brain disease. In one study, CSF lactate levels were used to differentiate individuals with brain stem lesions from those with cortical lesions. Other studies show that CSF lactate and adenylate kinase levels can be used to predict the outcome of patients after cardiopulmonary arrest. However, although continuous sampling of CSF can be achieved with subarachnoid catheters, CSF analysis is not routinely used in neurologic monitoring.

ELECTROENCEPHALOGRAPHY

The electroencephalogram (EEG) records at the skin surface the electrical activity of multiple cortical neurons.

Electrophysiology often can measure, and occasionally can monitor, cerebral function. During states of alertness or mental activity, the EEG shows a desynchronized pattern, with no obvious dominant frequency. During mental inactivity, sedation, or anesthesia, the EEG becomes synchronized, with characteristic waves (alpha, beta, theta, and delta) of varying frequency and amplitude. Alterations in EEG frequencies and their relative amplitudes may reflect improvement or decline in cortical function. For example, characteristic changes are seen after reductions in cerebral blood flow to the ischemic threshold. The EEG can also be used to detect focal seizure activity.

Unfortunately, the standard EEG generates large amounts of data that can be interpreted only by skilled personnel, thereby limiting the development of several techniques of automated EEG analysis for clinical purposes. The oldest and simplest technique is cerebral function monitoring, in which cortical electrical activity is sensed by two electrodes on opposite sides of the patient's head while the signal passes through a frequency filter that minimizes artifacts. The signal is then rectified to eliminate its biphasic nature and is displayed on a chart recorder as a line with perturbations reflecting changes in brain activity. The cerebral function monitor provides graphic evidence of gross changes, such as those caused by global ischemia following cardiopulmonary collapse. However, it appears to be less useful in documenting subtle and regional abnormalities and fails to localize seizure foci.

Whereas the cerebral function monitor compresses the frequency and amplitude information of the EEG into a single value, power spectrum analysis retains almost all the information available in the original EEG. This technique digitizes the standard EEG at frequent intervals, known as epochs, and analyzes each epoch of data into a number of component waves of different amplitudes, whose sum equals the original waveform. The power spectrum is calculated by squaring the amplitudes of the individual frequency components. Patterns are then identified by analyzing a number of epochs in succession. Power spectrum analysis can be displayed on a bar graph, linearly, and by gray scale. This technique, which comes close to being a continuous monitoring technique, has proved to be useful in the operating room setting. However, the potential for the application of power spectrum analysis in the critical care unit remains unknown.

EVOKED POTENTIAL RECORDING

In addition to assessing spontaneous neuronal activity, electrophysiologic studies also can be used to measure the body's response to sensory or motor stimulation. For example, stimulating a peripheral nerve (usually the ulnar nerve at the wrist or elbow) and visually observing contraction of the fingers can detect the magnitude and type of neuromuscular blockade in patients. A portable electromyograph also allows the twitch response to be recorded continuously on a dial or strip chart, without observation of the patient's fingers being necessary.

Just as muscle potentials produced by motor nerve stimulation can monitor neuromuscular blockade, so potentials elicited by sensory stimulation can assess sensory receptors and pathways. These potentials also serve as general indicators of function in adjacent structures. Sensory evoked potentials are usually recorded on the scalp following visual, auditory, or peripheral nervous stimulation. They may be used to determine the extent and location of nervous system injury in patients with conditions such as spinal cord compression and head trauma. Sensory evoked potentials can also be employed to determine the depth of anesthesia and the activity of the spinal cord during surgery. In more recent years, the recording of evoked potentials has been recommended for predicting outcome in comatose patients and for confirming brain death. However, although such recording may be used serially to follow up patients in the critical care unit, major changes in nervous system function must occur before potentials change dramatically. Because these changes occur too late to allow therapeutic intervention, recording of evoked potentials cannot be recommended as a routine monitoring tool.

MEASUREMENT OF CEREBRAL PERFUSION PRESSURE

Blood flow to body organs relates directly to the perfusion pressure across them and inversely to the organs' vascular resistance. The perfusion pressure of distensible organs is the difference between the arterial inflow pressure and the venous outflow pressure measured in a draining vein. For example, coronary perfusion pressure equals aortic root pressure minus pressure in the coronary sinus or right atrium. The brain,

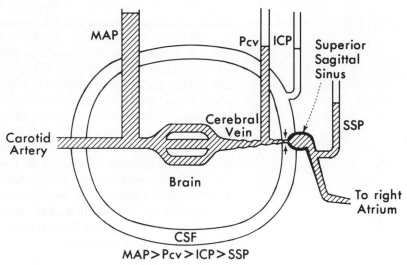

MAP > Pcv > ICP > SSP

FIGURE 15–1: A Starling resistor effect where the cerebral veins enter the sagittal sinus governs cerebral venous outflow. Increases in intracranial pressure (ICP) caused by increases in sagittal sinus pressure (SSP) due, for example, to positive end-expiratory pressure are transmitted to the cerebral veins, causing cerebral venous pressure (Pcv) to rise above ICP. Cerebral arteriolar resistance decreases as cerebral venous resistance increases, and a perfusion pressure gradient for cerebral blood flow is maintained. In this scheme, mean arterial pressure (MAP) is the effective inflow pressure for cerebral perfusion; ICP, which can be measured more readily than Pcv and in fact determines Pcv, is the effective outflow pressure. The cerebral perfusion pressure is MAP minus ICP. CSF, cerebrospinal fluid. (From Luce JM. Neurologic monitoring. Respir Care 30:471–480, 1985.)

Intracranial pressure (ICP)—pressure within the CSF

Given a normal MAP of 90 mm Hg and an ICP of 10 mm Hg or less, CPP should be approximately 80 mm Hg.

however, is enclosed in a nondistensible bony vault, and pressure in the extracranial right atrium and the jugular veins, and even in the sagittal sinus draining the vault, is not the same as pressure in the intracranial cerebral veins. Although pressure in the cerebral veins is difficult to measure, it closely resembles and is in fact established by the pressure within the CSF. The reason for this is that the brain behaves like a Starling resistor, in which the effective venous outflow pressure is the pressure around the cerebral veins (Fig. 15–1). Cerebral perfusion pressure (CPP) therefore equals mean arterial pressure (MAP) minus ICP (Table 15–3).

Assuming normal cerebral metabolism and arterial blood gas values, the body maintains a constant cerebral blood flow (CBF) of 50 mL/min/100 g tissue by adjusting cerebrovascular resistance over CPPs that

TABLE **15–3:** Normal Values for Cerebral Pressures, Blood Flow, and Metabolic Rates

Mean arterial pressure	90 mm Hg
Intracranial pressure	10 mm Hg
Cerebral perfusion pressure*	80 mm Hg
Brain weight	1200 g
Cerebral blood flow	50 mL/min/100 g tissue
Ischemic threshold for cerebral blood flow	15–20 mL/min/100 g tissue
Cerebral tissue oxygen tension	10 mm Hg
Cerebral arterial-venous oxygen content difference	3–6 mL O_2/100 mL blood
Cerebral metabolic rate of oxygen	3 mL/min/100 g tissue
Minimal cerebral metabolic rate of oxygen for aerobic metabolism	0.2 mL/min/100 g tissue
Cerebral metabolic rate of glucose	4.5 mg/min/100 g tissue

*Cerebral perfusion pressure = mean arterial pressure − intracranial pressure.

range from 50 to 150 mm Hg; this mechanism is called autoregulation. However, autoregulation is lost in many, if not most, patients with brain injury, in whom CBF varies linearly with CPP. Thus, CBF may fall below 50 mL/min/100 g tissue and reach an ischemic threshold between 15 and 20 mL/min/100 g tissue if CPP falls below 50 mm Hg. CBF may also run above normal levels if CPP exceeds 50 mm Hg. If the resultant increase in cerebral blood volume is not accompanied by a reciprocal decrease in the other intracranial contents (water, solids, and CSF), ICP will rise. This rise will be especially pronounced if intracranial volume and ICP are increased to begin with, as occurs with many brain diseases, including those that cause cerebral edema (Fig. 15–2). CPP falls without a compensatory increase in MAP, and cerebral ischemia ensues.

Lundberg and colleagues (1965) first demonstrated that continuous monitoring of ICP with a catheter in the cerebral ventricles provides important diagnostic information and a rational basis for therapy. The same catheters can be used to reduce ICP by draining CSF and to determine the intracranial compliance or volume-pressure relationship by injection of small amounts of saline or CSF. Because the possibility of insertion-related trauma and a subsequent infection rate of 2 to 5% exists with the use of the ventricular catheter, other investigators have recorded ICP either with subarachnoid screws that lie just beneath the dura, with miniature transducers in the epidural space, or with miniaturized fiberoptic devices in the brain parenchyma. These last devices are associated with fewer infections but may measure local rather than general ICP changes; in addition, they do not allow assessment of the volume-pressure relationship or drainage of CSF. Nevertheless, these

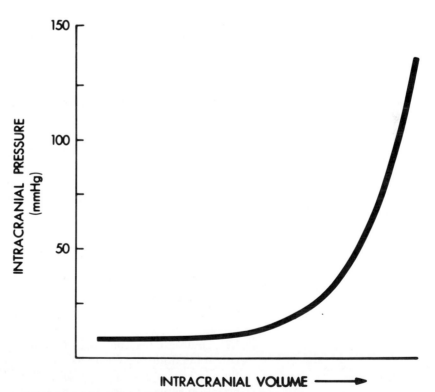

FIGURE 15–2: Intracranial compliance or volume-pressure response curve. Pressure increases little when volume is low but rises abruptly when volume is high, as in patients with cerebral edema or an increased intracranial blood volume. (From Luce JM. Neurologic monitoring. Respir Care 30:471–480, 1985.)

TABLE **15–4:** Comparison of Four Methods of Monitoring Intracranial Pressure

Method	Insertion	Accuracy	Infection Rate	VPR and CSF Drainage?
Ventricular catheter	Problem with small ventricles	Excellent	2–5%	Yes
Subarachnoid screw	Little difficulty	Good	1–2%	No
Epidural transducer	Little difficulty	Variable	Negligible	No
Parenchymal probe	Little difficulty	Good	Negligible	No

VPR, volume-pressure relationship; CSF, cerebrospinal fluid.

and other kinds of catheters are used today in concert with intra-arterial catheters to monitor CPP and, by inference, CBF. Table 15–4 compares the four methods of ICP monitoring.

ICP monitoring allows assessment of the effects of hyperventilation, the use of osmotic agents, diuretics administration, and other measures employed to reduce ICP. The impact of positive end-expiratory pressure and other therapies that may elevate ICP by increasing right atrial pressure and decreasing venous return from the brain can also be assessed. Similarly, one can evaluate the actions of techniques that may alter MAP, such as barbiturate loading for ICP reduction. Patients receiving these and other therapies may be candidates for hemodynamic monitoring with right atrial or pulmonary artery catheters as well. Despite the physiologic information gained by CPP monitoring and the dramatic immediate effects of therapy on MAP and ICP, the long-term benefits of monitoring and therapy are unclear. The identification of intracranial hypertension is of prognostic value. Neurologic recovery is less likely in a patient with head trauma whose ICP rises on admission. An improved outcome from severe head injury with early diagnosis and treatment was also suggested in one study. Nevertheless, such improvement has never been demonstrated by a randomized trial. A trial of this sort seems unlikely because clinicians now use ICP monitoring in many comatose or potentially unstable patients with head trauma, intracerebral masses, subarachnoid hemorrhage, hydrocephalus, and the metabolic encephalopathy associated with Reye's syndrome. Monitoring has also been recommended for comatose patients with massive stroke, encephalitis and meningitis, and anoxic encephalopathy following cardiopulmonary arrest, although its usefulness in these situations is unclear.

EVALUATION OF ARTERIAL BLOOD GAS VALUES

The arterial carbon dioxide tension (Pa_{CO_2}) and the arterial oxygen tension (Pa_{O_2}) have profound effects on CBF. Harper (1965) demonstrated that a 1-mm Hg increase or decrease in Pa_{CO_2} within the range of 20 to 80 mm Hg results in an increase or a decrease in CBF of 1 mL/min/100 g tissue while cerebral metabolism is unchanged (Fig. 15–3). The CBF changes immediately; the change is thought to occur secondary to changes in the pH of brain extracellular fluid surrounding arterioles. CBF plateaus as the Pa_{CO_2} increases above 80 mm Hg, presumably because maximal cerebral vasodilatation has been achieved. Minimal blood flow is reached at a Pa_{CO_2} of 20 mm Hg because the resultant vasoconstriction causes tissue ischemia and hypoxia (cerebral tissue oxygen tension of less than 10 mm Hg), which tends to cause vasodilatation. Vasodilatation and an increase in CBF also follow a fall in the Pa_{O_2} below 60 mm Hg.

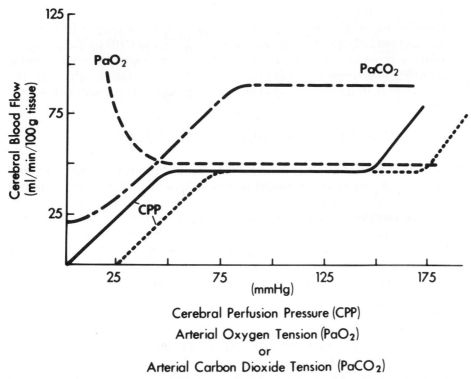

FIGURE 15–3: Changes in cerebral blood flow in response to changes in cerebral perfusion pressure (CPP), arterial oxygen tension (Pa_{O_2}), or arterial carbon dioxide tension (Pa_{CO_2}). If cerebral metabolism and arterial blood gas values are normal and autoregulation is present, cerebral blood flow remains constant when CPP varies between 50 and 150 mm Hg. Cerebral blood flow is affected by a higher CPP if CPP is chronically elevated. The relationship between blood flow and CPP becomes more linear if autoregulation is impaired. (From Luce JM. Neurologic monitoring. Respir Care 30:471–480, 1985.)

The Pa_{CO_2} should be used for medicolegal purposes to confirm brain death by apnea testing.

The profound impact of Pa_{CO_2} and Pa_{O_2} on CBF should prompt frequent measurement of these variables in most neurologic patients. In place of Pa_{O_2}, the arterial oxygen saturation may be measured continuously by oximetry techniques. Transcutaneous carbon dioxide tension and oxygen tension also may prove to be useful, and end-tidal carbon dioxide tensions may be sampled continuously and measured by mass spectrophotometry. The end-tidal carbon dioxide tension and Pa_{CO_2} correlate closely in patients with normal lung function.

ASSESSMENT OF CEREBRAL OXYGENATION

Although direct measurement of cerebral tissue oxygenation is not possible at present, indirect assessment can be performed with the use of cerebral optical spectroscopy. This technique relies on the fact that light in the infrared and near-infrared range passes through extracranial tissue into the brain and returns to a sensor, where its intracerebral attenuation can be computed. Such attenuation is due almost solely to light-absorbing molecules, including oxyhemoglobin, deoxyhemoglobin, and oxidized cytochrome *c. oxidase*. Because the vascular beds encountered in the brain are primarily venous, the saturations of hemoglobin measured by cerebral optical spectroscopy represent mainly the venous compartment. Cerebral mixed venous saturation by itself should be an excellent indicator of the adequacy of cerebral oxygen delivery, just as central mixed venous saturation measured in the pulmonary arteries is an indicator of the adequacy of systemic oxygen delivery. In addition, cerebral optical spectroscopy can be used to assess CBF by depicting the influx and decay of signals given off by indocyanine green and other nondiffusable tracers injected into the central circulation. Although this technique is in its infancy, it shows great promise as a monitoring tool.

MEASUREMENT OF CEREBRAL ARTERIAL FLOW

Transcranial Doppler is an ultrasound technique that measures central flow in major intracranial arteries. This technique uses a pulsed Doppler system with low frequencies (1 to 2 MHz) that allows the operator to sense blood velocities in vessels, such as the middle cerebral artery, that are accessible through various cranial foramina or thin portions of the skull. This information can then provide calculations of peak and mean velocities and pulsatile indices. Transcranial Doppler is accurate in detecting severe stenosis in major intracranial arteries, in assessing the extent of the collateral circulation, in studying arteriovenous malformations, and in documenting brain death. One of the widest applications of transcranial Doppler is in the evaluation of cerebral vasospasm in patients with subarachnoid hemorrhage. Transcranial Doppler is particularly useful in detecting changes in velocity that correlate with alterations in vessel size or configuration; it is less useful in measuring absolute values of CBF. Nevertheless, because it is effective, noninvasive, and inexpensive and because it can be repeated often without concern for safety, it will probably occupy an important place in neurologic monitoring.

ESTIMATION OF CEREBRAL BLOOD FLOW AND METABOLISM

Although CBF and metabolism can be inferred from CPP, direct measurement of flow and metabolic activity would seem to be desirable. The oldest technique for measuring CBF is the inert gas clearance method of Kety and Schmidt (1948). This is based on the principle that the amount of tracer taken up by the brain in a given period equals the amount delivered by the arterial blood minus that removed in cerebral venous blood (the Fick principle). Tracer concentration in the brain is assumed to be proportional to that in venous blood if sufficient time is allowed for tissue-blood equilibration. Nitrous oxide, inhaled over 15 minutes to achieve equilibration between brain and cerebral venous blood, was used as the tracer by Kety and Schmidt, although radioactive gases may be used today. Samples taken intermittently from a peripheral artery and the jugular bulb are used to create curves of arterial and venous concentrations, and the area between the curves is used to compute CBF. In addition, simultaneous assessment of cerebral oxygen consumption ($CMRO_2$) and glucose consumption (CMRG) can be obtained if arterial and jugular venous oxygen and glucose concentrations are measured; arterial-venous differences in oxygen content ($CAVDO_2$) and lactate (CAVDL) concentrations can also be obtained from paired arterial and jugular venous samples. The inert gas clearance technique gives reliable information about hemispheric blood flow and metabolic activity and remains the standard against which other methods are compared. However, this method does not yield information about regional flow and metabolism, and the need for arterial and jugular venous sampling precludes its wide clinical application.

The intra-arterial radioactive inert gas clearance technique of Lassen and coworkers (1981) is also based on the Fick principle. This method involves measuring the clearance of radioactive gas tracers following their injection as a bolus into the carotid artery. Assuming that the tracer is almost completely exhaled on passage through the lungs and has minimal recirculation, the change in brain concentration over time, and hence in CBF, can be described by a simple exponential equation. Either radioactive krypton (^{85}Kr) or radioactive xenon (^{133}Xe) is used because both are relatively insoluble and hence are rapidly excreted by the lungs. As gamma-emitting isotopes, they can also be detected through the skull by one or more cameras that measure regional as well as hemispheric CBF. The flow itself is resolved into fast (gray matter) and slow (white matter) compartments. Studies of $CMRO_2$ and CMRG can also be performed with arterial and venous samples. Because the technique requires arterial puncture, its use is generally limited to patients requiring carotid arteriography. In addition, because isotope is delivered to only part of the brain, global function cannot be evaluated.

Despite their limitations, the techniques of Kety and Schmidt and Lassen and coworkers are not complicated by extracranial flow because the jugular bulb does not drain the scalp and the internal carotid does not supply it. Furthermore, the rapid entry into and clearance from the body of the radioactive tracers used today in both techniques prevent significant recirculation. In addition, they do not require the incorporation of arterial concentrations into the washout equations, the solutions of which require computer assistance. Such assistance is used in the inhaled or intravenous radioactive chest gas clearance technique of Obrist and associates (1967). This method uses a 2-minute period of ^{133}Xe inhalation followed by a 40- to 60-minute washout period. This allows separation of flow into fast, slow, and slowest compartments, the last of which is assumed to represent extracranial recirculation. Arterial samples can be obtained directly (along with jugular bulb samples to assess metabolic function), or values can be estimated indirectly by sampling end-tidal expired gases. This technique appears to be an ideal clinical tool in that total and regional CBF over both hemispheres can be measured noninvasively. At the same time, serial studies are limited only by cumulative radiation exposure. Nevertheless, questions remain about the accuracy of the Obrist method. Its long washout period precludes its steady-state use, and expired gas samples cannot be substituted for arterial samples in patients with pulmonary disease.

The newest technique for assessing CBF and metabolism is positron emission tomography (PET). This method uses isotopes such as $C^{15}O_2$, $^{15}O_2$, and ^{18}F-deoxyglucose. Given intravenously or by inhalation, these isotopes decay into two positrons emitted 180 degrees apart. By using two electronically linked coincidence detectors that record only events seen simultaneously, one can locate the source of the positrons in one dimension. Similarly, a three-dimensional change can be obtained with computer-assisted rotating or stationary isotope detectors. PET potentially offers precise imaging of CBF, $CMRO_2$, and CMRG. However, this expensive technique requires short-lived isotopes generated by an on-site cyclotron. Although imaging quality may suffer somewhat, the disadvantages of PET may be overcome by single photon emission computed tomography, using isotopes such as ^{81}Kr for measuring perfusion and N-

If CBF is known, $CMRO_2$ can be calculated from the equation

$$CMRO_2 = CBF \times CAVDO_2$$

isopropyl-$p[^{123}I]$-iodoamphetamine for metabolic studies. Although both PET and single photon emission computed tomography are as yet experimental, they may prove to have clinical application.

Despite the advent of new techniques to measure CBF, CBF assessment is not yet available in most clinical situations. Nevertheless, as noted earlier, paired samples of arterial and jugular venous blood can be used to calculate the CAVDO$_2$ and the CAVDL. Arterial blood can be sampled from the radial artery or another source; jugular blood can be obtained from a catheter inserted into the internal jugular vein and directed cephalad into the jugular bulb. Although clearly invasive, jugular bulb catheterization is a relatively safe procedure that has been performed in many infants and children as well as in adults.

As is true across vascular beds elsewhere in the body, the CAVDO$_2$ may be expected to decrease from its normal range of about 3 to 6 mL O$_2$/100 mL blood when cerebral hyperemia is present and less oxygen is extracted from the CBF. This situation would be accompanied by a normal (i.e., nonexistent) CAVDL because the brain would not be ischemic. On the other hand, cerebral ischemia induced either by severe brain injury or by excessive hyperventilation would tend to increase the CAVDO$_2$, producing a proportional increase in jugular venous lactate. Determination of CAVDO$_2$ and CAVDL thus provides a ready estimation of CBF that can augment measurement of CPP in the critically ill patient.

SUMMARY

The advent of techniques for measuring CBF, CMRO$_2$, and CMRG provides hope for sophisticated noninvasive neurologic monitoring. Nevertheless, most of these techniques are only experimental at present. Furthermore, although methods of determining cerebral anatomy and electrophysiologic function are of proven clinical utility, they remain cumbersome and costly. As a result, neurologic monitoring currently consists largely of

- Recording vital signs serially
- Administering repeated physical examinations
- Measuring CPP
- Determining arterial blood gas values
- Perhaps determining CAVDO$_2$ and CAVDL

These techniques are very useful in evaluating neurologic changes and should be applied widely in critical care.

Suggested Readings

Barelli A, Valente MR, Clemente A, et al. Serial multimodality-evoked potentials in severely head-injured patients: Diagnostic and prognostic implications. Crit Care Med 19:1374–1381, 1991.

Bruce DA, Langfitt TW, Miller JD, et al. Regional cerebral blood flow, intracranial pressure, and brain metabolism in comatose patients. J Neurosurg 38:131–144, 1973.

Enevoldsen EM, Cold G, Jensen FT, Malmros R. Dynamic changes in regional CBF, intravascular pressure, CSF pH and lactate levels during the acute phase of head injury. J Neurosurg 44:191–214, 1976.

Harper AM. The inter-relationship between a PCO$_2$ and blood pressure in the regulation of blood flow through the cerebral cortex. Acta Neurol Scand 41(Suppl):94–103, 1965.

Jennett B, Teasdale G. Aspects of coma after severe head injury. Lancet 1:878–881, 1977.

Judson JA, Cant BR, Shaw NA. Early prediction of outcome from cerebral trauma by somatosensory evoked potentials. Crit Care Med 18:363–368, 1990.

Kety SS, Schmidt CF. The nitrous oxide method for the quantitative determination of cerebral blood flow in man: Theory, procedure and normal values. J Clin Invest 27:476–483, 1948.

Lassen NA. Control of cerebral circulation in health and disease. Circulation 34:749–760, 1974.

Lassen NA, Henriksen L, Paulson O. Cerebral blood flow in stroke by [133]Xenon inhalation and emission tomography. Stroke 12:284–288, 1981.

Luce JM, Huseby JS, Kirk W, Butler J. A Starling resistor regulates cerebral venous outflow in dogs. J Appl Physiol 53:1496–1503, 1982.

Lundberg N, Troupp H, Lorin H. Continuous recording of the ventricular-fluid pressure in patients with severe acute traumatic brain injury. J Neurosurg 22:581–590, 1965.

McCormick PW, Stewart M, Goetting MG, et al. Noninvasive cerebral optical spectroscopy for monitoring cerebral oxygen delivery and hemodynamics. Crit Care Med 19:89–97, 1991.

McDowall DG. Monitoring the brain. Anesthesiology 45:117–134, 1976.

Miller JD, Becker DP, Ward JD, et al. Significance of intracranial hypertension in severe head injury. J Neurosurg 47:503–516, 1977.

Naidich TP, Moran CJ, Pudlowski RM, Hanaway J. Advances in diagnosis: Cranial and spinal computed tomography. Med Clin North Am 63:849–895, 1979.

Obrist WD, Thompson HK, King HC, Wang SH. Determination of regional cerebral blood flow by inhalation of [133]Xenon. Circ Res 20:124–135, 1967.

Pitts LH, Andrews BT. Intracranial pressure monitoring and treatment of intracranial hypertension. *In* Hall JB, Schmidt GA, Wood LDH (eds). Principles of Critical Care Medicine. New York, McGraw-Hill, 1992, pp 443–452.

Plum F, Posner JB. The Diagnosis of Stupor and Coma, 3rd ed. Philadelphia, FA Davis, 1980.

Robertson CS, Narayan RK, Gokaslan ZL, et al. Cerebral arteriovenous oxygen difference as an estimate of cerebral blood flow in comatose patients. J Neurosurg 70:222–230, 1989.

Seiler RW, Grolimund P, Aaslid R, et al. Cerebral vasospasm evaluated by transcranial ultrasound correlated with clinical grade and CT-visualized subarachnoid hemorrhage. J Neurosurg 64:594–600, 1986.

Sharbrough FW, Messick JM, Sundt TM. Correlation of continuous electroencephalograms with cerebral blood flow measurements during carotid endarterectomy. Stroke 4:674–683, 1973.

Teasdale G, Jennett B. Assessment of coma and impaired consciousness: A practical scale. Lancet 2:81–84, 1974.

16

Electrocardiography

Steven J. L. Evans, M.D., and
Stephen Blumberg, M.D.

Many of the disorders of the heart's electrical system can be diagnosed from the surface ECG.

The heart is composed of several different types of tissue. The muscle tissue of the heart, or myocardium, is responsible for the pumping action that delivers blood to the rest of the body. The valves of the heart, composed of fibrous tissue, ensure that blood flows only in the proper (forward) direction. The electrical conduction system of the heart allows all of the various parts of the heart to act in concert. By carrying the impulses to the various parts of the heart in an orderly fashion, the electrical conduction system permits organized cardiac function to occur synchronously with each heartbeat.

The heart generates an electrical signal (voltage) with each beat. This signal may be easily measured on the surface of the body with a special type of voltmeter adapted for patient use, the electrocardiogram (ECG). When the electrical system of the heart is diseased, the heart can beat too fast or too slow, seriously harming a patient.

ELECTRICAL PROPERTIES OF THE CARDIAC MUSCLE CELL

The membrane of the cardiac cell generates and maintains different ionic concentrations inside and outside the cell. The different concentrations of electrically charged ions (potassium, sodium, calcium, and others) inside and outside the cell cause an ionic gradient to be formed. Ionic gradients create an electrochemical potential (relatively negative and positive charges, similar to a battery). When the cardiac cell is in the resting state, the cell membrane is relatively impermeable to these ions, and the inside of the cell remains negatively charged relative to the outside of the cell (Fig. 16–1).

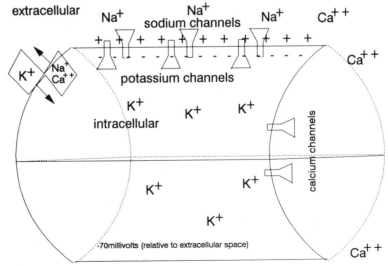

FIGURE 16–1: When the cardiac cell is in the resting state, the cell membrane is relatively impermeable to ions. The inside of the cell remains negatively charged relative to the outside of the cell.

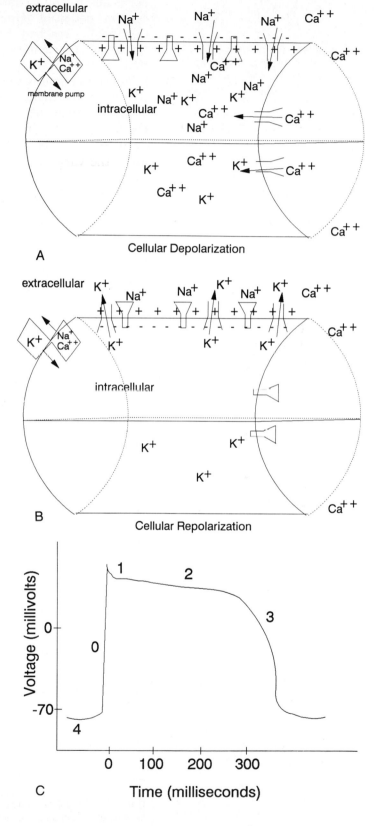

FIGURE 16–2: *A*, Stimulation of the cell causes an alteration in the cell membrane's ionic permeability, initiating ionic flow across the membrane. Initiation of the action potential causes the ionic gates of the membrane to open. Rapid inward movement of sodium and calcium causes the cell to depolarize and become positively charged intracellularly. *B*, After depolarization, rapid outward potassium flow causes the cell to repolarize and again become negatively charged intracellularly. *C*, Recording of voltages by a microelectrode inside the cell during an action potential. Phase 0 represents rapid depolarization, whereas phases 1, 2, and 3 represent repolarization. Phase 4 is the resting state of the cell.

Sufficiently strong mechanical or electrical stimulation of the cell membrane can cause a slight alteration in the cell membrane's ionic permeability and initiate ionic flow across the cell membrane. The intracellular potential becomes more positive, until the action potential threshold is reached. Initiation of the action potential causes the ionic "gates" of the membrane to burst open. The rapid inward movement of sodium and calcium along their electrochemical gradient causes the cell to depolarize and become positively charged intracellularly. After depolarization, the rapid outward flow of potassium along its electrochemical gradient causes the cell to repolarize and again become negatively charged intracellularly (Fig. 16–2). Between repolarization and the next depolarization, ionic "pumps" in the membrane move potassium inward and sodium and calcium outward, thereby maintaining the gradient so that further cycles of depolarization and repolarization can occur.

ELECTRICAL CONDUCTION SYSTEM OF THE HEART

In the normal heart, the sinus node, located in the upper part of the right atrium, initiates each beat (Fig. 16–3). The first cellular depolarization at the start of each new cardiac cycle (each new heartbeat) automatically commences in the sinus node. From there, the depolarization wave front sweeps throughout both atria. The wave front arrives at the atrioventricular (AV) node and travels slowly across it. After traversing the AV node, the impulse is transmitted down the His bundle and the left and right bundle branches, over what is termed the His-Purkinje system. Most left bundle conduction systems are divided into three separate anatomic fascicles: the anterosuperior, the posteroinferior, and the centriseptal. The right bundle conduction system is thinner and divides into right ventricular septal and free wall fibers at the base of the right ventricular papillary muscle.

The His-Purkinje system rapidly distributes the depolarization wave front to the ventricular myocardium; then the wave front depolarizes the ventricles. Rapid impulse conduction via the normal His-Purkinje system allows essentially simultaneous right and left ventricular activation. After ventricular depolarization occurs, the ventricular myocardium

The muscle of the heart is composed of millions of cardiac cells. The cardiac cell contracts during depolarization and relaxes during repolarization. The synchronous contraction and relaxation of these cells causes the heart to function normally to pump blood throughout the body.

The sinus node is responsible for the normal heart rhythm (normal sinus rhythm).

The His-Purkinje system is composed of specialized, rapidly conducting cardiac cells.

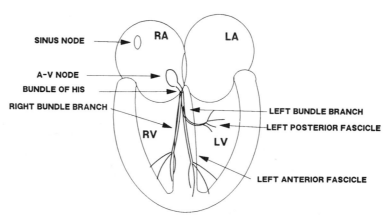

FIGURE 16–3: The sequence of activation during a normal cardiac cycle is sinus node depolarization followed by atrial depolarization, atrioventricular (AV) nodal depolarization, His–bundle branch–Purkinje depolarization, and finally ventricular depolarization. RA, LA, right and left atria; RV, LV, right and left ventricles.

- Repolarizes
- Accepts another impulse
- Repeats the cardiac cycle

Hence, to summarize, the sequence of activation during a normal cardiac cycle is

- Sinus node depolarization
- Atrial depolarization
- AV node depolarization
- His–bundle branch–Purkinje depolarization
- Ventricular depolarization

Repolarization occurs after depolarization.

P Wave, QRS Complex, and T Wave

Although many cardiac tissues depolarize and repolarize during each cardiac cycle, as described previously, not all of the cardiac electrical activity is seen on the surface ECG. This is because certain cardiac tissues do not generate a large enough electrical charge (a high enough voltage) to be measured by standard ECG techniques. AV node activity, His-Purkinje activity, and atrial repolarization are usually not of high enough voltage to be seen on the surface ECG. Hence, only atrial depolarization, ventricular depolarization, and ventricular repolarization are normally visualized on the surface ECG. Atrial depolarization creates the P wave seen on the surface ECG; ventricular depolarization, the QRS complex; and ventricular repolarization, the T wave (Fig. 16–4).[1]

Electrodes and Leads

By positioning electrodes on the body in various configurations, different "electrical views" of the heart may be obtained (Fig. 16–5). The limb lead tracings (I, II, III, aVR, aVL, and aVF) are bipolar cardiac recordings derived from electrodes placed on the arms and legs. The

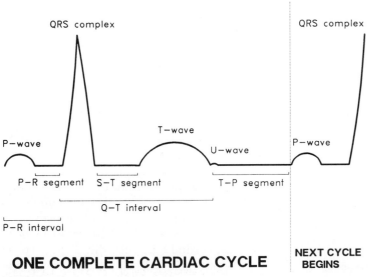

ONE COMPLETE CARDIAC CYCLE   **NEXT CYCLE BEGINS**

FIGURE 16–4: The cardiac cycle.

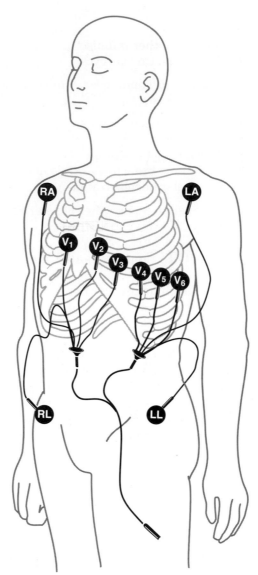

FIGURE 16–5: The position of the electrocardiographic leads on the surface of the body.

electrodes positioned on the arms and the left leg create a frontal plane recording triangle centered around the heart, whereas the electrode on the right leg serves as an electrical ground. In lead I, the left arm is positive and the right arm is negative. In lead II, the left leg is positive and the right arm is negative. In lead III, the left leg is positive and the left arm is negative. Leads aVR, aVL, and aVF are mathematical derivations of leads I, II, and III affording differing views of the heart's electrical activity. The precordial lead tracings (V_1 through V_6) are unipolar recordings derived from an electrode placed in various positions on the left precordium (chest wall) and an indifferent electrode. The indifferent electrode used is a common central terminal, which is created by connecting all three limb electrodes through a 5000-Ω resistance.

The standard 12-lead ECG is composed of the six frontal and six precordial lead recordings (Fig. 16–6). The ECG is recorded on standard 1-mm grid paper at a standard paper speed rate of 25 mm/sec. Hence, every 1-mm box on the horizontal axis represents 0.04 second, and divi-

The standard 12-lead ECG permits clinical interpretation of rhythm, rate, axis, conduction, chamber enlargement, arrhythmia, and myocardial ischemia or infarction.

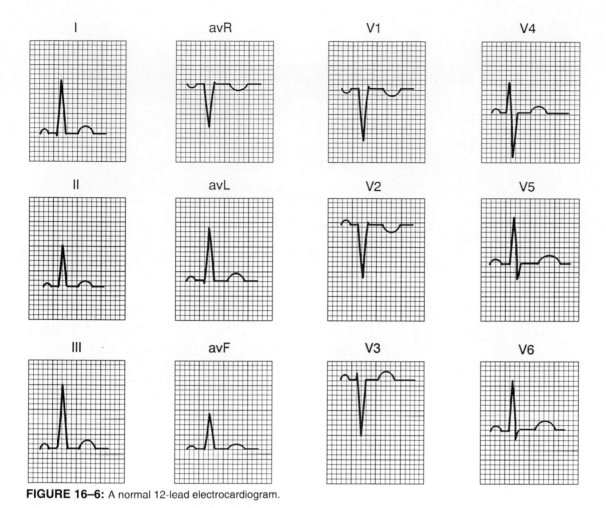

I   avR   V1   V4

II   avL   V2   V5

III   avF   V3   V6

FIGURE 16–6: A normal 12-lead electrocardiogram.

sions of five boxes represent 0.2 second. The vertical axis is calibrated such that 1 mm (one box) corresponds to a 1-mV amplitude (Fig. 16–7A).

Rhythm and Rate

It is best to approach the standard ECG by first noting the rhythm and rate. The sinus node is the principal pacemaker of the normal heart. Its ability to generate impulses at rates varying from 60 to 100 beats per minute, under normal conditions, determines the basic heart rate. This is called normal sinus rhythm (Fig. 16–8).

Rhythm regularity and initiation site should be noted. If the rhythm is irregular, it should be determined whether there is a pattern to the irregularity (e.g., paired beats, group beating, regularly dropped beats, bigeminal beats, or trigeminal beats) or if the rhythm is chaotic (e.g., atrial or ventricular fibrillation). The initiation site should be noted as sinoatrial, AV junctional, idioventricular, or ventricular in origin.

Rapid rate estimation for regular rates may be made by counting the number of QRS complexes that lie between two 3-second markers on the paper (6 seconds) and multiplying by 10. Alternatively, the number of "five-box" groups that lie between two consecutive QRS complexes may be measured, and Figure 16–7A having been committed to memory, the estimated heart rate can be determined. In ECGs demonstrating an irregular rate, an accurate rate calculation may be made by counting the

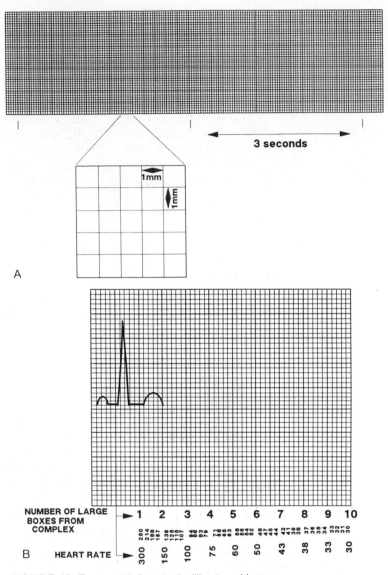

3 seconds

A

NUMBER OF LARGE BOXES FROM COMPLEX

	1	2	3	4	5	6	7	8	9	10
	260 214 188 167	136 125 115 107	86 83 79	71 65 63	58 56 52	48 47 45 44	42 41 39 38	37 36 34	33 32 31	30

B **HEART RATE** → 300 150 100 75 60 50 43 38 33 30

FIGURE 16–7: *A* and *B*, Standard millimeter grid paper.

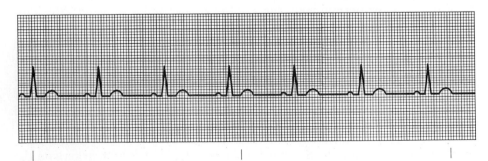

FIGURE 16–8: Normal sinus rhythm.

number of QRS complexes during a 6-second interval and multiplying that number by 10.

Electrical Axis

For an electrical impulse to move in any given direction, it must form what is known as a dipole. The ionic gradient across the cell membrane is an example of a dipole. Once a dipole has been achieved, an impulse can flow along the dipole like water flowing downhill.

Figure 16–9 represents an isolated strip of myocardium. On the left side of the strip, at time zero, the dipole enters this area and the muscle tissue depolarizes. As the tissue depolarizes, it becomes relatively negative because the inflow of positive ions into the cells leaves a paucity of positive charges in the area relative to the nondepolarized areas. This creates a moving dipole with a positive "leading" edge and a negative "following" edge. The dipole then moves through the nondepolarized myocardium from left to right, depolarizing the tissue as it passes through.

As the positive edge of the dipole moves toward the positive pole of a lead pair, it causes a positive voltage to be recorded. If it moves away from the positive pole and toward the negative pole, a negative voltage is recorded.

As the electrical impulse travels throughout the myocardium, it has

A dipole is simply an area in which part of the impulse is relatively positive and part of the impulse is relatively negative, similar to the positive and negative poles on a battery.

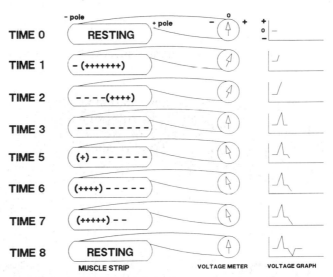

FIGURE 16–9: Electrical dipole activation. A strip of myocardium is represented, with a positive and negative monitoring electrode pair attached to a meter. At time 0, the muscle is in the resting state and the meter registers 0 (no voltage). At time 1, as the muscle starts to depolarize from the left, the area of depolarization becomes relatively negative as positive ions flow into the cells and leave a relative paucity of positive ions in the area. This is now measured as a positive voltage because the muscle strip has a relatively positive charge on the side with the positive electrode. As depolarization continues (time 2), the voltage is increased. Time 3 represents complete depolarization. Because there is no relative imbalance in charge here, no voltage is measured. Repolarization commences at time 5, with a reversal of the above sequence as positive ions flow out of the cell. By time 8, the cell is back in the resting state.

a direction. In the isolated strip of myocardium, the impulse spreads from left to right and represents a voltage moving along a one-dimensional axis. However, in the intact heart, the impulse spreads in all three dimensions. Because the front-to-back depth of the body is not nearly as large as the side-to-side or the top-to-bottom measurements, the electrical axis of the heart may be simplified by being considered as a two-dimensional, x- and y-axis system (Fig. 16–10).

Because the electrical impulse traveling through the myocardium has both a voltage and a direction, it is considered to be a vector. This vector may be broken down into its component parts of voltage and direction along the x and y axes. Alternatively, if the voltage and direction are known, the vector may be reconstructed and evaluated. These concepts set the stage for understanding the determination of the QRS axis.

The QRS axis determination uses a frontal plane, compass-like grid derived from the Einthoven triangle (Fig. 16–11A). Lead I constitutes the horizontal plane, with a positive orientation leftward at 0 degrees. Lead aVF denotes the vertical plane, with a positive downward orientation at 90 degrees. Leads II and III are positive at 60 and 120 degrees. Leads aVR and aVL are positive at −150 and −30 degrees. To calculate the axis (vector) of the QRS complex, the quadrant in which the axis is located must first be determined by examining leads I and aVF. For example, if the complex is upright in lead I and in lead aVF, the axis will lie within quadrant one (Fig. 16–12A). If it is upright in lead I and downward in lead aVF, it will lie in quadrant two. The exact axis may be determined by measuring the voltage in leads I and aVF and drawing lines perpendicular to the corresponding axes at these voltages. Then, another line is drawn from the origin (center of the graph) to the point of intersection. This line is the angle of the axis of the QRS complex (see Fig. 16–12B). Determination of the P wave and T wave axes is performed in a similar manner.

A normal axis falls between +110 and −30 degrees (see Fig. 16–11B). A left axis deviation is designated when the axis falls between −30 and −90 degrees. An axis falling between +110 and +180 degrees is a

Right axis deviation may be associated with

- Right ventricular hypertrophy
- Right bundle branch block
- Chronic emphysema
- Left posterior hemiblock
- Ventricular arrhythmias

Left axis deviation can be seen in

- Left bundle branch block
- Left anterior hemiblock
- Congenital heart disease
- Ventricular arrhythmias[2]

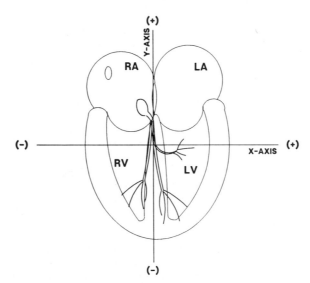

FIGURE 16–10: Electrical system of the heart superimposed on a two-dimensional, x- and y-axis system. RA, LA, right and left atria; RV, LV, right and left ventricles.

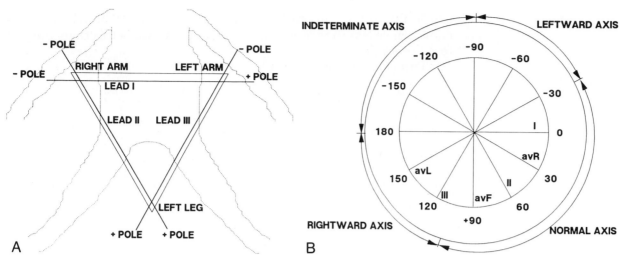

FIGURE 16–11: *A,* Einthoven's triangle superimposed on the body. *B,* Electrical axis system derived from frontal leads.

right axis deviation. The territory between −90 and −180 degrees is "no man's land," where it is impossible to determine a left versus a right axis deviation.

COMPLEXES, INTERVALS, AND SEGMENTS

P Wave

The P wave, which corresponds to atrial depolarization (see Fig. 16–4), starts with sinus node depolarization and ends when all of the atrial tissue (both the left and the right atrium) depolarizes. The normal P wave is rounded, not peaked or notched. It is upright in leads I, II, aVF,

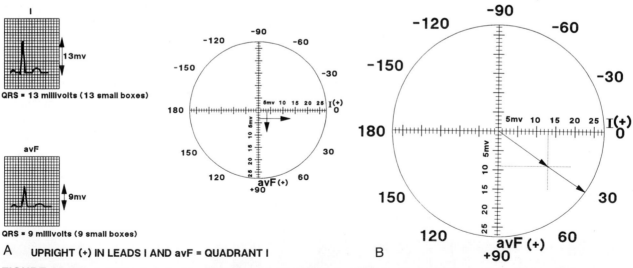

FIGURE 16–12: *A,* QRS axis derivation. In this example, the QRS is upright in lead I, placing the axis leftward along the lead I line. The QRS is also upright in lead aVF, placing the axis downward along the aVF line. In this manner, the quadrant in which any QRS complex lies may be easily determined. *B,* Determination of the exact electrical axis. First, the voltage is measured in leads I and aVF. In this example, the QRS voltage in lead I is 13 mV, and in lead aVF it is 9 mV. Then a line perpendicular to each corresponding axis at that voltage is drawn. Another line may then be drawn from the origin (center of the graph) to the point of intersection. This line is the angle of the axis of the QRS complex.

and V₄ through V₆; inverted in aVR; and variable in all other leads. The amplitude is less than or equal to 2.5 mm. Its width is less than or equal to 0.11 second.

Pathologic P waves may be

- Inverted, as in atrial depolarization from a low atrial site because of an ectopic atrial or AV junctional rhythm (Fig. 16–13)
- Peaked or of large amplitude, as in right atrial hypertrophy or dilatation secondary to valvular heart disease, right ventricular hypertension, cor pulmonale, or congenital heart disease
- Wide or diphasic, implying left atrial enlargement, which may be due to hypertension, mitral or aortic valvular disease, or ventricular diastolic dysfunction

PR Interval

The normal PR interval is between 0.12 and 0.20 second in duration (see Fig. 16–8).

The PR interval, which is measured from the onset of the P wave to the onset of the QRS, represents the time from sinus node depolarization to the start of ventricular depolarization.

Abnormal prolongation (first-degree AV block) may be seen as a normal variation, in coronary or rheumatic disease, and occasionally in hyperthyroidism (Fig. 16–14). Shortened PR intervals occur in

- AV junctional and low atrial rhythms
- Wolff-Parkinson-White syndrome
- Normal variants and occasionally hypertension

QRS Complex

The QRS complex (see Fig. 16–4) represents ventricular depolarization. Any positive deflection is called an R wave. If there are two positive deflections, the first is called an R wave and the second an R′ wave (Fig. 16–15A). If the initial part of the QRS complex is negative, it is called a Q wave. Any subsequent negative deflection that follows either a Q wave or an R wave is termed an S wave. A Q wave may be followed by an R wave or by an S wave. However, if the initial deflection of the QRS complex is positive (an R wave), any subsequent negative deflection is called an S wave. Hence, a Q wave can exist in the QRS complex only if the initial deflection is negative, and there can be a QRS complex without the "Q." The relative amplitude of the waves of the QRS complex is denoted by lower case or capital letters. For example, a QRS complex

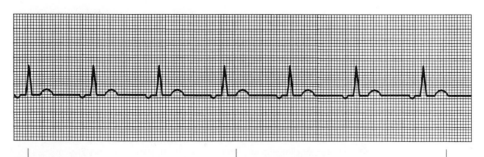

FIGURE 16–13: Inverted P waves from a low atrial ectopic focus.

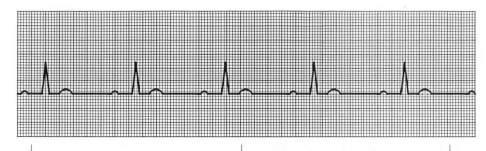

FIGURE 16–14: First-degree atrioventricular block. Note the prolonged PR interval of 0.28 second.

with a large Q wave, a small R wave, and a large S wave would be designated "QrS" (see Fig. 16–15B), whereas a complex with a small Q wave, a large R wave, and no S wave would be designated as a "qR" complex (see Fig. 16–15C).

The normal QRS duration varies from 0.5 to 0.10 second. Limb lead amplitude is normally greater than 5 mm. Precordial amplitude is normally greater than or equal to 10 mm in V_1 through V_6 and is less than 25 to 30 mm in V_1 or V_2 plus V_5 or V_6. Q waves of less than 0.03 second in duration may be seen ("insignificant" Q waves). The normal frontal plane QRS axis falls between -30 and $+110$ degrees.

Abnormally prolonged QRS complexes occur in intraventricular conduction delays, bundle branch block, and ventricular arrhythmias. Low voltage (an amplitude of less than 5 mm leads in I, II, or III or of less than 10 mm in leads V_1 through V_6) can be seen in diffuse coronary disease, heart failure, pericardial effusion, myxedema, emphysema, generalized edema, or obesity. High voltage (greater than or equal to 25 to 30 mm in V_1 or V_2 plus V_5 or V_6) may occur in left ventricular hypertrophy.

Q waves of greater than or equal to 0.03 second signify probable myocardial infarction. Axis deviations of less than -30 degrees or greater than $+110$ degrees may be seen in conduction system disease, ventricular arrhythmias, and congenital heart disease.

ST Segment

The ST segment occurs from the offset of the QRS to the onset of the T wave (see Fig. 16–4); therefore, it falls between the end of ventricular depolarization and the beginning of ventricular repolarization. The segment is normally isoelectric (i.e., at baseline) with the TP segment. Early

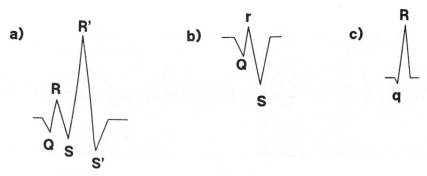

FIGURE 16–15: *A* to *C,* Classification of the QRS complex.

repolarization (upsloping elevated ST elevation) may be seen in young black males as a normal variant.

ST segment flattening implies myocardial ischemia. ST segment elevation can be seen in coronary artery spasm, myocardial infarction, and acute pericarditis and can be seen transiently after electrical cardioversion. ST segment depression occurs in myocardial ischemia.

T Wave

The T wave represents ventricular repolarization (see Fig. 16–4). It is normally upright in leads I, II, V_5, and V_6; inverted in a VR; and variable elsewhere. The wave is rounded and mildly asymmetrical, with an amplitude of less than or equal to 5 mm in the limb leads and of less than or equal to 10 mm in the precordial leads. Pathologic inversion may be seen in myocardial ischemia or infarction, chronic pericarditis, repolarization abnormalities associated with conduction disease or myocardial hypertrophy, and occasionally central nervous system events such as stroke. Tall T waves (greater than 5 mm in the limb leads or greater than 10 mm in the precordium) may be seen in myocardial infarction or ischemia, hyperkalemia, ventricular overloading, and stroke. T wave flattening is associated with obesity.

QT Interval

For determination of an accurate QT interval, a simple mathematical formula should be used to correct for heart rate. The measured QT interval is divided by the square root of the preceding RR interval; the number derived from this is called the corrected QT interval, or QT_c. The normal QT_c in men is 0.39 second; in women, it is 0.41 second.

The QT interval starts with the onset of the QRS and ends with the offset of the T wave (see Fig. 16–4). The normal interval varies with the heart rate, age, and sex of the patient. The normal QT interval is less than one half of the preceding RR interval.

Prolonged QT intervals imply delayed ventricular repolarization (Fig. 16–16). Conditions that prolong the QT interval include congestive heart failure; ischemia; rheumatic heart disease; myocarditis; cerebrovascular disease; electrolyte abnormalities, such as hypokalemia or hypocalcemia; use of drugs, such as type IA antiarrhythmic agents (e.g., quinidine and procainamide) and phenothiazines; hypothermia; severe dieting; and mitral valve prolapse. A prolonged QT interval may also be genetic in nature. Prolongation of the QT interval predisposes to ventricular tachyarrhythmias, syncope, and sudden death.[3] Shortened QT intervals are induced by digitalis use, hypercalcemia, and hyperkalemia.

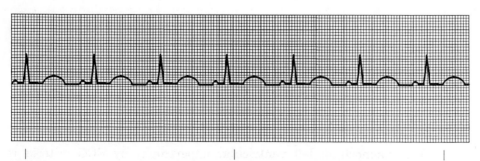

FIGURE 16–16: Prolonged QT interval. The QT interval measures 0.48 second.

V1   V5

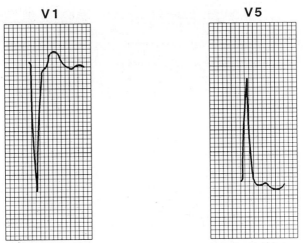

FIGURE 16–17: Leads V₁ and V₅ from a patient with left ventricular hypertrophy. Note the high voltages.

U Wave

The U wave, which occurs after the T wave (see Fig. 16–4), is often not visible on the ECG. The etiology of the U wave is uncertain. It is possibly due to repolarization of the papillary muscles or the Purkinje system. If present, it is a small, low-voltage wave with a polarity identical to that of the T wave.

TP Segment

The segment from the offset of the T wave to the onset of the P wave (the TP interval) represents the resting potential and serves as the true isoelectric reference point on the ECG.

RR Interval

The interval between consecutive QRS complexes is called the RR interval. During normal sinus rhythm, the RR interval is regular and does not vary by more than approximately 0.04 second.

CHAMBER ENLARGEMENT

The ECG measures the net sum of electrical voltage created during myocardial depolarization and repolarization. The contribution of each cardiac chamber to the total voltage recorded is relative to its myocardial mass. Increased ventricular wall thickness and mass will prolong the impulse conduction time (QRS duration) toward the upper limit of normal and increase the QRS voltage.[4]

Left Ventricular Hypertrophy

Left ventricular hypertrophy is commonly caused by long-standing untreated hypertension. Other causes include valvular heart disease and cardiomyopathy.

The diagnosis of left ventricular hypertrophy by ECG criteria is usually made by observing an increased voltage of the QRS complex in one or more leads (Fig. 16–17). Various scoring systems (e.g., Estes' and

TABLE **16–1:** Scott's Criteria for Left Ventricular Hypertrophy

Wave and Lead	Amplitude (mm)
R (I) + S (III)	> 25
R (aVL)	> 7.5
R (aVF)	> 20
S (aVR)	> 14
S (V_1 or V_2) + R (V_5 or V_6)	> 35
R (V_5 or V_6)	> 26
R + S (V_1–V_6)	> 45

Scott's) have been proposed to diagnose left ventricular hypertrophy from the surface ECG (Table 16–1).[5] The presence of any or all of either of these criteria on an ECG should be interpreted as left ventricular hypertrophy by ECG criteria. The association of ST-T wave abnormalities implies the presence of myocardial "strain"—ST segments are depressed, with an upward convexity, and run into an inverted T wave. Slight widening of the QRS complex may also be present.

Right Ventricular Enlargement

As left ventricular hypertrophy distorts the normal precordial QRS pattern, right ventricular hypertrophy predominantly affects the right precordial (V_1 and V_2) leads. Right ventricular hypertrophy characteristics include an initial q wave and a tall R wave in V_1 or V_2, with an R/S ratio of greater than 1.0 and a deep S wave in V_5 or V_6 (Fig. 16–18). The QRS duration is usually normal. There is an associated right axis deviation. The ST segment is depressed, with an upward convexity, and is associated with inverted T waves in V_1 and V_2.

Right ventricular hypertrophy can be seen in acquired valvular lesions, such as mitral stenosis and tricuspid insufficiency, and in congenital lesions, such as tetralogy of Fallot, pulmonic stenosis, and transposition of the great vessels.

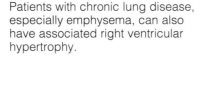

Patients with chronic lung disease, especially emphysema, can also have associated right ventricular hypertrophy.

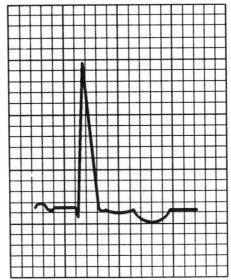

FIGURE 16–18: Lead V_1 from a patient with right ventricular hypertrophy. Note the initial q wave and the high R wave voltage.

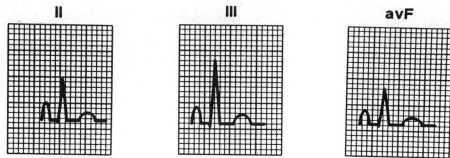

FIGURE 16–19: Leads II, III, and aVF from a patient with right atrial enlargement. Note the tall, peaked P waves.

Right Atrial Enlargement

Right atrial enlargement may result from right ventricular diastolic dysfunction associated with right ventricular hypertrophy (e.g., "P-pulmonale," "P-congenitale," and "P-tricuspidale").

Right atrial enlargement is marked by a P wave right axis deviation and an amplitude of greater than 2.5 mm, best seen in leads II, III, and aVF (Fig. 16–19).

Left Atrial Enlargement

Left atrial enlargement may be associated with hypertension or valvular disease (e.g., "P-mitrale").

Left atrial enlargement is characterized by a P wave width of 0.12 second or more; notching in leads II, III, or aVF; or a biphasic configuration with a negative terminal portion of 0.04 second or more in lead V_1 (Fig. 16–20).

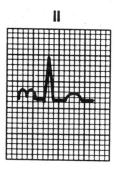 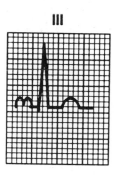 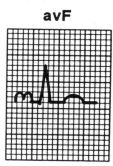

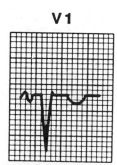

FIGURE 16–20: Leads II, III, aVF, and V_1 in left atrial enlargement. Note the notching of the P wave.

BUNDLE BRANCH BLOCK

Disease in one of the bundle branches causes the impulse to be blocked in that conduction pathway and to travel rapidly down the other, normal pathway. The ventricles then activate sequentially rather than simultaneously. The impulse propagates from the ventricle first activated through the septal muscle to the other ventricle. The relatively slow impulse conduction across the myocardium, which is much slower than via the His–bundle branch–Purkinje system, is reflected on the ECG recording as a wide QRS and an ST-T wave axis opposite to the main QRS deflection.

Left bundle branch block is usually characterized by a QS complex in V_1, an R or RR′ (no Q waves) in V_6, and an R or RR′ (no Q waves) in leads I and aVL (Fig. 16–21). Right bundle branch block has a RSR′ pattern in lead V_1 and a wide S in leads I and V_6 (Fig. 16–22). Right bundle branch block can be associated with a normal right or left axis deviation.[6]

The association of a T wave axis concordant with (in the same direction as) a bundle branch block's terminal QRS deflection implies the presence of associated myocardial disease, such as myocardial ischemia, infarction, or cardiomyopathy. When either right or left bundle branch block configurations are noted in the presence of QRS durations between 0.09 and 0.11 second, the diagnosis of incomplete bundle branch block is made.

ATRIOVENTRICULAR BLOCK

The concept of AV block refers to either a delay in or a complete interruption of an impulse transmitted over the normal conduction pathway linking the atrial and ventricular myocardium.

A bundle branch block will have a QRS duration of greater than or equal to 0.12 second.

Right and occasionally left bundle branch block may be seen in younger patients without organic heart disease; however, the onset of either type of bundle branch block in the majority of older patients may be associated with evidence of coronary artery disease.

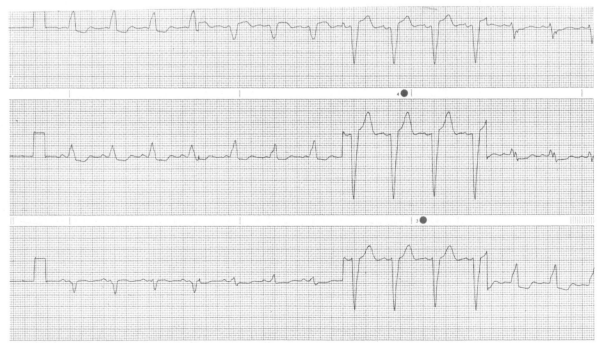

FIGURE 16–21: Left bundle branch block.

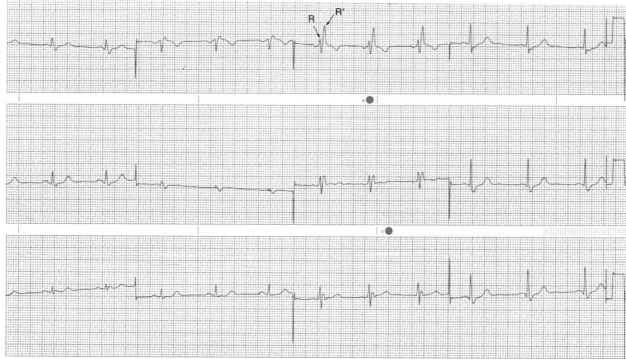

FIGURE 16–22: Right bundle branch block.

First-Degree Atrioventricular Block

An impulse conduction delay between the atria and the ventricles that may cause a prolonged PR interval, termed first-degree AV block, is usually caused by abnormalities affecting the AV node conduction tissue. A PR interval of greater than or equal to 0.21 second is considered to be a first-degree AV block (see Fig. 16–14). In most cases, isolated first-degree AV block is considered to be a benign finding.

Second-Degree Atrioventricular Block

Second-degree block occurs when one or more of the atrial impulses fail to be conducted to the ventricles because of block at any level of the AV node or His-Purkinje conduction system. This type of AV block has been subdivided into type I or AV node block (Wenckebach) and type II AV block.

Type I Second-Degree Atrioventricular Block (Wenckebach)

The conduction abnormality in type I second-degree block is usually localized in the AV node. It is frequently associated with reversible conditions, such as rheumatic fever, digitalis or beta-blocker effect, and acute inferior wall myocardial infarction. Chronic Wenckebach may be seen in aortic valve disease, ischemic heart disease, mitral valve prolapse, atrial septal defect, and even highly trained athletes. It carries a relatively benign prognosis, only rarely progressing to complete heart block.

Classically, an initially normal PR interval undergoes a progressive prolongation with each successive beat until an atrial impulse is blocked.

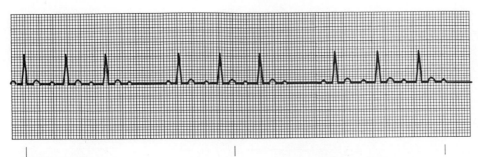

FIGURE 16–23: Type I second-degree atrioventricular block (Wenckebach phenomenon).

Group beating—repetitive groups of two, three, or more ventricular complexes between dropped complexes

This is seen as a P wave without a following QRS complex on the ECG. The next PR interval is "reset," conduction restored after the dropped complex, and the process repeats itself once again. While the PP intervals are lengthening, the RR intervals are shortening. The longest RR interval containing the dropped ventricular complex is less than two times the shortest cycle length. The presence of one or all of these characteristics along with "group beating" enables recognition of Wenckebach beating (Fig. 16–23).[7,8]

Type II Second-Degree Atrioventricular Block

Type II second-degree AV block is suspected when ECG patterns of two or more normally conducted P waves precede a nonconducted P wave and an associated dropped ventricular complex P (no QRS) (Fig. 16–24). The next atrial impulse, however, is again transmitted to the ventricle (P-QRS) via a restored conduction pathway. The pattern may then repeat itself. However, the diagnosis of type II second-degree AV block is established by identifying constant PR intervals in all complexes immediately preceding and following the nonconducted P waves and by recognizing that the longest RR interval containing the dropped ventricular complex is equal to two times the shortest RR interval. This is as opposed to the classic type I second-degree AV block, in which the PR intervals lengthen before the dropped ventricular complex and the RR intervals containing the dropped ventricular beat are less than two times the shortest interval.

Although type II second-degree AV block is considerably less frequent than Wenckebach, it has a high risk of evolving to complete heart block and syncope.

Complete Heart Block or Third-Degree Atrioventricular Block

Complete heart block occurs when all atrial impulses are blocked, preventing transmission to the ventricles. The usual cause is trifascicu-

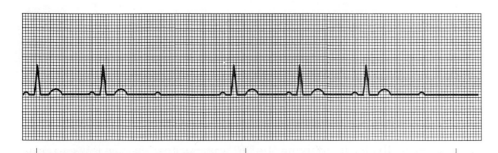

FIGURE 16–24: Type II second-degree atrioventricular block.

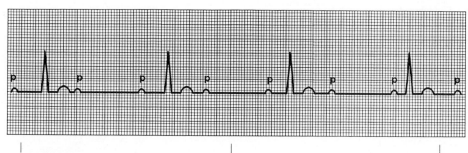

FIGURE 16–25: Atrioventricular dissociation.

lar block or bilateral bundle branch block. AV node block or His bundle block may also be the cause.

The recognition of AV dissociation is key to the diagnosis. The ECG recording usually demonstrates a regular atrial rate that is independent of a regular junctional (narrow QRS) or ventricular (wide QRS) escape rhythm (Fig. 16–25).

HEMIBLOCKS, BIFASCICULAR BLOCKS, AND TRIFASCICULAR BLOCKS

Hemiblock

Conduction disease affecting the left anterosuperior or posteroinferior fascicles may be readily interpreted on the ECG. Conduction block in these fascicles has been designated as either left anterior hemiblock or left posterior hemiblock (the term *fascicular block* may also be used in place of the term *hemiblock*).

In a left anterior hemiblock, a block in the anterosuperior fascicle causes a change in the normal activation sequence of the left ventricle, which is reflected on the ECG as a left axis deviation of greater than or equal to − 30 degrees; a qR in leads I and aVL; an rS in leads II, III, and aVF; and normal QRS duration (Fig. 16–26). The activation sequence with a left posterior hemiblock is reversed, causing a right axis deviation of + 120 degrees or more; an rS in leads I and aVL; a qR in leads II, III, and aVF; and normal QRS duration (Fig. 16–27). It is not uncommon to discover an anterior hemiblock in otherwise normal hearts. A left posterior hemiblock is usually abnormal, implying underlying heart disease.

Bifascicular and Trifascicular Block

Conduction disease is generally the consequence of a diffuse disease process affecting the entire conduction system. Thus, it is not uncommon to have ECG evidence of bifascicular and multi- or trifascicular disease or block. A left anterior hemiblock is commonly associated with a right bundle branch block, creating one type of bifascicular block (Fig. 16–28). In addition, a left posterior hemiblock is often seen with a right bundle branch block, causing a different bifascicular block combination. The hemiblock and bundle branch block criteria are both present on the ECG recording.

Conduction block affecting the left anterior fascicle, the left posterior fascicle, and the right bundle branch is termed trifascicular block (Fig. 16–29). Complete block involving all of the fascicles will cause complete

The greatest danger of sudden cardiac death due to complete heart block is from ventricular asystole—only P waves are seen on the ECG when the ventricular escape rhythm is absent. Permanent pacemaker implantation is strongly indicated.

Longevity and prognosis are usually unaffected by the presence of a left anterior hemiblock.

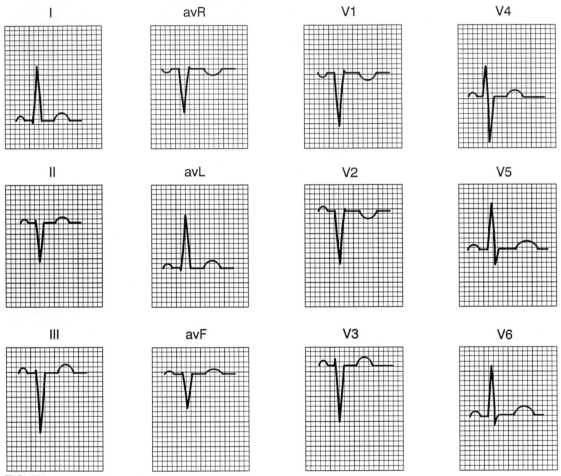

FIGURE 16–26: Left anterior hemiblock.

I   avR   V1   V4

II   avL   V2   V5

III   avF   V3   V6

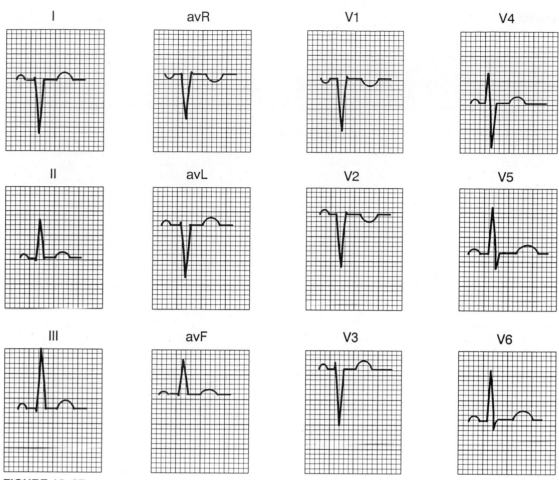

FIGURE 16–27: Left posterior hemiblock.

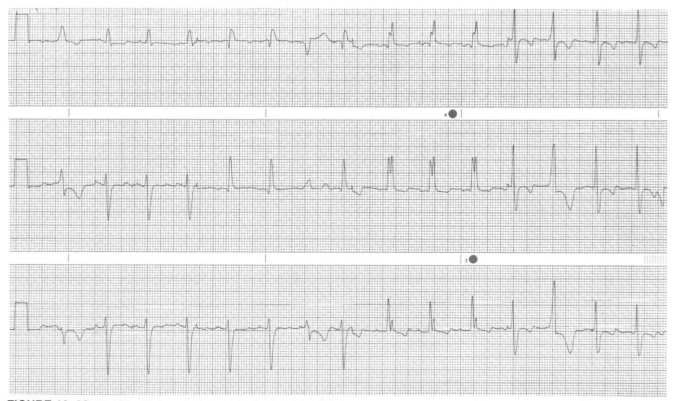

FIGURE 16–28: Right bundle branch block and left anterior hemiblock.

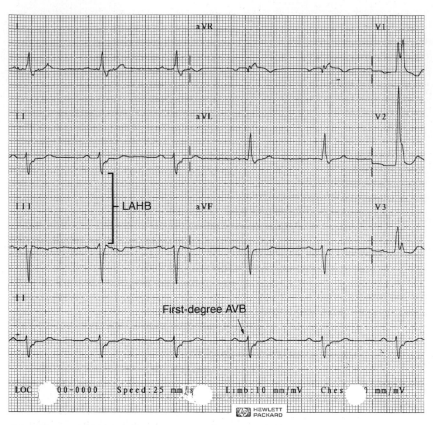

FIGURE 16–29: Trifascicular block. LAHB, left anterior hemiblock; AVB, atrioventricular block.

heart block. Therefore, the presence of AV conduction with trifascicular block implies that one or more of the fascicles have a relative degree of incomplete block, allowing impulse transmission between the atria and the ventricles.

EXTRASYSTOLES

Extrasystoles are beats created by an impulse formed at a region or focus of the heart other than the sinus node (i.e., an ectopic focus) that appear earlier than expected. These premature complexes may originate in the atrium (premature atrial complexes [PACs]), in the AV node or junction (premature junctional complexes), or in the ventricle (premature ventricular complexes [PVCs]).

Premature Atrial Complexes

Premature atrial complex (PAC) characteristics include the presence of an early or a premature ectopic P wave (P′), a QRS morphology unchanged from the predominant sinus rhythm, and a post-PAC pause allowing sinus rhythm recovery (Fig. 16–30). Ectopic atrial foci may fire in a bigeminal or trigeminal pattern similar to the ventricular mechanisms described below.

Nonconducted PACs are occasionally seen (i.e., a P′ wave without an associated QRS). This occurs when the PAC falls very early after the preceding sinus complex, in the AV nodal refractory period. Its conduction to the ventricles is blocked at the AV node.

Extrasystoles, whether atrial or ventricular, may lead patients to experience a sensation of "skipped" or "extra" beats.

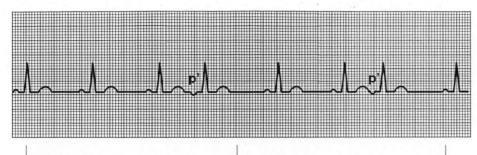

FIGURE 16–30: Rhythm strip with premature atrial contractions.

Premature Ventricular Complexes

A PVC is recognized as a wide (greater than 0.12 second) and bizarre QRS complex with a T wave axis opposite the main QRS axis. There are no preceding P waves associated with the QRS complex, but there may occasionally be P waves (P′) that closely follow the QRS because of "retrograde" or ventriculoatrial conduction. Retrograde conduction occurs when the initial impulse generated in the ventricle is conducted backward up the His-Purkinje conduction system and through the AV node to the atrium, thereby generating a retrograde P wave.

PVCs are most often followed by a "compensatory pause": that is, a pause following the extrasystole that compensates for the extrasystolic early firing and allows the sinus node to reset (Fig. 16–31). Occasionally, PVCs have no compensatory pauses and are "interpolated" between consecutive complexes. The dominant rhythm is unaltered by the "extra" beat (interpolated PVC).

If PVCs have different morphologies in a given ECG lead (i.e., varied shapes or forms), they are described as "multifocal" or "multiform" premature complexes (Fig. 16–32). The changing morphology may be due to either different impulse-initiating foci or the same focal impulse taking alternate myocardial conduction pathways.

Ventricular extrasystoles (ES) as well as atrial extrasystoles, may demonstrate self-perpetuating repetitive bigeminal (P-QRS:ES, P-QRS:ES) (Fig. 16–33A), trigeminal (P-QRS, P-QRS:ES; P-QRS, P-QRS:ES) (see Fig. 16–33B), or even quadrigeminal (P-QRS, P-QRS, P-QRS:ES; P-QRS, P-QRS, P-QRS:ES) patterns. It is generally agreed that ventricular bi- or trigeminy, and uniform or multiform PVCs (even frequent PVCs) in the "normal" heart are benign, even if they are symptomatic (felt by the patient). Therapy would be indicated only to control symptoms.

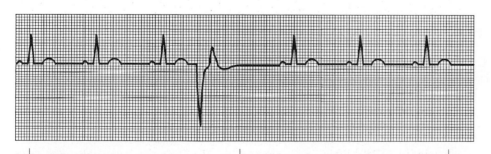

FIGURE 16–31: Premature ventricular contraction with compensatory pause.

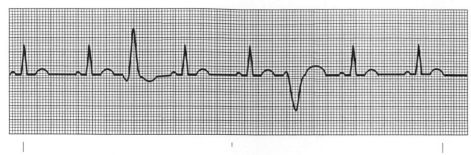

FIGURE 16–32: Multiform premature ventricular complexes.

Premature Junctional Complexes

Extrasystoles originating in the AV node region (or junction) generate QRS complexes similar to the predominant QRS complex because the impulse created in the AV node follows the normal anterograde conduction pathway to the ventricles. The impulse is also conducted in a retrograde manner to the atrium, creating "inverted" P′ waves, as compared with normal P waves (Fig. 16–34).

SUPRAVENTRICULAR TACHYCARDIA

Clinically, a supraventricular tachycardia may be paroxysmal (occasional, with acute onset and offset), persistent (stubbornly recurring), or chronic (permanent).

Supraventricular tachycardia is a generic term grouping rapid heart rates (tachycardia) in which the originating impulse begins above the ventricles. This group may be subdivided into various classifications and diagnoses regarding the site or focus of initiation (sinoatrial node, atrium, AV node, AV node bypass tract, or accessory pathway [Wolff-Parkinson-White syndrome]) or the mechanism of initiation and perpetuation of a tachycardia (reentry or automatic).

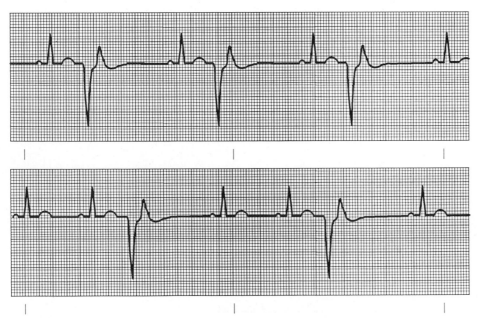

FIGURE 16–33: *A,* Ventricular bigeminy. *B,* Ventricular trigeminy.

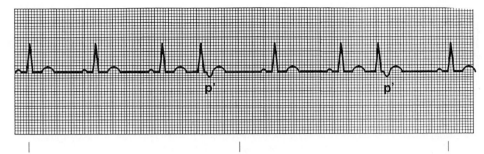

FIGURE 16–34: Junctional extrasystolic beats with retrograde P waves.

Atrial Flutter

Atrial flutter has a characteristic "sawtooth" or "picket fence" baseline pattern caused by rapid P′ flutter waves ("F waves"), best seen in leads II, III, and aVF on the ECG (Fig. 16–35). The baseline is rarely isoelectric or level between atrial complexes in these leads, in contrast to an atrial or sinus tachycardia. Lead V_1 usually reveals discrete positive F waves, which frequently confirm the diagnosis. Negative F waves may often be seen in V_5 and V_6.

The F wave rate can vary from approximately 240 to 370 beats per minute and more, but it is usually closer to a rate of 300 beats per minute. The most common AV conduction ratio is 2:1, with two P′ flutter waves to one ventricular complex. This is due to the normal properties of the AV node, which acts as a conduction rate–limiting "filter." AV conduction ratios can vary from moment to moment in the same patient. Ratios of 3:1, 4:1, and higher are seen in patients with AV node conduction disease and those receiving medication that affects the atrial rate or controls the ventricular response rate (e.g., digoxin). A 1:1 ratio is extremely rare and potentially life threatening because of the rapid ventricular response rate.

> Atrial flutter, although infrequent in the adult, can be precipitated by almost any form of heart disease, especially ischemic heart disease.

Atrial Fibrillation

The atrial fibrillatory wave ("f wave") baseline can vary from a very "coarse" to a very "fine" appearance and is best seen in leads II and V_1. When one is confronted with a very fine or an almost flat baseline, the diagnosis of atrial fibrillation depends on recognizing an irregularly irregular ventricular response rate.

A normal AV node can conduct atrial fibrillatory impulses at rates of up to 200 per minute. A diseased AV node or the use of digitalis,

> An irregular wavy baseline with no evidence of P waves and an "irregularly irregular" ventricular rhythm (Fig. 16–36) is diagnostic of atrial fibrillation.

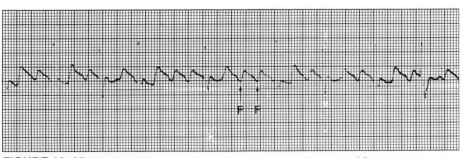

FIGURE 16–35: Rhythm strip of atrial flutter. Note the sawtooth pattern of flutter waves.

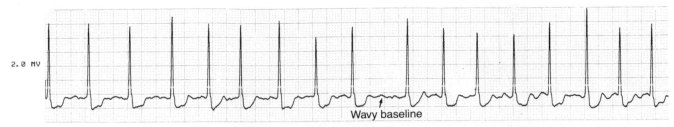

FIGURE 16–36: Rhythm strip of atrial flutter. Note the wavy, wandering baseline with no discernible P waves and the "irregularly irregular" ventricular response.

calcium, or beta-blockade will limit the maximal ventricular response rate. Atrial fibrillation is often associated with mitral valve disease, ischemic myocardial disease, hypertension or hyperthyroidism, pericarditis (especially after cardiac surgery), and acute and chronic cardiomyopathies.[9]

Atrial Tachycardia

Atrial tachycardia is a distinct ectopic atrial rhythm between 100 and 250 beats per minute that returns to baseline between P′ waves. The P′ wave morphology is usually different from that of the underlying sinus P waves; however, they can seem identical (Fig. 16–37). AV conduction can be 1:1, 2:1, or more, depending on the conduction properties of the AV node.

Multiform or multifocal atrial tachycardia is an atrial tachycardia of between 100 and 130 beats per minute (Fig. 16–38) that has at least three P wave morphologies (multiple ectopic foci) and varying PR intervals. The varying P wave morphologies depend on the different atrial ectopic foci that are firing independently of the sinus node. The varying PR intervals relate to the distance of the ectopic atrial focus from the AV node. Multifocal atrial tachycardia is often seen in severe lung disease with right ventricular overload due to pulmonary hypertension.

VENTRICULAR TACHYCARDIA

Ventricular tachycardia is defined as three or more consecutive ventricular complexes occurring at rates of greater than 100 beats per minute.

PVCs generated by impulses originating in the ventricles can initiate sustained ventricular arrhythmias, provided that the proper cardiac substrate is present. The diagnosis of ventricular tachycardia stems from the recognition of three or more beats of a wide complex (ventricular QRS complexes of more than 0.14 second in duration) rhythm at a rate

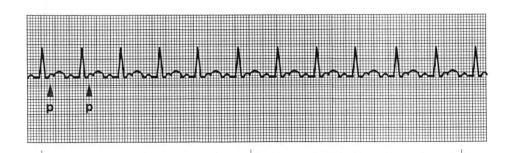

FIGURE 16–37: Atrial tachycardia.

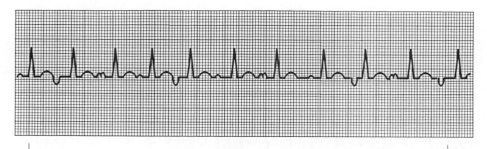

FIGURE 16–38: Multifocal atrial tachycardia. Note the differing P wave morphologies and PR intervals.

of greater than 100 beats per minute that is usually associated with a significant change in QRS morphology or axis shift (change in the QRS axis—often a left superior axis between −30 and −180 degrees) as compared with the baseline ECG (Fig. 16–39). It is usually a regular rhythm.

Three criteria, if present, help to confirm the diagnosis of ventricular tachycardia:

- First, there may be evidence of ventriculoatrial dissociation (ventricular complexes totally independent from atrial complexes). P waves may be seen to occur regularly during the tachycardia, but at different intervals from the QRS complexes, sometimes deforming the appearance of the QRS complexes themselves (Fig. 16–40A).
- Second, capture beats may occur, appearing as a QRS complex with

I

V1

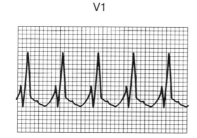

avF

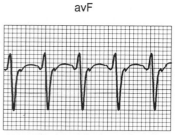

FIGURE 16–39: Ventricular tachycardia, shown in leads I, aVF, and V₁. The tachycardia rate is 185 beats per minute. Note the right bundle branch block and the left superior axis configuration.

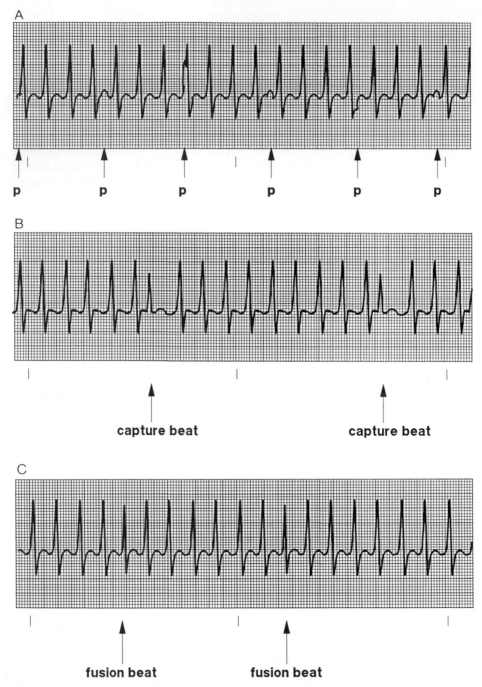

FIGURE 16–40: *A*, Ventricular tachycardia with atrioventricular dissociation, as evidenced by the P waves "marching through" the tachycardia. *B*, Ventricular tachycardia with occasional "capture" beats. *C*, Ventricular tachycardia with "fusion" beats.

the same morphology as the patient's complex during sinus rhythm (see Fig. 16–40*B*). These are caused by a P wave that is transmitted through the AV node and "captures" the ventricles for one beat during the tachycardia.

• Third, fusion complexes causing QRS morphology variation may be seen (see Fig. 16–40*C*). This is due to partial capture of the ventricular myocardium by a transmitted P wave, with the rest of the ventricles being depolarized by the ventricular tachycardia.

Although these criteria, if present, are useful to confirm the diagnosis of ventricular tachycardia, their absence does not imply that a fast, wide-complex rhythm is not ventricular tachycardia. Indeed, any wide-complex tachycardia should be considered to be ventricular tachycardia unless proved otherwise.[10]

Ventricular tachycardia can be nonsustained (three or more consecutive ventricular complexes lasting less than 30 seconds at rates of greater than 100 beats per minute) or sustained (lasting longer than 30 seconds).

Ischemic heart disease, especially after myocardial infarction with impaired left ventricular function or aneurysm, is the most frequent cause of ventricular tachycardia. Additional associations include cardiomyopathy, myocarditis, long QT syndrome, mitral valve prolapse, rheumatic heart disease, and metabolic or electrolyte abnormalities.

VENTRICULAR FIBRILLATION

Ventricular fibrillation is most often preceded by ventricular tachycardia. It can also be a primary event, especially during an acute myocardial infarction. The ECG characteristics include a completely irregular and chaotic wavy baseline on which there is no evidence of distinct ventricular or atrial complexes (Fig. 16–41).

ACCELERATED IDIOVENTRICULAR RHYTHM

The presence of three or more consecutive ventricular complexes at a regular rate of 50 to 100 beats per minute is termed an accelerated idioventricular rhythm. This rhythm is usually hemodynamically stable and has little tendency to evolve to a malignant ventricular arrhythmia. It usually requires no treatment.

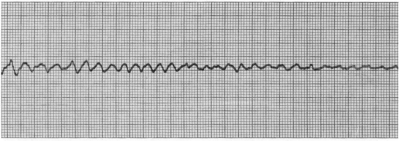

FIGURE 16–41: Rhythm strip of ventricular fibrillation. Note the irregular, wavy baseline with no evidence of synchronized ventricular activity (no QRS complexes).

PRE-EXCITATION

Approximately two in 1000 persons are born with an abnormal bridge of muscle tissue that crosses from the left or the right atrium to the corresponding ventricle. This congenital abnormality, termed an accessory pathway or a bypass tract, can conduct impulses from the atria to the ventricles independently of the normal conduction system of the heart. The direct activation of ventricular myocardium by a conduction pathway other than the normal AV node–His-Purkinje conduction system is termed pre-excitation.[11]

The Wolff-Parkinson-White syndrome is the most frequent example of pre-excitation. Its characteristics include a short PR interval (less than 0.12 second) with a slurred QRS onset or "delta wave," which often causes a widening of the overall QRS duration (greater than 0.12 second) (Fig. 16–42). The short PR interval results from rapid AV conduction down the accessory pathway (bypassing the slower AV node). The delta wave and increased QRS duration are due to ventricular activation by the slow intramyocardial conduction at the ventricular insertion site of the accessory pathway, bypassing the more rapid His-Purkinje system that sequentially activates the ventricles.

Wolff-Parkinson-White syndrome can be complicated by atrial fibrillation with very rapid conduction rates down the accessory pathway (ventricular response rates can exceed 250 beats per minute). These rates can cause profound hypotension, syncope, and sudden cardiac death because ventricular fibrillation can be induced by very rapid ventricular response rates during atrial fibrillation.

ECTOPIC SUPRAVENTRICULAR RHYTHMS

Supraventricular rhythms, originating from an ectopic atrial or junctional (AV node region) focus, can assume a cardiac "pacemaker" role by firing faster (an abnormally accelerated intrinsic rate) than the normal sinus node ("overdrive" suppression of the sinus node) or by intrinsically

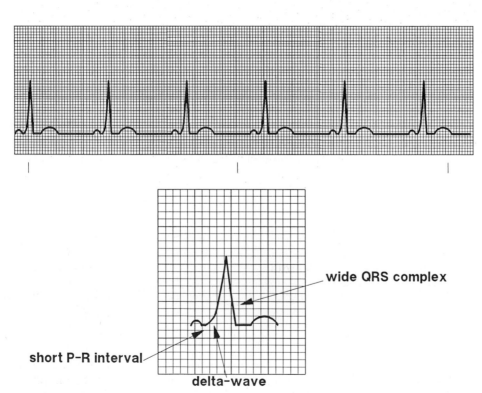

wide QRS complex

short P–R interval

delta-wave

FIGURE 16–42: Rhythm strip of Wolff-Parkinson-White syndrome and schematic of the QRS complex found in this disease.

generating impulses (normal intrinsic rate) that are faster than the abnormally slow firing sinus node.

Junctional Rhythm

AV node tissue properties allow the AV node to generate impulses at an intrinsic rate of between 45 and 60 beats per minute. The characteristics of these junctional complexes have been described previously (premature junctional complexes). A junctional rhythm may appear as a secondary or backup ("escape") rhythm when the sinus rate is slow or absent (e.g., in sinus bradycardia, sinus arrest, or sinoatrial block).

Accelerated Junctional Rhythm

Junctional rhythm rates that fall between 60 and 100 beats per minute are referred to as accelerated junctional rhythms. When the junctional rate exceeds the sinus rate, the QRS rate appears different and independent from the P wave rate (i.e., AV dissociation).

Wandering Pacemaker

When two or more P′ wave morphologies with respective varying PR intervals have similar rates (competing supraventricular rhythms), the diagnosis of a "wandering pacemaker" is made. The rhythms are usually of both sinus and junctional etiologies.

Ectopic Atrial Rhythms

An atrial rhythm with a different P′ wave morphology, as compared with the sinus-generated P wave, at rates of between 60 and 100 beats per minute falls into the category of ectopic atrial rhythms. P′ waves may be from a low atrial focus (inverted P′ waves [II, III, aVF, V_5, and V_6] due to a retrograde atrial activation pattern) or a mid or high atrial ectopic site with varying P′ wave morphologies.

SINUS-RELATED ARRHYTHMIA

Sinus Tachycardia

The normal sinus node generates a heart rate from 60 to 100 beats per minute. Sinus tachycardia usually occurs in reaction to an underlying physiologic or pathologic process: it is not a primary event.

Sinus Bradycardia

Sinus rhythm at a rate of less than 60 beats per minute is termed sinus bradycardia (Fig. 16–44). Sinus bradycardia may result from physiologic influences (e.g., sleep, vagal responses, or athletic training), underlying noncardiac disease, myocardial infarction, medication use, or primary sinus node disease (e.g., sick sinus syndrome).

Sinus tachycardia is defined as a sinus node–generated rate of between 100 and 180 beats per minute (Fig. 16–43).

Causes of sinus tachycardia:

- Emotion
- Exercise
- Pain
- Infection
- Fever
- Hyperthyroidism
- Volume depletion (severe bleeding or dehydration)
- Myocardial ischemia or infarction
- Medication use

Sinus bradycardia is defined as a sinus rhythm of less than 60 beats per minute.

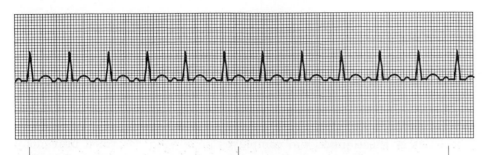

FIGURE 16–43: Rhythm strip of sinus tachycardia at a rate of 107 beats per minute.

Sinus Arrhythmia

Irregularity of the sinus rhythm is referred to as sinus arrhythmia.

Sinus arrhythmia is more pronounced in the younger population, especially during respiration. This finding is considered normal regardless of patient age.

Sinoatrial Block

Periodic dropped P waves should raise a suspicion of sinoatrial (SA) block, partial SA block, sinus pause, or sinus arrest (complete SA block). Partial SA block is present when the PP interval containing the intermittently dropped P wave or waves is a multiple of the shorter PP intervals (Fig. 16–45A). Sinus pause refers to intervals of dropped P waves that are not even multiples of the shorter baseline PP intervals (see Fig. 16–45B). These phenomena occur when some of the sinus node impulses are unable to exit the perinodal tissue (blocked in the perinodal tissue) and are not conducted to the atrial myocardium. Sinus arrest or complete SA block occurs when all sinus node impulses are blocked in the perinodal tissue, which results in atrial asystole (no P waves). The patient is then dependent on either a junctional or a ventricular escape rhythm (secondary or backup rhythm) to take over. Increased vagal tone, coronary artery disease, and medication use can induce SA block.

Sick Sinus Syndrome

Although sick sinus syndrome can refer to significant sinus bradycardia, sinus arrest, and SA block, it also includes the "tachycardia-bradycardia" syndrome. This syndrome comprises episodes of rapid atrial rhythms (commonly atrial fibrillation) alternating with episodes of slow

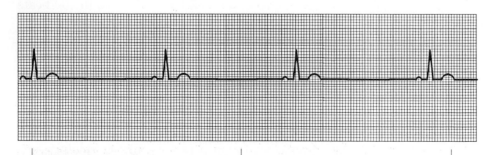

FIGURE 16–44: Sinus bradycardia at a rate of 26 beats per minute.

A

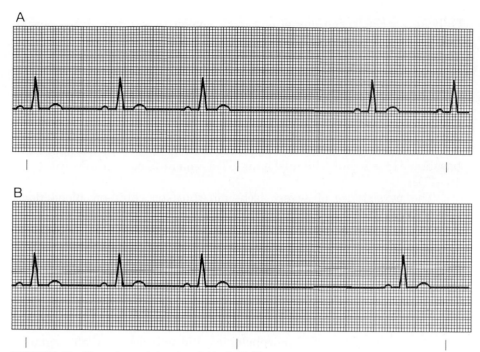

B

FIGURE 16–45: *A*, Sinoatrial node exit block. *B*, Sinus pause.

atrial rhythms. Sick sinus syndrome is more frequent in the elderly population, but it may affect patients of any age.[12]

MYOCARDIAL ISCHEMIA AND INFARCTION

Myocardial ischemia results from a critical reduction in coronary blood flow that induces hypoxia of the myocardial tissue. Myocardial infarction is due to either a total or a near-total blockage of coronary blood flow that causes myocardial tissue death. Ischemia can be transient, causing no tissue death, or severe and of long duration, leading to infarction.

Myocardial Ischemia

The ECG signature of myocardial ischemia ("ischemic pattern") includes ST segment depression below the baseline TP segment (horizontal or downward sloping), often associated with T wave inversion (Fig. 16–46). T wave inversions may occasionally be the only sign of ischemia.

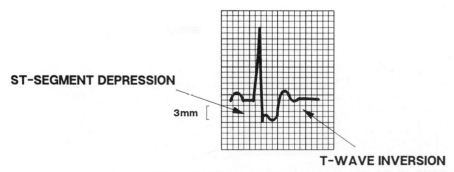

ST-SEGMENT DEPRESSION

3mm

T-WAVE INVERSION

FIGURE 16–46: ST segment depression and an inverted T wave are the hallmarks of myocardial ischemia.

Only in special situations of coronary spasm (variant or Prinzmetal's angina) will ischemia induce ST segment elevation and not depression. This is the exception, not the rule.

Myocardial Infarction

An acute myocardial infarction in early evolution is recognized by an "injury pattern," seen initially as an ST segment elevation above the baseline TP segment (the upsloping ST segment is convex upward) (Fig. 16–47).

The persistence of severe ischemia (blocked coronary blood flow) causes tissue damage or infarction. The QRS complex changes, becoming inverted and developing an initial Q wave. The Q wave or QS pattern can develop early or take up to several days to manifest. The presence of a QS or a Q wave ("Q wave myocardial infarction") denotes permanent myocardial tissue death, necrosis, or scarring. The ECG of an old Q wave myocardial infarction will have a permanent residual Q or QS pattern. Q waves must be greater than or equal to 0.03 second wide to meet infarction criteria. The injury pattern, however, will progressively revert back to the baseline ST-T morphologies and polarity. The ST segment often returns to baseline after several hours or days; however, T wave changes can persist up to several weeks.

The various ECG patterns described help to determine the size or localization of myocardial ischemia, infarction, or scar of the left ventricle (anterior, inferior, lateral, or posterior walls).

Because of the overwhelming left ventricular mass and the resulting contribution to the QRS complex, only ischemia or infarction of the left ventricle is easily identified on the standard 12-lead ECG. Other techniques are required to recognize atrial or right ventricular infarction.

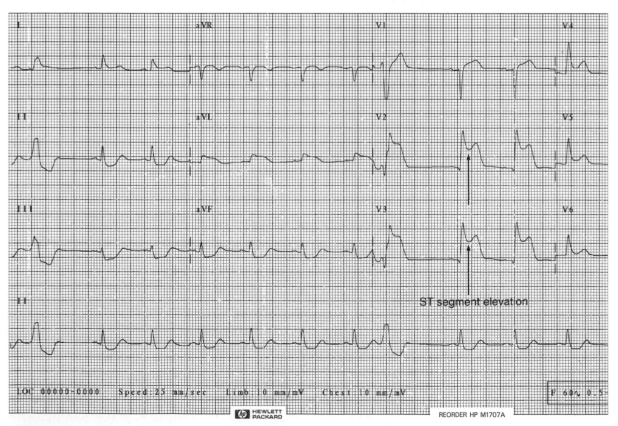

FIGURE 16–47: ECG of an acute anterior wall myocardial infarction.

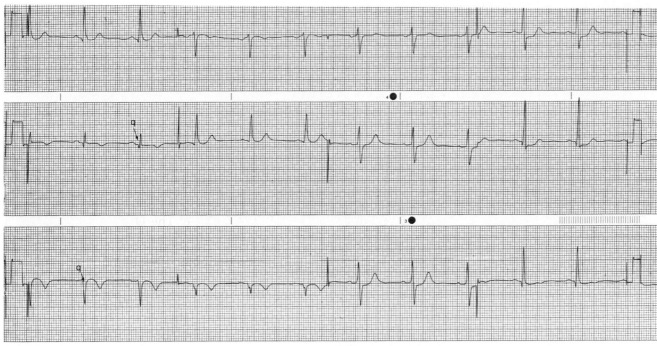

FIGURE 16–48: ECG of a chronic, old inferior wall myocardial infarction.

Ischemia, injury, or infarction patterns in leads II, III, and aVF signal the presence of inferior wall ischemia or infarction (Fig. 16–48). An anteroseptal wall myocardial infarction would be seen in leads V_1, V_2, V_3, and V_4. An anterior wall myocardial infarction affects leads V_1 through V_6. An infarction pattern in leads I, aVL, and V_1 through V_6 is described as an anterolateral wall myocardial infarction. A lateral wall myocardial infarction is noted in leads I, aVL, V_5, and V_6, and a high lateral wall myocardial infarction is noted in only leads I and aVL. Infarctions involving the posterior wall (true posterior wall myocardial infarction) are the most difficult to recognize. One sees a "mirror image" pattern of infarction in lead V_1 (i.e., an R or Rs pattern commonly associated with an ST segment depression and an upright T wave). Posterior wall myocardial infarctions are most frequently associated with inferior wall myocardial infarctions—rarely are they isolated.

Myocardial infarctions without evidence of Q waves are described as non–Q wave myocardial infarctions. Persistent ST segment depression or inverted T waves are often the only markers of infarction in this subset of patients. This arbitrary classification of Q wave versus non–Q wave myocardial infarction aids in the identification, risk stratification, and treatment of patients who have had myocardial infarction.[13]

SUMMARY

The heart generates an electrical signal with each heartbeat. By measuring this electrical signal from different areas of the body and recording the results on paper, one can construct an ECG that has recognizable characteristics. The ECG acts as a window into the electrical activity of the heart. If one understands the characteristics of the normal ECG, many diseases of the heart may be diagnosed by evaluating of an abnormal ECG. Diseases that may be diagnosed include myocardial infarction (heart attack), arrhythmia (irregular heartbeat), and ischemia (ongoing obstruction of blood flow to the heart muscle). In this chapter, the electrical activity of the heart is presented conceptually, from the single heart cell to the whole heart, and many abnormal ECGs are shown to help diagnose specific heart disease entities.

References

1. Hiss RG, Lamb LE. Electrocardiographic findings in 122,043 individuals. Circulation 25:947, 1962.
2. Marriot HJL. Practical Electrocardiography, 7th ed. Baltimore, Williams & Wilkins, 1983.
3. Jackman WM, Friday KL, Anderson JL, et al. The long Q-T syndromes: A critical review, new clinical observations and a unifying hypothesis. Prog Cardiovasc Dis 31:115, 1988.
4. Surawicz B. Electrocardiographic diagnosis of chamber enlargement. J Am Coll Cardiol 8:714, 1986.
5. Scott RC. Ventricular hypertrophy. Cardiovasc Clin 5(3):220, 1973.
6. Chou TC. Electrocardiography in Clinical Practice, 2nd ed. Orlando, FL, Grune & Stratton, 1986.
7. Friedman HS, Gomes JAC, Haft JI. An analysis of Wenckebach periodicity. J Electrocardiol 8:307, 1975.
8. Fisch C. Electrocardiography of Arrhythmias. Philadelphia, Lea & Febiger, 1989.
9. Zipes DP, Jalife J (eds). Cardiac Electrophysiology: From Cell to Bedside. Philadelphia, WB Saunders, 1990.
10. Josephson ME, Almendral JM, Buxton AE, et al. Mechanisms of ventricular tachycardia. Circulation 75:41, 1987.
11. Prystowsky EN. Diagnosis and management of the preexcitation syndromes. Curr Probl Cardiol 13:227, 1988.
12. Bigger JT, Reiffel JA. Sick sinus syndrome. Annu Rev Med 30:91, 1979.
13. Klein LW, Helfant RH. The Q-wave and non-Q-wave myocardial infarction: Differences and similarities. Prog Cardiovasc Dis 29:205, 1986.

17 Pulmonary Function Testing

Jane Luchsinger, M.S., R.P.F.T., and
Harry Steinberg, M.D.

Key Terms

Diffusing Capacity
Exercise Testing
Expiratory Flow Rates
Lung Volumes
Spirometry

Pulmonary function tests measure various properties of the lung, such as volume, elasticity, ventilation, and gas exchange. Testing procedures may be performed on a subject at rest, during exercise, or under specific controlled conditions. Pulmonary function tests generally provide quantitative information about the adverse effects of diseases on the lungs but usually do not yield a definitive pathologic diagnosis. However, combined with a clinical history, pulmonary function data can be useful

- To determine the existence of pulmonary abnormalities
- To quantitate the abnormalities
- To determine the efficacy of therapy
- To monitor disease progression
- For preoperative screening
- For employment screening
- For epidemiologic studies

Since the 1950s, pulmonary function testing technology has rapidly expanded. Labor-intensive studies have been replaced by computerized studies. In an effort to standardize both the equipment and the techniques, the American Thoracic Society (ATS) has set guidelines for pulmonary function testing, thus improving intra- and interlaboratory reproducibility.[1-3] Laboratory personnel qualifications, computer guidelines, and quality assurance standards have also been adopted through ATS position papers.[4-6]

The personnel carrying out the testing must be formally trained in the performance of these tests. Training may be acquired through higher education respiratory therapy programs. Certified programs or more comprehensive programs leading to an associate's or a bachelor's degree are available.

NORMAL VALUES

Studies of large groups of subjects have been performed in order to develop normal values for each of the pulmonary functions. These studies have shown that lung function varies with sex, age, race, height, and weight. These dependent variables have become part of regression equations used to predict values for normal lung function. Traditionally, the lower limits of normal values have been set as 80% of predicted values. This approach is somewhat controversial because it does not follow the standard statistical approach defining a 95% confidence level for normal values. The standard statistical approach assumes that normal subjects' lung functions fall within a bell-shaped curve. This information has generally not been provided by the large population studies that have been used to develop regression equations. At this time, neither the traditional

315

80% lower-limit approach nor the standard statistical approach is best for defining what is normal or average for all lung function parameters.

Before a prediction equation is chosen for a particular laboratory, it is recommended that

1. The testing method used to determine predicted values closely resemble the laboratory's methods
2. The patient populations be similar
3. The tests first be performed on a representative sample of a normal population (10 to 20 samples)
4. If more than 30% of the laboratory's normals fall outside of the normal range of the chosen equation, the equations, the testing protocol, or both be reviewed and the tests repeated
5. If once again 30% of the normals fall outside of range, the process be repeated using other equations[7]

LUNG VOLUMES

Definitions

The volume of gas in the lungs is subdivided into compartments (Fig. 17–1). It is simplest to remember that a volume is one compartment of the lung, whereas lung capacities are more than one compartment.

All lung volumes are expressed at body conditions: body temperature, ambient pressure, and saturation with water vapor at these conditions (BTPS).

Lung Volumes

Tidal volume (V_T)—the volume of gas inhaled or exhaled during a resting normal breath.

Inspiratory reserve volume (IRV)—the maximal volume of gas that can be inspired from the end of a resting inspiration.

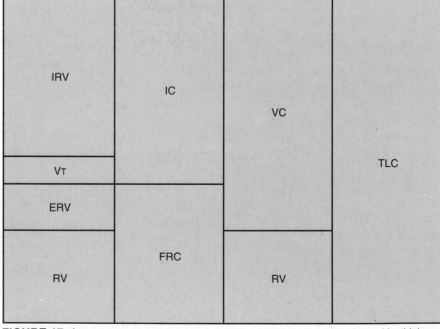

FIGURE 17–1: Lung volumes and capacities. IRV, inspiratory reserve volume; V_T, tidal volume; ERV, expiratory reserve volume; RV, residual volume; IC, inspiratory capacity; FRC, functional residual capacity; VC, vital capacity; TLC, total lung capacity.

Expiratory reserve volume (ERV)—the maximal volume of gas that can be expired at the end of a resting expiration.

Residual volume (RV)—the volume of gas remaining in the lungs after a maximal expiration.

Lung Capacities

Vital capacity (VC)—the maximal volume of gas that can be expelled from the lungs after a maximal inspiration. The VC includes the V_T, IRV, and ERV.

Inspiratory capacity (IC)—the maximal volume of gas that can be inspired from the end-tidal expiration. The IC includes the V_T and IRV.

Functional residual capacity (FRC)—the volume of gas remaining in the lungs at the end of a resting expiration. The FRC includes the RV and ERV.

Total lung capacity (TLC)—the volume of gas in the lungs at the end of a maximal inspiration. The TLC includes the V_T, IRV, ERV, and RV.

Methods of Measurement

Three methods exist to determine static lung volumes:

- Dilution techniques measure the volume of gases in the lung that communicate with the airways.
- Body plethysmography measures the volume of compressible gases within the thorax.
- Radiographic techniques mathematically measure the intrathoracic gas volume.

The last two methods measure both communicating and noncommunicating airspaces. Although there are other methods of measuring partial lung volume (i.e., spirometry), total lung volume may be measured only through one of the previously mentioned methods. In normal subjects, these volume measurement techniques yield similar results, but this may not be true for subjects with pulmonary disease. Therefore, the method of measurement should be considered in making clinical interpretations.

Dilution Techniques

Lung volume measurements are determined either by diluting the gas within the lung with a nonphysiologic (inert) reference gas or by eliminating a physiologic reference gas from the lungs. The former method uses helium as the tracer gas; the latter uses nitrogen. Both techniques utilize a principle of proportionality relating volume and gas concentrations.

Helium Equilibration

Spirometer—a device that measures the volume of gas inhaled or exhaled from the lungs

The helium equilibration method is a closed-circuit (sealed-system) measurement of the FRC. The subject begins the test at end-expiration and breathes from a volume of gas in a spirometer containing a known concentration of helium, oxygen, and air. A carbon dioxide absorber is placed in the breathing circuit, eliminating the rebreathing of carbon dioxide. Oxygen is titrated into the spirometer to maintain a constant volume as carbon dioxide is absorbed and oxygen is consumed by the patient. When the subject's lungs have reached a helium equilibration with the spirometer (concentration is the same), the FRC may be calculated from the following proportion. (Remember: concentration × volume = amount of gas.)

Pretest	Post-test
He sys + He L	= He sys + He L
$(C_1 \times V\ sys) + 0$	$= (C_2 \times V\ sys + (C_2 \times V_L)$
$\dfrac{C_1\ V\ sys - C_2\ V\ sys}{C_2}$	$= V_L$

where

He sys = amount of helium in the system
He L   = amount of helium in the lungs
C_1 = helium concentration of the system (pretest)
V sys   = volume of the system
C_2 = helium concentration of the system (post-test)
V_L = volume of the lung at FRC

The subject is asked to perform a slow VC maneuver while breathing on the closed circuit; the ERV may then be subtracted from the FRC, yielding the RV. The IC may be added to the FRC to determine the TLC.

Care must be taken during the testing procedure to have the subject use nose clips and to maintain a tight seal around the mouthpiece. If a leak occurs, equilibration will not be reached during the testing procedure.

Nitrogen Washout

The nitrogen washout technique of measuring lung volumes is an open-circuit method (exhalation to the room).

If the patient breathes 100% oxygen, nitrogen is washed out or removed from the lungs. The volume of exhaled gas is measured as the nitrogen is replaced by the oxygen. Because the nitrogen concentration of ambient air is approximately 80%, it is assumed that this same concentration exists in the lungs. The test begins at FRC and continues until the nitrogen concentration of the exhaled gas is below 1.0%. The volume and the nitrogen concentration of the exhaled gases are measured, and a proportion is made to calculate the FRC. After the subject performs a slow VC maneuver, all lung volumes may again be calculated.

As with the helium equilibration method of lung volume measurement, care must be taken to prevent leaks from the patient or the system.

Pretest	Post-test
$N_2 sys + N_2 L$	$= N_2 sys + N_2 L$
$0 + (80\% \ V_L)$	$= (5\% \times 60{,}000 \text{ mL}) + 0$
$0.8\ V_L$	$= 3000$
V_L	$= 3750 \text{ mL}$

where

$N_2 sys$ = amount of nitrogen in the system (nitrogen concentration × exhaled volume)
$N_2 L$ = amount of nitrogen in the lungs
V_L = volume of the lung at FRC
80%   = concentration of nitrogen in ambient air

Body Plethysmography

A body plethysmograph measures total compressible thoracic gas volume by employing a method of measurement using Boyle's law, which

Boyle's law states that at a constant temperature

$$Pressure_1 \times volume_1 = pressure_2 \times volume_2$$

defines the relationship between changes in gas pressure and volume. Thoracic gas volume measurement is obtained by having the subject sit in an airtight chamber resembling a telephone booth. Transducers measuring box pressure, mouth pressure, and flow at the mouth are components of the box assembly. While in the box, the subject breathes through a mouthpiece-shutter assembly. When the subject reaches end-expiration (FRC), the shutter is closed and an inspiratory effort is made. As the effort to inspire is made, the diaphragm descends and the chest expands, but no gas enters the lungs because the shutter to room air has been occluded. The result is that the gas that was in the lungs at end-exhalation decompresses, filling the expanded thoracic volume. Simultaneously, the gas in the box surrounding the subject is compressed because of the expansion of the subject's thorax. The pressure rise in the box is proportional to the volume change in the thorax and is electrically measured. The pressure at the mouth (which is equal to alveolar pressure) is measured simultaneously. At end-expiration or FRC, no gas flows in or out of the lungs. Therefore, no pressure gradient exists between the lungs and the atmosphere, and alveolar pressure equals ambient pressure. Measurements are made while the subject pants at FRC:

Shutter Open		Shutter Closed
$P \times V$	$=$	$P_1 \times V_1$

where

P = alveolar pressure, which is equal to ambient pressure at FRC
V = unknown thoracic volume
P_1 = mouth pressure, which is equal to alveolar pressure when the shutter is closed
V_1 = unknown thoracic volume + thoracic volume change[8]

Radiographic Techniques

Two common radiographic measurement techniques are the planimetry method described by Harris and coworkers[9] and the ellipsoid method described by Barnhard and associates.[10] Both methods use frontal and lateral chest radiographs taken at maximal inspiration. Measured sections are summed, and TLC is calculated.

Radiographic measurement techniques are time consuming and are therefore rarely used. They may provide retrospective information in the absence of prior pulmonary function tests.

Interpretation

The measurement of lung volumes results in three patterns: restrictive, obstructive, and normal (Fig. 17–2). A restrictive pattern indicates a reduction in lung volumes. Conditions leading to restrictive patterns include

- Decreased chest wall compliance, such as in kyphoscoliosis or obesity
- Respiratory muscle weakness, such as in myasthenia gravis or neuromuscular disease
- Increased lung recoil (increased transpulmonary pressure), such as in interstitial pulmonary fibrosis
- Space-occupying abnormalities, such as pneumonia or tumor

An obstructive pattern indicates an increase in lung volumes. Conditions leading to this pattern include

The RV should occupy approximately 30% of the normal TLC. Hyperinflation is present when the RV/TLC ratio exceeds 30%.

- Increased airway resistance, such as in chronic bronchitis

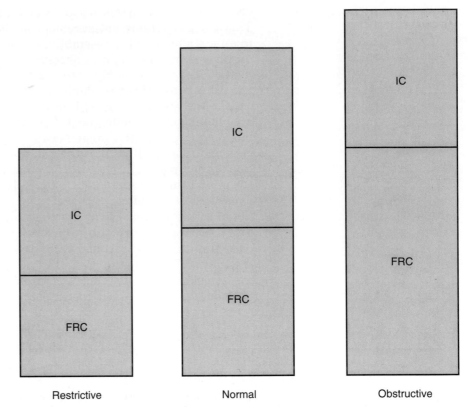

Restrictive   Normal   Obstructive

FIGURE 17–2: Patterns of lung volumes. IC, inspiratory capacity; FRC, functional residual capacity.

- Decreased lung recoil or increased lung compliance, such as in emphysema

In severely obstructed lung disease or bullous emphysema, lung volumes measured by plethysmography may exceed those measured by dilution techniques because plethysmography can detect noncommunicating airspaces.

EXPIRATORY FLOW RATES

Definitions

A rapid assessment of lung function achieved by measuring exhaled volume and flow rates can be accomplished with spirograms and flow-volume loops. Both airflow and forced vital capacity (FVC) are measured with one breath. Current technology permits testing to be performed in a laboratory, at the bedside, in the physician's office, or in the field for epidemiologic studies. Volume displacement devices, spirometers (wedge, bellows, bell, dry rolling seal), or flow-sensing devices (pneumotachometer) are used to obtain data.

Methods of Measurement

Spirometry

During spirometry, the subject is instructed to breathe normally into a spirometer or through a pneumotachometer, then to inhale quickly to

Three acceptable, reproducible maneuvers should be performed for valid testing.[1]

TLC, and immediately thereafter to perform a rapid and complete forced exhalation (FVC). On the spirogram (Fig. 17–3), time is plotted on the abscissa and volume on the ordinate.

Measurements obtained from spirometry include both volume and flow rate measurements. Lung volumes measured by spirometry include V_T, IC, ERV, and FVC.

The forced exhaled volume in a specified unit of time is also measured (FEV_t). The FEV_1 is the volume of gas forcefully expelled from the lungs in 1 second. Before the FEV_t is measured, the start of the test or "time zero" must be determined.[1]

Mean flow rates over volume segments are calculated from spirograms. The initial flow rate is expressed by determining the mean forced expired flow (FEF) over the exhaled volume from the first 200 to 1200 mL of the FVC ($FEF_{200-1200mL}$). The mean flow rate over the midportion of the FVC is referred to as the $FEF_{25-75\%}$. Both flow rates are determined by calculating a "best-fit" line between points of the FVC. All volumes and flow rates are expressed in BTPS.

Flow-Volume Loops

The flow-volume loop plots volume on the abscissa and integrates the volume with time to determine flow rate, which is then plotted on the ordinate (Fig. 17–4). The x-axis represents zero flow. By convention, flow rates above the x-axis represent expiratory flow rates, whereas points below represent inspiratory flow rates. Maximal flow rates are

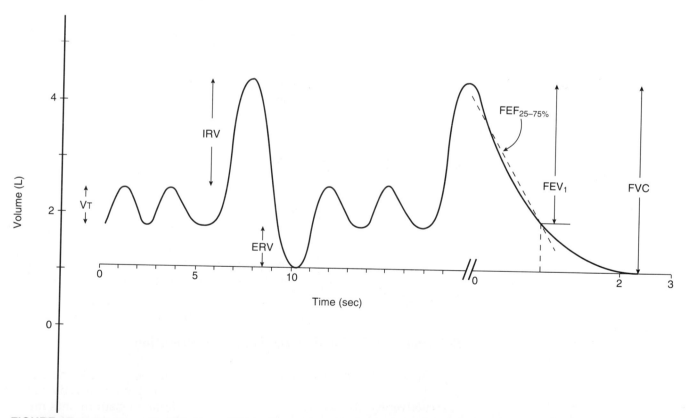

FIGURE 17–3: Spirogram. V_T, tidal volume; IRV, inspiratory reserve volume; ERV, expiratory reserve volume; FVC, forced vital capacity; FEV_1, volume expired in 1 second; $FEF_{25-75\%}$, mean flow rate (midportion of FVC).

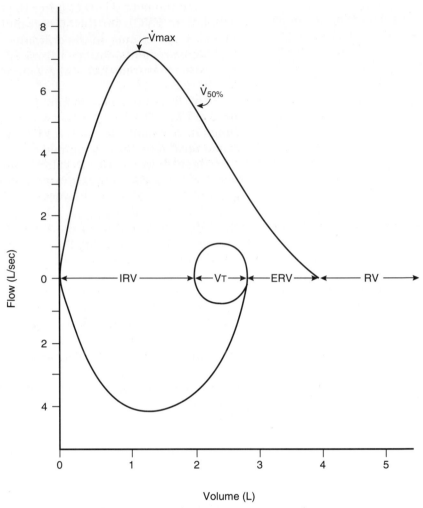

FIGURE 17–4: Flow-volume loop. $\dot{V}max$, maximal flow rate; $\dot{V}_{50\%}$, flow rate at 50% of the forced vital capacity; IRV, inspiratory reserve volume; V_T, tidal volume; ERV, expiratory reserve volume; RV, residual volume.

easily determined at any given volume. All values are expressed in BTPS.

Maximal Voluntary Ventilation

The maximal voluntary ventilation is the maximal volume of gas that can be inspired and expired in a given period. The subject is instructed to take deep, fast breaths for 12 to 15 seconds. The measured exhaled volume is extrapolated to the volume (in liters) exhaled in 1 minute (BTPS).

Spirometry and Flow-Volume Loop Interpretation

VC, as with all lung volumes, depends on the height, age, race, and sex of the subject. The FVC may be reduced in both restrictive and obstructive ventilatory patterns. Total lung volume measurements must be made to determine the pattern of lung function responsible for a reduced FVC. In patients with obstructive lung disease, the FVC may be

An FEV$_1$/FVC ratio lower than 75 may be indicative of an obstructive pattern, whereas an FEV$_1$/FVC ratio of greater than 80 indicates an absence of airway obstruction. (This value is actually age related.)

less than the slow VC owing to airway collapse as a result of increased intrathoracic pressures generated during the forced exhalation maneuver. The ratio of the FEV$_1$ to the FVC (FEV$_1$/FVC) is often viewed as a delineation of restrictive versus obstructive ventilatory patterns.

Flow is directly proportional to driving pressure and inversely proportional to resistance ($\dot{V}$ = P/R). The driving pressure for exhaled gas from the lungs is generated by the lung recoil pressure. The resistance to airflow is airway resistance. The exhaled flow rate during approximately the initial 60% of a FVC maneuver is subject to patient effort, whereas the remaining portion is independent of effort and is related directly to lung airway resistance and recoil pressure. This is evident when FVC maneuvers performed at varying efforts are superimposed. Inspiratory flow rates, however, depend on patient effort at all lung volumes.

Expiratory flow rates are reduced in obstructive lung diseases such as asthma, chronic bronchitis, and emphysema. The reduction in flow rates may be due to increased airway resistance (as a result of bronchospasm, airway edema, or increased mucus production) or to reduced recoil pressure (as a result of parenchymal lung destruction). Sometimes, in asthma, there is an increase in recoil pressure, but because resistance increases to a greater extent, expiratory flow rates fall. Obstructive patterns are also frequently detected in patients with cystic fibrosis, bronchiolitis, and bronchiectasis. The severity of obstruction is frequently assessed as "mild," "moderate," or "severe." These terms may vary between laboratories. The reader is referred to a review citing different interpretative strategies.[3]

Assessment of Airway Reactivity

Bronchodilator Therapy

The expiratory flow rates in patients with asthma commonly improve after bronchodilator medication. To assess the efficacy of bronchodilator medication, airflow measurements are made before and after bronchodilator administration. A positive bronchodilator response is considered significant when the FEV$_1$ increases by at least 200 mL or 12 to 15% of the predilator study. A negative response to bronchodilator medication does not preclude the presence of bronchospasm or heightened airway reactivity.

Bronchial Provocation

Bronchial provocation studies are usually performed when bronchial hyperreactivity is suspected from the patient's history and reversibility of airflow obstruction has not been demonstrated with bronchodilator agents. The stimulants that have been used in the laboratory for bronchial provocation include histamine, methacholine, allergens, and subfrigid air.

Before a bronchial provocation test is started, baseline measurements of volume and flow rates are made (by spirometry or flow-volume loop). The provocation stimulus is then administered, after which retesting is done. Specific protocols are followed depending on the stimulus administered.[11-13] Spirometry or flow-volume loop measurements are made after administration of each dose. Bronchodilator therapy is always available before the commencement of testing procedures. If a response is elicited, reversal, if necessary, is achieved through the administration of bronchodilator.

Sources of Spirometry and Flow-Volume Loop Error or Artifact

Performance of spirometry or flow-volume loop measurements requires a cooperative patient capable of understanding and following instructions. Sometimes several trials are necessary before the subject is fully able to repeat the manuever. The ATS recommends that three reproducible tests be obtained before the results are considered to be acceptable.[1] To be acceptable, a test must

1. Have a good "start of test" (a minimal delay from the initiation of exhalation to peak expiratory flow—less than 5% FVC or 0.1 L) of exhalation
2. Be free of cough during the 1st second of the test
3. Be made while the glottis is open
4. Have complete expiration (at least 6 seconds)
5. Have no leakage
6. Have no obstruction of the mouthpiece (e.g., with the tongue or false teeth)

A common source of error is inadequate patient performance. Reproducibility is best assessed with the actual data rather than with a computer simulation. Personnel must be able to recognize an acceptable trial and be able to reinstruct the patient when unacceptable trials occur. Bronchodilator responses may result in false-negative test results if the bronchodilator was inhaled incorrectly (metered dose inhalers) or because of poorly functioning aerosol equipment.

> To be considered reproducible, the largest FVC and FEV_1 should not vary more than 5% or 0.1 L from the second largest values.

DIFFUSING CAPACITY

Definitions

The lungs' ability to transfer gas across the alveolar surface into the pulmonary capillary is customarily measured by the carbon monoxide diffusing capacity (DL_{CO}). CO is chosen as the reference gas because its properties of binding to hemoglobin resemble oxygen's. CO, however, has approximately 210 times the affinity for hemoglobin, thereby making it a diffusion-limited gas. Essentially, no CO exists in the mixed venous blood. These properties, therefore, make it possible to use very small amounts of CO (0.3%) for testing purposes. In the simplest terms, the diffusion properties of the lung are measured by knowing the amount of gas (CO) inspired, allowing time for diffusion (breath holding), and measuring the amount of gas (CO) exhaled.

> Diffusing capacity is a rate of gas transfer, and the units are mL CO (STPD)/min/mm Hg.

Methods of Measurement

The instrumentation required for testing purposes includes a CO and helium analyzer (helium is used to determine the alveolar volume and thus the initial dilution of CO in the FRC), a timer, inspiratory and expiratory gas sample bags, and a rapidly rotating valve facilitating inspiratory sampling and expiratory gas collection.

The single-breath technique, which is the most commonly used technique at this time, requires the subject to exhale to RV, then inhale test gas to TLC (the inhaled volume should equal at least 90% of the measured VC), perform a 10-second breath hold, and rapidly exhale. The first 750 to 1000 mL is discarded as dead space, followed by the collection of alveolar gas. The average of two acceptable trials should be reported. Calculations are made by using the following formula:[2]

$$D_{L_{CO}} = V_A \times (60/t) \times [1/(P_B - 47)] \times \ln (FA_{CO_0} / FA_{CO_t})$$

where

$$V_{A(STPD)} = V_{I(STPD)} \times (FI_{He} / FA_{He})$$

and where

$$FA_{CO_0} = FI_{CO} \times (FA_{He} / FI_{He})$$

Interpretation

The amount of gas transferred across a tissue is in part directly proportional to the tissue area and inversely proportional to the tissue thickness. Lung pathology resulting in either a decrease in tissue area or an increase in tissue thickness will therefore result in a reduced diffusion capacity.

Lung resection is an obvious cause of reduced tissue area. Tissue area is also reduced in emphysematous patients as a result of alveolar septal rupture and destruction of capillary beds. Because this destruction does not occur in asthma and chronic bronchitis, the $D_{L_{CO}}$ is often helpful in differentiating patients with obstructive patterns in lung function. Pulmonary vascular disease causes a reduction in the pulmonary capillary bed area, and a reduction in oxygen binding sites is present with anemia. Either of these conditions will result in a reduced diffusing capacity.

Few pathologic entities result in an increased $D_{L_{CO}}$. Occasionally, an increase may be observed in conditions resulting in an increased pulmonary blood volume, such as a left-to-right cardiac shunt. Polycythemia or alveolar hemorrhage may also contribute to an elevation in $D_{L_{CO}}$.[14]

DISTRIBUTION OF VENTILATION

Methods of Measurement

Single-Breath Nitrogen Test

The single-breath nitrogen test involves a maximal inspiration of 100% oxygen following expiration to RV. Because the distribution of ventilation varies within the lung and the initial portion of the inspiratory gas (nitrogen-containing dead space gas) will be distributed to the apex, many of the alveolar units at the lung bases are actually closed or flow limited at the onset of the breath. The remainder of the inspiratory gas, containing 100% oxygen, will go to the lung bases. A measurement of the nitrogen concentration during exhalation to RV preceded by a single breath of 100% oxygen results in a characteristic pattern related to the distribution of the inhaled oxygen.

As can be seen in Figure 17–5, phase I will contain no nitrogen because the first gas to be exhaled is from the anatomic dead space containing 100% oxygen. Phase II represents mixed gases (both gas from the dead space and alveolar gas), whereas phase III represents the alveolar plateau, only alveolar gas. As exhalation approaches RV, the basal units, richer in oxygen, begin once again to close, leaving the remainder of exhaled gas to come from the apical portion of the lung, the portion richer in nitrogen at the beginning of the testing procedure. Phase IV represents this rise in nitrogen concentration.

The single-breath nitrogen test must be performed at inspiratory and expiratory flow rates of less than 0.5 L/sec. The exhaled nitrogen concentration is plotted against volume. The mean value of three acceptable tracings is ideal.

Measurements derived from the single-breath nitrogen test include[15]

Closing volume—the volume of phase IV.
Closing capacity—the volume comprised of the closing volume plus the RV. This is usually expressed as a percentage of the TLC.
Slope of phase III—the best-fit line between 70% of the VC and the onset of phase IV, expressed as the percentage of nitrogen per liter. (The less acute the slope, the more uniform the distribution of ventilation.)

Multiple-Breath Tests

The time necessary to reach equilibration during the measurement of FRC using helium may be employed as a measure of the distribution of ventilation. For example, someone with obstructive lung disease will take longer to equilibrate because of areas of poor or low ventilation. Similarly, the time to exhale nitrogen from the lung during a multiple-breath nitrogen washout test may also be used as an indication of the distribution of ventilation. Although not strictly a pulmonary function

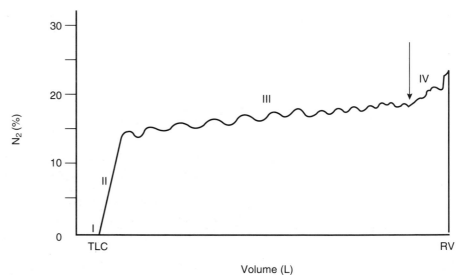

FIGURE 17–5: Single-breath nitrogen test. Phase I is dead space gas, phase II is mixed gas (dead space and alveolar), phase III is alveolar gas, and phase IV is closing volume. TLC, total lung capacity; RV, residual volume.

test, evaluation of the distribution of radioactive gases, such as xenon or krypton, can be used to assess regional ventilation.

Interpretation

When the single-breath nitrogen test is performed in combination with other pulmonary function tests, the results may confirm suspected abnormalities in the distribution of ventilation. An increased closing volume may be an early sign of obstructive disease appearing when other pulmonary function test results are normal.

CONTROL OF VENTILATION

Definitions

A host of physiologic processes must occur to complete even one ventilatory cycle of inspiration and expiration. Chemical receptors (central and peripheral) and mechanoreceptors (pressure and stretch) play a part in the regulation of breathing. Brain stem activities coordinated by these receptors respond by signaling efferent respiratory muscle contraction or relaxation. Abnormalities at any step in the cycle will affect the drive to ventilation.

Methods of Measurement

An overall assessment of ventilatory drive is accomplished by having the subject breathe either a hypercapnic or a hypoxic gas mixture while the minute ventilation response is measured. Abnormal results do not provide information about the location of the problem (e.g., the brain stem or phrenic nerves), but they alert the observer to the presence of an abnormality. Results must be interpreted with caution because an abnormality in lung function can also affect minute ventilation.

Another way to assess ventilatory drive is the $P_{0.1}$ test. The inspiratory pressure of an occluded airway is measured 0.1 second after the onset of inspiration. This measurement is thought to represent an estimate of central ventilatory drive.[16]

COMPLIANCE

Definitions

Compliance of the lung is defined as the change in lung volume for a change in transpulmonary pressure or elastic recoil pressure. Compliance measurements are used more commonly for research than as clinical tools. Compliance measurements answer the question What elastic recoil pressure must be overcome to inflate the lungs at a given volume?

Methods of Measurement

Elastic recoil pressure is approximated from esophageal pressure because the esophagus is

$$\text{Compliance} = \frac{\Delta V}{\Delta P}$$

where

V = volume
P = pleural pressure

- Subject to intrapleural pressure changes similar to those in the lung
- More accessible for testing purposes

Testing is accomplished by passing a balloon attached to a catheter through the nostril of the subject. The proximal end of the catheter is connected to a pressure transducer. Care is taken to position the balloon in the midportion of the esophagus. The balloon is then inflated to a point at which a transducer can detect changes in pleural pressure. As the subject breathes through a mouthpiece into a spirometer or pneumotachometer, simultaneous measurements of volume and pressure can be made and compliance can be calculated.

Interpretation

Compliance measurements are not performed routinely but may be useful in evaluating patients with suspected parenchymal disease. For example, reduced compliance measurements may be present in patients with interstitial lung disease, and increased compliance may be seen in patients with emphysema.

AIRWAY RESISTANCE

Definitions

Airway resistance (RAW) is a measurement of the opposing forces to airflow. Airway conductance (GAW) is the inverse of airway resistance. Total respiratory resistance equals the sum of airway resistance, tissue resistance, and chest wall resistance. Total respiratory resistance is difficult to measure, but it may be useful for diagnostic purposes to measure these components.

Methods of Measurement

Pulmonary resistance is the sum of airway resistance and tissue resistance. This is measured with the insertion of an esophageal balloon similar to that described in the compliance section. Pleural pressures are measured via the transducer; flows, via a spirometer or pneumotachometer. Pulmonary resistance may then be calculated ($R = P/\dot{V}$). Airway resistance alone may be measured with the plethysmograph, which permits measurement of flow and pressure simultaneously.

Interpretation

Airway resistance or conductance (1/RAW) measurements may aid in the diagnosis of obstructive airway disease and may be useful in determining the efficacy of responses to medication. In practice, however, these questions are frequently answered by spirometric measurement.

MAXIMAL INSPIRATORY AND EXPIRATORY PRESSURES

Definitions

Respiratory muscle strength may be assessed by measuring maximal inspiratory pressure (MIP) and maximal expiratory pressure (MEP).

Methods of Measurement

The method described by Black and Hyatt requires the subject to breathe through a tight-fitting mouthpiece attached to a cylinder.[17] Two manometers at the distal end of the cylinder measure negative inspiratory pressure and positive expiratory pressure. A small leak at the distal end of the cylinder prevents facial muscles from generating significant pressure, which may interfere with respiratory pressure measurements. With nose clips in place, the subject performs a maximal inspiration followed by a maximal expiration.

MIP is measured near RV, and MEP near TLC.

Interpretation

Expiratory pressures are necessary to generate a cough, and adequate inspiratory pressures are necessary for normal ventilation and maintenance of gas exchange. For these reasons, MIPs and MEPs are frequently used as weaning parameters for mechanically ventilated patients. Successful weaning requires respiratory muscle strength and may be assessed by these measurements.

Patients with neuromuscular disease also exhibit reduced MIPs and MEPs. Serial measurements may be performed to monitor the stage of the disease process or the response to therapy.

EXERCISE TESTING

The tests described thus far in this chapter have examined the lungs of subjects at rest. However, resting measurements of lung function may not adequately reflect the functional ability of a subject's cardiopulmonary status because physiologic gas exchange involves the heart and the peripheral circulation as well as the lungs. For example, the metabolic demand for oxygen increases 20 times for walking and 40 times for jogging. For a more complete discussion of exercise testing, the reader is referred to several excellent texts.[18, 19]

Methods of Measurement

During exercise, muscles are stressed, and the cardiac and pulmonary systems respond to these increased demands. Exercise testing has been developed to measure cardiac and pulmonary responses directly while indirectly assessing peripheral gas exchange. Exercise tests commonly employ stationary ergometers or treadmills while measurements of exhaled gas (volume, and oxygen and carbon dioxide concentrations), heart rate, and blood pressure are obtained. Exercise tests are usually performed for 6 to 12 minutes, allowing the subject to reach the maximal attainable work.

During exercise testing, the following direct measurements are made.

Measurement	Equipment
Exhaled gas concentrations of O_2 and CO_2	Gas analyzers
V_T and respiratory frequency, thus V_E	Pneumotachometer or spirometer
Blood pressure	Sphygmomanometer
Heart rate	Electrocardiographic monitor
Oxygen saturaton	Oximeter or arterial blood gases
Workload	Cycle ergometer or treadmill

Calculated parameters may include

$\dot{V}O_{2max}$	Maximal oxygen consumption
$\dot{V}CO_2$	Carbon dioxide production
O_2 pulse	Oxygen consumption/heart rate
RQ	Respiratory quotient
VD/VT	Dead space volume/tidal volume

The cardiac and ventilatory responses to increased work are measured during exercise testing. As workload increases, ventilation, heart rate, oxygen consumption, and carbon dioxide rise in a linear fashion (Fig. 17–6). When oxygen demand increases beyond supply, anaerobic metabolism supplements energy production. Excess hydrogen ions enter the bloodstream, where they are sensed by chemoreceptors. Ventilation increases more rapidly at this point, resulting in a rise in end-tidal O_2 because O_2 consumption continues to increase only linearly and therefore O_2 consumption per breath actually decreases. The point at which this alinear response to increasing workload appears is termed the anaerobic threshold. In normal subjects, the anaerobic threshold occurs at a point greater than 40% of predicted maximal oxygen consumption ($\dot{V}O_{2max}$). There is increasing evidence that these relationships may be more complex and occasionally lead to difficulty in interpretation.

Cardiopulmonary fitness is related to $\dot{V}O_{2max}$, maximal heart rate, and anaerobic threshold. The response to exercise testing in subjects with sedentary lifestyles may mimic abnormal responses. Limitations of either cardiac, pulmonary, or peripheral vascular systems affect exercise capacity. Through the integration of measured responses during exercise testing, the limiting system may be defined.

Formal exercise testing requires sophisticated equipment and trained personnel to operate this equipment. A simple way of assessing exercise performance is with a 12-minute walking test. This can be performed in any hospital corridor by timing the subject as he or she covers the greatest distance possible in the allotted 12 minutes. The results of

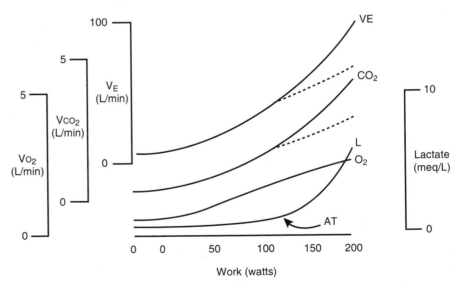

FIGURE 17–6: Data obtained from incremental exercise using cycle ergometry. The anaerobic threshold (AT) occurs when lactate (L) increases. $\dot{V}E$, minute ventilation; $\dot{V}O_2$, O_2 consumption; $\dot{V}CO_2$, CO_2 output.

this test, described by Cooper, have been shown to correlate well with $\dot{V}O_{2max}$ during treadmill exercise testing.[20]

PREOPERATIVE EVALUATION

Because pulmonary complications are a common cause of postoperative morbidity, evaluation of pulmonary function has become an integral part of the preoperative management of many patients. A number of studies have attempted to address which patients require preoperative pulmonary function tests and which tests are the best predictors of postoperative morbidity. In general, the greater the pulmonary risks of the surgery for the patient, the more likely he or she is to need preoperative pulmonary function testing. These risk factors include age, obesity, type of anesthesia, underlying disease processes, and type of surgery. The elderly patient clearly has an increased morbidity after most surgical procedures. Although lung volumes, expiratory flow rates, Pa_{O_2}, and airway reflexes decline with age, these changes are not the entire explanation for this morbidity.[21]

In obesity, there is a reduction in FRC due principally to a reduction in ERV. Therefore, closing volume may exceed ERV, resulting in airway closure during normal tidal breathing (Fig. 17–7). Interestingly, abdominal surgery results in a similar sequence of physiologic events, predisposing these same patients to basilar atelectasis, decreased $\dot{V}/\dot{Q}$ ratios, and hypoxemia.

General anesthesia results in a 20% reduction in FRC that may be due to a loss of tonic activity of chest wall muscles and the diaphragm, resulting in a cephalad shift of the diaphragm.[22] Others have explained the diminished FRC by the appearance of atelectasis demonstrable on computed tomography of the thorax during anesthesia. Hypoxia, which has also been observed, has been explained by the loss of hypoxic vasoconstriction during anesthesia. However, this abnormality could be equally well explained by a reduction in FRC. Some of these same physiologic abnormalities have also been seen with regional anesthesia.[23]

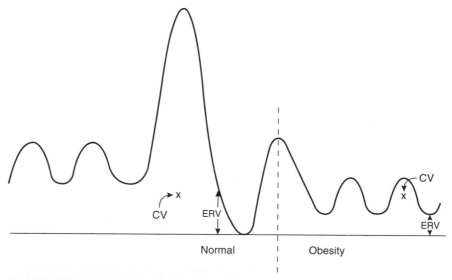

FIGURE 17–7: Closing volume exceeding expiratory reserve volume in obesity. CV, closing volume; ERV, expiratory reserve volume.

The greatest reduction in postoperative pulmonary function seems to occur after surgical procedures adjacent to the diaphragm, such as thoracic and upper abdominal surgery. Although it was once thought that postoperative pain was the major contributing factor, more recently diaphragmatic dysfunction has been implicated.[24] The cause of the impairment is not known. Incisions in the abdomen that cut across muscle groups seem to cause the greatest pulmonary dysfunction. Although all of the previously mentioned factors increase the risk of surgery, in general, if the surgical procedure is corrective and the postoperative cardiorespiratory care is adequate, the patient's pulmonary function usually returns to the preoperative state.

Patients undergoing lung resection present unique problems. At present, most of these resections are for lung cancer. These patients usually suffer from coexistent chronic obstructive lung disease because cigarette smoking is a risk factor for both emphysema and cancer. In addition to routine pulmonary function tests, special studies, including differential bronchospirometry, lung scanning, pulmonary function tests in the lateral position, and pulmonary artery occlusion, have been used as predictors of postoperative morbidity and pulmonary function.[24] Although physiologic abnormalities such as pulmonary hypertension (at rest or during exercise), hypercapnia, or an FEV_1 of less than 1 L should alert the physician to the potential for serious postoperative problems (Table 17–1), criteria have not yet been established to define which patients are unfit for resectional surgery.[25] The introduction of laparoscopy and thoroscopy procedures will have a significant impact on these criteria.

NEONATAL AND PEDIATRIC PULMONARY FUNCTION TESTING

Pulmonary function measurement in neonates and children has represented a challenge because

- Testing usually depends on the cooperation of the subject
- Instrumentation must have minimal dead space and be sensitive enough to measure small volumes and flow rates
- Normal values need to be established

Currently, inspiratory and expiratory flow rates and associated volumes are measured by three techniques:

- Passive tidal volume flow-volume loop[26]
- Partial forced expired curve (hug or squeeze technique)[27]

TABLE **17–1:** Pulmonary Function Criteria Suggesting High Risk of Morbidity and Mortality for Thoracic Surgery

Spirometry	
FVC	<1.7 L
FEV_1	<1.2 L
FEV_1/FVC	<35%
MVV	<50% of predicted or <28 L/min
Gas Exchange	
DL_{CO}	<50% of predicted
CO_2	>45 mm Hg

Adapted from Tisi G. Preoperative evaluation of pulmonary function. Am Rev Respir Dis 119:293–310, 1979; and Gass GD, Olsen G. Preoperative pulmonary function testing to predict postoperative morbidity and mortality. Chest 89:127–135, 1986.
MVV, maximal voluntary ventilation.

- Deflation curve (FVC)[28]

Almost all infant pulmonary function testing is performed while the subject is asleep; therefore, most testing requires sedative administration before testing. Mechanically ventilated infants may also be tested with these methods.

A passive tidal volume flow-volume loop is obtained by placing a pneumotachometer over the infant's nose and mouth. Flow and volume values of the tidal breath are recorded and analyzed.

During the partial forced expired curve, the infant is wrapped in a pneumatic jacket surrounding the thorax and abdomen. At end-inspiration, the jacket inflates, forcing the gas out of the lungs by exerting pressure around the compliant chest wall. Flow is measured with a pneumotachometer via a face mask.

The deflation curve is performed on intubated infants only. After a manual inflation to TLC, a negative pressure is applied, forcing the gas from the lungs through a pneumotachometer.

Dynamic respiratory mechanics measurements are obtained by using an esophageal balloon for pressure measurements and a pneumotachometer for simultaneous volume and flow measurement. Both compliance and resistance values may be obtained with this technique.

Functional residual volume (FRC) measurements are obtained with methods similar to those used on adults.[29, 30] Helium dilution, nitrogen washout, and body plethysmography techniques are used for volume measurements.

Currently, techniques for measuring carbon monoxide diffusing capacity are still being investigated.

SUMMARY

Pulmonary function testing is used to assess an individual's pulmonary status while monitoring disease activity and efficacy of therapy. It may also be used for employment screening, epidemiologic studies, and preoperative evaluation. This chapter reviews methods of testing commonly performed in pulmonary function laboratories, such as measurements of expiratory flow, diffusing capacity, and lung volume, as well as the more specialized tests including measurement of compliance, resistance, and control of ventilation. Testing procedures performed at rest and during exercise are presented. Some physiologic explanations for abnormal test results are given after descriptions of testing procedures. The final section describes the burgeoning field of neonatal and pediatric testing, in which the technology and the methodology continue to evolve.

References

1. American Thoracic Society. Standardization of spirometry—1987 update. Am Rev Respir Dis 136:1285–1298, 1987.
2. American Thoracic Society. Single breath carbon monoxide diffusing capacity (transfer factor). Recommendations for a standard technique. Am Rev Respir Dis 136:1299–1307, 1987.
3. American Thoracic Society. Lung function testing: Selection of reference values and interpretative strategies. Am Rev Respir Dis 144:1202–1218, 1991.
4. American Thoracic Society. Pulmonary function laboratory personnel qualifications. Am Rev Respir Dis 134:623–624, 1986.
5. American Thoracic Society. Computer guidelines for pulmonary laboratories. ATS position paper. Am Rev Respir Dis 135:628–629, 1986.

6. American Thoracic Society. Quality assurance in pulmonary function laboratories. ATS position paper. Am Rev Respir Dis 134:625–627, 1986.
7. Clausen J, Zarins L. Pulmonary Function Testing Guidelines and Controversies, Equipment, Methods and Normal Values. New York, Academic Press, 1982.
8. Comroe JH, Forster RE, DuBois AB, et al. The Lung: Clinical Physiology and Pulmonary Function Tests. Chicago, Year Book Medical Publishers, 1962.
9. Harris TR, Pratt PC, Kilburn KH. Total lung capacity measured by roentgenograms. Am J Med 50:756–763, 1971.
10. Barnhard HJ, Pierce JA, Joyce JW, et al. Roentgenographic determination of total lung capacity. Am J Med 28:51–60, 1960.
11. Chai H, Farr RS, Froehlich LA, et al. Standardization of bronchial inhalation challenge procedures. J Allergy Clin Immunol 56:323–327, 1975.
12. Scharf SM, Heimer D, Walters M. Bronchial challenge with room air temperature isocapnic hyperventilation—A comparison with histamine challenge. Chest 88:584–593, 1985.
13. Heaton RW, Henderson AF, Gray BJ, Costello JF. The bronchial response to cold air challenge: Evidence for different mechanisms in normal and asthmatic subjects. Thorax 38:506–511, 1983.
14. Ewan PW, Jones HA, Rhodes CG, et al. Detection of intrapulmonary hemorrhage with carbon monoxide uptake: Application in Goodpasture's syndrome. N Engl J Med 295:1391, 1976.
15. Buist AS, Ross BB. Predicted values for closing volumes using a modified single breath nitrogen test. Am Rev Respir Dis 107:744–752, 1973.
16. Whitelaw WA, Derenne J, Milic Emili J. Occlusion pressure as a measure of respiratory center output in conscious man. Respir Physiol 23:181–199, 1975.
17. Black LF, Hyatt RE. Maximal respiratory pressures: Normal values and relationship to age and sex. Am Rev Respir Dis 99:696–702, 1969.
18. Wasserman K, Hansen JE, Sue DY, Whipp BJ. Principles of Exercise Testing and Interpretation. Philadelphia, Lea & Febiger, 1987.
19. Jones NL. Clinical Exercise Testing. Philadelphia, WB Saunders, 1988.
20. Cooper KH. A means of assessing maximal oxygen intake. JAMA 203:135–138, 1968.
21. Tisi G. Preoperative evaluation of pulmonary function. Am Rev Respir Dis 119:293–310, 1979.
22. Busmar B, Hedenstierna G, Strandberg A, et al. Pulmonary densities during anesthesia with muscular relaxation. A proposal for atelectasis. Anesthesiology 62:422–428, 1985.
23. Ravin MB. Comparison of special and general anesthesia for lower abdominal surgery in patients with chronic obstructive pulmonary disease. Anesthesiology 35:319–322, 1971.
24. Ford GT, Whilelaw WA, Rosenal TW, et al. Diaphragm function after upper abdominal surgery in humans. Am Rev Respir Dis 127:431–436, 1983.
25. Gass GD, Olsen G. Preoperative pulmonary function testing to predict postoperative morbidity and mortality. Chest 89:127–135, 1986.
26. Abramson AL, Goldstein MN, Stenzler A, Steele A. The use of the tidal breathing flow volume loop in laryngotracheal disease of neonates and infants. Laryngoscope 92:922–926, 1982.
27. Wall MA, Misley MC, Dickerson D. Partial expiratory flow volume curves in young children. Am Rev Respir Dis 129:557–562, 1984.
28. Motoyama EK. Pulmonary mechanics during early postnatal years. Pediatr Res 11:220–223, 1977.
29. Gerhardt T, Hehred, Feller R, et al. Pulmonary mechanics in normal infants and young children during first 5 years of life. Pediatr Pulmonol 3:309–316, 1987.
30. Gaultier C. Lung volumes in neonates and infants. Eur Respir J 2:130S–134S, 1989.

18

Clinical Application of Laboratory Examinations

Suzanne M. Burns, R.N., M.S.N., R.R.T., C.C.R.N.

Leukocytes—WBCs
Polycythemia vera—an overproduction of RBCs
Aplastic anemia—decreased RBCs characterized by defective bone marrow function

For respiratory care practitioners to provide comprehensive pulmonary care to the acutely ill patient, a working knowledge of laboratory tests is necessary. Although all laboratory tests are important tools for use in the diagnosis and treatment of disease, certain tests are essential as screening indices and as a monitor of physiologic function. This chapter reviews laboratory studies commonly performed in acute care settings.

COMPLETE BLOOD COUNT

The maintenance of adequate oxygenation is an important goal of respiratory care. Although oxygen supply can be enhanced through the delivery of inspired gases and the use of selected ventilatory modes, the most important element in tissue oxygenation is the red blood cell (RBC); its main function is to carry oxygen. For the respiratory care practitioner to assess, plan, and intervene intelligently in potential or actual alterations in oxygenation, an understanding of the RBC and its components is necessary.

The complete blood count, one of the most frequently ordered laboratory tests, consists of RBC studies; white blood cell (WBC) counts with differentials; and in many laboratories, platelet counts. Understanding how these cells are formed, in addition to understanding their function, is essential to interpretation.

Hematopoiesis, the maturation and proliferation of the cellular constituents of blood, occurs predominantly in the bone marrow. Normally, only mature cells enter the circulation; however, with some diseases, immature cells can be found. For example, leukemia is characterized by an excessive number of leukocytes. The type of leukemia is determined by identifying the cells present (e.g., increased numbers of myelocytes may indicate a myelocytic leukemia). Referring to Figure 18–1 for the components of the complete blood count will give a more thorough understanding of the significance of the tests.

Red Blood Cell Count (Erythrocyte Count)

The erythrocyte, a mature RBC, has a life span of approximately 120 days. The erythrocyte is formed in the bone marrow and is removed by the spleen, liver, and red bone marrow. Its main function is to carry hemoglobin. Steady-state production and differentiation of RBCs occurs in the bone marrow, with mediation by the hormone erythropoietin,

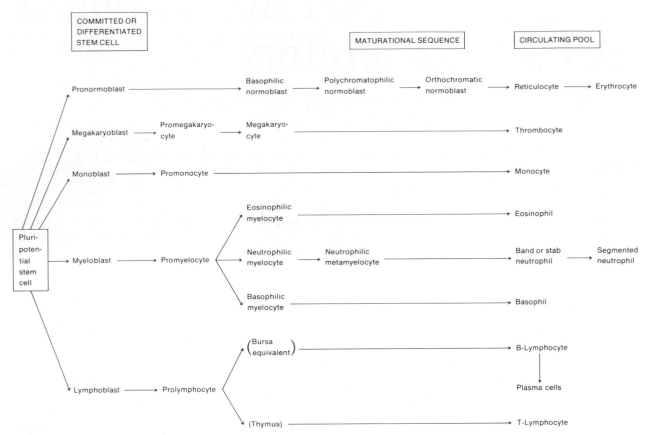

FIGURE 18–1: Theory of formation and maturation of blood cells (hematopoiesis). (From Price SA, Wilson LM. Pathophysiology, 3rd ed. New York, McGraw-Hill Book Company, 1986, p 1981. Copyright © 1986 by McGraw-Hill, Inc. Used by permission of McGraw-Hill Book Company.)

RBC count (erythrocyte count)

Male: 4.6 to 6.2 million/mm³
Female: 4.2 to 5.4 million/mm³

Reticulocyte count

Male: 0.5 to 1.5% of total erythrocytes, or 0.005 to 0.015
Female: 0.5 to 2.5%, or 0.005 to
0.025

which is released from the kidney.[1] Erythropoietin also stimulates the increased erythrocyte production found in chronic hypoxemic states.[2] In these conditions, an excess of RBCs can result, which is called polycythemia. Hemoconcentration secondary to dehydration can falsely elevate the erythrocyte count. Decreases are seen in acute hemolytic anemia (blood cell destruction), in acute and chronic blood loss, and in conditions in which blood cell production is affected (e.g., certain drug therapies). Fluid overload with resulting hemodilution can falsely decrease the erythrocyte count.

Although an erythrocyte count is helpful as an initial screen, it is inclusive of all components of the RBC. Therefore, further differentiation is necessary.

Reticulocyte Count

Reticulocytes, immature RBCs, are normally released in small numbers into the circulation from the bone marrow. These non-nucleated cells, which mature in 1 to 2 days, are called reticulocytes because reticulum (mitochondria and other organelles) is present. Reticulocytes indicate how actively the bone marrow produces RBCs because they are formed during erythropoiesis. They can increase after an acute blood loss or hemolytic process by a factor of three to six. Decreased levels indicate decreased production, as seen in iron deficiency anemia, chronic infections, and radiation therapy. In underproduction anemias, when iron, vitamin B_{12}, or folic acid is given, the reticulocyte count should begin to increase in approximately 1 week.

Hematocrit and Hemoglobin

Hematocrit

Male: 40 to 50%
Female: 38 to 47%

Hemoglobin

Male: 13.5 to 18 g/dL
Female: 12 to 16 g/dL

The hematocrit, a measurement of packed RBCs, or the RBCs separated from the plasma, is expressed as the percentage of RBCs in a volume of whole blood. The hematocrit is normally three times the hemoglobin level. Hematocrit and hemoglobin levels increase and decrease for similar reasons. Therefore, they are usually interpreted together.

Hemoglobin is made up of two substances, heme and globin. Heme is a substance composed of porphyrin (a red pigment) and iron atoms (which combine with oxygen). Globin, a protein, is made up of four distinct amino acid chains (two alpha and two beta). The resultant hemoglobin, with a unique ability to bind oxygen, carries the majority of oxygen to the tissues.

Oxygen supply is a function of hemoglobin level, saturation, and cardiac output, with the hemoglobin level being a major determinant of oxygen-carrying capacity. Therefore, to evaluate oxygenation states, the hemoglobin level must be measured.

Tissue oxygenation occurs when oxygen dissociates from hemoglobin into the plasma and then into the tissues. This occurs more readily when the host is hyperthermic or acidic or has increased levels of 2,3-diphosphoglyccrate (2,3-DPG). However, oxygen loading onto the hemoglobin decreases in these conditions. The converse is true with alkalosis, hypothermia, or low levels of 2,3-DPG: oxygen loads readily, but there is decreased dissociation from the hemoglobin.[3]

Occasionally, an abnormal inherited hemoglobin pattern (autosomal recessive) is responsible for a globin that has a substituted amino acid on the beta-chain (sickle cell anemia). When these abnormal cells deoxygenate, the cell changes shape (sickles), occludes vessels, and infarcts tissues.

Other disorders of hemoglobin include those involving the heme portion. In these situations, elements other than oxygen combine with the heme to form substances that are harmful and occasionally fatal to the patient. Two examples include methemoglobin and carboxyhemoglobin.

Methemoglobin forms when the iron in the heme portion of deoxygenated hemoglobin oxidizes to a ferric form rather than a ferrous form. Oxygen and iron cannot combine in the ferric form; thus, the patient has symptoms of anoxia and cyanosis without evidence of cardiac or pulmonary disease. The condition can be inherited or acquired. The most common cause of acquired methemoglobinemia is toxic exposure to drugs or chemicals (e.g., nitrates, nitrites, some sulfonamides, and chlorates), but it is also associated with infections such as clostridial infection and malaria.[4]

Toxic levels of carboxyhemoglobin are generally those above 20%. The carboxyhemoglobin level can be mildly elevated (6 to 10%) with smoking or with exposure to automobile exhaust fumes.[5]

The formation of carboxyhemoglobin occurs when hemoglobin is exposed to carbon monoxide. Because hemoglobin's affinity for carbon monoxide is 200 times greater than that for oxygen, the receptor sites become saturated with carbon monoxide instead of oxygen. Further complicating the situation is the fact that the remaining oxygen bound to the hemoglobin is not readily unloaded for tissue use.

Assessing hemoglobin and hematocrit levels is essential to understanding tissue oxygenation. However, for a complete interpretation to occur, the clinician must understand the complex properties of hemoglobin and those conditions affecting cellular function. This is especially true because the optimal level of hemoglobin or hematocrit is unknown.

Today, the threshold for blood replacement is much higher than in the past. Even in the most complex surgical cases, autotransfusion may be used exclusively, allowing hematocrits of 25% or less to exist postoperatively. Therefore, hematocrit and hemoglobin levels must be interpreted in conjunction with clinical findings and a careful evaluation of oxygenation supply and demand. For example, in the weaning patient, the work of breathing may greatly increase oxygen demand. When the level of hemoglobin decreases, oxygen supply is less, and the imbalance between supply and demand can result in weakness, dyspnea, fatigue, and weaning failure.[6] In this patient situation, increasing the oxygen-carrying capacity before initiating weaning trials may be prudent.

Increased levels of hemoglobin and hematocrit are found with high-altitude living, in chronic hypoxic states, with dehydration, and in polycythemia vera. Decreased values are present with hemodilution and fluid overload; in anemic states; and with leukemia, hyperthyroidism, cirrhosis, renal failure, hemorrhage, and hemolytic anemia.

WHITE BLOOD CELL COUNT (LEUKOCYTE COUNT) AND DIFFERENTIAL

Respiratory care practitioners frequently work with patients who have infectious or altered immune systems. An understanding of WBC function is therefore important in order to give comprehensive care. For example, an acutely ill patient (e.g., one who is infected, has an elevated WBC count, or is febrile) should not be submitted to a weaning trial until the acute episode has resolved. This type of activity may exhaust and demoralize the patient, making future trials less promising. A knowledgeable respiratory care practitioner, able to perform a basic interpretation of a WBC differential, can apply knowledge related to the acute infection to an appropriate and effective care plan for the patient. Further, an understanding of WBC function is essential for understanding the immunocompromised or immunosuppressed state so prevalent in hospitalized patients. Nosocomial infections can be prevented through education and diligent use of aseptic technique. The role of the clinician in preventing infection cannot be overstated. A description of WBC function and differentiation follows.

Leukocytes—WBCs

Numerous types of WBCs exist, each of which has a specific role in the immune system. WBCs, formed in the bone marrow (granulocytes and monocytes-macrophages) and the lymphatic tissue (lymphocytes), are sent via the circulatory system to areas of the body where they are needed. A careful evaluation of the type, quantity, and stage of development of the leukocytes can help to diagnose disease and determine appropriate therapies. Figure 18–1 shows the progressive evolution of the WBC to maturity. Immature cells are normally found only in the bone marrow or the lymphatic tissue. Mature cells are seen in the circulating blood and in infected organs or tissues.

White Blood Cell Count

The WBC count indicates the total number of leukocytes per cubic millimeter of blood. Leukocytosis is seen with infections, inflammation,

WBC count

5 to 10³/mL *or*
5 to 10⁹/L

Leukocytosis—elevated WBC count
Leukopenia—decreased WBC count

Granulocytes

Band neutrophils: 0 to 5%
Neutrophils: 60 to 70%
Eosinophils: 1 to 4%
Basophils: 0.5 to 1%

Nongranulocytes

Lymphocytes: 20 to 40%
Monocytes: 2 to 6%

leukemias, and parasitic infections. Leukopenia is seen in malnutrition, bone marrow depression, and severe infections, as well as in some viral infections, autoimmune diseases, and malignancies.

Differential

The WBC differential distinguishes between the types of leukocytes present; the components are expressed as percentages. To determine the absolute number of each cell present, the percentage for each cell is multiplied by the total WBC count.

Segmented Neutrophils or Polymorphonuclear Neutrophils

Segmented neutrophils or polymorphonuclear neutrophils, known as the cells of acute inflammation, appear within 4 to 6 hours at the site of infection in response to complement activation to phagocytose. With a life span of approximately 24 hours, they respond to virulent organisms such as streptococci, staphylococci, pneumococci, *Haemophilus influenzae*, and meningococci, as well as to necrosis, infarction, and hemolysis.[7,8] In an effort to produce and release enough cells to control the acute process, the bone marrow also releases immature cells into the peripheral blood. The WBC count then shows an increased number of bands (immature neutrophils) and metamyelocytes (juveniles) and is called a shift to the left. (This term is a throwback to the days when these cells were listed on the left side of the laboratory slip.)

Basophils

The function of the basophil is not clearly understood. These granulocytes are known to phagocytose as well as to store and produce heparin, histamine, and serotonin. Basophils are counted to study anaphylactic and allergic reactions (they appear in different quantities in the tissue and blood of afflicted individuals). Basophil counts are also increased in some leukemias, in Hodgkin's disease, and in polycythemia vera.

Eosinophils

Eosinophils are phagocytic granulocytes. Their numbers are most commonly increased in allergic responses and parasitic infections.

Monocytes and Macrophages

Monocytes: 2 to 6%

The monocytes (in the circulation) or macrophages (in the tissue) are responsible for phagocytosing the debris and foreign proteins found in infected and necrotic processes. Therefore, they are referred to as the cells of chronic inflammation. These cells appear within 2 to 4 days. Macrophage activation occurs through the release of macrophage-activating lymphokines from T lymphocytes specifically sensitized to antigens from the infecting organism.[9] The antiviral agent called interferon (a substance that helps to identify and reject foreign cells) is an especially important macrophage-activating lymphokine.[10]

Lymphocytes

Lymphocytes: 20 to 40%

Two groups of lymphocytes exist: T (thymus derived) and B (first described in chicken bursas) cells. However, they are not differentiated in a WBC count. Instead, a total number is reported. These agranulocytes, a source of serum immunoglobulins, are responsible for immune memory and response. When a second contact with an antigen (e.g., bacteria, viruses, or parasites) occurs, the specifically sensitized lymphocytes rapidly produce a large quantity of antibody to fight the infection. The majority of lymphocytes appear in peripheral lymphoid tissues and the spleen.[11]

Generally, serum lymphocyte levels increase in infections, leukocytosis, infectious mononucleosis, during the recovery stage of disease, and with numerous other viral and bacterial infections.

Deficiencies of lymphocyte function and production have been studied in great detail, prompted in large part by the appearance and rapid spread of the human immunodeficiency virus (HIV) and the acquired immunodeficiency syndrome (AIDS) (described later). Lymphopenia occurs in immunosuppressed states such as those caused by steroid use, AIDS, Cushing's disease, and radiation therapy. Lymphocyte levels also decrease in Hodgkin's disease, lupus erythematosus, and chronic uremia.

B and T Lymphocytes

Antigen—foreign substance

B lymphocytes make up 30% of the circulating lymphocytes. When presented with an antigen, these cells turn into plasma cells, which then permanently produce antibodies to that specific antigen. From then on, when an antigen appears, the specific antibody binds to the antigen and causes rapid activation of inflammatory and other immune defense responses.[12] Called immunoglobulins, these antibodies are differentiated by function and labeled arbitrarily (IgA, IgD, IgE, IgG, and IgM).

The majority (70%) of all lymphocytes are T lymphocytes originating in the thymus gland. There are three different types of T cells: killer (T3), helper (T4), and suppressor (T8). Killer T cells release substances known as lymphokines, which are responsible for the identification and rejection of foreign cells. Helper T cells orchestrate the immune system, or turn the immune system "on." These cells secrete the immune system enhancer interleukin-2, as well as augment the function of B lymphocytes and killer T lymphocytes. Suppressor T cells, also known as "off" cells, keep the body from reacting to itself (an autoimmune response).[13] In AIDS, the total number of helper T lymphocytes is reduced and the helper-suppressor ratio changes from a normal value of greater than 1.0 to less than 1.0.

Interferon is a kind of lymphokine.

T cells: 640–2200 cells/mL
Helper cells:490–1190 cells/mL
Suppressor T cells: 180–785 cells/mL
B cells: 92–392 cells/mL
Lymphocyte ratio: TH/Ts ratio > 1.0

Whereas B cells are primarily responsible for the initial immune response to many bacterial pathogens and antigens such as dust, mold, dander, pollen, and ragweed, T cells provide the primary defense against viruses, fungi, and protozoans. Patients with AIDS or immunocompromise secondary to antirejection drug regimens (i.e., following transplantation) are especially prone to opportunistic infections, infections by organisms of lower pathogenicity resulting from abnormal host defenses. In view of the prevalence of these organisms in the health care setting, a brief description of common opportunistic infections follows.

Opportunistic Infections in Acquired Immunodeficiency Syndrome

Opportunistic infections are the primary mode of presentation in AIDS. The infections most often associated with T cell abnormalities predominate.

Pneumocystis carinii pneumonia is the most common opportunistic infection seen in AIDS patients, occurring in 60 to 80% of adults and in 39% of children.[14, 15] The causative organism was originally classified as a protozoan.[16] However, researchers have since suggested that this organism is a fungus.[17] The diagnosis is made by the presence of the organism in bronchial secretions, in lung tissue obtained with bronchoalveolar lavage, or in biopsy specimens obtained during bronchoscopy. Trimethoprim-sulfamethoxazole or aerosolized pentamidine isethionate is given to treat the infection.

Cytomegalovirus, a member of the herpesvirus family, is present in virtually all patients with AIDS but does not usually cause clinical disease.[18-20] However, when disseminated, the organism is associated with encephalitis, chorioretinitis, and pneumonitis, and infection with it may be treated with ganciclovir. The diagnosis is made by the examination of bronchoalveolar lavage fluid, blood, saliva, and urine by cytology, culture, and immunofluorescence. An association between cytomegalovirus infection, birth defects, and mortality has been demonstrated.[21]

Candida albicans, a ubiquitous fungus, can cause esophageal candidiasis, oral lesions, and disseminated fungemia. The diagnosis is made by endoscopy with biopsy of the affected esophageal tissue and blood cultures. Ketoconazole and amphotericin B (for more debilitating cases) are used to treat candidiasis.[22, 23]

In addition to fungal, protozoan, and viral opportunistic infections, infection with low-virulence bacteria, such as *Mycobacterium avium-intracellulare* and *Mycobacterium tuberculosis*, can also result in significant illness in the immunocompromised host.

M. avium-intracellulare, an organism found in dust, water, poultry, and livestock, can cause disseminated disease with multiorgan involvement.[24] The disease is diagnosed with chest films, cultures of blood and sputum, and biopsies of specific tissues. Treatment consists of multidrug regimens, such as that of amikacin, clofazimine, rifampin, ethambutol, and ciprofloxacin.[25-27]

Tuberculosis, for many years considered all but eradicated in the United States, has emerged as a serious problem in AIDS patients, intravenous drug abusers, and the homeless.[28, 29] Tuberculosis can be latent for many years and pose no serious health risk, but in patients with AIDS, it can be devastating. In fact, HIV infection is considered to be the highest known risk factor for progression from infection to active disease. The diagnosis can be made with skin testing; however, often the immunocompromised host is anergic, so chest x-ray studies and sputum analysis are necessary. Treatment usually consists of isoniazid, rifampin, and pyrazinamide. Reports of multidrug-resistant strains of tuberculosis have appeared.[30]

Health care workers frequently care for immunocompromised patients. Given the prevalence of AIDS and immunosuppressive drug regimens associated with transplantation, the respiratory care practitioner must understand immune dysfunction and the resultant risk of opportunistic infections.

Platelet Count (Thrombocytes)

Platelets, which are round, oval, flat, or dish-shaped nuclear cells, are formed in the bone marrow and are necessary for blood clotting. When an injury occurs, the platelet initiates a plug at the site of the trauma. Coagulation depends on the presence of numerous clotting factors, which work in a stepwise series of interactions called cascade pathways. These pathways are initiated either in the vessel (intrinsic) or in

Pregnant health care workers are cautioned to follow Centers for Disease Control and Prevention isolation precautions carefully in caring for these patients because cytomegalovirus infection may pose a serious risk to the unborn fetus.

Platelet count (thrombocytes): 150,000 to 350,000/mm³

the tissue (extrinsic). Common elements of the coagulation process occur in the common pathway (Fig. 18–2).

The circulating blood contains two thirds of the body's platelets, and one third remain in the spleen. The spleen also removes old or damaged platelets from the circulation. With hypersplenism, excessive numbers of platelets can be trapped in the spleen, resulting in few circulating platelets and bleeding. Conditions that result in low platelet counts include infectious mononucleosis, lupus erythematosus, some leukemias, and cirrhosis. Thrombocytopenia can also be a result of drug therapy (toxic thrombocytopenia) in which cells are either damaged or underproduced, anemias, or conditions such as DIC. Another cause of a decreased platelet count is heparin use. In some patients receiving heparin, antibodies develop that bind to the platelets in the presence of heparin and result in platelet activation. The activated platelets form thrombi that can result in numerous catastrophic occlusive phenomena, such as stroke or heart attack.[31-33] When the platelet count falls below 50,000/mm^3, the clinician must be alert to the potential for increased bleeding. If the value falls below 20,000/mm^3, even routine invasive procedures, such as blood drawing and suctioning, can result in a profound hemorrhage. Emergency platelet replacement is often necessary and is occasionally given in addition to fresh frozen plasma (which contains other important coagulation factors). Thrombocythemia or thrombocytosis can be found in cases of advanced or disseminated malignancy, trauma, some acute infections, splenectomy, polycythemia vera, and leukemia.

In addition to resulting from decreases in total numbers of platelets, bleeding can also be caused by platelet malfunction. Platelet aggregation requires the presence of ionized calcium, fibrinogen, and a protein called von Willebrand's factor. Deficiencies of any of these substances affect platelet function. Adherence of the platelet plug improves the release of prostaglandins, which are generated by the platelets.[34] Aspirin inhibits prostaglandin synthesis and therefore prolongs bleeding. Aspirin has been recommended for use in individuals at risk for coronary occlusion and stroke to decrease the thrombotic element. To determine whether platelet dysfunction is the reason for prolonged bleeding, other studies of coagulation are often necessary. For example, bleeding time, which measures how long it takes for bleeding to stop after a small, clean incision is made in the skin, may be prolonged even with a platelet count of 100,000/mm^3. The prolonged bleeding time (or platelet adherence time) can be the result of a drug (e.g., aspirin) or an inherited deficiency (e.g., von Willebrand's factor).

DIC—disseminated intravascular coagulation

Thrombocytosis—an increased number of platelets

COAGULATION STUDIES

Many procedures commonly performed by respiratory care practitioners, such as suctioning, arterial blood gas drawing, and chest physical therapy, can result in hemorrhage in patients with increased bleeding tendencies. By understanding the tests used to determine coagulation function, the knowledgeable clinician can prevent the occurrence of catastrophic events through careful assessment and care planning.

The most common screening tests for coagulation function are the platelet count, bleeding time, prothrombin time (PT), and partial thromboplastin time (PTT) or activated partial thromboplastin time (APTT). Because the platelet count and bleeding time were discussed earlier, this

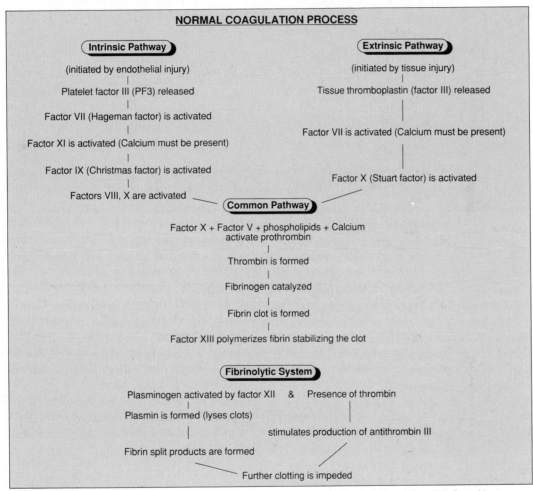

FIGURE 18–2: Normal coagulation process. (From Young LM. DIC: The insidious killer. Crit Care Nurse 10:28, 1990.)

section focuses on PT, PTT, and APTT, as well as on the studies performed to diagnose DIC.

Prothrombin Time and Partial Thromboplastin Time or Activated Partial Thromboplastin Time

PT and PTT or APTT

PT: 10 to 14 seconds
PTT: 30 to 45 seconds
APTT: 16 to 25 seconds

PT and PTT or APTT are used together to evaluate the extrinsic and intrinsic coagulation pathways (see Fig. 18–2) and to monitor anticoagulation therapy. By comparing the test results, the clinician can determine which coagulation factors are deficient, thereby diagnosing congenital coagulation disorders.

Prothrombin Time

Prothrombin, a precursor to thrombin formation that is produced by the liver, depends on the presence of vitamin K. The PT test detects problems associated with components of the extrinsic pathway. Because PT measurement does not test the clotting factors involved in the intrinsic pathway, it cannot detect hemophilia A ("classic" hemophilia, or factor VIII deficiency) or hemophilia B (Christmas disease, or factor IX deficiency).

Warfarin, an anticoagulant, prolongs the PT by inhibiting hepatic synthesis of vitamin K–dependent factors (II, VII, IX, and X). Vitamin K can reverse a prolonged PT. Increased PTs are found in liver disease, DIC, anticoagulant therapy, vitamin K deficiency, and prothrombin deficiency.

Partial Thromboplastin Time and Activated Partial Thromboplastin Time

PTT is used to detect deficiencies in the intrinsic pathway (hemophilia A and hemophilia B) and to monitor anticoagulant therapy with heparin. By comparing the PTT with the PT, one can differentiate which factors are responsible for bleeding disorders. For example, when the PT is normal and the PTT is prolonged, factors XII, XI, IX, and VIII may be deficient.

Some clinicians prefer to monitor APTT instead of PTT in heparinized patients because APTT is thought to be more sensitive than PTT. Increased PTTs and APTTs are found in liver disease, DIC, anticoagulant therapy, disorders of the intrinsic pathway (hemophilia), and polycythemia. The antidote for a prolonged PTT or APTT is protamine sulfate.

Disseminated Intravascular Coagulation and Associated Laboratory Tests

DIC is characterized by uncontrolled widespread bleeding.

The syndrome of DIC is precipitated by numerous serious conditions, such as sepsis, traumatic injuries, allergic reactions, cirrhosis, obstetric emergencies (e.g., abruptio placentae), and many others.

In this disorder, uncontrolled fibrin thrombi formation and deposition cause vascular occlusions and necrosis. This enhanced clotting depletes the coagulation factors, resulting in an increased bleeding tendency. Further complicating this tendency is the fact that fibrinolysis is activated. As a result, findings in numerous tests of coagulation are abnormal: PT, PTT (or APTT), bleeding time, and fibrin split product levels increase, whereas platelet count and fibrinogen levels decrease.[35, 36] PT, PTT, APTT, bleeding time, and platelet count have previously been discussed.

Fibrinogen

Fibrinogen: 150 to 450 mg/dL

Fibrinogen (factor I) is converted to fibrin by thrombin in the common final coagulation pathway. In DIC, the process of clot formation and breakdown is enhanced, and the fibrinogen level decreases in the plasma.

Fibrin Split Products or Fibrin Degradation Products or D-Dimers

Fibrin split products or fibrin degradation products or D-dimers

Fibrin split products:
  less than 5 μg/mL
D-dimers: 250/mg/mL

The fibrinolytic system prevents excessive clotting. Plasmin breaks down fibrin and fibrinogen to form fibrin split or degradation products. These products greatly increase in DIC. Fibrin degradation product measurement has been found to be an extremely sensitive, if not specific, indicator of DIC. A new test, called the D-dimer test, has been found to be highly specific. When used in conjunction with fibrin degradation product measurement, this test can confirm the presence of these end-products of degradation.[37] These tests, in combination with the other coagulation studies, are diagnostic of DIC.

ELECTROLYTE STUDIES

Electrolytes, electrically charged molecules, play a large part in the functioning of all cells, especially in muscular and nervous system function. Made up of cations, which carry a positive charge, and anions, which carry a negative charge, these molecules help to identify specific organ abnormalities and evaluate the results of therapies. Generally, the electrolyte abnormalities are viewed in conjunction with other chemical and clinical findings before a diagnosis is made. Although respiratory care practitioners play a very small part in the actual diagnosing of such disorders, an understanding of the effect of electrolyte imbalance on various body systems is imperative if thoughtful care planning is to occur.

Sodium (Na$^+$)

Sodium (Na$^+$)

135 to 148 mmol/L *or*
135 to 148 mEq/L

Sodium, the most abundant cation in extracellular fluid, is responsible for the bulk of serum osmolality, assisting in acid-base balance (through association with bicarbonate and chloride) and the transmission of nerve impulses. Control of Na$^+$ is chiefly through the kidneys.

With high blood flow through the kidneys, excretion of sodium and chloride increases, whereas with low flow (e.g., shock), the body retains sodium and chloride. Renin, produced in the kidneys, regulates renal blood flow, glomerular filtration rate, and salt and water excretion. Renin stimulates aldosterone production, which affects sodium reabsorption. Hyperaldosteronism results in sodium retention and potassium excretion, causing hypertension and hypokalemia. Antidiuretic hormone (vasopressin), a posterior pituitary hormone, controls water reabsorption at the distal tubules of the kidney. Lastly, other steroids, controlled by the anterior pituitary gland, can cause salt and water retention. Examples include estrogen and progesterone.[38]

Hypernatremia is rare, but it is found in conditions promoting a deficit of intravascular fluid volume (i.e., dehydration or insufficient water intake) and in conditions in which the autoregulating mechanisms of the kidney are malfunctioning. Examples include diabetes insipidus (not enough antidiuretic hormone) and Cushing's disease (increased adrenal release of steroids).

Hyponatremia is generally associated with excessive body fluid volume (dilution) or with any condition that contributes to rapid, excessive body fluid loss in which electrolytes are wasted with the fluid loss. Some conditions that promote hyponatremia include the syndrome of inappropriate antidiuretic hormone, diuretic use, profuse sweating, severe burns, diarrhea, excessive vomiting, Addison's disease, and diabetic acidosis.

Because one of the main functions of Na^+ is to maintain serum osmolality, evaluation of Na^+ abnormalities often necessitates a concurrent evaluation of serum osmolality.

Osmolality

Osmolality: 275 to 295 mOsm/kg

Serum osmolality is a measure of the net osmotic action of all the blood-borne molecules. Osmotic pressure is, in general, a function of the size of the molecule: the larger the molecule, the lower the pressure. Serum osmolality increases with dehydration and decreases with overhydration. It is measured to evaluate conditions that affect hydration status and antidiuretic hormone function. When osmolality increases, antidiuretic hormone is secreted and water is reabsorbed at the renal tubules in an effort to make the serum less concentrated. Urine osmolality, on the other hand, becomes higher as a result. Reasons for increased and decreased values of osmolality are similar to those of sodium.

Potassium (K^+)

Potassium (K^+)

3.5 to 5 mEq/L *or*
3.5 to 5.0 mmol/L

Most K^+ is contained within the cell itself (90%), with potassium bicarbonate being the primary intracellular buffer. In conditions such as acute diabetic acidosis, K^+ is driven out of the cell, intracellular potassium bicarbonate is depleted, and intracellular acidosis can be profound. The respiratory center compensates for this acidosis by increasing the respiratory rate and depth, thus lowering Pa_{CO_2} and raising pH. A low serum K^+ level in acute diabetic ketoacidosis can be a medical emergency requiring immediate potassium replacement.

Potassium is especially important for skeletal and cardiac muscle contraction. Because potassium affects cardiac impulse conduction, cardiac patients and those receiving digitalis need close monitoring. In conjunction with calcium and magnesium, potassium controls the force of muscular contraction. Thus, in the weak pulmonary patient, such imbalances can lead to respiratory muscle fatigue, weaning intolerance, and respiratory failure.[39]

The most common causes of hyperkalemia include renal failure, conditions in which hemolysis occurs (e.g., trauma, burns, and DIC), and acidosis (K^+ is driven out of the cells and into the blood). Increased levels are also associated with Addison's disease, acute renal failure, and hypoaldosteronism.

Decreased levels of potassium are associated with gastrointestinal fluid loss, diuretic therapy, intravenous supplementation without K^+ replacement, diarrhea, severe vomiting, severe burns, primary aldosteronism, malabsorption, starvation, acute tubular necrosis, and steroid therapy.

Chloride (Cl^-)

Chloride (Cl^-)

98 to 106 mEq/L *or*
98 to 106 mmol/L

The chloride anion, which exists primarily in the extracellular space, usually combines with sodium (NaCl) or hydrogen to form gastric hydrochloric acid (HCl). This acid assists in digestion and enzyme activities. With changes in the concentration of other anions, such as bicarbonate, chloride increases or decreases so that electrical neutrality is maintained. When bicarbonate levels fall and chloride levels remain normal, an anion gap acidosis exists (see later discussion).

The chloride level increases in dehydration, Cushing's syndrome, hyperventilation, eclampsia, anemia, and some kidney disorders, and it decreases most commonly during massive diuresis (e.g., diabetic ketoacidosis, diuretic therapy, and severe burns) and gastrointestinal losses (e.g., diarrhea and vomiting). Hypochloremia is also found in Addison's disease, dehydration, and pyloric obstruction.

Serum Bicarbonate (HCO_3^-, CO_2 Content, and Serum CO_2)

Serum bicarbonate (HCO_3^-, CO_2 content, and serum CO_2): 19 to 25 mEq/L

The serum bicarbonate test measures the acidity or alkalinity of the blood. Although the carbon dioxide level measured in this test is sometimes confused with the carbon dioxide level measured by blood gas analysis, arterial blood gas analysis measures dissolved CO_2 gas (regulated by the lungs). Bicarbonate, on the other hand, is the major extracellular buffer in the blood (regulated by the kidneys). HCO_3^- exists first as CO_2 and then as carbonic acid, H_2CO_3.

Elevated CO_2 content levels occur with chronic hypercapnia, severe vomiting or gastrointestinal suctioning, and aldosteronism, and with the use of some diuretics. Decreased levels are found with diabetic ketoacidosis, severe diarrhea, acute renal failure, salicylate overdose, some diuretic therapy, and starvation (as discussed in the next section).

Anion Gap

In cases of metabolic acidosis in which the etiology of the acidosis is unclear, measurement of an anion gap may be helpful. Normally, the difference between the measured cations, Na^+ and K^+, and the measured anions, Cl^- and HCO_3^-, is less than 16 mEq/L (less than ± 12 mEq/L if K^+ is not used). Unmeasured anions, which increase in many acidic states, include proteins, PO_4^-, SO_4^-, ketones, and lactic acid. Therefore, when metabolic acidosis exists, the anion gap increases because no compensatory rise in the chloride level occurs. Causes include alcoholic ketoacidosis, diabetic ketoacidosis, fasting and starvation, lactic acidosis, salicylate overdose, and ethylene glycol or methanol ingestion. Acidosis with a nonanion gap (or normal gap) is associated with diarrhea, renal tubular acidosis, hyperalimentation, ureteroileostomy, ureterosigmoidostomy, external drainage of pancreaticobiliary fluids, and use of NH_4Cl and other drugs.

Glucose

Nonfasting glucose: 85 to 125 mg/dL

Hemoglobin A_{1c}

Normal: 4.0 to 7.0%
Diabetic: greater than 7%

The glucose test monitors glucose metabolism disorders, such as diabetes. It also evaluates nutritional and pharmacologic interventions, such as central hyperalimentation and steroid therapy.

When the blood sugar level is as low as 50 mg/dL and the patient is unresponsive, intravenous 50% dextrose must be given immediately because glucose levels of less than 30 mg/dL can result in brain damage. For an alert patient, an oral source of glucose may be given. Blood sugar levels of greater than 300 mg/dL can lead to coma and ketoacidosis. In the critically ill patient, insulin coverage is provided intermittently by a sliding scale or by continuous infusion. With a continuous infusion of insulin, very frequent glucose monitoring (every hour) is necessary until the glucose level stabilizes.

In diabetics, hemoglobin A_{1c} (glycosylated hemoglobin) is measured periodically (monthly or less frequently) because it reflects long-term glucose control. The more glucose exposed to the hemoglobin over its life span of 120 days, the higher the hemoglobin A_{1c} value. This test, a valuable outpatient monitoring tool, may be used in the acute care setting to provide a historical perspective to the diabetic patient's condition.

Hyperglycemia—an elevated blood sugar level
Hypoglycemia—a low blood sugar level

An elevated blood sugar level is found in diabetes, Cushing's syndrome, acute stress, pancreatitis, steroid therapy, nutritional replacement with central hyperalimentation, pheochromocytoma, pancreatic adenoma (increased glucose production), and chronic liver disease.

Examples of conditions in which hypoglycemia is found include too much insulin (overdose), Addison's disease, sepsis, and islet cell carcinoma of the pancreas (too much insulin is produced).

Calcium, Magnesium, and Phosphorus

Calcium, magnesium, and phosphorus are not always measured with routine screens ("chem 7's" include only Na, K, Cl, CO_2, blood urea nitrogen, creatinine, and glucose); instead, they are ordered separately or as part of a more inclusive metabolic screen. In the patient being weaned from mechanical ventilation, deficiencies of these electrolytes can result in respiratory muscle weakness and fatigue, weaning intolerance, and respiratory failure.[40–42] An understanding of the importance of these electrolytes, together and in combination, can help to assess the pulmonary patient comprehensively.

Calcium (Ca²⁺)

Calcium (Ca²⁺)

Total: 8.5 to 10.5 mg/dL
Ionized: 4.2 to 5.4 mg/dL

Calcium exists in two forms:

- Bound to protein
- Circulating in an ionized form

Ionized calcium, the active form, is used for the coagulation process, nerve impulse transmission, muscular contraction, and cardiac function. Serum calcium measurement includes both the ionized and the protein-bound calcium. When protein is low, the measurement of calcium will be artificially low. Therefore, the total calcium level is always viewed in conjunction with the protein level. A bedside calculation can sometimes determine whether the calcium level is normal. The formula is as follows: for each gram change in serum albumin (below the normal of 4), an alteration of 0.8 to 1.2 mg/dL of calcium is expected.

Calcium is the body's most abundant cation. The parathyroid glands and vitamin D regulate the calcium level, with bone being the electrolyte's major reservoir. Other factors influencing calcium levels include calcitonin, estrogens, androgens, carbohydrates, and lactose. An inverse relationship exists between calcium and phosphate: when calcium decreases, phosphate increases, and vice versa. This relationship is often seen in renal failure.[43]

Increased levels of calcium are seen in hyperparathyroidism, some carcinomas, bone metastasis, dehydration, sarcoidosis, prolonged immobilization, and Addison's disease. Decreased levels of calcium are seen in low-protein states, renal insufficiency with high phosphorus, vitamin D deficiency, pancreatitis, and hypomagnesemia, and with the administration of some drugs.

Magnesium (Mg²⁺)

Magnesium: 1.3 to 2.1 mEq/L

Magnesium, important for muscular contraction, nerve impulse conduction, cardiac function, and coagulation, also plays a role in modulating smooth muscle contractility. The infusion of intravenous magnesium may assist in the relief of acute and unrelenting bronchospasm.[44,45] Magnesium and calcium depend on one another: the presence of magnesium assists in the reabsorption of calcium in the intestines, whereas a lack of magnesium results in the movement of calcium out of bone.[43] In renal insufficiency and failure, magnesium is retained. Increased levels of magnesium are seen in renal failure, antacid use (those with magnesium salts), Addison's disease, and hemolysis.

Although dietary deficiency of magnesium is rare, hypomagnesemia is occasionally seen in chronic alcoholism. Other causes of low magnesium levels include hypocalcemia, hypokalemia, hyperalimentation (long term), intravenous therapy, diabetes mellitus, hyperparathyroidism, diuretic therapy, pregnancy, and hyperaldosteronism.

Phosphorus (P or PO₄)

Phosphorus: 3.0 to 4.5 mg/dL

The majority of total phosphorus is combined with calcium in the bone, with the rest stored intracellularly. Phosphate levels, like calcium levels, are controlled by parathyroid hormone, and phosphate levels are always evaluated in conjunction with calcium levels. As noted earlier, the two exist in an inverse relationship.

Phosphate, which is essential for bone metabolism, for the regulation of calcium, and as a buffer in the maintenance of acid-base balance, is also necessary for the formation of 2,3-DPG. When 2,3-DPG is low, oxygen unloading decreases (shift to the left). Phosphate's presence promotes renal tubular reabsorption of glucose, aids in fat transport, and is essential in the maintenance of energy stores (i.e., adenosine triphosphate).

Increased levels are seen with exercise, dehydration, acromegaly, hypoparathyroidism, bone metastasis, hypervitaminosis D, sarcoidosis, cirrhosis, and renal failure. Low phosphorus levels are frequently seen in conditions in which there is hypercalcemia. Hypophosphatemia is also found in renal tubular acidosis, vitamin D deficiency, hyperparathyroidism, carbohydrate ingestion, malnutrition, hypothyroidism, alcoholism, and rickets.

Blood Urea Nitrogen and Creatinine

Blood urea nitrogen and creatinine levels, most commonly measured to interpret kidney function, are usually considered together. An understanding of each separately, however, assists in accurate interpretation.

Blood Urea Nitrogen

Blood urea nitrogen: 6 to 20 mg/dL

Urea, a nonprotein nitrogenous product formed in the liver from ammonia, is excreted by the kidney. Normally, the production and excretion of urea are balanced; however, levels may be altered with liver function abnormalities, kidney dysfunction, fluid imbalance, and changes in protein intake. For example, with dehydration, the blood urea nitrogen (BUN) level may increase. To determine whether kidney function is the reason for an elevated BUN level, the BUN level must be assessed in conjunction with creatinine. With elevated levels of BUN, encephalopathic changes can include confusion and coma.

Increased BUN levels are seen with impaired renal function, dehydration and shock, gastrointestinal hemorrhage, overwhelming infections, crushing injuries, diabetes, excessive protein breakdown or intake, gout, and some malignancies. Decreased BUN levels are found in conditions such as liver failure, malnutrition, and overhydration.

Creatinine

Creatinine

Male: 0.7 to 1.3 mg/dL
Female: 0.6 to 1.2 mg/dL

Creatinine is the end-product of creatine phosphate breakdown (found in skeletal muscle). Because the formation and excretion of creatinine remain fairly constant, the creatinine level is a more sensitive indicator of renal function than is the BUN level. The creatinine balance is less affected by changes in fluid balance and blood flow. With trauma (and muscle injury) and degenerative diseases, excessive amounts can appear in the blood. When the creatinine level is elevated in the absence of such conditions, renal dysfunction may exist.

Other reasons for increased creatinine levels include obstruction of the urinary tract and chronic nephritis. Decreased levels of creatinine are rare but are seen with muscular dystrophy.

Bilirubin

Bilirubin

Total: 0.2 to 1.0 mg/dL
Conjugated: 0.0 to 0.2 mg/dL
Indirect unconjugated: 0.2 to 0.8
  mg/dL

Bilirubin, a product of the breakdown of the pigmented heme portion of hemoglobin is normally removed from the body by the liver and excreted into the bile. The pigments of the bilirubin provide the yellowish color in urine and bile and the brown color of stool. When serum bilirubin levels increase, the skin appears jaundiced.

Two forms of bilirubin exist, conjugated and unconjugated. Bilirubin attaches to albumin (unconjugated) and circulates in the plasma until it reaches the liver. Here, it separates from the albumin and joins (conjugates) with glucuronic acid. Finally, it is secreted into the intestines as bile, converted to urobilinogen, and excreted into the stool. A small amount is recycled to the liver.

Elevations in the bilirubin level occur secondary to hepatic (hepatitis or cirrhosis), obstructive (bile or liver duct stones), or hemolytic causes (e.g., sickle cell anemia or transfusion reactions). Increases in unconjugated bilirubin are frequently associated with hemolysis, whereas in-

Enzymes **351**

creases in the conjugated form are often associated with liver obstruction or dysfunction.

ENZYMES

Enzymes are complex molecules that serve as catalysts for most biologic clinical reactions. The ones discussed here exist intracellularly. They are released into the bloodstream when cellular damage or necrosis occurs, and their presence often indicates a specific organ tissue necrosis or injury.

Various molecular forms of the same enzyme in different tissues (isoenzymes) also exist. Detection of the isoenzymes serves to differentiate the location of the insult further.

Creatine Kinase (Creatine Phosphokinase) and Isoenzymes

Creatine kinase

Male: 40 to 174 U/L
Female: 96 to 140 U/L

Isoenzymes

MM: 100%
MB: 0%
BB: 0%

Creatine kinase (CK) is located in skeletal, heart, and brain tissues. Because CK elevations can occur with any tissue injury (surgical or traumatic), further differentiation is necessary.

Two distinct CK isoenzymes exist (M for muscle and B for brain), and they appear in different combinations depending on where the tissue injury occurs. With skeletal muscle injury, CK-MM increases, and with brain injury, CK-BB elevation occurs. Both CK-MB levels and CK-MM levels increase with heart damage. CK-MB levels of greater than 4% are associated with acute myocardial infarction. CK and CK-MB levels rise within 3 to 5 hours after acute myocardial infarction. They peak at 6 hours and remain elevated in the serum for 24 to 36 hours. Total CK decreases in 3 days.[46, 47] Determination of the CK level is often diagnostic in the early detection of muscular dystrophy.

Lactic Acid Dehydrogenase

Total LDH (this varies considerably between laboratories)

80 to 120 U (Wacker)
71 to 207 IU/L
150 to 450 U (Wroblewski)

Isoenzymes

LDH_1: 22 to 36%
LDH_2: 35 to 46%
LDH_3: 13 to 26%
LDH_4: 3 to 10%
LDH_5: 2 to 9%

Lactic acid dehydrogenase (LDH), important in the breakdown of glycogen for energy, is present in practically all cells. As noted earlier, isoenzymes exist in different tissues; thus, differentiation is possible as follows:

LDH_1 Heart muscle, red blood cells, and renal cortex
LDH_2 Normal serum (because this enzyme is normally more prevalent in serum than LDH_1, a reversal indicates significant myocardial damage, renal cortex insult, or hemolysis)
LDH_3 Lungs (elevation may indicate lung infarction)
LDH_4 Pancreas and placenta
LDH_5 Liver and skeletal muscle

In myocardial disease, total levels of LDH rise slowly between 24 and 72 hours and remain elevated for 2 weeks. Thus, if CK isoenzymes were not drawn early, this test, in conjunction with clinical and electrocardiographic findings, may be diagnostic.[48]

Serum Glutamic-Oxaloacetic Transaminase (Aspartate Aminotransferase) and Serum Glutamic-Pyruvic Transaminase (Alanine Aminotransferase)

SGOT

Male: 7 to 21 m/L
Female: 6 to 18 m/L

Serum glutamic-oxaloacetic transaminase (SGOT) exists in large concentrations in the heart and the liver, with lesser concentrations found in skeletal muscle, the kidney, and the red blood cells. Because it is not as specific for myocardial damage as is CK or LDH, it is usually assessed in combination with serum glutamic-pyruvic transaminase (SGPT) to determine liver involvement. In myocardial disease, the enzyme level peaks in 24 to 48 hours and returns to normal in approximately 4 to 6 days.[49]

SGPT

Male: 7 to 24 U/L
Female: 6 to 24 U/L

Because SGPT is found primarily in the liver, an elevation in its level is a sensitive indicator of acute hepatocellular injury. It is also used to follow the course of hepatitis and other liver disorders.[49]

Alkaline Phosphatase and Acid Phosphatase

Alkaline phosphatase: 25 to 92 U/L
Acid phosphatase

Male: 2.5 to 11.7 U/L
Female: 0.3 to 9.2 U/L

Alkaline phosphatase, an important enzyme for the production of bone by osteoblasts, is found in bone and liver but is associated primarily with hepatobiliary system function. Bile duct abnormalities affect the serum alkaline phosphatase level. In early obstructive disease of the major bile ducts (i.e., gallstones), the alkaline phosphatase may rise to diagnostic levels.[49] Acid phosphatase, found primarily in the prostate, is a marker for prostatic cancer.

Amylase and Lipase

Amylase: 50 to 150 U/L or 50 to 130 IU/L
Lipase (varies with method): 4 to 24 U/L

The activity of amylase is mostly extracellular: the changing of starch to sugar. The parotid and pancreatic glands, as well as the liver and fallopian tubes, produce and store amylase. Its presence in the blood and excretion in the urine indicates inflammation in or damage to these cells. Urine and serum amylase levels are measured to diagnose pancreatitis, peptic ulcer disease, empyema of the gall bladder, intestinal obstruction, ectopic pregnancy, and peritonitis. In acute pancreatitis, amylase levels can rise to 2000 IU/L in 12 hours, but they fall rapidly, returning to normal within 48 to 72 hours. Lipase levels, which parallel amylase levels, are often also followed in acute pancreatitis. The lipase level rises sooner than the amylase level, and the lipase elevation persists longer in the serum than does the amylase increase.

SUMMARY

The respiratory care practitioner must have a working knowledge of the common laboratory tests performed in the acute care setting. With accurate evaluation of the results of the tests, in conjunction with information on the patient's clinical status and other assessment data, comprehensive and effective patient care planning can occur.

References

1. Erslev A. Humoral regulation of red cell production. Blood 8:349, 1953.
2. Christensen RD. Recombinant erythropoietin. Pediatr Rev 12:244, 1991.

3. Shapiro BA, Harrison RA, Trout CA. Clinical Application of Respiratory Care, 3rd ed. Chicago, Year Book Medical Publishers, 1985.
4. Baker SA, Young DJ. Methemoglobinemia: The hidden diagnosis. Crit Care Nurse 10:50, 1990.
5. Rutherford KA. Principles and application of oximetry. Crit Care Nurs Clin North Am 1:649, 1989.
6. Rochester DF, Arora NS. Respiratory muscle failure. Med Clin North Am 67:573, 1983.
7. Golde DW, Cline MJ. Regulation of granulopoiesis. N Engl J Med 291:1388, 1974.
8. Malech HL, Gallin JI. Immunology: Neutrophils in human diseases. N Engl J Med 317:687, 1987.
9. Johnston RB. Current concepts: Immunology monocytes and macrophages. N Engl J Med 318:747, 1988.
10. Nathan CF, Prendergast TJ, Wiebe ME, et al. Activation of human macrophages: Comparison of other cytokines with interferon-γ. J Exp Med 160:600, 1984.
11. Rowlands DT, Daniele RP. Surface receptors in the immune response. N Engl J Med 293:26, 1975.
12. Cooper MD. B lymphocytes: Normal development and function. N Engl J Med 317:1452, 1987.
13. Tami JA, Parr MO, Thompson JS. The immune system. Am J Hosp Pharm 43:2483, 1986.
14. Sanders-Laufer D, DeBruin W, Edelson PJ. Pneumocystis carinii infections in HIV-infected children. Pediatr Clin North Am 38:69, 1991.
15. Bartlett MS, Smith JW. Pneumocystis carinii, an opportunist in immunocompromised patients. Clin Microbiol Rev 1:137, 1991.
16. Hughes WT. Pneumocystis carinii: Taxing taxonomy. Eur J Epidemiol 5:265, 1989.
17. Stringer SL, Stringer JR, Blase MA, et al. Pneumocystis carinii: Sequence from ribosomal RNA implies a close relationship with fungi. Exp Parasitol 68:150, 1989.
18. Miles PR, Baughman RP, Linnemann CC. Cytomegalovirus in the bronchoalveolar lavage fluid of patients with AIDS. Chest 97:1072, 1990.
19. Merigan TC, Resta S. Cytomegalovirus: Where have we been and where are we going? Rev Infect Dis 12(Suppl 7):693, 1990.
20. Rook AH. Interactions of cytomegalovirus with the human immune system. Rev Infect Dis 10(Suppl 3):S460, 1988.
21. Frenkel LD, Gaur S, Tsolia M, et al. Cytomegalovirus infection in children with AIDS. Rev Infect Dis 12(Suppl 7):S820, 1990.
22. Whelan WL, Kirsch DR, Kwon-Chung KJ, et al. Candida albicans in patients with the acquired immunodeficiency syndrome: Absence of a novel of hypervirulent strain. J Infect Dis 162:513, 1990.
23. Matthews R, Burnie J, Smith O, et al. Candida and AIDS: Evidence for protective antibody. Lancet 2:263, 1988.
24. Horsburgh CR, Havlik JA, Ellis DA, et al. Survival of patients with acquired immune deficiency syndrome and disseminated mycobacterium avium complex infection with and without antimycobacterial chemotherapy. Am Rev Respir Dis 144:557, 1991.
25. Horsburgh CR, Selik RM. The epidemiology of disseminated nontuberculosis mycobacterial infection in the acquired immunodeficiency syndrome (AIDS). Am Rev Respir Dis 139:4, 1989.
26. Chiu J, Nussbaum J, Bozzette S, et al. Treatment of disseminated mycobacterium avium complex infection in AIDS with amikacin, ethambutol, rifampin, and ciprofloxacin. Ann Intern Med 113:358, 1990.
27. Benson CA, Kessler HA, Pottage JC, et al. Successful treatment of acquired immunodeficiency syndrome-related mycobacterium avium complex disease with a multiple drug regimen including amikacin. Arch Intern Med 151:582, 1991.
28. Jordan TJ, Lewit E, Montgomery RL, et al. Isoniazid as preventive therapy in HIV-infected intravenous drug abusers: A decision analysis. JAMA 265:2987, 1991.
29. Tuberculosis outbreak among persons in a residential facility for HIV-infected persons—San Francisco. MMWR 40:649, 1991.
30. Nosocomial transmission of multidrug-resistant tuberculosis among HIV-infected persons—Florida and New York, 1988–1991. MMWR 40:585, 1991.
31. Schneiderman E. Thrombocytopenia in the critically ill patient. Crit Care Nurs Q 13:1, 1990.
32. Cola C, Ansell J. Heparin-induced thrombocytopenia and arterial thrombosis: Alternative therapies. Am Heart J 119(2 Pt 1):368, 1990.
33. Brady J, Riccio JA, Yumen OH, et al. Plasmapheresis. A therapeutic option in the management of heparin associated thrombocytopenia with thrombosis. Am J Clin Pathol 96:394, 1991.
34. Weiss HJ. Platelet physiology and abnormalities of platelet function (Parts I and II). N Engl J Med 293:531, 580, 1975.
35. Green D. Disseminated intravascular coagulation. Crit Care Nurs Q 13:7, 1990.
36. Young LM. DIC: The insidious killer. Crit Care Nurs 10:26, 1990.
37. Carr JM, McKinney M, McDonagh J. Diagnosis of disseminated intravascular coagulation: Role of D-dimer. Am J Clin Pathol 91:280, 1989.
38. Isley WL. Serum sodium concentration abnormalities. Crit Care Nurs Q 13:82, 1990.
39. Calhoun KA. Serum potassium concentration abnormalities. Crit Care Nurs Q 13:34, 1990.

40. Dhingra S, Solven F, Wilson A, McCarthy DS. Hypomagnesemia and respiratory muscle power. Am Rev Respir Dis 129:497, 1984.
41. Agusti AGN, Torres A, Estopa R, Agustividal A. Hypophosphatemia as a cause of failed weaning: The importance of metabolic factors. Crit Care Med 12:142, 1984.
42. Newman JH, Neff TA, Ziporin P. Acute respiratory failure associated with hypophosphatemia. N Engl J Med 296:1101, 1977.
43. Graves L. Disorders of calcium phosphorus and magnesium. Crit Care Nurs Q 13:3, 1990.
44. Rolla G, Bucca C. Hypomagnesemia and bronchial hyperreactivity. Allergy 44:519, 1989.
45. Gold ME, Buga GM, Wood KS, et al. Antagonistic modulatory roles of magnesium and calcium on release of endothelium–derived relaxing factor and smooth muscle tone. Circ Res 66:355, 1990.
46. Doran GR, Flech A. Limitation of serum creatine kinase assay in diagnosis of acute myocardial infarction. Lancet 336:697, 1990.
47. Fisher ML, Plotnich GD. Diagnostic tests for MI: Efficacy and cost containment. Hosp Pract 11:195–213, 1984.
48. Hamfelt A, Moller BHJ, Soderhjelm L. Use of biochemical tests for myocardial infarction in the county of Vasternorrland, a clinical chemistry routine for the diagnosis of myocardial infarction. Scand J Clin Lab Invest 50(Suppl 200):20, 1990.
49. Bozzuto TM. Other enzymes: Creatinine phosphokinase, lactate dehydrogenase, serum glutamic oxaloacetic transaminase, serum glutamic pyruvic transaminase, and alkaline phosphatase. Emerg Med Clin North Am 4:329, 1986.

Suggested Readings

Cella JH, Watson J. Nurse's Manual of Laboratory Tests. Philadelphia, FA Davis, 1989.
Dolan JT. Critical Care Nursing: Clinical Management Through the Nursing Process. Philadelphia, FA Davis, 1991.
Fischbach F. A Manual of Laboratory Diagnostic Tests. Philadelphia, JB Lippincott, 1988.
Griffin JP. Hematology and Immunology Concepts for Nursing. Norwalk, CT, Appleton-Century-Crofts, 1986.
Hillman RS, Finch CA. Red Cell Manual, 5th ed. Philadelphia, FA Davis, 1985.
Jacobs DS, Kasten BL, DeMott WR, Wolfson WL. Laboratory Test Handbook. Cleveland, Lexi Comp/Mosby, 1988.
Kinney MR, Packa DR, Dunbar SB. AACN Clinical Reference for Critical-Care Nursing, 2nd ed. New York, McGraw-Hill Book Company, 1988.
Pittiglio DH. Clinical Hematology and Fundamentals of Hemostasis. Philadelphia, FA Davis, 1987.
Rifkind RJ, Bank A, Marks PA, et al. Fundamentals of Hematology, 3rd ed. Chicago, Year Book Medical Publishers, 1986.

19

Blood Gas and Acid-Base Measurement

George H. Hicks, M.S., R.R.T.

Arterial blood gas determinations are the most common laboratory measurements ordered for patients in the intensive care unit, emergency department, and operating room environments.[6]

Blood was first described to be slightly alkaline by Des Plantes in 1776, and oxygen and carbon dioxide were detected by Davy in 1799.[1] Since these discoveries, the techniques used to quantify blood gas and hydrogen ion concentrations have continued to evolve. From the mid-1800s into the early 1900s, there was considerable debate between Ludwig, Pfluger, and others about the exact mechanism of gas movement between alveolar gas, blood, and tissue.[1] To reach accurate conclusions, the precise analysis of oxygen and carbon dioxide was perfected. This set the stage for the clinical use of blood gas and acid-base analysis for the understanding and treatment of patients with respiratory, cardiovascular, and metabolic abnormalities.

In the first half of the 1900s, chemical techniques were refined by Van Slyke, Scholander, and others for the precise manometric or volumetric detection of gases.[2-5] These methods, however, are cumbersome and slow, require exacting precision, and pose potential health hazards to the person performing the measurement. These drawbacks, coupled with advances in oxygen therapy, ventilatory support, and extracorporeal gas exchange over the second half of this century, have driven the development of easily used, highly accurate, and fast response analyzers.

Today, blood gas and pH determinations are routine measurements. These measurements provide a cornerstone in the diagnosis and management of the patient in cardiopulmonary distress. Frequently, blood gas results, rather than bedside physical findings, signal the presence and magnitude of an oxygenation, ventilation, and acid-base disorder. However, each step in the measurement process can introduce errors that can mislead the clinician and direct him or her to potential therapeutic misadventures. For these reasons, the accuracy of blood gas and acid-base balance measurements carries more potential impact on immediate patient care than most other laboratory determinations and types of monitoring.

INVASIVE MEASUREMENT TECHNIQUES

Indications for Invasive Sampling and Analysis

Arterial blood sampling and determination of P_{O_2}, P_{CO_2}, pH, and other variables represent a "snapshot" of the patient's respiratory gas and acid-base status. These measurements are considered indispensable in determining a patient's condition and response to treatment. Repeated sampling from unstable, critically ill patients who require intensive care is not uncommon. This approach reveals trends in the patient's condition. Although there are many benefits from routine and frequent analysis, this approach to monitoring respiratory function is expensive and not always necessary. The development of both noninvasive (e.g., pulse ox-

355

imetry) and invasive (e.g., fiberoptic oxyhemoglobin saturation catheter) monitors provides ongoing "real-time" information and reduces the need for more frequent arterial sampling. These technologic advances, coupled with the development of guidelines for sampling (Table 19–1) and the use of an intensive care unit "stat blood gas laboratory" controlled by respiratory care practitioners, have improved the appropriate use of blood gas analysis from 53 to 75% in retrospective studies.[7, 8] This rational approach to sampling, along with the use of noninvasive monitors, will become increasingly important in the development of quality improvement programs that guide the need for blood gas sampling and analysis.

Knowledge of the Patient's Condition

Before collecting blood for analysis and interpretation, the clinician must have an understanding of the patient's current condition. Table 19–2 summarizes the major factors that should be known.

A review of the patient's chart for the physician's order and the current diagnosis should precede any sampling. The chart should then be checked for any information indicating if the patient may carry an infectious disease that may be transmitted by contact with blood. In all

Infections transmitted by blood include human immunodeficiency virus infection (HIV types 1 and 2), viral hepatitis (types A, B, and C), infection with Epstein-Barr virus (the cause of mononucleosis), syphilis, bacterial septicemia, and the rare Jakob-Creutzfeldt virus–induced neurologic disease.

TABLE **19–1:** Guidelines for Appropriate Sampling for Blood Gas and pH Analysis

Yes to one or more of the following suggests the need for sampling:

Procedural Indicators
1. Is the patient on ventilatory support a new admission to the intensive care unit?
2. Is the $F_{I_{O_2}} > 0.60$ and has it been > 3 hr since the last ABG or Sp_{O_2} analysis?
3. Is the PEEP or CPAP > 10 cm H_2O and has it been > 3 hr since the last ABG or Sp_{O_2} analysis?
4. Is the patient to be extubated and has it been > 1 hr since the last ABG analysis?

Clinical Indicators
1. Does the patient exhibit any of the following?
   a. Absence of breath sounds
   b. Asynchronous breathing
   c. Cyanosis
   d. Diaphoresis
   e. Pallor
   f. Unexpected dysrhythmia
   g. Unexpected change in mental status
2. Has there been an unexpected change of ± 20% in respiratory rate, or > 35 or < 5 breaths per minute?
3. Has there been an unexpected change of ± 30% in heart rate?
4. Has there been an unexpected change of ± 30% in systolic blood pressure?
5. Has there been an unexpected change of ± 20% in cardiac output?
6. Has there been an unexpected and sustained increase of > 5 mm Hg in ICP or an absolute ICP of > 25 mm Hg?
7. Does the patient's previous ABG report or oximetry findings show any of the following?
   a. $Pa_{O_2} < 60$ or > 125 mm Hg?
   b. $Sa_{O_2} < 85\%$?
   c. $Pa_{CO_2} > 65$ or < 20 mm Hg?
   d. pH > 7.55 or < 7.30?

Therapeutic Indicators
1. Has there been an extubation or a change in a respiratory support variable ($F_{I_{O_2}}$, V_T, f, PEEP or CPAP, mode)?
2. Has there been a change in bronchodilator or vasoactive medication?

Modified from Beasley KE, Darin JM, Durbin CG Jr. The effect of respiratory care department management of a blood gas analyzer on the appropriateness of arterial blood gas utilization. Respir Care 37:343, 1992.

ABG, arterial blood gas; CPAP, continuous positive airway pressure; ICP, intracranial pressure; PEEP, positive end-expiratory pressure.

TABLE **19–2:** Factors That Should Be Known Before Sampling Blood

Patient's diagnosis
Patient's infectious disease status
Patient's blood coagulation status
Patient's vital signs and values from noninvasive monitors
Current respiratory care modalities in use
Amount of time the patient has been in a steady state

Hemophilia—a genetic defect that results in an inability to synthesize coagulation factor XIII
Thrombocytopenia—a blood platelet count of less than 200,000/mm³

Blood sampling by needle puncture may need to precede administration of the next anticoagulant or thrombolytic by 30 minutes to help avoid excessive bleeding.

Patients with chronic obstructive pulmonary disease require more than 20 minutes to reach a steady state after F_{IO_2} adjustments.[12] The recommended practice is to wait 20 to 30 minutes after any oxygen therapy, ventilator use, or other therapy to reach steady-state conditions.[13]

cases, universal body fluid precautions *must* always be practiced, whether the infectious disease information is available or not.

Blood coagulation disorders and medications that interfere with the clotting mechanism should be evaluated. Sampling blood from a patient who has a coagulation defect or is receiving an anticoagulant leads to greater bleeding from needle puncture sites, which results in large hematomas. Hemophilia, thrombocytopenia, and other clotting factor deficiencies (e.g., from liver failure) are conditions that prolong clotting time and promote excessive bleeding. Either of these conditions may require a noninvasive approach to determine blood gases (e.g., pulse oximetry, transcutaneous Po_2 and Pco_2, or capnometry).

The drugs that the patient is currently receiving should be reviewed for evidence of anticoagulant or thrombolytic therapies that may be in use. Commonly used anticoagulants include heparin, warfarin (Coumadin), and aspirin. Streptokinase (Streptase), a potent bacterial enzyme with thrombolytic action, is used as a clot "buster" in the treatment of vascular occlusive disorders (e.g., coronary artery disease).

Understanding the patient's current vital signs and psychological status is very useful in interpreting the data. The components of the vital signs (heart rate, blood pressure, respiratory rate, and temperature) are broad indicators of physiologic stability and response to stress. The patient's temperature is frequently desired so that "corrections" can be made in the blood gas and pH results. However, these corrected values may actually give the clinician the wrong impression and lead to the wrong therapeutic decisions (e.g., accepting "normal" corrected blood pH and Pco_2 values from a patient with a core temperature of 25°C). Of greater importance, the vital signs record gives the clinician an indication of the patient's stability over time—the patient's steady-state status. Patients who are anxious or in pain frequently hyperventilate or breath hold and distort the results from a true steady state.

The type and adjustments of respiratory care in use should also be evaluated. Oxygen concentration (F_{IO_2}), ventilatory rate, exhaled minute ventilation, and level of positive end-expiratory pressure should be recorded for the blood gas report. Values from other respiratory monitors (e.g., pulse oximetry findings, end-tidal CO_2, and transcutaneous O_2 and CO_2) should be recorded. The current settings and conditions should be stable or at steady-state conditions long enough for the conditions at sample collection to resemble steady-state conditions. If a patient is free of significant lung disease and stable for as little as 3 to 10 minutes, blood gas and acid-base values will reach steady-state conditions following adjustments in F_{IO_2}.[9–11] If samples are taken before a steady state is reached, the results give an inaccurate picture of the patient's true steady-state condition. Some patients will be very unstable when sample collection is necessary, and the results should be evaluated in the light of their unstable condition. This can result in values that make them appear either better or worse than they actually are. A requisition slip

TABLE **19–3:**   Data the Complete Requisition Slip Should Contain

Patient's name, code number, or both
Location of patient
Date and time of sampling
Sampling site
Ventilation parameters
   Spontaneous breathing rate
   Mechanical ventilation mode, set rate, total rate, V_T and $F_{I_{O_2}}$
   PEEP or CPAP level
Data from noninvasive respiratory monitors
   Pulse oximetry
   Transcutaneous P_{O_2} and P_{CO_2}
   End-tidal P_{CO_2}
Body temperature and location of measurement
Activity: quiet, asleep, under anesthesia, comatose, anxious, crying, agitated, or
   convulsing
Diagnosis
Name of physician requesting the measurement
Name or initials of the clinician who obtained the sample

Modified from National Committee for Clinical Laboratory Standards. Percutaneous Collection of Arterial Blood for Laboratory Analysis [Approved standard]. Villanova, PA, National Committee for Clinical Laboratory Standards, 1985. NCCLS publication H11-A.
   CPAP, continuous positive airway pressure; PEEP, positive end-expiratory pressure.

that documents sampling conditions must be prepared at the time of blood sampling. It should contain the information listed in Table 19–3.

Blood Sampling Techniques

A variety of periodic and continuous invasive sampling techniques are available to the clinician. Periodic sampling of blood followed by in vitro analysis in a remote laboratory is the usual method for determining respiratory gas tension, saturation, and pH. Periodic sampling techniques have been refined since the mid-1970s to reduce preanalytic and analytic errors, but they still have some major disadvantages. They provide a snapshot of the patient's condition, which can change within minutes after sampling. Significant time delays (e.g., 10 to more than 60 minutes) often occur between sampling and reporting of the data, which can delay necessary therapeutic adjustments. The neonatal patient can lose significant amounts of blood from serial sampling. An extensive amount of expensive clinician time is necessary for sampling and analysis. Despite these reasons, periodic sampling continues to play an important role in the initial and ongoing assessment of the patient. This protocol will remain the gold standard with which other methods will be compared.

Continuous sampling or monitoring employs invasive sensors, noninvasive sensors, or both for in vivo measurements. Continuous sampling is indicated for patients who are at high risk for decompensation or for those who are unstable in whom the benefits outweigh the risks. This approach permits the clinician to "see" the patient's real-time condition. Early warning signs of deterioration can be detected before significant physiologic alterations occur. The patient's response to therapeutic changes can be seen immediately, which allows greater therapeutic precision. This approach also reduces blood loss and the risk of exposing the clinician to blood samples.

Continuous sampling is not without disadvantages. The invasive techniques require intravascular catheters, which increase the risks to the patient and introduce calibration difficulties and potential analytic errors. These disadvantages can give erroneous data that may lead to inaction or result in inappropriate therapeutic decisions.

Arterial Puncture

Systemic arterial blood gas and acid-base composition is the product of lung, cardiovascular, kidney, and metabolic functions. This blood is chemically the same throughout the arterial circuit and therefore is the preferred sample to analyze for evaluating gas exchange and acid-base balance.

Having all the necessary equipment at hand when the sample is to be collected allows the process to proceed smoothly and quickly. The items needed include

Needle
Needle protection device (e.g., Needle-Pro, Concord/Portex)
Syringe
Anticoagulant
Capping device for the syringe
Antiseptic swabs (iodine, chlorhexidine, or alcohol)
Sterile gauze pads (e.g., 2 × 2 inch)
Band-Aid or tape
Syringe identification label
Container holding ice for transport[14]

The smaller needles frequently require some gentle aspiration by pulling back on the syringe plunger to assist blood collection.[15] When smaller needles are used, careful attention to technique results in little effect on blood gas composition.[16]

A very sharp, short-beveled 20- to 25-gauge needle with a clear hub for visualization of blood entry should be used. Although a 1-inch-long 22- or 23-gauge needle is the size more commonly used in adults, a ⅝-inch-long 25-gauge needle should be used with small children, infants, and patients who may bleed easily.[14]

To avoid excessive dilution of the sample with anticoagulant, the syringe size (1, 3, or 5 mL) should be no larger than the sample size to be collected.[14] Its smooth filling action and easy ability to clear air bubbles make the glass syringe the preferred collection container. Glass syringes also provide a gas-impermeable barrier to the atmosphere so that sample gases remain unaltered. Special plastic syringes have been designed for smooth spontaneous filling and come prepackaged with heparin. More attention is necessary to clear air bubbles from the sample because they appear to stick to the walls of plastic syringes. Plastic syringes may alter the gas composition of the specimen to a minor degree because of the ability of the gases to diffuse through the syringe wall. At normal partial pressures, these changes are greater for carbon dioxide than for oxygen.[17, 18] Sampling of blood with a very low P_{O_2} (e.g., from the pulmonary artery) and leaving the sample stored for a prolonged period can actually result in diffusion of oxygen from the atmosphere into the sample and cause the P_{O_2} to be artifactually high.[19] When routine arterial samples are collected with plastic syringes and analyzed within 10 to 15 minutes, the differences in gas tensions are clinically insignificant.[16, 20, 21] These findings, coupled with the availability of these syringes in low-cost, commercially prepared kits for single patient use, make the plastic syringe the preferred arterial blood collection device in many hospitals.

Evacuated blood collection tubes are routinely used for numerous clinical laboratory tests. A special tube developed with 100% nitrogen at subatmospheric pressure for the collection of arterial blood for blood gas determination was found to be effective.[22] However, the evacuated tube is not recommended for routine arterial blood gas collection because of its potential for subatmospheric-induced blood gas tension changes.[13]

Collected blood begins to clot shortly after exposure to the foreign surface of a syringe. Contact with the syringe initiates the intrinsic clotting mechanism, which starts with activation of the Hageman factor (factor XII). Clot formation needs to be completely avoided in collecting and analyzing blood gases. Clots interfere with blood collection, plug the fine plumbing of the blood gas analyzer, and alter or halt the performance of the analyzer. Heparin salts are considered to be the best anticoagulants for blood gas analysis.[13] An aqueous solution of heparin salt is slightly acidic and contains gases that are in equilibrium with air. When large amounts of a sodium heparin solution are mixed with blood, the gas tensions, pH, and Na^+ values can be substantially altered.[16, 23, 24] This is especially important when very small samples (e.g., 0.2 mL) are collected in syringes. Fifty international units of heparin is sufficient to anticoagulate 1 mL of blood. Thus, a syringe should contain 0.05 mL of a 1000-IU/mL solution of aqueous heparin per milliliter of blood to be collected. A standard 5-mL syringe with a 1-inch-long 22-gauge needle has a dead space volume of 0.2 mL. When this dead space is filled with a 1000-IU/mL solution of heparin, this will prevent coagulation and avoid heparin dilution errors.[13] Lithium heparin is the heparin of choice when the blood sample will be split for analysis of gases, pH, and electrolytes.

Some commercially prepared blood gas sample kits have syringes that contain 100 to 200 IU of lyophilized or dry lithium heparin that coats the needle and syringe barrel. This approach reduces syringe preparation time, effectively prevents clot formation, and eliminates heparin dilution–induced errors.

Blood, which is metabolically active, continues to consume oxygen and produce carbon dioxide in the syringe after collection. These changes are clinically insignificant if the sample is analyzed within 10 minutes.[16] These changes can be intensified if the sample is taken from a patient with a leukocytosis (e.g., leukemia), which causes the oxygen tension to drop more rapidly as a result of the numerous aerobic leukocytes.[25] To reduce these changes, the metabolic activity of blood can be quenched by cooling the sample down to 0 to 5°C for analysis up to 1 or 2 hours later. This cooling can be achieved by placing the sample-filled syringe in a container (cup, basin, or zip-lock bag) filled with finely chipped ice or a slurry of ice chips and water that covers the syringe.

The hazards of arterial puncture include arteriospasm, bleeding and hematoma formation, thrombosis, puncture injuries to surrounding tissues (e.g., nearby nerves), infection, pain, anxiety, and fainting.[26–28] For these reasons, the sampling site is selected on the basis of sufficient collateral circulation, accessibility, and the risk of injury to periarterial tissues.[14]

Arterial blood is collected anaerobically by inserting a sharp beveled needle with an attached syringe into the selected artery. The system should be leak-proof and free of any air bubbles. The arterial blood pressure is sufficient to force blood into a low-drag or well-lubricated syringe. Table 19–4 outlines the steps used for percutaneous arterial blood sampling, as shown in Figure 19–2.

Sample Sites

The radial artery best meets the previously mentioned criteria and is the site of first choice.[14, 29] Although relatively small, it is easily palpated in the wrist over the lateral edge and distal end of the radius. In

In the adult, the most common sample sites include the radial, brachial, femoral, and dorsalis pedis arteries (Fig. 19–1). The carotid artery is highly accessible, but using it is very dangerous because of the risks of introducing air or clot emboli during or after sampling and potential injury to numerous surrounding vital tissues.

Collateral circulation of the hand is provided by the ulnar artery in most individuals.

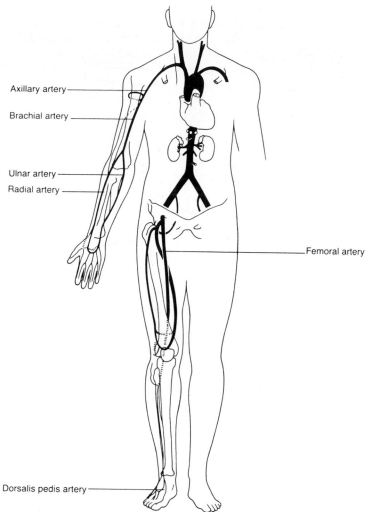

Axillary artery

Brachial artery

Ulnar artery

Radial artery

Femoral artery

Dorsalis pedis artery

FIGURE 19–1: The common arterial puncture sites used in the collection of blood for blood gas and pH determination. (Modified from Jacob SW, Francone CA. Structure and Function in Man, 2nd ed. Philadelphia, WB Saunders, 1970, p 456.)

infants, a transillumination light has been found to be useful in localizing the radial artery.[30] Because of its superficial location, it is easily compressed to prevent hematoma formation after the puncture. The modified Allen test (Fig. 19–3) or the use of a Doppler ultrasonic blood flow detector is effective in determining the ability of the ulnar artery to provide collateral blood flow.[31] If collateral flow is poor or nonexistent, another site should be evaluated.

The brachial artery, which is larger than the radial artery, should be the second selection site if both radial arteries are found to be unacceptable. Collateral circulation is usually adequate.[14, 27] However, this artery is more difficult to puncture successfully because of its deeper location between muscle and connective tissue. This is often true in attempting to take a sample from a patient with very fleshy arms, in whom the pulse is more difficult to palpate. Because of its deep location, it is also more difficult to compress sufficiently, and as a consequence, a greater chance of hematoma formation exists.[27]

The brachial artery is located by palpating over the anterior bend of the elbow toward the median aspect at the distal end of the biceps brachii muscle.

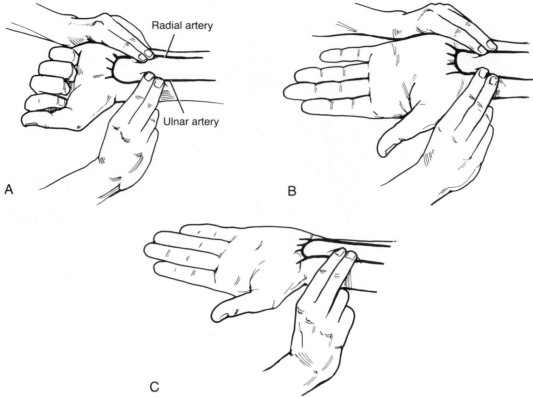

FIGURE 19–2: The modified Allen test. *A,* The radial and ulnar arteries are occluded by applying pressure to them while the patient's hand is clenched into a tight fist two or three times. *B,* The hand is opened while pressure is maintained on the arteries. The clinician should note the blanched palm color. *C,* Pressure is released from the ulnar artery, and the palm should flush with color within 5 to 15 seconds. This is a positive Allen test finding and indicates acceptable collateral circulation through the ulnar artery. If the hand flushes poorly in more than 15 seconds, an alternative site should be chosen. (*A* to *C,* From Malley WJ. Clinical Blood Gases—Application and Noninvasive Alternatives. Philadelphia, WB Saunders, 1990, p 14.)

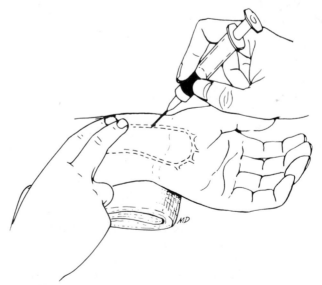

FIGURE 19–3: The radial artery puncture. The wrist is extended approximately 30 degrees over a rolled towel, and the puncture is made at a 45-degree angle, with the bevel of the needle up and directed into the oncoming arterial flow. (From Malley WJ. Clinical Blood Gases—Application and Noninvasive Alternatives. Philadelphia, WB Saunders, 1990, p 16.)

TABLE **19–4:** Steps for Percutaneous Arterial Blood Sampling

1. Locate, greet, and identify the patient. Explain the procedure and have the patient sit or place him or her in a semi-Fowler position. Complete the requisition and information slip.
2. Wash your hands, put on gloves, and select the site for puncture through evaluation of the pulse.
3. Anesthetize the puncture site with a local anesthetic (0.25 mL of 0.5% lidocaine) with a 25-gauge needle after cleansing the site with an antiseptic swab. Many clinicians, however, do not believe that this is necessary.
4. Prepare the sampling syringe by aseptically drawing up 0.5 mL of a 1000-IU/mL lithium heparin solution into the syringe, wetting the entire inside of the syringe barrel. Carefully remove the needle used to draw up the heparin solution and replace it with the needle to be used for the puncture, and (while holding the syringe with the needle up in a vertical orientation) expel the air and excess heparin solution, leaving heparin in the needle and syringe dead space. No air bubbles should be left in the syringe. If a commercial blood gas sampling kit is to be used, carefully follow the manufacturer's instructions for preparing the syringe.
5. Clean the puncture site with an antiseptic swab (e.g., iodine), and maintain asepsis by using sterile gloves and needle. With the prepared syringe in one hand, palpate the site with the other hand to determine the exact puncture site. Visualize the artery in your mind as you determine its pulsing location. Extending the patient's hand over a folded towel is often helpful. The syringe is held at a 45-degree angle, with the bevel of the needle up and directed toward the upstream pathway of the artery (see Fig. 19–3). Puncture the skin over the artery about 5 mm below the site where you are palpating the pulse. The needle is advanced until blood is observed to "flash" into the clear hub of the needle. If you miss, withdraw the needle until the tip is just below the skin (do not withdraw it completely), pivot the needle toward the location of the pulse, and advance until you see the "flash" of blood. Blood will spontaneously fill the syringe. Assist it by gently pulling on the syringe plunger if necessary. After a sufficient volume has been collected (2 to 3 mL from adults, 0.5 to 1.0 mL from children, and 0.2 mL from infants), the needle is quickly withdrawn, a sterile gauze pad is firmly pressed over the puncture site for a minimum of 5 min, and the needle protection device is safely closed over the needle. If the patient is on anticoagulants or you are sampling from the femoral or brachial sites, pressure over the site should be increased (for as long as 20 min when anticoagulants are being used). Pressure bandages should not be used as a substitute. Inspect the puncture site 2 min after relieving the pressure for evidence of hematoma formation, and cover the site with a Band-Aid. Check for a downstream pulse before you leave the patient.
6. Carefully remove the needle within the protection device from the syringe, expel any air bubbles that are present, and cap the syringe. Careful attention is necessary during these steps to avoid an accidental needle stick or any kind of exposure to blood. Mix the sample by rolling the syringe between your hands, attach the patient label to the syringe, and place it in the transport container that has the ice water slurry.

Adapted from National Committee for Clinical Laboratory Standards. [Approved standard]. Villanova, PA, National Committee for Clinical Laboratory Standards, 1985. NCCLS publication H11-A.

The femoral artery, which is a large artery that is easily palpated just below the inguinal ligament in the groin, has virtually no collateral circulation. Its location makes aseptic technique difficult. Its deep location also makes compression of the puncture site less effective and increases the risk of excessive bleeding into the fascial planes of the leg, which can go undetected. In addition, because the femoral vein is located in the same area, there is an increased incidence of accidental venous sampling. This site should be used only when the radial and brachial sites are not palpable and there is an emergency need for sampling.

The dorsalis pedis artery is a superficial artery that can easily be palpated on the superior surface of the foot midway between the great toe and the ankle. Although easily punctured, it is not commonly used as a sampling site.

The temporal artery, which is sometimes used as a sampling site in small children and infants,[14] is located almost directly above the auditory meatus and at about eye level. This small artery can be successfully punctured with a 25-gauge butterfly scalp vein needle plus a syringe attached to the adapter of the short polypropylene connecting tube.

Arterialized Capillary Stick

Sampling from the radial, temporal, dorsalis pedis, and posterior tibial arteries has been performed effectively in infants.[32] A more common method of blood collection in the infant and small child is the capillary sampling technique. Capillary sampling is simple and is less hazardous in this size patient than is the arterial puncture method just described. Frequent capillary sampling is less necessary now for the evaluation of oxygenation and ventilation because there is widespread availability of the pulse oximeter and transcutaneous oxygen and carbon dioxide electrodes. Capillary sampling is still useful for occasional spot checking of oxygenation, ventilation, and acid-base balance.

The reliability of this technique is based on the ability to dilate and arterialize the capillary bed by warming. Theoretically, this results in flushing of the capillary bed with arterial blood. Numerous studies comparing arterial and arterialized capillary PO_2, PCO_2, and pH values[33-37] show a strong correlation in pH and PCO_2 when the patient has good blood pressure and good technique is used. Capillary PO_2 values are generally lower than arterial ones. Heel stick sampling produces general correlation for PO_2 but becomes less reliable as the arterial value exceeds 60 mm Hg. Samples collected from the fingers or toes appear to have a stronger correlation for PO_2 than do those collected from heel sticks.

The supplies needed include a sterile lance, a heparinized 100-μL capillary tube, an antiseptic swab, a sterile gauze pad (2 $\times$ 2 inch), a Band-Aid, tube caps, a metal mixing "flea," a mixing magnet, and a transport container with ice water slurry.

Table 19–5 outlines the steps for the capillary sampling shown in Figure 19–4.

Systemic Artery Catheter Sampling

The indwelling arterial catheter, or A line, provides continuous access to direct measurement of systemic blood pressure and arterial blood sampling. When the patient's blood pressure drops, it becomes more

---

TABLE **19–5:** Steps for Arterialized Capillary Sampling

1. Locate, identify, and reassure the patient. Place the patient in a supine or semi-Fowler position and complete the requisition and information slip.
2. Wash your hands, put on gloves, and select the site for puncture (earlobe, lateral heel, great toe, or fingertip). Warm the site to 42°C for 10 min with a heated compress, heat lamp, or commercially prepared exothermic chemical pack. Clean the skin with an antiseptic swab.
3. Puncture the site to a depth of no more than 2.5 mm. Wipe the first drop of blood away and then place one end of a level heparinized capillary tube into the blood that flows out of the wound. Blood will be collected in the tube by capillary action. Avoid squeezing blood from the site or it will result in contaminating the free-flowing arterial blood with venous blood. Care should also be directed to preventing air bubbles from being collected with the blood. When the tube is at least 75% full, cap one end.
4. Clean the puncture site with an alcohol swab and cover it with a Band-Aid. Place the steel mixing "flea" in the capillary tube and run it back and forth through the tube with the aid of a magnet for 10 sec to mix the sample with the heparin. Remove the flea, cap both ends of the tube, and place it in the transport container with the ice water slurry.

Adapted from National Committee for Clinical Laboratory Standards. Percutaneous Collection of Arterial Blood for Laboratory Analysis [Approved standard]. Villanova, PA, National Committee for Clinical Laboratory Standards, 1985. NCCLS publication H11-A; and Schreiner RL, Lemons JA, Kisling JA, Meyer CL. Techniques of obtaining arterial blood. *In* Schreiner RL, Kisling JA (eds). Practical Neonatal Respiratory Care. New York, Raven Press, 1982.

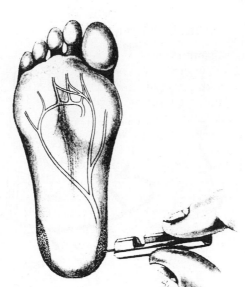

FIGURE 19–4: Heel sticks for arterialized capillary sampling can be collected from the lateral aspects of the plantar surface of the foot. (From Goldsmith JP, Karotkin EH. Assisted Ventilation of the Newborn, 2nd ed. Philadelphia, WB Saunders, 1988, p 221.)

difficult to obtain an arterial sample by the percutaneous technique described previously. Thus, the arterial catheter is the ideal tool for an unstable patient who requires continuous blood pressure monitoring and frequent blood gas and pH determinations.

Any of the arteries described earlier can be catheterized. The radial artery is the most common choice for catheter placement in the adult and the child. The umbilical and temporal arteries are preferred with the neonate. The length of time the catheter can be used can vary from short-term monitoring during exercise studies to longer periods of up to 7 days in the critically ill.[38] The use of a pressurized heparin low-flow infusion system (Fig. 19–5), which is necessary for long-term maintenance of a patent catheter, reduces the risk of thrombosis. The major complications associated with radial artery catheterization include

Hemorrhage
Thrombosis
Gangrenous extremity
Infection
Pain[28]

Temporary occlusion of the radial artery is fairly common after initial placement of the catheter; however, it results in little or no clinical changes in the extremity.[39] Smaller catheters are associated with less frequent occlusion.[40] If the hand becomes cool, the catheter should be removed immediately. A study of arterial catheter use in critically ill patients demonstrated an 18% infection rate at the catheter site and 5% developed septicemia.[41] With proper care, the overall rate of major complications has been reported to be approximately 1%.[42]

After the appropriate peripheral artery site has been located and the catheter system has been assembled, an 18- or 20-gauge Teflon catheter can be introduced into the artery by several techniques. The National Committee for Clinical Laboratory Standards has described a number of

It was also determined that the infection rate was related to the duration of catheter placement, with the more severe infections associated with placements that exceeded 4 days.

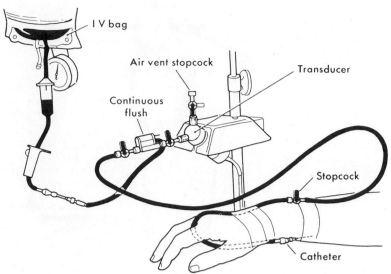

FIGURE 19–5: The components of a pressurized continuous-infusion arterial catheter include a 20- or 22-gauge Teflon catheter, a high-pressure connecting tube, stop cocks, an intraflow infusion device, a high-pressure connecting tube to a pressure transducer, a connecting tube to a heparinized solution bag (e.g., containing normal saline with 5000 IU heparin/L), and a pressure bag (kept at 50 mm Hg greater than systolic blood pressure). IV, intravenous. (From Daily EK, Schroeder JS. Techniques in Bedside Hemodynamic Monitoring. St. Louis, CV Mosby, 1981, p 99.)

For umbilical artery catheter use, the committee recommends a 3.5 Fr catheter for infants weighing less than 1200 g and a 5 Fr catheter for infants weighing more than 1200 g.

catheter placement techniques,[14] including over an inserted needle, through an inserted needle, and through a plastic cannula.

Umbilical artery catheterization is frequently performed shortly after birth for the neonate in respiratory distress. This is the preferred technique for systemic blood pressure monitoring and arterial blood sampling in this population of patients. A thorough description of the umbilical catheterization technique has also been given by the National Committee for Clinical Laboratory Standards.[14] The initial distance the catheter is advanced is determined with Dunn's method, which relates catheter distance to the distance from the umbilicus to the shoulder.[43] The catheter is frequently positioned in the aorta in a "low" position, below the renal arteries at a level adjacent to lumbar vertebra 3 or 4 when viewed on a radiograph.[32] Some clinicians prefer a "high" placement, above the diaphragm.

Although the incidence of complications from umbilical artery catheterization is low in the institutions in which these catheterizations are frequently used, they can produce significant complications. Hemorrhage (from aortic or iliac artery puncture), infection, thromboembolism (to the kidneys, gastrointestinal system, and lower extremities), air embolism, vasospasm, peritoneal perforation, leg hypoperfusion, and electrical hazards have all been documented.[44–47]

Table 19–6 outlines the steps for sampling blood from an indwelling vascular catheter such as that shown in Figure 19–5.

Pulmonary Artery Catheter Sampling

Critically ill patients with unstable cardiac performance frequently need a pulmonary artery catheter to monitor their hemodynamics. Samples of mixed venous blood can be collected from this catheter to evaluate tissue oxygenation and acid-base balance better.[48–50] The sampling tech-

TABLE **19–6:**   Steps for Sampling From Indwelling Vascular Catheters

1. Locate, identify, and reassure the patient while placing the patient in a supine or semi-Fowler position. Complete the requisition and information slip, wash your hands, and put on gloves.
2. With sterile technique, a waste syringe is attached to the stopcock closest to the interflow device (see Fig. 19–5). The stopcock is opened to the waste syringe (closed to the pressurized heparin source); infusion solution and blood are pulled into the waste syringe until a volume of 8 to 10 mL with adults and 2 mL with infants is removed. It is imperative that all the infusion fluid be removed to prevent significant blood gas and pH artifaction.[48]
3. The sample syringe is attached to the stopcock closest to the arterial catheter (see Fig. 19–5), the stopcock is opened to the catheter and syringe, and the sample of blood is pulled into the sample syringe (2 to 3 mL for adults, 0.5 to 1 mL for children, and 0.2 mL for infants). The sample syringe is removed after the stopcock has been closed; is cleared of air bubbles; and is capped, labeled, and placed in the transport container with the ice water slurry. In situations in which the sample is collected in an unheparinized syringe, the sample should be placed in the analyzer within 2 to 3 min to avoid clotting and the analyzer should be flushed immediately.
4. The waste syringe with the blood-infusion solution is carefully removed from its closed stopcock and disposed of in a biohazard or sharps container. The plunger "pigtail" of the intraflow device is gently pulled to allow heparinated infusion solution to flush the catheter clear of any blood. In the neonatal intensive care unit setting, the waste blood is frequently returned to the patient to avoid iatrogenic anemia.

Adapted from Malley WJ. Clinical Blood Gases—Application and Noninvasive Alternatives. Philadelphia, WB Saunders, 1990.

nique is essentially identical to that described for the systemic artery catheter. When blood is drawn into both the waste and the sample syringes, it has been suggested that it be withdrawn slowly to avoid "pulling" pulmonary capillary blood back into the artery and mixing it with pulmonary artery blood.[27]

Venous Catheter Sampling

Peripheral systemic venous catheters, which are used primarily for fluid and drug administration, are rarely used in the adult care setting for blood gas sampling. Peripheral venous samples have widely different P_{O_2} values that can range from 30 to 75 mm Hg when samples are collected from different sites.[51, 52]

However, taking samples from these sites is becoming more common in both the neonatal and the pediatric acute care settings. This sampling site is frequently available and less likely to disturb the patient. The acid-base and P_{CO_2} data reflect arterial values fairly well, whereas venous P_{O_2} underestimates arterial values significantly and is variable depending on the site of sampling.[51, 52] The same precautions described for sampling from an arterial catheter are necessary for good sample collection from a peripheral venous catheter.

Sample Handling

After collection of a blood sample, careful handling, storage, and transport are necessary to preserve the composition of the gas and the acid-base values. The correct patient label should be affixed to the syringe or capillary tube before transport. In addition, the blood specimen must *always* be treated as if it were from a patient with an infectious disease and must therefore be handled with *universal precautions.*[53] Gloves must be worn when the sample is being handled, and the sample should not be transported uncapped or with an attached needle.

Air bubbles should be removed from the sample as soon as possible.

Room air has a P_{O_2} of approximately 155 mm Hg and a P_{CO_2} of essentially zero at sea level.

The presence of air bubbles in the syringe or capillary tube will allow gas exchange between these two mediums as a result of the gas tension gradients present. The P_{O_2} value may be increased or decreased depending on the gas tension gradient between the blood and the air bubble. The P_{CO_2} would decrease on exposure to air, and the pH would increase as a result. When air bubbles are present in arterial specimens, the P_{O_2} value is primarily altered.[54-58] The magnitude of change depends on the P_{O_2} in the sample, the air bubble size, and the duration of blood-air exposure.[57, 58] Samples contaminated with more than minor air bubbles should be discarded if the duration of exposure is unknown.[27]

Transporting the specimen to the laboratory for analysis should be direct, taking as little time as possible. Pneumatic tube systems are used in some institutions to transport the specimen to the laboratory. Transport by this method can result in opening or breakage of the syringe from the increased gravitational forces. If the syringe or capillary tube remains intact and red blood cells remain whole, little or no change in gas tension and pH should occur.[13] However, no evidence is available about the effects of pneumatic tube transport on blood gas and pH values.

Ideally, samples should be analyzed immediately on collection. In reality, the sample may have to wait some time before it arrives in the laboratory, and more time may elapse before its actual analysis. The metabolic activity of blood, which is due primarily to the highly aerobic leukocytes, continues after its collection. This results in gas tension and pH changes.[16, 59] Table 19–7 shows the magnitude of gas tension and pH changes as a result of storing a normal arterial blood sample at different temperatures. This indicates that a sample stored at room temperature would change very little if analyzed within 10 minutes. If the sample is stored in an ice water slurry at 4°C, the sample changes very little over an hour. The degree of change, however, is greater in samples with a very high P_{O_2}. For example, the Pa_{O_2} can drop from 400 to below 250 mm Hg in 1 hour if the sample is stored at room temperature.[27]

Leukocytosis—leukocyte count of greater than 10,000/mm³

During conditions of leukocytosis, blood gas changes can be even more pronounced when analysis is delayed. Fox and colleagues have given the term *leukocyte larceny* to the phenomenon of a rapid P_{O_2} drop during leukocytosis.[60] They described a case in which a patient with leukemia had a leukocyte count of 276,000/mm³ and demonstrated a drop in the P_{O_2} of a stored sample from 130 to 58 mm Hg in just 2 minutes. Other investigators have seen similar declines, with some values reaching a P_{O_2} of zero by the time the analysis was made.[61]

TABLE **19–7:** Effects of Time Delay in Analysis on Blood Gas and pH Values

Time Delay (min)	Storage Temperature (°C)	Magnitude of Change*		
		P_{O_2}	P_{CO_2}	pH
	37			
10		−2	+1	−0.01
30		−8	+3	−0.03
60		−20	+5	−0.06
	20			
10		−1	+0.5	−0.005
30		−5	+1	−0.01
60		−10	+3	−0.03
	4			
10		−0.5	+0.1	−0.001
30		−2	+0.3	−0.003
60		−3	+0.6	−0.006

Data from references 16, 27, and 56.
*Magnitude of change in millimeters of mercury or pH units in a normal arterial sample.

Continuous Invasive Monitoring

Placing sensors for continuous blood gas, oxyhemoglobin saturation, and pH measurement in special vascular catheters has met with improving success.[62] These indwelling devices, which rely on direct contact with blood, can by placed in either systemic or pulmonary arteries for continuous monitoring. However, these devices have had problems with accuracy because of protein deposition on the catheter and sensor instability over time. Newer-generation devices that incorporate advances in fiber-optic fluorescence-based sensors and microprocessor technology now provide improved signal stability and accuracy during continuous use over 72 hours.[62]

Blood Sample Analysis: Measured and Derived Values

The modern in vitro blood gas analyzer (Table 19–8) incorporates a variety of sensors for highly accurate measurement of Po_2, Pco_2, and pH. The sensors are maintained at 37°C. Many models have the capability of automatic sensor recalibration (e.g., every 30 minutes) to maintain stable accuracy. Samples of correct size are delivered to the sensor sites by automatic pumping followed by automatic flushing of the sample lines. They also have extensive internal diagnostics for quick detection of errors and automatic trouble shooting. Some have the ability to measure hemoglobin content, the percentage of oxyhemoglobin saturation, and various other hemoglobin derivatives (e.g., carboxyhemoglobin). More often, hemoglobin analysis is carried out by stand-alone analyzers (e.g., the CO-oximeter). In addition to measured values, a large number of derived values are calculated by these analyzers.

TABLE **19–8:**   Modern Blood Gas and Acid-Base Analyzers

	ABL 520*	AVL 995Hb†	IL BG3‡	Corning 288§
Measured parameters				
Po_2, Pco_2, and pH	Yes	Yes	Yes	Yes
Barometric pressure	Yes	Yes	Yes	Yes
Total hemoglobin	Yes	Yes	CO-OX	Yes
Percentage saturation of hemoglobin derivatives	Yes	CO-OX¶	CO-OX	CO-OX
Derived parameters				
HCO_3^-, total CO_2, and base excess	Yes	Yes	Yes	Yes
Percentage saturation of oxyhemoglobin	Yes	Yes	Yes	Yes
P_{50}	Yes	No	CO-OX	CO-OX
O_2 content and O_2 capacity	Yes	Yes	CO-OX	CO-OX
Sample size requirements				
Normal sample	85 μL	40 μL	90 μL	200 μL
Microsample	35 μL	25 μL	70 μL	100 μL
Automatic calibration	Yes	Yes	Yes	Yes
Automatic sample introduction	Yes	Yes	Yes	Yes
Automatic flushing	Yes	Yes	Yes	Yes

*Radiometer, Westlake, OH.
†AVL Scientific, Roswell, GA.
‡Instrumentation Laboratories, Lexington, MA.
§Ciba Corning Diagnostics, Medfield, MA.
¶Requires interphasing with a CO-oximeter.

Electrical current flows from a negatively charged cathode to a positively charged anode through a conductor. The amount of current flow through a conductor is proportional to the charge or potential difference that exists between cathode and anode. Electrical current flow is expressed in units of amperes and is measured with a device called an ammeter. The electrical potential difference (equivalent to the pressure drop across a pneumatic system) is expressed in units of volts and is measured with a device called a voltmeter.

Electrodes

The measurement of respiratory gas tension and hydrogen ion concentration in blood is carried out by exposing a blood sample to electrochemical sensors. These sensors are more commonly referred to as electrodes. The sensing capacity of a chemical-specific electrode is based on the ability of the electrode to change its electrical properties on exposure to the chemical. The two primary electrical changes used in blood gas and pH electrodes are the detection of current and the voltage changes.

The generic electrode (Fig. 19–6) incorporates two electrode terminals, which are metal or special glass contacts that are exposed to an electrolyte medium. These terminals are commonly referred to as half-cells. Each electrode has one measuring half-cell and one reference half-cell. The measuring half-cell is placed in contact with the blood sample. The reference half-cell is in contact with a reference electrolyte solution. The two half-cells are connected by a conductor to form a circuit within which is housed an ammeter or a voltmeter to detect electrical changes. Voltage or current changes occur when the blood sample causes an electrochemical reaction at the measuring half-cell. These changes are proportional to the amount of chemical the measuring half-cell is exposed to.

pH Electrode

The blood pH electrode in use today was developed by Sanz.[63] It has a rapid response time, requires a very small amount of blood (e.g., 25 μL), and is heated to 37°C. Figure 19–7 shows the components of a typical pH electrode system. It includes a specimen chamber, a pH-sensitive glass measuring half-cell, a conductive circuit with a sensitive voltmeter, a reference half-cell, and a potassium chloride liquid junction.[27, 28] The measuring half-cell is frequently composed of a silver–silver chloride wire that is bathed by an electrolyte of constant pH (e.g., 6.840). The silver–silver chloride wire and bathing electrolyte are separated from the blood sample by pH-sensitive glass. A voltmeter is placed in the circuit between the measuring half-cell and the reference half-cell. The reference half-cell is usually a calomel half-cell. A calomel half-cell consists of a glass tube housing a platinum wire that is extended into a calomel paste of mercury–mercurous chloride. The calomel paste is in contact with a solution of potassium chloride. The reference half-cell is

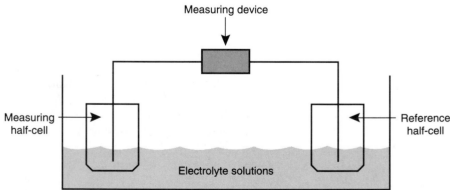

FIGURE 19–6: The generic chemical-detecting electrode consists of a measuring half-cell and its sample, a sensor circuit (with a measuring device, either an ammeter or a voltmeter), a battery, a reference half-cell, and a reference electrolyte.

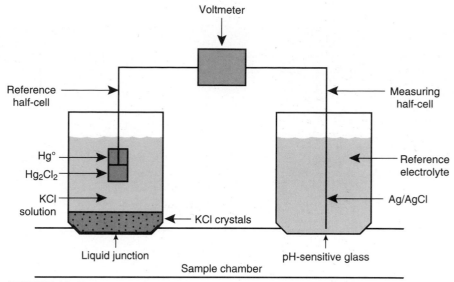

FIGURE 19–7: The basic components of a blood pH measuring and reference half-cell electrode system.

placed in contact with the blood specimen through a potassium chloride solution "bridge." Blood comes into contact with both half-cells to complete the circuit.

The H^+ ions in the blood sample chamber exchange with metallic ions in the pH-sensitive glass of the measuring half-cell. This generates an electrical potential difference across the pH-sensitive glass and through the rest of the circuit. This potential difference is expressed as a voltage that is proportional to the difference between the pH of the blood sample and the known pH (e.g., 6.840) bathing the silver–silver chloride wire in the measuring half-cell. If the pH of the blood sample were 6.840, there would be no potential difference between it and the pH of the electrolyte inside the measuring half-cell, and the display (actually a voltmeter) would show a pH value of 6.840. If the H^+ concentration were higher (or lower), a potential difference would be generated, and the voltmeter would indicate a lower (or a higher) pH according to the degree of potential difference generated. This relationship is described by the modified Nernst equation, which equates a 1.0 pH unit change with a 61.5-mV potential difference generated across the pH-sensitive glass.[27] The accuracy of the electrode is approximately ±0.02 pH units.

P_{CO_2} Electrode

The present-day P_{CO_2} electrode was first developed by Stow and later modified by Severinghaus to provide a reliable and rapid method of blood carbon dioxide detection.[64, 65] Before the development of the Stow-Severinghaus electrode, the Astrup CO_2 equilibration method was used.[66] This method, which is slow, allows more errors because of its reliance on proper gas-blood equilibration, multiple pH measurements, and manual plotting of the results.

The Stow-Severinghaus P_{CO_2} electrode (Fig. 19–8) consists of a pH electrode that is covered by a carbon dioxide–permeable membrane (usually of silicon or Teflon). The membrane prevents H^+ ions from reaching the pH-sensitive glass. The membrane is separated from the pH elec-

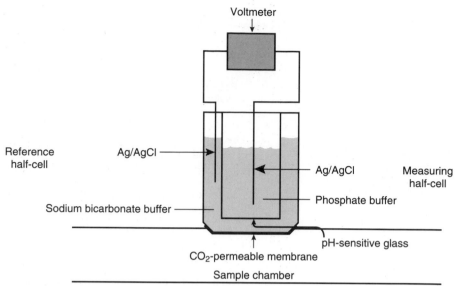

FIGURE 19–8: The basic components of a P_{CO_2} electrode.

trode face by a nylon spacer. The space between the membrane and the pH-sensitive glass is filled with a sodium bicarbonate electrolyte solution. When a blood sample is in contact with the electrode's membrane, CO_2 diffuses through the membrane at a rate proportional to the partial pressure of CO_2. As CO_2 enters the electrolyte solution, the following reaction occurs:

$$\text{Blood } CO_2 \longrightarrow\!\!\!| \longrightarrow CO_2 + H_2O \leftrightarrow H_2CO_3 \leftrightarrow H^+ + HCO_3^-$$
$$\text{(membrane)}$$

The net effect is an alteration in the H^+ concentration in the electrolyte solution of the electrode. The P_{CO_2} in the blood sample causes a proportional change in the H^+ concentration (according to the Henderson-Hasselbalch equation). The resulting pH change of the electrolyte solution causes an electrical potential (voltage) difference to be generated between the measuring and the reference half-cells. The voltage generated by the electrode is displayed as a P_{CO_2} value. The accuracy of the electrode is approximately ± 2 mm Hg.

P_{O_2} Electrode

Clark developed the present-day polarographic P_{O_2} electrode out of the need for rapid determination of oxygen content in tissue and for use in monitoring blood oxygen levels provided by heart-lung machines.[67, 68] The electrode (Fig. 19–9) consists of an oxygen-permeable membrane (polypropylene, polyethylene, Mylar, or Teflon), a platinum measuring half-cell (cathode) mounted in a glass rod, a silver–silver chloride reference half-cell (anode), and a potassium chloride and phosphate buffer solution. The platinum cathode is maintained at a fixed polarizing voltage with respect to the silver–silver chloride anode. Oxygen diffuses through the membrane and undergoes a reduction reaction (requiring electrons) at the platinum cathode to form hydroxyl ions. The electrons are provided by an oxidation reaction at the anode as anions (e.g., chloride ions) from the bathing electrolyte solution react with the silver to form silver chloride. The reduction reaction at the cathode drives the

Cathode reaction:

$$\text{Blood } O_2 \longrightarrow\!\!\!| \longrightarrow O_2 + 2 H_2O + 4 \text{ electrons} \rightarrow 4 OH^-$$
$$\text{(membrane)}$$

Anode reaction:

$$4 KCl + 4 Ag \rightarrow 4 K^+ + 4 Cl^+ + 4 Ag \rightarrow 4 AgCl + 4 \text{ electrons}$$

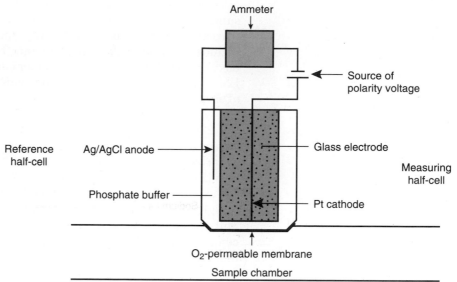

FIGURE 19–9: The basic components of a P_{O_2} electrode.

oxidation reaction at the anode, enhancing a current flow from the anode to the cathode. The established polarizing voltage of 600 mV between the two terminals provides rapid response and minimizes interference from other gases that may participate in the reaction at the cathode. Because the reaction consumes oxygen, a relatively impermeable membrane is used to allow a stable but small amount of oxygen diffusion from the sample to the electrode interior. The membrane also prevents reactions at the cathode with other chemicals (e.g., protein) that would cause considerable error. The current generated is proportional to the amount of oxygen diffusing through the membrane at a given partial pressure. Thus, the current flow is proportional to the partial pressure of oxygen dissolved in the plasma. The current is quantified and displayed by an ammeter as a P_{O_2}. The accuracy of the electrode is approximately ±2 to 5 mm Hg with a range of 40 to 100 mm Hg. Special calibration is necessary when the accuracy needs to be improved outside of this range.

CO-Oximeter

Light, of known wavelengths, may be transmitted through a colored specimen (e.g., blood) and then analyzed for the amount of light absorbed by the specimen. The color of a specimen determines what wavelengths of light will be absorbed, whereas the concentration of the specimen influences the amount of light absorbed. The amount of light transmitted through the sample can be detected by a photodetector cell (usually an oxide-coated metallic surface), which generates an electrical current proportionate to the amount of light reaching it. According to the photoelectric effect, the amount of light transmitted from a light source (e.g., a thallium cathode lamp) can be compared with the amount reaching the photodetector cell after it passes through an unknown and a reference specimen. These principles describe the technique of spectrophotometry.

Spectrophotometry was first employed in 1932 by Nicolai to determine oxygen saturation in tissues.[1] The term *oximeter* was coined by Milliken in 1942 to describe a noninvasive analyzer for determining oxyhemoglobin saturation with a spectrophotometric sensor that was

With the use of the Lambert-Beer law, the concentration of an unknown specimen can be determined with the following relationship:

$$c = (\log_{10} Io/Ix)/(Kd)$$

where c is the concentration of the light-absorbing substance, Io is the intensity of the incident light on the specimen, Ix is the intensity of the light transmitted through the specimen, K is a constant for the characteristics of the specimen and the wavelength of light used, and d is the length in centimeters of the light pathway from the light source to the photodetector cell.[28]

attached to the earlobe.[1] Laboratory benchtop oximeters for analyzing samples of blood (CO-oximeters) are used today to determine the concentration of the various hemoglobin forms or derivatives. These derivatives include reduced or deoxyhemoglobin (HHb), oxyhemoglobin (O$_2$Hb), carboxyhemoglobin (COHb), methemoglobin (MetHb), and sulfhemoglobin. Each one of these hemoglobin derivatives has its own unique color and absorption spectra (Fig. 19–10), which are used for its detection.

Modern CO-oximeters (e.g., Instrumentation Laboratory 482, Corning 270, Radiometer OSM3, and AVL 912 CO-oximeters) measure the concentrations of the various hemoglobin derivatives by determining the absorbance of specific wavelengths of light by in vitro blood sample analysis (Fig. 19–11). These devices use a single light source (e.g., a thallium cathode lamp) and multiple filters to produce up to 7 specific wavelengths of light. Each specific wavelength is passed to a reference photodetector and through a blood sample chamber with a second photodetector for comparison to determine the amount of light absorbed. For accurate detection, the hemoglobin derivatives are released from the erythrocyte by a hemolyzer before placement in the sample chamber. The specific wavelengths of light used by the oximeter are those that result in large differences in light absorption for each of the hemoglobin derivatives to be identified.

When a hemolyzed sample of blood is exposed to the various wavelengths of light in the sample chamber, an absorbance value is detected (at the sample detector) for each wavelength. A corresponding zero reference absorbance is detected (at the reference photodetector) and is

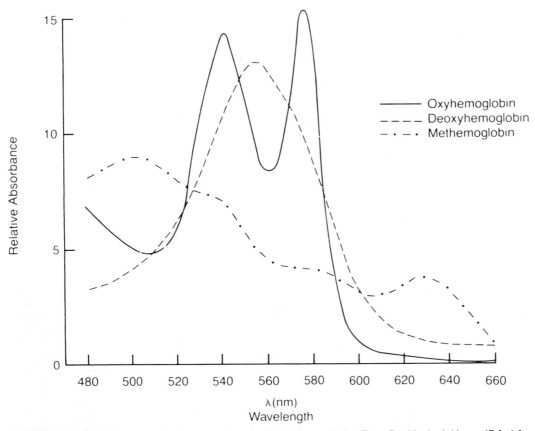

FIGURE 19–10: Absorption spectra for various species of hemoglobin. (From Davidsohn I, Henry JB [eds]. Todd-Sandford Clinical Diagnosis by Laboratory Methods, 17th ed. Philadelphia, WB Saunders, 1984, p 581; and Bunn HF, Forget BG, Ranney HM. Human Hemoglobins. Philadelphia, WB Saunders, 1977.)

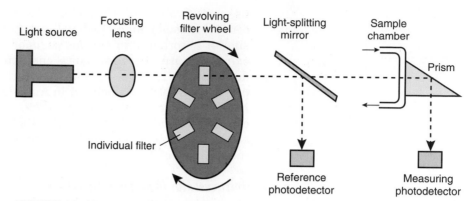

FIGURE 19–11: The components of a multiwavelength CO-oximeter for in vitro determination of various hemoglobin derivative concentrations.

subtracted from the sample absorbance to produce a true sample absorbance at each wavelength. Each true sample absorbance is multiplied by an appropriate extinction coefficient (derived from established references) for each of the hemoglobin derivatives. The concentration (in grams per 100 mL of blood) of each of the hemoglobin derivatives is then calculated with a matrix equation. The following equations are used by a 7-wavelength CO-oximeter:

$$[O_2Hb] = C_{O_2Hb}1A1 + C_{O_2Hb}2A2 + \ldots + C_{O_2Hb}7A7$$
$$[HHb] = C_{HHb}1A1 + C_{HHb}2A2 + \ldots + C_{HHb}7A7$$
$$[COHb] = C_{COHb}1A1 + C_{COHb}2A2 + \ldots + C_{COHb}7A7$$
$$[MetHb] = C_{MetHb}1A1 + C_{MetHb}2A2 + \ldots + C_{MetHb}7A7$$

where C is the extinction coefficient for each of the hemoglobin derivatives at each of the projected wavelengths of light (wavelengths 1 through 7) and A is the true absorbance value at each wavelength of light (wavelengths 1 through 7).[69] The total hemoglobin concentration (THb) is then calculated with the following equation:

$$[THb] = [O_2Hb] + [HHb] + [COHb] + [MetHb]$$

The percentage saturation is the customary method of expressing the concentration of each of the hemoglobin derivatives. The oximeter calculates this fractional hemoglobin as a ratio between the derivative in question and all of the major derivatives measured. Another approach is to determine the functional O_2Hb concentration. This is a ratio between the amount of hemoglobin carrying oxygen and the total amount that can. However, this method results in an overestimation of the amount of O_2Hb present when dyshemoglobins (e.g., COHb and MetHb) are present.

Thus, the CO-oximeter can both differentiate the type of hemoglobin derivatives present and determine the concentration or percentage saturation of the various hemoglobins by using a variation of Beer's law and the matrix formula.

This assumption, however, may lead to a variety of errors. Incomplete hemolysis of the erythrocytes or the presence of lipids can cause light scatter in the sample cuvette and erroneously low measurements.[70, 71] Intravenous dyes such as methylene blue strongly absorb light in the red and infrared wavelengths, which causes falsely low O_2Hb determinations made in this region of the spectrum.[72] Oximeters that

$$\text{Fractional XHb (\%)} = \frac{[XHb]}{[O_2Hb] + [HHb] + [COHb] + [MetHb]} \times 100\%$$

$$\text{Functional } O_2Hb \text{ (\%)} = \frac{[O_2Hb]}{[O_2Hb] + [HHb]} \times 100\%$$

use only two different wavelengths of light (e.g., pulse oximeters) indicate erroneously high O_2Hb values when COHb is present because of its similar absorbance in various parts of the spectrum.[73] In addition, most oximeters use the absorbance characteristics of adult hemoglobin for determining the type and concentrations of hemoglobin present. The presence of fetal hemoglobin in a sample will cause some oximeters to indicate a false COHb of up to 7%.[74, 75] Some CO-oximeters have the capability of determining fetal hemoglobin concentrations, whereas others make corrections if the known fetal hemoglobin saturation is entered into the device.[74, 75]

Intravascular Reflectance Oximeters

The microprocessor of the intravascular reflectance oximeter calculates a functional O_2Hb percentage with the following relationship:

$$O_2Hb (\%) = A - B (EI/ER)$$

where A is a specific constant for each catheter, B is a constant for the light intensity ratio, EI is the intensity of the infrared light reflected, and ER is the intensity of the red light reflected.[76]

The intravascular fiberoptic oximeter was first introduced in the early 1970s for the continuous determination of functional O_2Hb saturation.[76–79] The current systems employ two or three light-emitting diodes (LEDs), fiberoptic bundles for transmission and reflection of light, a silicon photodetector, and a microprocessor for processing the information. The different LEDs produce red (685 nm) and infrared (920 nm) light, which are better reflected by HHb and O_2Hb, respectively. The system switches the different-colored LEDs on and off in rapid succession. The light is transmitted down the catheter to the tip, where it interacts with the different derivatives of hemoglobin flowing by. The reflected light is channeled back to the photodetector, which produces electrical currents that are proportional to the amount of light being reflected.

A number of factors limit the reliability of this system. Optical fibers can be broken during placement of the catheter, which will degrade its accuracy.[76] The tip of the catheter may be accidentally placed up against the wall of the vessel, which will cause erroneous readings,[77] although repositioning the catheter can easily correct this problem. Clot formation over the optical ports can reduce accuracy, but clots can be prevented from forming by continuous fluid infusion through an infusion channel in the catheter.[76] Because the system determines a functional O_2Hb, it will not detect COHb or MetHb and thus will report a factitiously high value for the percentage of total hemoglobin present as O_2Hb.[78] Although the system is calibrated before insertion, its accuracy can drift over time. For these reasons, the system should be checked and recalibrated on a daily basis by adjusting it to the value reported by an in vitro determination of the O_2Hb percentage by a multiwavelength CO-oximeter.

Errors of more than 5% have been reported when these systems have been used in patients with hematocrits below 30%.[77]

Intravascular oximeters have been used in conjunction with noninvasive pulse oximeters for the determination of both mixed venous and arterial saturation. This dual oximetry approach to monitoring oxygenation has been found useful in the management of patients in severe respiratory and cardiovascular failure.[80]

Optodes

Advances in fiberoptics and photochemistry have led to the development of the optode, a sensor that responds to the presence of a specific chemical through optical detection. These devices use microprocessors, photodetectors, fiberoptic channels, and sensing sites. Optode sensors are classified into three categories: fluorescence optodes, energy-transference optodes, and transmission optodes.

A fluorescent optode uses a fluorescent dye that emits a small amount of light energy (luminescence) as the electrons in it return to a basal energy state after exposure to an excitation light of proper wavelength and intensity. Fluorescent dyes produce different wavelengths of light when a specific ion or molecule chemically interacts with them. These dyes are placed on the tip of a fiberoptic sensor and covered with a semipermeable membrane to make them chemically specific. The dye fluoresces different light intensities as the specific chemical concentration changes in the immediate environment following excitation. The resulting fluorescence is transmitted back through a fiberoptic channel, and the changes are detected by a photodetector and analyzed by a microprocessor. A variety of O_2, CO_2, and pH fluorescence optodes have been developed.[81] Most of these advances have been in the area of continuous in vivo monitoring systems, with a number of devices being marketed (e.g., Gas Stat, CDI System 1000, Optex Biosentry, and Puritan-Bennett PB 3300 intra-arterial blood gas monitor). Their accuracy is improving, and in some cases it is comparable to in vitro analysis.[82, 83] More recent developments are taking these sensors to the bedside in the form of miniature blood gas analyzers that can analyze in vitro samples on demand by withdrawing samples into them from an arterial catheter and completing the analysis in 90 seconds (e.g., the CDI 2000 system).

The relatively small number of chemical-specific fluorescence dyes limits the utility of the fluorescence optode. Energy-transference optodes use a combination of colorimetric reagents with fluorescent indicators, which broadens the field of chemicals that can be detected. Optical sensors utilizing this principle have been developed for the measurement of blood Na^+, K^+, and pH.[84]

The transmission optodes sense attenuation of the light beam being transmitted through the sensor site. Attenuation of the light may occur as a result of absorption, scattering, or reflection due to the chemical interaction at the sensing site. An absorbance-based transmission optode has been developed for blood pH measurement.[85]

These types of new sensors and their applications represent the dawn of the next generation of blood gas analyzers.

Derived Oxygen and Acid-Base Indices

A plethora of calculated parameters of oxygenation and acid-base balance have been developed over the past century. These calculations can provide values for those variables that are not directly measured. Implicit in any calculation of a variable is the assumption that all the needed information that would change the value of the variable to be calculated is available. Obviously, all the conditions that would alter the value of a variable cannot be known; thus, the following calculations present the clinician with data that closely approximate the true value of the variable. All of the following equations assume a normal body temperature of 37°C.[86]

Oxyhemoglobin Saturation

$$O_2Hb\,(\%) = 100 \times (Z^{2.60}/[26.6]^{2.60} + Z^{2.60})$$

where

$$Z = Po_2 \times 10^{-0.48(7.40 - pH)}$$

Oxygen Content of Blood

$$O_2\text{ content (mL }O_2/100\text{ mL blood)} = (1.39 \times THb \times [\%O_2Hb/100]) + (0.003 \times Po_2)$$

Oxygen-Carrying Capacity of Blood

$$O_2\text{-carrying capacity (mL }O_2/100\text{ mL blood)} = (1.39 \times THb) + (0.003 \times Po_2)$$

This equation assumes the calculation of normal adult hemoglobin with a P_{50} of 26.6 mm Hg. It does not account for any other hemoglobin derivative, such as COHb. Thus, it would result in an overestimation of the true percent saturation of hemoglobin with oxygen.

P$_{50}$

P$_{50}$ (in millimeters of mercury) can be derived after measuring Po$_2$ and O$_2$Hb and determining K, an equilibrium constant of O$_2$Hb in the modified Hill equation:

$$\text{Log K} = \log (O_2Hb/100 - O_2Hb) - 2.6 \log (Po_2)$$

After solving for K, the equation is rearranged to solve for the Po$_2$ (P$_{50}$) when the O$_2$Hb saturation is 0.50 (50%).

Plasma HCO$_3^-$ Concentration

$$[HCO_3^-]\,(mEq/L) = 0.03 \times Pco_2 \,(\text{antilog } [pH - 6.1])$$

or

$$[HCO_3^-] = (0.03 \times Pco_2 \times 6.1)/[H^+]$$

Total CO$_2$ Concentration in Plasma

$$[CO_2]\,(mEq/L) = (0.03 \times Pco_2) + [HCO_3^-]$$

Base Excess (BE) of Blood

$$BE_{blood}\,(mEq/L) = (1 - 0.014\,[THb])([HCO_3^-] - 24 + ((1.43\,[THb] + 7.7)(pH - 7.40))$$

Extracellular Fluid Base Excess (BE$_{ECF}$)

$$BE_{ECF}\,(mEq/L) = (1 - 0.014\,[5])([HCO_3^-] - 24 + ((1.43\,[5] + 7.7)(pH - 7.40))$$

The calculation of different acid-base parameters can be carried out graphically with the aid of various alignment nomograms. Figure 19–12 shows the Siggard-Andersen nomogram, which was used extensively until microprocessor-equipped analyzers carried out the calculations.[87] The term *alignment nomogram* indicates that calculations are carried out by placing a straight line through the measured values of Pco$_2$ and pH. This line is extended through the corresponding values of base excess, plasma [HCO$_3^-$], and total [CO$_2$].

Temperature Correction

Whereas the sensors of the blood gas analyzer are heated to a normal body temperature of 37°C, some patients may have a core temperature above or below this value. One approach would be to heat or cool the sensors to the patient's temperature. This is impractical in the busy blood gas laboratory when numerous samples are arriving from patients with different temperatures and when there is the need for a 30-minute sensor restabilization period at a new temperature. Blood gas tension and pH values change when the blood samples (in a closed container) are heated or cooled to the analyzer's temperature (Table 19–9). Because of this change, it is common practice to apply mathematical factors to "correct" the 37°C in vitro values back to the approximate in vivo value of the patient.[88–90]

TABLE **19–9:** Effects of Temperature Variation on Gas Tensions and pH of Blood

Temperature (°C)	Po$_2$ (mm Hg)	Pco$_2$ (mm Hg)	pH
25	37	24	7.58
35	70	37	7.43
37	80	40	7.40
40	97	45	7.36

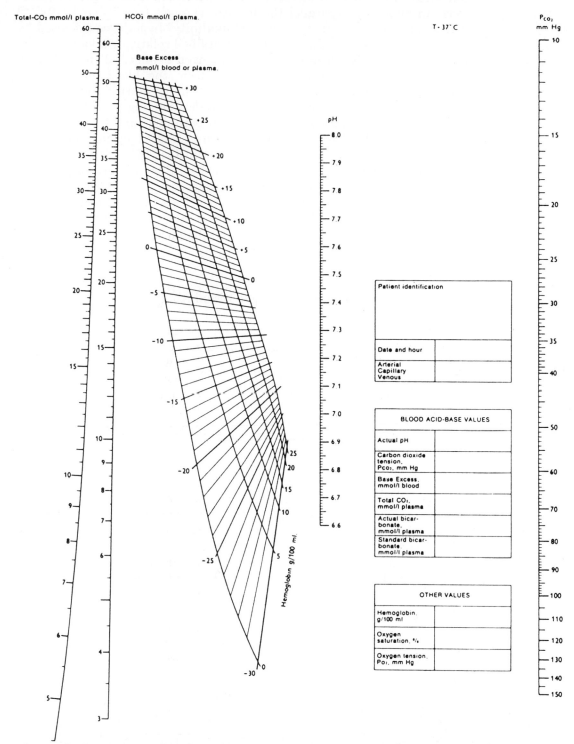

FIGURE 19–12: The Siggard-Andersen blood acid-base alignment nomogram. (From Siggard-Andersen O. Blood acid-base alignment nomogram. Scand J Clin Lab Invest 15:211, 1963.)

A question immediately arises: what are the *normal* Po_2, Pco_2, pH, and $[HCO_3^-]$ values for a given temperature? Studies of ectothermic (cold-blooded) animals at various temperatures show that blood gas and acid-base in vivo values parallel the in vitro changes (see Table 19–9).[91-93] These findings support the "relative alkalinity" hypothesis proposed by Rahn, which suggests that blood is maintained relatively alkaline to the neutral value of water over a wide temperature range.[94] Thus, it is now suggested that the uncorrected values from the blood gas analyzer (heated to 37°C) should be used to guide the interpretation and therapeutic decisions.[27, 89, 95-97] This is supported by the findings of better cardiovascular function during hypothermia in both dogs and human infants when cardiopulmonary support maintains blood at normal values, as reported by a blood gas analyzer maintained at 37°C.[98-100] A study of acid-base management during hypothermia in open heart surgical patients, however, found no significant differences in cardiovascular and neurophysiologic variables when arterial pH was maintained with "uncorrected" or "corrected" values.[101] These findings support the idea that either approach to managing acid-base balance is acceptable during short-term moderate hypothermia.

Ensuring the Accuracy of Invasive Blood Analysis

Sources of Error

The critical importance of blood gas and acid-base measurement in acute care medicine demands that these measurements be very accurate and precise. The reliability of a sensor is the ability of that sensor to be both accurate and precise. Figure 19–13 illustrates these concepts by using the analogy of "hitting" a target or known value.

To improve measurement accuracy and precision, the sources of error must be identified and reduced to acceptable limits. Positive and negative errors can occur in no detectable pattern (random errors) as a result of accidental variations in technique (e.g., air bubbles in the sample) or equipment performance (e.g., poor sample introduction or inconsistent sensor calibration). A series of errors can result in a consistent positive or negative pattern (systematic errors) as a result of consistent technical errors (e.g., consistent heparin dilution) or equipment performance (e.g., calibration of a sensor with contaminated reagents). Errors can occur in three phases of measurement and reporting: preanalytic, analytic, and postanalytic.

Accuracy is the term used to describe how close the measured value of a sample is to the true value of that sample. *Precision* refers to how close a series of measurements of the same sample are to the true value.

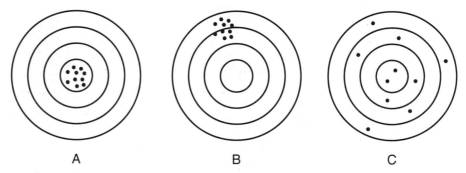

FIGURE 19–13: Analytical accuracy and precision are illustrated by the ability to "hit" a known target. *A,* Very good accuracy and precision. *B,* Poor accuracy but good precision. *C,* Occasional accuracy but poor precision.

The types of preanalytic errors include

- Collecting the wrong information about the patient's condition
- Accidental venous sampling
- Air bubble contamination of the sample
- Heparin dilution
- Contaminating a sample with catheter infusion solution
- Excessive time delays between sampling and analysis
- Clot formation in the sample
- Leukocytosis (leukocyte larceny)
- Insufficient sample size
- Mixing up unlabeled patient samples or labeling the sample with the wrong patient identification tag[102]

Analytic errors can result from

- Sensor accuracy drift (too much time between calibrations)
- Improper sensor calibration (contaminated or inaccurate calibrants)
- Clot introduction or formation in the analyzer
- Introduction of air bubbles into the analyzer
- Oxygen consumption by the Po_2 electrode
- Protein buildup on the sensor membrane or window
- Malfunctioning sensor
- Improper data entry into the analyzer
- Inaccurate barometric pressure measurements
- Not maintaining sensors at 37°C[13, 27]

Postanalytic errors can occur when

- Data are transcribed or transmitted incorrectly
- Incorrect data are reported for the right patient
- Data are lost

Quality Assurance

The key tasks of a quality assurance program include

- Accurate patient data collection
- Correct sample collection and handling
- Regular analyzer maintenance
- Sensor calibration and following a quality control program
- Development of action plans to improve and maintain overall laboratory performance

Interpretation of blood gas and acid-base data should always be done with some suspicion that errors have been made. An unexpected change in blood gas results should signal the possibility of errors. A quality assurance program is necessary to monitor, document, and improve the accuracy, precision, and reporting of measured values. The driving forces behind quality assurance programs are the Health Care Financing Administration's Clinical Laboratory Improvement Amendments (CLIA 1967 and 1988), the standards established by the Joint Commission for the Accreditation of Hospitals, and various state health agencies.[103–105]

Analyzer Maintenance

For proper function, the sample pathway and blood gas, pH, and hemoglobin sensors must be maintained in a proper condition, as described by the manufacturer. This includes flushing the sample pathway after each analysis to avoid clot formation. Protein deposition frequently occurs and requires flushing of the sample pathway with a deproteinizing solution (e.g., hydrochloric acid, pepsin, and a surfactant solution) periodically. The pathway should also be occasionally flushed with an antibacterial agent (e.g., potassium hydroxide solution) to minimize bacterial and fungal infections of the analyzer. Electrode membranes should be replaced at proper intervals or when the electrode's performance becomes sluggish or develops a systematic error pattern. The internal electrolyte solution of the electrodes should also be periodically changed. Any maintenance actions taken and the results of those actions must be recorded in a log book for each analyzer.

Calibration

Calibration of sensors should be carried out frequently to avoid having a sensor's accuracy drift to an unacceptable range over time. This process establishes the proper relationship between the sensor's electrical output (voltage or amperage) and the actual amount of an analyte (e.g., oxygen, carbon dioxide, H^+, or O_2Hb percentage saturation) present. Calibration is carried out by exposing the sensors to standardized gases or solutions (calibrant) that contain known amounts of analyte. This can be performed manually or in automated analyzers, where this is done by a microprocessor. After a short stabilization period, the sensor output or readout is adjusted (manually or under microprocessor control) to the value of the calibrant.

A sensor should be calibrated with one- and two-point calibration standards. The one-point calibration should be done before each measurement or every 30 minutes. The one-point calibrant is frequently a standard gas mixture (from a tank of precision gas with an established accuracy of $\pm 0.01\%$) and a liquid standard buffer solution of known pH (conforming to the standards of the National Institutes of Standards and Technology). The typical standards used for one-point calibration are

P_{O_2} = 85.6 mm Hg (12% of [barometric pressure − water vapor pressure])
P_{CO_2} = 35.7 mm Hg (5% of [barometric pressure − water vapor pressure])
pH = 7.384

A two-point calibration refers to using two different standard calibrants. Two-point calibration should be done (1) if the one-point calibration results in excessive adjustment due to sensor drift (e.g., more than 2 to 5 mm Hg in P_{O_2} and P_{CO_2} and more than 0.01 pH unit), (2) when the sensor response during the one-point calibration is excessive, or (3) every 8 hours. The typical two-point calibration includes the one-point standards (frequently referred to as the cal) plus a second set of standards (the slope):

P_{O_2} = 0.0 mm Hg (0.0% of [barometric pressure − water vapor pressure])
P_{CO_2} = 71.3 mm Hg (10% of [barometric pressure − water vapor pressure])
pH = 6.380

The one-point calibration adjusts the sensor to a normal physiologic point, whereas the two-point calibration improves the accuracy to a range that spans the two different standards used. Periodically (e.g., every 6 months), the sensor's linearity needs to be verified by using four different reagent levels of known values that would span the sensor range of measurement.

The sensor is said to be linear if it reports values accurately over a range defined by the low and high points of the two standards.

Quality Control

The goal of a quality control program is to determine if the analyzer is operating with acceptable accuracy and precision. This can be done by comparing the measured values of a control reagent with its known values. At first glance, this appears to be the same as using a calibration standard. However, the analyzer is not adjusted to the values of the control reagent, as would be done with the calibration standard. The control reagent is used solely to evaluate how accurately and precisely the analyzer is performing.

Internal quality control programs use daily analysis of either commercial quality control reagents or laboratory-prepared solutions. The results are evaluated, and appropriate actions are taken to improve analyzer performance if indicated. In addition, the laboratory must participate in an external quality control or proficiency testing program to maintain its accreditation for acceptable procedures and practice. These programs screen the performance of the analyzer for the presence of random or systematic errors and form an essential program for maintenance of laboratory accuracy and precision.

The internal quality control program begins with selecting a control reagent. Various quality control reagents are available for blood gas, pH, and hemoglobin analysis.[106] They include gases, perfluorinated emulsions, aqueous buffers, glycerin solutions, human and animal serum, and human and animal blood. All of these reagents are commercially available or can be prepared by tonometry (a technique of equilibrating liquids with precision gases of known concentration). The different levels of control reagent are used to evaluate the accuracy of the sensor over the physiologic range that the analyzer will test. For example, a set of aqueous buffer controls from a commercial source (BIO RAD, ECS Division, Anaheim, CA) for evaluation of the pH sensor found in the Radiometer ABL 500 blood gas analyzer would provide the following values:

Level I = 7.20 ± 0.03
Level II = 7.42 ± 0.03
Level III = 7.64 ± 0.03

Each of the control levels is initially analyzed at least 20 to 30 times. The mean value ($\overline{X}$), standard deviation (SD), and coefficient of variance are determined for each sensor at each control level. If the results fall within the specifications determined by the manufacturer, the reagent is suitable as an internal quality control reagent.

The internal quality control program continues as an ongoing series of measurements. Typically, three different control levels are analyzed two or three times each day. The results must be logged and reviewed for indications of analyzer errors. These logs must be archived for 2 years to maintain the laboratory's certificate of accreditation. The results are also plotted for rapid identification of errors.

The use of a plotting system allows rapid detection of out-of-control conditions, which in turn would indicate unacceptable accuracy, precision, or both. Out-of-control conditions have been defined by Westgard and coworkers through the use of a multirule technique.[108, 109] This technique evaluates the number of times a measured control value falls outside the known mean for that control level and the measured value's degree of variation from the mean (how many SDs). It is also useful in detecting both random and systematic errors with a reduced probability of false alarms for technique- and sensor-generated errors. The rules are abbreviated through the symbol A_L, where A represents the number of controls measured and L represents the degree of variation in SDs. Thus, 1_{1S} indicates that one control measurement was 1 SD outside the known mean value for that control level. The set of conditions recommended by Westgard and coworkers is listed in Table 19–10.

The Levey-Jennings chart (Fig. 19–14) is one of the more straightforward methods of determining the presence of an error.[107] The charts are constructed to show the individual results from each sensor for each control level. The measured value for the control is found on the y-axis, and successive measurements are plotted along the x-axis. The typical sensor is considered to be within control limits if the measured values are within ±2 SD with a random pattern about the mean (see Fig. 19–14). This would indicate acceptable accuracy and precision.

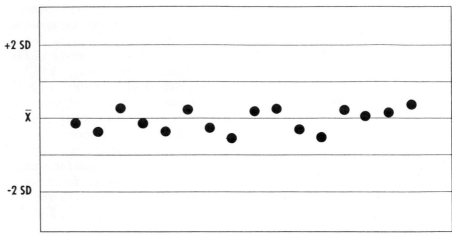

FIGURE 19–14: Levey-Jennings plot of a series of control measurements that illustrates a sensor with acceptable accuracy and precision.

The multirule can be employed by using the following decision flow chart:

Control level measured
↓
1_{2S} no→ within control, sensor working acceptably
↓ yes (warning, but OK to continue using instrument)
1_{3S} yes→ out of control, take corrective action
↓ no
2_{2S} yes→ out of control, take corrective action
↓ no
R_{4S} yes→ out of control, take corrective action
↓ no
4_{1S} yes→ out of control, take corrective action
↓ no
10_X yes→ out of control, take corrective action
↓ no
Within control, sensor working acceptably

TABLE **19–10:**   Westgard's Rules for Laboratory Quality Control

1_{2S}	Warning: one control measurement is outside the known mean value by ± 2 SDs; closely monitor next controls (Fig. 19–15)
1_{3S}	Stop and take corrective action on the sensor when the control measurement is outside the known mean value for that control by more than ± 3 SDs (Fig. 19–16)
2_{2S}	Stop and take corrective action on the sensor when two consecutive control measurements are outside the known mean value by more than ± 2 SDs (Fig. 19–17)
R_{4S}	Stop and take corrective action on the sensor when the range of difference between two consecutive control measurements is more than 4 SDs (Fig. 19–18)
4_{1S}	Stop and take corrective action on the sensor when four consecutive control measurements are more than ± 1 SD from the known mean (Fig. 19–19)
10_X	Stop and take corrective action on the sensor when 10 consecutive control measurements are within 1 SD of the mean but all fall on one side of the known mean (Fig. 19–20)

Adapted from Statland BE, Westgard JO. Quality control: Theory and practice. *In* Henry JB (ed). Clinical Diagnosis and Management by Laboratory Methods. Philadelphia, WB Saunders, 1984.

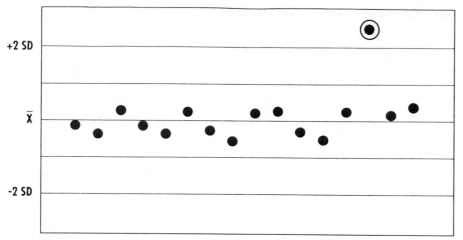

FIGURE 19–15: Violation of the 1_{2S} rule shows one measurement more than 2 SDs outside the expected mean. This would indicate a random error that was corrected.

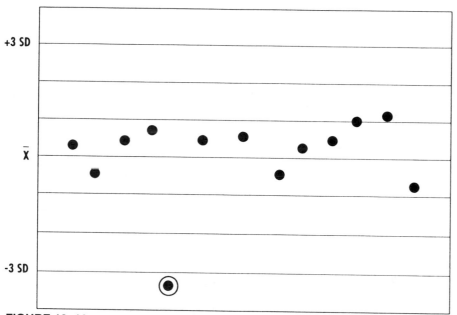

FIGURE 19–16: Violation of the 1_{3S} rule shows one measurement more than 3 SDs outside the expected mean. This would also indicate a random error.

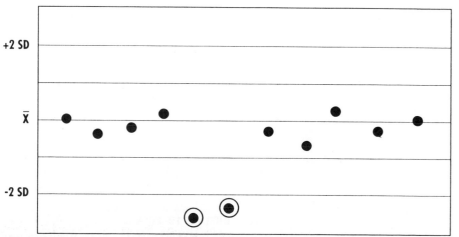

FIGURE 19–17: Violation of the 2_{2S} rule shows two consecutive measurements that are more than 2 SDs from the expected mean. This indicates the presence of a systematic error.

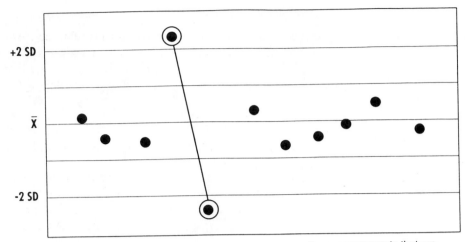

FIGURE 19–18: Violation of the R_{4S} rule shows two consecutive measurements that are more than 4 SDs apart. This indicates the development of reduced precision through dispersion.

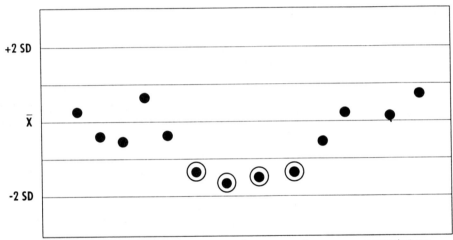

FIGURE 19–19: Violation of the 4_{1S} rule shows four consecutive measurements that are more than 1 SD from the expected mean. This shifted pattern indicates the development of a systematic error.

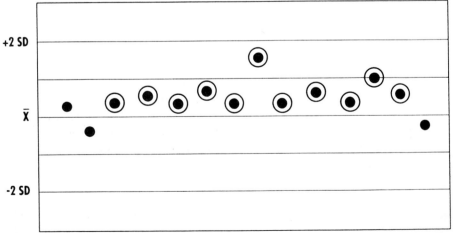

FIGURE 19–20: Violation of the 10_x rule shows 10 consecutive measurements that are on one side of the expected mean. This also is a shifted pattern that suggests the presence of a systematic error.

The first step in using the multirule system is to determine if a control is outside 2 SDs. The operator then progresses through each of the rules until a "yes" is encountered, indicating an out-of-control condition. At this point, the electrode should be recalibrated and the control attempted again. If a rule is violated again, the operator needs to consult the laboratory action plan for trouble shooting and correcting the problem. All rule violations, corrective actions, and continuing maintenance actions need to be logged for proper quality control. If no rule is broken, the sensor is considered to be within control parameters and is free to be used.

Proficiency testing involves periodic analysis (e.g., 3 times per year) of unknown controlled samples that are produced by an approved independent agency (e.g., the College of American Pathologists, the California Thoracic Society, or the American Thoracic Society). The laboratory conducts measurements of Po_2, Pco_2, and pH on five unknown control samples and reports the results to the agency for outside evaluation of accuracy. Laboratories are not required to be 100% acceptable on all samples tested. Minimal acceptability is accomplished if 80% of Po_2, Pco_2, or pH determinations are performed acceptably during analysis of the five samples provided for each testing event.

Acceptable performance for a blood gas analyzer would require

pH = target value ± 0.04 units
Pco_2 = target value ± 5 mm Hg or 8%
Po_2 = target value ± 3 of the group's SD (typically ±10 mm Hg)

Personnel Requirements

The CLIA rules also define the type of education and credentials needed by personnel to operate and supervise the laboratory.[105] The basis for the various levels of education and credentialing is defined by the type of blood gas analyzer used by the laboratory. The complexity classification given to a testing device is based on (1) the needed level of skill for proper operation and (2) the potential for mismeasurements to harm the patient. Erroneous blood gas and pH determinations hold high risks for patients because of the potential for making the wrong decisions about life support. Analyzers that have automatic calibration and automated sample introduction and flushing (e.g., those listed in Table 19–8) are classified as moderately complex. Analyzers that require considerable manual operation and calibration are classified as highly complex devices.

Operating personnel for the moderately complex devices need at least a high school diploma and adequate training and experience. Highly complex analyzers require operators with at least an associate's degree plus adequate training in pulmonary function testing or a bachelor's degree in respiratory care plus adequate training and experience (by September of 1997). The laboratory also needs a director (holding at least a bachelor's degree in clinical laboratory or biologic sciences) who is responsible for overall operation, administration, quality assurance, and documentation of laboratory activities. In addition, the laboratory must have a technical consultant (with at least a bachelor's degree) to carry out quality assurance and education programs and a clinical consultant (a physician) to ensure proper utilization and interpretation of test results. The rationale behind the CLIA rules is to help ensure patient safety by requiring adequate education and experience for the level of testing to be performed.

NONINVASIVE MONITORING

Patients are monitored for two basic reasons: (1) to detect adverse events and (2) to optimize their care. Hudson[110] and Hess[111] have put forth a definition of monitoring that ties these basic reasons together:

Monitoring is a continuous, or nearly continuous evaluation of the physiologic function of a patient in real time to guide management decisions—including when to make therapeutic interventions—and assessment of those interventions.

Noninvasive monitoring refers to techniques that detect ongoing physiologic events through the use of sensors that are applied to the surface of the skin or exposed to inhaled and exhaled gases.

Many factors are driving the interest in noninvasive monitoring. Invasive techniques have numerous complications for the patient.[26, 31, 39–47, 112] In addition, invasive techniques carry the added risk of possible infection for the health care provider.[53] Intermittent blood sampling has the potential to miss important changes, whereas a continuous technique will better detect them. Noninvasive monitoring (e.g., transcutaneous O_2 determination and pulse oximetry) can lead to reduced use of invasive blood gas analysis and reduced costs.[113–115] However, this cost savings may not be real.[111] For these reasons, noninvasive respiratory monitoring will remain an essential part of acute care medicine.

Transcutaneous and Transconjunctival Blood Gas Monitoring

The phenomenon of O_2 and CO_2 exchange across the skin was first described by Gierlach in 1851. In the 1960s, with the development of the rapid-response blood gas electrodes, Severinghaus[115] and Evans and Naylor[117] exploited this phenomenon. They measured transcutaneous partial pressures (Ptc_{CO_2} and Ptc_{O_2}) that accurately reflected arterial PCO_2 and PO_2 values when the electrodes were placed in direct contact with skin.[116, 117] The present-day transcutaneous electrodes have evolved into miniaturized forms of the larger electrodes found in the standard in vitro blood gas analyzer.[118]

The electrodes are equipped with heating elements to heat the application site to 42°C, which greatly increases local blood flow in the dermis. This effectively flushes the capillary bed with arterial blood and improves O_2 delivery to the epidermal layer of the skin and the attached electrode. Heating also partially melts the lipid matrix of the outer epidermal layer (stratum corneum), further enhancing gas diffusion and electrode accuracy. However, heating causes increased dermal metabolism, which in turn results in elevated O_2 consumption and CO_2 production. These metabolic changes can lead to corresponding errors in estimating arterial blood values unless corrective steps are taken.

The Ptc_{O_2} electrode is a modified Clark electrode that uses a silver anode and a platinum or gold cathode with a polarizing voltage of approximately 600 mV.[119] The Ptc_{CO_2} electrode is a modified Severinghaus electrode consisting of a chlorinated silver wire pH-sensitive glass measuring half-cell and silver–silver chloride reference cell.[119] The surface of the Ptc_{O_2} electrode is covered with a polyethylene or polypropylene membrane, whereas the Ptc_{CO_2} uses Teflon or Silastic membranes. These membranes maintain the necessary internal electrolytes and provide a selective barrier to enhance their accuracy. The internal heating element and monitoring thermistor are capable of maintaining temperatures of up to 45°C, although 42°C is an effective and safer operating temperature. The electrodes are available as individual units or as dual O_2-CO_2 electrodes (Fig. 19–21).

The use of the electrodes, which is relatively straightforward, requires attention to details.[119, 120] The electrodes are two-point calibrated

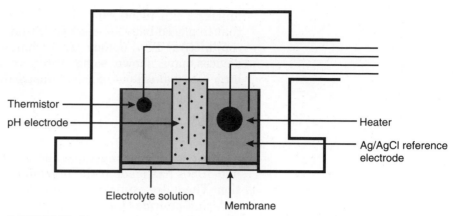

FIGURE 19–21: The basic components of a transcutaneous CO_2 electrode.

The sites for transcutaneous
monitoring include

Upper chest
Abdomen
Inner thigh
Lower back

Extremities are occasionally used
for the evaluation of peripheral
perfusion.

with precision gases before placement. Because of its heating the tissue and increasing CO_2 production, the Ptc_{CO_2} electrode requires a correction factor during calibration or activation of the monitor's correction feature to reduce the values back toward the arterial range.[121] For optimal performance, the electrode should be placed over a flat area of well-perfused skin. Areas with bony prominences or hair should be avoided. Electrodes are attached to the skin with double-sided adhesive tape and a small drop of contact solution to enhance electrode performance. Care is necessary in making a complete seal or the electrode will be contaminated with air, thus giving erroneous values. The electrode then requires 15 to 20 minutes to stabilize and equilibrate with blood before the values can be used. The electrode should be removed every 3 to 4 hours, recalibrated, and placed on another site to maintain accuracy and to avoid burning the skin. Occasional blood sampling and in vitro gas analysis are necessary to verify the system's accuracy.

The ability of these electrodes to report the arterial values correctly is influenced by a variety of patient and electrode factors (Table 19–11). The Ptc_{CO_2} electrode has been found to be reasonably accurate (± 5 to 8 mm Hg) in all age groups.[122] The Ptc_{O_2} electrode, on the other hand, is most accurate in a limited population of neonates with arterial values below 80 mm Hg.[122, 123] In adults, Ptc_{O_2} values consistently fall 20 mm Hg or more below Pa_{O_2} values, making transcutaneous PO_2 monitoring less useful in this population.[122-125] With these limitations and the development of accurate pulse oximeters, the demand for Ptc_{O_2} has dropped, and Ptc_{CO_2} monitoring remains more common in the care of the critically ill neonate and pediatric patient.

Miniature Clark electrodes have also been developed for transcon-

TABLE 19–11: Factors That Affect the Ability of the Transcutaneous Electrode to Report Arterial Values Accurately

	Patient Factors	**Electrode Factors**
Ptc_{O_2}	Epidermal thickness	Electrode condition
	Perfusion status	Membrane condition
	Vascular dilating agents	Calibration
	Age	Site selection
		Temperature
		Electrode adhesion
Ptc_{CO_2}	Perfusion status	Same factors as above
		Acidosis

junctival PO_2 monitoring through the use of a conforming scleral ring that is placed between the eyelid and the eye.[126, 127] In addition, a transconjunctival PCO_2 optode sensor has been developed.[128] Although these devices have shown some utility in the adult population, they have largely remained out of the mainstream of acute care monitoring.

Pulse Oximetry

The phenomenal growth and acceptance of pulse oximetry since the mid-1980s has made it the preeminent noninvasive monitor of oxygenation. The pulse oximeter was developed by Aoyagi in 1974 on the basis of isolating and measuring the light absorption of pulsing blood noninvasively.[129] Through evaluation of the pulsing portion (Fig. 19–22) of the absorbance spectrum in an intact tissue bed of the earlobe, the measurement of O_2Hb pulse saturation (Sp_{O_2}) was found to reflect the value of O_2Hb saturation in arterial blood accurately.

The modern pulse oximeter (Fig. 19–23) is a transmission spectrophotometer that uses a red (660 nm) and an infrared (940 nm) LED as light sources, a broad-spectrum photodetector, and a microprocessor to analyze and compute the Sp_{O_2}.[130] The LEDs are positioned on one side of the tissue bed, and the photodetector is placed on the other side. The LEDs are individually turned on and off rapidly in succession hundreds of times per second. The microprocessor analyzes the output of the photodetector when each LED is flashed on to determine the absorbance of light by the tissues when each LED is flashed on. The absorbance of the pulsing portion of the signal is isolated, and the Sp_{O_2} is derived by

The following equation is used to determine the pulse saturation:

$$Sp_{O_2} (\%) = K_1 (AC_{660}/AC_{940})^2 + K_2 (AC_{660}/AC_{940}) + K_3$$

where K_1, K_2, and K_3 are calibration constants; AC_{660} is the pulsing absorbance value during 660-nm illumination; and AC_{940} is the pulsing absorbance value during 940-nm illumination.[131]

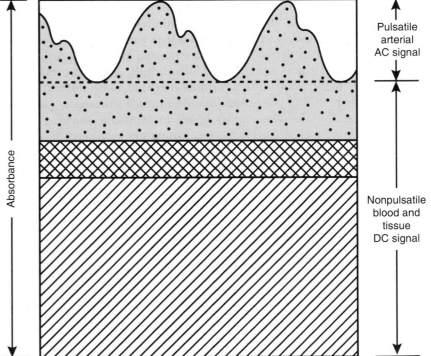

Pulsatile arterial AC signal

Nonpulsatile blood and tissue DC signal

Absorbance

FIGURE 19–22: The absorption signal received by a pulse oximeter showing the pulsatile alternating current (AC) component from arterial blood and the direct current (DC) component from venous and tissue absorption.

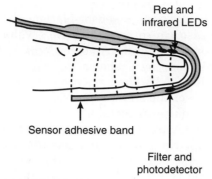

FIGURE 19–23: The basic components of a transmission pulse oximeter sensor. LED, light-emitting diode.

comparing the measured absorbance to reference values taken from studies of volunteers.

Reflectance pulse oximeters have been developed but remain unpopular.

The simple operation of the transmission pulse oximeter is one of the major reasons for its popularity. The device is calibrated at the factory and undergoes a self-diagnostic check when it is first powered up. Factory control over sensor LED quality is critical to the performance of the monitor. Sensors have been developed in various sizes and configurations for use with neonates, children, and adults. Sensors for the earlobe, finger, toe, neonatal foot, and bridge of the nose have been successfully developed. Most sensors are mounted in an adhesive bandage–like appliance that is simply taped to the selected monitoring site and easily adjusted for optimal pulse detection.

The accuracy (95% confidence limits) of the transmission pulse oximeter is generally within ±4% of the actual value when saturations are greater than 70% and is ±6% when they fall below 70%.[132] This disparity is thought to be due in large part to the reference values generated from volunteers, who are normal and in whom few values below 75% saturation are generated. The degree of inaccuracy in normal subjects can also be attributed to the engineering design, quality control of LEDs, microprocessor programming, condition of study subjects, and evaluation methodology.[133]

Various clinical factors have been found to influence accuracy (Table 19–12). Poor hemodynamics and subsequently the arterial pulsation will limit the accuracy of Sp_{O_2}.[132, 133] The pulse oximeter attempts to search for the pulse and to amplify it when it is weak. Unfortunately, this may also result in amplification of background noise, which can produce an inaccurate reading. Many of the devices on the market have the ability to notify the clinician of poor pulse strength and not to display readings

TABLE 19–12: Factors Affecting the Accuracy of Pulse Oximetry During Clinical Use

Poor hemodynamics	Temperature variation
Edematous sensor site	Presence of vascular dyes
Motion	Dark skin pigmentation
Ambient light artifaction	Nail polish
Dysfunctional hemoglobins	

during these conditions. During poor-perfusion states, the earlobe may be a better site for sensor placement.[134] Patient movement of the sensor may also cause erroneous Sp_{O_2} values and require immobilization to improve accuracy.[135] Ambient light from fluorescent, infrared, and xenon lamps has been shown to cause inaccuracies and require proper shielding.[136, 137] The presence of COHb causes falsely high Sp_{O_2} readings because of the similar absorbance properties in the light spectrum used by the pulse oximeters.[138] Patients with methemoglobinemia, such as those who are receiving sodium nitroprusside or dapsone therapy, may have the Sp_{O_2} driven artifactually toward 85% secondary to the unique light absorption properties of methemoglobin at both the red and the infrared wavelengths.[139] If patients are suspected of having abnormally elevated dysfunctional hemoglobin levels, they should have their blood analyzed by a multiwavelength CO-oximeter to determine the value of O_2Hb and any other hemoglobin derivatives accurately. Temperature variations above or below body temperature can cause the LEDs to shift their spectral outputs (0.2 nm/°C), which in turn results in additional errors of 1 to 4%.[133] The use of vascular dyes (e.g., methylene blue, indigo carmine, or indocyanine green) in diagnostic studies is known to cause erroneously low Sp_{O_2} values.[133, 140] Although dark skin pigmentation can lead to inaccuracies in measuring through the earlobe, it generally does not affect accuracy.[130, 141] In addition, the dark exogenous dyes in blue, green, or black nail polish are capable of absorbing some light and result in inaccurately low Sp_{O_2} measurements.[142]

Although both transcutaneous P_{O_2} monitoring and pulse oximetry have their distinct advantages (Table 19–13), the pulse oximeter has largely replaced the transcutaneous P_{O_2} electrode as the preferred noninvasive monitor of oxygenation in all age groups.

Capnometry and Capnography

Analyzing gas from the patient's airway can be accomplished with either sidestream or mainstream CO_2 detector systems.[143, 144] The sidestream system continuously collects a small sample of gas from the patient's airway by aspirating gas at 150 mL/min. The sample is then directed to the detector. This approach to sampling enables the monitoring of gas from patients who may or may not be intubated and from a variety of exhaled gas collectors. The limitations of a sidestream sampler include blockage of the sample tubing, contamination of the detector with aspirated water or ambient air, and lag time between sampling and

Capnometry—measuring CO_2 in the inhaled and exhaled gas and reporting its value as a partial pressure or percentage

Capnogram—displaying of the rise and fall of the concentration of CO_2 over time

Capnography—analysis of the rise and fall of the concentration of CO_2 over time

TABLE **19–13:** Comparison of Noninvasive Oxygen Monitoring Techniques

Advantages of Ptc$_{O_2}$ Monitoring
Will detect hyperoxemia
Accurately estimates Pa_{O_2} in neonatal respiratory distress
Less distorted by motion
Can better detect pre- versus postductal oxygen disparities

Advantages of Pulse Oximetry
No membrane to replace or complicated calibration
Rapid readings
No risk of thermal injury
Measures pulse rate
More effective in monitoring oxygenation in older patients

Adapted from Martin RJ. Transcutaneous monitoring: Instrumentation and clinical application. Respir Care 35:577, 1990.

reporting values. These problems can be avoided by the use of traps, purging of the sample tubing, proper placement as close to the airway as possible, and the use of short sample tubing. The mainstream system places the detector at the airway and thus requires an artificial airway for effective attachment. Although this provides a very rapid response, the windows that the detector is "viewing" through can be contaminated with sputum or water, which would lead to inaccuracies. Some of the mainstream detectors are relatively large and heavy, which can place substantial torque on the airway and increase the amount of mechanical dead space. Newer mainstream detectors are smaller, lighter, and more robust than their predecessors.

The most popular detector used in clinical medicine today is based on the rapid-response infrared analyzers first described by Luft[145] and Fowler[146] in the 1940s. This method is based on the property of CO_2 to absorb light in the infrared region of the spectrum. Most infrared capnometers use a wavelength of 4250 nm. With the use of this specific wavelength, the sensor will better detect CO_2 and avoid detecting water vapor, carbon monoxide, and nitrous oxide (N_2O), which absorb light better at other wavelengths. However, these gases do absorb light very close to this wavelength, which can lead to inaccuracies. To improve the sensor's accuracy, the light is carefully filtered to the desired wavelength, and correction factors are employed to correct for the effect (collision broadening) of other gases (notably N_2O) on CO_2 absorbance.[143]

The nondispersive double-beam, positive-filter detector (Fig. 19–24) is commonly found in sidestream capnometers.[143] Infrared light is reflected through a spinning wheel (chopper) that allows intermittent transmission of light through the sample chamber and the reference chamber and then on to the detector. CO_2 in the sample chamber absorbs some of the light, allowing less to travel on to the measuring half-cell of the detector. The reference chamber allows a fixed amount of light through to the reference half-cell of the detector. The measuring and reference half-cells are filled with CO_2 and are separated by a moveable diaphragm. Greater amounts of CO_2 in the sample chamber absorb more light, which in turn causes less light to reach the measuring half-cell. Less light reaching the measuring half-cell results in less thermal expansion of the gas, which causes the diaphragm to move. This movement can be detected and translated into a CO_2 value. The chopper improves the accuracy of the sensor by allowing equal amounts of light to reach the sample chamber and the reference chamber. The chopper also provides a zero light (dark) reference.

Some mainstream capnometers use single-beam, negative-filter sensors (Fig. 19–25).[143] Infrared light is passed through windows (sapphire

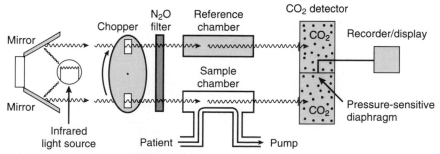

FIGURE 19–24: The basic components of a nondispersive double-beam, positive-filter infrared CO_2 detector used in many sidestream sampling systems.

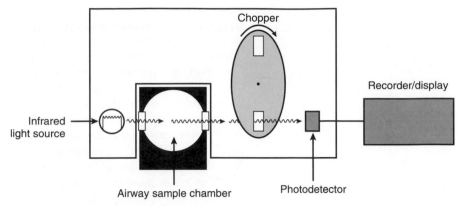

FIGURE 19–25: The basic components of a single-beam, negative-filter infrared CO_2 detector used in some mainstream sampling systems.

glass) of an adapter that is attached to the patient's airway. The space between the windows forms the sample chamber. The light is chopped after leaving the chamber by a spinning wheel with small cells of CO_2 and N_2 embedded in it. This results in the generation of two different signals by a photodetector. The ratio of the detector output is proportional to the amount of CO_2 in the sample chamber. A zero reference is provided during the inspiratory phase of breathing, when the partial pressure of CO_2 is virtually zero. This, however, can lead to inaccuracies when CO_2 is present during the inspiratory phase.

Mass spectrometry has been used successfully in the clinical environment for monitoring CO_2, O_2, N_2, and various anesthetic agents.[147-149] The medical gas mass spectrometer (Fig. 19–26) uses sidestream sampling. Gas samples are aspirated into a vacuum chamber and ionized by exposure to an electron beam. The ionized gas molecules enter and spread out in a dispersion chamber and fall in various trajectories according to their mass. The detectors for each gas respond as each charged gas molecule strikes them, a count is made, and gas concentration is determined. Most mass spectrometers used in critical care and anesthesia are centralized monitors that rely on computer-controlled sampling systems and data analysis to monitor multiple patients.

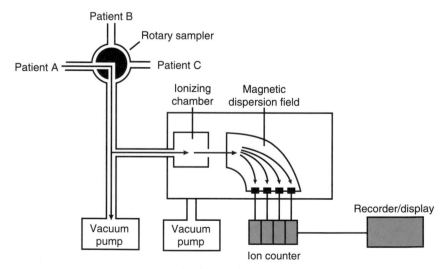

FIGURE 19–26: The basic elements of a medical gas mass spectrometer.

In practice, the analyzer is calibrated with high- and low-precision gases before and during use. Some are equipped with automatic calibrating features, whereas others have to be calibrated manually. Once attached to the patient's airway, the monitor begins to show breath-to-breath changes in CO_2 concentration.

The normal capnogram (Fig. 19–27) shows the changes in the partial pressure of CO_2 that occur during the respiratory cycle. As exhalation begins (midway between A and B), the first gas to pass the sensor is upper airway (anatomic dead space) gas with no CO_2 in it. The recording rapidly climbs (from B to C) as gas from alveoli begins to be exhaled. The slightly sloped plateau that follows (C to D) is the CO_2 concentration in alveoli as exhalation continues. The end-tidal CO_2 (PET_{CO_2}) is found at the end of alveolar emptying (D) and reflects an averaging of gas concentration. With the beginning of inspiration, the CO_2 rapidly declines to inspiratory gas values (D to E), which are normally 0.003% or 0.02 mm Hg.

The normal value of PET_{CO_2} is 35 to 45 mm Hg (5 to 5.5%), which is generally 2 to 5 mm Hg lower than the Pa_{CO_2}.[150–153] This has led to the widespread belief that PET_{CO_2} is an accurate reflection of the Pa_{CO_2}. However, poor gas sampling, contaminated sampling chambers, and failure to correct the readings to 37°C can lead to errors. In addition, the $P(a - ET)CO_2$ difference has been found to be greater in patients with cardiopulmonary disease (with variations in tidal ventilation, $\dot{V}/\dot{Q}$ mismatching, and increased dead space) and in some patients during anesthesia.[154, 155] In patients with lung disease, the gradient can be both increased and variable as the disease process evolves. In patients with airway obstruction, the PET_{CO_2} difference can be reduced by having the patient maximally exhale.[156] Occasionally, the PET_{CO_2} may be greater than the Pa_{CO_2}.[157, 158] This is thought to be the result of large tidal exhalation from lungs with low $\dot{V}/\dot{Q}$ ratios.[144] Thus, these findings suggest that PET_{CO_2} is useful in tracking Pa_{CO_2} in patients with relatively healthy lungs but becomes less reliable in those with lung disease.

Ironically, the noninvasive techniques described here are not held to the same quality control standards described for the in vitro analysis of blood. Although the degree of quality control may not be necessary, the data produced by these monitors is acted on so that patient care changes. This suggests that an appropriate quality control program is probably needed to strengthen the accuracy of these devices.

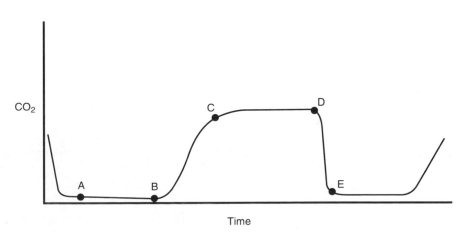

Time

FIGURE 19–27: The normal capnogram (see text for description).

SUMMARY

The determination of blood gas and acid-base parameters is central to the assessment of the patient in respiratory distress. Invasive and noninvasive techniques are available in both periodic and continuous sampling methodologies. Periodic invasive sampling of blood with in vitro analysis is the primary method for measuring Po_2, Pco_2, pH, and other parameters. Sampling methods for arterial, venous, and capillary blood have been developed to provide the clinician with various options in different clinical situations. With periodic sampling, the radial artery is the preferred site for collection in the adult, whereas capillary and venous sites are favored in the newborn and small pediatric patient, respectively. Care is needed to ensure the chemical integrity of the blood sample after its collection. This can be done by using a gas-tight syringe, placing the sample syringe in an ice bath if more than 10 minutes will elapse before analysis, and avoiding contamination of the sample with air bubbles and excessive heparin.

Continuous in vivo sampling and analysis techniques are available through the use of special intravascular catheters, which are equipped with sensors for the measurement of gases, acid-base balance, and oxyhemoglobin saturation. Electrodes and optodes are used to measure respiratory gases and pH, whereas oxyhemoglobin saturation is determined by spectrophotometry. Numerous derived values, such as oxygen content, plasma $[HCO_3^-]$, and base excess, are determined by the use of equations that are programmed into the typical automated analyzers. Both attention to sampling and analysis technique and the use of quality assurance programs are essential for reporting accurate values.

Various noninvasive technologies are available for both periodic and continuous monitoring. Miniaturized electrodes have been developed to measure transcutaneous and transconjunctival Po_2 and Pco_2. Oxyhemoglobin saturation can be accurately measured transcutaneously with the use of a pulse oximeter. Rapid-response infrared analyzers and mass spectrometry are used to measure end-tidal Pco_2. Although noninvasive methods are attractive alternatives to invasive methods, the noninvasive methods lack the degree of quality assurance that the in vitro blood analysis methods are required to have in place. This, coupled with the inherent limitations of the various noninvasive methods, renders them less accurate and precise than the periodic in vitro analytic method. On the other hand, continuous noninvasive methods uncover many more events and reveal trends that are important in understanding the patient's condition. Invasive and noninvasive measurement systems continue to evolve in ways that expand their utility and improve their accuracy.

References

1. Astrup P, Severinghaus JW. The History of Blood Gases, Acids and Bases. Copenhagen, Munksgaard International Publishers, 1986.
2. Van Slyke DD, Neill JM. The determination of gases in blood and other solutions. J Biol Chem 61:523, 1924.
3. Scholander PF. Analyzer for accurate estimation of respiratory gas in one half cubic centimeter samples. J Biol Chem 167:235, 1947.
4. Natelson S. Routine use of ultramicro methods in the clinical laboratory. Am J Clin Pathol 21:1153, 1951.
5. Lloyd BB. A development of Haldane's gas analysis apparatus. J Physiol (Lond) 143:6, 1958.
6. Mauakkassa FF, Rutledge R, Fakhry SM, et al. ABGs and arterial lines: The relationship to unnecessarily drawn arterial blood gas samples. J Trauma 30:1087, 1991.

7. Browning JA, Kaiser DL, Durbin CG Jr. The effect of guidelines on the appropriate use of arterial blood gas analysis in the intensive care unit. Respir Care 34:269, 1989.
8. Beasley KE, Darin JM, Durbin CG Jr. The effect of respiratory care department management of a blood gas analyzer on the appropriateness of arterial blood gas utilization. Respir Care 37:343, 1992.
9. Howe JP, Alpert JS, Rickman FD, et al. Return of arterial PO_2 values to baseline after supplemental oxygen in patients with cardiac disease. Chest 67:256, 1975.
10. Hess D, Good C, Didyoung R, et al. The validity of assessing arterial blood gases 10 minutes after an FIO_2 change in mechanically ventilated patients without chronic pulmonary disease. Respir Care 30:1037, 1985.
11. Mathews PJ. The validity of PaO_2 values 3, 6, and 9 minutes after an FIO_2 change in mechanically ventilated heart-surgery patients. Respir Care 32:1029, 1987.
12. Sherter CB, Jabbour SM, Kount DM, Snider GI. Prolonged rate of decay of arterial PO_2 following oxygen breathing in chronic airways obstruction. Chest 67:259, 1975.
13. National Committee for Clinical Laboratory Standards. Blood Gas Preanalytical Considerations: Specimen Collection, Calibration, and Controls [Tentative guideline]. Villanova, PA, National Committee for Clinical Laboratory Standards, 1989. NCCLS publication C27-T.
14. National Committee for Clinical Laboratory Standards. Percutaneous Collection of Arterial Blood for Laboratory Analysis [Approved standard]. Villanova, PA, National Committee for Clinical Laboratory Standards, 1985. NCCLS publication H11-A.
15. Sabin S, Taylor JR, Kapalan AI. Clinical experience using a small-gauge needle for arterial puncture. Chest 69:437, 1976.
16. Bageant RA. Variations in arterial blood gas measurement due to sampling technique. Respir Care 20:565, 1975.
17. Bryant MTT. Gases stored in disposable syringes. A study of changes in their concentrations. Anesthesia 32:784, 1977.
18. Scott PV, et al. Leakage of oxygen from blood and water samples stored in plastic and glass syringes. Br Med J 3:512, 1971.
19. Restall RVF, et al. Plastic or glass syringes: A comparison of the changes in oxygen tension when blood or water samples are stored in iced water. Br J Anaesth 47:636, 1975.
20. Evers W, Racz GB, Levy AA. A comparative study of plastic (polypropylene) and glass syringes in blood-gas analysis. Anesth Analg 51(1):92, 1972.
21. Winkler JB, Huntington CG, Wells DE, Befeler B. Influence of syringe material on arterial blood gas determinations. Chest 66:518, 1974.
22. Mueller RG, Lang GE. Phase equilibria of oxygen in "nitrogen filled Vacutainers." Clin Chem 19:1198, 1973.
23. Hansen JE, Simmons DH. A systematic error in the determination of blood PCO_2. Am Rev Respir Dis 115:1061, 1977.
24. Gauer P, et al. Effects of syringe and filling volume on analysis of blood pH, oxygen tension and carbon dioxide tension. Respir Care 25:558, 1980.
25. Hess CE, et al. Pseudohypoxemia secondary to leukemia and thrombocytosis. N Engl J Med 301:361, 1979.
26. Mortensen JD. Clinical sequelae from arterial needle puncture, cannulation, and incision. Circulation 35:1118, 1967.
27. Shapiro BA, Harrison RA, Cane RD, Kozlowski-Templin R. Clinical Applications of Blood Gases, 4th ed. Chicago, Year Book Medical Publishers, 1989.
28. Malley WJ. Clinical Blood Gases—Application and Noninvasive Alternatives. Philadelphia, WB Saunders, 1990.
29. Sackner MA, Avery WG, Sokolowski J. Arterial puncture by nurses. Chest 59:97, 1971.
30. Cole FS, Todres ID, Shannon DC. Technique for percutaneous cannulation of the radial artery in the newborn infant. J Pediatr 92:105, 1978.
31. Allen EV. Thromboangiitis obliterans: Method of diagnosis of chronic occlusive arterial lesions distal to the wrist with illustrative cases. Am J Med Sci 178:237, 1929.
32. Schreiner RL, Lemons JA, Kisling JA, Meyer CL. Techniques of obtaining arterial blood. *In* Schreiner RL, Kisling JA (eds). Practical Neonatal Respiratory Care. New York, Raven Press, 1982.
33. Gandy G, Grann L, Cunningham N, et al. The validity of pH and PCO_2 measurements in capillary samples in sick and healthy newborn infants. Pediatrics 34:192, 1964.
34. Hunt CE. Capillary blood sampling in the infant: Usefulness and limitations of two methods of sampling, compared with arterial blood. Pediatrics 51:501, 1973.
35. Powers WF. Digital capillary sampling. J Pediatr 93:729, 1978.
36. Karna P, Poland RL. Monitoring critically ill newborn infants with digital capillary blood samples: An alternative. J Pediatr 92:270, 1978.
37. Folger GM, Kouri P, Sabbah H. Arterialized capillary blood sampling in the neonate: A reappraisal. Heart Lung 9:521, 1980.
38. Gurman GM, Kriemerman S. Cannulation of big arteries in critically ill patients. Crit Care Med 13:217, 1985.
39. Slogoff S, Keats AS, Arlund C. On the safety of radial artery cannulation. Anesthesiology 59:42, 1983.

40. Bedford RF. Radial arterial function following percutaneous cannulation with 18 and 20-gauge catheters. Anesthesiology 47:37, 1977.
41. Band JD, Maki DG. Infections caused by arterial catheters used for hemodynamic monitoring. Am J Med 67:735, 1979.
42. Horowitz JH, Luterman A. Postoperative monitoring following critical trauma. Heart Lung 4:269, 1975.
43. Dunn PM. Localization of the umbilical artery catheter by post-mortem measurement. Arch Dis Child 41:69, 1966.
44. Miller D, Kirkpatrick BV, Kodroff M, et al. Pelvic exsanguination following umbilical artery catheterization in neonates. J Pediatr Surg 14:264, 1979.
45. Krauss AN, Albert RF, Kannan MM. Contamination of umbilical catheters in newborn infant. J Pediatr 77:965, 1970.
46. Bard H, Albert G, Teasdale F, et al. Prophylactic antibiotics in chronic umbilical artery catheterization in respiratory distress syndrome. Arch Dis Child 48:630, 1973.
47. Goetzman BW, Stadalnik RC, Bogren HG, et al. Thrombotic complications of umbilical artery catheters: A clinical and radiographic study. Perinatal Med 6:15, 1975.
48. Dennis RC, Ng R, Yeston NS, Statland B. Effect of sample dilutions on arterial blood gas determinations. Crit Care Med 13:1067, 1985.
49. Tung SH, Bettice J, Wang B, Brown EB Jr. Intracellular and extracellular acid-base changes in hemorrhagic shock. Respir Physiol 26:229, 1976.
50. Griffith KK, McKenzie MB, Peterson WE, Keyes JL. Mixed venous blood-gas composition in experimentally induced acid-base disturbances. Heart Lung 12:581, 1983.
51. Gambino SR, Thiede WH. Comparison of pH in human arterial, venous and capillary blood. Am J Clin Pathol 32:298, 1959.
52. Jung RC, Balchum OJ, Massey FJ. The accuracy of venous and capillary blood for the prediction of arterial pH, PCO_2 and PO_2 measurements. Am J Clin Pathol 45:129, 1965.
53. National Committee for Clinical Laboratory Standards. Protection of Laboratory Workers From Infectious Disease Transmitted by Blood, Body Fluids, and Tissues [Approved guideline]. Villanova, PA, National Committee for Clinical Laboratory Standards, 1991. NCCLS publication M29-T2.
54. Ishikawa S, Fornier A, Borst C, Segal MS. The effects of air bubbles and time delay on blood gas analysis. Ann Allergy 33:72, 1974.
55. Mueller RG, et al. Bubbles in samples for blood gas determination. A potential source of error. Am J Clin Pathol 65:242, 1976.
56. Madiedo G, Sciacca R, Hause L. Air bubbles and temperature effect on blood gas analysis. J Clin Pathol 33:864, 1980.
57. Mueller RG, Lang GE. Blood gas analysis: Effect of air bubbles in syringe and delay in estimation [Letter]. Br Med J 285:1659, 1982.
58. Biswas CK, Ramos JM, Agroyannis B, Kerr DNS. Blood gas analysis: Effect of air bubbles in syringe and delay in estimation. Br Med J 284:923, 1982.
59. Kelman GR, Nunn JF. Nomogram for correction of blood PO_2, PCO_2, pH and base excess for time and temperature. J Appl Physiol 21:1484, 1966.
60. Fox MJ, Brody JS, Weintraub LR. Leukocyte larceny: A cause of spurious hypoxemia. Am J Med 67:742, 1979.
61. Robin ED. Pathophysiology of hypoxia. Semin Respir Med 3:112, 1981.
62. Shapiro BA. In-vivo monitoring of arterial blood gases and pH. Respir Care 37:165, 1992.
63. Sanz MC. Ultramicro methods and standards of equipment. Clin Chem 3:406, 1957.
64. Stow RW, Randall BF. Electrical measurement of the PCO_2 of blood. Am J Physiol 179:678, 1954.
65. Severinghaus JW, Stupfel M, Bradley AF. Accuracy of blood pH and PCO_2 determinations. J Appl Physiol 9:189, 1956.
66. Astrup P. A simple electrometric technique for the determination of carbon dioxide tension in blood and plasma, total content of carbon dioxide in plasma and bicarbonate content in "separated" plasma at a fixed carbon dioxide tension. Scand J Clin Lab Invest 8:33, 1956.
67. Clark LC Jr, Wolf R, Granger D, Taylor Z. Continuous recording of blood oxygen tensions by polarography. J Appl Physiol 6:189, 1953.
68. Clark LC. Monitor and control of blood tissue oxygen tension. Trans Am Soc Artif Intern Organs 2:41, 1956.
69. Benesch RE, Benesch R, Yung S. Equations for the spectrophotometric analysis of hemoglobin mixtures. Anal Biochem 55:245, 1973.
70. Nilsson NJ. Oximetry. Physiol Rev 40:1, 1960.
71. Cane RD, Harrison RA, Shapiro BA, et al. The spectrophotometer absorbance of Intralipid. Anesthesiology 53:53, 1980.
72. Sidi A, Rush WR, Paulus DA, et al. Effect of fluorescein, indocyanine green and methylene blue on the measurement of oxygen saturation by pulse oximetry. Anesthesiology 65:A132, 1986.
73. Barker SJ, Tremper KK. The effect of carbon monoxide inhalation on pulse oximetry and transcutaneous PO_2. Anesthesiology 66:677, 1987.
74. Operator's Manual 482: Co-Oximeter. Lexington, MA, Instrumentation Laboratory.
75. Corning 2500 Co-Oximeter Operator's Manual. Ciba Corning.

76. Cole JS, Martin WE, Cheung PW, et al. Clinical studies with a solid state fiberoptic oximeter. Am J Cardiol 29:383, 1972.
77. Taylor JB, Lown B, Polanyi M. In-vivo monitoring with a fiber optic catheter. JAMA 221:667, 1972.
78. Martin WE, Cheung PW, Johnson CC, et al. Continuous monitoring of mixed venous oxygen saturation in man. Anesth Analg 52:784, 1973.
79. Divertie MB, McMichan JC. Continuous monitoring of mixed venous saturation. Chest 85:423, 1984.
80. Rasen J, Downs JB, Dehaven B. Titration of continuous positive airway pressure by real time dual oximetry [Abstract]. Crit Care Med 15:395, 1987.
81. Peterson JL, Vurek GG. Fiber-optic sensors for biomedical applications. Science 224:123, 1984.
82. Shapiro BA, Cane RD, Chomaka CM, et al. Preliminary evaluation of an intra-arterial blood gas system in dogs and humans. Crit Care Med 17:455, 1989.
83. Mahutte CK, Sassoon CSH, Muro JR, et al. Progress in the development of a fluorescent intravascular blood gas system in man. J Clin Monit 6:147, 1990.
84. Angel SM. Optodes: Chemically selective fiber-optic sensors. Spectroscopy 2:38, 1987.
85. Saari LA, Seitz WR. pH sensor based on immobilized fluoresceinamine. Anal Chem 54:821, 1982.
86. National Committee for Clinical Laboratory Standards. Tentative Standards for Definitions of Quantities and Conventions Related to Blood pH and Gas Analysis. Villanova, PA, National Committee for Clinical Laboratory Standards, 1982. NCCLS publication C12-T.
87. Siggard-Andersen O. Blood acid-base alignment nomogram. Scand J Clin Lab Invest 15:211, 1963.
88. Severinghaus JW. Blood gas calculation. J Appl Physiol 21:1108, 1966.
89. Ashwood ER, Kost G, Kenny M. Temperature correction of blood gas and pH measurement. Clin Chem 29:1977, 1983.
90. Andritsch RF, Muravchick S, Gold MI. Temperature correction of arterial blood-gas parameters: A comparative review of methodology. Anesthesiology 55:311, 1985.
91. Howell BJ, Baumgardner FW, Bondi K, Rahn H. Acid-base balance in cold-blooded vertebrates as a function of body temperature. Am J Physiol 218:600, 1970.
92. Randall DJ, Cameron JN. Respiratory control of arterial pH as temperature changes in rainbow trout, *Salmo guirdneri*. Am J Physiol 225:997, 1973.
93. Hicks GH, Stiffler DF. Patterns of acid-base regulation in urodele amphibians in response to variations in environmental temperature. Comp Biochem Physiol 77A:693, 1984.
94. Rahn H. Gas transport from the external environment to the cell. *In* de Reuk AVS, Porter R (eds). Development of the Lung. Boston, Little, Brown and Company, 1967.
95. Rahn H, Reeves RB, Howell BJ. Hydrogen ion regulation, temperature and evaluation. Am Rev Respir Dis 112:165, 1975.
96. Hansen JE, Sue DY. Should blood gas measurements be corrected for the patient's temperature? [Letter]. N Engl J Med 303:341, 1980.
97. Ream AR, Reitz BA, Silverberg G. Temperature correction of PCO_2 and pH in estimating acid-base status. Anesthesiology 56:41, 1982.
98. McConnel D, White F, Nelson RL, et al. Importance of alkalosis in maintenance of "ideal" blood pH during hypothermia. Surg Forum 26:263, 1975.
99. Ohmura A, Wong KC, Westenskow DR, et al. Effect of hypocarbia and normocarbia on cardiovascular dynamics and regional circulation in the hypothermic dog. Anesthesiology 50:293, 1979.
100. Matthews AJ, Stead AL, Abbott TR. Acid-base control during hypothermia. Anesthesia 39:649, 1984.
101. Bashein G, Townes BD, Nessly ML, et al. A randomized study of carbon dioxide management during hypothermic cardiopulmonary bypass. Anesthesiology 72:7, 1990.
102. Moran RF. External factors influencing blood gas analysis: Quality control revisted. Am J Med Tech 45:1009, 1979.
103. Medicare, Medicaid and CLIA programs: Regulations implementing the Clinical Laboratory Improvement Amendments of 1988 (CLIA '88)—Proposed rule with requests for comments. Federal Register 55(50):9538, 1990.
104. Medicare, Medicaid and CLIA programs: Regulations implementing the Clinical Laboratory Improvement Amendments of 1988 (CLIA '88)—Proposed rule. Federal Register 55(98):20896, 1990.
105. Clinical Laboratory Improvement Amendments of 1988: Final rule. Federal Register 57(40):7001, 1992.
106. Elser RC. Quality control of blood gas analysis: A review. Respir Care 31:807, 1986.
107. Levey S, Jennings ER. The use of control charts in the clinical laboratory. Am J Clin Pathol 20:1059, 1950.
108. Westgard JO, Barry PL, Hunt M, Groth T. A multi-rule Shewhart chart for quality control in clinical chemistry. Clin Chem 27:493, 1981.
109. Statland BE, Westgard JO. Quality control: Theory and practice. *In* Henry JB (ed). Clinical Diagnosis and Management by Laboratory Methods. Philadelphia, WB Saunders, 1984.

110. Hudson LD. Monitoring of critically ill patients. Conference summary. Respir Care 30:628, 1985.
111. Hess D. Noninvasive monitoring in respiratory care—Present, past, and future: An overview. Respir Care 35:482, 1990.
112. Lemen RJ, Quan SF. Intravascular line placement in critical care patients. In Fallat RJ, Luce JM (eds). Cardiopulmonary Critical Care Management. New York, Churchill Livingstone, 1988.
113. Peevy KJ, Hall MW. Transcutaneous oxygen monitoring: Economic impact on neonatal care. Pediatrics 75:1065, 1985.
114. King K, Simon RH. Pulse oximetry for tapering supplemental oxygen in hospital patient. Evaluation of protocol. Chest 92:713, 1987.
115. Bone RC, Balk RA. Noninvasive respiratory care unit: A cost effective solution for the future. Chest 93:390, 1988.
116. Severinghaus JW. Methods of measurement of blood and gas carbon dioxide during anesthesia. Anesthesiology 21:717, 1960.
117. Evans NTS, Naylor PRD. The systemic oxygen supply to the surface of human skin. Respir Physiol 3:21, 1967.
118. Huch A, Huch R, Lubbers DW. Transcutaneous PO_2. New York, Thieme-Stratton, 1981.
119. Martin RJ. Transcutaneous monitoring: Instrumentation and clinical application. Respir Care 35:577, 1990.
120. Taylor W. Transcutaneous and transconjunctival blood gas monitoring. Probl Respir Care 2:240, 1989.
121. Peabody JL, Emery JR. Noninvasive monitoring of blood gases in the newborn: Symposium on noninvasive neonatal diagnosis. Clin Perinatol 12:147, 1985.
122. Palmisano BW, Severinghaus JW. Transcutaneous PCO_2 and PO_2: A multicenter study of accuracy. J Clin Monit 6:189, 1990.
123. Martin RJ, Robertson SS, Hopple MM. Relationship between transcutaneous and arterial oxygen tension in sick neonates during mild hypoxemia. Crit Care Med 10:670, 1982.
124. Mahutte CK, Michiels TM, Hassel KT, et al. Evaluation of a single transcutaneous PO_2-PCO_2 sensor in adult patients. Crit Care Med 12:1063, 1984.
125. Green GE, Hassel KT, Mahutte CK. Comparison of arterial blood gas with continuous intra-arterial and transcutaneous PO_2 sensor in adult critically ill patients. Crit Care Med 15:491, 1987.
126. Fatt I, Bieber MT. The steady state distribution of oxygen and carbon dioxide in the in vivo cornea. Exp Eye Res 7:103, 1968.
127. Kwan M, Fatt I. A noninvasive method of continuous arterial oxygen tension estimation from measured palpebral conjunctival oxygen tension. Anesthesiology 35:309, 1971.
128. Vurek GG, Feustel PJ, Severinghaus JW. A fiberoptic PCO_2 sensor. Ann Biomed Eng 11:499, 1983.
129. Aoyagi T, Kishi M, Yamaguchi K, et al. Improvements of the earpiece oximeter [in Japanese]. Abstr 13th Annu Meeting Jpn Soc Med Electronics Biol Eng 90, 1974.
130. Welsh JP, DeCesare R, Hess D. Pulse oximetry: Instrumentation and clinical application. Respir Care 35:584, 1990.
131. Ohmeda Biox 3700 Pulse Oximeter Service Manual. Boulder, CO, Ohmeda, 1986.
132. Tremper KK, Barker SJ. Pulse oximetry. Anesthesiology 70:98, 1989.
133. Craig KC. Clinical application of pulse oximetry. Probl Respir Care 2:255, 1989.
134. Evans ML, Geddes LA. An assessment of blood vessel vasoactivity using photoplethysmography. Med Instrum 22:29, 1988.
135. Pologe JA. Pulse oximetry: Technical aspects. Int Anesthesiol Clin 25:137, 1987.
136. Amar D, Neidswski J, Wald A, Pinck AD. Fluorescent light interferes with pulse oximetry. J Clin Monit 5:135, 1989.
137. Costarino AT, Davis DA, Keon TP. False normal saturation reading with the pulse oximeter. Anesthesiology 67:830, 1987.
138. Barker SJ, Tremper KK. The effect of carbon dioxide inhalation on pulse oximeter signal detection. Anesthesiology 67:599, 1987.
139. Watch MF, Connor MT, Hing AV. Pulse oximetry in methemoglobinemia. Am J Dis Child 143:845, 1989.
140. Sidi A, Paulus DA, Rush W, et al. Methylene blue and indocyanine green artificially lower pulse oximetry reading of oxygen saturation: Studies in dogs. J Clin Monit 3:249, 1987.
141. Ries AL, Prewitt LM, Johnson JJ. Skin color and ear oximetry. Chest 96:287, 1989.
142. Cote CJ, Goldstein EA, Fuchsman WH, Hoaglin DC. The effect of nail polish on pulse oximetry. Anesth Analg 67:683, 1989.
143. Gravenstein JS, Paulus DA, Hayes TJ. Capnography in Clinical Practice. Boston, Butterworths, 1989.
144. Hess D. Capnometry and capnography: Technical aspects, physiologic aspects, and clinical applications. Respir Care 35:557, 1990.
145. Luft K. Über eine neue Methode der registrierenden Gasanalyse mit Hilfe der Absorption ultraroter Strahlen ohne spektrale Zerlegung. Z Techn Phys 24:97, 1943.
146. Fowler RC. A rapid infra-red gas analyzer. Rev Sci Instr 20:175, 1949.

147. Fowler KT, Hugh-Jones P. Mass spectrometry applied to clinical practice and research. Br Med J 1:1205, 1957.
148. Ayers SM. Use of mass spectrometry for evaluation of respiratory function in the critically ill patient. Crit Care Med 4:219, 1976.
149. Ozanne GM, Young WG, Mazzei WJ, Severinghaus JW. Multipatient anesthetic mass spectrometry: Rapid analysis of data stored in long catheters. Anesthesiology 55:62, 1981.
150. Nunn JF, Hill DW. Respiratory dead space and arterial to end-tidal CO_2 tension in anesthetized man. J Appl Physiol 15:383, 1960.
151. Whitsell R, Asiddao C, Gollman D, et al. Relationship between arterial and peak expired carbon dioxide pressure during anesthesia and factors influencing the difference. Anesth Analg 60:508, 1981.
152. Perrin F, Perrot D, Hotzapfel L, Robert D. Simultaneous variations of $PaCO_2$ and $PACO_2$ in assisted ventilation. Br J Anaesth 55:525, 1983.
153. Weinger MB, Brimm JE. End-tidal carbon dioxide as a measure of arterial carbon dioxide during intermittent mandatory ventilation. J Clin Monit 3:73, 1987.
154. Hatle L, Rokseth R. The arterial to end-expiratory carbon dioxide tension gradient in acute pulmonary embolism and other cardiopulmonary diseases. Chest 66:352, 1974.
155. Raemer DB, Frances D, Philip JH, et al. Variation in PCO_2 between arterial blood and peak expired gas during anesthesia. Anesth Analg 62:1065, 1983.
156. Tulou PP, Walsh PM. Measurement of alveolar carbon dioxide tension at maximal expiration as an estimate of arterial carbon dioxide tension in patients with airway obstruction. Am Rev Respir Dis 102:921, 1970.
157. Moorthy SS, Losasso AM, Wilcox J. End-tidal PCO_2 greater than $PaCO_2$. Crit Care Med 12:534, 1984.
158. Shankar KB, Moseley H, Kumar Y. Arterial to end tidal carbon dioxide tension differences during caesarean section anesthesia. Anesthesia 41:678, 1986.

Therapeutic Techniques

20 Cardiopulmonary Resuscitation

Nicholas G. Bircher, M.D., F.C.C.M.

Cardiopulmonary resuscitation (CPR) ought to comprise an important part of the skills of every health care professional. However, many of the key aspects of CPR are performed poorly by those with limited airway management experience. Thus, the respiratory therapist becomes an essential member of the team, for without adequate airway management, any patient experiencing cardiac arrest will surely die. For each of the interventions discussed in the following sections, optimal patient care requires a complete knowledge of the techniques, as well as the evidence concerning their use. CPR is divided into three phases, each of which has three steps, as illustrated in Table 20–1. This discussion includes both scientific and clinical principles of resuscitation. This chapter is not designed to present basic skills; these have been reviewed in greater detail elsewhere.[1–4]

EMERGENCY AIRWAY CONTROL

Airway control and artificial ventilation are necessary adjuncts to chest compressions in cardiac arrest because chest compressions do not provide ventilation.[5] Although arterial oxygen tension does remain adequate for up to 30 minutes during complete cardiac arrest, initiation of chest compressions without ventilation results in severe arterial hypoxemia within minutes.

Manual Methods Without Equipment

The combination of head tilting, forward displacement of the jaw, and opening of the mouth is termed the triple airway maneuver or jaw thrust maneuver.

In the unconscious patient, backward tilting of the head and forward displacement of the mandible usually prevent hypopharyngeal obstruction by the base of the tongue.[6] Lifting of the chin also prevents hypopharyngeal obstruction and keeps the mouth open.[7] Head tilt produced by lifting the chin is not demonstrably different from that produced by lifting the neck.[8]

However, in some unconscious patients, backward tilting of the head is not by itself sufficient to open the airway, and additional forward displacement of the jaw may be necessary.[7] Excessive opening of the mouth can compromise airway patency, as can the epiglottis.[8]

Positive Pressure Ventilation Attempts

Because the chances of successful resuscitation decline rapidly with increasing arrest time, the initiation of resuscitation should never be delayed while equipment is awaited. Medical personnel who may have to perform resuscitation should keep a complete array of equipment readily at hand.

Airway patency is verified by positive pressure ventilation attempts. There is no evidence to support the use of "staircase" ventilation as the initial ventilatory maneuver.[3] Furthermore, even a brief period of positive end-expiratory pressure can severely compromise hemodynamics during CPR, whereas high inflation pressures can inflate the stomach.[9] The initial attempts to ventilate an unintubated patient must be of

405

TABLE **20–1:** Phases and Steps of Resuscitation

Phase	Step
I. Basic life support	A. Airway control
	B. Breathing support
	C. Circulation support
II. Advanced life support	D. Drugs and fluids
	E. Electrocardiography
	F. Fibrillation treatment
III. Prolonged life support	G. Gauging
	H. Human mentation
	I. Intensive care

adequate volume but with low inflation pressures.[10] Both inflation of the stomach and passive regurgitation may be reduced by cricoid pressure.[11]

Manual Methods With Equipment

Placement of an oropharyngeal or a nasopharyngeal airway may facilitate lifting the tongue off of the posterior wall of the pharynx. The tongue is the most common cause of airway obstruction in the comatose or anesthetized patient. Cuffed pharyngeal tubes[12, 13] offer a greater likelihood of protecting the airway, although no reduction in the incidence of aspiration or change in outcome has been demonstrated. Aspiration, which remains a common complication of conventional ventilatory techniques used before endotracheal intubation, is significantly associated with mortality.

Esophageal Obturator Airway

The esophageal obturator airway is suitable for use by those not trained to perform endotracheal intubation, but its use is clearly inferior to endotracheal intubation.[3] In a modified form, the esophageal obturator airway allows a gastric decompression but does not provide definitive airway control. The rate of unrecognized tracheal intubation is up to 3%. A wide range of other complications attend the use of this device. Although no study has shown a definitive change in outcome with the use of this device as compared with endotracheal intubation, experts recommend that all in-hospital personnel and paramedics receive training in the latter, with esophageal obturator airway or esophageal gastric tube airway training being discouraged.

Endotracheal Intubation

Endotracheal intubation, the definitive means of airway control during resuscitation, should be performed as soon as feasible in all patients who need CPR. As stated previously, this should not delay the institution of ventilation by any immediately available means. No data exist on the delay of intubation and its contribution to mortality or morbidity. However, aspiration is a common and highly morbid if not fatal complication. A wide variety of paramedical personnel can be trained to safely and successfully intubate patients, and this skill is mandatory for any physician charged with the care of critically ill patients. Although the data concerning foreign body obstruction of the airway and difficult endotracheal intubation in humans are almost exclusively anecdotal, the unequivocal conclusion is that failure to establish an airway is uniformly fatal and that delay in establishing an airway adversely influences outcome. A full spectrum of techniques and equipment should be in the armamentarium of all acute care facilities, especially intensive care units.

EMERGENCY VENTILATION AND OXYGENATION

Ventilation Patterns

Intermittent positive pressure ventilation remains the principal means of artificial respiration during resuscitation. The use of positive end-expiratory pressure is an essential element of the management of most critically ill patients receiving intermittent positive pressure ventilation. However, although hypoxemia is a frequent antecedent of cardiac arrest and a common occurrence during CPR,[15] the use of positive end-expiratory pressure during CPR can either augment or depress cardiac output.[15] The mechanism of the latter effect is not entirely clear, but it is probably related to a reduction in venous return to the chest. On the other hand, pulmonary edema, which is seen frequently during CPR, may limit resuscitation. As a consequence, 100% oxygen should always be administered during the immediate phase of resuscitation, with reduction occurring only under controlled circumstances in the intensive care unit.

Although ventilation may produce some circulation, it is rarely sufficient to restart the heart once it has arrested. Simultaneous ventilation and compression, either manually, mechanically, or with a vest, have given variable results.[16] Independent or asynchronous ventilations provide oxygenation and ventilation comparable to those of interposed or alternating ventilations (delivered in between compressions). The ratio of interposed ventilations to chest compressions has little impact on oxygenation or ventilation until the interval between ventilations exceeds 15 seconds.[17]

Mouth-to-Mouth or Mouth-to-Nose Ventilation

The superiority of mouth-to-mouth ventilation over the wide variety of alternative manual methods has long been recognized.[14, 18, 19] Exhaled air must be delivered at approximately twice the normal tidal volume in order to maintain satisfactory oxygenation and ventilation. Ventilation should never await the arrival of adjuncts. The essential clinical criterion for adequacy of ventilation is that the chest must rise and fall with each and every ventilatory attempt. No technique or piece of equipment can be expected to provide ventilation unless it is used properly. If one technique fails, the problem must be rapidly corrected or another technique quickly adopted.

Low ventilatory pressures, as well as cricoid pressure, may limit gastric insufflation.[9–11] Although gastric distention is a real danger in children, it rarely poses a problem in adults.[19] Mouth-to-nose ventilation may be of use in the patient with trismus, arthritic fixation of the jaw, facial or oral scarring, facial fractures, or extensive lacerations of the mouth, but it is not uniformly successful in the hands of the minimally trained.[6]

The manual methods of artificial ventilation (Holger Nielsen and Silvester's) are obsolete for the management of cardiac arrest because they neither control the airway nor provide adequate tidal volume.[14]

Asynchronous ventilations are delivered randomly with respect to chest compressions.

The two essential advantages of mouth-to-mouth ventilation are the ability to maintain a patent airway and the delivery of positive pressure ventilation.

Mouth-to-Adjunct Ventilation

Mouth-to-airway ventilation, using any of the airway adjuncts described previously as well as the S tube (two Guedel airways connected at their proximal ends), avoids direct contact with the patient, maintains a patent airway, and thereby improves success in ventilation, especially by untrained laymen.[14] However, all pharyngeal tubes carry a risk of laryngospasm and the induction of vomiting in the stuporous patient. Mouth-to-mask ventilation also obviates direct patient contact but does not improve ventilatory efficacy over mouth-to-mouth ventilation, and mask leaks may detract from success in ventilation. If equipped with an oxygen nipple, a mask allows delivery of 40 to 54% oxygen during mouth-to-mask ventilation and 98% oxygen during intermittent occlusion of the breathing port of the mask with a 30-L/min oxygen inflow.

Bag-Valve-Mask Ventilation With Oxygen

In inexperienced hands, bag-valve-mask manual ventilation is fraught with hazards, principally because of difficulties in establishing a satisfactory seal between the mask and the face.[20-22] Although mouth-to-mask ventilation may be less effective than mouth-to-mouth ventilation in the inexperienced, with minimal training and the use of both hands to secure the mask and maintain head tilt and with the rescuer's vital capacity to compensate for leaks, mouth-to-mask ventilation becomes clearly more effective than bag-valve-mask ventilation. The efficacy of bag-valve-mask ventilation may also be improved by enlisting the assistance of a second rescuer,[23] by changing masks,[24] or by using an oxygen-powered, manually triggered positive pressure ventilation device.

Although the mask seal is the main limitation in the hands of those with limited training, the design of the bag for ventilation is critical for all rescuers. The capability to deliver 100% oxygen during CPR is contingent on the use of a reservoir of adequate size and flow rates sufficient to keep it filled.[25, 26] Pediatric bag-valve units[27] also require higher flows than Mapleson D anesthetic circuits to maintain the $F_{I_{O_2}}$ above 90%. The only limitation on the latter is that fresh gas flow must exceed 100 mL/kg/min to prevent rebreathing. If a pressure-limiting ("pop-off") valve is present, the $F_{I_{O_2}}$ becomes rate sensitive;[27] occluding this valve may be necessary to achieve adequate ventilatory pressures and a satisfactory $F_{I_{O_2}}$. Operator skill does influence delivered tidal volume, even if the mask seal is not in question;[28] thus, sufficient training of providers and adequate supervision of trainees is well advised. Because modern equipment still occasionally malfunctions, back-up equipment should be readily available, and if all else fails, mouth-to-mouth or mouth-to-adjunct ventilation should be initiated.

Mechanical Ventilators

Although it has never been studied with respect to outcome, severe hyperventilation carries the risk of exacerbating cerebral ischemia during CPR.

Early mechanical ventilators were not adequate for the management of cardiac arrest; currently available mechanical ventilators can theoretically come close to what an operator can do by hand. Unfortunately, this degree of sophistication in equipment and virtuosity in use are rarely available for the treatment of cardiac arrest. However, the vast majority of experimental models of CPR employ mechanical ventilation with satisfactory results. High-pressure ventilation via an endotracheal tube results in severe arterial respiratory alkalemia during CPR despite carbon dioxide admixture. At present, the safest approach is manual ventilation guided by arterial blood gas findings, which allow assessment of both oxygenation and ventilation.

High-Frequency Jet Ventilation

High-frequency ventilation, whether delivered by a jet ventilator (either transtracheally or via a specially configured endotracheal tube to achieve a jet effect) or by a conventional ventilator, provides adequate ventilation and oxygenation during CPR. This has been investigated for transtracheal ventilation for both ventricular fibrillation and asphyxial cardiac arrest.[15] There was no difference in hemodynamics between high-frequency jet ventilation and conventional positive pressure ventilation; in addition, the transtracheal route offers protection against aspiration in the unintubated animal. The necessary techniques and equipment can be mastered by emergency medical technicians.

Varying frequencies in jet ventilation does not appear to change ventilation or oxygenation; increased frequency in conventional ventilation results in arterial hypocarbia but does not alter mixed venous blood gas tensions.

EMERGENCY CIRCULATION

No variety of artificial circulation offers tissue preservation on an indefinite basis with impunity. Resuscitative efforts must therefore be focused on the rapid restoration of spontaneous circulation. This and other resuscitative measures may be facilitated by the use of algorithms or protocols.

Causes of Cardiac Arrest

The primary and secondary causes of cardiac arrest have been reviewed elsewhere.[29] The cause, if it can be determined, may have very important therapeutic implications, but this determination should never delay institution of life-support maneuvers. The most common electrocardiographic diagnosis associated with cardiac arrest both inside and outside hospitals is ventricular fibrillation. Ventricular fibrillation may be primary (as is common in the prehospital setting) or secondary (i.e., associated with noncardiac disease or injury). Other causes of primary cardiac arrest, in either ventricular fibrillation, asystole, or electromechanical dissociation, include acute myocardial infarction, heart block, electrical shock to the heart, cardiac toxicity of drugs, and cardiogenic shock. Common secondary causes of cardiac arrest include asphyxia and exsanguination, as well as severe hypoxemia or respiratory acidosis from pulmonary disease, metabolic acidosis from septic shock, and brain stem failure with intractable hypotension.

Recognition of Cardiac Arrest

Sudden arrest of the circulation results in a loss of consciousness within 15 seconds, an isoelectric electroencephalogram in 15 to 30 seconds, and agonal gasping for up to 60 seconds.

The prompt and accurate diagnosis of cardiac arrest is extremely important. Delay in diagnosis prolongs the arrest interval, which is one of the principal determinants of outcome, both experimentally and clinically. Cardiac arrest is defined clinically as the absence of a palpable

If an arterial line is in place, a pulse pressure of less than 5 mm Hg constitutes cardiac arrest, although the prognostic and therapeutic implications of a weakly beating heart have not been thoroughly investigated.

pulse in a large artery (i.e., the carotid, femoral, or brachial artery). If the patient is truly in cardiac arrest, unconsciousness will follow rapidly. However, the patient who is profoundly hypotensive may be able to sustain consciousness. The diagnosis of pulseless electrical activity is made imprecisely because the absence of a pulse does not necessarily mean cessation of mechanical activity of the heart. Fluctuations in intrathoracic pressure, such as those produced by both positive pressure ventilation and chest compressions, may either augment or impede the function of the failing heart.[15]

Closed-Chest Cardiopulmonary Resuscitation

Fundamental Physiology

There is now no doubt whatsoever that fluctuations in intrathoracic pressure can cause blood flow during cardiac arrest in a variety of circumstances.[15, 30] Debate remains about the extent to which direct cardiac compression contributes to flow and if so, when. Kouwenhoven's[31] hypothesis regarding compression of the heart was challenged almost immediately, but definitive experimental evidence took more than a decade to be amassed. A diffuse rise in intrathoracic pressure cannot, in and of itself, account for blood flow because it cannot produce a pressure gradient for flow inside the chest. The peripheral vasculature plays a critical role in the generation of pressure gradients giving rise to forward flow during CPR. The valves of the jugular venous system attenuate but do not ablate pressure transmission to the peripheral veins of the head. Because arteries transmit an unattenuated pressure, there is a peripheral arteriovenous perfusion gradient and consequent flow.

Relatively few hemodynamic data are available on human external CPR. Aortic pressures and cardiac output are inferior to those of direct cardiac massage,[32, 33] and measurements of arterial and venous pressures tend to support the thoracic pump mechanism of blood flow.[15] The duration of compression is a major determinant of flow in adult humans.[34] A rate of compression of between 40 and 80 compressions per minute does not appear to influence carotid blood flow[34] in adult humans, nor does increasing the compression rate from 60 to 140 alter end-tidal CO_2 during CPR.[35] Experimentally, the depth of compression shows a threshold of effectiveness,[36] so the depth of compression should always be evaluated clinically to ensure that it is sufficient to produce a femoral or carotid pulse.

The Brain During Cardiopulmonary Resuscitation

As noted earlier, high central venous pressures during chest compressions are transmitted to peripheral veins, and the sagittal sinus is no exception.[30, 37] Similarly, the coupling between vena cava pressure and cerebral venous pressure in the steady state was recognized long ago, as was the relationship between intrathoracic and intracranial pressure (ICP). During CPR, the large fluctuations in intrathoracic pressure are reflected in the intracranial space,[15, 30, 37] although intracranial compliance is not altered by cardiac arrest per se. However, in dogs with normal intracranial compliance, ICP is only modestly elevated by chest compressions,[15, 30, 37] through both direct transmission via cerebrospinal fluid and nonvalved vertebral veins.

Cerebral blood flow (CBF) during CPR is a critical concern because

Arrest time (total circulatory arrest) before the institution of CPR is a major determinant of the maximal CBF generated by chest compressions; maximal CBF falls very rapidly with increasing arrest time.[38, 39]

the goal in resuscitation is to return the patient home without any neurologic sequelae of resuscitation. The maintenance of cerebral perfusion pressure is essential because cerebral autoregulation cannot increase CBF if cerebral perfusion pressure is too low and is compromised by hypoxia or by cerebral ischemia itself. Cerebral perfusion pressure during CPR may be the difference of arterial pressure and either ICP or cerebral venous pressure; the greater of the latter two is the subtrahend.

CBF during standard CPR can be adequate to maintain cerebral venous oxygen tension[37] above levels thought to cause irreversible damage, but it is not reliable in this regard. Although the difference in outcome with complete ischemia versus very low flow has been debated, the preponderance of evidence suggests that minimal blood flow is better than no flow at all. Cerebral perfusion can be improved during standard CPR by epinephrine,[40] is improved or unchanged by other alpha-adrenergic agonists,[41] and is made worse by isoproterenol and by volume loading.[42] Alternative means of performing CPR variably improve or reduce CBF, but none has been demonstrated to improve outcome. In particular, despite very promising findings in the laboratory,[43, 44] simultaneous ventilation-compression CPR failed to improve outcome in a randomized, prospective clinical trial.[45] CBF is typically elevated along with ICP in the immediate postresuscitation period, but the cerebral hyperemia is rapidly replaced with cerebral hypoperfusion and normalization of ICP.

The Heart During Cardiopulmonary Resuscitation

Coronary blood flow is usually exceedingly poor during standard CPR.[40, 41, 46] The elevation in right atrial pressure produced by chest compression in humans is nearly equal to the elevation in aortic pressure.[47] Consequently, the perfusion pressure across the heart is nearly zero during chest compression. During the relaxation phase (CPR "diastole"), perfusion pressures are higher and predict outcome, and coronary perfusion can be markedly improved by epinephrine.[15]

The Lung During Cardiopulmonary Resuscitation

Little work has been done to elucidate pulmonary function during CPR. End-tidal CO_2 is known to be markedly depressed because of the profound low-flow state,[37, 48, 49] but no studies have directly measured CO_2 production. Dead space is estimated to be quite high,[37] and V_D/V_T is estimated to be 0.59.[48] In dogs with initially normal lungs, Pa_{O_2} can be maintained around 80 mm Hg with room air;[37] however, because arterial hypoxemia is a common finding in clinical resuscitation, 100% oxygen should always be administered when available. Shunt fraction during human CPR has not been studied, although instances in which a satisfactory arterial oxygen tension cannot be achieved with 100% oxygen are rare.

Combinations of Ventilations and Chest Compressions

The early investigations in the area of combinations of ventilations and chest compressions established the outer limits of the ratio of compressions to ventilations[17] but did not exhaustively map out optima for this ratio. It is, however, clear that chest compressions alone cannot provide ventilation[5] and require the addition of positive pressure venti-

Although CBF values as high as 90% of control (spontaneous circulation) have been reported during standard CPR, the majority of reported flows are in the range of 0 to 33% of control.

lation and that protracted periods between ventilations result in arterial desaturation.

One-Rescuer Cardiopulmonary Resuscitation

Current recommendations[3] call for a rate of 80 to 100 compressions per minute, a ratio of two slow (i.e., taking 1 to 2 seconds to deliver to minimize peak inspiratory pressure) ventilations to every 15 compressions, a minimal tidal volume of 800 mL, and a 50% duty cycle and 1.5- to 2-inch depth for compressions. This set of recommendations is specifically designed for the education of lay persons, who are unlikely to enjoy the luxury of a second trained rescuer.

Recommendations for one-rescuer CPR in infants (the 1st year of life) and children (aged 1 to 8 years) are similar to those for adults, except that for infants the pulse is evaluated in the brachial rather than the carotid artery, the rate of chest compression is greater than 100, the ratio of compressions to ventilations is 5:1, tidal volume is the minimum required to make the chest rise, and compressions are delivered with the index and middle fingers in the middle of the sternum, with a depth of 0.5 to 1 inch. Differences in children are that compressions are performed with the heel of one hand and to a depth of 1 to 1.5 inches.

Two-Rescuer Cardiopulmonary Resuscitation

Current recommendations[3] call for the rate of compression for adult CPR to be 80 to 100 compressions per minute, a brief pause after every fifth compression to deliver a slow ventilation, and a ratio of five compressions to every ventilation. The energy cost to the rescuer of performing CPR has never been measured, but CPR is a rapidly fatiguing activity. Once the trachea has been intubated, interposition of ventilations between compressions yields better oxygenation and ventilation[17] than ventilation at ordinary pressure simultaneous with chest compression. As discussed earlier, high-pressure ventilations can overcome this problem but have variable effects on cardiac output and on coronary and cerebral perfusion.

Monitoring the Effectiveness of Cardiopulmonary Resuscitation

Essential and Desirable Monitoring Equipment

No special devices are required for evaluating the effectiveness of artificial ventilation, oxygenation, and circulation. Careful attention must be paid, however, to inspection and palpation. Inspection determines whether or not the chest rises and falls with ventilation, the depth of chest compression proves to be adequate, and the rescuer's hands remain properly positioned. Palpation establishes the clinical diagnosis of cardiac arrest, locates landmarks, and helps to evaluate the quality of the pulse generated by chest compressions. Although simple means of assessing the quality of CPR are useful in avoiding poor performance, they are not reliable: it is possible to meet the recommended criteria and still have an extremely low cardiac output. For this reason, technologic assessment should be employed whenever possible.

Health care professionals are encouraged to learn both the one- and two-rescuer techniques because two or more rescuers are frequently available in both prehospital and in-hospital settings.

Because both chest compressions and ventilations are physically taxing, rescuers should seek help whenever feasible and should know organized means of switching roles in order to avoid interruption of artificial perfusion.[3]

Ventilations

The essential clinical criterion is that the chest must rise and fall with every ventilatory effort. Auscultation of breath sounds before and after intubation is a useful indicator of air exchange, but it neither guarantees adequate ventilation during CPR nor definitively establishes endotracheal intubation. Capnography confirms endotracheal intubation and provides a useful assessment of cardiac output as well.[49, 50] Although the absence of arterial blood gas capability does not preclude successful resuscitation, direct measurement of arterial blood gases should be considered an essential item for all in-hospital resuscitations. Abnormalities of oxygenation, ventilation, and metabolic acid-base status are common.[15, 18, 37, 51–54]

The chemically treatable component of acidosis (i.e., the metabolic component) is essentially the same on the arterial and venous sides of the circulation, as is the lactate concentration, even though there may be a substantial difference in pH because of venous hypercarbia. Therefore, the use of arterial blood gas measurements should be encouraged, but administration of sodium bicarbonate, as discussed later, should be limited to the correction of severe metabolic acidosis (i.e., a base deficit of greater than 10 mEq/L). Pulse oximetry, which relies on the delivery of oxygenated blood to tissue in a pulsatile fashion, can be used during CPR to assess the adequacy of both oxygenation and circulation; however, this technique is not entirely reliable.

Repetitive sampling of arterial blood is an indication for arterial cannulation, and because the femoral artery is frequently punctured for this purpose during CPR, placement of an arterial line using the Seldinger technique may be a useful option. Radial artery cutdown is also reliable.[35]

Circulation

Clinical assessment of the quality of the circulation by palpation of the pulse serves only to ensure that the chest compressions delivered are of sufficient depth[36] or force to generate a palpable arterial pressure wave. Because the intrathoracic perfusion pressures are small and the extrathoracic perfusion pressures are difficult to predict, the presence of a pulse may or may not be indicative of flow. An arterial line may be a useful indicator of the adequacy of chest compressions, allows immediate recognition of the return of a pulse pressure, and permits repetitive sampling of arterial blood. Pulse oximetry may give some indication of the quality of the circulation, but end-tidal CO_2 is a much more sensitive indicator. Direct measurement of cardiac output during CPR is feasible but technically difficult because of the profound low-flow state.[32, 33]

Flow is typically too low to allow auscultation of arterial pressure with a cuff, although flow may be detectable with a Doppler device.

Neurologic Function

Neurologic assessment during CPR is a very poor predictor of outcome, and decisions to continue or to stop resuscitative efforts should not be made on this basis. The absence of specific neurologic signs during basic life support does not preclude their prompt return on restoration of spontaneous circulation.

Mechanical Cardiopulmonary Resuscitation

Mechanical devices may offer some advantages during clinical CPR. Early versions had a wide variety of problems, but currently available devices offer consistent compressions and higher arterial pressures in humans.[55] They have never, however, been shown to influence outcome in patients.

Complications of Cardiopulmonary Resuscitation

The complications of CPR are legion,[15] but unavoidable complications are acceptable compared with an otherwise certain death. On the other hand, many potentially fatal complications are avoidable. Hepatic trauma, for instance, which seems to have been common early in the modern era of CPR, can lead to rapid exsanguination. The more recently reported incidence is lower. Gastroesophageal damage, which was also a remarkably frequent complication, carries the risk of fatal mediastinitis or hemorrhage despite the restoration of circulation and consciousness. Reduced gastric damage may have resulted from attention to landmark location, limiting of gastric insufflation by cricoid pressure, earlier intubation, or gastric decompression. Inadvertent esophageal intubation is not uncommon and is a risk factor for gastric distention and rupture, although pneumoperitoneum does not always indicate visceral rupture. Similarly, kidney, pancreas, colon, spleen, and mesenteric vessel trauma are rare complications in present-day CPR.

Cardiac trauma presumably falls into the unpreventable category, but this should be tempered by degree. Mild cardiac contusions are routine in the laboratory and clinical setting, as are small hemopericardia or pericardial effusions, but laceration or rupture of the heart or the great vessels is rare, as are papillary muscle rupture, atheromatous emboli, and subclavian thrombosis. Direct mechanical trauma to the lung is ordinarily limited to the hilum, but barotrauma tends to be parenchymal. Rupture of the diaphragm is fortuitously rare. Aspiration of gastric contents or blood, pneumonia, and adult respiratory distress syndrome are also common.

Bony trauma, a very common problem, typically involves the ribs and sternum but rarely the vertebrae. However, not all patients receiving chest compressions have rib fractures. Hemothoraces secondary to rib fractures can be substantial and can contribute to the relative or absolute hypovolemia of the patient. Bone marrow emboli are common sequelae of CPR but may be from other causes. Infectious complications related to rescuers contracting disease from their CPR patients have received a great deal of attention in the lay press. Although there is no sound epidemiologic basis for this conclusion, universal precautions are justified during CPR because of the possibility of seropositivity in patients.

PHARMACOLOGY

Routes for Drugs and Fluids

The intramuscular, sublingual, and intralingual routes have no role during CPR.

Virtually any secure peripheral intravenous route will allow a successful resuscitation to be conducted.[56] Central venous access is not a necessity during CPR but offers the advantages of more rapid drug delivery and higher peak levels, although these are not consistent findings. Delay in restarting the heart should not be caused by a lack of intravenous access. Alternatives include intratracheal,[57] intraosseous,[58] intra-arterial, and intracardiac administration.

Drugs

Epinephrine

Aside from oxygen, epinephrine is the single most useful drug currently available for the treatment of cardiac arrest. An enormous body of evidence now supports the use of epinephrine during CPR,[3, 4, 15, 16, 41, 59–73] and withholding this drug if CPR and defibrillation fail to restore spontaneous circulation can only rarely be justified. The optimal use of epinephrine requires that all other components of an ongoing resuscitation be conducted efficiently. Both metabolic and respiratory acidosis limit its effectiveness, as does hypoxia. Although epinephrine does not alter the rate of successful defibrillation after brief periods of cardiac arrest, it does increase the rate of return of spontaneous circulation.[64] This effect appears to be a combination of the increased myocardial perfusion provided during CPR and the increase in myocardial contractility that accrues immediately after restarting of the heart.[64] Although there is a dramatic increase in coronary blood flow with epinephrine, the beta-adrenergic stimulus can limit the degree of improvement in the ratio of either subendocardial to epicardial blood flow or myocardial oxygen supply to demand.[74]

Alternative alpha-adrenergic agents that have been compared with epinephrine include phenylephrine,[15, 40, 60, 61] metaraminol, and methoxamine.[59, 60, 70] None of these has been demonstrated to offer any advantage in outcome compared with epinephrine. Coronary vasoconstriction remains a risk of any agent with alpha-adrenergic activity, as is an excessive hypertensive response after restarting of the heart, which may influence cerebral outcome for better or worse or may precipitate rearrest from coronary ischemia. However, higher doses of epinephrine are not more efficacious than those presently used clinically.[3, 4, 41] In pigs, raising the dose from 0.02 to 0.2 mg/kg improves myocardial blood flow.[68] Clearly, increasing the dose from 0.01 to 0.1 mg/kg provides a much more dramatic elevation in epinephrine levels over those endogenously available, but three randomized clinical trials in adults[75–77] have failed to demonstrate improved outcome. Epinephrine is the drug most commonly administered via the endotracheal tube during CPR, but this route of administration is not reliable.[72]

Atropine

Atropine is an essential adjunct to the resuscitation of children, in whom profound bradycardia, even in the presence of a pulse, signals a nearly complete cessation of circulation. Their higher degree of vagal tone renders them more susceptible to circulatory compromise than adults, but the latter are not immune. Atropine has no known hemodynamic effects during CPR. It is reportedly efficacious in epinephrine-refractory asystole,[78] although its effect is not consistent. It is of no value for experimental electromechanical dissociation. It can be administered intravenously, intraosseously, or endotracheally.[3]

Sodium Bicarbonate

Investigations of carbon dioxide (CO_2) transport during CPR[35, 49, 50] unfortunately have been widely misinterpreted to mean that there is no indication for the administration of sodium bicarbonate during CPR. So-called selective venous hypercarbia[53] is a necessary result of a profound low-flow state:[79] that is, it follows directly from the Fick principle that if CO_2 production remains constant and cardiac output decreases, the arteriovenous difference in CO_2 content must rise. Although it is erroneous to automatically use bicarbonate, especially for arrests of brief duration[80] or in an attempt to correct acidosis of respiratory origin, the correction of severe metabolic acidosis after prolonged periods of complete circulatory arrest does improve outcome in animals.[15, 51, 81, 82]

Severe metabolic acidosis is well documented to exist in some patient populations.[15] However, the vast majority of cardiac arrests in critical care areas are witnessed and are therefore unlikely to be associated with severe metabolic acidosis. Experimentally, if CPR is initiated after a brief period of arrest, pH falls slowly in dogs.[37, 83, 84] On the other hand, a prolonged arrest time can lead to a substantial acidosis. Unwitnessed cardiac arrest associated with severe acidosis is a frequent phenomenon on hospital wards[15] and in the prehospital setting.[52] Similarly, prolonged resuscitation efforts require bicarbonate to maintain physiologic blood gas levels despite early CPR and aggressive hyperventilation.[85] In very rare situations, ventilator therapy fails to correct pH even with a beating heart, and bicarbonate is required to prevent cardiac arrest.[86] Severe acidosis of either respiratory or metabolic origin depresses the myocardium,[15] although the beating heart can tolerate extreme hypercarbia remarkably well.[87] Mild metabolic or respiratory acidosis may slightly improve hemodynamics, protect the hypoxic myocardium, or limit hypoxic and posthypoxic myocardial contracture.[15] In animals with an initially normal pH, bicarbonate infusion produces a decrease followed by an increase in myocardial contractility. Metabolic acidosis renders the heart more susceptible to ventricular fibrillation, whereas mild metabolic alkalosis protects against fibrillation and respiratory alteration of pH may have little effect. Mild acidosis and hypoxia do not influence the rate of successful defibrillation in animals,[88] but they may do so in clinical cardiac arrest.[89]

Although it has long been known that changing the extracellular bicarbonate concentration changes intracellular pH even if CO_2 is held constant, the optimal treatment of metabolic acidosis of ischemic or hypoxic origin remains controversial.[4, 15, 76, 80] Exogenous infusion of lactic or other acid (extracellular "metabolic" acidosis) and exogenously administered CO_2 (extracellular respiratory acidosis, for which the time frame for resolution of the extracellular-intracellular gradient is very short) are fundamentally different than acidosis that is generated by ischemia or hypoxia (intracellular metabolic acidosis). In the last instance, the intracellular pH is considerably less than the extracellular pH, and this type of acidosis produces damage to cellular components by itself. Secondly, when exogenous metabolic acid is used to bathe normal cells with an intact cell membrane, the cell membrane provides the intracellular components with substantial protection because the acid gets into the cell slowly as compared with CO_2. On the other hand, although CO_2 gets into the cell very quickly, it does relatively little damage to cells by itself.[87] Cerebrospinal fluid acidosis accrues during CPR if bicarbonate is administered every 5 minutes irrespective of arterial pH,[90] but not if one or two doses are given.[54, 91] Clinical administration of sodium bicarbonate must therefore be done judiciously, titrated to the treatment of severe metabolic acidosis documented by arterial blood gas measurement. It cannot be given endotracheally, but it can be given intravenously or intraosseously.

Alternative buffering agents include 2-amino-2-(hydromethyl)-1,3-propanediol, which is also known as tris(hydroxymethyl)aminomethane and "tris buffer," dichloroacetate, sodium lactate, and Carbicarb. None has been shown to yield outcome superior to that of bicarbonate in severe metabolic acidosis due to cardiac arrest and resuscitation.[15] Compared with saline, dichloroacetate does accelerate clearance of lactate after

Risks of bicarbonate therapy include

Hyperosmolarity
Exacerbation of pre-existing hypoventilation
Alkalemia
Hypernatremia
Hemodynamic compromise, especially if hypoxia remains uncorrected
Mixed venous hypercarbia[53]

resuscitation from asphyxial cardiac arrest, but the therapeutic implication of this result remains unclear.[15]

Antidysrhythmics

Lidocaine is not known to alter the hemodynamics of CPR. It does, however, raise the energy requirement for defibrillation, but this effect is modulated by the anesthetic used in experimental work. It can facilitate treatment of refractory ventricular fibrillation when it is administered by either the intravenous or the endotracheal route. In the setting of myocardial infarction, it may lower the incidence of primary or recurrent fibrillation but can also cause asystole. Hepatic blood flow is inadequate to clear lidocaine during CPR; infusions therefore ought to be started after the heart has been restarted. The antidysrhythmic efficacy of lidocaine is determined by concentrations of lidocaine in ischemic myocardium rather than by blood levels, so a higher dose may be required. The hemodynamic effects of procainamide on CPR have not yet been investigated. After brief periods of cardiac arrest, it does not facilitate successful defibrillation compared with epinephrine alone.[92] Bretylium is known to have a biphasic effect on the sympathetic nervous system during spontaneous circulation. It cannot be relied on to produce chemical defibrillation. It does not significantly alter the defibrillation threshold and does not offer any advantage over lidocaine in the management of cardiac arrest.

Adrenergic Agonists Other Than Epinephrine

Norepinephrine can provide more cerebral blood flow during CPR than epinephrine,[4, 41] but the impact on outcome after CPR has yet to be demonstrated. It functions best in a nonacidotic milieu but is currently regarded as a last resort in the pharmacologic support of the ischemic heart. Dopamine and epinephrine are equally effective in the treatment of both asphyxial and fibrillatory cardiac arrest in dogs.[61] Dopamine's principal utility is in the support of the beating heart; however, this requires correction of severe metabolic acidosis for optimal effect. Because dobutamine is essentially a pure beta-adrenergic agonist, it offers no advantage during CPR and may worsen outcome compared with alpha-adrenergic agents.[61] Multiple comparisons of isoproterenol and epinephrine have shown that the latter is vastly superior for the treatment of cardiac arrest.[16, 59, 61] During CPR, isoproterenol shunts blood away from vital organs. Catecholamine cardiomyopathy is a real risk with this drug; therefore, in the setting of myocardial ischemia, it should be carefully titrated to achieve the desired chronotropic effect in atropine-refractory block and bradycardia. Even asthmatics with healthy hearts can experience fatal myocardial damage during isoproterenol infusion.[93]

Calcium Chloride

Ever since Ringer's serendipitous discovery of calcium's inotropic effect, there has been interest in its use for resuscitation. It has proved to be a useful adjunct to direct cardiac massage for fibrillation controlled with potassium salts and the reversal of perioperative myocardial depression. Calcium has also long been known to be of only moderate efficacy in other resuscitative circumstances.[59, 66] In the critical care and perioperative settings, ionized calcium is an important determinant of myocardial function. Low levels of ionized calcium are observed more commonly in patients in the prehospital setting than in those in intensive care units. It does not appear to be of any value in asystole[94, 95] or experimental electromechanical dissociation.[15] The response to calcium is limited in clinical electromechanical dissociation but it appears to be effective in some patients in the prehospital setting.[94] Administration of calcium has risks, both in the patient with a beating heart and during cardiac arrest. The effect of epinephrine depends on available calcium but is impaired only at very low calcium levels.

Calcium Entry Blockers

The calcium entry blockers are, in general, potent negative inotropes and vasodilators. Consequently, they have no role during standard CPR and serve to defeat the therapeutic advantages offered by epinephrine. Although cardioprotective and antifibrillatory, they are of no value in the treatment of asystole or electromechanical dissociation. They may be of value in refractory ventricular tachycardia or hypercalcemia, but they carry the risk of profound hypotension in recently resuscitated patients and of inducing ventricular fibrillation in patients with Wolff-Parkinson-White syndrome.

SUMMARY

CPR is a set of skills essential to preventing sudden, unexpected death from occurring and to minimizing the morbidity of an episode of pulselessness. The three life-support phases of CPR are (1) basic, (2) advanced, and (3) prolonged. Basic life support consists of airway control, artificial ventilation, and manual circulation of blood flow with chest compressions. Definitive airway control is accomplished through endotracheal intubation, which provides superior airway protection and optimizes the use of positive pressure ventilation. Chest compressions circulate blood but are no substitute for adequate spontaneous circulation. Basic life support, if well performed, slows the progression of damage during cardiac arrest, but for optimal patient outcome, it must be rapidly accompanied by advanced life support.

Advanced life support focuses on restarting the heart and consists of electrocardiographic diagnosis, defibrillation, and drug therapy. Although present-day algorithms stress defibrillation as the first priority, initial countershocks still frequently require adjunctive pharmacotherapy (especially epinephrine) to be effective. Rapid and reliable intravenous access is the optimal means of delivering drugs. Once the heart has been restarted, the patient must be rapidly stabilized and prolonged life support must be instituted if indicated.

Prolonged life support involves not only ongoing resuscitation to optimize cerebral and systemic oxygen transport but also rational consideration of the prognosis. Intensive care means precise control of physiologic variables. This control must be rapidly instituted with invasive monitoring and judicious use of pressor, inotropic, and antidysrhythmic agents. This is usually best done in the intensive care unit. The overall prognosis is governed by extracranial organ systems, but this must be coupled with prognostic information regarding cerebral outcome. Finally, the broad spectrum of long-term life-support measures applied in the intensive care unit is also essential for optimizing patient outcome.

To achieve the optimal outcome after an episode of sudden cardiac arrest, all of these skills must be applied with deliberate speed but not with precipitous haste. Careful and proficient resuscitation requires a thorough knowledge of techniques and strategies. Only through alacrity can the best patient outcome be reached.

References

1. Albarran-Sotelo R, Atkins JM, Bloom RS, et al. Textbook of Advanced Cardiac Life Support. Dallas, TX, American Heart Association, 1987.
2. Safar P, Bircher NG. Cardiopulmonary Cerebral Resuscitation: An Introduction to Resuscitation Medicine. London, WB Saunders, 1988.
3. Emergency Cardiac Care Committee, American Heart Association. Guidelines for cardiopulmonary resuscitation and emergency cardiac care. JAMA 268:2135, 1992.
4. Brown CG, Paraskos JA (eds). Proceedings of the 1992 National Conference on Cardiopulmonary Resuscitation and Emergency Cardiac Care. Ann Emerg Med 22:275, 1993.
5. Safar P, Brown TC, Holtey WJ, Wilder RJ. Ventilation and circulation with closed-chest cardiac massage in man. JAMA 176:574, 1961.
6. Safar P, Aguto-Escarraga L, Chang F. Upper airway obstruction in the unconscious patient. J Appl Physiol 14:760, 1959.
7. Elam JO, Greene DG, Schneider MA, et al. Head-tilt method of oral resuscitation. JAMA 172:812, 1960.
8. Morikawa S, Safar P, DeCarlo J. Influence of the head-jaw position upon upper airway patency. Anesthesiology 22:265, 1961.
9. Ruben H, Knudsen EJ, Carugati G. Gastric inflation in relation to airway pressure. Acta Anaesthesiol Scand 5:107, 1961.
10. Melker RJ. Alternative methods of ventilation during respiratory and cardiac arrest. Circulation 74(Suppl IV):IV-63, 1986.
11. Sellick BA. Cricoid pressure to control regurgitation of stomach contents during induction of anesthesia. Lancet 2:404, 1961.
12. Niemann JT, Rosborough JP, Myers R, Scarberry EN. The pharyngeotracheal lumen airway: Preliminary investigation of a new adjunct. Ann Emerg Med 13:591, 1984.
13. Frass M, Frenzer R, Zdrahal F, et al. The esophageal tracheal combitube: Preliminary results with a new airway for CPR. Ann Emerg Med 16:768, 1987.
14. Safar P, Escarraga LA, Elam JO. A comparison of the mouth-to-mouth and mouth-to-airway methods of artificial respiration with the chest-pressure arm-lift methods. N Engl J Med 258:671, 1958.
15. Bircher NG. Physiology and pharmacology of standard cardiopulmonary resuscitation. *In* Kaye W, Bircher NG (eds). Cardiopulmonary Resuscitation. New York, Churchill Livingstone, 1989, pp 55–86.
16. Chandra NC: Mechanisms of blood flow during CPR. Ann Emerg Med 22:281, 1993.
17. Harris LC, Kirimli B, Safar P. Ventilation-cardiac compression rates and ratios in cardiopulmonary resuscitation. Anesthesiology 28:806, 1967.
18. Elam JO, Brown ES, Elder JD, et al. Artificial respiration by mouth-to-mask method. A study of the respiratory gas exchange of paralyzed patients ventilated by operator's expired air. N Engl J Med 250:749, 1954.
19. Gordon AS, Frye CW, Gittleson L, et al. Mouth-to-mouth versus manual artificial respiration for children and adults. JAMA 167:320, 1958.
20. Harrison RR, Maull KI, Keenan RL, Boyan CP. Mouth-to-mask ventilation: A superior method of rescue breathing. Ann Emerg Med 11:74, 1982.
21. Elling R, Politis J. An evaluation of emergency medical technicians' ability to use manual ventilation devices. Ann Emerg Med 12:765, 1983.
22. Hess D, Baran C. Ventilatory volumes using mouth-to-mouth, mouth-to-mask, and bag-valve-mask techniques. Am J Emerg Med 3:292, 1985.
23. Jesudian MCS, Harrison RR, Keenan RL, Maull KI. Bag-valve-mask ventilation; Two rescuers are better than one: Preliminary report. Crit Care Med 13:122, 1985.
24. Stewart RD, Kaplan R, Pennock B, Thompson F. Influence of mask design on bag-mask ventilation. Ann Emerg Med 14:403, 1985.
25. Barnes TA, Watson ME. Oxygen delivery performance of old and new designs of the Laerdal, Vitalograph, and Ambu adult resuscitators. Respir Care 28:1121, 1983.
26. Campbell TP, Stewart RD, Kaplan RM, et al. Oxygen enrichment of bag-valve-mask units during positive-pressure ventilation: A comparison of various techniques. Ann Emerg Med 17:232, 1988.
27. Finer NN, Barrington KJ, Al-Fadley F, Peters KL. Limitations of self-inflating resuscitators. Pediatrics 77:417, 1986.
28. Augustine JA, Seidel DR, McCabe JB. Ventilation performance using a self-inflating anesthesia bag: Effect of operator characteristics. Am J Emerg Med 5:267, 1987.
29. Safar P, Bircher NG. Pathophysiology of dying and reanimation. *In* Schwartz GR, Cayten CG, Mangelson MA, et al (eds). Principles and Practice of Emergency Medicine, 3rd ed. Philadelphia, Lea & Febiger, 1992, pp 3–41.
30. Bircher NG, Safar P, Eshel G, Stezoski W. Cerebral and hemodynamic variables during cough-induced CPR in dogs. Crit Care Med 10:104, 1982.
31. Kouwenhoven WB, Jude JR, Knickerbocker GG. Closed-chest cardiac massage. JAMA 173:1064, 1960.

32. Del Guercio LRM, Coomaraswamy RP, State S. Cardiac output and other hemodynamic variables during external cardiac massage in man. N Engl J Med 269:1398, 1963.
33. Del Guercio LRM, Feins NR, Cohn JD, et al. Comparison of blood flow during external and internal cardiac massage in man. Circulation 31/32(Suppl I):I–171, 1965.
34. Taylor GJ, Tucker WM, Greene HL, et al. Importance of prolonged compression during cardiopulmonary resuscitation in man. N Engl J Med 296:1515, 1977.
35. Ornato JP, Gonzalez ER, Garnett AR, et al. Effect of cardiopulmonary resuscitation compression rate on end-tidal carbon dioxide concentration and arterial pressure in man. Crit Care Med 16:241, 1988.
36. Babbs CF, Voorhees WD, Fitzgerald KR, et al. Relationship of blood pressure and flow during CPR to chest compression amplitude: Evidence for an effective compression threshold. Ann Emerg Med 12:527, 1983.
37. Bircher NG, Safar P, Stewart R. A comparison of standard, "MAST"-augmented, and open-chest CPR in dogs. A preliminary investigation. Crit Care Med 8:147, 1980.
38. Lee SK, Vaagenes P, Safar P, et al. Effect of cardiac arrest time on cortical cerebral blood flow during subsequent standard external cardiopulmonary resuscitation in rabbits. Resuscitation 17:105, 1989.
39. Szmolenszky T, Szoke P, Halmagyi G, et al. Organ blood flow during external heart massage. Acta Chir Acad Sci Hung 15:283, 1974.
40. Schleien CL, Dean JM, Koehler RC, et al. Effect of epinephrine on cerebral and myocardial perfusion in an infant animal preparation of cardiopulmonary resuscitation. Circulation 73:809, 1986.
41. Brown CG, Werman HA. Adrenergic agonists during cardiopulmonary resuscitation. Resuscitation 19:1, 1990.
42. Ditchey RV, Lindenfeld J. Potential adverse effects of volume loading on perfusion of vital organs during closed-chest resuscitation. Circulation 69:181, 1984.
43. Luce JM, Ross BK, O'Quin RJ, et al. Regional blood flow during cardiopulmonary resuscitation in dogs using simultaneous and non-simultaneous compression and ventilation. Circulation 67:258, 1983.
44. Koehler RC, Chandra N, Guerci AD, et al. Augmentation of cerebral perfusion by simultaneous chest compression and lung inflation with abdominal binding after cardiac arrest in dogs. Circulation 67:266, 1983.
45. Krischer JP, Fine EG, Weisfeldt ML, et al. Comparison of prehospital conventional and simultaneous compression-ventilation cardiopulmonary resuscitation. Crit Care Med 17:1263, 1989.
46. Ditchey DV, Winkler JV, Rhodes CA. Relative lack of coronary blood flow during closed-chest resuscitation in dogs. Circulation 66:297, 1982.
47. Sanders AB, Ogle M, Ewy GA. Coronary perfusion pressure during cardiopulmonary resuscitation. Am J Emerg Med 3:11, 1985.
48. Bircher N, Safar P. Cerebral preservation during cardiopulmonary resuscitation. Crit Care Med 13:185, 1985.
49. Sanders AB, Ewy GA, Bragg S, et al. Expired PCO_2 as a prognostic indicator of successful resuscitation from cardiac arrest. Ann Emerg Med 14:948, 1985.
50. Falk JL, Rackow EC, Weil MH. End-tidal carbon dioxide concentration during cardiopulmonary resuscitation. N Engl J Med 318:607, 1988.
51. Sanders AB, Ewy GA, Taft TV. Resuscitation and arterial blood gas abnormalities during prolonged cardiopulmonary resuscitation. Ann Emerg Med 13:676, 1984.
52. Ornato JP, Gonzalez ER, Coyne MR, et al. Arterial pH in out-of-hospital cardiac arrest: Response time as a determinant of acidosis. Am J Emerg Med 3:498, 1985.
53. Weil MH, Rackow EC, Trevino R, et al. Difference in acid-base state between venous and arterial blood during cardiopulmonary resuscitation. N Engl J Med 315:153, 1986.
54. Sessler D, Mills P, Gregory G, et al. Effects of bicarbonate on arterial and brain intracellular pH in neonatal rabbits recovering from hypoxic lactic acidosis. J Pediatr 111:817, 1987.
55. McDonald JL. Systolic and mean arterial pressures during manual and mechanical CPR in humans. Ann Emerg Med 11:292, 1982.
56. Kaye W, Bircher NG. Access for drug administration during cardiopulmonary resuscitation. Crit Care Med 16:179, 1988.
57. Quinton DN, O'Byrne G, Aitkenhead AR. Comparison of endotracheal and peripheral intravenous adrenaline in cardiac arrest. Is the endotracheal route reliable? Lancet 1:828, 1987.
58. Smith RJ, Keseg DP, Manley LK, Standeford T. Intraosseous infusions by prehospital personnel in critically ill pediatric patients. Ann Emerg Med 17:491, 1988.
59. Pearson JW, Redding JS. Influence of peripheral vascular tone on cardiac resuscitation. Anesth Analg 44:746, 1965.
60. Redding JS, Pearson JW. Resuscitation from ventricular fibrillation. Drug therapy. JAMA 203:255, 1968.
61. Yakaitis RW, Otto CW, Blitt CD. Relative importance of alpha and beta adrenergic receptors during resuscitation. Crit Care Med 7:293, 1979.
62. Otto CW, Yakaitis RW, Redding JS, Blitt CD. Comparison of dopamine, dobutamine, and epinephrine in CPR. Crit Care Med 9:366, 1981.
63. Otto CW, Yakaitis RW, Blitt CD. Mechanism of action of epinephrine in resuscitation from asphyxial arrest. Crit Care Med 9:364, 1981.

64. Otto CW, Yakaitis RW, Ewy GA. Effect of epinephrine on defibrillation in ischemic ventricular fibrillation. Am J Emerg Med 3:285, 1985.
65. Koehler RC, Michael JR, Guerci AD, et al. Beneficial effect of epinephrine infusion on cerebral and myocardial blood flows during CPR. Ann Emerg Med 14:744, 1985.
66. Niemann JT, Adomian GE, Garner D, Rosborough JP. Endocardial and transcutaneous cardiac pacing, calcium chloride, and epinephrine in postcountershock asystole and bradycardias. Crit Care Med 13:699, 1985.
67. Gonzalez ER, Ornato JP, Garnett AR, et al. Dose-dependent vasopressor response to epinephrine during CPR in human beings. Ann Emerg Med 18:920, 1989.
68. Brown CG, Werman HA, Davis EA, et al. The effect of graded doses of epinephrine on regional myocardial blood flow during cardiopulmonary resuscitation in swine. Circulation 75:491, 1987.
69. Spivey WH, Schoffstall JM, Davidheiser S, Kirkpatrick R. Correlation of plasma catecholamines with blood pressure during cardiac arrest. Ann Emerg Med 17:413, 1988.
70. Turner LM, Parsons M, Luetkemeyer RC, et al. A comparison of epinephrine and methoxamine for resuscitation from electromechanical dissociation in human beings. Ann Emerg Med 17:443, 1988.
71. Goetting MG, Paradis NA. High dose epinephrine in refractory pediatric cardiac arrest. Crit Care Med 17:1258, 1989.
72. Orlowski JP, Gallagher JM, Porembka DT. Endotracheal epinephrine is unreliable. Resuscitation 19:103, 1990.
73. Paradis NA, Koscove EM. Epinephrine in cardiac arrest. A critical review. Ann Emerg Med 19:1288, 1990.
74. Ditchey RV, Lindenfeld JA. Failure of epinephrine to improve the balance between myocardial oxygen supply and demand during closed-chest resuscitation in dogs. Circulation 78:382, 1988.
75. Stiell IG, Hebert PC, Weitzman BN, et al. High-dose epinephrine in adult cardiac arrest. N Engl J Med 327:1045, 1992.
76. Brown CG, Martin DR, Pepe PE, et al. Multicenter High-Dose Epinephrine Study Group. A comparison of standard-dose and high-dose epinephrine in cardiac arrest outside the hospital. N Engl J Med 327:1051, 1992.
77. Callaham M, Madsen CD, Barton CW, et al. A randomized clinical trial of high-dose epinephrine and norepinephrine vs standard-dose epinephrine in prehospital cardiac arrest. JAMA 268:2667, 1992.
78. Brown DC, Lewis AJ, Criley JM. Asystole and its treatment: The possible role of the parasympathetic nervous system in cardiac arrest. JACEP 8:448, 1979.
79. Wiklund L, Soderberg D, Henneberg S, et al. Kinetics of carbon dioxide during cardiopulmonary resuscitation. Crit Care Med 14:1015, 1986.
80. Guerci AD, Chandra N, Johnson E, et al. Failure of sodium bicarbonate to improve resuscitation from ventricular fibrillation in dogs. Circulation 74(Suppl IV):IV–75, 1986.
81. Bircher NG. Sodium bicarbonate improves immediate survivorship and 24 hour neurological outcome after ten minutes cardiac arrest in dogs. Crit Care Med, 19:S87, 1991.
82. Vukmir RB, Bircher NG, Radovsky A, Safar P. Sodium bicarbonate improves hemodynamics and perfusion in canine cardiac arrest. Crit Care Med 21:S272, 1993.
83. Bishop RL, Weisfeldt ML. Sodium bicarbonate administration during cardiac arrest. Effect on arterial pH, PCO_2, and osmolality. JAMA 235:506, 1976.
84. Sanders AB, Otto CW, Kern KB, et al. Acid-base balance in a canine model of cardiac arrest. Ann Emerg Med 17:667, 1988.
85. Martin DR, Aufderheide TP, Olson DW, et al. Prehospital bicarbonate use in cardiac arrest: A three-year experience. Ann Emerg Med 16:514, 1987.
86. Menitove SM, Goldring RM. Combined ventilator and bicarbonate strategy in the management of status asthmaticus. Am J Med 74:898, 1983.
87. Steinhart CR, Permutt S, Gurtner GH, Traystman RJ. Beta-adrenergic activity and cardiovascular response to severe respiratory acidosis. Am J Physiol 244:H46, 1983.
88. Yakaitis RW, Thomas JD, Mahaffey JE. Influence of pH and hypoxia on the success of defibrillation. Crit Care Med 3:139, 1975.
89. Kerber RE, Sarnat W. Factors influencing the success of ventricular defibrillation in man. Circulation 60:226, 1979.
90. Berenyi KJ, Wolk M, Killip T. Cerebrospinal fluid acidosis complicating therapy of experimental cardiopulmonary arrest. Circulation 52:319, 1975.
91. Sanders AB, Otto CW, Kern KB, et al. The effect of bicarbonate on cerebral spinal fluid acidosis during cardiac arrest. Ann Emerg Med 16:1102, 1987.
92. Redding JS, Pearson JW. Evaluation of drugs for cardiac resuscitation. Anesthesiology 24:203, 1963.
93. Kurland G, Williams J, Lewiston NJ. Fatal myocardial toxicity during continuous infusion intravenous isoproterenol therapy of asthma. J Allergy Clin Immunol 63:407, 1979.
94. Stueven HA, Thompson B, Aprahamian C, et al. Lack of effectiveness of calcium chloride in refractory asystole. Ann Emerg Med 14:630, 1985.
95. Stueven HA, Thompson B, Aprahamian C, et al. The effectiveness of calcium chloride in refractory electromechanical dissociation. Ann Emerg Med 14:626, 1985.

21

Key Terms

Cough

"Huff" Coughing

Mucus

Positive Expiratory Pressure (PEP)

Postural Drainage Therapy

The daily production of mucus, which ranges from 10 to 100 mL, provides an airway lining 2 to 5 μm thick from the alveoli to the trachea.[3, 4]

Bronchial Hygiene

Eric D. Bakow, M.A., R.R.T.

Postural drainage, percussion, cough, and related airway clearance techniques have become a mainstay of modern respiratory care. The use of these techniques has been shown to result in often dramatic improvement in many patients. When performed well, therapy can be very labor intensive; it is therefore important to monitor the appropriateness of these procedures in light of scarce inpatient resources.

The clinical practice guidelines published by the American Association of Respiratory Care replaced the previous designation of chest physical therapy with postural drainage therapy (PDT).[1] The clinical practice guidelines define PDT as therapeutic interventions designed to

- Improve the mobilization of secretions
- Improve the matching of ventilation and perfusion
- Normalize the functional residual capacity[2]

PDT includes turning, postural drainage, percussion, vibration, and cough. This much-needed change in terminology more accurately defines the scope and focus of therapy.

This chapter deals with components of bronchial hygiene therapy: positive expiratory pressure and PDT, which includes turning, cough, and postural drainage. The chapter begins with a functional description of the root of retained secretion problems: airway mucus. A basic understanding of airway structure and function related to mucus hypersecretion is a useful introduction to the treatment of these clinical problems.

RESPIRATORY MUCUS

The lung is an efficient organ that is obviously essential to homeostasis in a large portion of the animal kingdom. Its large surface area facilitates the exchange of respiratory gases and requires an equally effective mechanism to protect this vital function. Airway mucus provides one such protective function. Table 21–1 lists the protective, barrier, and transport functions of mucus in the airways. In a normal state, these functions do not interfere with gas transport and other vital func-

TABLE **21–1:** Functions of Respiratory Mucus

Protective functions
Lubrication
Humidification
Waterproofing
Insulation
Provides an appropriate environment for ciliary action
Barrier functions
Selective macromolecular sieve
Entrapment of microorganisms
Extracellular surface for immunoglobulin actions
Extracellular surface for enzyme actions
Neutralizes nontoxic gases
Transport function
Covering sheet for disposal of trapped materials (along with cilia)

From Kaliner M. Human respiratory mucus. J Allergy Clin Immunol 73:318–323, 1984.

Respiratory Mucus **423**

tions of the lung. In diseases such as asthma, bronchitis, and cystic fibrosis, this system becomes pathogenic and further exacerbates the patient's clinical condition.

Many cells are responsible for airway secretions, including alveolar type II cells, Clara's cells, goblet cells, plasma cells, mucous and serous glandular cells, and duct cells from submucous glands.[3] These secretions form two general layers: the sol phase, a serous, nonviscous substance that bathes the cellular environment of the cilia, and the gel phase, a viscous substance above the periciliary fluid. The gel portion of respiratory secretions, a noncontinuous layer of discrete plaques, tends to coalesce in the upper airway.[5] The viscoelastic property of mucus is due to mucus glycoprotein (MGP), which is formed by a protein core and oligosaccharide side chains and apparently displays a significant heterogeneity in size.[6] MGP can bind with serum proteins (either by electrostatic or disulfide bonding) to render the gel phase less movable by the ciliary structure.[8] Goblet cells, so called because of their characteristic shape, are found adjacent to columnar epithelial cells in all areas of the tracheobronchial tree to the level of alveolar ducts, whereas the submucosal glands are thought to exist from the nose to airways containing cartilage. Submucosal glands outnumber goblet cells by a 40:1 ratio and communicate with the luminal surface of the airway via a hollow, tubular projection from the base of the gland.[9] Although the focus on MGP is in a description of mucus, many substances exist in this complex fluid. Table 21–2 lists the constituents of airway secretions and their cellular origins.

MGP:

- 70 to 80% carbohydrate
- 20% protein
- 1 to 2% sulfate[7]
- primary sources are goblet cells and submucosal glands, which contain both serous and mucosal cells

TABLE **21–2:** Constituents of Airway Secretions and Their Cellular Origins

Mucus Glycoproteins

Droplets, sheet or blanket (gel)	Mucous cell
Periciliary fluid (sol)	Serous, ciliated cell or transudate
Surface mucosubstance	All epithelial cells (glycocalyx)
Surfactant hypophase	Clara or type II cell

Proteins and Peptides

Lysozyme (muramidase)	Serous cell and alveolar macrophage
Lactoferrin	Serous cell and neutrophil
Secretory piece (component)	Surface epithelium and submucosal glands
Regulatory neuropeptides	Dense, core-granulated cell and nerves
Fibronectin	Alveolar macrophages

Glycosaminoglycans (Polysaccharides and Proteoglycans)

Heparan sulfate	Luminal cell membrane (? releasable)
Heparin	Mast cell
Chondroitin sulfates	? Cell membranes and connective tissue
Hyaluronate	Intercellular matrix

Lipids

Triglycerides	Storage lipids (all cells)
Glycolipids	Cell membrane
Phospholipids	Type II alveolar cell (surfactant) and ? Clara cell
Sphingolipids	Cell membranes
Steroids	? Clara cell
Terpenes	Cell membrane

Antiproteases and Antioxidants

Bronchial protease inhibitor	Serous and Clara cells
Alpha$_2$-macroglobulin	Macrophage
Alpha$_1$-antitrypsin	Transudate
Antioxidants	Type II alveolar cell and macrophage

Other "Secretions"

Ions and water	Surface epithelium and submucosal glands
Mediators of inflammation	Mast cell granules and all membranes
Serum proteins	Transudate

From Killburn KH. A hypothesis for pulmonary clearance and its implications. Am Rev Respir Dis 98:449–463, 1968.

The beating of the cilia is affected by

- Temperature
- Presence of inflammation
- Oxygen
- Toxic substances[5]

Mucus is transported throughout the lung via ciliary movement, which carries the secretions in a cephalad direction for further clearance by the cough reflex. This directional movement is facilitated by the presence of ciliary "claws," as identified by electron microscopy. These structures, on the uppermost ends of the cilia, contact the gel layer during their forward stroke and then recoil through the sol fluid to repeat the process.[5] Each ciliated cell accounts for approximately 250 cilia, which have a beat frequency of 12.5 ± 1.3 Hz. Mucus transport, although difficult to measure, ranges from 4 to 10 mm/min in the tracheas of nonsmokers.[10] Clearly, many factors precipitate an alteration in mucociliary function, and Table 21–3 lists a wide range of known causative agents.

Figure 21–1 illustrates the complex topic of the neural control of mucus production. The predominant neural control of the secretion of MGP is through the vagus nerve, but the nonadrenergic, noncholinergic nervous system (neuropeptides such as substance P and endorphins) and the sympathetic nervous system may also play a role in the release of MGP.[11, 12] In fact, the resultant secretion of MGP may occur by direct autonomic stimulation or by an interaction of adrenergic and cholinergic fibers.[12] In addition, C fiber reflexes have been identified as possible sources of mucus hypersecretion in diseases that are characterized by airway inflammation.[11, 13]

Lundgren and Shelhamer summarize the cumulative effect of disease, infection, and inflammation on the mucus-secreting cells of the lung in Figure 21–2. Disease entities such as acute and chronic bronchitis, asthma, and cystic fibrosis are depicted, all of which result in an increase in mucus production by secretory cells (resulting in gland hypertrophy) and an increase in the number of cells that produce MGP (hyperplasia).

TABLE **21–3:**   Factors That Can Adversely Affect Mucociliary Function

Airway disorders	Cigarette smoke
Asthma	Air pollutants
Chronic bronchitis	Sulfur dioxide
Bronchiectasis	Nitrogen dioxide
Allergic bronchopulmonary	Ozone
aspergillosis	Other gases and aerosols
Congenital defects	Ammonia, chlorine
Cystic fibrosis	Hydrochloric acid, sulfuric acid
Primary ciliary dyskinesia syndrome	Formaldehyde, hydrogen sulfide
Young's syndrome	Cyanide, smoke inhalation
Hypogammaglobulinemia	Lung transplantation
Medications	Increasing age
Narcotics	Sleep
Ethyl alcohol	Blood and tissue factors
Atropine	Serum
Acetylsalicylic acid (aspirin)	Complement factors (C3a, C5a)
Beta-adrenergic antagonists	Neutrophil elastase
Inhaled and intravenous anesthetics	Monocyte-derived mucus secretagogue
Acute respiratory tract infections	Mast cell products (histamine, prostaglandins
Mycoplasma pneumoniae	$[A_2, D_2, E_1, F_{2\alpha}]$, and leukotrienes $[C_4, D_4]$)
Influenza virus	
Other airway viruses	
Acute bacterial bronchitis	
Physical mechanisms	
Hyperoxia	
Dehydration	
Low humidity	
Hypercapnia	
Tracheal intubation	
Tracheal suctioning	

From Burton GG, Hodgkin JE, Ward JJ (eds): Respiratory Care: A Guide to Clinical Practice, 3rd ed. Philadelphia, JB Lippincott, 1991, p 636.

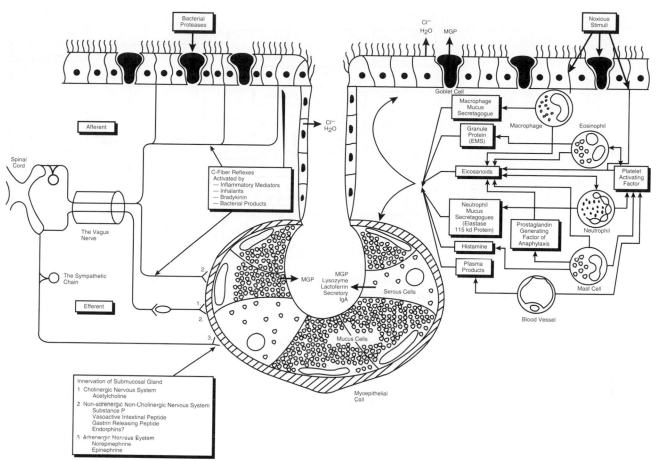

FIGURE 21–1: Mechanisms by which acute mucus hypersecretion from the airways may occur. MGP, mucus glycoprotein; EMS, eosinophil mucus secretagogue. (From Lundgren JD, Shelhamer JH. Pathogenesis of airway mucus hypersecretion. Allergy Clin Immunol 35(2):399–413, 1990.)

The resultant mucus hypersecretion, then, is a physiologic response due to multiple neurohumoral mechanisms. The full scope and nature of each mechanism is not well understood, and potential therapeutic implications await research into this process. Regardless of the mechanism, many clinical sequelae result from mucus hypersecretion: atelectasis, infection, increased airway resistance, increased work of breathing, increased cough with its resultant complications, and ultimately, hypoxemia and tissue hypoxia.

This chapter deals with a narrow array of therapeutic options for the treatment of mucus hypersecretion, but a more global perspective can be found in Table 21–4.

Clearly, the cornerstone of managing the patient with mucus hypersecretion is the treatment of the patient's primary disease entity. It is important to retain this perspective and to avoid too narrow a focus on airway secretions only. Admittedly, there may be few options for the patient with severe chronic lung disease, but attention to the specifics of Table 21–4 is a necessary starting point in designing a comprehensive care plan for the patient with retained secretions.

POSTURAL DRAINAGE THERAPY

Previously referred to as chest physiotherapy, chest physical therapy, and postural drainage and percussion, PDT is designed to

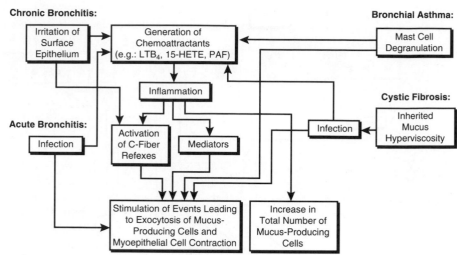

FIGURE 21–2: Pathogenesis of mucus hypersecretion. LTB_4, leukotriene B_4; 15-HETE, hydroxyeicosatetraenoic acid; PAF, platelet-activating factor. (From Lundgren JD, Shelhamer JH. Pathogenesis of airway mucus hypersecretion. Allergy Clin Immunol 35(2):399–413, 1990.)

The components of PDT, as defined by the American Association of Respiratory Care clinical practice guidelines, are

- Turning
- Postural drainage
- External manipulation of the thorax (percussion and vibration)
- Cough

- Improve the mobilization of bronchial secretions
- Improve the matching of ventilation and perfusion
- Normalize functional residual capacity (FRC)[2]

A substantial body of literature now exists on the clinical use of PDT in a variety of settings and disease entities. However, the literature does not support the routine use of PDT in patients without significant lung dysfunction (to be defined later).

Turning

Routine turning of patients in bed is a mainstay of good care; many reasons exist for this practice. It is well known that frequent changes in body position occur during sleep. Patients who are unable to perform this basic function develop decubital ulcers that occur from the interruption of circulation when soft tissue is compressed by its own weight. It is also recognized that pulmonary secretions respond to body position because the effect of gravity results in the movement of these secretions to the gravity-dependent areas of the lung.

TABLE **21–4:**   Treatment of Mucus Hypersecretion

1. Treat the primary disorder
2. Remove exogenous factors (pollutants, allergens)
3. Improve mucociliary clearance (increase ciliary beat frequency): beta-agonists, methylxanthine
4. Improve airway dynamics (increase expiratory flows to enhance clearance): beta-agonists, methylxanthine
5. After the gel phase: mucolytics*
6. Reduce inflammation: agents to treat infection, steroids
7. Perform postural drainage therapy
8. Use cough or the forced expiratory technique
9. Suction the airways
10. Perform positive expiratory pressure therapy

*This practice must be applied with caution because of the paucity of clinical investigations that document the efficacy of this technique.

Changing of body position also has a profound effect on the relationship of alveolar ventilation ($\dot{V}A$) and pulmonary circulation ($\dot{Q}$), or $\dot{V}/\dot{Q}$. West describes the distribution of ventilation on the basis of varying transpulmonary (alveolar-intrapleural) pressure across the vertical axis of the lung.[14] Figure 21–3 depicts the differences in intrapleural pressures at the base and apex for a vertical lung at both functional residual volume (FRC) and residual volume. The pressure at the apex of the lung is more negative than at the base; because of this difference in pressure, alveoli in these zones are on different parts of the pressure-volume curve. Because the weight of the lung tissue superior to their position compresses the alveoli at the base of the lung, their volume is considerably smaller than that of the alveoli at the top of the lung. Therefore, there is a larger change in volume per unit of pressure applied to the lung at the base of a vertical lung than at its apex. This results in an increase in ventilation per unit of alveolar volume at the base of the upright lung compared with the apex.[15] In Figure 21–3, a larger change in the volume of the alveoli at the base (at FRC, letter A) occurs compared with that in lung zones at the apex.

Blood flow to the lung is also highly variable in different zones of the lung. Figure 21–4 shows that the base of the lung receives the lion's share of both ventilation and blood flow. As a result, the relationship of these two variables, the $\dot{V}/\dot{Q}$, is also changed at different points along the upright lung. However, these relationships do not apply only to the vertical lung.

Although theoretically gas exchange should be improved in the sitting position, clinical studies do not demonstrate a consistent advantage for this position versus the supine position. Marti and Ulmer found Pa_{O_2} to be higher in the sitting position in both normal subjects and patients with chronic obstructive pulmonary disease.[16] Dalrymple and coworkers[17] and Russell[18] published data that confirm the opposite to be true, whereas Gui and associates[19] found no difference in Pa_{O_2} for the two positions.

Similarly, lateral placement of the patient could have a significant

> Changes in body position from upright to supine, lateral, or prone positions have all been associated with alterations in clinically measurable changes in gas exchange.

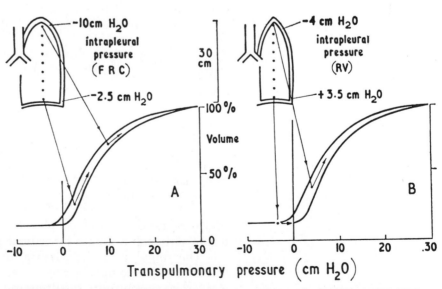

FIGURE 21–3: Intrapleural pressures across a vertical lung at both FRC and RV. FRC, functional residual capacity; RV, residual volume. (From West JB. Ventilation/Blood Flow and Gas Exchange. Oxford, Blackwell Scientific Publications, 1971, pp 30–31.)

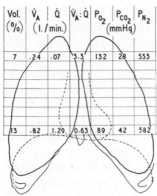

FIGURE 21–4: Distribution of ventilation, blood flow, and gas pressures in an upright lung. (From West JB. Ventilation/ Blood Flow and Gas Exchange. Oxford, Blackwell Scientific Publications, 1971, pp 30–31.)

Careful monitoring of outcomes, such as Pa_{O_2}, Pa_{CO_2}, Sp_{O_2}, blood pressure, and Sv_{O_2}, should be incorporated into any intervention that involves a change in body position for this group of patients.

effect on gas exchange in view of the ramifications of this position for the distribution of ventilation and blood flow to the lung. Clauss and colleagues found a significant improvement in Pa_{O_2} with patients in a lateral position compared with supine.[20] This was true for normal subjects, patients with chronic obstructive pulmonary disease, and patients who had had thoracotomy. Zack and coworkers compared the effect of positioning in patients with normal lung function, bilateral disease, and unilateral disease.[21] This group reported that in patients with unilateral lung disease, the Pa_{O_2} is higher with the normal lung down and the diseased lung up. This point was also confirmed by Syracuse and coworkers, who studied oxygenation in patients with unilateral lung disease.[22] Syracuse and coworkers placed patients in a supine or a lateral position that resulted in the "good" lung as being down and noted a uniform improvement in oxygenation with the lateral-positioning group. Several studies have reached similar conclusions about the effect of lateral positioning in patients with unilateral disease: Pa_{O_2} is uniformly best when the diseased lung is positioned in the nondependent ("up") position.[23–27] From these data, it is clear that the practitioner must exercise caution in the movement of body position for critically ill patients with unilateral lung disease.

Postural Drainage

As noted earlier, PDT is the preferred term encompassing postural drainage, turning, positioning, percussion, and vibration.

A wealth of information exists on postural drainage in various disease states, with a myriad of variations in this practice grouped under the loose heading of chest physiotherapy. Therefore, a clarification of terms, although it makes for tedious reading, is absolutely necessary.

The singular goal of postural drainage, the mobilization of airway secretions, is accomplished by enlisting the effect of gravity on a body of a given mass (sputum), resulting in the movement of sputum toward the gravity-dependent area of the lung. Many secondary effects of this process can be appreciated: the subsequent reversal of atelectasis following movement of secretions, the subsequent improvement in arterial oxygen levels that occurs because of increased ventilation, and a reduced work of breathing, which may result from a reduction in the resistive load to the respiratory muscles. The literature is not, however, uniform in its support for these effects; significant hazards of this procedure warrant close attention by the practitioner.

Most practitioners agree that patients with copious secretions benefit from this procedure (see the bibliography in reference 2). This encompasses patients with cystic fibrosis, bronchiectasis, and infectious processes that produce abundant secretions i.e., at least 30 mL of sputum per day.

The merit of postural drainage has been documented in patients with lobar atelectasis[28, 29] or with foreign body aspiration.[30] However, no evidence suggests the use of postural drainage as a routine therapeutic measure in patients with chronic or acute lung disease who are not producing large quantities of sputum.[31] Documentation must indicate the clear need for postural drainage in patients with conditions such as pneumonia or chronic bronchitis.

The use of techniques that involve external manipulation to the chest have become popular over the years. Specifically, percussion, vibration, and clapping are used by many as a routine method of sputum mobilization. However, these techniques have little in the way of convincing evidence that supports their use. Sutton and associates studied the effects of percussion (clapping the chest at a frequency of 5 Hz), vibration (administered at 12 to 16 Hz), and shaking (performed at 2 Hz) in a population of eight patients, all of whom had severe airway obstruction and copious mucus production (mean, 44 ± 23 g/day of sputum).[32] A radioaerosol technique was employed, and no significant differences were found in baseline pulmonary function studies and radioaerosol clearance (both whole lung and regional). The dry weight of sputum produced was significantly greater when each of the therapies was compared with the control, but no statistically significant differences existed between the therapies. Sutton and associates concluded that postural drainage and the forced expiratory technique account for the majority of mucus mobilization. Radford and colleagues presented a theoretical argument for the use of "percussion-augmented" clearance of secretions from the pulmonary system.[33] Their conclusions were based on observations of the movement of mucus in both in vivo and in vitro animal preparations. Although their findings suggest an improved rate of clearance with percussion and an optimal percussion energy range of 25 to 35 Hz, studies of patient outcomes employing mechanical adjuncts to postural drainage have not demonstrated significant improvement over drainage and cough alone.[34, 35] This conclusion is true for both mechanical and manual techniques to improve sputum mobilization.

The previously mentioned studies used patients with chronic lung disease in their study design. In distinction, Holody and Goldberg studied the effect of vibrators in a group of patients who were bound to ventilators and had acute lung disease.[36] They demonstrated a small (10 to 15 mm Hg) but statistically significant improvement in Pa_{O_2} in patients after the use of a mechanical vibrator. These authors argued that the thixotropic property of sputum renders the substance more liquid on mechanical disruption (vibration or shaking). This conflicts with a study by Connors and associates, in which a sharp decline in Pa_{O_2} (mean, 16.8 mm Hg) was observed immediately after postural drainage and percussion (clapping and vibration).[37] Both studies employed acutely ill patients, but Connors and associates used Trendelenburg positioning, whereas Holody and Goldberg employed a sitting or semi-Fowler posi-

Pneumonia and chronic bronchitis do not warrant the use of postural drainage unless they are accompanied by sputum production of at least 30 mL/day.

tion. A rational conclusion reconciling these two studies is difficult. Clearly, the routine use of these interventions should be discouraged until supporting evidence warrants it. When using these techniques, the practitioner must closely follow objective markers of outcome in an effort to define their success in a specific patient's care.

The various positions for postural drainage are well noted in many sources and are not reproduced here. The reader should review the supplemental readings at the end of this chapter for details of drainage positions and segmental anatomy. However, it should be noted that the earlier comments about the altered matching of perfusion and blood flow arising from positional changes become very important in this situation.

Cough

Few therapeutic interventions seem so natural as cough, but at the same time, attention to detail with this maneuver is important in the removal of retained secretions. The mechanics of the cough are divided into four distinct phases:

- Deep inspiration, optimally to total lung capacity
- Closure of the glottis
- Contraction of the expiratory muscles against the closed glottis to generate high transpulmonary pressures as the thoracic volume is compressed by the muscle contraction
- Opening of the glottis, allowing for the rapid flow of gas that propels secretions from the airways

The period of muscular contraction in the cough process pressurizes the pleural space and creates a point at which the pressures around the airway equal those in the airway. This has been termed the equal pressure point.

Measurements of cough mechanics by Langlands[38] and by Loudon[39] indicate that maximal pressures in the airway during cough may exceed 160 cm H_2O, peak expiratory flow may range from 155 (bronchitic) to 654 L/sec, and exhaled volume may extend across a range of 0.5 (bronchitic) to 5.1 L in normal subjects. Of particular interest in the cough process is the phenomenon of airway compression. The forced expiratory maneuver creates a compression of the airway that moves more peripherally (toward the alveoli) as the lung volume decreases. At this point, small airways tend to collapse, resulting in diminished expired flows and reduced clearance of bronchial secretions. Lawson and Harris, however, postulate that some airway compression acts to accelerate airflow through a tube (given the volume of gas is the same) and that this may result in a "scrubbing action" on the wall of the airway.[40]

Cough alone has been compared with chest physiotherapy with mixed results. de Boeck and Zinman found no difference in sputum production, flow rates, or lung volumes between controlled cough only and a regimen of percussion and vibration in 11 different drainage positions.[41] However, Bateman and associates recorded conflicting results in their investigation comparing controlled cough with cough plus a sequence of drainage, vibration, shaking, and percussion.[42] Their design incorporated the use of radiolabeled aerosol to define the movement of secretions in either the peripheral, central, or intermediate zones of the lung. They found that cough cleared only the central lung zone, whereas chest physiotherapy and cough increased the clearance of the central and peripheral lung zones. Sputum production was also greater in the cough plus physiotherapy group. It is difficult to draw many conclusions on the basis of these studies. Clearly, the subjects in the de Boeck study were younger than those in the Bateman study (11.6 versus 60 $\pm$ 16 years) and had a higher FEV_1/FVC ratio (65 $\pm$ 12% versus 52 $\pm$ 6%). The practitioner must consider the relative merit of the premise that sputum production immediately after therapy is a sensitive measure of these therapeutic interventions. In fact, a study of radiolabeled aerosol clearance by Hasani and coworkers demonstrated that unproductive coughing still results in the cephalad movement of secretions from the central regions of the lung.[43] It seems prudent, then, to withhold generalizations about the efficacy of one intervention versus another and to base a care plan for the treatment of mucus hypersecretion on short- and long-term patient outcomes to the degree that the specific patient condition allows.

The high intrathoracic pressures associated with the cough maneuver may be associated with complications. Care must be exercised in patients with suspected cerebral hypertension or myocardial infarction in order to avoid further exacerbation of these clinical problems due to sequelae of the elevated intrathoracic pressures.

A variation of the cough maneuver described previously is the forced expiratory technique (FET), also known as "huff" coughing, which is widely espoused by Pryor.[46] The FET is an expiratory maneuver that does not compress the thoracic gas volume because the glottis remains open throughout the procedure. An effective huffing maneuver is described as an expiratory maneuver that

- Sounds like a forced sigh
- Makes use of an open mouth
- Contracts both the chest wall and the abdominal musculature
- Individualizes the rate of expiratory gas flow
- Is usually performed at mid to low lung volumes[47]

The presence of the open glottis in this maneuver is an attractive feature because the significantly elevated intrathoracic pressures associated with the cough maneuver may be greatly avoided, as may some of the complications mentioned earlier. Patients with chronic obstructive pulmonary disease, who may be susceptible to the deleterious effects of airway compression with the controlled cough, may have more effective clearance of secretion with this technique. An investigation by van der Schans and coworkers documented an improvement in the clearance of mucus from the peripheral lung zones in patients with chronic bronchitis who used FET as compared with controlled cough.[48] Patients with emphysema, however, did not show evidence of this same benefit from FET. The authors concluded that reduced lung recoil pressure, as found in the emphysema group, was a determinant in the movement of mucus. Because the differences in mucus production did not correlate with the initial FEV_1 in the two groups, it is difficult to understand the role of dynamic airway compression in explaining these data. The open glottis involved in this technique should also be important in reducing postoperative pain in patients who have had thoracic or upper abdominal surgery.[46]

FET has also been shown to be a valuable adjunct to conventional chest physiotherapy. Pryor and associates, who studied patients with cystic fibrosis, were able to demonstrate an increase in the volume and rate of sputum production in the therapy combined with FET.[49, 50] Sutton and associates evaluated patients with airway obstruction and noted both greater sputum production and greater clearance of inhaled radiolabeled particles in the group treated with FET plus chest physiotherapy compared with the group that received FET alone.[51]

Cough is a technique that requires muscular effort for the successful clearance of secretions from the airway. Therefore, clinical conditions that affect muscle strength, such as nutrition, electrolyte levels, and

---

Cough complications:

- Reduced coronary perfusion[44]
- Reduced cerebral perfusion
- Lightheadedness
- Visual disturbances
- Paresthesia
- Spontaneous pneumothorax
- Chest pain
- Rib fracture[45]

Chest physiotherapy is defined as postural drainage, breathing exercises, percussion, and chest compression.

Measures of muscle strength, such as the vital capacity,[52] the maximal inspiratory pressure,[53] and the maximal expiratory pressure,[54] may prove to be useful in assessing the patient's ability to cough effectively.

neuromuscular disease, clearly limit the effectiveness of coughing in a given patient.

POSITIVE EXPIRATORY PRESSURE

Pressurizing the airway during spontaneous breathing is a concept that dates back to 1936 and the use of a positive pressure mask to treat congestive heart failure. Positive expiratory pressure (PEP) is a variation on this same theme, with the application now in the mobilization of mucus. An excellent historical perspective found in an article by Mahlmeister and associates traces the use of this technique to its current level of investigation as an alternative to PDT.[55] The therapeutic effect of PEP is believed to be due to

- The improved distribution of inspired volume in the lung due to collateral air channels
- The prevention of expiratory airway collapse
- The ability to generate pressure on exhalation in an area distal to the site of mucus obstruction

Patients with cystic fibrosis are the most studied patient population in the use of PEP therapy. Taken collectively, the data show favorable results when PEP is compared with common measures of sputum mobilization, such as chest physiotherapy, FET, and autogenic drainage, in this group of patients (see reference 37 for a review of extant literature). However, care must be taken in interpreting these data because a commonly used dependent variable is sputum production. It is not clear that a statistically significant increase in dry or 24-hour sputum samples actually translates into a concomitant reduction in morbidity or attenuation in symptoms. A study of 14 patients with cystic fibrosis by Falk and coworkers compared postural drainage (treatment A), postural drainage with PEP (treatment B), and PEP only (treatment C).[56] The mean weight of 24-hour sputum samples ($\pm$ the standard error of the mean) was 63.3 ± 9.16 g for A, 54.5 ± 9.72 g for B, and 42.3 ± 5.12 g for C. Although these mean values are statistically different from each other, it is difficult to know if this difference represents a reduction in pneumonia, number of hospital days, or other symptoms. In contradistinction, a study by Christensen and colleagues compared chest physiotherapy plus PEP therapy with PEP only in 43 patients who had chronic bronchitis.[57] The authors found the PEP only group to have a significant reduction in the rate of acute exacerbations, the number of sick days from work, and the use of antibiotics and mucolytics. In addition, the PEP only group showed small but statistically significant improvements in lung function studies, compared with observed decreases in pulmonary function for the control (chest physiotherapy) group.

The use of PEP therapy in adult postoperative patients has received much less attention in the more recent literature, but this patient population is a fertile area for future investigation. Ricksten and coworkers studied 43 patients who had had upper abdominal surgery and compared incentive spirometry, intermittent continuous positive airway pressure by face mask, and PEP, also by face mask.[58] They noted the PEP and continuous positive airway pressure groups to have the smallest increase in $P(A-a)O_2$, the highest forced vital capacity postsurgically, and the lowest incidence of atelectatic consolidation. Frolund and Madsen evaluated the role of PEP in 56 patients after thoracic surgery.[59] Compared with chest physiotherapy (which consisted of walking the patient, deep breathing, and coughing exercises), PEP plus chest physiotherapy offered no clinical benefit for this study population. However, the PEP therapy was self-administered (i.e., unsupervised), and the median level of PEP was 10 cm H_2O, with a range of 9 to 12 cm H_2O (see the following recommendations for pressure range).

The technique of PEP therapy is variable, but Mahlmeister and associates reported good success using PEP via either a mask or a mouthpiece at pressures from 10 to 20 cm H_2O. They instruct the patient to perform 10 to 20 breaths through the device, followed by several huff coughs. This sequence is then repeated four to six times per session, with each session performed one to four times per day. In addition, beta-agonist therapy can be simultaneously incorporated into this procedure with either a conventional updraft nebulizer or a metered dose inhaler that is attached to the PEP system. Care must be exercised in patients susceptible to barotrauma or hemodynamic compromise in evaluating the need for PEP therapy.

As mentioned previously, the adult postoperative patient population warrants further attention in clinical studies involving PEP therapy. A review of postoperative care of the thoracotomy patient by Forshag and Cooper offers the recommendation that chest physiotherapy, incentive spirometry, or both be continued until the time of hospital discharge.[60] Although the authors claim that this is a "reasonable guideline," they do so in light of the "paucity of studies on this patient population" that support their conclusion. The burden is on all practitioners to develop and publish the clinical data that will guide these decisions in the future (Table 21–5).

Two central themes of this chapter should be obvious. First, there is a need to continually assess the merit of using PDT techniques in the treatment of a specific clinical problem, with the use of meaningful objective criteria of outcome being the most desirable procedure. Second, in unstable patients, the process of positioning, percussing, and coughing can lead to several serious and undesirable outcomes. The principal concerns are listed in Table 21–5, and a short description of each follows. Being prepared for any of the following seems to be prudent. Quick access to oxygen, bronchodilators, and suction devices, for example, may make the difference in responding to unanticipated outcomes of PDT.

Hypoxemia

The monitoring of arterial oxygen saturation and Pa_{O_2} during PDT procedures is well reported in the literature. Various mechanical adjuncts to postural drainage have associated falls in Pa_{O_2}. Other studies confirm a reduction in arterial oxygen content during and after PDT,[61–63] but this may not imply a concomitant reduction in oxygen transport.[64] However, monitoring and reporting of measures of arterial oxygen con-

Practitioners should consider the following as possible contraindications to PEP therapy:

- Acute sinusitis
- Ear infection
- Epistaxis
- Recent facial, oral, or skull injury or surgery
- Active hemoptysis

TABLE **21–5:** Published Adverse Effects of Postural Drainage Therapy

Reduced Pa_{O_2}, Sa_{O_2}	Reduced FEV_1, wheezing
Reduced cardiac output	Pulmonary hemorrhage
Cardiac arrhythmias	Pain, injury to chest wall
Increased intracranial pressure	Vomiting and aspiration

FEV_1, forced expiratory volume in 1 second.

tent are difficult because of the dynamic character of the measurement: it is very much the "moving target." To illustrate, Barrell and Abbas published data showing the change in Pa_{O_2} and $P\bar{v}_{O_2}$ during and after PDT (Fig. 21–5).[65] Note the variability of these measures over time and as each intervention is performed. Did the improvement in Pa_{O_2} and the reduction in Pv_{O_2} occur because of the therapeutic interventions, the change to sitting position, or both? These questions are difficult to answer, but this figure demonstrates characteristic, moment-to-moment changes that are seen in critically ill patients. Clearly, monitoring of cardiopulmonary variables is a necessary adjunct to the safe administration of PDT.

Hemodynamic Effects

Changing body position alters the preload of the ventricles, thereby providing a potentially deleterious effect on cardiac output. The possibility of reduced cardiac output during PDT should be closely monitored in critically ill patients. The key to successful management is the early identification of risk factors coupled with close monitoring.

Patients at risk for cardiovascular complications are those who

- Present with low intravascular blood volume
- Have had myocardial infarction
- Have recently had cardiothoracic surgery
- Have cardiac arrhythmias[66]

Neurologic Effects

The relationship of the Trendelenburg position to changes in intracranial pressure is well documented.[67] Patients with suspected or known intracranial hypertension should be carefully evaluated for PDT. Because, along with positioning, coughing and suctioning are recognized sources of intracranial hypertension, they should also be cautiously used in this patient population. Direct monitoring of the intracranial pressure is the most direct method of clinical evaluation, but the availability of this invasive procedure may be limited.

An intracranial pressure in excess of 20 mm Hg is regarded as a relative contraindication to PDT.[68] The absence of neurologic signs, such as decorticate or decerebrate posturing, does not preclude the presence of an elevated intracranial pressure; therefore, there must be an easily identifiable indication for PDT to be applied to these high-risk patients. In patients presenting with head and neck injury, PDT is absolutely contraindicated.[68]

Wheezing

The clinical sign of wheezing can be associated with PDT, with or without a reduction in expiratory flow rates. In one study, the presence of wheezing occurred only in PDT that included percussion: it was not observed with drainage and coughing only.[69] It is unclear that pretreatment with a beta-agonist is indicated in all susceptible patients. However, it would not be unreasonable to premedicate patients who either are actively wheezing or have a strong history of wheezing.

Pulmonary Hemorrhage

Active pulmonary hemorrhage is an absolute contraindication to PDT,[68] and one case report describes a fatality that was possibly due to PDT in a patient with hemoptysis who was being treated for pneumonia after radiation therapy for a lung tumor.[70] Therefore, patients with cavitating lung disease, carcinoma of the lung, and lung abscess should be carefully evaluated for hemoptysis when PDT is being considered.

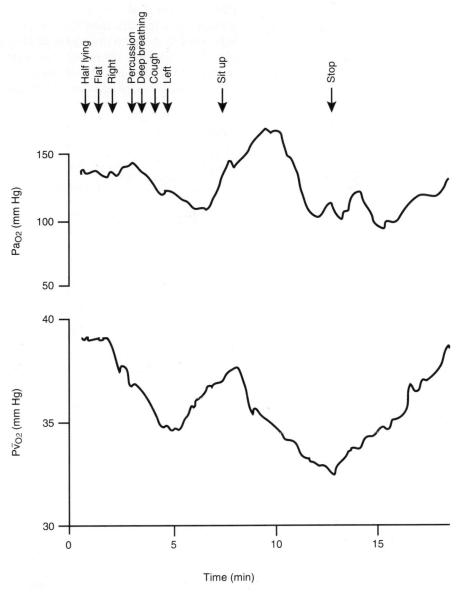

FIGURE 21–5: Variability of P$\bar{v}_{O_2}$ and Pa$_{O_2}$ during patient movement and cough. (From Barrell SD, Abbas HM. Monitoring during physiotherapy after open heart surgery. Physiotherapy 64(9):272–273, 1978.)

SUMMARY

This chapter has presented a basic overview of the therapeutic interventions involved in bronchial hygiene. It is hoped that these data challenge some deep-seated practices by some practitioners who have little in the way of corroborative studies to support the continued use of these methods. The routine use of drainage and percussion following surgery and the use of vibration are two examples of practices that merit serious review for widespread use. This is not the same as declaring these practices to be ineffective in all patients. Clearly a controlled initiation of therapy combined with monitoring of objective outcomes can be quite effective for a given patient. Lastly, therapy that might not be considered to be mainstream by some practitioners merits attention. For example,

PEP therapy has yet to be thoroughly tested in a variety of patient groups in which it may be helpful (e.g., postoperative patients). Few interventions are as quintessential to respiratory care as postural drainage therapy. It is therefore imperative that practitioners proceed with both a healthy skepticism of the past and an openness to new approaches in the future use of postural drainage therapy.

References

1. AARC Clinical Practice Guidelines for Postural Drainage Therapy. Respir Care 36:1418–1426, 1991.
2. AARC Clinical Practice Guidelines for Postural Drainage Therapy. Respir Care 36:1418, 1991.
3. Kaliner M, Shelhamer H, Borson B, et al. Human respiratory mucus. Am Rev Respir Dis 134:612–621, 1986.
4. Killburn KH. A hypothesis for pulmonary clearance and its implications. Am Rev Respir Dis 98:449–463, 1968.
5. Konietzko N. Mucus transport and inflammation. Eur J Respir Dis 69(Suppl 147):72–79, 1986.
6. Shelhamer J. *In* Kaliner M, Shelhamer JH, et al. Human respiratory mucus. Am Rev Respir Dis 134:612–621, 1986.
7. Kaliner M, Shelhamer JH, Borson B, et al. Human respiratory mucus. Am Rev Respir Dis 134:614, 1986.
8. Lundgren JD, Shelhamer JH. Pathogenesis of airway mucus hypersecretion. Allergy Clin Immunol 35(2):399–413, 1990.
9. Meyrick B, Sturgess JN, Reid L. A reconstruction of the duct system and secretory tubules of the human bronchial submucosal gland. Thorax 24:729–735, 1969.
10. Yates DB. Mucociliary tracheal transport rate in man. J Appl Physiol 497:39, 1975.
11. Lundgren JD, Shelhamer JH. Pathogenesis of airway mucus hypersecretion. Allergy Clin Immunol 35(2):402, 1990.
12. Kaliner M, Shelhamer JH, Borson B, et al. Human respiratory mucus. Am Rev Respir Dis 134:614–617, 1986.
13. Davis U, Roberts AM, Coleridge HN, Coleridge JCG. Reflex tracheal glands secretion evoked by stimulation of bronchial C-fibers in dogs. J Appl Physiol 53:985–991, 1982.
14. West JB. Ventilation/Blood Flow and Gas Exchange. Oxford, Blackwell Scientific Publications, 1971, pp 30–31.
15. West JB. Ventilation/Blood Flow and Gas Exchange. Oxford, Blackwell Scientific Publications, 1971, p 30.
16. Marti C, Ulmer WT. Absence of effects of the body position on arterial blood gases. Respiration 43:41–44, 1982.
17. Dalrymple DG, MacGowan SW, MacLeod GF. Cardio respiratory effects of the sitting position in neurosurgery. Br J Anaesth 51:1079–1082, 1979.
18. Russell WJ. Position of patient in respiratory function in immediate post-operative period. Br Med J 283:1079–1082, 1981.
19. Gui D, Tazza L, Boldrini G, et al. Effects of supine vs. sitting bedrest upon blood gas tensions, cardiac output, venous admixture and ventilation: Perfusion ratio in man after upper abdominal surgery. Int J Tissue Reac 4:67–72, 1982.
20. Clauss RH, Scalabrini BY, Ray JF, Vreed GE. The effects of changing body position upon improved ventilation-perfusion relationships. Circulation 37(Suppl 2):214–217, 1968.
21. Zack MB, Pontoppidan H, Pazemi H. The effect of lateral positions on gas exchange in pulmonary disease: A prospective evaluation. Am Rev Respir Dis 110:39–45, 1974.
22. Syracuse DC, Hyman AI, King TC. Postural influences on arterial blood gases in patients with unilateral pulmonary consolidation. Surg Forum 30:173–174, 1979.
23. Patz JD, Barash PG. Positional hypoxemia following post traumatic pulmonary insufficiency. Can Anaesth Soc J 24:346–352, 1977.
24. Remolina C, Kahn AU, Santiago TV, Evelman NH. Positional hypoxemia in unilateral lung disease. N Engl J Med 304:523–525, 1981.
25. Ibanez J, Raurich JM, Abizanda R, et al. The effects of lateral positions on gas exchange in patients with unilateral lung disease during mechanical ventilation. Intensive Care Med 7:231–234, 1981.
26. Rivara D, Articio H, Arcos J, Hiriart C. Positional hypoxemia during artificial ventilation. Crit Care Med 112:436–438, 1984.
27. Sonnenblick M, Melzer D, Rosin AJ. Body positional effect on gas exchange in unilateral pleural effusion. Chest 83(5):784–786, 1983.
28. Hammon WE, Martin RJ. Chest physical therapy for acute atelectasis. Physical Ther 61(2):217–220, 1981.
29. Stiller K, Geake T, Taylor J, et al. Acute lobar atelectasis, a comparison of two chest physio-therapy regimens. Chest 98(6):1336–1340, 1990.

30. Raghu G, Pierson DJ. Successful removal of an aspirated tooth by chest physio-therapy. Respir Care 31:1099–1101, 1986.
31. Graham WJB, Bradley DA. Efficacy of chest physio-therapy and intermittent positive pressure breathing in the resolution of pneumonia. N Engl J Med 299:624–627, 1978.
32. Sutton TP, Lopez-Didriero MP, Pavia D, et al. Assessment of percussion, vibratory shaking and breathing exercises in chest physio-therapy. Eur J Respir Dis 66:147–152, 1985.
33. Radford R, Barutt J, Billingsley JG, et al. The rational basis for percussion-augmented mucociliary clearance. Respir Care 27(5):556–563, 1982.
34. Pavia D, Thomson ML, Phillipakos D. A preliminary study of the effects of a vibrating pad on bronchial clearance. Am Rev Respir Dis 113:92–96, 1976.
35. Maxwell M, Redmond A. Comparative trial of manual and mechanical percussion technique with gravity-assisted bronchial drainage in patients with cystic fibrosis. Arch Dis Child 54:542–544, 1979.
36. Holody B, Goldberg HS. The effect of mechanical vibration physio-therapy on arterial oxygenation in acutely ill patients with atelectasis or pneumonia. Am Rev Respir Dis 124:372–375, 1981.
37. Connors AF, Hammon WE, Martin RJ, Rogers RM. Chest physical therapy: The immediate effect on oxygenation in acutely ill patients. Chest 78:559–564, 1980.
38. Langlands J. The dynamics of cough in health and disease. Am Rev Respir Dis 114:1033–1036, 1976.
39. Loudon RG. Cough: A symptom and a sign. Respir Care 26(8):767–774, 1981.
40. Lawson TV, Harris RS. Assessment of the mechanical efficiency of coughing in healthy young adults. Clin Sci 33:209–224, 1967.
41. DeBoeck C, Zinman R. Cough vs. chest physio-therapy, a comparison of acute effects on pulmonary function in patients with cystic fibrosis. Am Rev Respir Dis 129:182–184, 1984.
42. Bateman JRN, Newman ST, Daunt KN, et al. Is cough as effective as chest physio-therapy in the removal of excessive tracheal bronchial secretions. Thorax 36:683–687, 1981.
43. Hasani A, Pavia D, Agnew JE, Clarke SD. The effect of unproductive coughing/FET on regional mucus movement in the lungs. Respir Med 85(Suppl A): 23–26, 1991.
44. Kern MJ, Gudipati C, Tatimeni S, et al. Effect of abruptly increased intrathoracic pressure on coronary blood flow velocity in patients. Am Heart J 119:863–870, 1990.
45. Stern RC, Horwitz SJ, Doershuk CF. Neurologic symptoms during coughing paroxysms in cystic fibrosis. J Pediatr 112(6):909–912, 1988.
46. Pryor JA. The forced expiration technique. Respiratory Care. New York, Churchill Livingstone, 1981, pp 79–100.
47. Partridge C, Pryor J, Webber B. Characteristics of the forced expiration technique. Physiotherapy 75(3):193–194, 1989.
48. van der Schans CP, Piers DA, Beekhuis H, et al. Effect of forced expiration from mucus clearance in patients with chronic air flow obstruction: Effects of lung recoil pressure. Thorax 45:623–627, 1990.
49. Pryor JA, Webber BA. An evaluation of the forced expiration technique as an adjunct to postural drainage. Physiotherapy 65(10):304–307, 1979.
50. Pryor JA, Webber BA, Hodson ME, Batten JC. Evaluation of the forced expiration technique as an adjunct to postural drainage in the treatment of cystic fibrosis. Br Med J 2:417–418, 1979.
51. Sutton TP, Parker RA, Webber BA, et al. Assessment of the forced expiration technique, postural drainage and directed coughing in chest physio therapy. Eur J Respir Dis 64:62–68, 1983.
52. Shapiro BA, et al. EDS. Clinical Application of Respiratory Care. Chicago, Year Book Medical Publishers, 1979, p 158.
53. Black LF, Hayatt RE. Maximal static pressures in generalized neuromuscular disease. Am Rev Respir Dis 103(5):641–650, 1971.
54. Szinberg A. Cough capacity in patients with muscular dystrophy. Chest 94:1232–1235, 1988.
55. Mahlmeister MJ, Fink JB, Hoffman GL, Fifer LF. Positive expiratory pressure mask therapy: Theoretical and practical considerations and review of literature. Respir Care 36(11):1218–1230, 1991.
56. Falk M, Kelstrup M, Andersun JB, et al. Improving the ketchup bottle method with positive expiratory pressure, PEP, in cystic fibrosis. Eur J Respir Dis 65:423–432, 1984.
57. Christensen EF, Nedergard T, Dahl R. Long term treatment of chronic bronchitis with positive expiratory pressure mask and chest physio therapy. Chest 97:645–650, 1990.
58. Ricksten SE, Bengtsson A, Soderberg C, et al. Effects of periodic positive airway pressure by mask on post-operative pulmonary function. Chest 89:774–781, 1986.
59. Frolund L, Madsen F. Self administered prophylactic post operative positive expiratory pressure in thoracic surgery. Acta Anaesthesiol Scand 30:381–385, 1986.
60. Forshag MS, Cooper AD. Post operative care of the thoracotomy patient. Clin Chest Med 13(1):33–45, 1992.
61. Moody LE, Martindale CL. Effect of pulmonary hygiene measures on levels of arterial oxygen saturation in adults with chronic lung disease. Heart Lung 7:315–319, 1978.
62. Huseby J, Hudon L, Stark K, Tyler ML. Oxygenation during physiotherapy. Chest 70:430, 1976.

63. Tyler ML, Hudson LD, Grose BL, Huseby JS. Prediction of oxygenation during chest physio therapy in critically ill patients. Am Rev Respir Dis 121(2):218, 1980.
64. Tyler ML, Hudson LD, Hurn PD, et al. Systemic oxygen transport during chest physical therapy. Clin Res 30(1):76A, 1982.
65. Barrell SD, Abbas HM. Monitoring during physio therapy after open heart surgery. Physiotherapy 64(9):272–273, 1978.
66. Hammon WE, Kirmeyer PC, Connors AF, McCaffree DR. Cardiac arrhythmias during postural drainage and percussion of the critically ill patient [Abstract]. Respir Care 25:1244, 1980.
67. Moss E, Gibson JS, McDowall GD. The effect of nitrous oxide, althesin and thiopentone on intracranial pressure during chest physio therapy in patients with severe head injuries. In Shulman K, Mararow A, Miller JD (eds). Intracranial Pressure IV. New York, Springer-Verlag, 1980, pp 605–609.
68. AARC Clinical Practice Guidelines, Postural Drainage Therapy. Respir Care 36(12):1419, 1991.
69. Cambell AH, O'Connell JM, Wilson F. The effect of chest physio-therapy upon the FEV1 in chronic bronchitis. Med J Aust 1:133–135, 1975.
70. Hammon WE, Martin RJ. Fatal pulmonary hemorrhage associated with chest physical therapy. Physical Ther 59(10):1247–1248, 1979.

22

Key Terms

Gas Exchange

Perfusion

Permissive Hypercapnia

Ventilation

Ventilatory Failure

Ventilatory failure is a failure of the respiratory system to adequately move gas between alveoli and the environment.

Mechanical Ventilatory Support

Neil R. MacIntyre, M.D.

The purpose of the cardiorespiratory system is providing O_2 to and removing CO_2 from the tissues. This process can conceptually be broken into several steps, which have been depicted as a series of interlocking cogs (Fig. 22–1). Ventilation is the process of moving gas between the environment and the alveoli. Gas exchange is the process of moving gas between the alveoli and the pulmonary capillaries. Circulation is the process of moving gas between the pulmonary capillaries and the tissues.

This chapter discusses mechanical support of ventilation. Subsequent chapters deal with support strategies for alveolar-capillary gas exchange and circulation.

VENTILATORY FAILURE AND THE NEED FOR VENTILATORY SUPPORT

Ventilatory failure results in abnormalities in both Pa_{O_2} and Pa_{CO_2}. However, it is usually defined and quantitated by an abnormal Pa_{CO_2} (and resulting acidemia) because CO_2 transport is predominantly determined by ventilation and is much less affected by ventilation-perfusion matching ($\dot{V}/\dot{Q}$) and diffusion than is O_2 (see later discussion).

Ventilatory failure exists when an elevation in Pa_{CO_2} results in an arterial pH of 7.25 or less. This corresponds to a Pa_{CO_2} of 55 mm Hg in patients with normal baseline values for Pa_{CO_2}. In patients with chronic CO_2 elevations, however, ventilatory failure would be defined by much higher values for Pa_{CO_2}. Ventilatory failure can result from several factors with different manifestations and potential causes (Table 22–1). Regardless of the cause, ventilatory failure is a primary indication for mechanical ventilatory support.

CONVENTIONAL MECHANICAL VENTILATOR DESIGN PRINCIPLES (Fig. 22–2)

Conventional mechanical ventilation uses positive pressure breaths to provide ventilatory assistance. Gas transport is thus by bulk flow.

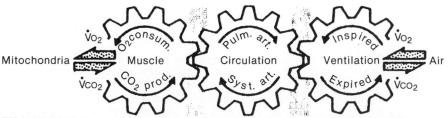

FIGURE 22–1: Essential elements in gas exchange between the cell mitochondria and the external environment. (Reprinted, by permission, from Wasserman, K. Breathing during exercise. N Engl J Med 298:780–785, 1978.)

TABLE **22-1:** Ventilatory Failure

Pathophysiology	Clinical Criteria	Potential Causes
Decreased respiratory drive	↑ Pa_{CO_2} (>55 mm Hg) Bradypnea → apnea	Neurologic dysfunction, drugs
Ventilatory muscle fatigue resulting from working on stiff or obstructed lungs	↑ Pa_{CO_2} (>55 mm Hg) Tachypnea (>35 breaths per minute) Muscle weakness (<25 cm H_2O negative inspiratory force) ↓ C_L ↑ R_{AW}	Obstructed lung disease, restricted lung disease
Ventilatory muscle fatigue resulting from large dead space ventilation requirements	↑ Pa_{CO_2} (>55 mm Hg) Tachypnea (>35 breaths per minute) ↑ V_D/V_T (>0.6)	Pulmonary vascular disease

C_L = lung compliance; R_{AW} = airway resistance.

Devices to deliver these positive pressure breaths have a number of important features.

Gas Delivery System

The important components of the gas delivery system are the positive pressure breath controller, the demand sensors, and the mode controller.

Positive Pressure Breath Controller

Most modern adult ventilators use piston-bellows systems or controllers of high-pressure sources to drive gas flow. Inspiratory breaths are generated by this gas flow and can either be controlled entirely by the ventilator or be interactive with patient efforts. Generally, with pneumatic, electronic, or microprocessor systems, four breath types are available. These can be classified by what initiates (triggers) the breath, what governs (limits) the breath during inspiratory flow, and what terminates (cycles) the breath (Tables 22–2 and 22–3). Triggers are generally set timers (controlled breaths) or patient efforts (assisted, supported, or spontaneous breaths). Limits are generally flow (pressure variable) or

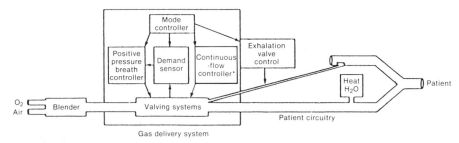

FIGURE 22–2: Ventilator design principles. Modern mechanical ventilatory support systems take blended fresh gas and regulate its flow through complex valving systems (which may include pistons or bellows). The positive pressure breath controller sets the characteristics for machine-delivered breaths. The demand sensor serves as the trigger for both assisted and unassisted breaths. A continuous-flow circuit for unassisted breathing exists on some systems *(asterisk)*. The mode controller sets the desired combination of controlled, assisted, supported, and spontaneous breaths. The exhalation valve control interacts with the valving system and the mode control to determine expiratory pressure. The patient circuitry delivers these gases to the patient. Heat and moisture are added to the delivered gases.

TABLE **22–2:** Breath Types Defined by Specific Combinations of Machine and Patient Control Over Phase Variables

	Trigger	Limit	Cycle
Mandatory	Machine	Machine	Machine
Assisted	Patient	Machine	Machine
Supported	Patient	Machine	Patient
Spontaneous	Patient	Patient	Patient

From American Respiratory Care Foundation Consensus Statement on the Essentials of Mechanical Ventilators. Respir Care 1992, 37:1000–1008.

pressure (flow variable). Cycles are generally volume, set timer, or flow. The current generation of mechanical ventilators provides wide versatility. Breathing frequencies of up to 150 breaths per minute, tidal volumes of up to 2500 mL, peak inspiratory pressures of up to 150 cm H_2O, flow rates of up to 180 L/min, inspiratory-expiratory timing ratios ranging from 1:5 to 4:1, and various inspiratory flow profiles (i.e., accelerating, decelerating, square wave, or sine wave) are commonly available. These delivery systems should be equipped with pressure relief valves to avoid dangerously high airway pressures.

Demand Sensors

Sensitivity refers to how much patient effort must be generated to open the valve. Responsiveness refers to the delay in initiating adequate gas flow after the valve starts to open.

Interactive breaths require the ventilator to sense patient effort ("demand"). This effort is usually sensed as a change in pressure or continuous flow (if present) in the ventilatory circuitry. Demand sensors are characterized by their sensitivity and responsiveness. Both properties are critical in providing a proper response to patient efforts. Unfortunately, sensitivity may be less than optimal for two reasons. First, sensitivity settings may have to be set low in order to avoid autocycling. Second, because the sensor is usually in the ventilator circuitry (and not in the pleural space), considerable patient effort may be required to effect the necessary pressure or flow changes for triggering. Likewise, the re-

TABLE **22–3:** Classification of Commonly Used Modes of Ventilation

Mode (Common Names)	Mandatory			Assisted			Supported			Spontaneous			Conditional Variable
	Trigger	Limit	Cycle	Trigger	Limit	Cycle	Trigger	Limit	Cycle	Trigger	Limit	Cycle	
CMV/VCV	Time	Flow	Volume*	—	—	—	—	—	—	—	—	—	—
ACV/VACV	Time	Flow	Volume*	Patient†	Flow	Volume*	—	—	—	—	—	—	Patient effort/time
IMV	Time	Flow	Volume*	—	—	—	—	—	—	Patient†	Pressure'	Pressure'	—
SIMV	Time	Flow	Volume*	Patient†	Flow	Volume*	—	—	—	Patient†	Pressure	Pressure	Patient effort/time
PCV	Time	Pressure	Time	—	—	—	—	—	—	—	—	—	—
PACV	Time	Pressure	Time	Patient†	Pressure	Time	—	—	—	—	—	—	Patient effort/time
PIMV	Time	Pressure	Time	—	—	—	—	—	—	Patient†	Pressure	Pressure	—
PSIMV	Time	Pressure	Time	Patient†	Pressure	Time	—	—	—	Patient†	Pressure	Pressure	Patient effort/time
APRV	Time	Pressure	Time	—	—	—	—	—	—	Patient†‡	Pressure	Pressure	—
Assist APRV	Time	Pressure	Time	Patient†	Pressure	Time	—	—	—	Patient†‡	Pressure	Pressure	Patient effort/time
PSV	—	—	—	—	—	—	Patient	Pressure	Flow§	—	—	—	—
MMV	Time	Flow	Volume*	Patient†	Flow	Volume*	—	—	—	Patient†	Pressure	Pressure	Minute volume

From American Respiratory Care Foundation Consensus Statement on the Essentials of Mechanical Ventilators. Respir Care 1992, 37:1000–1008.
*Cycling can also be due to set inspiratory time in the setting of a fixed flow, with or without a pause.
†May be patient-generated pressure or flow in the circuit.
‡Allows spontaneous breathing during both the mandatory inspiratory and expiratory time.
§Flow reflects interaction of patient effort, respiratory system impedance, and ventilator flow rate.
'Pressure limited only on demand valve systems where ventilator limits and cycles to maintain constant airway pressure (i.e., this applies to all modes in this column).
CMV/VCV, controlled mechanical ventilation/volume-controlled ventilation; ACV, assisted-controlled ventilation; VACV, volume assisted-controlled ventilation; IMV, intermittent mandatory ventilation; SIMV, synchronized IMV; PCV, pressure-controlled ventilation; PACV, pressure ACV; PIMV, pressure IMV; PSIMV, pressure SIMV; APRV, airway pressure-release ventilation; PSV, pressure support ventilation; MMV, mandatory minute ventilation.

sponsiveness of valve systems may be less than optimal because of inherent delays in mechanical valve functioning. The work imposed on a patient as a consequence of demand valve function is discussed later, in the section on complications.

A high-flow continuous flow circuit provides an alternative to a demand valve system for spontaneous breaths. In these systems, fresh gas sufficient to meet or exceed patient demand constantly flows through the gas delivery circuitry. Spontaneous breaths with continuous flow thus require no valve actuation.

Mode Controller

The desired combination of mandatory, assisted, supported, and spontaneous breaths is termed the mode of mechanical ventilatory support. The mode controller is an electronic, pneumatic, or microprocessor-based system designed to provide the proper combination of breaths according to set algorithms and feedback data (conditional variables) (see Table 22–3). Newer designs can incorporate advanced monitoring and feedback functions into these controllers to allow for continuous adjustments in mode algorithms as patient conditions change. Factors involved in mode selection are discussed later.

Subsystem of Mechanical Ventilators

In addition to the gas delivery system, several additional components exist in modern mechanical ventilators.

Gas Blenders

Gas blenders mix air and O_2 to produce a delivered FI_{O_2} from 0.21 to 1.0. Blenders may also be needed in the future to allow He or NO to be added to delivered gas.

Humidifiers

With the upper airway bypassed by tracheal intubation, sufficient heat and moisture must be added to the inspired gas mixtures to avert mucosal desiccation. Used effectively, humidifiers can adjust blended gas mixtures to near-body conditions. Although most systems warm the gas to increase water vapor content, particulate nebulizers have also been employed. Simple and inexpensive heat and moisture exchange humidifiers ("artificial noses") reutilize moisture trapped from the expiratory stream.

Expiratory Pressure Generator

Positive airway pressure can be sustained throughout expiration (positive end-expiratory pressure [PEEP]) to help maintain alveolar patency and improve $\dot{V}/\dot{Q}$ matching (see Chapter 23). PEEP is usually applied by regulating pressure in the expiratory valve of the ventilator system, but a continuous flow of source gas during the expiratory phase can provide a similar effect.

Gas Delivery Circuit

The gas delivery circuit usually consists of flexible tubing that often has the airway pressure tap and exhalation valve included. Significant

---

Disadvantages of a continuous high-flow system:

- Large gas volume usage
- Difficulty in maintaining the desired airway pressures

Disposable artificial noses usually supply adequate heat and moisture (i.e., greater than 28 to 30°C and greater than 25 mg H_2O/L of ventilation) for many patients, particularly those requiring mechanical ventilation for only short periods.

Some expiratory valves, even when fully open, have measurable resistance, which may result in some inadvertently applied PEEP.

Remember that this tubing has measurable compliance (4 mL/cm H_2O is a representative figure).

amounts of delivered gas may serve only to distend this circuitry rather than enter the patient's lungs when high airway pressures are encountered.

EFFECTS OF POSITIVE PRESSURE VENTILATION

A positive pressure breath has a number of important effects on the lung-thorax system (Fig. 22–3). These effects allow proper ventilatory support to be given and serve as sources for a number of complications.

Alveolar Ventilation and Ventilation Distribution

Relationship of $\dot{V}_A$, Pa_{CO_2}, and $\dot{V}_{CO_2}$

Alveolar ventilation ($\dot{V}_A$) is the ability of the lungs to remove CO_2. This relationship of $\dot{V}_A$ to Pa_{CO_2} and CO_2 production ($\dot{V}_{CO_2}$) is expressed by

$$\dot{V}_A = \dot{V}_{CO_2}/Pa_{CO_2} \times k$$

where $k \approx 800$ when gas flow is mL/min and gas tension is mm Hg.

Conventional mechanical ventilation provides fresh gas by periodically inflating the lungs with positive pressure. Such "bulk flow" or "convective transport" results in alveolar or "effective" ventilation ($\dot{V}_A$), which is often defined by the ability to remove CO_2. $\dot{V}_A$ is also quantified mechanically by the following expression:

$\dot{V}_A$ = breathing frequency (f)
  × (tidal volume [V_T] − wasted or dead space volume [V_D]).

For given values of $\dot{V}_{CO_2}$ and V_D, changes in Pa_{CO_2} can be predicted by changes in delivered f or V_T using these relationships. Note, however, that $\dot{V}_{CO_2}$ and V_D may change depending on both the underlying disease and the mechanical ventilatory support parameters used. For example, $\dot{V}_{CO_2}$ can change because the patient's work of breathing and comfort significantly affect the overall metabolic requirement, whereas V_D can

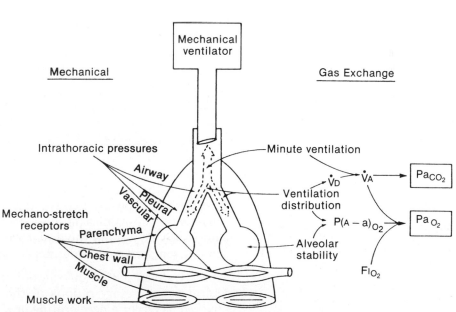

FIGURE 22–3: Physiologic effects of mechanical ventilation. Gas exchange is influenced by the delivered minute ventilation, the distribution of that ventilation with respect to perfusion, the alveolar stability, and the $F_{I_{O_2}}$. Mechanical effects result from the developed intrathoracic pressures, the ventilatory pattern interaction with thoracic mechanoreceptors, and the ventilatory pattern interactions with the inspiratory muscle efforts.

change as a consequence of airway pressures producing regional decreases in blood flow.

Delivered $\dot{V}_A$ and the V_T-f Relationship

The overall amount of ventilation supplied by the ventilator is the product of V_T and f. Minute ventilation requirements in sick patients, however, are often higher than normal because of increased metabolic needs (i.e., $\dot{V}_{O_2}$ and $\dot{V}_{CO_2}$) and increased V_D. Supplying adequate ventilatory support thus often requires a higher than normal V_T, f, or both. To increase minute ventilation, increases in V_T (rather than f) offer the advantage of a lower V_D/V_T ratio (given a constant V_D) and thus a lower total f times V_T requirement. However, a large V_T necessarily increases the maximal alveolar distending pressures. Common practice is generally to supply a V_T of 8 to 10 mL/kg and then adjust the f for the desired $\dot{V}_A$.

The goal of the V_T-f pattern is to provide an adequate $\dot{V}_A$. This often means a $\dot{V}_A$ necessary to normalize Pa_{CO_2} and pH. However, in patients in whom normal Pa_{CO_2} and pH values result in high airway pressures, strategies to provide less ventilation (i.e., "permissive hypercapnia"), while still maintaining acceptable values for pH and Pa_{O_2}, may spare the lung unnecessary pressures. In addition, target values for ventilatory support in patients with chronic CO_2 retention should also be aimed at the baseline, rather than a "normal" Pa_{CO_2}.

Inspiratory Flow Pattern

The inspiratory flow pattern affects both the distribution of delivered gases and the synchrony of ventilatory support to patient effort during assisted or supported breaths.

The distribution of gases refers to the matching of delivered gas and blood flow (ventilation-perfusion or $\dot{V}/\dot{Q}$ matching). Optimal distribution provides matched ventilation and perfusion ($\dot{V}/\dot{Q} = 1$). The distribution of gas from a positive pressure breath is a complex interaction of delivered flow and regional compliance and resistance that is difficult to predict. However, a few general clinical points can be made about inspiratory flow and ventilation distribution:

- The longer the inspiratory time, the more even the gas distribution, especially among high-resistance units, and the lower the peak airway pressure.
- On the other hand, the longer the inspiratory time, the shorter the expiratory time and thus the greater the potential for air trapping (see later discussion).
- Although the pattern (square versus sine versus decelerating versus accelerating) appears to have only small effects on overall ventilation effectiveness in clinical studies, decelerating patterns with high initial flows provide a more rapid alveolar filling pattern when gas is delivered through narrow endotracheal tubes.

In practice, ventilation distribution goals are generally met when the inspiratory-expiratory ratio is in the physiologic 1:2 range and flow is delivered as either a decelerating or a square wave.

Synchrony refers to the matching of ventilator-delivered flow to patient-demanded flow during assisted or supported breaths. Flow below that demanded by the patient can result in significant imposed work on the patient, with further worsening of Pa_{O_2} and Pa_{CO_2} (see later discus-

Minute ventilation = $V_T \times$ f

Normal values are 5 to 7 mL/kg times 12 to 20 breaths per minute.

The use of pressure-volume plots can help to provide the most mechanically efficient V_T (see Chapter 2).

Inspiratory flow pattern—flow magnitude and flow patterns during either flow-limited or pressure-limited breaths

Ventilation to bloodless units ($\dot{V}/\dot{Q} = \infty$) is dead space (V_D); perfusion to gasless units ($\dot{V}/\dot{Q} = 0$) is shunt (see Chapter 23).

sion). To address this, delivered flow should be appropriate to patient demand. This may require either (1) high set flows in conjunction with patient sedation or (2) automatic ventilator responses to match flow (i.e., the variable flows of pressure-limited breaths).

With modern ventilators, the clinician has several ways to manipulate delivered flow. Perhaps the most important option is the choice between flow-limited, volume-cycled breaths and pressure-limited breaths (Fig. 22–4). Flow-limited, volume-cycled breaths deliver gas according to the clinician-set flow magnitude and pattern (i.e., sine, square, decelerating, or accelerating). These breaths are delivered until a set volume has been achieved. Note that with these types of breaths, flow and volume are independent variables, whereas pressure is the dependent variable. In contrast, pressure-limited breaths deliver gas according to a clinician-selected pressure throughout the breath. This serves to maintain a "square wave" of airway pressure. These breaths are maintained either until a set inspiratory time has elapsed (pressure-assisted or pressure-controlled breath) or until flow has decreased to a certain minimum (pressure-supported breath). Note that with these pressure-limited breaths, pressure is the independent variable and flow and volume are the dependent variables. New breath designs that can be pressure limited but can also be volume cycled if a minimal V_T is not delivered may combine the best features of both of these breath types.

Total Versus Partial Ventilatory Support

Positive pressure breaths can be used to supply either all or part of the $\dot{V}_A$. In supplying all of the $\dot{V}_A$, these breaths perform all of the work of breathing and thereby rest the ventilatory muscles. This is termed total mechanical ventilatory support. Total support is guaranteed with

Flow-limited, volume-cycled breaths offer the advantage of a guaranteed V_T; pressure-limited breaths offer the advantage of adjustable decelerating flows, which may enhance gas mixing and patient synchrony.

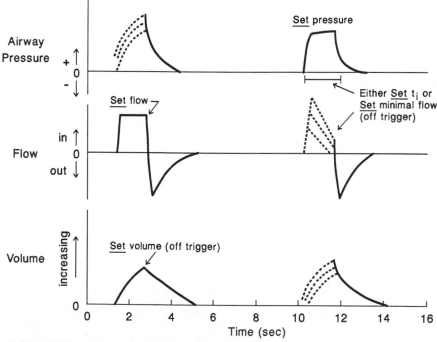

FIGURE 22–4: Pressure, flow, and volume tracings over time in flow-limited, volume-cycled breaths *(left)* and pressure-limited breaths *(right)*. Solid lines reflect clinician-set parameters; dashed lines reflect variable parameters. Both breath types can be patient- or machine-triggered. Pressure-limited breaths can be time- or flow (patient)-cycled.

modes of ventilation providing only controlled breaths in sedated or paralyzed patients (see Table 22–3). Near-total support is also delivered when modes providing mixtures of assisted and controlled breaths are used (see Table 22–3) if the assisted breaths are properly synchronized to patient demand. Near-total support can also be delivered with modes providing supported breaths (see Table 22–3) if the level of support provides all the work of each breath. On the other hand, if positive pressure breaths are used to supply only part of the $\dot{V}A$ and thus only part of the work of breathing (with the patient supplying the remainder), this is termed partial ventilatory support. Partial support is generally provided in one of two ways:

- Using modes that allow intermittent spontaneous (or low level supported) breaths among assisted-controlled breaths (see Table 22–3)
- Using supported breaths that provide a level of support for each breath that is less than that required for total support (see Table 22–3)

Total support is usually used in the initial phases of severe respiratory failure, when muscles are fatigued. Total support is also used when the ventilatory drive is either absent or unreliable. Partial support is usually used during the weaning process (see Chapter 39). Partial support is also used in patients who require substantial ventilatory support (i.e., those not ready for active weaning) but who have a reliable ventilatory drive and relatively stable mechanics. In this setting, partial ventilatory support results in:

- Less airway pressure being delivered by the ventilator (and thus perhaps a lower risk of barotrauma)
- Some level of patient muscle activity (which may forestall muscle atrophy)

COMPLICATIONS OF POSITIVE PRESSURE VENTILATION

A number of hazards associated with positive pressure mechanical ventilatory support can result in significant morbidity and mortality if they are not appropriately recognized and minimized by clinicians. Although many of these topics are discussed in other chapters, important aspects relating to ventilatory support are discussed in the following sections.

Hazards Associated With Endotracheal Tubes

A detailed discussion of intubation hazards and mucosal injury is found in Chapter 29. However, several other potential hazards are associated with the artificial airway. First, endotracheal tube dislodgment can occur in as many as 5 to 10% of all patients. If monitored and alarmed properly, this usually poses no serious threat to the patient. However, an unrecognized ventilator disconnection can be fatal. Endotracheal tubes also bypass the normal gas-conditioning process of the upper airway. Thus, the mechanical ventilatory support system must supply appropriate heat and humidity, as described earlier. Inadequate heat and humidity can result in tracheal mucosal injury, as well as in plugging of the endotracheal tube and airways with dried secretions. Another hazard of endotracheal tube use is the imposition of a significant resistive load to spontaneous breaths. This obviously becomes worse with narrow tubes and high patient demand. This form of imposed muscle load has been reported to increase the normal baseline work of breathing several-fold under certain conditions. This imposed work should always be considered when the clinician is assessing a patient who is difficult to wean from the mechanical ventilator.

Mechanical Malfunctions

The modern generation of mechanical ventilators is remarkably reliable. Nevertheless, any component of any mechanical system can fail. In ventilators, the component that most commonly fails is the exhaled flow transducer (up to a 2% failure rate per year). This is not surprising because the exhaled flow transducer is the one part of the machine that is exposed to patient secretions and nebulized solutions. Modern microprocessor systems usually have a variety of self-checks available. Along with these are numerous alarm systems that rarely fail. Of more concern is the fact that alarms are often turned off. This may be a consequence of too many alarms set too tightly, thus creating so many false alarms that the normal reaction is to shut down the system.

> Clinicians must know which alarms are important and which alarms may serve only to annoy.

Patient-Ventilator Dyssynchrony

A mechanical ventilator must interact with patient efforts during assisted, supported, and spontaneous breaths. This interaction exists during all three phases of the breath: trigger, limit, and cycle. As noted previously, inappropriate demand sensors (poor sensitivity or responsiveness) can impose significant loads on patients during triggering. Equally important is that during breath delivery to a patient with an active ventilatory drive, the machine limit and cycling settings can also impose significant loads if they are not properly "synchronized" to the patient's muscular efforts. This appears to be particularly true with flow-limited, volume-cycled breaths, especially in patients with very active ventilatory drives (Fig. 22–5).

Synchrony with these types of breaths can sometimes be improved by adjusting the flow pattern, increasing the machine breath rate, or sedating the patient. Perhaps a better approach to improving synchrony is to utilize the variable flows that exist with a pressure-limited breath (see Fig. 22–5 *right*). Patient-ventilator dyssynchrony ought to be considered in all cases of patient agitation, weaning difficulty, or both.

Air Trapping or Intrinsic Positive End-Expiratory Pressure

As noted previously, inadequate expiratory time can result in air trapping and the development of so-called intrinsic PEEP or auto-PEEP. This can have profound effects on delivered ventilation and airway pressures (Figs. 22–6 and 22–7). Although intrinsic PEEP is sometimes used as a goal in strategies designed to lengthen inspiratory time (see Chapter 23), usually this phenomenon is undesirable, both because it is difficult to monitor and because it can be the cause of unrecognized pressure-related hazards. One of the best ways to monitor the development of inadequate expiratory time is to follow a flow graphic. When expiratory

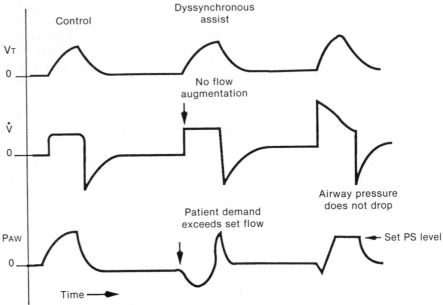

FIGURE 22–5: Patient-ventilator synchrony and dyssynchrony. *Left,* A flow-limited, volume-cycled controlled (i.e., no patient activity) breath. *Center,* The same flow-limited, volume-cycled breath, but this time assisted (i.e., patient activity). Note that the set flow in this example is less than patient demand, such that the airway pressure graphic is literally "sucked" downward, reflecting a large imposed muscle load. *Right,* This same patient activity during a pressure-limited, pressure support (PS) breath. Note that the variable flow of this breath is able to match demand and thus maintain a positive airway pressure.

Clinically, the development of intrinsic PEEP from inadequate expiratory time has manifestations similar to those of applied PEEP

- Barrel chest
- High peak airway pressures in volume-cycled modes
- Patient discomfort
- Cardiac compromise
- Loss of tidal volume in pressure-limited modes

time is inadequate, the expiratory flow signal does not return to the zero baseline (see Figs. 22–6 and 22–7). In the absence of a flow graphic, the clinician should suspect inadequate expiratory time in patients with high ventilatory demands, especially those patients with airway dysfunction. Monitoring airway pressures and volumes can be helpful (see Figs. 22–6 and 22–7), as can expiratory hold techniques (Fig. 22–8). Ventilator adjustments to reduce intrinsic PEEP from inadequate expiratory time include using a shorter inspiratory time (from either faster flows or lower tidal volumes) or a slower breath rate. These adjustments may result in hypercapnia as a tradeoff ("permissive" hypercapnia).

Air trapping can also develop as a consequence of dynamic airway collapse, even in the presence of a reasonable expiratory time. In addition to the previously mentioned effects of intrinsic PEEP, this type of air trapping is often associated with a difficulty in triggering assisted or supported breaths (Fig. 22–9). Under these circumstances, a small amount of applied PEEP (less than the intrinsic PEEP) can reduce this imposed load. If applied appropriately, the functional residual capacity will not increase, the peak pressure of a volume-cycled breath will not change, and the patient will have less difficulty triggering the ventilator.

Barotrauma

Barotrauma refers to lung damage caused by positive pressure and is discussed extensively in Chapter 34. A few comments about how it relates to positive pressure breaths, however, are in order here. Barotrauma is thought to be caused by two mechanisms: shearing and alveo-

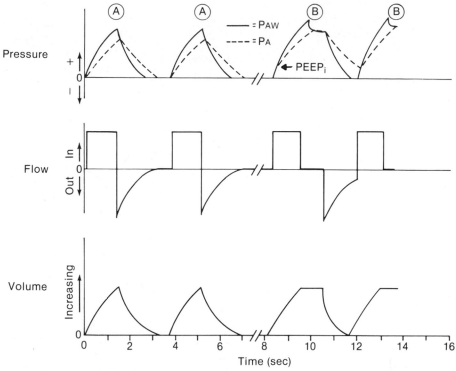

FIGURE 22–6: Intrinsic positive end-expiratory pressure (PEEP$_i$) developing during volume-controlled ventilation with an inspiratory hold. *Top,* Airway pressure *(solid line)* and alveolar pressure *(dotted line)* are plotted. *Center,* Flow is plotted. *Bottom,* Volume is plotted. Volume-controlled breaths are delivered either without (A) or with (B) inspiratory holds. In the A curves, expiratory flow is zero before the next inspiration; there is no air trapping, and PEEP$_i$ is zero. In the B curves, expiratory flow is greater than zero before the next inspiration; there is air trapping, and PEEP$_i$ is greater than zero. Note that PEEP$_i$ in volume-controlled ventilation raises peak pressure but keeps delivered volume constant (cf. Fig. 22–7). (From MacIntyre NR. Complications of mechanical ventilation. *In* Fulkerson W, MacIntyre NR (eds). Problems in Respiratory Care. Philadelphia, JB Lippincott, 1991.)

When high pressures are being used to ventilate and oxygenate diseased alveoli, overdistention of the remaining normal alveoli is often a consequence.

lar overdistention (Fig. 22–10). Shearing refers to the process of one region of the lung changing its shape faster than another, which in turn creates a tearing along the common interface. Alveolar overdistention reflects the fact that normal lung tissue overinflates with high intrathoracic pressures. Damage is inflicted by the physical stretching. Overdistention is related to alveolar pressure, which is estimated clinically by the inspiratory plateau or pause pressure.

There are two important manifestations of barotrauma. The most obvious is alveolar rupture, which results in mediastinal emphysema, subcutaneous emphysema, and pneumothorax. The risk for this is high when peak alveolar pressures exceed 60 cm H$_2$O. A less appreciated form of barotrauma, however, is tissue injury without rupture. This form of tissue injury can mimic many features of the infant and adult respiratory distress syndromes and thereby worsen the underlying lung disease. This injury is associated with alveolar distending pressures of 30 to 40 cm H$_2$O and may be potentiated by concurrent oxygen injury. Because this is more likely to occur in the remaining normal alveoli of an injured lung, some authorities argue for aggressively holding overall inspiratory plateau pressures below 30 to 40 cm H$_2$O in order to prevent iatrogenic damage.

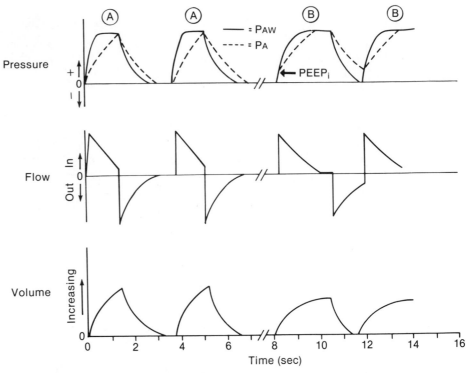

FIGURE 22–7: Intrinsic positive end-expiratory pressure (PEEP$_i$) during pressure-controlled ventilation with a long inspiratory time (t$_i$). The variables plotted are similar to those in Figure 22–6. The A curves have a short t$_i$ and a long t$_e$, and the B curves have a long t$_i$ and a short t$_e$. In the A curves, expiratory flow is zero before the next inspiration; there is no air trapping, and PEEP$_i$ is zero. In the B curves, expiratory flow is greater than zero before the next inspiration; there is air trapping, and PEEP$_i$ is greater than zero. Note that PEEP$_i$ in pressure-controlled ventilation maintains peak pressure but lowers delivered volume (cf. Fig. 22–6). (From MacIntyre NR. Complications of mechanical ventilation. *In* Fulkerson W, MacIntyre NR (eds). Problems in Respiratory Care. Philadelphia, JB Lippincott, 1991.)

Infections

Pulmonary infections are also a common complication of mechanical ventilatory support (estimates range from 15 to 40% of all ventilated patients). The reasons for this are several:

- The endotracheal tube impairs the lungs' physical defense against invading organisms and also impairs cough and mucus clearance.
- Cough is often decreased by disease and sedation.
- Atelectasis occurs frequently in patients on mechanical ventilators.

A common source of infecting organisms is the gastrointestinal tract; thus, prophylactic antibiotic use, gut sterilization, and maintaining acidity in the stomach have been advanced as ways to protect against infectious complications. Contaminated circuits and humidifiers are also a potential source of infecting organisms.

One of the best ways to prevent nosocomial infections is the simple step of hand washing when working with the patient's ventilator circuitry.

Cardiovascular Function

As intrathoracic pressures increase, cardiovascular function deteriorates. Although many mechanisms for this have been proposed, the fact that an elevation in intrathoracic pressure impedes venous return and

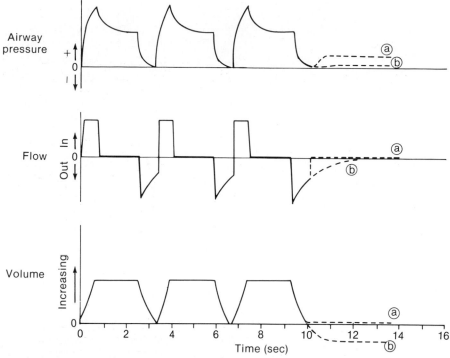

FIGURE 22–8: Expiratory hold techniques to estimate intrinsic positive end-expiratory pressure (PEEP$_i$). Curve a represents tracings that occur during an expiratory hold with the exhalation valve closed at the end of set expiration. With flow equal to zero, airway pressure rises to PEEP$_i$. Curve b represents tracings that occur with the exhalation valve open at the end of set expiration. Flow continues, and the additional exhaled volume equals the volume of trapped gas. (From MacIntyre NH. Complications of mechanical ventilation. *In* Fulkerson W, MacIntyre NR (eds). Problems in Respiratory Care. Philadelphia, JB Lippincott, 1991.)

thus cardiac filling appears to be the most important. Indeed, it has been known for years that to compensate for a reduction in cardiac output associated with high ventilatory pressures, the intravascular volume should be increased. The airway pressure measurement that seems to correlate best with cardiovascular filling difficulties is the mean airway pressure. One of the more interesting approaches to manipulating airway pressure to affect cardiac function is the use of a ventilator breath synchronized to cardiac systole. If the positive airway pressure is timed to occur during systole and the airway pressure is released during diastole, cardiac output can sometimes be increased such that the ventilator, rather than being a hindrance to cardiac function, actually serves as a partial ventricular assist device. Although this approach is still experimental, it does offer an interesting and important lesson in the physiology of heart-lung interactions.

NONINVASIVE TECHNIQUES FOR VENTILATORY SUPPORT

Two fundamental approaches to providing ventilatory support without the use of an artificial airway include

- Techniques designed to expand the thorax by negative pressure
- Techniques designed to inflate the chest with positive pressure applied through a mask

Because these approaches are often awkward to use and are usually

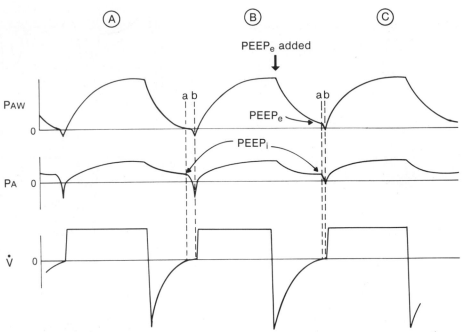

FIGURE 22–9: Tracings of airway pressure (Paw), alveolar pressure (Pa), and gas flow ($\dot{V}$) during assisted breathing in the presence of dynamic airway collapse and consequent intrinsic positive end-expiratory pressure (PEEP$_i$). In breath A, PEEP$_i$ is evident in the Pa tracing at end-expiration. Note that this PEEP$_i$ must be overcome before Paw is lowered such that the next assisted breath can be triggered (points a to b are the "phase delay"). In breath B, a small amount of applied or extrinsic PEEP$_e$ (less than PEEP$_i$) has been applied. This pressure serves to counteract dynamic airway collapse. At end-expiration, this causes Paw to rise, but not Pa. Subsequent Pa changes needed to trigger breath C are thus reduced. (From MacIntyre NR. Complications of mechanical ventilation. *In* MacIntyre NR (eds). Problems in Respiratory Care. Philadelphia, JB Lippincott, 1991.)

incapable of providing high levels of ventilatory support, they are generally used as either intermittent partial support (e.g., nocturnal ventilation) or as a short-term technique to "buy time" in an acute situation.

Negative Pressure Approaches

Negative pressure approaches range from iron lungs to chest wraps to rocking beds.

Although negative pressure applied to the thorax can provide some degree of lung inflation, negative pressure devices generally are cumbersome, are incapable of any synchrony with patient efforts, and provide no airway protection. Because of this, negative pressure approaches are generally limited to patients with neuromuscular dysfunction in whom some nocturnal assistance and muscle "rest" results in improved ventilatory function during the day.

Positive Pressure Mask Approaches

Ventilatory support or continuous positive airway pressure can be provided by positive pressure applied through mask systems. Full-face mask ventilation using either pressure-limited or flow-limited breaths can be provided through tight-fitting masks. However, leaks are common, and gastric overdistention can result in vomiting and aspiration. Such

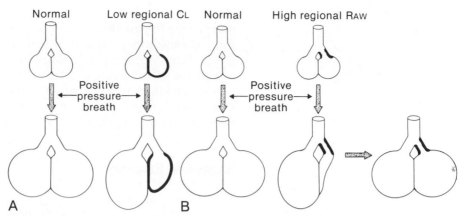

FIGURE 22–10: How overdistention of more normal alveoli and interface shearing can occur when positive pressure breaths are used in inhomogeneous lungs. *A,* Uneven compliance. *B,* Uneven resistance.

The use of these systems appears to be a reasonable strategy for short-term support in acute respiratory failure if the system is monitored properly. The role of this technique in long-term support without close monitoring (e.g., home care) is less clear because of concerns over leaks, undetected circuit occlusions, and gastric distention.

The nasal mask approach to providing continuous positive airway pressure has been very effective in managing obstructive sleep apnea.

systems can respond to patient efforts to provide either assisted or supported breaths.

Positive airway pressure can also be provided by nasal masks. Continuous gas flows can compensate for the inevitable mouth leakage. Continuous baseline pressure elevation (continuous positive airway pressure) is effective in managing obstructive sleep apnea. This technique probably also has a role in noninvasively restoring functional residual capacity and improving $\dot{V}/\dot{Q}$ mismatch in mild to moderate pulmonary edema (see Chapter 23). It may also have a role in compensating for some intrinsic PEEP due to dynamic airway collapse in patients with airway dysfunction (see the previous discussion of intrinsic PEEP and Fig. 22–9). The role of positive pressure breaths to provide ventilatory support through a nasal mask (generally using pressure-limited breaths) is less clear. Mask function, leakage tolerance, and patient synchrony with these systems vary; thus, these systems usually require close monitoring to be effective for short-term support in dyspneic patients. However, because the mouth is open with a nasal system, there is less concern about vomiting and aspiration and the danger of undetected circuit occlusion. Long-term use is thus a potential application of such systems (e.g., nocturnal support), and indeed, treatment of some patients with obstructive sleep apnea appears to be enhanced when positive pressure during inspiration is added to the elevation in baseline pressure. However, the long-term role of such systems in patients with intrinsic lung disease and dyspnea is unknown.

SUMMARY

Mechanical ventilatory support uses positive pressure breaths to provide ventilatory assistance to patients. Current systems make available a variety of inspiratory flow patterns, expiratory pressures, supplemental oxygen, and patient interactive features. The goal of mechanical ventilation is to provide adequate gas exchange. At the same time, complications relating to elevated alveolar pressures and elevated inspired oxygen concentrations are to be avoided. The usual settings for total mechanical support include tidal volumes of 8 to 10 mL/kg and a frequency adjusted to achieve the desired P_{CO_2} and pH. To protect the lung from unnecessary pressures, an elevated P_{CO_2} may be tolerated (so-called permissive hypercapnia), provided that the pH and P_{O_2} are acceptable. Partial ventilatory support is usually provided for patients who require a less than total level of ventilatory assistance, usually during the recovery phase of lung injury. Partial ventilatory support requires patient-ventilator interactions during the triggering, flow delivery, and termination of the mechanical breaths. Dyssynchrony during these phases can result in significant imposed workloads on the patient.

Suggested Readings

American Respiratory Care Foundation Consensus Conference on the Essentials of Mechanical Ventilators. Respir Care 37:1000–1008, 1992.

Boysen PG, Kacmarek RM. Mechanical ventilation—Part I and part II. Respir Care 32(6):403–479 and 33(1):517–616, 1987.

Chatburn RL. A new system for understanding mechanical ventilators. Respir Care 36:1123–1131, 1991.

Fulkerson W, MacIntyre NR (eds). Complications of mechanical ventilation. *In* Fulkerson W, MacIntyre NR (eds). Problems in Respiratory Care. Philadelphia, JB Lippincott, 1991.

Hickling KG. Ventilatory management of ARDS: Can it affect the outcome? Intensive Care Med 16:219–226, 1990.

Kacmarek RM, Pierson DJ. Positive end-expiratory pressure (PEEP). Respir Care 33:419–638, 1988.

Kolobow T, Moretti M, Fumagalli R, et al. Severe impairment in lung function induced by high peak airway pressure during mechanical ventilation. Am Rev Respir Dis 135:312–315, 1987.

MacIntyre NR. Respiratory function during pressure support ventilation. Chest 89:677–683, 1986.

Marini JJ, Smith TC, Lamb VJ. External work output and force generation during synchronized intermittent mechanical ventilation. Am Rev Respir Dis 138:1169–1179, 1988.

Morganroth ML. Mechanical ventilation. Clin Chest Med 9(1):1–147, 1988.

Pingleton SK. Complications of acute respiratory failure. Am Rev Respir Dis 137:1463–1493, 1988.

Plummer AL, Gracey DR. Consensus conference on artificial airways in patients receiving mechanical ventilation. Chest 96:178–180, 1989.

Sassoon CS. Positive pressure ventilation: Alternate modes. Chest 100:1421–1429, 1991.

Steier M, Ching N, Roberts E, et al. Pneumothorax complicating continuous ventilatory support. J Thorac Cardiovasc Surg 67:17–23, 1974.

Weisman IM, Rinaldo JE, Rogers RM, et al. Intermittent mandatory ventilation. Am Rev Respir Dis 127:641–647, 1983.

Zwillich CW, Pierson DJ, Creagh CE, et al. Complications of assisted ventilation. A prospective study of 354 consecutive episodes. Am J Med 57:161–170, 1974.

23

Oxygenation Support

Neil R. MacIntyre, M.D.

Hypoxemia can result from impairment of oxygen transport anywhere along the path from the environment to the pulmonary capillary (Fig. 23–1). Generally speaking, two major mechanisms exist:

- Decreases in the alveolar oxygen tension ($P_{A_{O_2}}$)
- Impairment in the alveolar-arterial transport of oxygen ($P(A - a)O_2$)

Oxygenation support refers to techniques used to improve arterial oxygen content. These techniques can either be independent from ventilatory support (e.g., simple $F_{I_{O_2}}$ enrichment by nasal cannula or constant positive airway pressure masks) or be incorporated with techniques that also supply positive pressure ventilation to produce a total "respiratory" support system (see Chapter 22). Oxygenation support strategies can be categorized by which step in oxygen transport they address (see Fig. 23–1).

TECHNIQUES TO INCREASE $P_{A_{O_2}}$

There are essentially two ways to increase the $P_{A_{O_2}}$:

- Increase the $P_{I_{O_2}}$ through increases in the $F_{I_{O_2}}$ (or, less commonly, through increases in barometric pressure). (See Chapters 26 and 27.)
- Increase the $\dot{V}_A$

The relationship among these factors is expressed in a rearrangement of the alveolar air equation:

$$P_{A_{O_2}} \propto P_{I_{O_2}} - \dot{V}_{O_2}/\dot{V}_A$$

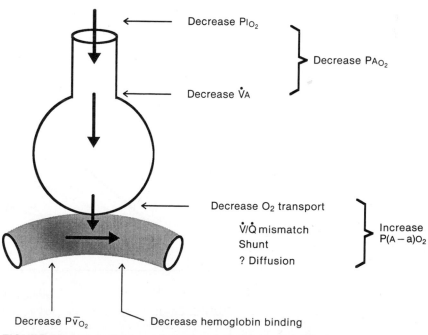

FIGURE 23–1: Potential sources of reduced arterial oxygen content.

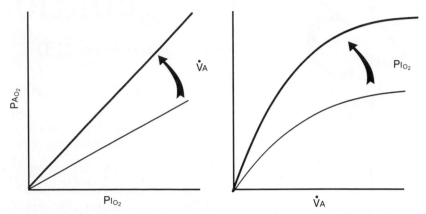

FIGURE 23–2: Relationship of alveolar P_{O_2} (PA_{O_2}) to inspired P_{O_2} ($PI_{O_2} \propto PB$ and FI_{O_2}) and to alveolar ventilation ($\dot{V}A$). Note that the relationship of PA_{O_2} to PI_{O_2} is linear and that $\dot{V}A$ affects the slope. On the other hand, the relationship of PA_{O_2} to $\dot{V}A$ is a curvilinear one that asymptotically approaches the PI_{O_2}.

Effects of changes in FI_{O_2}:

- FI_{O_2} of less than 0.4 can be tolerated for prolonged periods
- FI_{O_2} of greater than 0.6 increases the risk for oxygen toxicity
- FI_{O_2} approaching 1.0 can result in absorption atelectasis and oxygen toxicity

Note from these relationships that increases in PI_{O_2} have a linear relationship with PA_{O_2}, whereas the effects of an increase in $\dot{V}A$ are curvilinear (Fig. 23–2).

The effect of an increase in PA_{O_2} on ultimate arterial oxygen content depends on the other factors in oxygen transport affecting the $P(A - a)O_2$, especially ventilation-perfusion mismatch and shunt (Fig. 23–3). Thus, predicting the effects of a change in FI_{O_2} on Pa_{O_2} is an approximation at best. Raising the PA_{O_2} can also cause alveolar capillary injury through the toxic effects of oxygen radicals. Depending on the baseline

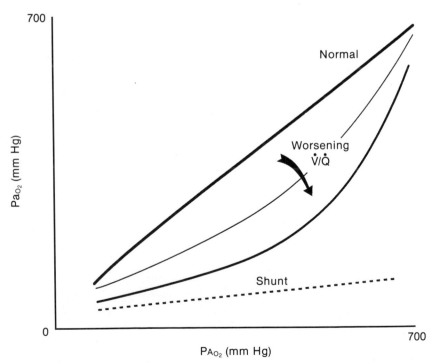

FIGURE 23–3: Relationship of PA_{O_2} to Pa_{O_2}. Note that although the normal relationship is linear, increasing $\dot{V}/\dot{Q}$ mismatching and shunts distort this and make an increase in PA_{O_2} less effective in increasing Pa_{O_2}.

lung pathology, the presence of certain drugs, and perhaps mechanical forces from positive pressure breaths, even mild increases in $F_{I_{O_2}}$ and $P_{A_{O_2}}$ have been associated with oxygen toxicity.

TECHNIQUES TO IMPROVE ALVEOLAR-ARTERIAL OXYGEN TRANSPORT

Impaired oxygen transport from the alveolus to the capillary in patients with respiratory failure is usually a consequence of impaired ventilation-perfusion $(\dot{V}/\dot{Q})$ matching (including shunts). This is manifest as a widening of the alveolar-arterial oxygen difference $(P(A - a)O_2)$ and worsening of the Pa_{O_2}/PA_{O_2} (or Pa_{O_2}/FI_{O_2}) ratio (see Fig. 23–3). One of the most important causes of these low $\dot{V}/\dot{Q}$ units and shunts is alveolar collapse due to loss of surfactant and alveolar edema. This alveolar collapse concept is depicted schematically in Figure 23–4. The mechanical properties of the alveoli depicted in Figure 23–4 are characterized in Figure 23–5. Two basic approaches can be taken to improve the $\dot{V}/\dot{Q}$ mismatch and shunts that occur as a consequence of alveolar collapse:

- Manipulation of baseline or expiratory pressures
- Manipulation of the positive pressure breath

Manipulation of Baseline or Expiratory Pressures

A commonly used technique to counteract the effects depicted in Figures 23–4 and 23–5 is the application of an elevated baseline or expiratory pressure. When used in a spontaneously breathing patient, this pressure can be applied either during expiration only (EPAP) or else

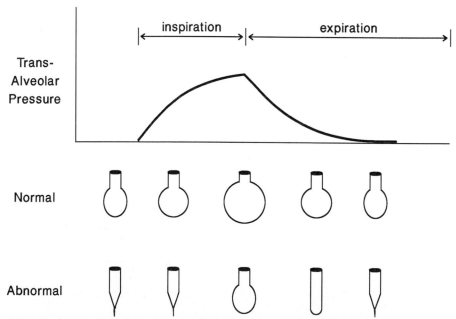

FIGURE 23–4: Alveolar behavior over the ventilatory cycle. Note that in the normal situation, alveolar patency exists throughout. On the other hand, lung abnormalities associated with surfactant loss, alveolar edema, and the like result in alveolar collapse during much of the ventilatory cycle. The consequence is low $\dot{V}/\dot{Q}$ relationships and shunts.

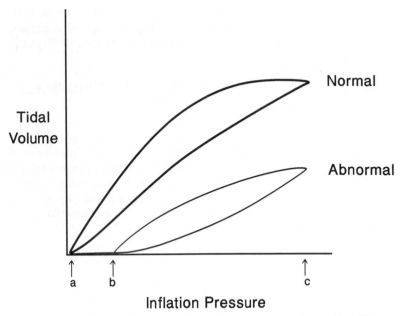

FIGURE 23–5: Mechanical properties of alveoli depicted in Figure 23–4. Note that the abnormal alveolus is characterized by both a period of initial closure (i.e., no volume change during the initial pressure change from point a to point b) and a reduced compliance (volume/pressure) at end-inspiration (point c).

as part of continuous positive airway pressure application (CPAP) (Fig. 23–6). The CPAP approach minimizes the inspiratory pressure drop (and thus muscle work) that must occur to provide a tidal breath. EPAP is thus rarely used. When used in mechanically ventilated patients, the

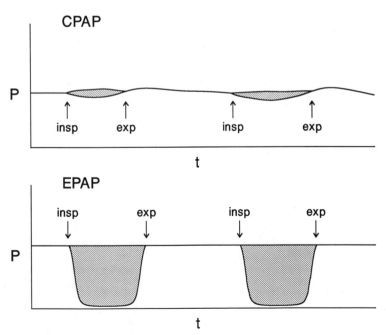

FIGURE 23–6: Airway pressure (P) in a spontaneously breathing patient receiving expiratory pressure either as part of a continuous elevation in pressures (CPAP) or during expiration only (EPAP). Note that EPAP requires considerable inspiratory work *(shaded area).* insp, inspiration; exp, expiration.

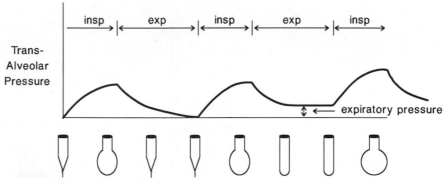

FIGURE 23–7: Behavior of the abnormal alveoli depicted in Figure 23–4 when expiratory pressure is applied. Note that alveolar collapse is prevented and the functional residual capacity is thus restored. Note that for the same transalveolar inflation pressure, the application of expiratory pressure increases both maximal transalveolar pressure and volume. insp, inspiration; exp, expiration.

elevated baseline pressure is referred to as positive end-expiratory pressure (PEEP). The addition of this pressure prevents a return to zero of the transalveolar pressure and serves to maintain alveolar patency throughout the ventilatory cycle (Fig. 23–7). The baseline lung volume is thus increased by this pressure, thereby improving $\dot{V}/\dot{Q}$ mismatching and shunts. Figure 23–8 depicts this shift in the "operating pressure" of the alveolus to a more effective position with appropriate PEEP (curve A to B) and to an overdistended position with excessive PEEP (curve B to C).

The baseline pressure that puts alveoli on the steep part of the pressure-volume curve is often considered to be the ideal baseline pres-

> The baseline lung volume is the functional residual capacity.

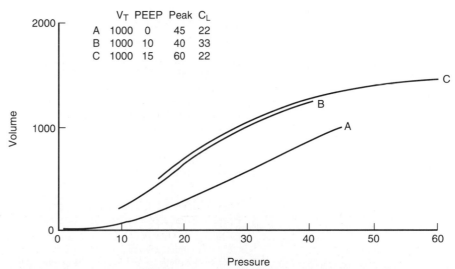

FIGURE 23–8: Mechanical changes in collapsed alveoli when ventilated with increasing levels of end-expiratory pressure (PEEP). Curve A represents alveoli that remain collapsed until 5 to 10 cm H_2O pressure is applied (opening pressure). Subsequent delivery of a 1000-mL tidal volume (V_T) produces a peak pressure of 45 cm H_2O and a calculated compliance (C_L) of 22 mL/cm H_2O. Preventing alveolar collapse with 10 cm H_2O PEEP improves C_L *(curve B)*. Levels of PEEP above this opening pressure, however, serve only to overdistend the alveoli, thereby worsening C_L *(curve C)*.

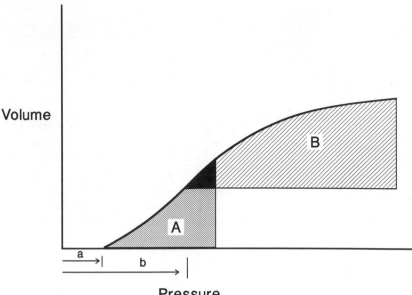

FIGURE 23–9: Example of appropriate (a) and excessive (b) expiratory pressure on the abnormal alveolus in Figure 23–5 and Figure 23–8, curve A. Both pressures eliminate closure, but because the pressure-volume curve becomes flatter as higher pressures are used, expiratory pressure a results in a much lower inspiratory work ($\int$ PdV of A is less than that of B, indicated by shading) and lower maximal pressure for the same tidal volume as expiratory pressure b.

sure for the alveoli (Fig. 23–8, curve B). At this point, not only does alveolar collapse not occur, but inspiratory work (i.e., $\int$PdV) is minimized (Fig. 23–9).

The previous discussion relates to pressure effects in a lung with homogeneous alveolar injury. In fact, lung injury is usually heterogeneous, and thus what may be ideal in one unit may not be so in another. Ideally applied CPAP or PEEP balances between the overall beneficial oxygenation effects and the adverse work and intrathoracic pressure effects. Several approaches to striking this balance have been proposed (Table 23–1). Our approach is to provide at least "minimal" PEEP but not exceed the PEEP providing "best" compliance.

Baseline pressures below ideal

- Provide suboptimal alveolar stabilization

Baseline pressures too high above ideal

- Demand too much inspiratory work
- Overdistend the alveoli
- Unnecessarily impede venous return

Manipulation of the Positive Pressure Breath to Improve $\dot{V}/\dot{Q}$ Mismatch and Shunt

There are two conceptual approaches to "shaping" the positive pressure breath that may affect $\dot{V}/\dot{Q}$ matching and shunts:

TABLE **23–1:** Different Approaches to Optimizing Continuous Positive Airway Pressure and Positive End-Expiratory Pressure

Normalize the $P(A - a)O_2$ and generally either ignore other pressure effects or compensate for them (e.g., give fluids to improve cardiac filling and use prophylactic chest tubes) ("maximal" PEEP)

Provide minimal pressure to keep $Pa_{O_2} > 60$ mm Hg and $FI_{O_2} < 0.4$ ("minimal" PEEP)

Balance increased Pa_{O_2} with other factors ("best" PEEP) by increasing PEEP until
    Best compliance is found (pressure-volume curve)
    Best O_2 delivery is found ($CO \times Sa_{O_2} \times$ hemoglobin)
    Best Pv_{O_2} is found

PEEP, positive end-expiratory pressure.
CO, cardiac output.

- Manipulating the delivered inspiratory flow pattern
- Adjusting the inspiratory time

Inspiratory Flow Pattern

As noted in the discussion on ventilation distribution (see Chapter 22), the inspiratory flow pattern as it interacts with regional compliance and resistance determines the distribution of the delivered positive pressure breath. Conceptually, the high initial flows of a decelerating pattern may fill alveoli more rapidly at the beginning of the breath. However, in clinical studies different flow patterns appear to have only small effects on ultimate arterial oxygenation. The selection of flow pattern is thus usually based on patient synchrony and the appropriateness of expiratory time rather than on its effects on $\dot{V}/\dot{Q}$ matching and shunts. Decelerating and square flow patterns are the most commonly used.

Inspiratory Time

As depicted in Figure 23–4, alveolar instability, especially in expiration, is believed to be a major source of the widened $P(A - a)O_2$ in respiratory failure. Expiratory pressure through applied CPAP and PEEP helps to open and stabilize these alveoli through elevation of baseline pressures and lung volumes (see Figs. 23–6 and 23–7). An alternative approach to managing this alveolar instability is to prolong the inspiratory time and shorten the expiratory time. This accomplishes several purposes:

- Alveoli will have a longer duration of inflation pressure and thus a longer time for mixing of fresh gases in the conducting airway with residual alveolar gas.
- Slow time constant units will have a longer opportunity to inflate.

If expiratory time is adequate for the lung to return to functional residual capacity, these two effects increase mean alveolar pressure and improve $\dot{V}/\dot{Q}$ matching without a concomitant rise in overall peak alveolar pressure.

Longer inspiratory times are thus an alternative strategy to applied PEEP to improve $\dot{V}/\dot{Q}$ without necessarily increasing peak alveolar pressures (Fig. 23–10). If, however, the shorter expiration time will not allow complete emptying of alveolar units, air trapping and intrinsic PEEP develop (Fig. 23–11). This intrinsic PEEP effect will *not* be reflected in circuit expiratory pressure but will increase peak alveolar pressures for the same tidal volume (volume-cycled ventilation; see solid lines in Figs. 23–11 and 23–12) or decrease the tidal volume for the same peak airway pressure (pressure-limited ventilation; see dotted lines in Figs. 23–11B and 23–12). Intrinsic PEEP appears to improve $\dot{V}/\dot{Q}$ mismatch and shunts in respiratory failure, but whether it is any better than applied PEEP for the same *mean* alveolar pressure is not clear. A disadvantage to intrinsic PEEP, as compared with applied PEEP, is the fact that intrinsic PEEP is *not* reflected in the routine measurements of airway pressure (see baseline airway pressures in Fig. 23–11). More careful attention to ventilation parameters is thus required when this strategy is being used. In addition, long inspiratory-expiratory time ratios are uncomfortable for many patients and may require substantial sedation or paralysis. At present, no data exist that report improved outcome or reduced complications with the use of long inspiratory times as an alternative to applied PEEP. However, for an empiric trial of this strategy,

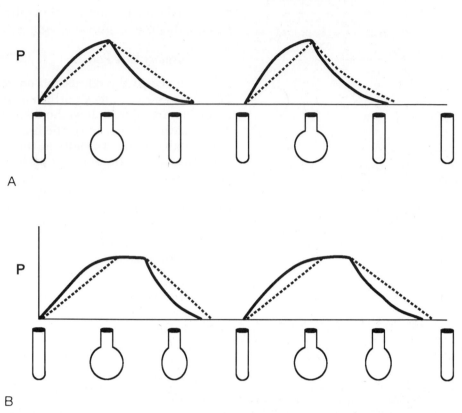

FIGURE 23–10: Effect of a longer inspiratory time on airway pressure (solid line), alveolar pressure (dotted line), and alveolar volume in the absence of air trapping. In this example, tidal volume and rate are kept constant. Note that by lengthening inspiratory time from *A* to *B*, mean airway pressure will increase, but because expiratory time is sufficient for alveolar pressure to equilibrate with airway pressure, no air trapping or "intrinsic" positive end-expiratory pressure develops. Peak pressures and tidal volume thus do not change.

Table 23–2 gives one approach to using long inspiratory time in managing oxygenation failure.

NONRESPIRATORY SUPPORT TECHNIQUES TO IMPROVE OXYGEN TRANSPORT

Patient Position

Gravitational effects can have an important influence on V̇/Q̇ mismatching in patients with large regional abnormalities. In general, blood flow tends to distribute toward dependent regions. Thus, patients with regional airspace disease might improve V̇/Q̇ matching if the well-ventilated regions are placed dependently. Turning the patient to shift gravity-related edema may also have some benefit.

Reduce Oxygen Consumption

An agitated or febrile patient can have significant oxygen demands, thereby reducing Pv_{O_2} and compromising arterial oxygenation. An important source of this agitation can be patient-ventilatory dyssynchrony (see

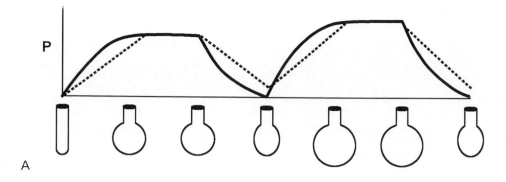

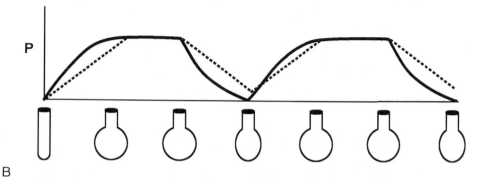

FIGURE 23–11: Effects of a longer inspiratory time on airway pressure (solid line), alveolar pressure (dotted line), and alveolar volume in the presence of air trapping. *A,* Flow-limited, volume-cycled ventilation. *B,* Pressure-limited, time-cycled ventilation. In both examples, inspiratory time is such that an inadequate expiratory time for alveolar-airway equilibration develops and air trapping (intrinsic positive end-expiratory pressure) is produced. With a constant tidal volume *(A),* the peak airway and alveolar pressure will thus increase; with a constant inspiratory pressure *(B),* the tidal volume decreases.

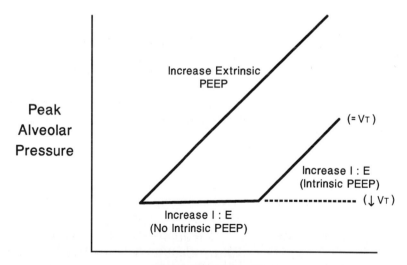

FIGURE 23–12: Relationship of peak alveolar pressure to various strategies to increase mean alveolar pressure. With increases in extrinsic or applied positive end-expiratory pressure (PEEP) above opening pressure, the relationship is linear. With increases in inspiratory time that do not produce air trapping (or intrinsic PEEP), mean airway pressure is increased without increases in peak alveolar pressure. However, when air trapping and intrinsic PEEP develop, either a higher peak alveolar pressure is needed for a constant V_T *(solid line)* or else V_T diminishes for a constant peak alveolar pressure *(dotted line).*

TABLE **23–2:**   A Stepwise Approach to Using Pressure Control Along With Prolonged Inspiratory Time to Improve V̇/Q̇

Patient selection: those in whom normal inspiratory time ventilation and applied PEEP have resulted in peak *alveolar* pressures exceeding 35 to 40 cm H_2O without satisfactory oxygenation

Steps (assess oxygenation goals after each step before advancing to the next):

1. Switch to pressure-controlled mode (if it is not already being used) with the same V_T, f, and t_i
2. Lengthen t_i to increase the mean P_{AW} to the point of air trapping (i.e., *no loss of* V_T)
3. Choice:
   a. Push t_i past the point of air trapping; to maintain V_T, maximal alveolar pressures must also increase (see Chapter 22 for monitoring of air trapping and intrinsic PEEP)

      or

   b. Maintain t_i and increase extrinsic PEEP

PEEP, positive end-expiratory pressure; t_i, inspiratory time.

Chapter 22). Adjustments of ventilator parameters can sometimes alleviate this, but sedation, paralysis, or both may be necessary.

Increase Oxygen-Carrying Capacity

Hemoglobin is a major determinant of oxygen content in the blood. The other important variable in oxygen delivery is cardiac output. Indeed, heroic efforts to improve P_{AO_2} and Pa_{O_2} will be rendered useless if the hemoglobin concentration or cardiac output is low.

In properly managing respiratory failure, *all* factors responsible for oxygen delivery must be considered:

- Hemoglobin oxygen saturation
- Hemoglobin concentration
- Cardiac output

Improve Alveolar Stability Through Surface-Active Material

Because normal alveoli require surface-active material for maintenance of patency, it seems reasonable to use either natural or artificial surfactant to help stabilize lungs in disease in which surfactant is either absent (e.g., prematurity) or abnormal (e.g., adult respiratory distress syndrome). Indeed, one or two intratracheal doses of surfactant in premature infants produce a striking improvement in both mechanics and gas exchange. Although currently under investigation, the role of surfactant replacement in adult disease is less clear.

SUMMARY

Goals of Oxygenation Support

The simplest goal of oxygenation support is to maintain an adequate Pa_{O_2} with minimal toxicity. However, oxygenation goals are probably best assessed when considered in the context of oxygen delivery to the tissues.

$$D_{O_2} = CO \times \text{hemoglobin} \times Sa_{O_2}$$

This relationship emphasizes the importance of hemoglobin and blood flow along with arterial oxygenation in oxygen transport. It also reminds the clinician that when one component in this equation is seriously compromised (e.g., Sa_{O_2}), compensation can be made by addressing other

An adequate Pa_{O_2} is greater than 55 to 60 mm Hg.

components (e.g., hemoglobin or CO). A detailed discussion of these concepts is given in Chapter 9. In general, however, oxygen delivery goals of 400 to 600 mL/min/m^2 are reasonable, although some would argue for even higher goals in trauma patients. In addition, a minimal Pa$_{O_2}$ of 55 mm Hg should be maintained to minimize pulmonary vasoconstriction and other hypoxemic reflexes.

Suggested Readings

Ashbaugh DG, Bigelow DB, Petty TL, Levine BE. Acute respiratory distress in adults. Lancet 2:319–323, 1967.

Cole AGH, Weller SF, Sykes MK. Inverse ratio ventilation compared with PEEP in adult respiratory failure. Intensive Care Med 10:227–232, 1984.

Connors AF, McCaffree DR, Gray BA. Effect of inspiratory flow rate on gas exchange during mechanical ventilation. Am Rev Respir Dis 124:537–543, 1981.

Danek SJ, Lynch JP, Weg JG, Dantzker DR. The dependence of oxygen uptake on oxygen delivery in the adult respiratory distress syndrome. Am Rev Respir Dis 122:387–395, 1980.

Dantzker DR, Brook CJ, Dehart P, et al. Ventilation-perfusion distributions in the adult respiratory distress syndrome. Am Rev Respir Dis 120:1039–1052, 1979.

Dantzker DR, Gutierrez G. The assessment of tissue oxygenation. Respir Care 30(6):456–462, 1985.

Duncan SR, Rizk N, Raffin TA. Inverse ratio ventilation. PEEP in disguise? Chest 3:391–392, 1987.

Gilbert EM, Haupt MT, Mandanas RY, et al. The effect of fluid loading, blood transfusion, and catecholamine infusion on oxygen delivery and consumption in patients with sepsis. Am Rev Respir Dis 134:873–878, 1986.

Gregory GA, Kitterman JA, Phibbs RH, et al. Treatment of the idiopathic respiratory distress syndrome with continuous positive airway pressure. N Engl J Med 284:1333–1340, 1971.

Herman S, Reynolds FOR. Methods for improving oxygenation in infants mechanically ventilated for severe hyaline membrane disease. Arch Dis Child 48:613–617, 1973.

Kacmarek RM, Pierson DJ (eds). AARC Conference on Positive End Expiratory Pressure. Respir Care 33:419–527, 1988.

Pepe PE, Marini JJ. Occult positive end-expiratory pressure in mechanically ventilated patients with airflow obstruction. The auto-PEEP effect. Am Rev Respir Dis 126:166–170, 1982.

Shoemaker WC. Hemodynamic and oxygen transport patterns in septic shock: Physiologic mechanisms and therapeutic implications. In Sibbald WJ, Sprung CL (eds). Perspectives on Sepsis and Septic Shock. Fullerton, CA, Society for Critical Care Medicine, 1986, 203–234.

Tyler DC. Positive end-expiratory pressure: A review. Crit Care Med 11:300–308, 1983.

Vincent JL, Roman A, De Backer D, Kahn RI. Oxygen uptake/supply dependency. Am Rev Respir Dis 142:2–7, 1990.

24

■

Key Terms

Apneic Ventilation

Coaxial Flow

Extracorporeal

High-Frequency Ventilation (HFV)

Intravascular Oxygenation (IVOX)

Liquid Lung Ventilation

HFV—greater than 100 breaths per minute in the adult and greater than 300 breaths per minute in the neonate or the pediatric patient

Usual jet settings:

- Frequency
- Pulse ("jetted") volume
- Entrainment volume
- Inspiratory time
- Baseline pressure

Unconventional Support Techniques for Ventilation and Oxygenation

Neil R. MacIntyre, M.D.,
and R. Alan Leonard, R.R.T.

Current approaches to mechanical ventilatory support generally attempt to duplicate the normal bulk-flow ventilatory pattern (i.e., tidal volumes and rates in the physiologic range) in conjunction with elevations in baseline pressures and FI_{O_2}. Unfortunately, in diseased lungs these strategies may not provide adequate CO_2 clearance or O_2 delivery. In addition, they may require the production of very high alveolar pressures, which can be deleterious both to the lung and to the cardiovascular system. This chapter reviews a number of approaches to using nonconventional techniques. For some of these techniques, enough data have been accumulated to warrant their approval by the US Food and Drug Administration for clinical use in specific circumstances. Other techniques are still in the experimental phase, awaiting more data before they find a clinical application. This chapter covers the following techniques:

- Various forms of high-frequency ventilation (HFV)
- Apneic ventilation and oxygenation
- Liquid ventilation
- Extracorporeal systems

HIGH-FREQUENCY VENTILATION

Broadly speaking, HFV is defined as mechanical ventilatory support using higher than normal breathing frequencies. For the purposes of this chapter, however, our comments are restricted to those techniques that utilize breathing frequencies several-fold higher than normal. Delivery of gas at these frequencies is generally impossible for conventional ventilators with standard valves and circuits. Different systems must be used, generally consisting of either jets or oscillators.

Jets (Fig. 24–1) operate on the principle of a nozzle or an injector creating a high-velocity "jet" of gas directed into the lung. Because of the inertia of jetted gas, exhalation valves and cuffed airway tubes are unnecessary (although they can be used to manipulate mean and baseline airway pressures). Exhalation with jet ventilation is passive (i.e., due to lung recoil).

Oscillators (Fig. 24–2) operate with a "to-and-fro" application of pressure on the airway opening, using either pistons or microprocessor

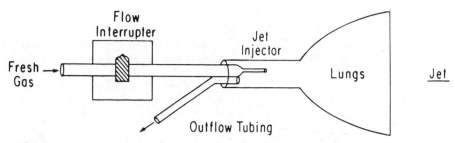

FIGURE 24–1: Jet ventilator for delivering high-frequency ventilation. Source gas is supplied to a controlling valve, which then provides jet pulses at the desired pressure, inspiratory duration, and frequency. The delivered pulse may be injected into the distal endotracheal tube or directly into the tracheal catheters. In addition, injected pulses can be augmented through entrainment (as shown). Exhalation is passive and does not involve an expiratory valve. Positive expiratory pressure can be applied, if desired, in the exhalation circuit. Airway pressure must be measured distal to the jet injector for accuracy. (From MacIntyre NR. New forms of mechanical ventilation in the adult. Clin Chest Med 9:47–54, 1988.)

Usual oscillator settings:

- Oscillator frequency
- Oscillator displacement (volume)
- Inspiratory to expiratory time
- Bias flow

gas controllers. Fresh gas is supplied into the ventilator circuit as a "bias flow," and mean airway pressure is adjusted by the relationship between fresh gas inflow and any negative pressure (i.e., vacuum) placed on the gas outflow from the bias-flow circuit. Important differences between jets and oscillators include their different flow profiles; in fact, the oscillator outstroke produces an active ventilator expiratory phase.

Mechanisms of Gas Transport

Coaxial flow—gas in the center of the airway having a net inflow, and gas in the periphery of the airway having a net outflow

The usually small jet or oscillator tidal breaths may approach (or even be smaller than) anatomic dead space. For effective CO_2 and O_2 transfer to take place between alveoli and the environment under these circumstances, mechanisms other than conventional bulk-flow transport must be invoked. This is because the traditional relationship between effective alveolar ventilation ($\dot{V}_A$) and the frequency (f), tidal volume (V_T)

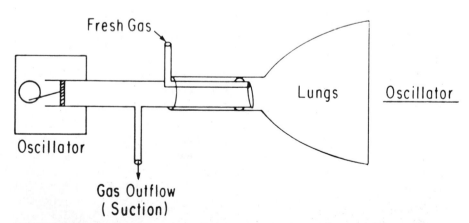

FIGURE 24–2: High-frequency oscillator for delivering high-frequency ventilation. Airway pressure oscillations are produced by a piston or membrane moving at a selected rate and displacement. Fresh gas inflow (bias flow) is set as close to the carina as possible. Gas outflow and circuit pressures are regulated by adjusting a vacuum source or the exhalation port. (From MacIntyre NR. New forms of mechanical ventilation in the adult. Clin Chest Med 9:47–54, 1988.)

and dead space volume (V_D)(i.e., $\dot{V}_A = f \times [V_T - V_D]$) becomes meaningless when V_T is less than V_D.

At least five different mechanisms exist to explain gas transport under these seemingly "unphysiologic" conditions:

- Bulk flow can still provide conventional gas delivery to proximal alveoli with very low regional dead space volumes.
- Coaxial flow can develop because of the asymmetrical flow profile of high-velocity gases.
- Taylor's dispersion can produce a mixing of fresh and residual gas along the "front" of a flow of gas through a tube.
- Pendelluft can mix gases between lung regions that have different impedances.
- Augmented molecular diffusion can occur in the alveolar regions of the lungs.

All of these mechanisms may operate simultaneously during various HFV settings in various disease states (Fig. 24–3). Therefore, predicting $\dot{V}_A$ from the f and V_T settings of HFV can be very difficult. Nevertheless, it is clear that the required product of f times V_T is generally much higher than that required during conventional ventilation and that V_T appears to have more influence on gas transport than f with non–bulk-flow mechanisms.

Airway pressures during HFV are a consequence of the applied baseline pressure along with the interactions of delivered volume, respiratory system impedances, and the development of gas trapping (dynamic hyperinflation or intrinsic positive end-expiratory pressure). In general, however, peak airway pressures during HFV are lower than those observed during a comparable level of conventional ventilation, reflecting primarily the small delivered V_T. Mean airway pressures may also be

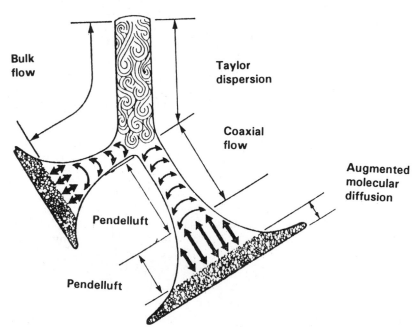

FIGURE 24–3: Lung regions where various gas transport mechanisms of high-frequency ventilation are thought to be operative. (From Chang HK. Mechanisms of gas transport during ventilation by high frequency oscillation. J Appl Physiol Respir Environ Exercise Physiol 56:553–563, 1984.)

lower, but they are often comparable to those observed during conventional ventilation.

Applications

Two conceptual advantages of HFV exist:

1. Lower peak pressures may reduce complications.
2. Non–bulk-flow mechanisms may improve ventilation-perfusion matching.

Clinical data supporting these advantages vary but appear to be strongest in the pediatric population. Indeed, HFV (both jets and oscillators) has found its greatest applicability in the support of neonates at risk for barotrauma because of high ventilatory pressures. In this population, breathing frequencies in the range of 500 to 1000 breaths per minute with effective volumes of 1 to 5 mL per breath produce mean airway pressures comparable to (or lower than) those observed during conventional therapy, with substantially reduced peak airway pressures. With this ventilator pattern, the manifestations of barotrauma (e.g., pulmonary interstitial emphysema and pneumothoraces) appear to be fewer, and the outcome seems improved.

Adult experience with HFV is generally limited to the use of jets with frequencies of up to 300 breaths per minute that use primarily bulk-flow gas transport. In this range of frequencies, HFV applications in the adult appear to be fewer than in the neonate. Indeed, in several controlled studies of adult respiratory failure, HFV was shown to provide reasonable gas transport with lower peak airway pressures; however, no improvement in outcome and no reduction in complications with HFV as compared with conventional therapy occurred.

Several specific applications for adult HFV do exist. First, the reduced peak pressure and faster rate can alter ventilation distribution and improve gas exchange in patients with very large pulmonary air leaks. However, no available data demonstrate improved survival in such patients with HFV. Most clinicians would argue that routine bronchopleural fistulas can be adequately ventilated with conventional mechanical ventilation. Second, although cardiac function generally is not affected by HFV as compared with conventional ventilation at a given mean airway pressure, synchronizing the HFV pressures with cardiac systole appears to benefit stroke volume in patients with severe cardiac dysfunction. Third, reduced thoracoabdominal motion during anesthesia with the use of HFV has been useful in extracorporeal shock wave lithotripsy by minimizing stone motion and thus procedure time. Finally, the open system provided by the jet ventilator (i.e., a system without a need for an exhalation valve or a tight-fitting endotracheal tube) offers additional advantages in two areas. First, this system allows airway surgical procedures (e.g., bronchoscopy or laryngoscopy) to be performed with adequate ventilatory support and low airway pressures. Second, transtracheal jet ventilation can be used by trained individuals in emergency situations.

Complications

Several potential problems exist with the use of HFV. Adequate humidification can be difficult to achieve when high gas flows and delivered minute volumes are being used. Appropriate systems to provide heat and humidity are therefore needed, along with frequent assessment of airway function and sputum consistency. The high gas velocity of HFV may also cause direct physical airway damage. This, along with inadequate humidification, is thought to be responsible for the necrotizing tracheobronchitis observed in some neonates receiving HFV. There is also a theoretical concern that the high gas flows of HFV can cause shearing at the interfaces of different lung regions that have different impedances. This may cause barotrauma to both airways and alveoli. Air trapping can also develop during HFV because of the large delivered volumes and short expiratory times. In general, air trapping during HFV behaves in a fashion similar to air trapping during conventional ventilation (i.e., hyperinflation, reduced cardiac output, and loss of delivered volume if HFV is pressure regulated or increasing airway pressures if HFV is volume regulated). Air trapping is discussed in more detail in Chapter 22. The potential for intraventricular hemorrhage in neonates during HFV may be related to the reduced cardiac output resulting from air trapping.

APNEIC VENTILATION AND OXYGENATION

Apneic ventilation and oxygenation refers to the technique of gases moving between the environment and the alveoli without any lung motion. The mechanism of gas transport is essentially one of diffusion, although this diffusion may be augmented through the creation of turbulence in the major conducting airways. Gases move along a partial pressure gradient such that O_2 moves from the environment to the alveoli and CO_2 moves from the alveoli to the environment.

A number of techniques have been used to maximize this diffusion mechanism. The simplest approach is the placement of the lung in a very high O_2 environment (often with hyperbaric conditions). However, although this can provide an adequate O_2 diffusion gradient, CO_2 transport in the opposite direction is limited by the physiologic levels of CO_2 in the blood. Thus, the technique is often referred to as merely apneic oxygenation, because ventilation (i.e., CO_2 removal) must be accomplished through other means (e.g., extracorporeal).

A technique that seems to augment this diffusion phenomenon involves placing catheters either in the trachea or in the mainstem bronchi. If a high fresh gas flow is delivered (e.g., up to 1 L/kg/min), enough turbulence occurs that both CO_2 removal and O_2 delivery can be effective. This technique has been demonstrated to be effective for long periods of time in animal models, in which lung motion was not used except for periodic sighs to prevent atelectasis. Much less human experience exists, although reports of several hours of support using this technique in surgical settings have appeared. Under these conditions, the peak alveolar pressures are obviously very small, although a small amount of stabilizing pressure (e.g., continuous positive airway pressure) may be used to prevent atelectasis. Although this technique holds promise in the sense that gas exchange takes place without much distention of the alveoli, a theoretical concern is that of lung damage from the turbulence created in the airways. Clinical application for long-term respiratory care must await many more data.

LIQUID LUNG VENTILATION

Liquid lung ventilation refers to the technique of using a gas-soluble liquid (usually a perfluorocarbon that has a low surface tension and a high solubility for O_2 and CO_2) to either replace or augment gas ventilation. Several techniques include

- Totally filling and emptying the lung of this fluid several times per minute (i.e., perfluorocarbons completely replacing gas ventilation)
- Using smaller amounts of this material in conjunction with superimposed gas ventilation (either at conventional or high frequency)
- Using a combination of these techniques

A number of animal studies have demonstrated that liquid ventilation can increase effective compliance and provide reasonable gas exchange. A limited number of reports have described the use of liquid ventilation as a "rescue" strategy in neonates (none of whom survived). Potential complications are related to the high specific gravity of the material, which can reduce preload and increase afterload on the right ventricle. Concern also exists about the potential adverse effects of systemic absorption of these perfluorocarbons if they are used for extended periods. Whether this technique will work for prolonged periods or affect survival in larger animals or humans obviously awaits considerably more data.

EXTRACORPOREAL SYSTEMS

The concept of extracorporeal support is not new. Heart-lung bypass to support life while the heart and lungs undergo surgical procedures has been in existence for a number of years. The obvious advantages of extracorporeal approaches include adequate gas exchange with lower inspired O_2 concentrations and ventilatory pressures. Potential complications involve the cannulation risks (especially arterial), clot formation, systemic anticoagulation with consequent bleeding, blood transfusions, cerebral blood flow alterations, and (with venoarterial bypass) greatly reduced blood flow through the lungs (Table 24–1). However, as clinical experience with extracorporeal support grows and as technologic advances occur in equipment, techniques, and circuits (especially intraluminal anticoagulant bonding), fewer complications from performing extracorporeal support will occur. In the intensive care unit, extracorporeal support is being offered to a variety of different patients (Tables 24–2 to 24–4). Several techniques are currently available in the clinical environment, and a number of others are undergoing experimental work.

Venoarterial Bypass

Venoarterial bypass is complete (Fig. 24–4) cardiopulmonary bypass because blood from the venous circulation is put through a device in which all O_2 and CO_2 transport takes place. Blood is then pumped back into the arterial circulation for delivery to the rest of the body. The system consists of six basic components: an extracorporeal circuit, a blood-circulating pump, a membrane lung or oxygenator, a heat exchanger, monitoring devices, and a patient cannula. The extracorporeal circuit consists of a series of Tygon tubes and access adapters to circulate "venous" blood from the patient through the membrane lung and to

Advantages of venoarterial extracorporeal support:

- Total control of oxygenation, ventilation, and perfusion

TABLE **24–1:** Selected Complications During Extracorporeal Life Support for Neonatal and Pediatric Cases

Type of Complication	Complications Reported (%)
Physiologic complications	
Hemorrhage	
Intracranial	6–13
Operative site	7–28
Gastrointestinal	3–6
Hemolysis	8
Seizures	10–13
Infection with positive culture	5–18
Renal dysfunction	14–28
Hypotension requiring inotropes	28
Hypotension with vasodilator	9–11
Mechanical complications	
Oxygenation failure	4–18
Tubing rupture	1–7
Pump failure	2–5
Cannulation kinks	1
Heat exchanger malfunction	1
Clots within circuitry	15
Air in circuitry	4
Cannula placement	9–14

TABLE **24–2:** Neonatal Extracorporeal Life Support Diagnoses and Survival Rates

Diagnosis	No. of Cases	Survival (%)
Meconium aspiration syndrome	2431	93
Respiratory distress syndrome	843	86
Congenital diaphragmatic hernia	1202	61
Sepsis or pneumonia	900	77
Persistent pulmonary hypertension	792	86
Air leak syndrome	26	62

Data from ELSO Neonatal ECLS Registry, Extracorporeal Life Support Organization. Six Year Data Summary. Ann Arbor, MI, ELSO, 1992.

TABLE **24–3:** Pediatric Extracorporeal Life Support Diagnoses and Survival Rates

Diagnosis	No. of Cases	Survival (%)
Bacterial pneumonia	34	47
Viral pneumonia	128	49
Intrapulmonary hemorrhage	6	67
Aspiration	45	60
Pneumocystis	7	29
Adult respiratory distress syndrome	113	45
Others	79	44

Data from ELSO Pediatric ECLS Program, Extracorporeal Life Support Organization. Six Year Data Summary. Ann Arbor, MI, ELSO, 1992.

TABLE **24–4:** Adult Extracorporeal Life Support Diagnoses and Survival Rates

Diagnosis	No. of Cases	Survival (%)
Intrapulmonary hemorrhage	1	0
Bacterial pneumonia	9	11
Viral pneumonia	12	67
Aspiration	5	0
Adult respiratory distress syndrome	16	50
Other respiratory conditions	14	36
Bridge to cardiac transplantation or cardiac support	59	36

Data from ELSO Adult ECLS Registry, Extracorporeal Life Support Organization. Six Year Data Summary. Ann Arbor, MI, ELSO, 1992.

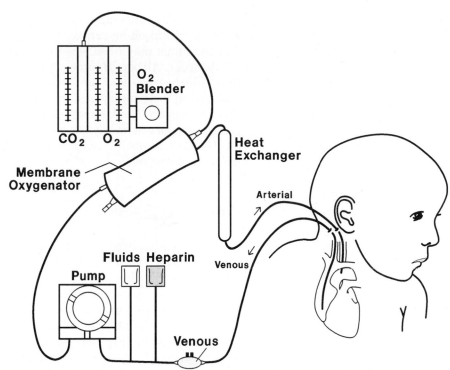

FIGURE 24–4: Venoarterial extracorporeal membrane oxygenation in a neonate.

Disadvantages of venoarterial extracorporeal support:

- Significant reduction in pulmonary blood flow
- Ligation of the common carotid artery in neonatal and some pediatric patients

return oxygenated blood back to the patient. The membrane lung is a hollow-fiber silicone oxygenator highly permeable to CO_2 and O_2 gas exchange. The surface area of the membrane lung, selected according to patient size, and the flow of ventilating gases across the membrane determine the rate of this gas exchange. The blood pump provides the driving pressure from the patient's venous circulation across the membrane lung and back to the arterial circulation. Two types of extracorporeal pumps are commonly used, the rollerhead displacement pump and a centrifugal pump. Circuit "cardiac" output is a function of blood volume (either within the extracorporeal circuit in contact with the pump rollerhead or within the chamber of the centrifugal pump) and the speed of pump revolutions. A water bath heat exchanger proximal to the patient's arterial return warms the circulating blood volume to body temperature to prevent hypothermia from the ambient cooling of extracorporeal blood volumes. Appropriately sized cannulas access the circuit to the patient. Specific monitors within the circuit provide information on circuit integrity, function, and performance.

Venoarterial extracorporeal support generally accesses the right atrium via cannulation of the internal jugular vein and the common carotid artery in both neonatal and pediatric patients. Adult patients typically require alteration of this technique, either by direct access to the atrium and aorta with thoracotomy or by femoral access sites. Venoarterial extracorporeal support is almost complete cardiopulmonary bypass, draining venous return in the right atrium, circulating the blood volume through the extracorporeal circuit, and returning blood volume to the aortic arch. The lung receives only small amounts of ventilatory support, primarily for protection against atelectasis. Because extracorporeal gas exchange is very effective, the patient can be supported for a number of days with this technique.

Currently, this approach is used in neonatal respiratory failure when oxygenation or ventilation is impossible through other techniques and the lungs may need several days to heal themselves of the underlying disorder. Although some centers are attempting to use this in adults, it should be reserved for patients who are likely to recover from the underlying lung injury and need only a few days of "lung rest" to allow this to happen. Ventilatory management during venoarterial extracorporeal support is minimal, with reductions of inspired O_2 to ambient levels and the use of ventilatory pressures and rates sufficient only to prevent atelectasis.

Venovenous Bypass

Venovenous bypass (Fig. 24–5), which is simpler than venoarterial bypass, takes only a portion (e.g., 30 to 60%) of the cardiac output from the venous circulation, puts it through a membrane oxygenator, and returns it to the major veins. Venovenous extracorporeal support accesses venous return in neonatal and some pediatric patients by placement of a double-lumen cannula into the right atrium through the internal jugular vein (Fig. 24–6). Venous return circulates from the right atrium through the extracorporeal circuit and returns to the right atrium. Cannula outflow is placed proximal to the tricuspid valve to minimize recirculation of oxygenated blood from the extracorporeal system. Cardiac output is provided entirely by the native heart, and patients must thus receive inotropic support if cardiac insufficiency develops.

In the neonate and pediatric populations, this technique is gaining popularity for patients who were previously considered for venoarterial

Advantages of venovenous extracorporeal support:

- Ease of vascular access
- Use of the native pulmonary circulation
- Salvage of the common carotid artery

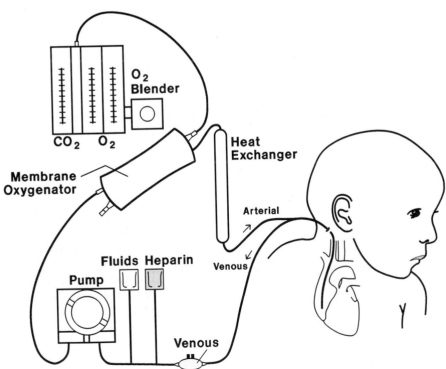

FIGURE 24–5: Venovenous extracorporeal membrane oxygenation via a double-lumen cannula in a neonate.

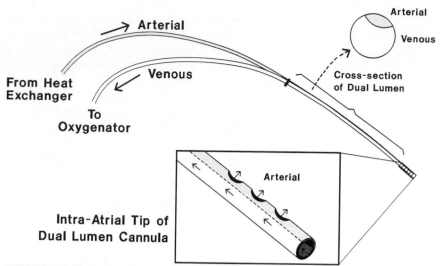

FIGURE 24–6: Details of the double-lumen cannula used in venovenous extracorporeal membrane oxygenation.

Disadvantages of venovenous extracorporeal support:

- Reduction in the efficiency of O_2 and CO_2 transport because of the recirculation of oxygenated extracorporeal blood in the right atrium
- Increased need for significant levels of conventional ventilatory support

bypass. This technique is also being investigated quite actively for use in adults. Sometimes referred to as extracorporeal CO_2 removal, this technique reflects the fact that CO_2 removal is quite effective but that oxygenation is less so. Extracorporeal CO_2 removal is usually accompanied by both low-frequency positive pressure ventilation and placement of a catheter near the carina to deliver 5 to 10 L/min of fresh gas. This transtracheal gas insufflation provides a level of apneic oxygenation (see earlier discussion) as well as clears the anatomic dead space during the ventilation expiratory cycle. Vascular access in the adult is generally through cannulation of the femoral vein, with cannula placement in the inferior vena cava.

Intravascular Oxygenation

The novel approach of intravascular oxygenation actually places the oxygenator inside the patient's major veins. Fresh gas is delivered through thousands of hollow tubes in the venous system, and gas transport takes place across the membranes into the venous blood. Thus, no bypass exists. Rather, this technique can be thought of as the use of a partial "implantable" lung. The current technology limits gas transport to 30 to 50% of what is usually needed by most patients. Nevertheless, this amount of support may make an important difference in the patient who requires high levels of traditional ventilatory support. Complications include air embolism (although this is minimized because the gas is usually under a negative pressure), cannulation risks, and bleeding (because patients are usually anticoagulated for this technique). Intravascular oxygenation is currently under active investigation.

SUMMARY

Although these exciting new techniques provide effective gas transport without necessarily placing high pressures or O_2 concentrations inside the diseased lung, it is important to remember that any form of oxygenation or ventilation support is just that, support. These techniques are rarely (if ever) therapeutic; thus, they should be used only for patients in whom effective therapy for the underlying lung disease exists. They should not be used merely to keep alive patients who have irreversible underlying disease.

In addition, experimental techniques should be used only as part of investigational protocols, preferably before lung injury related to high pressures or high O_2 concentrations has developed. Only then can we learn if the iatrogenic complications of conventional mechanical ventilatory support will be reduced with alternative approaches.

Suggested Readings

Bartlett RH. Extracorporeal life support for cardiopulmonary failure. Curr Probl Surg 27:621–705, 1990.

Bohn D. The current role of ECMO in paediatric practice. Int Care World 8:162–165, 1991.

Branson RD, Hurst JM, Davis K. Alternate modes of ventilatory support. Probl Respir Care 2, Philadelphia, JB Lippincott, 1989.

Carlton GC, Howland WS, Ray C, et al. High frequency jet ventilation: A prospective randomized evaluation. Chest 84:551–559, 1983.

Chang HK. Mechanisms of gas transport during ventilation by high frequency oscillation. J Appl Physiol Respir Environ Exercise Physiol 56:553–563, 1984.

Coghill CH, Haywood JL, Chatburn RL, et al. Neonatal and pediatric high-frequency ventilation: Principles and practice. Respir Care 36:596–612, 1991.

Extracorporeal Life Support Organization. Neonatal, Pediatric, and Adult ECLS Registry. Ann Arbor, MI, ELSO, 1992.

Fredburg JJ, Glass GM, Boynton BR, Frantz ID. Factors influencing mechanical performance of neonatal high frequency ventilators. J Appl Physiol 62:2485–2490, 1987.

Froese AB, Bryan AC. High frequency ventilation. Am Rev Respir Dis 135:1363–1374, 1987.

Fuhrman BP, Paczan PR, DeFrancisis M. Perfluorocarbon-associated gas exchange. Crit Care Med 19:712–722, 1991.

Greenspan JS, Wolfson MR, Rubenstein D, Shaffer TH. Liquid ventilation of human preterm neonates. J Pediatr 117:106–111, 1990.

HIFI Study Group. High-frequency oscillatory ventilation compared with conventional mechanical ventilation in the treatment of respiratory failure in preterm infants. N Engl J Med 320:88–93, 1989.

Kylstra JA, Tissing MO, Maen A. Of mice as fish. Trans Am Soc Artif Intern Organs 8:378–388, 1962.

MacIntyre NR, Follett JV, Deitz JL, et al. Jet ventilation at 100 BPM in adult respiratory failure. Am Rev Respir Dis 134:897–901, 1986.

Smith RB. Continuous-flow apneic ventilation. Respir Care 32:458–465, 1987.

Zapol WM, Snider MT, Hill DJ, et al. Extracorporeal membrane oxygenation in severe acute respiratory failure: A randomized prospective study. JAMA 242:2193–2196, 1979.

25

Key Terms

Bronchoalveolar Lavage
(BAL)

Nosocomial

Respiratory Syncytial Virus
(RSV)

Factors contributing to nosocomial
infections:

- Aspiration
- Supine position
- Gastric reflux
- Presence of nasogastric or
  endotracheal tube

Additional risk factors for
pneumonia:

- Surgery of the head, neck,
  chest, or abdomen
- Mechanical ventilation

Nosocomial Respiratory Tract Infection: Perspectives for Prevention and Respiratory Care

Donald E. Craven, M.D.,
and Kathleen A. Steger, R.N., M.P.H.

Nosocomial or hospital-acquired respiratory tract infections are not incubating on admission and usually occur 48 to 72 hours after admission to the hospital.[1–3] Despite extraordinary progress in patient care over the past 40 years, the incidence and case fatality rates of nosocomial pneumonia remain high.[1–4] Hospital-acquired pneumonia is at present the second most common nosocomial infection in the United States and results in the most deaths from hospital-acquired infection.[5, 6] Rates of pneumonia are highest in critically ill, mechanically ventilated patients.[7–10]

Oropharyngeal colonization with nosocomial gram-negative bacilli or staphylococci appears to be a prerequisite to the development of nosocomial pneumonia.[11–14] Aspiration of bacteria from the oropharynx is important in the pathogenesis of pneumonia.[15, 16] In addition, the supine position of the patient, gastric reflux, and the presence of a nasogastric or an endotracheal tube may increase oropharyngeal colonization and pneumonia.[17–21]

Because of the high rates of pneumonia and associated mortality in mechanically ventilated patients, despite treatment with antibiotics, the focus should be on prevention.[1–3, 9, 22–26] This chapter reviews current concepts of the epidemiology, pathogenesis, and prevention of nosocomial respiratory infection, with special emphasis on bacterial pathogens, infection control, and respiratory care.

EPIDEMIOLOGY

Nosocomial pneumonia is the second most common nosocomial infection, occurring in 0.6 to 1% of hospital admissions in the United States.[5, 26] Rates of pneumonia increase six- to 21-fold in mechanically ventilated patients.[7, 8, 10] Surgery of the head, neck, chest, or abdomen is a well-known risk factor for pneumonia. Postoperative pneumonia occurs in approximately 18% of the patients undergoing elective upper abdominal, lower abdominal, or thoracic surgery.[27]

Crude mortality rates for patients with nosocomial pneumonia may vary from 20 to 60%.[7, 24, 25, 28, 29] In a study of 200 consecutive hospital deaths, nosocomial pneumonia contributed to 60% of the fatal infections.[6] In one study, fatality rates were 50% for intensive care unit (ICU) patients with hospital-acquired pneumonia, compared with 3.5% for ICU patients without pneumonia.[28] Furthermore, in mechanically ventilated patients at our hospital, the mortality rate for patients with pneumonia was 55%, compared with 25% for patients without pneumonia.[24] Others have reported similar results.[25]

Although ventilator-associated pneumonia was univariately associated with mortality at our hospital, it did not remain significant after multivariate analysis.[24] Other investigators have reported high-risk organisms, bilateral infiltrates on chest x-ray studies, and respiratory failure to be among six independent risk factors for mortality due to nosocomial pneumonia.[7] Data suggest that the "attributable mortality," or the contribution of hospital-acquired pneumonia versus underlying disease in patient mortality, is 33%.[29]

Nosocomial pneumonia may increase a patient's length of stay by 7 to 9 days.[29, 30] Based on an estimated 40 million hospitalizations per year in the United States, the annual cost of diagnosing and treating nosocomial pneumonia exceeds $2 billion per year.[23, 26]

ETIOLOGIC AGENTS

Nosocomial pneumonia may be caused by viruses, bacteria, or fungi; bacteria are the most common and most frequently studied (Table 25–1).

TABLE **25–1.**   Possible Pathogens Causing Nosocomial Pneumonia

Pathogen	Overall Frequency (%)	Sources
Early-onset bacteria pneumonia		
Streptococcus pneumoniae	5–10	Endogenous
Haemophilus influenzae	<5	Endogenous
Early- and late-onset pneumonia		
Anaerobic bacteria	0–35	Endogenous
Legionella pneumophila	0–10	Water
Late-onset bacterial pneumonia		
Aerobic gram-negative bacilli	≥30–60	
Pseudomonas aeruginosa		Endogenous
Enterobacter species		Other patients
Acinetobacter species		Food and water
Klebsiella pneumoniae		Enteral feeding
Serratia marcescens		Hospital personnel
Escherichia coli		Equipment and devices
Gram-positive cocci		
Staphylococcus aureus	20–30	Endogenous
Acid-fast organisms		Hospital personnel, environment
Mycobacterium tuberculosis	<1	Host, patient, staff
Viruses		
Influenza A and B	Variable	Patients or staff (in winter)
Respiratory syncytial virus	Variable	Patients or staff (in winter)
Fungi and protozoa		
Aspergillus species	Rare	Air, construction
Pneumocystis carinii	Rare	

From Craven DE, Steger KA, Duncan RA. Prevention and control of nosocomial pneumonia. *In* Wenzel RP (ed). Prevention and Control of Nosocomial Infections. Baltimore, Williams & Wilkins, 1992. ©1992, the Williams & Wilkins Co., Baltimore. Rates of pneumonia are taken in part from Horan T, Culver D, Jarvis W, et al. Pathogens causing nosocomial infections. Antimicrob Newsletter 5:65–67, 1988.

Etiologic agents vary with the populations studied, the severity of underlying disease, and the clinical method used to diagnose pneumonia. Approximately 60% of cases of clinically diagnosed nosocomial pneumonia are caused by aerobic gram-negative bacilli.[5] *Staphylococcus aureus* has been isolated in nearly 20% of cases. Anaerobic bacteria have been cultured in approximately 30% of cases and are more common in nonventilated patients.[31] *Legionella pneumophila* is common in some hospitals in which the organism is present in the hospital water supply or cooling towers.[32, 33] Most of these data were obtained from expectorated sputum or from transtracheal or tracheal aspirates; lower rates of gram-negative bacilli have been reported in mechanically ventilated patients having bronchoscopy with protected specimen brushes or bronchoalveolar lavage.[34–40] Data have also compared lung histology at postmortem with cultures obtained by "mini-bronchoalveolar lavage."[41]

Mycobacterium tuberculosis, an uncommon cause of nosocomial pneumonia, should be considered as an etiologic agent in high-risk patients or in patients not responding to antimicrobial therapy. Respiratory therapists and other health care workers should have their tuberculin (purified protein derivative) skin reactivity monitored every 6 to 12 months and avoid directly inhaling large-droplet nuclei.[42] The concern is magnified by reports of multidrug-resistant strains of *M. tuberculosis* and unusual presentations occurring primarily among human immunodeficiency virus–infected patients in New York City and Miami.[43–45] Although most nosocomial pneumonia is bacterial in origin, epidemic viral pneumonia caused by influenza or respiratory syncytial virus occurs in the hospital setting.[46–48] Respiratory therapists are alerted to the high rates of respiratory syncytial virus on pediatric wards and in the pediatric ICU, particularly during the winter months.

Fungi are uncommon causes of nosocomial pneumonia, except in immunocompromised patients, although colonizing *Candida albicans* may appear in endotracheal cultures.[5] *Aspergillus fumigatus* should be considered if the patient is neutropenic or otherwise immunocompromised, especially if there is construction nearby.[49] Nosocomial pneumonia due to *Pneumocystis carinii* may occur in patients infected with human immunodeficiency virus who have T4 (helper) lymphocyte counts of less than 200/mm³, but nosocomial pneumonia due to gram-negative bacilli or *S. aureus* is more common.[50, 51]

DIAGNOSIS

Accurate data on etiologic agents and the epidemiology of bacterial nosocomial pneumonia are limited by the lack of a gold standard for diagnosing infection. Isolation of a potential pathogen from pleural fluid or blood cultures helps to confirm the clinical diagnosis of pneumonia.[1–3] However, these criteria are often absent, or culture results are unavailable for 24 to 48 hours. In the intubated patient, serial Gram's stains, when correlated with culture results and changes in the clinical status of the patient, often provide a clue for the initial choice of antibiotics.[2] All patients with suspected pneumonia should be evaluated for changes in temperature, mental status, oxygenation, respiratory symptoms, and arterial oxygen concentrations. Although clinical criteria may lack sensitivity and specificity, they are the only parameters available in most hospitals.[52, 53] In one study, 80% of new infiltrates in ICU patients could be eliminated within 8 hours with the use of vigorous chest physical

Gram-negative bacteria:

- *Pseudomonas aeruginosa*
- *Klebsiella pneumoniae*
- *Acinetobacter calcoaceticus*
- *Escherichia coli*

The following may mimic the clinical criteria for pneumonia.

- Atelectasis
- Pulmonary edema
- Pleural effusions
- Pulmonary emboli

therapy only.[53] Thus, the problem of accurate diagnosis of VAP remains troublesome, particularly in ventilated patients with adult respiratory distress syndrome.[54, 55]

Cultures of endotracheal aspirates have been commonly used to diagnose pneumonia. Although this technique detected 89% of the patients with pneumonia, the specificity was only 14%.[37] Clearly, additional diagnostic methods are necessary for optimal management of ventilated patients.[34–41, 56–58] Bronchoscopy with a protected specimen brush (PSB) or bronchoalveolar lavage (BAL) has been useful for the diagnosis of pneumonia in mechanically ventilated patients,[34–41, 56–58] with sensitivities in the range of 60 to 95% and specificities ranging from 80 to 100%.[37, 38] Early results of a meta-analysis of 15 studies suggested an overall sensitivity of 91% and a specificity of 95% for PSB.[34] Sensitivities for BAL ranged from 86 to 100%, whereas specificity was 100%. Further refinement of these methods may be possible with a balloon-tipped catheter for protected BAL.[59] Despite these seemingly high numbers, false-negative and false-positive rates of 10 to 30% represent a substantial opportunity for misdiagnosis. Of great concern is prior antibiotic use, which may have a dramatic effect on quantitative cultures obtained by BAL and PSB.[37, 59] Because bronchoscopy is a relatively costly and specialized technique, often requiring advanced scheduling, nonbronchoscopic quantitative "blind" sampling of the lower respiratory tract may provide a simpler and nearly comparable diagnostic technique.[60–64]

Studies of BAL and PSB should be interpreted with caution because of differences in study design, patient populations, definitions of pneumonia, and the effect of prior antibiotic use. Clear guidelines are needed for the use of bronchoscopic diagnosis in mechanically ventilated patients. Of note is that good correlation has been observed between bronchoscopic diagnosis and the clinical pulmonary infection score,[62] and the use of quantitative endotracheal aspirates, if validated, may provide an alternative to bronchoscopic diagnosis.

PATHOGENESIS

Pulmonary Aspiration and Intubation

Bacteria may enter the lung by bacteremia or translocation;[65] however, bacteria aspirated from the oropharynx cause most cases of pneumonia (Fig. 25–1). Although approximately 70% of healthy subjects aspirate during sleep, aspiration occurs even more frequently in patients with pathologically altered consciousness, abnormal swallowing, depressed gag reflexes, delayed gastric emptying, or decreased gastrointestinal motility.[15, 16, 66] The number and virulence of aspirated bacteria are important determinants of the development of pneumonia. Tracheal intubation of the patient (Fig. 25–2) increases colonization by bypassing the oropharynx and allowing leakage of bacteria around the cuff.[16, 66–68]

Colonization of the Oropharynx

Hospitalized patients tend to have high rates of oropharyngeal colonization with aerobic gram-negative bacilli. Johanson and coworkers demonstrated gram-negative bacillary colonization rates of 16% in moderately ill and 57% in critically ill patients.[12] In a follow-up study, pneu-

The clinical pulmonary infection score incorporates quantitative assessment of

- Patient's temperature
- Leukocyte count and differential
- Oxygenation
- Presence of infiltrates on chest radiography
- Gram's stain results
- Quantitative culture of tracheal secretions

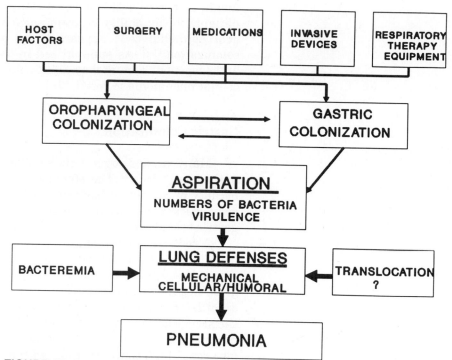

FIGURE 25-1: Mechanisms for colonization of the oropharynx and stomach. The development of pneumonia depends on the virulence and the numbers of bacteria aspirated into the lung and on the ability of pulmonary host defenses to protect against infection. (Adapted from Craven DE, Steger KA, Barber TW. Preventing nosocomial pneumonia: State of the art and perspectives for the 1990's. Am J Med 91[Suppl 3B]:44S–53S, 1991.)

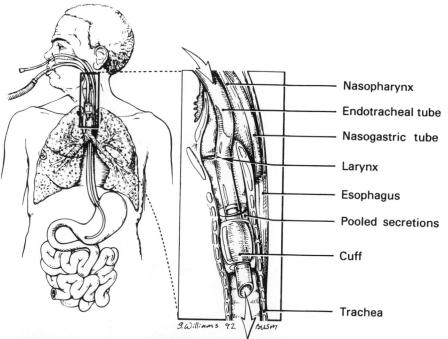

FIGURE 25-2: Routes of oropharyngeal colonization in the intubated patient with a nasogastric tube. In the presence of gastric colonization, the nasogastric tube may increase reflux by making the lower esophageal sphincter incompetent or acting as a conduit for nosocomial pathogens. Note the pooled secretions above the cuff of the endotracheal tube. (Adapted from Craven DE, Barber TW, Steger KA, Montecalvo MA. Nosocomial pneumonia in the 90's: Update of epidemiology and risk factors. Semin Respir Infect 5:157–172, 1990.)

monia occurred in 23% of colonized patients versus 3.3% of uncolonized patients.[11] The ability of gram-negative bacilli to adhere to oropharyngeal epithelial cells appears to be pivotal in determining successful colonization.[13, 69] As summarized in Table 25–2, numerous endogenous and exogenous factors may affect colonization and susceptibility to nosocomial pneumonia.[11, 12, 70, 71]

Gastric Colonization

Many studies suggest the stomach as a potential source of bacterial pathogens.[19, 20, 72–75] The stomach is normally sterile when the pH is 1 because of the potent bactericidal activity of hydrochloric acid.[76, 77] When gastric acid is absent or neutralized, the risk of respiratory infection and gastric colonization may increase.[19, 20, 72, 73, 78]

A reduced amount of gastric acid in the intubated patient may result from impaired acid production, neutralization with antacids, or decreased secretion with histamine type 2 (H_2) blockers.[79] Levels of aerobic gram-negative bacteria may increase several logs when the gastric pH is alkaline (Fig. 25–3). At a gastric pH of 5 or 6, the numbers of bacteria in the stomach may reach 1 to 100 million aerobic gram-negative bacilli per milliliter of gastric fluid. Gram-positive cocci and *Candida* species may also reach high concentrations with an elevated gastric pH.

The position of the patient may be important in reducing the frequency of reflux or aspiration from the stomach.[17, 80] Reflux and pneumonia may be more common in the presence of gastric tube feeding, which can increase volume and alter gastric pH.[18, 66, 81] Data from Torres and coworkers indicate that lying flat in bed and the duration of the supine position may increase the risk of aspiration.[17] Thus, elevating the head of the bed 45 degrees, unless contraindicated, may be a simple and effective method of reducing reflux, aspiration, and nosocomial respiratory tract infection.

TABLE **25–2.** Endogenous and Exogenous Factors That May Alter the Dynamic Equilibrium of the Oropharynx and Respiratory Tract*

Endogenous Factors	Exogenous Factors
Host factors	Environmental factors
Genetics (?)	Seasonal trends
Age	Cross-contamination
Male sex	Air flow
Chronic cardiopulmonary disease	Water supply
Malnutrition	Hospitalization
Obesity	Teaching hospital
Smoking	Critical care unit
Alcohol abuse	Medical-surgical wards
Upper gastrointestinal disease	Prolonged length of stay
AIDS; immunosuppression	Therapeutic
Depressed consciousness	Sedative or hypnotic drugs
Aspiration	Immunosuppressive therapy
Prior infection	Antacids or H_2 blockers
Prior surgery	Antibiotics
Head and neck	Invasive devices
Thoracic	Endotracheal tube
Abdominal	Tracheostomy tube
	Nasogastric tube
	Intracranial pressure monitor

*The presence of one or more of these risk factors may alter oropharyngeal or gastric colonization and increase the risk of nosocomial pneumonia.

Adapted from Craven DE, Steger KA, Barber TW. Preventing nosocomial pneumonia: State of the art and perspectives for the 1990's. Am J Med 91(Suppl 3B):445–535, 1991.

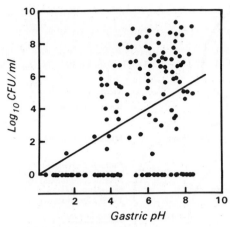

FIGURE 25–3: Correlation between gastric pH and log (base 10) concentrations of aerobic gram-negative bacilli per milliliter of gastric fluid from critical care patients receiving stress ulcer prophylaxis. The linear regression line is calculated by the least-squares method. The coefficient of correlation is 0.4073 with 133 degrees of freedom ($P <$ .001). CFU, colony-forming units. (From du Moulin GC, Hedley-Whyte J, Patterson DG, Lisbon A. Aspiration of gastric bacteria in antacid-treated patients: A frequent cause of postoperative colonization of the airway. Lancet 1:242–245, © by The Lancet Ltd, 1982.)

Different regimens for stress bleeding prophylaxis in the mechanically ventilated patient produce variable rates of pneumonia. Several studies have found significantly lower rates of pneumonia in patients given stress bleeding prophylaxis with sucralfate versus antacids or H_2 blockers.[20, 82–85] The rate of colonization with gram-negative bacilli was significantly lower in patients treated with sucralfate than in those treated with antacids with or without H_2 blockers.[20, 82, 84] In a meta-analysis of the efficacy of stress bleeding prophylaxis in ICU patients treated with sucralfate versus H_2 blockers (nine studies) or antacids (eight studies), respiratory tract infection was significantly less frequent ($P <$ .05) in patients treated with sucralfate than in patients receiving either H_2 blockers or antacids.[84] This result may be due to the effect of these agents on gastric pH or colonization or to undefined effects.[19, 20, 75, 82–84]

IMMUNE DEFENSES IN THE LUNG

The pulmonary host defense response to the invading microorganisms plays an integral part in the pathogenesis and outcome of infection.[14, 86–89] Mucociliary and mechanical clearance in the upper airway are reinforced by cellular and humoral factors in the lower airway (Fig. 25–4).

At present, the effect of airway colonization with different pathogens is not well understood. In vitro data suggest that certain types of bacteria may have specific colonization factors.[13, 69, 90] The scanning electron micrographs shown in Figure 25–5 demonstrate ciliated epithelium from a

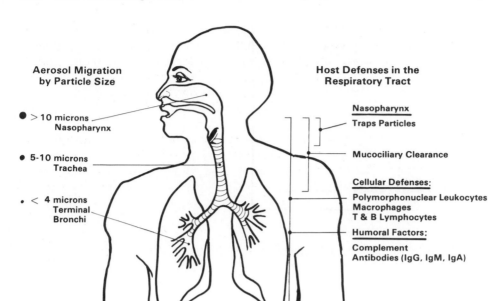

Aerosol Migration by Particle Size

- \> 10 microns Nasopharynx
- 5-10 microns Trachea
- < 4 microns Terminal Bronchi

Host Defenses in the Respiratory Tract

Nasopharynx
Traps Particles

Mucociliary Clearance

Cellular Defenses:
Polymorphonuclear Leukocytes
Macrophages
T & B Lymphocytes

Humoral Factors:
Complement
Antibodies (IgG, IgM, IgA)

FIGURE 25–4: *Right,* The host defenses in the upper and lower respiratory tract. *Left,* The degree of penetration of various-sized bacterial aerosols. (From Craven DE, Driks MR. Pneumonia in the intubated patient. Semin Respir Infect 2:20–33, 1987.)

normal monkey trachea in tissue culture before and after bacterial inoculation. After infection, the cilia begin to beat more slowly and irregularly and finally stop. Note that the ciliated cells also become displaced from the epithelial surface. It is unclear to what extent these in vitro observations can be extrapolated to bacterial colonization of the trachea in human infection.

Humoral factors, such as antibody with or without complement, may directly kill bacteria or enhance killing by polymorphonuclear leukocytes or macrophages (see Fig. 25–4). The pulmonary macrophage acts as a scavenger and antigen-presenting cell to the T helper lymphocyte. When local defense mechanisms are overwhelmed by a large or particularly

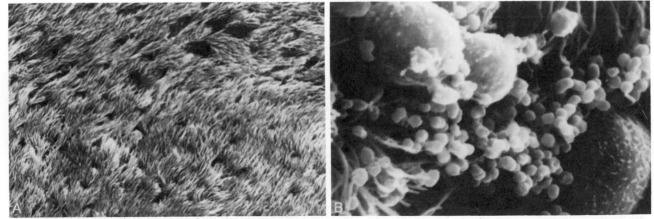

FIGURE 25–5: Scanning electron micrographs of normal monkey trachea in tissue culture *(A)* and after in vitro infection with *Neisseria meningitidis (B).* The cilia beat more slowly and irregularly. When the cilia stop beating, they are displaced from the epithelium.

virulent inoculum of bacteria, macrophages recruit circulating neutrophils to produce a more exudative inflammatory reaction.[14]

Cytokines, such as tumor necrosis factor-alpha and interleukin-1, appear to be early mediators of acute inflammation. In addition to its phagocytic and oxidative functions, the macrophage exposed to bacterial lipopolysaccharide produces tumor necrosis factor-alpha and interleukin-1, which in turn stimulate production of interleukin-8, a potent inflammatory cell chemoattractant that draws monocytes and neutrophils to the lung.[86, 88] Leukotrienes, complement components, and platelet-activating factor also assist in the inflammatory response. A better understanding of these complex immune mechanisms may provide targets for future therapy.[88, 89, 91]

ANTIBIOTIC PROPHYLAXIS AGAINST COLONIZATION

Aerosolized Antibiotics

Several investigators have suggested antibiotic prophylaxis as a strategy for preventing pneumonia or eliminating bacterial colonization of the oropharynx or trachea. Lepper and associates used aerosolized polymyxin B to prevent tracheal colonization with *P. aeruginosa*.[92] Later, Feeley and colleagues reported that daily use of polymyxin B aerosolized into the trachea decreased the incidence of pneumonia due to *P. aeruginosa,* but colonization and pneumonia with resistant gram-negative bacilli developed.[93] Local administration of aminoglycosides into the trachea has also been successfully employed for treatment of patients.[94]

Unertl and coworkers administered a solution of polymyxin B, gentamicin, and amphotericin B into the nose, oropharynx, and stomach of 19 intubated patients and compared the outcomes with those in 20 control patients.[95] Colonization of the oropharynx and trachea was significantly lower ($P < .001$) in the antibiotic prophylaxis group, and there was only one case of pneumonia in the prophylaxis group, versus nine in the control group.

Antibiotic Prophylaxis

Selective decontamination of the digestive tract (SDD) with systemic and local antibiotics has been advocated to prevent or reduce nosocomial pneumonia.[96–103] SDD is aimed at preventing oropharyngeal and gastric colonization by aerobic gram-negative bacilli without disturbing the anaerobic flora. The SDD regimen usually includes systemic antibiotics, such as cefotaxime, trimethoprim, or a quinolone, and nonabsorbable local antibiotics, such as an aminoglycoside, polymyxin B, and amphotericin B. The local antibiotics are usually applied as a paste (Orobase) in the oropharynx and are given either orally or through the nasogastric tube. Several studies using SDD have demonstrated dramatically decreased rates of nosocomial respiratory tract colonization and infection, but few have found significant differences in duration of mechanical ventilation, length of stay in the ICU, or mortality.[98–103]

At present, the following questions remain:

What patient populations should receive SDD?
Which regimen is most effective?

What types of antimicrobial selection and resistance will emerge?

Although some of the preliminary data were encouraging,[96, 97] larger prospective, randomized, double-blind studies are needed to assess the efficacy, costs, and benefits of SDD for mechanically ventilated patients.

INFECTION CONTROL

Infection control is aimed at identifying potential reservoirs of infection, interrupting transmission between patients and personnel, and preventing or reducing colonization in the host.[104–106] The importance of surveillance of infections, tracking of nosocomial pathogens, and elimination of devices associated with nosocomial pathogens cannot be overemphasized (Table 25–3).

Data from the Study on the Efficacy of Nosocomial Infection Control suggested that hospitals with effective surveillance and infection control programs had rates of pneumonia that were 20% lower than those in hospitals without such programs.[107] Staff education programs may also be helpful. Britt and associates reported a drop in pneumonia rates from 4.0 to 1.6% following the institution of an awareness program that consisted of surveillance, identification of high-risk patients, and staff education.[108]

Colonization of the hands of hospital workers with gram-negative bacilli or *S. aureus* is a common source of the transfer of nosocomial pathogens between patients.[104, 105, 109, 110] Hand colonization, although usually transient, may persist in persons with dermatitis. Although hand washing before and after patient contact is an effective means of removing transient bacteria, this practice is often ignored or inadequately performed.[104] In one study, hand washing was performed by nurses 43% of the time and by doctors 28% of the time after contact with ICU patients.

In a more recent study in a pediatric ICU, rates of nosocomial infection were significantly reduced by the use of gowns and gloves for patient contact.[111] Staff contact with patients was not impaired by the use of gowns and gloves. In a similar study, transmission of respiratory syncytial virus was significantly reduced with the use of gowns and gloves.[112] Although similar studies are needed in adult medical and surgical ICUs, these data, coupled with the poor staff compliance and inconsistent hand-

Special note: Gloves may become contaminated with nosocomial pathogens, which can easily be transferred between patients if the gloves are not discarded between patient contacts.[11]

TABLE **25–3.**   Host Effects of Endotracheal, Nasotracheal, and Nasogastric Tubes on Oropharyngeal Colonization and the Pathogenesis of Pneumonia

Endotracheal Tube	Nasogastric Tube
Acts as a foreign body, traumatizes epithelium	Acts as a foreign body
Impairs cilia clearance and cough	Impairs swallowing
Often requires suctioning to remove secretions	Causes pooling of oropharyngeal secretions
Impairs swallowing	Makes the lower esophageal sphincter incompetent
Changes mouth flora	Increases the risk of gastric reflux
Produces cuff ischemia	Acts as a conduit for bacterial migration
Causes leakage of secretions around the cuff	
Nasotracheal Tube	
Causes sinusitis	
Same as those for an endotracheal tube	

Adapted from Craven DE, Steger KA. Nosocomial pneumonia in the intubated patient: New concepts on pathogenesis and prevention. Infect Dis Clin North Am 3:843–866, 1989.

washing practices, suggest that nosocomial infection can be prevented with the routine use of gowns and gloves.

Most hospitals have strict guidelines for the isolation of infected patients.[113] Unfortunately, some patients are not properly classified or diagnosed.[114] Exposure to tuberculosis is a well-documented risk to health care workers.[115, 116] As stated previously, the acquired immunodeficiency syndrome epidemic and the emergence of multidrug-resistant strains have increased the concern about tuberculosis.[43-45] Coughing can transmit tuberculosis; respiratory therapists inducing sputum for diagnosis or giving aerosol treatments are at particular risk.[42-45, 115, 116] For these reasons, respiratory therapists should comply with infection control guidelines and tuberculosis skin testing through employee health services.

DEVICES AND PROCEDURES

Tracheal Suctioning

Nasotracheal suctioning may be used to obtain sputum or to remove sections from the lower airway. Care must be exercised not to introduce nosocomial pathogens into the lower airway via the catheter or to increase the patient's risk of aspiration. The mechanically ventilated patient is often debilitated and susceptible to colonization from contaminated local antiseptics, laryngoscopes, improper tracheobronchial suctioning, or contaminated solutions used to rinse the suction catheter.[117] Proper tracheal suctioning of the ventilated patient may prevent the introduction of nosocomial pathogens into the lower respiratory tract via the catheter or saline wash. Gloves should always be used to protect the health care worker and the patient. More recently, standard single-catheter suctioning of the ventilated patient has been compared with a closed, multiuse-catheter system.[118] Although more detailed data are needed, the closed tracheal suctioning system may prevent a drop in arterial oxygen levels, save personnel time, and decrease the likelihood of cross-contamination from condensate splashing when the circuit is opened.[119]

Endotracheal Tube

Several different mechanisms increase the risk of infection during patient intubation (Table 25-4). Special care should be taken to place the endotracheal tube without traumatizing the hypopharynx and to avoid aspiration. The cuff should be maintained at optimal pressure; efforts should be made to avoid leakage around the cuff when it is inflated and to prevent seepage of pooled secretions when the cuff is deflated (see Fig. 25-2). New endotracheal tubes have a suction port above the cuff to reduce upper airway colonization.

Because the endotracheal tube is not routinely changed, it may become a nidus for bacterial colonization. Sottile and coworkers studied endotracheal tubes by scanning electron microscopy.[120] Of the 25 tubes studied, 96% had partial bacterial colonization, and 84% were completely covered by bacteria enmeshed in biofilm or glucocalyx. The authors hypothesize that aggregates of bacteria, dislodged from the endotracheal tube during suctioning, may be aspirated into the tracheobronchial tree.

TABLE **25–4.** Methods to Prevent Nosocomial Pneumonia in Mechanically Ventilated Patients

---

General Principles
Treatment of the patient's underlying disease
Appropriate selection and use of antibiotics
Extubation and removal of the nasogastric tube as indicated
Stress bleeding prophylaxis
   Carefully assess the risk-benefit ratio
   Maintain the natural gastric acid barrier
Elevation of the patient's head (at least 30 degrees)
Assessment of the need for enteral versus parenteral feeding
Selective decontamination of the digestive tract

Infection Control
Surveillance
Awareness and education programs to reduce infection
Proper techniques for suctioning patients
Appropriate hand washing and infection control precautions
Use of gowns and gloves
Effective methods of disinfection
Controlled use of antibiotics

Respiratory Care Equipment
Discrimination between nebulizers and humidifiers
$\geq$48-hour circuit changes for mechanical ventilators
Proper removal of tubing condensate
No transfer of equipment between patients
Care of inline medication nebulizers
Proper disinfection of tubing, bags, and spirometers
Selective use of heat and moisture exchangers

Adapted form Craven DE, Steger KA. Nosocomial pneumonia in the intubated patient: New concepts on pathogenesis and prevention. Infect Dis Clin North Am 3:843–866, 1989.

Aggregates of bacteria in biofilm may be protected from killing by antibiotics or host immune defenses.[120, 121] Studies are underway to evaluate the role of endotracheal tube colonization in the pathogenesis of pneumonia.

Nasogastric Tube Use and Tube Feeding

The nasogastric tube may be beneficial for managing excess gastric secretions, preventing gastric distention, administering drugs, or tube feeding. Conversely, the tubes may increase the risk of nosocomial pneumonia, particularly if tube feedings are administered.[7, 18, 80, 122] Table 25–3 summarizes the possible mechanisms for changes in colonization and increased risk of pneumonia. In a trial of 38 patients randomized to gastric tube versus jejunal tube feeding, rates of pneumonia were similar. However, patients in the jejunal group received significantly more of their daily caloric goal and had significantly higher prealbumin levels.[122] All of these patients were in the upright position and received continuous, carefully monitored tube feeding. More data are needed to ascertain the contribution of tube feeding to nosocomial pneumonia, as well as to determine specific methods of prevention.

Resuscitation Bags

Each patient must have his or her own resuscitation bag!

Resuscitation bags are used for urgent ventilation and for ventilating patients during ventilator circuit changes. They may also be used to ventilate patients during chest physiotherapy, when large volumes of secretions may be mobilized. Several groups have reported that bedside resuscitation bags are a potential source of bacterial contamination.[123, 124] Resuscitation bags may become contaminated with secretions and may be difficult to decontaminate effectively. In addition, the transfer of bags between patients is a potential source of cross-contamination. The bags must be properly disinfected and must not be transferred between patients.

Spirometers and Oxygen Analyzers

The spirometer used to monitor gas flow is a well-known source of cross-contamination in an ICU. An increase in respiratory infections due to *Acinetobacter* species was traced to contaminated spirometers that were transferred between patients.[125] At Boston City Hospital, an outbreak of *Pseudomonas (Xanthomonas) maltophilia* sputum colonization occurred in two ICUs separated by six floors. A contaminated spirometer and oxygen analyzer T piece were the source of sputum colonization in the two ICUs.[126] A shortage of T pieces and a nonfunctioning spirometer led to a sharing of items between patients and between units. After correction of the problem, the outbreak abated. Because the mechanical ventilator circuit may be colonized with nosocomial pathogens, any device put into a patient's circuit can become contaminated. Therefore, these items should not be transferred between patients.[127]

Wall Oxygen Humidifiers

Reusable and disposable oxygen wall humidifiers are used regularly in hospitals. The Centers for Disease Control and Prevention (CDC) guidelines suggest that reusable units be washed daily, with the water left in the reservoir discarded before refilling. Disposable wall humidifiers should be used according to the manufacturer's recommendations.[127]

Nebulization Equipment

Many infection control personnel, respiratory therapists, physicians, and nurses fail to discriminate between different types of equipment in assessing the associated risk of infection.[1–3, 127] Nebulizers saturate the inspiratory-phase gas with water and disperse particles of less than 4 μm. As shown in Figure 25–4, the size of the particle determines the distance traveled. Larger particles (5 to 10 μm) are trapped in the nasopharynx, and smaller particles (less than 4 μm) float past host defenses into the patient's terminal bronchioles and alveoli.[128] Thus, careful attention is needed to prevent contamination of nebulization equipment, and patients who are intubated or have a tracheostomy are at greatest risk.

The rate of gram-negative necrotizing bacillary pneumonia increased 10-fold from 1952 to 1963, paralleling the increased use of nebulization equipment.[129] Classic studies by Reinarz and coworkers determined that equipment with contaminated mainstream nebulizers could generate bacterial aerosols, leading to a necrotizing gram-negative pneumonia.[128] Proper disinfection of nebulization equipment reduced the rates of gram-negative necrotizing pneumonia to levels present before the use of reservoir nebulizers.

Possible sources of nebulizer contamination include oxygen, room air compressed to power the nebulizer or entrained to dilute oxygen, hands of hospital personnel, use of contaminated water to fill the reservoir, reflux of contaminated condensate into the reservoir, and inadequate sterilization or disinfection of the equipment. Methods for proper decontamination and sterilization of nebulization equipment have been reviewed elsewhere and are beyond the scope of this chapter.[1-3, 127]

Mist Tents

Mist tents are usually used for newborns and infants with severe respiratory tract infections. Generally, most mist tents have unheated nebulizers and reservoirs. Properly filling the reservoir every 24 hours with sterile water in an aseptic manner and effectively cleaning the tent after use reduce the likelihood of bacterial contamination. The guidelines from the CDC[127] suggest that the residual water be discarded before water is added to the reservoir.

Mechanical Ventilators With Heated Humidifiers

The volume ventilators currently used in most US hospitals warm and humidify the inspiratory-phase gas (Fig. 25–6). Although the CDC's 1982 Guideline for the Prevention of Nosocomial Pneumonia recommends that mechanical ventilator breathing circuits be changed every 24 hours,[127] other published literature suggests that the interval can be extended to at least 48 hours. Levels of bacteria in the ventilator circuit

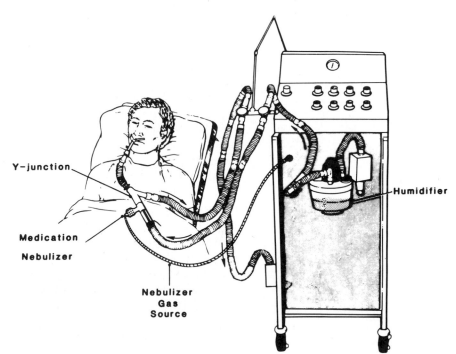

FIGURE 25–6: A mechanically ventilated patient maintained in the upright position. The patient's ventilator circuit has condensate in the dependent portion of the tubing and an inline medication nebulizer. (From Craven DE, Connolly MG Jr, Lichtenberg DA, et al. Contamination of mechanical ventilators with tubing changes every 24 or 48 hours. Reprinted, by permission of the New England Journal of Medicine 306:1505–1509, 1982.)

and the rate of nosocomial pneumonia were not affected by changing the ventilator tubing every 48 hours versus every 24 hours.[24, 130] More recent data suggest that the tubing can be routinely changed at intervals of greater than 48 hours.[131–133] The latest CDC Guideline for the Prevention of Nosocomial Pneumonia issued by the Hospital Infection Control Practices Advisory Committee endorses circuit changes at intervals no more frequent than 48 hours.[134] No recommendation is made for intervals greater than 48 hours.

Tubing Colonization and Condensate

Mechanical ventilators with humidifying cascades often have significant amounts of tubing colonization and condensate formation.[130, 135] Ventilator tubing often colonizes high numbers of bacteria, with concentrations of bacteria highest proximal to the endotracheal tube and the swivel adapter. In some patients, up to 1 million nosocomial pathogens could be cultured from a 2-cm area; minimal colonization was detected in the distal tubing or the humidifying cascade.[135, 136] During the first 24 hours after a circuit change, 33% were colonized at 2 hours, and 67% had colonization at 12 hours. The data indicate that the tubing is not sterile, that high levels of colonization may be present as soon as 2 hours after a circuit change, and that colonization in the circuit primarily originates from the patient. The highest level of bacterial contamination is present in the patient's endotracheal tube, but the endotracheal tube is not changed routinely with the circuit. Dreyfuss and coworkers have suggested that circuits can be changed at intervals of greater than 48 hours.[131]

Tubing condensate is a likely but not well-documented risk factor for pneumonia. The rate of condensate formation in the ventilator circuit relates to the temperature differences between the inspiratory-phase gas and the ambient temperature.[135] In unheated ventilator tubing, the mean level ($\pm$ standard deviation) of condensate formation may be 30.2 $\pm$ 11.9 mL/hr, whereas the median level of bacterial colonization in the condensate was 200,000 organisms/mL, mostly nosocomial gram-negative bacilli. Similar concentrations of nosocomial pathogens have been reported in the circuits of mechanically ventilated dogs with experimental pneumonia.[137] Heating ventilator tubing will markedly reduce the rate of condensate formation. Simple procedures such as turning the patient or raising the bed rail may accidentally wash contaminated condensate directly into the patient's tracheobronchial tree. Inoculation of large amounts of fluid with high concentrations of bacteria is an excellent method of overwhelming pulmonary defense mechanisms and of producing pneumonia in experimental animals.[87, 138]

Inappropriate disposal of contaminated condensate may lead to contamination of environmental surfaces and the hands of medical personnel. Several traps have been developed to reduce or eliminate tubing condensate, but these devices have not been examined critically in clinical trials. Inline devices with one-way valves to collect condensate may not fit well into disposable circuits and may not be able to handle high volumes of condensate.

Humidifier Colonization

Of 326 Puritan-Bennett cascade bubbling humidifier reservoirs cultured after 24 hours of mechanical ventilation and 140 sampled after 48 hours, no growth was present in 88% of the reservoirs, and the remaining 12% had levels of colonization of less than 100 organisms/mL.[136] The median temperature of the bubbling humidifiers at our hospital was 51°C, a temperature that rapidly kills nosocomial pathogens inoculated in vitro. Bacterial kill was less dramatic at 44°C and was absent at 37°C. The data help to explain why colonization in heated humidifiers is low and why they are therefore an unlikely source of nosocomial pathogens.

In contrast to wick humidifiers, bubbling humidifiers may aerosolize small water particles secondary to bursting bubbles.[139] These in vitro data, however, were obtained using a large inoculum of bacteria introduced into unheated reservoirs, which limits their relevance in clinical practice.

Heat and Moisture Exchangers or Hygroscopic Condenser Humidifiers

Heat and moisture exchangers or hygroscopic condenser humidifiers recycle exhaled heat and moisture, eliminating the need for a humidifier.[140–147] These devices consist of a filter or small sponge in a plastic casing inserted into the ventilator circuit between the swivel adapter and the Y junction. Heat and moisture exchangers and hygroscopic condenser humidifiers add dead space to the circuit, increase circuit resistance, and may not provide sufficient humidity for critically ill patients. A heat and moisture exchanger is capable of supplying necessary heat and moisture for at least a 24-hour period, but critically ill patients, patients with respiratory disease, and patients with heavy secretions may experience complications.[140, 147] To increase humidity, Suzukawa and coworkers have suggested attaching the heat and moisture exchanger to a circuit with a humidifier.[145] The efficacy of these devices must be carefully evaluated with regard to the risks and benefits for each patient.[146, 147]

Small-Volume Nebulizers

Medication nebulizers or small-volume nebulizers inserted into the inspiratory-phase tube of the mechanical ventilator circuit (see Fig. 25–6) may produce bacterial aerosols. Inline medication nebulizers may become contaminated by reflux of tubing condensate or contaminated solutions.[148] Cultures from the nebulizers often contained the same organisms present in the tubing condensate, suggesting that the reflux of condensate was the source of the contamination.

Because inline nebulizers have small reservoir volumes and because treatments are usually needed for only 15 to 20 minutes every 4 to 6 hours, the risk for pneumonia is probably low. However, every precaution should be taken to prevent aerosolizing bacteria directly into the lower respiratory tract of critically ill patients. Nebulized metaproterenol (Alupent) or isoetharine (Bronkosol) was not essential for most of the patients with contaminated nebulizers. When nebulized medications are needed, we recommend using inline nebulizers that can be opened, rinsed with sterile water or saline, and dried between treatments.

Outflow Traps and Filters

Nebulization equipment may also produce environmental contamination or cross-contamination between patients. Particles from pressure ventilators may travel as far as 32 feet from the exhalation valve.[149] The authors suggested that efficient filtering devices be placed on the exhalation valve to reduce environmental contamination. This suggestion is supported by data from a canine model of *P. aeruginosa* pneumonia, indicating that organisms could be recovered at distances as far as 15 feet from the animal.[137] Little dispersion of *P. aeruginosa* was noted in dogs connected to mechanical ventilators with humidifiers. In our experience, however, contaminated condensate and large particles may be emitted from certain types of mechanical ventilators, which may be a source of environmental contamination or cross-colonization of patients located close to the exhalation site. Further studies are needed to assess the importance of outflow traps in the pathogenesis of nosocomial infection.

SUMMARY

Mechanically ventilated patients have high rates of pneumonia compared with nonintubated patients. The presence of an endotracheal tube circumvents natural host defenses, causes local trauma and inflammation, and increases the risk for aspiration of nosocomial pathogens from the oropharynx. Because of the high mortality rate of nosocomial pneumonia and the poor outcomes despite the use of appropriate antibiotic therapy, efforts have been directed at the prevention of infection. They include

The discrete use of antibiotics
Compliance with standard infection control techniques
A knowledge of the risks associated with respiratory therapy equipment
Proper patient positioning to reduce gastric reflux
Reduction of gastric overgrowth with bacteria
In selected patients, the use of selective decontamination to reduce colonization in the oropharynx and gastrointestinal tract

The proper use of infection control practices is a cornerstone for preventing nosocomial pneumonia and protecting the health of the respiratory therapist.

Acknowledgment

We thank Maria Tetzaguic for her assistance in the preparation of the manuscript.

References

1. LaForce FM. Lower respiratory tract infections. *In* Bennett JV, Brachman PS (eds). Hospital Infections. Boston, Little, Brown and Company, 1992, pp 611–640.
2. Pennington JE. Nosocomial respiratory infection. *In* Mandell GL, Douglas RG Jr, Bennett JE (eds). Principles and Practice of Infectious Diseases, 3rd ed. New York, Churchill Livingstone, 1990, pp 2199–2204.
3. Craven DE, Steger KA, Duncan RA. Prevention and control of nosocomial pneumonia.

In Wenzel RP (ed). Prevention and Control of Nosocomial Infections. Baltimore, Williams & Wilkins, 1993, pp 580–599.

4. Daschner FD, Frey P, Wolff G, et al. Nosocomial infection in intensive care wards: A multicenter prospective study. Intensive Care Med 8:5–9, 1982.

5. Horan T, Culver D, Jarvis W, et al. Pathogens causing nosocomial infections. Antimicrob Newsletter 5:65–67, 1988.

6. Gross PA, Neu HC, Aswapokee P, et al. Deaths from nosocomial infection: Experience in a university hospital and a community hospital. Am J Med 68:219–223, 1980.

7. Celis R, Torres A, Gatell JM, et al. Nosocomial pneumonia: A multivariate analysis of risk and prognosis. Chest 93:318–324, 1988.

8. Cross AS, Roupe B. Role of respiratory assistance devices in endemic nosocomial pneumonia. Am J Med 70:681–685, 1981.

9. Craven DE, Barber TW, Steger KA, Montecalvo MA. Nosocomial pneumonia in the 90's: Update of epidemiology and risk factors. Semin Respir Infect 5:157–172, 1990.

10. Haley RW, Culver DH, White JW, et al. The nationwide nosocomial infection rate: A new need for vital statistics. Am J Epidemiol 121:159–167, 1985.

11. Johanson WG Jr, Pierce AK, Sanford JP, Thomas GD. Nosocomial respiratory infections with gram-negative bacilli: The significance of colonization of the respiratory tract. Ann Intern Med 77:701–706, 1972.

12. Johanson WG, Pierce AK, Sanford JP. Changing pharyngeal bacterial flora of hospitalized patients: Emergence of gram-negative bacilli. N Engl J Med 281:1137–1140, 1969.

13. Niederman MS. Gram-negative colonization of the respiratory tract: Pathogenesis and clinical consequences. Semin Respir Infect 5:173–184, 1990.

14. Reynolds HY. Normal and defective respiratory host defenses. *In* Pennington JE (ed). Respiratory Infections: Diagnosis and Management, 2nd ed. New York, Raven Press, 1989, pp 1–33.

15. Amberson JB. Aspiration bronchopneumonia. Int Clin 3:126–134, 1937.

16. Huxley EJ, Viroslav J, Gray WR, et al. Pharyngeal aspiration in normal adults and patients with depressed consciousness. Am J Med 64:564–568, 1978.

17. Torres A, Serra-Battles J, Ros E, et al. Pulmonary aspiration of gastric contents in patients receiving mechanical ventilation: The effect of body position. Ann Intern Med 116:540–542, 1992.

18. Ibanez J, Penafiel A, Raurich J, et al. Gastroesophageal reflux and aspiration of gastric contents during nasogastric feeding: The effect of posture [Abstract]. Intensive Care Med 14(Suppl 2):296, 1988.

19. du Moulin GC, Hedley-Whyte J, Paterson DG, Lisbon A. Aspiration of gastric bacteria in antacid-treated patients: A frequent cause of postoperative colonization of the airway. Lancet 1:242–245, 1982.

20. Driks MR, Craven DE, Celli BR, et al. Nosocomial pneumonia in intubated patients given sucralfate as compared with antacids or histamine type 2 blockers: The role of gastric colonization. N Engl J Med 317:1376–1382, 1987.

21. Cheadle WG, Vitale GC, Mackie CR, Cuschieri A. Prophylactic postoperative nasogastric decompression: A prospective study of its requirement and the influence of cimetidine in 200 patients. Ann Surg 202:361–366, 1985.

22. Craven DE, Steger KA, Barber TW. Preventing nosocomial pneumonia: State of the art and perspectives for the 1990's. Am J Med 91(Suppl 3B):44S–53S, 1991.

23. LaForce FM. Hospital-acquired gram-negative rod pneumonias: An overview. Am J Med 70:664–669, 1981.

24. Craven DE, Kunches LM, Kilinsky V, et al. Risk factors for pneumonia and fatality in patients receiving continuous mechanical ventilation. Am Rev Respir Dis 133:792–796, 1986.

25. Torres A, Aznar R, Gatell JM, et al. Incidence, risk, and prognosis factors of nosocomial pneumonia in mechanically ventilated patients. Am Rev Respir Dis 142:523–528, 1990.

26. Wenzel RP. Hospital-acquired pneumonia: Overview of the current state of the art for prevention and control. Eur J Clin Microbiol Infect Dis 8:56–60, 1989.

27. Garibaldi RA, Britt MR, Coleman ML, et al. Risk factors for postoperative pneumonia. Am J Med 70:677–680, 1981.

28. Stevens RM, Teres D, Skillman JJ, et al. Pneumonia in an intensive care unit: A thirty-month experience. Arch Intern Med 134:106–111, 1974.

29. Leu HS, Kaiser DL, Mori M, et al. Hospital-acquired pneumonia: Attributable mortality and morbidity. Am J Epidemiol 129:1258–1267, 1989.

30. Freeman J, Rosner BA, McGowan JE. Adverse effects of nosocomial infection. J Infect Dis 140:732–740, 1979.

31. Bartlett JG, O'Keefe P, Tally FP, et al. Bacteriology of hospital acquired pneumonia. Arch Intern Med 146:868–871, 1986.

32. Kirby BD, Synder KM, Meyer RD, et al. Legionnaires' disease: Report of sixty-five nosocomially acquired cases and review of the literature. Medicine 59:188–205, 1980.

33. Blatt SP, Parkinson MD, Pace E, et al. Nosocomial Legionnaire's disease: Aspiration as a primary mode of disease acquisition. Am J Med 95:16–22, 1993.

34. Pingleton SK, Fagon JY, Leeper KV. Patient selection for clinical investigation of ventilator-associated pneumonia. Criteria for evaluating diagnostic techniques. Chest (Suppl 1):S553–S556, 1992.

35. Fagon JY, Chastre J, Hance AJ, et al. Detection of nosocomial lung infection in ventilated patients: Use of a protected specimen brush and quantitative culture techniques in 147 patients. Am Rev Respir Dis 138:110–116, 1988.

36. Chastre J, Viau F, Brun P, et al. Prospective evaluation of the protected specimen brush for the diagnosis of pulmonary infections in ventilated patients. Am Rev Respir Dis 130:924–929, 1984.

37. Torres A, De La Bellacasa JP, Xaubet A, et al. Diagnostic value of quantitative cultures of bronchoalveolar lavage and telescoping plugged catheters in mechanically ventilated patients with bacterial pneumonia. Am Rev Respir Dis 140:306–310, 1989.

38. Chauncey JB, Lynch JP III, Hyzy RC, Toews GB. Invasive techniques in the diagnosis of bacterial pneumonia in the intensive care unit. Semin Respir Infect 5:215–225, 1990.

39. Meduri GU. Ventilator-associated pneumonia in patients with respiratory failure: A diagnostic approach. Chest 5:1208–1219, 1990.

40. Jimenez P, Torres A, Rodriguez-Roisin R, et al. Incidence and etiology of pneumonia acquired during mechanical ventilation. Crit Care Med 17:882–885, 1989.

41. Rouby JJ, Martin de Lassele E, Poete P, et al. Nosocomial bronchopneumonia in the critically ill. Histologic and bacteriologic aspects. Am Rev Respir Dis 146:1059–1066, 1992.

42. Centers for Disease Control. Guidelines for preventing the transmission of tuberculosis in health-care settings, with special focus on HIV-related issues. MMWR 39:RR-17, 1990.

43. Snider DE Jr, Roper WL. The new tuberculosis. N Engl J Med 326:703–705, 1992.

44. Fischl MA, Daikos GL, Uttamchandani RB, et al. Clinical presentation and outcome of patients with HIV infection and tuberculosis caused by multiple drug resistant bacilli. Ann Intern Med 117:184–190, 1992.

45. Barnes PF, Bloch AB, Davidson PT, Snider DE Jr. Tuberculosis in patients with human immunodeficiency virus infection. N Engl J Med 324:1644–1650, 1991.

46. Hoffman PC, Dixon RE. Control of influenza in the hospital. Ann Intern Med 87:725–728, 1977.

47. Valenti WM, Hall CB, Douglas RG, et al. Nosocomial viral infections: Epidemiology and significance. Infect Control 1:33–37, 1979.

48. Hall CB. Nosocomial viral respiratory infections: Perennial weeds on pediatric wards. Am J Med 70:670–676, 1981.

49. Arnow PM, Anderson RL, Mainous PD, et al. Pulmonary aspergillus infection during hospital renovation. Am Rev Respir Dis 118:49–53, 1978.

50. Witt DJ, Craven DE, McCabe WR. Bacterial infections in adult patients with the acquired immune deficiency syndrome (AIDS) and AIDS-related complex. Am J Med 82:900–906, 1987.

51. Cohn DL. Bacterial pneumonia in the HIV-infected patient. Infect Dis Clin North Am 5:485–507, 1991.

52. Bryant LR, Mobin-Uddin K, Dillon ML, et al. Misdiagnosis of pneumonia in patients needing mechanical respiration. Arch Surg 106:286–288, 1973.

53. Joshi M, Ciesla N, Caplan E. Diagnosis of pneumonia in critically ill patients [Abstract]. Chest 94:4S, 1988.

54. Andrews CP, Coalson JJ, Smith JD, Johanson WG Jr. Diagnosis of nosocomial bacterial pneumonia in acute, diffuse lung injury. Chest 80:254–258, 1981.

55. Bell RC, Coalson JJ, Smith JD, Johanson WG Jr. Multiple organ system failure and infection in adult respiratory distress syndrome. Ann Intern Med 99:293–298, 1983.

56. Bartlett JG. Invasive diagnostic techniques in pulmonary infections. In Pennington JE (ed). Respiratory Infections: Diagnosis and Management, 2nd ed. New York, Raven Press, 1989, pp 69–96.

57. Bartlett JG, Faling LJ, Willey S. Quantitative tracheal bacteriologic and cytologic studies in patients with long-term tracheostomies. Chest 74:635–639, 1978.

58. Chastre J, Fagon JY, Soler P, et al. Diagnosis of nosocomial bacterial pneumonia in intubated patients undergoing ventilation: Comparison of the usefulness of bronchoalveolar lavage and the protected specimen brush. Am J Med 85:499–506, 1988.

59. Meduri GU, Beals DH, Maijub AG, Baselski V. Protected bronchoalveolar lavage: A new bronchoscopic technique to retrieve uncontaminated distal airway secretions. Am Rev Respir Dis 143:855–864, 1991.

60. Piperno D, Gaussorgues P, Bachmann P, et al. Diagnostic value of nonbronchoscopic bronchoalveolar lavage during mechanical ventilation. Chest 93:223, 1988.

61. Gaussorgues P, Piperno D, Bachmann P, et al. Comparison of nonbronchoscopic bronchoalveolar lavage to open lung biopsy for the bacteriologic diagnosis of pulmonary infections in mechanically ventilated patients. Intensive Care Med 15:94–98, 1989.

62. Pugin J, Auckenthaler R, Mili N, et al. Diagnosis of ventilator-associated pneumonia by bacteriologic analysis of bronchoscopic and nonbronchoscopic "blind" bronchoalveolar lavage fluid. Am Rev Respir Dis 143:1121–1129, 1991.

63. el-Ebiary M, Torres A, Gonzalez T, et al. Quantitative cultures of endotracheal aspirates for the diagnosis of ventilator-associated pneumonia. Am Rev Respir Dis 148:1552–1557, 1993.

64. Pham LH, Brun-Buisson C, Legrand P, et al. Diagnosis of nosocomial pneumonia in mechanically ventilated patients. Am Rev Respir Dis 143:1055–1061, 1991.

65. Deitch EA, Berg R. Bacterial translocation from the gut: A mechanism of infection. J Burn Care Rehabil 8:475–480, 1987.
66. Olivares L, Segovia A, Revuelta R. Tube feeding and lethal aspiration in neurological patients: A review of 720 autopsy cases. Stroke 5:654–656, 1974.
67. Cameron J, Zuidema G. Aspiration pneumonia: Magnitude and frequency of the problem. JAMA 219:1194–1198, 1972.
68. Wynne JM, Modell JJ. Respiratory aspiration of stomach contents. Ann Intern Med 87:466–469, 1977.
69. Reynolds HY. Bacterial adherence to respiratory tract mucosa: A dynamic interaction leading to colonization. Semin Respir Infect 2:8–19, 1987.
70. Penn RG, Sanders WE, Sanders CC. Colonization of the oropharynx with gram-negative bacilli: A major antecedent to nosocomial pneumonia. Am J Infect Control 9:25–34, 1981.
71. Valenti WM, Trudell RG, Bentley DW. Factors predisposing to oropharyngeal colonization with gram-negative bacilli in the aged. N Engl J Med 298:1108–1111, 1978.
72. Atherton ST, White DJ. Stomach as a source of bacteria colonizing respiratory tract during artificial ventilation. Lancet 2:968–969, 1978.
73. Daschner F, Kappstein I, Engels I, et al. Stress ulcer prophylaxis and ventilation pneumonia: Prevention by antibacterial cytoprotective agents. Infect Control Hosp Epidemiol 9:59–65, 1988.
74. Donowitz LG, Page MC, Mileur BL, Guenthner SH. Alteration of normal gastric flora in critical care patients receiving antacid and cimetidine therapy. Infect Control 7:23–26, 1986.
75. Tryba M. The gastropulmonary route of infection—Fact or fiction? Am J Med 91(Suppl 2A):135S–146S, 1991.
76. Garrod LP. A study of the bacterial power of hydrochloric acid and of gastric juice. St Barth Hosp Rep 72:145–167, 1939.
77. Giannella RA, Broitman SA, Zamcheck N. Influence of gastric acidity on bacterial and parasitic enteric infections: A perspective. Ann Intern Med 78:271–276, 1973.
78. Arnold I. The bacterial flora within the stomach and small intestine: The effect of experimental alterations of acid-base balance and the age of the subject. Am J Med Sci 186:471–481, 1933.
79. Gourdin TG, Smith BF, Craven DE. Prevention of stress bleeding in critical care patients: Current concepts on risk and benefit. Perspect Crit Care 2:44–70, 1989.
80. Border J, Hassett J, LaDuca J, et al. The gut origin septic states in blunt multiple trauma (ISS + 40) in the ICU. Ann Surg 206:427–448, 1987.
81. Pingleton SK, Hinthorn DR, Liu C. Enteral nutrition in patients receiving mechanical ventilation: Multiple sources of tracheal colonization include the stomach. Am J Med 80:827–832, 1986.
82. Kappstein I, Friedrich T, Hellinger P, et al. Incidence of pneumonia in mechanically ventilated patients treated with sucralfate or cimetidine as prophylaxis for stress bleeding: Bacterial colonization of the stomach. Am J Med 91(Suppl 2A):125–131, 1991.
83. Tryba M. Risk of acute stress bleeding and nosocomial pneumonia in ventilated intensive care unit patients: Sucralfate versus antacids. Am J Med 83(Suppl 3B):117–124, 1987.
84. Prod'hom G, Leutenberger P, Koerfer J, et al. Nosocomial pneumonia in mechanically ventilated patients receiving antacid, rantidine or sucralfate as prophylaxis for stress ulcer: A randomized controlled clinical trial. Ann Int Med 120:653–662, 1994.
85. Tryba M. Sucralfate versus antacids or H_2-antagonists for stress ulcer prophylaxis: A meta-analysis on efficacy and pneumonia rate. Crit Care Med 19:942–949, 1991.
86. Kunkel SL, Strieter RM. Cytokine networking in lung inflammation. Hosp Pract 25:63–76, 1990.
87. Toews GB. Pulmonary clearance of infectious agents. In Pennington JE (ed). Respiratory Infections: Diagnosis and Management, 2nd ed. New York, Raven Press, 1989, pp 41–51.
88. Rose RM. Pulmonary macrophages in nosocomial pneumonia: Defense function and dysfunction, and prospects for activation. Eur J Clin Microbiol Infect Dis 8:25–28, 1989.
89. Fick RB. Lung humoral response to Pseudomonas species. Eur J Clin Microbiol Infect Dis 8:29–34, 1989.
90. Ramphal R, Small PM, Shands JW Jr, et al. Adherence of *Pseudomonas aeruginosa* to tracheal cells injured by influenza infection or by endotracheal intubation. Infect Immun 27:614–619, 1980.
91. Pennington JE. Immunological perspectives in prevention and treatment of nosocomial pneumonia. Intensive Care Med 18:545–560, 1992.
92. Lepper MH, Kofman S, Blatt N, et al. Effect of antibiotics used singly and in combination on the tracheal flora following tracheostomy in poliomyelitis. Antibiot Chemother 4:829–833, 1954.
93. Feeley TW, de Moulin GC, Hedley-Whyte J, et al. Aerosol polymyxin and pneumonia in seriously ill patients. N Engl J Med 293:471–475, 1975.
94. Klastersky J, Thys JP. Local antibiotic therapy for broncho-pneumonia. In Pennington JE (ed). Respiratory Infections: Diagnosis and Management. New York, Raven Press, 1983, p 481–489.

95. Unertl K, Ruckdeschel G, Selmann HK, et al. Prevention of colonization and respiratory infections in long-term ventilated patients by local antimicrobial prophylaxis. Intensive Care Med 13:106–113, 1987.

96. Stoutenbeek CP, van Saene HKF, Miranda DR, et al. The effect of selective decontamination of the digestive tract on colonization and infection rate in multiple trauma patients. Intensive Care Med 10:185–192, 1984.

97. Ulrich C, de Weerd W, Bakker NC, et al. Selective decontamination of the digestive tract with norfloxacin in the prevention of ICU-acquired infections: A prospective randomized study. Intensive Care Med 15:424–431, 1989.

98. Duncan RA, Steger KA, Craven DE. Selective decontamination of the digestive tract: Risks outweigh benefits for intensive care patients. Semin Respir Dis 1994, in press.

99. Pugin J, Auckenthaler R, Lew DP, Suter PM. Oropharyngeal decontamination decreases incidence of ventilator-associated pneumonia: A randomized, placebo-controlled, double-blind clinical trial. JAMA 265:2704–2710, 1991.

100. Gastinne H, Wolff M, Delatour F, et al. A controlled trial in intensive care units of selective decontamination of the digestive tract with nonabsorbable antibiotics. N Engl J Med 326:594–599, 1992.

101. Cockerill FR, Muller FM, Anhalt JP, et al. Prevention of infection in critically ill patients by selective decontamination of the digestive tract. Ann Intern Med 117:545–553, 1992.

102. Hammond JM, Potgieter PD, Sanders GL, et al. A double-blind study of selective decontamination in intensive care. Lancet 340:5–9, 1992.

103. Meta-analysis of randomised controlled trials of selective decontamination of the digestive tract. Selective Decontamination of the Digestive Tract Trialists' Collaborative Group. Br Med J 307:525–532, 1993.

104. Albert RK, Condie F. Handwashing patterns in medical intensive care units. N Engl J Med 304:1465–1466, 1981.

105. Maki DG. Control of colonization and transmission of pathogenic bacteria in the hospital. Ann Intern Med 89:777–780, 1978.

106. Flaherty JP, Weinstein RA. Infection control and pneumonia prophylaxis strategies in the intensive care unit. Semin Respir Infect 5:191–203, 1990.

107. Haley RW, Hooton TM, Culver DH, et al. Nosocomial infections in US hospitals, 1975–1976: Estimated frequency by selected characteristics of patients. Am J Med 70:947–959, 1981.

108. Britt MR, Schleupner CJ, Matsumiyi S. Severity of underlying disease as a predictor of nosocomial infection: Utility of the control of nosocomial infection. JAMA 239:1047–1051, 1978.

109. Steere AC, Mallison GF. Handwashing practices for prevention of nosocomial infections. Ann Intern Med 83:683–686, 1975.

110. Saltzman TC, Clark JJ, Klemm L. Hand contamination of personnel as a mechanism of cross-infection in nosocomial infections with antibiotic-resistant Escherichia coli and Klebsiella-Aerobacter. Antimicrob Agents Chemother 7:97–100, 1967.

111. Klein JJ, Watanakunakorn C. Hospital-acquired fungemia: Its natural course and clinical significance. Am J Med 67:51–58, 1979.

112. Leclair JM, Freeman J, Sullivan BF, et al. Prevention of nosocomial respiratory syncytial virus infections through compliance with glove and gown isolation precautions. N Engl J Med 317:329–334, 1987.

113. Williams WW. Guidelines for infection control in hospital personnel. Infect Control 4(Suppl):326–349, 1983.

114. Kantor HS, Poblete R, Pusateri SL. Nosocomial transmission of tuberculosis from unsuspected disease. Am J Med 84:833–838, 1988.

115. Centers for Disease Control. Nosocomial transmission of multidrug-resistant tuberculosis among HIV-infected persons—Florida and New York, 1988–1991. MMWR 40:585–591, 1991.

116. Ehrenkranz NJ, Kicklighter JL. Tuberculosis outbreak in a general hospital: Evidence of airborne spread of infection. Arch Intern Med 77:377–382, 1972.

117. Craven DE, Steger KA. Nosocomial pneumonia in the intubated patient: New concepts on pathogenesis and prevention. Infect Dis Clin North Am 3:843–866, 1989.

118. Deppe SA, Kelly JW, Thoi LL, et al. Incidence of colonization, nosocomial pneumonia, and mortality in critically ill patients using a Trach Care^R closed-suction system versus an open-suction system: A prospective, randomized study. Crit Care Med 18:1389–1394, 1990.

119. Mayhall CG. The Trach Care™ closed tracheal suction system: A new medical device to permit tracheal suctioning without interruption of ventilatory assistance. Infect Control Hosp Epidemiol 9:125–126, 1988.

120. Sottile FD, Marrie TJ, Prough DS, et al. Nosocomial pulmonary infection: Possible etiologic significance of bacterial adhesion to endotracheal tubes. Crit Care Med 14:265–270, 1986.

121. Inglis TJJ, Millar MR, Jones JG, Robinson DA. Tracheal tube biofilm as a source of bacterial colonization of the lung. J Clin Microbiol 27:2014–2018, 1989.

122. Montecalvo MA, Korsberg TZ, Farber HW, et al. Nosocomial pneumonia and nutritional status of critical care patients randomized to gastric versus jejunal tube feedings. Crit Care Med 20:1377–1387, 1992.

123. Thompson AC, Wilder BJ, Powner DJ. Bedside resuscitation bag: A source of bacterial contamination. Infect Control 6:231–232, 1985.
124. Weber DJ, Wilson MB, Rutala WA, Thomann CA. Manual ventilation bags as a source for bacterial colonization of intubated patients. Am Rev Respir Dis 4:892–894, 1990.
125. Irwin RS, Demers RR, Pratter MR, et al. An outbreak of Acinetobacter infection associated with the use of a ventilator spirometer. Respir Care 25:232–237, 1980.
126. Carroll AR, Goularte TA, McGinley KN, et al. An outbreak of Pseudomonas maltophilia in intensive care units traced to contaminated respiratory therapy equipment. Paper presented at the 12th Annual Conference of the Association of Practitioners in Infection Control, Las Vegas, 1985.
127. Simmons BP, Wong ES. Guidelines for prevention of nosocomial pneumonia. Am J Infect Control 11:230–243, 1983.
128. Reinarz JA, Pierce AK, Mays BB, et al. The potential role of inhalation-therapy equipment in nosocomial pulmonary infection. J Clin Invest 44:831–839, 1965.
129. Pierce AK, Sanford JP, Thomas GD, Leonard JS. Long-term evaluation of decontamination of inhalation-therapy equipment and the occurrence of necrotizing pneumonia. N Engl J Med 282:528–531, 1970.
130. Craven DE, Connolly MG Jr, Lichtenberg DA, et al. Contamination of mechanical ventilators with tubing changes every 24 or 48 hours. N Engl J Med 306:1505–1509, 1982.
131. Dreyfuss D, Djedaini K, Weber P, et al. Prospective study of nosocomial pneumonia and of patient and circuit colonization during mechanical ventilation with circuit changes every 48 hours versus no change. Am Rev Respir Dis 143:738–743, 1991.
132. Fink J, Mahlmeister M, York M, et al. A comparison of organism growth in ventilator circuits at 48 hours versus seven days. Am J Infect Control 20:103, 1992.
133. Boher M, Lohse S, Glasby C, et al. Impact of seven day ventilatory tubing changes on nosocomial lower respiratory tract infections. Am J Infect Control 20:103, 1992.
134. Hospital Infection Control Practice Advisory Committee. Recommendations for Prevention of Nosocomial Pneumonia. Feb 2, 1994, Federal Register 59:4980–5022.
135. Craven DE, Goularte TA, Make BJ. Contaminated condensate in mechanical ventilator circuits: A risk factor for nosocomial pneumonia? Am Rev Respir Dis 129:625–628, 1984.
136. Goularte TA, Craven DE. Bacterial colonization of cascade humidifier reservoirs after 24 and 48 hours of continuous mechanical ventilation. Infect Control 8:200–204, 1987.
137. Christopher KL, Saravoltz LD, Bush TL, et al. Cross-infection: A study using a canine model for pneumonia. Am Rev Respir Dis 128:271–275, 1983.
138. Toews GB, Gross GN, Pierce AK. The relationship of innoculum size to lung bacterial clearance and phagocytic cell response in mice. Am Rev Respir Dis 120:559–566, 1979.
139. Rhame FS, Streifel A, McComb C, et al. Bubbling humidifiers produce microaerosols which can carry bacteria. Infect Control 7:403–407, 1986.
140. MacIntyre NR, Anderson HR, Silver RM, et al. Pulmonary function in mechanically ventilated patients using 24-hour use of a hydroscopic condenser humidifier. Chest 84:560–564, 1983.
141. Cohen IL, Weinberg PF, Fein IA, et al. Endotracheal tube occlusion associated with the use of heat and moisture exchangers in the intensive care unit. Crit Care Med 16:277–279, 1988.
142. Martin C, Perrin G, Gevaudan MJ, et al. Heat and moisture exchangers and vaporizing humidifiers in the intensive care unit. Chest 97:144–149, 1990.
143. Misset B, Escudier B, Rivara D, et al. Heat and moisture exchanger vs heated humidifier during long-term mechanical ventilation: A prospective randomized study. Chest 100:160–163, 1991.
144. Roustan JP, Keinlen J, Aubas P, et al. Comparison of hydrophobic heat and moisture exchangers with heated humidifier during prolonged mechanical ventilation. Intensive Care Med 18:97–100, 1992.
145. Suzukawa M, Usuda Y, Numata K. The effects of sputum characteristics of combining an unheated humidifier with a heat moisture exchanger. Respir Care 34:976, 1989.
146. Branson RD, Chatburn RL. Humidification of inspired gases during mechanical ventilation [Editorial]. Respir Care 38:461–468, 1993.
147. Branson RD, Davis K, Campbell RS, et al. Humidification in the intensive care unit: Prospective study of a new protocol utilizing heated humidification and a hygroscopic condenser humidifier. Chest 104:1800–1805, 1993.
148. Craven DE, Lichtenberg DA, Goularte TA, et al. Contaminated medication nebulizers in mechanical ventilator circuits: A source of bacterial aerosols. Am J Med 17:834–838, 1984.
149. Dyer ED, Peterson DE. How far do bacteria travel from the exhalation valve of IPPB equipment? Anesth Analg 51:516–519, 1972.

26

Besides its medical use, oxygen has many other applications, such as in steel making, glass manufacture, and paper-pulp bleaching and as an oxidant in rocket fuel for space exploration.

Oxygen Therapy

Rich Malloy, R.R.T., and
Margarete Pierce, R.R.T., C.P.F.T.

No process is more fundamental to the homeostasis of human life than that of breathing oxygen. This chapter, dedicated to the therapeutic administration of oxygen, explores basic concepts related to equipment and physiology. The chapter also describes commonly used oxygen delivery systems along with protocols that enhance the effectiveness and efficiency of oxygen therapy.

OXYGEN: HISTORY AND CHEMISTRY

Oxygen, a colorless, odorless gas, sustains aerobic life and supports combustion (Table 26–1). It comprises 20.93% of the earth's atmosphere.[1, 2] In 1774, Priestley was credited with the discovery of "dephlogisticated air" (oxygen), a term he used because of his belief in the phlogiston theory of fire and combustion (i.e., that a nonexistent chemical was released during combustion). Scheele had independently discovered this "air" in 1772, but his findings were not published until 1777. In that same year, Lavoisier recognized oxygen as an element, along with its significance in respiration and combustion. His experiments discredited the phlogiston theory and forged the scientific basis of modern chemistry. He named the element oxygen, Greek for "acid former."[3-7]

MANUFACTURE OF OXYGEN

The most common method used to produce oxygen is called liquefaction. Air is liquefied by compression and expansion, and the components of liquid air are then separated by fractional distillation.

OXYGEN CYLINDERS AND REGULATORS

Cylinders

All gas cylinders, which are made from seamless steel, are manufactured, transported, and tested under the auspices of the Department of Transportation. Medical gas cylinders are manufactured by a spinning

TABLE **26–1:** Oxygen

Chemical symbol	O
Atomic number	8
Atomic weight	16
Molecular oxygen	O_2
Molecular weight	32
Boiling point	$-183°C$
Critical temperature	$-118.4°C$
Critical pressure	715 psig

TABLE **26–2:** Cylinder Facts

	Amount of Oxygen	
Cylinder Size	Cubic Feet	Liters
D	12.5	354
E	22.0	623
H	244.0	6905

Conversion: 1 cubic foot = 28.3 L

The Food and Drug Administration regulates the standards of purity for medical gases set by the United States Pharmacopeia, which states that medical oxygen shall be 99% pure. The National Fire Protection Agency establishes standards for safe storage of cylinders and specifications of piping systems.

Calculating the duration of cylinder flow is central to the safe administration of oxygen (Table 26–3). For example, with a cylinder at 10 L/min for a 30-minute trip to the x-ray department, would a single E cylinder suffice? If the cylinder is currently at 1500 psi, the equation becomes

$$\text{Time} = \frac{0.28 \times 1500 \text{psi}}{10 \text{ L/min}}$$

Therefore, at 10 L/min, the cylinder would last 42 minutes.

process or a "plug process," with the method of manufacture stamped on the shoulder of the cylinder.

Oxygen cylinders (Table 26–2) are required to have safety relief devices, which release gas if the pressure in the cylinder increases (e.g., owing to high temperatures). Two basic systems exist: a frangible disc designed to burst under excessive pressure and a fusible plug designed to melt and release gas if it is exposed to high temperatures, such as in a fire.[8, 9]

Regulators

High pressure from a cylinder needs to be reduced to a workable pressure (usually 50 psig) to operate much of the equipment used in gas administration. A regulator (sometimes referred to as a reducing valve) is used for this purpose. A single-stage regulator uses a spring and diaphragm to reduce cylinder pressure in one "step" (Fig. 26–1). The diaphragm separates the spring chamber on the top and the gas pressure chamber on the bottom of the regulator. As gas pressure drops, the spring tension forces the diaphragm down and allows gas to enter the pressure chamber until an equilibrium is met and the diaphragm returns to its flat position. The regulator also has a pressure relief mechanism (pop-off valve), which allows excess gas pressure to be released to the atmosphere in the event of a malfunction of the internal regulator assembly.

Multistage regulators operate on the same principle but reduce the gas pressure in stages, using more than one reducing valve. A pressure relief valve is present for each reducing chamber on the regulator.

FLOWMETERS

A flowmeter is a flow-regulating device that measures the volume of gas passing through it, usually in liters per minute. The most common flowmeter design is the Thorpe tube. Thorpe tubes can be classified as either back pressure compensated or non–back pressure compensated. The basic design of a Thorpe tube includes a clear vertical tube with a float suspended in the center, which rises and falls depending on the amount of gas passing around it. Flow is adjusted by a needle valve, and

TABLE **26–3:** Oxygen Cylinder Duration Equation

$$\text{Time (min)} = \frac{\text{conversion factor} \times \text{pressure (psig)}}{\text{flow rate (L/min)}}$$

Conversion factor for cylinder size: D, 0.16; E, 0.28; H, 3.14.

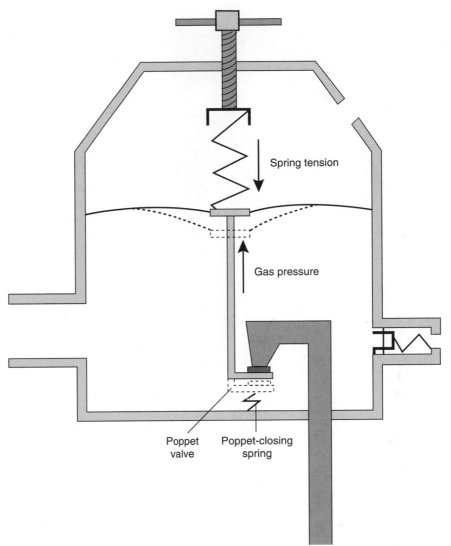

FIGURE 26–1: A typical single-stage regulator.

the location of the needle valve determines whether the flowmeter is compensated or noncompensated to back pressure (Fig. 26–2). In the pressure-compensated flowmeter, the needle valve is distal to the meter, and the flow-regulating device is calibrated at 50 psig and 70°F. This gives an accurate reading when back pressure is applied in the form of several lengths of additional tubing to a nasal oxygen setup. Each length of tubing generates significant back pressure to the flowmeter because of its reduced radius, but the actual flow delivered through the Thorpe tube continues to be displayed with this device. The flowmeter registers zero if the outlet becomes occluded.

The needle valve is proximal to the meter in the noncompensated flowmeter, and the meter is calibrated at atmospheric pressure. Non–pressure-compensated flowmeters should never be used with equipment that may cause back pressure because inaccurate readings may result.[10] Here, the placement of the needle valve will result in a reading that consistently overstates the actual flow through the tube.

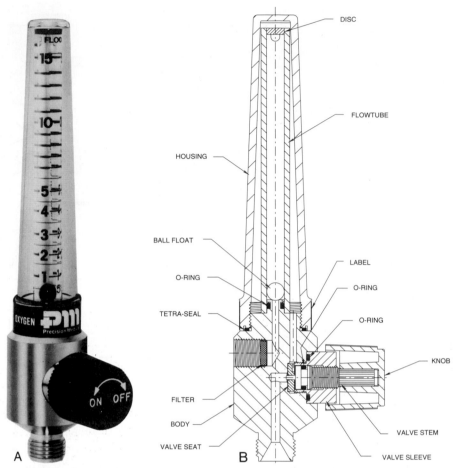

FIGURE 26–2: *A* and *B,* Flowmeters. (*A* and *B,* Courtesy of Precision Medical, Northampton, PA.)

OXYGEN ANALYZERS

Oxygen analyzers are generally classified by their principle of operation; some of the more common instruments are listed in the following paragraphs with a brief description of their operation.

Physical analyzers operate on Pauling's principle of paramagnetic susceptibility. Oxygen is paramagnetic (attracted by a magnetic field). In the Beckman D-2, for example, a glass dumbbell is suspended on a twisted quartz fiber. The dumbbell is filled with nitrogen, which is diamagnetic (repelled by a magnetic field). When oxygen is added to the sampling chamber, the magnetic field changes, forcing the dumbbell to rotate, which provides a reading of the oxygen percentage.

Electrical analyzers operate on the principle of thermal conductivity and a Wheatstone bridge. The analyzer contains a reference wire exposed to room air and a sampling wire. When oxygen enters the sampling chamber, the sampling wire cools. As it cools, the wire conducts more current. This change in current compared with the reference wire is read as the oxygen percentage. The Mira and the OEM models are examples of electrical analyzers.

Electrochemical analyzers can be categorized into the galvanic fuel cell and the polarographic electrodes. In the galvanic fuel cell, oxygen diffuses through a semipermeable membrane (Teflon) into a hydroxide

Chemical reaction of the galvanic fuel cell analyzer:

$$O_2 + H_2O + 4\ electrons \rightleftarrows 4\ OH + Pb \rightleftarrows 2H_2O + 2\ PbO_2 + 4\ electrons$$

bath, where it reacts with the cathode (usually a gold wire) to form hydroxyl ions. Electrons are gained in this reaction, which is called a reduction reaction. The hydroxyl ions diffuse to the anode (a lead wire), where they are oxidized. Loss of electrons in a chemical reaction is known as oxidation. The electron current generated in this process is proportional to the oxygen concentration and is read on the analyzer as the oxygen percentage.

The polarographic electrode (Clark's) uses a similar reaction formula, but a battery is used to polarize the electrodes to improve the response time of the analyzer. Examples of galvanic fuel cell analyzers are the Teldyne and the Biomarine. Examples of polarographic analyzers are the IL 207 and the IMI.

The previous sections briefly review oxygen manufacturing, oxygen cylinders, flow- and pressure-regulating devices, and devices to analyze the percentage of gaseous oxygen. Respiratory care practitioners must fully understand the operation of all equipment they are using in patient care. The reader is encouraged to refer to a respiratory therapy equipment text for a more detailed explanation of this equipment.[11]

CLINICAL OXYGEN THERAPY

Oxygen is a drug, and the safe administration of any drug is based on the premise of the "five rights." These rights are

- The right patient
- The right drug
- The right dosage
- The right route
- The right time

A sixth right for oxygen therapy, the *right indication,* is added for completeness.

The purpose of oxygen therapy is to increase the content of oxygen in arterial blood delivered to the tissues to facilitate aerobic metabolism. Like any drug, oxygen is to be given with caution. Oxygen therapy was viewed in the past by some health care providers as a benign therapy that could be administered by anyone for any reason. In this era of fiscal constraint, the cost of unnecessary care has become an important issue.[12, 13]

In a study published in 1992, Small and coworkers reported clinical carelessness in the application of oxygen.[14] Their study revealed that although errors in the administration of oxygen were numerous and significant, a simultaneous review of antibiotic administration revealed no errors. Errors that were observed with oxygen administration included the administration of oxygen to the wrong patient, the use of an incorrect dosage, the improper application of the delivery device, and the omission of documentation of therapy or indications for oxygen therapy.

With oxygen, as with any drug, there are acceptable doses. It is important to remember the proper components of an oxygen prescription:

- The percentage or flow of oxygen (in liters per minute)
- The duration of therapy
- The goals of therapy[15, 16]

A hospital-approved therapist-driven protocol or a care plan may simplify the proper prescription to avoid potential problems with oxygen delivery.

Basic Concepts

Room air (or any other source gas) moves through the lungs during inspiration. This volume then diffuses across the alveolar-capillary membrane because of differences in the partial pressures of the various gases between the alveoli and the mixed venous blood in the capillary. For example, in a person breathing room air, the alveolar partial pressure of

There are approximately 750 square feet of capillary surface area in the lungs, and significant loss of lung or destruction of alveolar walls that causes a decrease in the surface area available for gas exchange must occur before the patient becomes symptomatic.

oxygen is 110 mm Hg, whereas it is 40 mm Hg in the capillary; therefore, oxygen diffuses from the alveolus to the capillary.

The diameter of an average capillary is 5 μm. The red blood cell (about 7.7 μm) is physically distorted as it transits through the capillary, where 97% of the total oxygen content attaches to the hemoglobin of the red blood cell; the remaining 3% dissolves in plasma. The volume of gas moving across the alveolar-capillary membrane is approximately 21 mL of oxygen diffusing per minute for each unit of pressure difference between the alveolus and the capillary. Because this pressure difference is normally about 11 mm Hg, the total volume of gas moved across the membrane is 230 mL/min, or that amount of oxygen that is needed to sustain aerobic metabolism.

It is often helpful to relate the two components of oxygen content, arterial saturation (Sa_{O_2}) and the partial pressure of dissolved oxygen (Pa_{O_2}), because they are interdependent variables. This relationship is commonly expressed as the oxyhemoglobin dissociation curve. The normal curve is sigmoidal in shape and illustrates a nonlinear relationship between the hemoglobin saturation (percentage saturation) and the Pa_{O_2} (Fig. 26–3, a normal curve). This curve demonstrates that at low levels of oxygen content (which is effectively represented by low oxygen saturation), the curve is vertical in nature. At this point in the curve, large changes in Sa_{O_2} are associated with relatively small changes in Pa_{O_2}. This explains why small changes in Pa_{O_2} can result in significant improvements in oxygen content. Consider the patient with chronic obstructive pulmonary disease, who may have a low Pa_{O_2} on room air. A nasal cannula delivering oxygen at a rate of 1 L/min may increase the Pa_{O_2} by 15 mm Hg. This small improvement in Pa_{O_2} is associated with a 23%

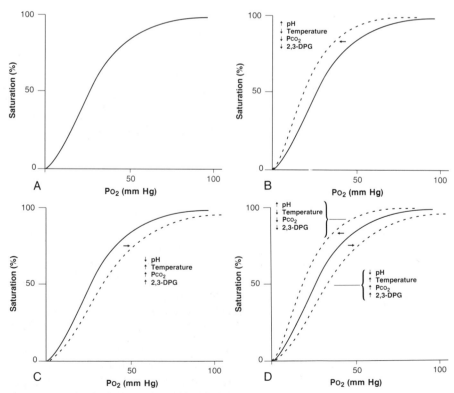

FIGURE 26–3: *A* to *D*, Oxyhemoglobin dissociation curves. DPG, diphosphoglycerate. Normal position with left and right shifts.

increase in saturation on the vertical portion of the oxyhemoglobin dissociation curve.

The "flat" portion of the curve also explains why there is little clinical benefit in maintaining a Pa_{O_2} in excess of 90 to 100 mm Hg. At this point in the curve, small improvements in content (Sa_{O_2}) are realized when the Pa_{O_2} is elevated to levels significantly above this range.

Many variables can shift the position of this curve; this change in the curve represents a difference in the affinity of bonding between the Fe^{2+} ion and molecular oxygen. These relationships ultimately drive the "unloading" of oxygen at the tissue level, so it is helpful to understand the concept because it may also determine the method of oxygen delivery. Shifting the curve to the right decreases the hemoglobin's affinity for oxygen (i.e., results in a weakened bond between the Fe^{2+} ion and the oxygen molecules). In this state, more oxygen is unloaded at the tissue level. Causes of the curve's shifting to the right include

↓ pH
↑ Temperature
↑ Pco_2
↑ 2,3-DPG

Perhaps more problematic for the patient is the notion of shifting the curve in the opposite direction. This shift to the left depicts an increased affinity for oxygen by Fe^{2+} and therefore, less oxygen is available to the tissues (i.e., the oxygen is more tightly bonded to the Fe^{2+} ion). Causes of the curve's shifting to the left are

↑ pH
↓ Temperature
↓ Pco_2
↓ 2,3-DPG
↑ Fetal hemoglobin
↑ Carbon monoxide

In cases of carbon monoxide poisoning, for example, a patient may need to maintain a clinically high Pa_{O_2}, beyond the realm of 80 to 100 mm Hg, to compensate for possible tissue hypoxia due to reduced oxygen unloading. This would be a consideration for the delivery of oxygen, in addition to the classic use of 100% oxygen that results in a 50% depletion of carboxyhemoglobin within 80 minutes.[18]

Clinical Indications

Hypoxemia, a reduction in the arterial oxygen tension, is the primary indication for oxygen therapy. In adults, this is demonstrated either by a Pa_{O_2} of less than 60 mm Hg or by an Sp_{O_2} (saturation of oxygen determined by pulse oximetry) of less than 88%.[17] Many causes of a reduced level of arterial oxygen exist. The following section describes some of the more important factors that determine the need for supplemental oxygen.

Pierson defines the following four causes of hypoxemia:[45]

- Low inspired oxygen concentration
- Alveolar hypoventilation (central nervous system depression, acute chronic obstructive pulmonary disease)
- Ventilation-perfusion ($\dot{V}/\dot{Q}$) mismatch (chronic obstructive pulmonary disease, pulmonary embolus)

2,3-Diphosphoglycerate (2,3-DPG) is a phosphorous enzyme that enhances dissociation of oxygen from the Fe^{2+} in the hemoglobin molecule.

Although hypoxemia may lead to tissue hypoxia, not all causes of tissue hypoxia are amenable to oxygen therapy.

- Right-to-left shunt (adult respiratory distress syndrome, atelectasis)

Each of these causes differs in the degree of clinical problems that might result. Shunting is the most serious mechanism.

Patients differ in their responses to hypoxemia and in the degree to which lowered amounts of arterial oxygen affect organ function. The principal issue is the degree of tissue hypoxia that results from hypoxemia. The following classic causes of hypoxia illustrate why some cases of hypoxia do not respond to oxygen therapy.

Hypoxic hypoxia is a reduction in the amount of oxygen in the inspired air or blood causing hypoxemia, as may be seen in $\dot{V}/\dot{Q}$ mismatch, diffusion defect, or alveolar hypoventilation. An example of this is the reduction in available oxygen at higher elevations.

Anemic hypoxia is a reduction in the oxygen-carrying capacity, which may be due to anemia, carbon monoxide poisoning, sickle cell anemia, or other hemoglobin abnormalities. For example, in carbon monoxide poisoning, hemoglobin has a higher affinity for carbon monoxide than for oxygen, resulting in carboxyhemoglobinemia and subsequent tissue hypoxia.

Stagnant hypoxia may be due to poor tissue perfusion or a reduction in the normal flow of blood, as in cardiac failure, shock, cardiac arrest, or peripheral vascular disease.

Histotoxic hypoxia is an inability to utilize oxygen at the cellular level, as in cyanide or alcohol poisoning.[19]

Obviously, patients who evidence hypoxic hypoxia are the most efficiently treated with oxygen therapy. Anemic and stagnant hypoxia may respond to oxygen in some circumstances (e.g., in the case of carbon monoxide poisoning). Clearly, however, little in the way of positive outcomes might be expected for patients afflicted with metabolic poisons that interfere with mitochondrial function.

Each organ system reacts in a specific manner to oxygen desaturation, which may or may not lead to overt signs and symptoms. Pierson stresses that "no single, clinically available monitoring technique is both sensitive and specific enough to provide an immediate and reliable warning of hypoxemia and hypoxia."[45] Careful monitoring is therefore the cornerstone of managing suspected hypoxemia.

In addition to hypoxia, other clinical indications for oxygen therapy exist. Following general anesthesia a patient may experience some degree of atelectasis that has its genesis in general anesthesia. Two mechanisms are important: the loss of skeletal muscle tone from anesthesia, which results in compression atelectasis, and the denitrogenation of the lung, which is commonly referred to as absorption atelectasis.[46] Higher concentrations of oxygen "wash out" nitrogen from the alveoli, and factors such as airway mucus reduce ventilation to the affected lung unit. This process then leads to a loss of pressure and volume in the alveolus, and the stage is set for progressive lung collapse. Oxygen is given after anesthesia to increase the Pa_{O_2} because there is a presumed $\dot{V}/\dot{Q}$ mismatch. Most studies suggest providing, and the common practice is to provide, oxygen therapy for 12 to 24 hours after anesthesia.[18–20] Oxygen therapy is also indicated in the patient with a suspected or confirmed myocardial infarction.[21] Hypoxemia may increase the work of myocardial tissue, thus increasing the demand for oxygen by this muscle. To meet this demand, oxygen is administered because there is some evidence that the increased Pa_{O_2} may decrease the size of the myocardial infarction.[47]

Trauma to the skeletal muscles resulting from an arterial puncture may lead to a release of enzymes that are measured for diagnostic purposes in a myocardial infarction. Therefore, it may be prudent to avoid this risk and to use pulse oximetry instead of the traditional arterial blood gas measurements in these patients.[21, 22] It should be noted that oxygen may also increase the systemic vascular resistance, which is not without some complications in a patient with a significantly depressed cardiac status who may not tolerate increases in afterload.

Oxygen therapy is indicated in the care of the terminally ill patient or the patient for whom oxygen offers some subjective relief of dyspnea. Analgesics given in increasing doses cause a reduction in minute ventilation and for some may cause the sensation of breathlessness. In general, the use of oxygen therapy should strongly be considered in terminally ill patients if this therapy offers any subjective relief in dyspnea, despite near-normal pulse oximetry readings.

Studies have suggested that oxygen may be beneficial in the treatment of acute cluster headaches. Some studies have suggested the use of 7 to 8 L/min of oxygen via a face mask for approximately 10 to 15 minutes.[24] Other studies have shown that 75% of patients experience some relief, which is thought to be secondary to the vasoconstrictive effect of oxygen in the cerebral circulation.[23, 25]

There are many other medical emergencies in which the use of oxygen may be beneficial. The use of oxygen is indicated if the patient displays clinical signs of dyspnea, hypoxemia, or shock, regardless of the etiology.

Goals of Therapy

The goal of oxygen therapy is defined as delivering the least amount of oxygen necessary to elevate the Pa_{O_2} to greater than 60 mm Hg or to elevate the Sp_{O_2} to greater than 90%. However, there is a question as to what to seek as an end-point for pulse oximetry. Jubran and Tobin studied 54 critically ill patients receiving mechanical ventilation to determine the reliability of Sp_{O_2} values as a substitute for Pa_{O_2} measurements.[41] They noted that an Sp_{O_2} of 92% accurately predicted a Pa_{O_2} of 60 mm Hg or greater in white patients. However, this same "target" Sp_{O_2} was frequently associated with significantly lower Pa_{O_2} values in black patients. In fact, the authors concluded that an Sp_{O_2} of 95% was required to predict a satisfactory Pa_{O_2} (60 mm Hg or greater) reliably in black patients.

Patient comfort should be ensured in the application of an appropriate oxygen delivery device. Observation of the patient's work of breathing and subjective comfort can be a guide for the practitioner to assess the adequacy of oxygen therapy. The work of breathing may be monitored by observing the respiratory musculature, the rate and pattern of ventilation, the heart rate, and the skin color. Because of sedation, patients may not experience a sensation of dyspnea, so it may not be wise to place much emphasis on this single subjective symptom.

Weaning from Oxygen

When the patient is receiving oxygen and is comfortable, the respiratory care practitioner should begin to anticipate the process of weaning the patient from oxygen. Ideally, this weaning process should occur on a daily basis and should begin with a bedside evaluation of skin color, respiratory rate, Sp_{O_2}, and heart rate to determine whether to continue therapy. However, caution must be exercised in the assessment process because the patient must be evaluated in the context of his or her overall disease process and not simply viewed as a source of a few objective data points. Is the patient's overall condition stable or deteriorating? Does exercise or the increased activity associated with the activities of daily life need to be factored into the equation of need for oxygen?

If the evaluation shows the patient's condition to be stable, it may be feasible to lower the patient's oxygen or discontinue it for approximately 15 to 30 minutes and then to re-evaluate the patient on room air. Comparison of the clinical observations mentioned previously becomes the cornerstone for evaluating the patient's tolerance for oxygen withdrawal. Such a practice was the subject of study by Albin and coworkers.[40] They implemented ongoing pulse oximetry to evaluate the continued need for oxygen in 274 patients, which resulted in 1084 individual assessments. Their data were startling in that an Sp_{O_2} of 92% or greater was documented in 75% of the assessments of patients who were not wearing oxygen but had active orders for this drug. They also noted that in 233 assessments, the Sp_{O_2} was 92% or greater on room air for patients who wore their oxygen but were successfully weaned to this end-point via the study protocol.

Documentation is the last piece of the weaning process. What is charted and how well it is charted will serve as a record of the weaning process. In addition, third-party payers often take the position that payment for services will not occur if documentation does not exist.

ADVERSE EFFECTS

With oxygen, as with any drug, side effects exist; therefore, some precautions must be observed in the delivery process.

In the Patient With Chronic Obstructive Pulmonary Disease

Oxygen therapy should be used with caution in any patient with known or suspected chronic obstructive pulmonary disease. At issue is whether the patient will be sensitive to increased oxygenation, which might alter the patient's drive to breathe. In normal patients, the stimulus for ventilation is regulated by carbon dioxide levels in the blood. In patients with chronic obstructive pulmonary disease, this regulatory function is altered, and lowered blood oxygen levels regulate breathing instead. Therefore, higher levels of oxygen in the arterial blood may blunt the patient's hypoxic respiratory drive. In the patient with a history of retaining carbon dioxide, it will be necessary to maintain the Pa_{O_2} at a low-normal range, from 50 to 60 mm Hg. This may necessitate monitoring these patients with arterial blood gas measurements as opposed to pulse oximetry. In the presence of a normal Pa_{O_2}, the hypoxia can be treated with oxygen. The risk of progressive respiratory acidosis must always be monitored in this patient population. The goal of achieving an Sp_{O_2} of 90% or a Pa_{O_2} of greater than 60 mm Hg is generally acceptable. The reason that this patient group is satisfactorily managed with a subnormal Pa_{O_2} is reflected in the group's position on the oxyhemoglobin dissociation curve along with the not uncommon finding of a compensatory polycythemia. Both tend to preserve tissue delivery of oxygen.

Oxygen Toxicity

With oxygen, as with any drug, too little can be given. In the case of oxygen, giving too little results in a continuation of the patient's hypoxemia, and giving too much can result in oxygen toxicity. In oxygen toxicity, biochemical and cytotoxic concerns lead to a chain reaction of events at the cellular level. This cascade of events, in turn, creates clinical changes resulting in lung tissue damage.

Cellular Toxicity or the Free Radical Theory

The free radical theory espouses the existence of free radicals that normally exist in a low oxygenated state. Exposure to a hyperoxygenated environment, as with an increased $F_{I_{O_2}}$ results in the increased production of radicals such as O_2^- (the superoxide anion or oxygen radical), H_2O_2 (hydrogen peroxide), and the hydroxyl radical (OH). It is believed that mitochondria and the endoplasmic reticulum are responsible for increasing the production of these free radicals. The end-product results in structural and metabolic alterations of the cell that may lead to cellular death.[26-28]

Other factors enhance oxygen toxicity, including drugs such as bleomycin and the herbicide paraquat. Additionally, some physiologic states may lead to increased susceptibility to oxygen toxicity. These include hyperthermia, hyperthyroidism, prematurity of the newborn, vitamin E deficiency, and protein deficiency.[29] In the presence of these drugs or factors, the use of oxygen must be very judicious. Although oxygen must always be maintained at a level commensurate with life, it is necessary in these patients to use as little supplemental oxygen as possible. We have had significant experience with bleomycin toxicity at our facility and have developed the policy of maintaining an $F_{I_{O_2}}$ of no higher than 0.25 if at all possible.

Generally, prolonged exposure to high concentrations of oxygen results in acute and chronic symptoms of oxygen toxicity. However, the literature has not defined well the duration of exposure or the exact concentration of oxygen that may precipitate these clinical changes. Studies in humans and in animal preparations have demonstrated that after 6 hours of breathing oxygen at an $F_{I_{O_2}}$ of 1.0, healthy subjects experience symptoms similar to those of tracheobronchitis.[30] In a study of 70 patients, Nash and associates defined two stages of toxicity: the exudative and the histologic stages.[34] The end-result of prolonged exposure to concentrations of oxygen at an $F_{I_{O_2}}$ of greater than 0.40 is damage to the lungs in all species, but the degree of damage is difficult to determine prospectively. Probably oxygen exposure of 72 hours or less will initiate cellular changes that are reversible within 1 week.

Other Adverse Effects

Other adverse effects are comfort and safety related. Safety problems that place the patient at risk include

- Combustion
- Infection
- Breakdown of epidermal integrity
- Drying of the mucous membranes
- Therapeutic misadventures (e.g., failure of equipment)

Oxygen supports combustion, so any open flame may be intensified in the presence of oxygen. No-smoking signs should be prominently displayed and the policy enforced, and careful attention should be given to the placement of electrical devices around the patient's bedside.

Sources of friction may also cause a spark and place the oxygen-enriched environment at risk of conflagration.

Oxygen is considered pure as it leaves the wall outlet and should not pose an infectious threat to the patient. However, devices that are used to deliver oxygen are sources of potential contamination; current practices of changing this equipment are quite diverse. Because some practitioners believe that colonization of a patient occurs within 72 hours, they change oxygen delivery equipment every 72 hours. However, cost and time constraints may lead to prolonging that time interval. Definitive scientific evidence that would cast light on specific recommendations for the routine changing of oxygen delivery equipment is lacking.

Skin integrity becomes an issue with long-term use of an oxygen device because the strap that secures the mask or cannula to the patient also applies pressure on the skin.[32] Factors contributing to skin breakdown include nutritional status, skin turgor, increased humidity, a bony prominence, and pressure applied to pressure-sensitive points. In applying any device, the practitioner needs to be mindful of the patient's "skin vital signs," including color, temperature, turgor, and contour. Routine monitoring of the patient should include examining the pressure-sensitive points that come into contact with the oxygen device. The most common points in question are the bridge of the nose and behind the ears. Commercially prepared sponge-like cushions are available for behind the ears, but both areas can be protected with gauze or a soft material that is comfortable for the patient.

The mucous membranes lining the nasal cavities and the pharynx may also become irritated with the addition of dry gas. In the average patient, this will not pose a major problem, but on occasion, epistaxis or a patient complaint of drying of the nose or throat may occur. This is usually remedied with the addition of a humidifier. However, there is no need for routinely adding humidity for flow rates of less than 4 L/min.[33]

LOW-FLOW DEVICES

This section omits descriptions that attempt to predict the $F_{I_{O_2}}$ of a given device at a specific liter flow because it is not advisable to "guess" what an $F_{I_{O_2}}$ will be. An $F_{I_{O_2}}$ can be determined from the patient's inspiratory flow rate, tidal volume, and inspiratory time. The clinical effectiveness of oxygen therapy can be determined by monitoring the Sp_{O_2}. If the exact amount of oxygen given is critical, for instance when oxygen toxicity is a concern, then devices that will deliver a specific $F_{I_{O_2}}$ (i.e., with an oxygen blender) should be used.

In general, some basic standards need to be observed in oxygen administration, regardless of the device used. First, the practitioner should explain to the patient what is being done and why. The practitioner must also make certain of the patient's identity and the right prescription. Standards of sterility and universal precautions should be observed in setting up equipment. This may mean the wearing of gloves and goggles if there is any potential for exposure of the mucous membranes to patient blood or bodily fluids. A careful explanation to the patient about safety precautions includes information on the necessity of a no-smoking environment and on monitoring the use of electrical items in the proximity of oxygen.

Nasal Catheter

Catheters are supplied in French sizes, usually 10, 12, and 14 Fr, with 14 Fr being the largest. The catheter is included in this chapter for completeness; however, its inclusion does not constitute an endorsement of its use. In fact, nasal catheters are rarely if ever used.

Nasal catheters are inserted directly into the nares. To insert the catheter properly, the distance from the tip of the nose to the lobe of the ear is measured, which allows placement in the posterior pharynx. The catheter should be lubricated with a water-soluble lubricant and then passed into the nares. Once placed, the catheter should be secured with tape to the nose. The catheter should always be used with a humidifier and should deliver flow in the range of 2 to 6 L/min. In theory, with the average patient, this should produce an $F_{I_{O_2}}$ in the range of 0.28 to 0.40. The actual catheter must be changed, alternating nares, every 8 hours. Complications with the catheter may include epistaxis, excessive drying of the nares, ulceration of the nares, discomfort, and obstruction to flow. In addition, the catheter may be a source of sepsis.

Nasal Cannula

The cannula is available in adult, pediatric, and neonatal sizes. The cannula is versatile, providing very low ranges of flow (1 to 4 L/min) to higher flows (6 to 8 L/min).

The cannula is by far the most commonly used delivery device because it is the most comfortable to the patient and generally meets the goal of increasing the $F_{I_{O_2}}$. It is secured, generally, with a lariat that loops behind the ears and under the chin. It may also be available with an around-the-head strap. For the rare patient with multiple allergies, ceramic cannulas are available, as opposed to the standard vinyl. The cannula may be routinely used without humidity at flow rates of less than 4 L/min. The ability to deliver the very low ranges depends on having a calibrated low-flow gauge because there is no way to ensure a liter flow *lower* than the lowest calibrated setting of a Thorpe tube. A cannula should deliver an $F_{I_{O_2}}$ in the range of 0.23 to 0.35. However, measurements of $F_{D_{O_2}}$ with a nasal cannula have shown up to a 40% variation in $F_{D_{O_2}}$ when minute ventilation is being altered.[37] This is due to the dilutional effect of mixing room air with a fixed amount of 100% oxygen. Obviously, extremes in tidal ventilation and inspiratory flow rates exert considerable influence on the delivered $F_{I_{O_2}}$; careful monitoring to avoid resultant hypoxemia is a critical factor in these patients.

Questions have always arisen about a possible variation in $F_{I_{O_2}}$ depending on whether the patient breathes through the mouth versus the nose. One study reviewed "normal" subjects and found that there was a significant difference between mouth and nose breathing in the concentration of oxygen.[35] This article authenticates the frequent observation that oxygen-dependent patients often place the cannula in their mouths during times of increased activity. Another study suggests that there may be a considerably higher $F_{I_{O_2}}$ with a nasal cannula than was originally thought. This study supports the belief that the most acceptable manner to titrate $F_{I_{O_2}}$ with a nasal cannula is to monitor Sp_{O_2} and Pco_2 values.[36] Complications with a cannula include skin breakdown, misapplication (specifically, the prongs may not be in the nares), and patient discomfort.[37]

Venturi Masks

The Venti mask, or Venturi mask, is really a series of exact concentration adapters that may be attached to a mask. The Venti mask is the only fixed-percentage, nonaerosol device available. The mask operates on the Bernoulli principle: by varying the size of the downstream orifice, specific air-oxygen entrainment ratios can be created (Table 26–4). Venti masks have fixed oxygen percentages, and although these may vary slightly with the manufacturer, they are generally 24, 28, 31, 35, 40, and 50% oxygen.

The Venturi mask is used to deliver a precise percentage of oxygen. Delivering a fixed percentage may be critical in a hypercapnic patient because the actual tracheal oxygen concentration will be insensitive to variations in the patient's minute volume, as is the case with the nasal cannula. Note in Table 26–4 that total flow rates with the more commonly used Venturi devices do not provide high flow rates to the patient when used in the 40 to 50% range. The thought that Venti masks are uniformly high-flow devices is misleading because of the delivery of gas flows of less than 40 L/min at an FI_{O_2} of 0.50. It is easy to imagine that the tachypneic patient, for example, will most likely not have his or her inspiratory flow needs met with these devices when this level of oxygen therapy is administered. In these cases, it is prudent to consider aerosol systems. The precision of the Venti mask has been examined by Woolner and Larkin, who found that the FI_{O_2} of these devices was affected when the inspiratory flow rates of a lung simulator exceeded 200 L/min.[42] They suggest that the Venti system is capable of generating delivered gas flows 30% greater than the patient's inspiratory flow demand. Other studies suggest that mask size may be an important variable in determining the delivered percentage of oxygen with these systems.[44]

The Venturi mask is used without particulate humidity because this may create a backflow that alters the entrainment ratio and may increase the FI_{O_2}. If humidity is critical, the Venturi mask may be used with a side-port adapter that allows placement of an aerosol generator. The advantage of the Venturi mask is its accuracy. The disadvantages are those associated with the use of a mask (i.e., the need for the patient to remove the mask for meals, expectoration, and so on) and the need for controlled flow rates, which may not meet the patient's flow demands.

Simple Oxygen Mask

Frequently, a nasal cannula will not meet the oxygen needs of the patient. In these instances, it is necessary to use mask systems for the

---

The Bernoulli principle stipulates that as fluid (gas) moves through a fixed orifice size, a predictable entrainment of surrounding fluid (gas) occurs. This mixing of fluids is thought to be due to the "dragging" of surrounding particles into the fluid stream, probably because of inherent intermolecular attraction (i.e., gas viscosity). The once-believed notion that a pressure drop at the fringes of the gas stream accounted for this mixing is not consistent with current understanding.[43]

The practitioner must make sure that nothing obstructs the entrainment port because less air entrained may lead to a higher concentration of delivered oxygen.

TABLE **26–4:** Total Flow from Venti Systems

FI_{O_2} (%)	Air-Oxygen Entrainment Ratio	Flow Rate (L/min)	
		Oxygen	*Total*
0.24	20:1	4	84
0.28	10:1	4	44
0.31	6:1	8	54
0.35	5:1	8	48
0.40	3:1	8	32
0.50	1.7:1	12	32

delivery of oxygen-enriched gas. The premise behind this method is to increase the reservoir for the patient's inspiratory needs. The nasal cannula makes use of the anatomic reservoir of the upper airway only. Adding a mask to the patient increases the reservoir from which the patient may breathe gas, which can result in an increased arterial oxygen content. This system can be further enhanced with the interposition of a second reservoir between the patient's mask and the source of oxygen. This typically takes the form of a reservoir bag, which is usually equipped with valving to permit breathing of room air in the event of accidental discontinuation of gas flow. The anatomic reservoir, the mask, and the reservoir bag all act synergistically to ensure that all of the patient's inspiratory needs are met by the delivery system. This is not to say that such a system works for all patients all the time. Clearly, the choice of flow device, the type and size of the mask, the fit of the mask to the face, and the patient's inspiratory flow all need to be factored into the design of a system that will meet the needs of a given patient.

The simple oxygen mask is a device that permits the delivery of a midrange of oxygen to the patient. An $F_{I_{O_2}}$ in the range of 0.35 to 0.50 can be expected with this appliance. If condensation appears in the mask, the flow rate should be increased. Again, this is a nonfixed concentration, so the exact $F_{I_{O_2}}$ will vary with the pattern of ventilation. The use of pulse oximetry to verify the goals of therapy is critical. Generally, humidifiers are not used with a simple mask.

Complications with the mask include discomfort, skin breakdown, and retention of exhaled carbon dioxide. Some patients will have a significant fear of suffocation associated with mask use. Masks generally share a problem with regard to the patient's having to remove the mask to drink, eat, or expectorate. Regardless of the flow rate used, the practitioner should make sure that the patient is comfortable. Anxiety may lead to hyperventilation, which may require increasing the oxygen flow rate to remove exhaled carbon dioxide.

The simple mask must be run at a liter flow sufficient to ensure removal of exhaled carbon dioxide, which should be no less than 6 L/min.

Partial Rebreathing and Nonrebreathing Masks

Although still dependent on patterns of ventilation for the exact concentration delivered, partial rebreathing and nonrebreathing masks allow the delivery of high concentrations of oxygen. Both types of mask are equipped with a reservoir bag that serves as a source of 100% oxygen from which the patient can breathe. On each side of the mask, between the reservoir bag and the mask (depending on whether it is a partial rebreathing or nonrebreathing mask), there will be a flap valve. The side flaps close during inspiration, thus allowing the patient to draw from the reservoir bag only. $F_{I_{O_2}}$ values as high as 0.90 can be achieved with this system. Removal of the valve between the mask and the bag creates a partial rebreathing mask. This allows some mixing of exhaled gas with the source gas, thus lowering the $F_{I_{O_2}}$ to perhaps 0.60 to 0.80. However, few data support the routine use of partial rebreathing systems. In fact, the possibility of significant carbon dioxide rebreathing exists with the interrupted flow of oxygen. Once again, the only accurate or meaningful assessment of $F_{I_{O_2}}$ occurs by viewing the end-result, the change in the patient's clinical status.

The most common use of a mask is in the form of an aerosol delivery system. As with the use of the Venti mask described previously, the use of an aerosol system must take into account the total flow of the delivery system. This concept stems from the fact that the common aerosol generators are entrainment devices that vary total flow from the system as a function of the FI_{O_2} setting. For example, gas flow to the patient may be in excess of 60 L/min at an FI_{O_2} of 0.30, but only 10 L/min at FI_{O_2} of 1.0. Obviously, this is an important consideration for the patient with acute lung disease who may be tachypneic. To this end, some use a system that places two nebulizers in "tandem" to achieve higher inspiratory flow rates for the delivery of an FI_{O_2} of greater than 0.50. This concept was examined by Foust and coworkers with a lung simulator that explored the efficacy of this system with varying breathing patterns.[39] They found the distal airway oxygen percentage to be consistently lower than the setting when the respiratory rate and the tidal volume were increased. This difference in the setting versus the actual FI_{O_2} exceeded 20% in some of their trials. They recommend a system that provides a consistent FI_{O_2} that is largely independent of the patient's breathing pattern. Blended oxygen, high-flow capability and a "closed" design (the use of a reservoir bag and flap valves) are the basic components of the system.

Humidification

Humidifying a gas implies the addition of molecular or particulate water to it. Gas, as it comes out of a wall, tank, or concentrator, is anhydrous. Historically, all gas was humidified. However, the current practice is to humidify gas delivered at a rate of greater than 4 L/min. Because gas from a nasal cannula is delivered into the nasal pharynx, which has a high absolute humidity, it is sufficiently saturated with water vapor by the time it enters the airway. The individual patient determines whether the delivered gas is too dry. A word of caution: most long-term patients always insist on humidification. It was common to humidify gas for these patients, so many will give nonspecific reasons why they "need" the extra humidity. It is also important to assess the need for humidity versus moisture. Humidity will not moisten the airway or deposit water vapor in it. If added water vapor is desirable in the airways, the practitioner needs to consider additional forms of therapy.

Special Oxygen Delivery Alternatives

A number of innovations are now available to the clinician. These newer modalities of oxygen delivery include

Elongated cannulas and oxygen tubing are available in lengths of 14, 25, and 50 feet, depending on the manufacturer.

- Elongated cannulas
- Concentrators
- Portable liquid systems
- Reservoir cannulas
- Transtracheal oxygen therapy
- Demand pulsators

Elongated Cannulas

Before the advent of elongated cannulas, linking together tubing using crude connections and eventually molded connectors to lengthen these devices was not uncommon. Manufacturers now make available elongated cannulas or oxygen tubing. There is no reason to increase the liter flow ordered when elongated tubing is used. By connecting a 50-foot cannula to a calibrated monitor, we have been unable to alter the actual flow on the basis of tubing length. However, there may be an increased risk of obstruction to flow in this tubing because of the added length.

Oxygen Concentrators

An oxygen concentrator is an electrical device, usually the size of a room humidifier, that extracts oxygen from room air and concentrates the oxygen until it reaches clinically appropriate concentrations (85 to 90%). The oxygen then delivered to the patient through the selected device is roughly 85 to 90% "pure." Usually, these units are limited to flows of no greater than 4 to 6 L/min. The two principles governing concentrators are the membrane oxygenator and the sieve bed, or sand bed. In general, oxygen concentrators offer a more convenient and affordable option to the patient committed to long-term oxygen therapy.

A certain period of time, usually 15 to 30 minutes, is required for the unit to achieve the desired concentration of oxygen. A concentrator must be regularly analyzed to ensure an FI_{O_2} greater than 0.85.

Portable Liquid Systems

Liquid oxygen delivery systems, a small version of the large liquid vessels found in health care facilities, are low-pressure systems that are supplied to the patient in the form of a large reservoir and a small portable unit to permit mobility. Some acute care facilities have initiated conversion to liquid systems for in-house patient transport. The advantages with liquid systems for the long-term patient include lower cost, the ability to store a larger volume of gas (in liquid form), and safety (low-pressure system). The disadvantages include safety (supports combustion); some dissipation of oxygen from the system, which is wasteful of gas, especially in the patient with only intermittent use; and the need for some manual dexterity to transfill the small vessel.

Reservoir Cannulas

A reservoir cannula is a conservation device that allows a buildup of oxygen in a reservoir or bladder, usually at the prongs, from which the patient may inspire. This allows a reduction in the liter flow of oxygen and thereby conserves gas.

Demand Systems

Demand systems, or pulsators, supply oxygen to the patient in "bursts" during the first 25% of inspiration. This allows considerable conservation of gas, as much as 50% in some studies. These systems are also limited to lower flows, usually of less than 6 L/min.[37]

Transtracheal Oxygen Therapy

First pioneered by Heimlich, transtracheal oxygen therapy is a method of delivering oxygen directly into the trachea by means of a small catheter inserted percutaneously. The primary value of this therapy is the conservation of oxygen achieved by reduced oxygen flow rates. Some secondary benefits include reduced work of breathing and increased exercise tolerance, although these are less well documented. Disadvantages include the invasiveness of the system, which can be a potential source of sepsis. Some problems have been reported with bleeding and obstruction of flow by mucous plugging. Daily maintenance is required to maintain catheter patency.

MONITORING THE PATIENT ON OXYGEN

The goal of oxygen therapy is to correct hypoxemia. A secondary goal is to correct the problem in a timely manner and with the use of noninvasive means whenever possible. The gold standard for measuring the effect of oxygen is arterial blood gas analysis. Because this is a painful and expensive procedure, the next best alternative is the Sp_{O_2}. Another monitor is usually the patient. The patient's subjective relief of dyspnea can sometimes define successful intervention.

Monitoring of the patient begins with a simple hello, a handshake, and a look. "Hello" elicits a response and provides a bare measurement of neurologic function. A handshake allows one to feel the temperature of the skin and to observe the color. It may also provide a measure of muscle strength. A quick look may reveal cyanosis, diaphoresis, or restlessness.

Pulse oximetry, or the Sp_{O_2} measurement, is the best noninvasive method of determining oxygenation status. In some situations, pulse oximetry may not be as useful as arterial blood gas analysis. These situations include when there is a decreased temperature or blood supply to the area used for monitoring. With pulse oximetry, as with any diagnostic procedure, the value obtained must be viewed with the patient's overall clinical status in mind. If the value appears to be questionable, question it and verify the results with a blood gas analysis.

Other monitoring tools available to the practitioner include the heart rate, respiratory rate, neurologic status, skin color, pattern of ventilation, and Sv_{O_2}.

HOME OXYGEN THERAPY

Home oxygen therapy is initiated when the physician decides that the patient's oxygenation status needs continued support. Beyond this, each third-party payer has a set of specific guidelines for reimbursement. It is important for practitioners to be aware of these guidelines. A patient who does not qualify for home oxygen therapy will probably be financially liable for the considerable cost of home oxygen therapy. Many carriers use the following guidelines, established and updated regularly by Medicare:

Pa_{O_2} of less than 55 mm Hg or Sp_{O_2} of less than 88% (taken at rest)
Pa_{O_2} of 56 to 59 mm Hg or Sp_{O_2} of less than 89% if one of the following also exists:
   Congestive heart failure with edema
   Cor pulmonale or pulmonary hypertension
   Erythrocythemia with a hematocrit of greater than 56%
Pa_{O_2} of greater than 60 mm Hg or Sp_{O_2} of greater than 90%

The Sp_{O_2} may be as acceptable as the blood gas analysis if there are no extenuating factors present, such as hypercapnia, low hemoglobin, or hemoglobin abnormalities.

Cyanosis, or the bluish tinting of the skin, which is most often seen in the lips or in the nail beds, may correlate with an Sp_{O_2} of less than 90%.

Sometimes the correlation of the pulse reported by the oximeter versus one measured by the practitioner can help in assessing the reliability of the oximetry reading.

A complete prescription that includes modality, flow or concentration, and duration per day, as well as anticipated total duration time, laboratory evidence, other forms of therapy tried, and indications, is required for home oxygen therapy.

Only with extensive physician documentation will there be a slight possibility of paid coverage. There must be a documented need for the patient to ambulate beyond 50 feet from the source gas for portable oxygen. These are strict guidelines given the clinical care provided in an acute environment. However, these are the established guidelines that must be observed. Frequently, a practitioner will be asked to exercise the patient to check on values after exercise.

MANAGING THE PATIENT ON OXYGEN THERAPY

Several types of therapist-driven protocols are in practice today. Two examples are

- Nasal cannula at 2 L/min as needed for shortness of breath. This is an order that requests that the patient have access to a nasal cannula delivering oxygen at a rate of 2 L/min when the patient is experiencing shortness of breath.
- Oxygen to maintain an Sp_{O_2} of greater than 91%. This is a request to deliver oxygen therapy to the patient in an amount sufficient to raise the Sp_{O_2} to a level of greater than 91%. This allows the clinician to determine the best method of doing this as well as to monitor the patient with specific goals in mind.

With the first example, which is the traditional method that physicians use to order oxygen therapy, several problems exist. First, there is no stated goal. Will the patient experience relief with the oxygen, how will this be determined, what factors will display shortness of breath, and so on? The second order is far more specific. Oxygen should be delivered in the most efficient manner to increase the patient's Sp_{O_2} to above 91%. There will be times when the Sp_{O_2} will not be clinically applicable.

Branching Logic

A branching logic diagram allows the practitioner to modify or discontinue oxygen therapy once it has been ordered. Usually, this is accomplished by a series of parameters with programmed responses. For example, if a patient's Sp_{O_2} is greater than 95%, wean oxygen and monitor the Sp_{O_2} every 30 minutes for 2 hours. Wean oxygen if the Sp_{O_2} is greater than 92%.

Open Loop or Care Plan

Our facility has developed a respiratory care plan that identifies a problem with the patient's respiratory system (e.g., hypoxemia).[38] The practitioner then evaluates the patient to determine the extent of the problem and decides on an appropriate course of action. This is loosely referenced to a series of clinical interventions that have been approved by the executive committee of the medical staff. The interventions set allows

- The practitioner to implement a response to the patient problem. This response is based on the existence and severity of the problem.

- A more timely and appropriate response to the problem than one that follows rigid guidelines.
- Proactive therapy and responses to the onset of problems. Under more traditional systems, the practitioner usually worked retroactively to ensure correct therapy, correcting problems after they had persisted for some time.

SUMMARY

This chapter provided an overview of the theory and process of clinical oxygen therapy. Clearly, other texts are more suited for readers needing in-depth explanations of the equipment for O_2 delivery. However, the practical material presented here regarding indications for therapy, adverse effects, and complications must be clearly understood by practitioners and therefore integrated into all aspects of clinical practice. The use of clinical protocols or care plans is a relatively new idea that shows much promise in the effective application of and weaning from this potent drug. It is conceivable that such protocols will become a national standard of practice for administering oxygen. Finally, as all new techniques of oxygen delivery gain acceptance, it is important that they, too, become fully incorporated into care plans to properly control and define their clinical use.

References

1. Greenwood NN, Earnshaw A. Oxygen. Chemistry of the Elements, 1st ed. Oxford, Pergamon Press, 1984, pp 698–707.
2. Emsley J. Oxygen. The Elements, 1st ed. Oxford, Clarendon Press, 1989, pp 134–135.
3. Germino VA. Medical history, Lavoisier: Disproving the phlogiston theory. Physicians Associates, July 1971, pp 84–86.
4. Richards CC. Oxygen—History, physics and chemistry. Inhalation Ther 13:5, 1968.
5. Encyclopaedia Britannica, Lavoisier, Antoine Laurent. Vol 10, 15th ed. Chicago, Helen Hemingway Benton, 1974, pp 713–714.
6. Encyclopaedia Britannica, Priestly, Joseph. Vol 14, 15th ed. Chicago, Helen Hemingway Benton, 1974, pp 1012–1014.
7. Encyclopaedia Britannica, Stahl, Georg Ernst. Vol 17, 15th ed. Chicago, Helen Hemingway Benton, 1974, p 566.
8. Garrett DF, Donaldson WP. Gas supply systems. *In* Physical Principles of Respiratory Therapy Equipment. Madison, Ohio Medical Products, 1975, pp 1–8.
9. McPherson SP, Spearman CB. Primary systems: Cylinders and piping systems. Respiratory Therapy Equipment, 2nd ed. St. Louis, CV Mosby, 1981, pp 33–68.
10. McPherson SP, Spearman CB. Primary systems: Gas administration devices. *In* Respiratory Therapy Equipment, 2nd ed. St. Louis, CV Mosby, 1981, pp 69–83.
11. McPherson SP, Spearman CB. Gas controlling devices and analyzing devices. *In* Respiratory Therapy Equipment, 2nd ed. St. Louis, CV Mosby, 1981, pp 153–160.
12. Ryerson GG, Block AJ. Oxygen as a drug: Clinical properties, benefits, modes, and hazards of administration. *In* Burton GG, Hodgkin JE, Ward JJ (eds). Respiratory Care, a Guide to Clinical Practice, 3rd ed. Philadelphia, JB Lippincott, 1991, pp 319–320.
13. Stoller JK. Misallocation of respiratory care services: Time for a change. Respir Care 38:263, 1993.
14. Small D, Duha A, Wieskopf B, et al. Uses and misuses of oxygen in hospitalized patients. Am J Med 92:591–595, 1992.
15. AARC. Oxygen therapy in the acute care hospital. Respir Care 36(12):1414, 1991.
16. Murray JF. Respiratory diseases. *In* Wyngaarden JB, Smith LH (eds). Cecil Textbook of Medicine, vol I, 18th ed. Philadelphia, WB Saunders, 1988, p 395–403.
18. Committee on Oxygen Therapy. Oxygen therapy in cardio-pulmonary diseases. Am Rev Respir Dis 101:332, 1970.
19. Kaplan RF. Postanesthetic problems. *In* Civetta JM, Taylor RW, Kirby RR (eds). Critical Care, 1st ed. Philadelphia, JB Lippincott, 1988, p 173.

20. Buran M. Oxygen consumption. *In* Snyder JV, Pinsky MR (eds). Oxygen Transport in the Critically Ill, 1st ed. Chicago, Year Book Medical Publishers, 1987, pp 16–20.
21. Guidelines for Medical Necessity. Chicago, Blue Cross and Blue Shield Association, 1982.
22. Uretsky BF, Lawless CE. Pharmacologic treatment of cardiogenic shock. *In* Snyder JV, Pinsky MR (eds). Oxygen Transport in the Critically Ill, 1st ed. Chicago, Year Book Medical Publishers, 1987, p 434–445.
23. Donegan JD (chairperson). Myocardial infarction. *In* Donegan JD, et al (eds). Textbook of Advanced Cardiac Life Support, 2nd ed. American Heart Association, 1990, p 12.
24. Kudrow L. Response of cluster headaches to oxygen inhalation. Headache 21:1, 1981.
25. Gallagher RM. Use of oxygen for headaches. *In* Drug Therapy for Headaches, 1st ed. Toronto, Marcel Dekker, 1991.
26. Fogan LA. A double blind comparison of oxygen versus air inhalation. Arch Neurol 42:362, 1991.
27. Fisher A (chairman). National Conference on Oxygen Therapy: Oxygen toxicity. Chest 86:2, 1984.
28. Jenkinson SG. Pulmonary oxygen toxicity. Clin Chest Med 3:1, 1982.
29. Comroe JH. Oxygen toxicity. *In* Physiology of Respiration. Chicago, Year Book Medical Publishers, 1965.
30. Ryerson GG, Block AJ. Oxygen as a drug: Clinical properties, benefits, modes, and hazards of administration. *In* Respiratory Care, 3rd ed. Philadelphia, JB Lippincott, 1991, pp 319–325.
31. Fischer AB. Oxygen therapy: Side effects and toxicity. Am Rev Respir Dis 5:2, 1980.
32. Pare JAP, Fraser RG. Synopsis of Diseases of the Chest. Philadelphia, WB Saunders, 1983, pp 597–599.
33. Kacmarek RM. Supplemental oxygen and other medical gas therapy. *In* Foundations of Respiratory Care, 1st ed. New York, Churchill Livingstone, 1992, pp 888–889.
34. Nash G. Pulmonary lesions associated with oxygen therapy and artificial ventilation. N Engl J Med 276:368, 1967.
35. Fulmer R, Snyder J. Report of the National Conference on Oxygen Therapy. Chest 86:2, 1986.
36. Dunleavey S, Tyl L. The effect of oral versus nasal breathing on oxygen concentration received from a nasal cannula. Respir Care 37:4, 1993.
37. Ooi R. An evaluation of oxygen delivery using nasal prongs. Anaesthesia 47:591, 1992.
38. Malloy R, Pierce M, McElroy PK, et al. Reduction of unnecessary care using a respiratory care plan. Respir Care 37:11, 1992.
39. Foust GR, Potter WA, Wilsons MD, Golden M. Shortcomings of using two jet nebulizers in tandem with an aerosol face mask for optimal therapy. Chest 99:1346, 1991.
40. Albin RJ, Criner GJ, Thomas S, Abou-Jaoude S. Pattern of non-ICU supplemental oxygen utilization in a university hospital. Chest 102:1672, 1992.
41. Jubran A, Tobin M. Reliability of pulse oximetry in titrating supplemental oxygen therapy in ventilator dependent patients. Chest 97(6):1420, 1990.
42. Woolner DF, Larkin J. An analysis of the performance of a variable type Venturi-type oxygen mask. Anaesth Intensive Care 8:44, 1980.
43. Sacci R. Air entrainment masks: Jet mixing is how they work; the Bernoulli and Venturi principles are how they don't. Respir Care 24:928, 1979.
44. Cox D, Gillbe C. Fixed performance oxygen masks: Hypoxic hazard of low capacity drugs. Anaesthesia 36:958, 1981.
45. Pierson D. Normal and abnormal oxygenation: Physiology and clinical syndromes. Respir Care 38(6):587, 1993.
46. Lindberg P, Gunnarson L. Atelectasis and lung function in the postoperative period. Acta Anaesthesiol Scand 36:546, 1992.
47. Maroko PR, Radvany P, Braunwald E. Reduction in infarct size by oxygen inhalation following acute coronary occlusion. Circulation 52:360, 1975.

27 Hyperbaric Oxygen Therapy

Richard E. Moon, M.D.

PRINCIPLES OF HYPERBARIC OXYGEN THERAPY

The goals of hyperbaric oxygen (HBO) therapy include

- Increasing the tissue P_{O_2} to levels higher than can be obtained at 1 atmosphere absolute (ATA).
- Increasing ambient pressure

With a blood hemoglobin level of 12 g/dL and an arterial P_{O_2} of 100 mm Hg, the total arterial O_2 content equals approximately 16.5 mL/dL, of which less than 2% is dissolved in the plasma. If the patient breathes 100% O_2 and attains an arterial P_{O_2} of 670 mm Hg, the total arterial O_2 content rises to 18.7 mL/dL, of which nearly 11% is dissolved. Under hyperbaric conditions, the amount of dissolved O_2 increases further. In a person at 3 ATA breathing 100% O_2, the arterial P_{O_2} is likely to be 1700 to 1800 mm Hg. The total arterial O_2 content rises to around 22 mL/dL, of which nearly 25% is dissolved in the plasma. Under these conditions, the amount of O_2 dissolved is approximately equivalent to the amount that would be carried in arterial blood under normal conditions at a hemoglobin concentration of 4 g/dL. Under hyperbaric conditions, it is therefore possible to sustain adequate O_2 delivery to tissues without any hemoglobin at all. Moreover, the additional O_2 carried in dissolved form in the plasma is not associated with increased blood viscosity, as normally occurs when the O_2 content increases by an equivalent amount with a blood transfusion.

An increased P_{O_2} in the pharmacologic range may have several therapeutic effects:

- Increased O_2 delivery to ischemic tissues may promote healing or granulation.
- An elevated P_{O_2} can also augment phagocytosis or antibiotic killing of bacteria or may have direct bacteriostatic or bactericidal properties, usually against anaerobic organisms.
- The vasoconstriction produced by pharmacologic hyperoxia can also reduce tissue edema.

Increased ambient pressure is useful to treat conditions in which there is pathologic tissue gas:

- Decompression sickness or arterial gas embolism in divers
- Accidental injections of gas during diagnostic or therapeutic procedures

Table 27–1 lists the range of pressures (and equivalent depths) that are commonly used in HBO therapy.

TABLE **27–1:**   Range of Pressures Used in Clinical Hyperbaric Oxygen Therapy

Ambient Pressure (ATA)	Equivalent Depth		
	Feet of Sea Water	*Meters of Sea Water*	
1	0	0	Sea level
2	33	10	⎫ Commonly used treatment
2.5	45	14	⎬ pressure range for chronic indications
2.8	60	18	Most commonly used initial treatment pressure for decompression illness
3.04	68	21	Duke treatment pressure for clostridial myonecrosis
6	165	50	Occasionally used for arterial gas embolism, using 21–50% O_2 patient breathing gas; produces significant nitrogen narcosis in tenders

ATA, atmospheres absolute.

INDICATIONS

Gas Bubble Disease

Breathing gas at increased ambient pressures results in inert gas uptake into tissue. During and after decompression, the tissues can become supersaturated, with gas bubbles developing in situ, leading to joint pain, neurologic symptoms, lymphedema, skin rash, or inner ear symptoms. During decompression, arterial gas embolism in divers occurs from pulmonary overexpansion due to breath holding or localized intrapulmonary gas trapping. Recompression therapy immediately reduces bubble size. Gas within bubbles can then be slowly eliminated if the pressure is reduced in a controlled fashion. Bubble shrinkage can be greatly augmented by having the patient simultaneously breathe 100% O_2. This additional benefit results from the washout of inert gas from the immediate environment of the bubble, thereby increasing the gradient for the diffusion of inert gas out of the bubble (Fig. 27–1).

HBO therapy remains the treatment of choice for gas bubble disease. Typically, a recompression schedule such as the one shown in Figure 27–2 is used. The patient is recompressed to 2.8 ATA. After a period of time, the chamber is then decompressed to 1.9 ATA. Periods of 100% O_2 breathing are interspersed with short "air breaks," which minimize pulmonary O_2 toxicity.

Carbon Monoxide

CO—carbon monoxide
HbCO—carboxyhemoglobin
HbO_2—oxyhemoglobin

M is a binding constant (approximately 200 to 250).
Pco is the partial pressure of CO.

Hemoglobin binds with CO 200 to 250 times more avidly than with O_2.

CO binds avidly to hemoglobin. At equilibrium, the ratio of HbCO to HbO_2 is described by the following equation:

$$\frac{[\text{HbCO}]}{[\text{HbO}_2]} = \frac{M P_{CO}}{P_{O_2}} \tag{27.1}$$

Indeed, the major mechanism for the toxic effect of CO is believed to be the occupation of hemoglobin by CO, which prevents its use in O_2 transport, and the increased affinity for O_2 of the remaining hemoglobin (shift

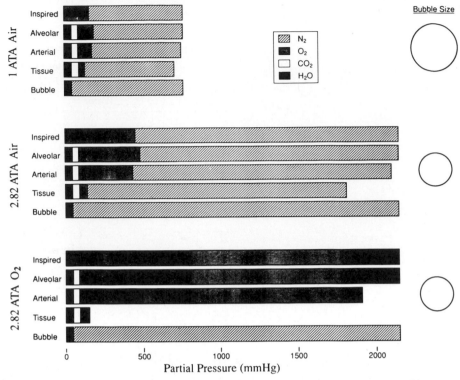

FIGURE 27–1: Treatment of bubbles with pressure and oxygen. Partial pressures of four gases in various locations are shown. The rate of resolution of a bubble depends on two factors: The diffusion of nitrogen from a bubble into adjacent tissue or blood, and the rate of transport of dissolved gas back to the lung (which may be related to tissue-phase diffusion, blood flow, and gas solubility). Tissue partial pressures are assumed to be equal to mixed venous values. Partial pressures within the bubble are shown at the time of or shortly after bubble formation (before O_2 and CO_2 have diffused into the bubble), at 1 ATA. While the patient is breathing air, there is a 142-mm Hg gradient tending to favor diffusion of nitrogen from bubble to tissue. If the ambient pressure is raised to 2.82 ATA (60 feet of sea water [fsw] equivalent depth) the bubble diameter is reduced by 29%, and the diffusion gradient for nitrogen increases to 432 mm Hg. If 100% O_2 is breathed, total tissue gas pressure is only 152 mm Hg. The resulting diffusion gradient for nitrogen is therefore increased dramatically to 2096 mm Hg, hastening bubble resorption. This is referred to as the "oxygen window." (From Moon RE. Treatment of gas bubble disease. Probl Respir Care 4:232–252, 1991.)

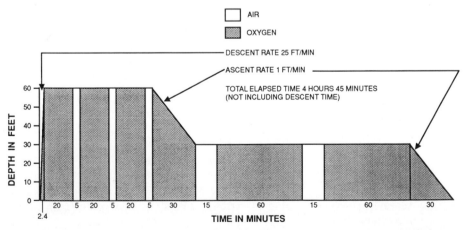

FIGURE 27–2: Recompression schedule (table) for treatment of neurologic decompression illness in patients with pain only or mild cutaneous symptoms that are not relieved within 10 minutes of reaching 60 feet breathing oxygen. This schedule can be extended at 60 feet and at 30 feet if symptoms have not been relieved within the first three oxygen cycles. A modified US Navy schedule has been designed at the Catalina Marine Science Center, allowing for up to five extensions at 60 feet. (From Moon RE. Treatment of gas bubble disease. Probl Respir Care 4:232–252, 1991.)

TABLE **27-2:**   Carbon Monoxide Elimination Half-Times Under Various Conditions

Breathing Gas	Ambient Pressure (ATA)	Mean Half-Life (min)*
Air	1	214
Oxygen	1	43
Oxygen	2.5	19

*Data from Pace N, Strajman E, Walker EL. Acceleration of carbon monoxide elimination in man by high pressure oxygen. Science 111:652, 1950.
ATA, atmospheres absolute.

of the HbO_2 dissociation curve to the left). CO also binds to other proteins, for example myoglobin and cytochrome aa_3. There is evidence that this binding results in direct tissue toxicity.

Inspection of Equation 27.1 reveals that at equilibrium, the fraction of hemoglobin that is occupied by CO is inversely proportional to the P_{O_2}. Because of this reciprocal relationship, an elevated blood P_{O_2} results in an acceleration of CO elimination. Table 27–2 shows the half-time of elimination of HbCO in persons breathing different gases. Presumably, a high P_{O_2} also hastens the elimination of CO from these other binding sites. Breathing O_2 at increased ambient pressure may also, by virtue of the increased plasma O_2 content, provide adequate O_2 delivery to tissues pending the removal of CO from the body.

Indeed, administration of HBO to patients with CO poisoning often results in a dramatic reversal of symptoms and neurologic signs. Evidence shows that HBO treatment of CO-poisoned patients with a history of impaired consciousness reduces the probability of long-term neurologic complications. Current controversy swirls around the appropriate selection of less severely poisoned patients for HBO treatment.

HBO therapy has also been used for both cyanide and hydrogen sulfide exposures, both of which impair cellular respiration by inhibition of cytochrome oxidase. Apparent improvement with HBO therapy has been reported, although the rationale for using HBO therapy for these exposures is less sound than that for CO poisoning.

Infections

Clostridial Myonecrosis

HBO therapy was suggested as a treatment for clostridial myonecrosis on the grounds that high tissue O_2 tension inhibits alpha-toxin production by clostridia while killing the organism. HBO treatment of patients with this condition often provides immediate clinical benefits, as evidenced by slowing of the spread of infection and a reduction in toxicity. Controlled animal studies support its efficacy. A typical treatment consists of exposure of the patient to 2.5 to 3 ATA for 90 minutes while the patient breathes 100% O_2. In conjunction with antibiotic therapy and surgical débridement, HBO treatments are given two to three times daily, for a total of five to 10 treatments.

Necrotizing Fasciitis and Other Mixed Aerobic and Anaerobic Infections

A similar rationale applies to the treatment of patients with mixed nonclostridial aerobic and anaerobic infections of the subcutaneous tissue or muscle. Because of the comparative rarity of these infections, no controlled studies exist. However, combined analysis clinical reports have suggested a beneficial effect of HBO therapy.

Chronic Infections

Human trials show the potential beneficial effect of HBO treatment as an adjunctive therapy for chronic osteomyelitis. The rationale for treatment is that osteomyelitic bone is hypoxic; the observed P_{O_2} in chronic osteomyelitic infection inhibits leukocytic killing of staphylococci and probably other microorganisms. Exposure of experimental animals to 2.5 ATA of O_2 normalizes the P_{O_2} in infected bone. Rhinocerebral mucomycosis has also been treated with HBO therapy, as an adjunct to surgery and antifungal chemotherapy. Treatment schedules for these disorders, as with most other nonacute indications, consist of multiple hyperbaric exposures once or twice daily, usually at 2 to 2.5 ATA for 90 to 120 minutes, for a total of 40 or more treatments.

Ischemic Wounds

Readings depend on edema, skin thickness, electrode temperature, patient position, and the use of vasoconstrictors (e.g., nicotine) or vasodilators (antihypertensive medications), all of which probably modulate the predictive value of Ptc_{O_2}.

For wounds in which the blood supply, and hence the tissue P_{O_2}, are insufficient to sustain neovascularization, intermittent HBO therapy may improve fibroblast proliferation and granulation. There is a correlation between healing and the transcutaneous P_{O_2} (Ptc_{O_2}) measurement at the site of the wound. At 1 ATA of breathing air, Ptc_{O_2} values of less than 15 to 20 mm Hg are associated with poor prognosis, indicating possible benefit from HBO therapy. Patients in whom the Ptc_{O_2} exceeds 100 mm Hg while they are breathing 100% O_2 at 2 to 2.5 ATA have a high likelihood of wound healing with HBO. Patients with wounds in which the Ptc_{O_2} exceeds 30 to 40 mm Hg while they are breathing air at 1 ATA are likely to heal without additional O_2 therapy. However, the Ptc_{O_2} is not a perfect predictor of failure or success.

Osteoradionecrosis and Soft Tissue Radiation Necrosis

Irradiated tissue may be chronically hypoperfused because of radiation-induced endarteritis. The tissue may have a sufficient blood supply for basal function but may be unable to complete healing in the event of injury or a surgical wound. In this disorder, intermittent HBO therapy usually results in an excellent clinical response. HBO therapy is also a valuable adjunctive therapy in individuals with osteoradionecrosis because it may, by virtue of its enhancement of neovascularization, permit subsequent surgical reconstruction.

Other Conditions

There is evidence for the efficacy of HBO therapy in several other conditions. A summary is given in Table 27–3.

THE HYPERBARIC ENVIRONMENT

When the ambient pressure is increased, the resultant increased partial pressure of each component gas results in several physical and biologic effects.

TABLE **27–3:** A Partial List of Conditions for Which There is Evidence of Efficacy for Hyperbaric Oxygen Therapy

Gas bubble disease
  Air embolism
  Decompression sickness
Poisoning
  Carbon monoxide
  Cyanide
  Hydrogen sulfide
Infections
  Clostridial myonecrosis
  Other soft tissue necrotizing infections
  Refractory chronic osteomyelitis
  Mucomycosis
Acute ischemia
  Crush injury
  Compromised skin flaps

Chronic ischemia
  Radiation necrosis (soft tissue radiation cystis and osteoradionecrosis)
  Ischemic ulcers, including diabetic ulcers
Central nervous system edema
Acute hypoxia
  Support of oxygenation during therapeutic lung lavage
  Exceptional blood loss anemia (when transfusion is delayed or unavailable)
Thermal injury (burns)

Altered Gas Physical Properties

Gas density increases in direct proportion to the ambient pressure. This results in increased resistance of gas flow within tubes, which includes the tracheobronchial tree and tracheal tubes and fluidic or pneumatic control devices. Pulmonary conductance (G) varies according to the following relationship:

$$G = G_0 r^{-k} \tag{27.2}$$

G_0 is conductance at 1 ATA.
r is gas density.
k is a constant (0.3 to 0.5).

Although there may be increased awareness of breathing, individuals with normal pulmonary mechanics will not experience respiratory difficulty under resting conditions. However, the increase in airway resistance can result in significant hypoventilation in spontaneously breathing individuals with severe obstructive lung disease. This factor, combined with the depressant effect of the elevated Po_2 on respiratory drive, can result in hypercapnia.

The altered density results in an altered voice ("Donald Duck voice"), which is nevertheless comprehensible with pressures in the usual clinical range (1 to 6 ATA). Altered function of fluidic ventilator circuitry is likely to cause a change in the delivered minute volume. Pressure-cycled ventilators are most likely to be affected. Volume-cycled ventilators are more reliable but should be monitored carefully during changes in ambient pressure because their operating characteristics may alter at these times. No significant changes in gas viscosity occur over the therapeutic pressure range (1 to 6 ATA).

Increased Partial Pressure of Nitrogen

At increased pressure, the narcotic properties of nitrogen become evident. Mild euphoria may be evident around pressures of 2.5 to 3 ATA, but at 4 to 6 ATA, significant performance decrements can be measured. Some individuals experience frank intoxication, with inappropriate laughter and difficulty in concentrating. Tasks such as setting a ventilator, zeroing a transducer, or inflating the balloon on a pulmonary artery catheter can be performed erroneously; confirmation by someone outside the chamber may be needed to ensure accuracy and appropriate technique.

Increased Partial Pressure of Oxygen

Increased P_{O_2} values can produce toxicity, which is most apparent in two forms. Central nervous system O_2 toxicity, although infrequent at ambient P_{O_2} values of less than 2 ATA (less than 0.02% of exposures), becomes rapidly more probable as P_{O_2} is increased. At an inspired P_{O_2} of 3.06 ATA, around 4% of HBO treatments result in convulsions. Provided that no secondary complications of the seizures (e.g., aspiration) occur, hyperoxic convulsions leave no permanent sequelae. Symptoms or signs of O_2 toxicity are effectively managed by having the patient breathe air for a few minutes until the symptoms resolve. Small doses of benzodiazepines can be used to control or prevent symptoms. Other anticonvulsants, such as phenobarbital or phenytoin, have also been effectively used as prophylaxis against hyperoxic seizures.

Pulmonary O_2 toxicity develops more slowly. Objective measurements may include a decrease in vital capacity. Prolonged exposure to a high P_{O_2} can ultimately result in adult respiratory distress syndrome and pulmonary fibrosis. The rate at which pulmonary O_2 toxicity develops depends on the inspired P_{O_2}. Although mild symptoms can occur after long treatments (e.g., see Fig. 27–2), clinical HBO protocols are designed to avoid more serious pulmonary O_2 toxicity. Intermittent rather than continuous exposure results in a slower onset of toxicity (Fig. 27–3). Susceptibility to O_2 toxicity varies with the individual; this susceptibility may also exhibit diurnal or day-to-day variability.

Central nervous system toxicity

- Muscular twitching
- Vertigo
- Nausea (with or without vomiting)
- Tremors
- Convulsions

Symptoms of pulmonary O_2 toxicity

- Retrosternal burning
- Pain on inspiration
- Cough

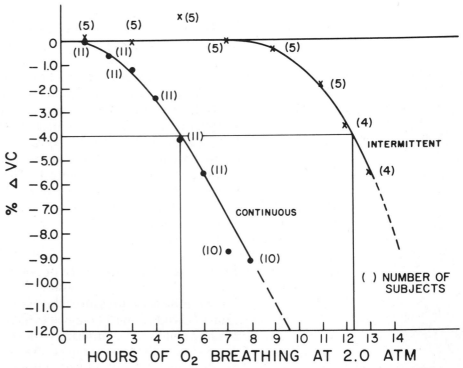

FIGURE 27–3: Rate of development of pulmonary oxygen poisoning in normal men during continuous and intermittent oxygen breathing at 2.0 ATA. VC, vital capacity. (From Clark JM. Oxygen toxicity. *In* Bennett P, Elliot DH [eds]. The Physiology and Medicine of Diving. 4th ed. Philadelphia, WB Saunders, 1993, pp 121–169.)

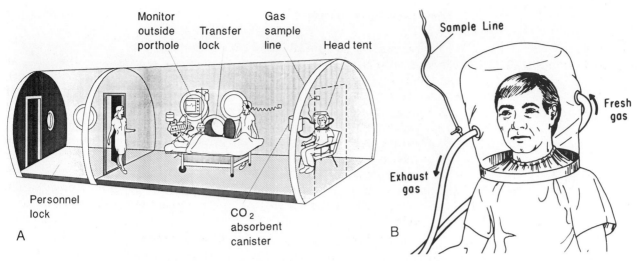

FIGURE 27–4: *A,* Hospital-based multiplace chamber. Patients may receive oxygen either using a tight-fitting oronasal mask (not shown) or a head tent or via endotracheal tube. Many patients may typically be treated simultaneously. Medical personnel (tenders) usually accompany the patient during treatment. Additional personnel may enter or leave the chamber while it is at pressure through a personnel lock. Supplies (drugs and food) may be locked in and out of the chamber through a transfer lock. Monitors are typically kept outside the chamber and may be viewed through a porthole. The chamber atmosphere is usually compressed air. *B,* Head tent used to deliver oxygen to awake patients in multiplace chambers. Oxygen flow at a rate of 30 to 60 L/min delivered at pressure will usually maintain a head tent O_2 concentration of greater than 98% and a CO_2 concentration of less than 0.1%. Patient treatment gas may be monitored with a sample line, preferably connected to the expired limb of the circuit. This will also facilitate the detection of leaks (manifested as low inspired O_2). (*A* and *B,* From Moon RE, Camporesi EM. Clinical care at altered environmental pressures. *In* Miller RD [ed]. Anesthesia. New York, Churchill Livingstone, 1994, p 2285.)

HYPERBARIC CHAMBER OPERATIONS

Hyperbaric chambers are classified by the number of individuals that can conveniently occupy them. Multiplace chambers, in which more than one individual can be recompressed (Figs. 27–4 and 27–5), may hold from two to 10 or more individuals. These chambers are compressed with air while the patient breathes 100% O_2 with either a face mask, a head tent, or an endotracheal tube. The patient is usually accompanied by a nurse, a physician, a respiratory therapist, or other medical personnel ("tenders") who monitor and provide immediate care for the patient. Usually manufactured of Plexiglas, monoplace chambers can hold only one individual (Figs. 27–6 to 27–8). Most commonly, monoplace chambers are compressed with 100% O_2, removing the necessity for an auxiliary gas supply. A monoplace chamber can not hold a tender unless the patient is an infant or a small child. Some monoplace chambers are fitted with masks that have a demand regulator (built-in breathing system), from which the patient may breathe air (for an air break) during prolonged treatment; alternatively, the chamber may be compressed with air while the patient breathes O_2 from the built-in breathing system supply. This latter configuration is somewhat safer: if the patient has a hyperoxic convulsion, the mask falls away from the patient's face, allowing the patient's inspired Po_2 to decrease to a safe level.

Care of critically ill patients is generally easier in a multiplace chamber because any practical intervention can be readily performed by an inside tender. At one time, it was considered mandatory to treat a critically ill individual in a multiplace rather than a monoplace chamber. However, the technology of monoplace chamber operations has advanced sufficiently so that intravenous fluid administration, hemodynamic mon-

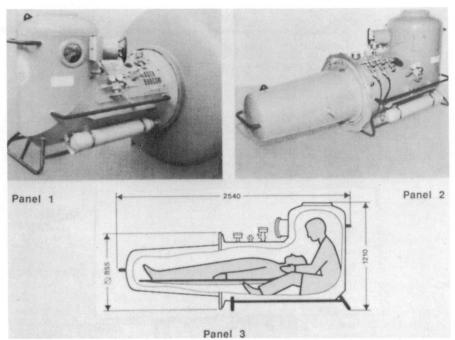

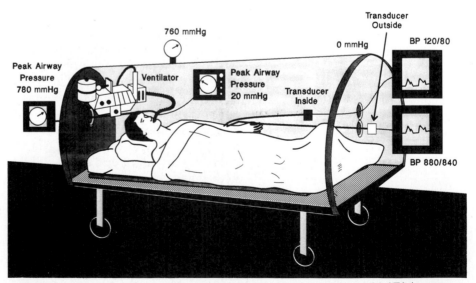

FIGURE 27–5: Portable multiplace chamber designed for transportation of divers. Depicted is the Dräger Duocom (manufactured by Dräger, Lübeck, Federal Republic of Germany; distributed in North America by National Draeger, Pittsburgh, PA). Entry into the chamber is accomplished by removing the tapered "boot" (panel 2). A diver and a tender can be accommodated, as shown in panel 3. There is a mating flange that will allow the Duocom to be connected to an appropriately fitted larger multiplace chamber (panel 1), permitting transfer of an injured diver under pressure. The chamber weighs 225 kg and can be compressed to 6 ATA. (Courtesy of National Draeger, Pittsburgh, PA.)

FIGURE 27–6: Monoplace chamber compressed to an absolute pressure of 2 ATA (gauge pressure, 1 ATA or 760 mm Hg). When measured with respect to atmospheric pressure, all pressures (e.g., blood pressure [BP] and airway pressure) are increased by 760 mm Hg. For example, if arterial pressure measured with respect to chamber pressure (transducer inside the chamber) is 120/80, the value recorded with respect to atmospheric pressure (transducer outside the chamber) would be 880/840. Sample values for peak airway pressure are similarly shown.

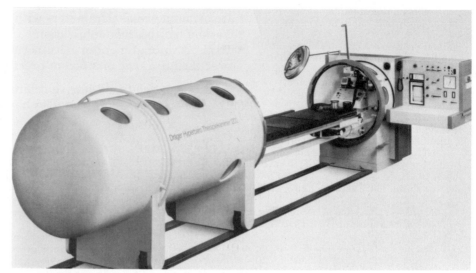

FIGURE 27–7: Draeger HTK 1200 monoplace hyperbaric chamber. (Courtesy of National Draeger, Pittsburgh, PA.)

itoring, mechanical ventilation, and chest tube management can all be performed inside a monoplace chamber (see the following sections).

Ventilators

An ideal ventilator for a hyperbaric environment includes the following features:

- Small size and portability
- No requirement for electrical power

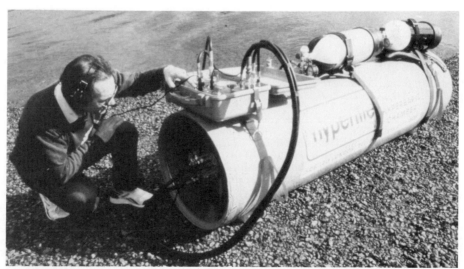

FIGURE 27–8: The SOS hyperbaric chamber. This monoplace chamber constructed of Kevlar is designed for treatment of decompression illness. It is compressed with air from a scuba tank. 100% O_2 can be delivered to the patient via an oronasal mask. Headset voice communication is incorporated. Unoccupied, the device weighs only 40 kg, and when not in use, it can be folded up in concertina fashion and placed with its accessories in a case small enough to be carried as "checked baggage" on a commercial aircraft. (Courtesy of SOS, London, England.)

- Invariant delivery parameters with changing ambient pressure
- Lack of hydrocarbon lubrication
- Expired volume monitor with accurate measurement of tidal volume over the full range of ambient pressures

Although relatively few ventilators have been specifically designed for hyperbaric use, a large number have been used or adapted (Table 27–4).

TABLE **27–4:** Ventilators Used in Hyperbaric Chambers

Ventilators	Comments	References
Bennett PR-2	Controlling circuitry can be separated from the actuator and kept outside the chamber	Weaver LK. Probl Resp Care 4:189, 1991
Bird	Pressure-cycled ventilators; operating characteristics vary significantly as ambient pressure changes	Gallagher TJ. Aviat Space Environ Med 49:375, 1978
Dräger Oxylog	Extremely compact fluidically controlled ventilator	
Dräger Hyperlog	Extremely compact fluidically controlled ventilator designed specifically for hyperbaric use	Pelaia P, Volturo P, Rocco M, et al. Minerva Anestesiol 56:1371, 1990
Logic 03		Deganque C, Lamy M, Stas M. Acta Anaesthesiol Belg 28:251, 1977
Monaghan 225	Fluidically controlled ventilator; satisfactory performance at least to 7 ATA with some slowing of rate at increasing ambient pressure; modification possible to allow compressed air actuation	Moon RE, Bergquist LV, Conklin B, et al. Chest 89:846, 1986
Ohio 550	Fluidically controlled ventilator; preliminary tests at Duke revealed satisfactory operation to 4 ATA	
Penlon Nuffield 200		Lewis RP, Szafranski J, Bradford RH, et al. Anaesthesia 46:767, 1991
Penlon Oxford	Successfully tested at 31 ATA	Saywood AM, Howard R, Goad RF, et al. Anaesthesia 37:740, 1982
Pneumatic Emerson	Controller; intermittent mandatory ventilation circuit may be added separately if needed; originally designed using leather bellows and mineral oil lubricant, which would require modification for safe hyperbaric use	Gallagher TJ: Aviat Space Environ Med 49:375, 1978
pneuPAC Variant HB	Compact ventilator designed for use in monoplace chambers	Spittal MJ, Hunter SJ, Jones L. Br J Anaesth 67:488, 1991
Sechrist 500A	Compact fluidically controlled ventilator designed for monoplace chamber use; some alteration of performance with changes in supply pressure, and thoracic compliance and at ambient pressures of higher than 2.2 ATA	Weaver LK. Probl Respir Care 4:189, 1991
Siemens 900C	Sophisticated, compact, electronically controlled ventilator; high O_2 levels near electrical components; expired volume monitor may not be accurate except at 1 ATA	Davis JC, Hunt TK (eds). Problem Wounds: The Role of Oxygen. New York, Elsevier, 1988, p 195

ATA, atmospheres absolute.

In order to prevent excessive O_2 leakage into a multiplace chamber, expired gas must be scavenged. Ventilators that use compressed O_2 in their control circuitry (e.g., the unmodified Monaghan 225) should also have scavenging tubing placed under the ventilator cowling. The Monaghan 225 ventilator can be modified for inspired hyperbaric performance, as shown in Figure 27–9.

Compression of the endotracheal tube cuff as the ambient pressure increases is likely to result in loss of seal. Filling the cuff with water avoids the need for continual adjustment of cuff volume during chamber compression and decompression. Expired volume can be measured with any device that does not alter its characteristics with changes in gas density. Screen-type pneumotachs, such as are used in the Siemens 900C, will lose their calibration under hyperbaric conditions. Simple monitors such as the Bennett or Wright spirometers can be readily used, although some Bennett spirometers will not cycle appropriately at ambient pressures of higher than about 4 ATA. The Ohmeda expired volume monitor has less than 5% error when used at ambient pressures of up to 6 ATA (its accurate range may be higher, but to my knowledge it has not been tested at greater than 6 ATA).

Monitoring

For reasons of safety, electronic instrumentation should be kept outside the chamber as much as possible. Bioelectrical or transducer signals can be transmitted from patient to preamplifier via through-hull penetrators. In particular, cathode ray tubes are potentially susceptible to implosion. However, monitors with liquid crystal displays have been successfully used in hyperbaric chambers.

Blood Gases

Values for arterial pH, P_{CO_2}, and bicarbonate are relatively unchanged during hyperbaric therapy, whereas P_{O_2} is generally elevated to between 1000 and 1800 mm Hg, depending on the treatment pressure and the patient's gas exchange efficiency. Table 27–5 shows mean values for a series of normal volunteers. Accurate measurement of pH, P_{CO_2}, and bicarbonate can be made on arterial blood samples anaerobically sealed and decompressed. However, P_{O_2} values measured in decompressed blood samples are likely to be inaccurate because (1) O_2 will be supersaturated at 1 ATA of ambient pressure and will tend to diffuse

TABLE **27–5:** Mean Blood Oxygen, Acid-Base, and Cardiovascular Responses to Hyperbaric Oxygenation

				Arterial Blood						Venous Blood*			
Atmospheric Pressure (ATA)	Inspired Gas	Inspired P_{O_2} (mm Hg)	$P_{A_{O_2}}$ (mm Hg)	P_{O_2} (mm Hg)†	pH†	P_{CO_2} (mm Hg)†	Ca_{O_2} (mL/dL)	Ca_{O_2} Dissolved (mL/dL)	O_2 Dissolved (%)	P_{O_2} (mm Hg)†	pH†	P_{CO_2} (mm Hg)†	Cardiac Output (L/min)†
1	Air	150	102	89	7.45	37	16.3	0.3	2	41	7.42	41	6.1
1	O_2	713	673	507	7.46	37	18.2	1.5	8	57	7.42	42	5.8
3.04	Air	475	427	402	7.45	39	17.9	1.2	7	68	7.41	44	5.7
3.04	O_2	2263	2223	1721	7.47	37	21.8	5.2	24	424	7.40	45	5.3

*Obtained from a catheter with the tip at the junction of the superior vena cava and the right atrium.

†Data from Whalen RE, Saltzman HA, Holloway DH, et al. Cardiovascular and blood gas responses to hyperbaric oxygenation. Am J Cardiol 15:638–646, 1965.

‡Calculated from measured arterial P_{O_2}, assuming a hemoglobin level of 12 g/dL.

ATA, atmospheres absolute.

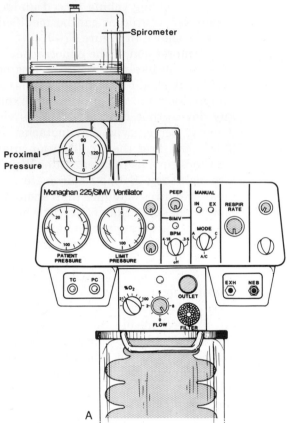

FIGURE 27–9: Monaghan 225 ventilator and modification for use in multiplace chambers. *A* shows the unmodified ventilator, with an added pressure gauge that is connected to the patient end of the ventilator circuit in order to monitor airway pressure. In order to allow the ventilator to be actuated with compressed air rather than oxygen and to obviate the use of the Venturi air–O_2 mixer (which cannot be relied on to deliver an accurate O_2 concentration while under pressure), the ventilator has been modified as shown in *B.* The Venturi control has been removed and the inspired O_2 setting has been permanently set at 21% so that all gas delivered to the patient is entrained through the filter, which usually admits room air. A gas-mixing circuit has been connected to this inlet with separate O_2 and airflow controls. A 5-L reservoir bag is used to buffer the gas requirement. A subambient pressure relief valve allows chamber air to be entrained if the gas supply fails. A positive pressure relief valve with flowmeter allows excess O_2 to be scavenged via the chamber overboard dump system. (*A* and *B,* From Moon RE, Bergquist LV, Conklin B, et al. Monaghan 225 ventilator use under hyperbaric conditions. Chest 89:846–851, 1986.)

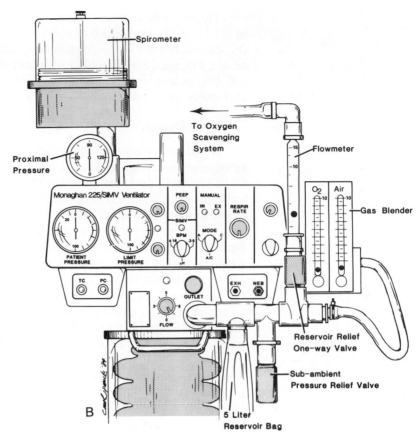

FIGURE 27–9: *Continued*

into small bubbles within the syringe, thereby decreasing the blood PO_2 and (2) PO_2 electrodes at 1 ATA cannot be accurately calibrated to values higher than around 700 mm Hg. However, if the blood gas measurement is made immediately after decompression, with a clinical blood gas analyzer, the PO_2 measurement may be acceptably accurate for clinical purposes. Indeed, such measurements made outside the chamber with a Radiometer ABL330 analyzer are only about 6% low. Provided that the interval between decompression and measurement is short, PO_2 measurements obtained at 1 ATA are sufficiently accurate for clinical purposes. More accurate PO_2 measurements can be obtained with a blood gas machine that is calibrated and operated inside the chamber.

If arterial PO_2 measurement is desirable for a given patient but not possible in practice, the estimated PO_2 can be calculated using a constant arterial-alveolar PO_2 ratio (Pa_{O_2}/PA_{O_2}). The following equation can be used to calculate alveolar PO_2:

PB is ambient pressure.

PH_2O is the saturated vapor pressure of water.

PA_{CO_2} is alveolar PCO_2 (usually assumed to equal arterial PCO_2).

FI_{O_2} is the inspired concentration of O_2.

R is the respiratory quotient (usually assumed to be equal to 0.8).

At 37°C, PH_2O is 47 mm hg.

$$PA_{O_2} = (PB - PH_2O) \times FI_{O_2} - PA_{CO_2} \times \left[FI_{O_2} + \frac{(1 - FI_{O_2})}{R} \right] \quad (27.3)$$

Predicted arterial PO_2 (PO_{2pred}) can then be calculated from Equation 27.4:

$$PO_{2pred} = a/A \times [(760 \times PATA - 47) - Pa_{CO_2}] \quad (27.4)$$

where PATA is the chamber pressure in atmospheres absolute, Pa_{CO_2} is the 1 ATA arterial PCO_2, and a/A is Pa_{O_2}/PA_{O_2} calculated from 1 ATA values.

These prediction equations have been validated over the range of 1 to 3 ATA. In the presence of baseline lung disease, the predicted arterial Po_2 calculated with the previous equations tends to underestimate the actual Po_2 because the effect of intrapulmonary shunt to decrease arterial Po_2 is less under hyperbaric conditions, when mixed venous Po_2 is extremely high (see Table 27–5) or approaches 100%.

Blood Pressure

Noninvasive measurement of blood pressure with a stethoscope and sphygmomanometer will work satisfactorily inside hyperbaric chambers. Only anaeroid pressure gauges should be used, however, because residual mercury from accidental spillage can provide a permanent source of chamber contamination with mercury vapor.

Although all pressures within the body increase in proportion to the ambient pressure (see Figure 27–6), intravascular pressures remain within usual clinical ranges when they are referenced to chamber atmosphere. Standard strain gauge pressure transducers work satisfactorily inside chambers, with no modification necessary. Intraflow devices, which provide a constant, low-level infusion of saline to prevent intraluminal clot formation, also function properly. However, if gas-pressurized bags are used, the pressure must be adjusted during compression and decompression to maintain the usual 300-mm Hg differential. Chamber compression and the attendant increase in ambient temperature tend to produce an offset error in large, nondisposable pressure transducers. The practitioner may therefore want to rebalance (rezero) such pressure transducers at the end of each stepwise change in ambient pressure. This does not appear to be necessary with the small, disposable transducers most commonly in use. Figure 27–10 shows a method of using arterial pressure transducers in monoplace chambers.

It is important to remember that all enclosed gas-containing spaces will be compressed or decompressed according to the ambient pressure of the chamber. For example, a bubble in the arterial transducer tubing enlarges during decompression. For this reason, the practitioner should ensure that the balloon channel of a pulmonary artery catheter remains open, with no syringe attached, during compression and decompression. Inadvertently leaving the inflation syringe on the balloon port during decompression usually results in rupture of the balloon and injection of gas into the patient.

Intravenous Fluid Administration

Gas within the drip chambers of intravenous administration sets compresses or expands according to the chamber ambient pressure. These changes may require constant adjustment, particularly during decompression, to prevent intravenous injection of air. Extreme care must be taken when glass intravenous containers are being used because failure of venting during decompression may result in explosion.

If possible, glass intravenous fluid containers should not be used in hyperbaric environments.

Infusion pumps require special care. Those that maintain the infusion rate by counting droplets may malfunction during compression and decompression of the chamber: the droplet count at the drip chamber may be significantly affected by changes in the drip chamber gas volume. Other types of infusion pumps (e.g., the Abbott Plum, Abbott Laboratories) work extremely well without adjustment of the settings over the therapeutic pressure range.

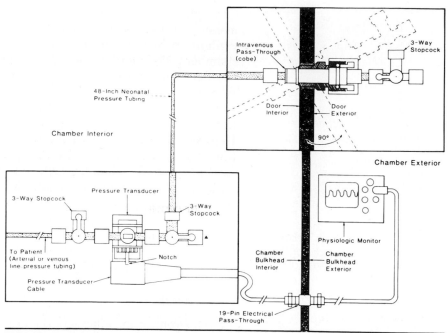

FIGURE 27–10: Pressure monitoring system that permits sampling of blood from a patient who is pressurized within the monoplace chamber. Either the intraflow can be removed or the three-way stopcock can be turned off to the intraflow. Neonatal pressure tubing minimizes the system dead space. The catheter needs to be periodically flushed from outside the chamber to keep it patent. (From Weaver LK. Clinical application of hyperbaric oxygen—monoplace chamber use. In Moon RE, Camporesi EM [eds]. Clinical Applications of Hyperbaric Oxygen. Probl Respir Care 4:189–214, 1991.)

Delivery of intravenous fluids to patients in monoplace chambers can be accomplished by an infusion pump inside the chamber, controlled from outside, or by an exterior pump. The latter method is preferred in most US monoplace facilities. In order to generate flow, the pump must develop sufficient pressure to overcome the resistance of the tubing, the patient's venous pressure, and the chamber ambient pressure. A pump designed for this purpose has been developed (IVAC 530, IVAC Corporation, San Diego, CA).

Atmosphere Control

Control of the atmosphere includes the following factors:

- Temperature
- O_2
- CO_2
- Pollutants

Rapid chamber compression results in an increase in temperature, whereas cooling occurs during decompression. These temperature changes over the clinical range of pressure are not dangerous, but they may be disconcerting to the uninitiated patient or tender. Rapid decompression can also result in the condensation of water droplets within the chamber, which can transiently impair visibility to a minor degree. Most large multiplace chambers have the ability to heat or cool the atmosphere to a comfortable temperature. Although the atmosphere of monoplace chambers is 100% O_2 by design, the practitioner must be vigilant about not allowing excessive O_2 accumulation within multiplace chambers. The main danger of a high ambient O_2 concentration is fire. If possible, the O_2 concentration inside multiplace chambers should not exceed 22 to 23%.

During short periods of hyperbaric therapy, CO_2 accumulation does not usually occur rapidly enough to result in clinically significant levels. However, occasionally patients with decompression illness will be maintained at a therapeutic pressure for several days (saturation treatment). In this event, the chamber CO_2 concentration should be monitored and maintained at safe levels (usually less than around 4 mm Hg of partial pressure) by using CO_2 scrubbing or by venting the chamber with fresh gas.

Because of the entirely enclosed atmosphere, trace contaminants can build up and reach toxic partial pressures. The source gas used for chamber compression should be analyzed periodically for impurities.

Barotrauma

Gas-containing spaces in the body, such as those in the lung, middle ear, paranasal sinuses, and gastrointestinal tract, are all subject to compression and decompression during hyperbaric treatment. Failure to equilibrate these gas spaces with ambient pressure can result in bleeding or fluid accumulation, rupture (e.g., of the tympanic membrane) during compression, or explosive rupture during decompression. Holding one's breath during decompression or air trapping within the lung due to local airway pathology can result in pneumothorax, pneumomediastinum, or arterial gas embolism. Although otic barotrauma and, to a lesser extent, sinus barotrauma are relatively common during hyperbaric therapy, pulmonary barotrauma is extremely rare. Despite the high frequency of lung pathology among patients requiring hyperbaric therapy, I am aware of only two instances of pulmonary barotrauma during decompression from therapeutic HBO exposure. Nevertheless, reversible airway obstruction should preferably be treated before hyperbaric therapy is used. The condition of patients with cystic or bullous lung disease or severe lung airway obstruction should be considered carefully before hyperbaric therapy is instituted.

Otic barotrauma can usually be managed by careful coaching of the patient in methods for equalizing pressure in the middle ear, by the nasal application of topical vasoconstrictors or by myringotomy. Although some physicians believe that in unconscious patients the middle ear automatically equilibrates via the eustachian tube, others perform routine myringotomy for such individuals.

Decompression Sickness

Tenders who breathe air are at potential risk for decompression sickness due to tissue bubble formation. Such instances are rare because depth-time exposures are usually insufficient to generate tissue bubbles, the chamber is kept warm during decompression, and decompression rates are slow. The risk of decompression sickness can be further minimized by having tenders breathe 100% O_2 during decompression. Duke guidelines call for O_2 breathing during all decompressions from 50 feet (2.5 ATA) to the surface or for 15 minutes, whichever is less. Because the patient breathes 100% O_2 throughout treatment, he or she will not develop decompression sickness.

Significant elevations in the CO_2 level may cause hyperpnea or respiratory acidosis and may contribute to narcosis.

Toxic substances include alcohol (from skin disinfectant solutions), mercury vapor (from broken glass thermometers or sphygmomanometers), sulfur dioxide (from lithium batteries), and hydrocarbons and CO (from compressor malfunction). Volatile substances, mercury, and batteries other than alkaline cells should be kept out of the chamber entirely.

Fire

Because of the elevated atmospheric P_{O_2}, combustion occurs significantly more quickly in hyperbaric environments. Fires in monoplace chambers compressed with 100% O_2 usually incinerate the chamber before any corrective action can be taken. A recent monoplace fire was caused by a sparking toy taken into the chamber by a child, who died of burns within a few seconds. Another fire occurred in a multiplace chamber when a prewarmed sheet was passed into a chamber at 2 ATA through the transfer lock: the additional heat engendered during compression caused the sheet to catch on fire.

To minimize this risk, all flammable materials should be removed from the patient before the patient enters the chamber. Sources of spark and heat should be minimized. If 110-V power is required, it should be delivered to the instrument via a connection that cannot easily be disconnected (e.g., Arktite Series, Crouse-Hines, Division of Cooper Industries, Syracuse, NY). Further safety can be ensured by purging the electrical housing of appliances with 100% N_2 at 3 to 4 L/min by attaching Luer or other convenient fittings to holes drilled in the instrument cowling.

If the patient requires defibrillation, all flammable material must be removed from the immediate environment. A low-resistance electrical gel (e.g., Signa gel, Parker Laboratories, Orange, NJ) is recommended to lower the electrical impedance between the paddles and the skin; the heat generated during defibrillation is thus minimized.

Flame-retardant treatment of clothing and bed linen may offer some additional safety. Patients should not be allowed to go into the chamber with greasy hair. The humidification of breathing gas helps to prevent the buildup of static charge and the potential for sparking within head tents. Hydrocarbon lubricants must be avoided. Hydrocarbons in contact with aluminum may spontaneously ignite in the presence of a high ambient P_{O_2}. Fluorocarbon lubricant is preferred for applications within the chamber.

SUMMARY

HBO therapy has many indications for use, including

- Gas bubble disease
- Poisoning
- Infections
- Acute and chronic ischemia
- Central nervous system edema
- Acute hypoxia
- Thermal injury

The use of HBO therapy requires knowledgeable practitioners, strict adherence to procedures and safety measures, and modifications to equipment to meet the physical changes encountered at higher atmospheres.

Suggested Readings

Bennett PB, Elliott DH (eds). The Physiology and Medicine of Diving, 4th ed. Philadelphia, WB Saunders, 1993.

Bove AA, Davis JC (eds). Diving Medicine. Philadelphia, WB Saunders, 1990.

Camporesi EM, Barker AC (eds). Hyperbaric Oxygen Therapy: A Critical Review. Bethesda, MD, Undersea and Hyperbaric Medical Society, 1991.

Edmonds C, Lowry C, and Pennefather J. Diving and Subaquatic Medicine. Boston, Butterworth-Heinemann, 1992.

Holcomb JR, Matos-Narrarro AV, Goldmann RW. Critical care in the hyperbaric chamber. *In* Davis JC, Hunt TK (eds). Problem Wounds: The Role of Oxygen. New York, Elsevier, 1988, pp 187–209.

Moon RE, Camporesi EM. Clinical Care at Altered Environmental Pressure. *In* Miller RD (ed). Anesthesia. New York, Churchill Livingstone, 1994, pp 2277–2306.

Moon RE, Camporesi EM (eds). Probl Respir Care 4(2), 1991.

Persels J. Hyperbaric medicine—Tools of the trade. J Hyperbaric Med 4:81–93, 1989.

U.S. Navy Department. U.S. Navy Dive Manual. Vol 1: Air Diving. NAVSEA 0994-LP-001-9010. San Pedro, CA, Best, 1993.

Youn BA, Gordon D, Moran C, et al. Fire in the multiplace hyperbaric chamber. J Hyperbaric Med 4:63–67, 1989.

28

Key Terms

Dead Volume

Diffusion

Inertial Impaction

Respiratory Syncytial Virus
(RSV)

Sedimentation

Stokes' Law

Physical factors affecting aerosol
penetration and deposition:

- Inertial impaction
- Sedimentation
- Diffusion

Clinical factors affecting aerosol
penetration and deposition:

- Particle size
- Ventilatory pattern
- Lung function

MDI—metered dose inhaler
SVN—small-volume nebulizer
DPI—dry powder inhaler

Aerosol Therapy

Dean Hess, M.Ed., R.R.T.

Therapeutic aerosols, the most common of which are the beta$_2$-agonist bronchodilators, are a familiar component in the treatment of patients with lung disease. Other aerosolized medications include anticholinergics, cromolyn sodium, steroids, pentamidine, and ribavirin. The use of aerosols to treat lung disease produces an ideal therapeutic ratio: that is, aerosols provide optimal therapy with minimal side effects. The use of sympathomimetic aerosols also produces greater and more rapid bronchodilation than drugs administered orally.

FACTORS AFFECTING AEROSOL PENETRATION AND DEPOSITION

To produce a therapeutic effect, aerosols must be deposited at an appropriate site in the respiratory tract. Bronchodilators must be deposited in the airways, whereas medications such as pentamidine and ribavirin should settle in the lung parenchyma.

Inertial impaction refers to the tendency of aerosol particles to deposit when the air stream changes direction. The size and the density of aerosol particles affect sedimentation, the deposition of aerosol particles in the lung due to the effect of gravity. Stokes' law states that the particle sedimentation rate equals the density times the diameter squared. Diffusion, the deposition of extremely small particles, occurs because of the brownian movement of surrounding gas molecules.

The mass median aerodynamic diameter (MMAD), usually used to specify clinical aerosol particle size, is the diameter around which the mass is equally divided. In other words, 50% of the mass is of particles smaller than the MMAD, and 50% of the mass is of particles greater than the MMAD. The geometric standard deviation measures the variability of the aerosol particle size; a high geometric standard deviation indicates a broad distribution of particles. Few aerosol particles larger than an MMAD of 5 μm penetrate the upper respiratory tract (Fig. 28–1). Aerosols with an MMAD of 1 to 2 μm tend to have maximal deposition in alveoli, whereas aerosols with an MMAD of 2 to 5 μm tend to be deposited in airways. Very stable aerosols with an MMAD of less than 1 μm tend to be exhaled.

In spontaneously breathing patients, the pattern of inhalation also affects the amount of aerosol deposited in the lower respiratory tract. The ideal ventilatory pattern is device specific, with lower inspiratory flows favored for MDIs and SVNs and more rapid inspiratory flows favored for DPIs. An increase in tidal volume may increase the volume of aerosol inhaled into the lungs, but this has a lesser effect on aerosol deposition patterns within the lung. An end-inspiratory pause may be beneficial, but this is also device specific and is probably less important with the DPI. Inhalation of aerosol through the mouth rather than the nose improves aerosol delivery into the lower respiratory tract.

Aerosol penetration and deposition are decreased in the presence of airway obstruction. Aerosol deposition into the lower respiratory tract decreases with chronic obstructive pulmonary disease and a decrease in

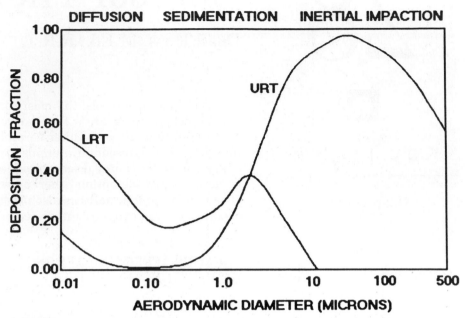

FIGURE 28–1: Aerosol deposition fraction as a function of aerodynamic diameter for the lower respiratory tract (LRT) and upper respiratory tract (URT).

FEV_1. Ironically, aerosol deposition decreases in those patients who might need it most. Partially for this reason, bronchodilators may need to be administered more frequently or in higher dosages to patients with acute airflow obstruction.

NEBULIZERS

Technical Aspects

Nebulizers are of two types: ultrasonic and jet. The electrically powered ultrasonic nebulizer (USN) consists of an electrical power unit and a nebulization unit (Fig. 28–2). The electrical power unit converts electrical power (110 V of alternating current at 60 Hz) to high-frequency

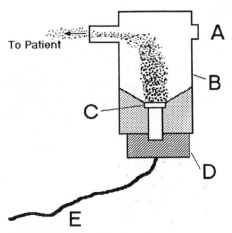

FIGURE 28–2: Ultrasonic nebulizer. A, air inlet; B, nebulization chamber; C, transducer; D, power unit; E, electrical cable.

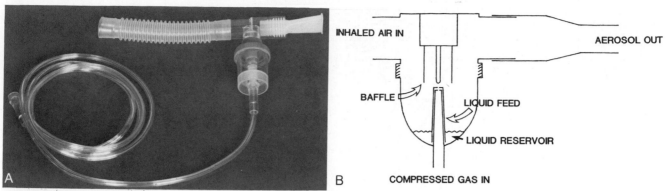

FIGURE 28–3: *A,* Typical small-volume nebulizer. *B,* Schematic illustration of a small-volume nebulizer. (*B,* From Newman SP. Aerosol generators and delivery systems. Respir Care 36:939–951, 1991.)

Disadvantages of the USN:

- Cost
- Mechanical malfunction

radio waves (1.35 MHz). The nebulization unit includes a piezoelectrical transducer that converts high-frequency radio waves to mechanical energy. The transducer vibrates at the frequency of the radio waves with displacement related to the amplitude of the radio waves. The manufacturer's preset and unchangeable frequency determines the aerosol particle size. The variable amplitude determines the output of the USN. The vibrations of the transducer transmit to the surface of the medication in the USN, creating an aerosol. Historically, the USN was used for bland aerosol therapy. The commercially available USNs for aerosol medication delivery are not commonly used.

The most commonly used nebulizers for aerosol medication delivery are jet nebulizers (Fig. 28–3), also referred to as SVNs, hand-held nebulizers, medication nebulizers, and wet nebulizers. The SVN uses the Bernoulli principle. Compressed gas passes through a Venturi, thus creating an area of low pressure. This low pressure draws medication solution from a reservoir through a liquid feed. The gas stream fragments the solution into an aerosol. The majority of aerosol particles impact on baffles and the walls of the nebulizer, so only the smallest particles reach the patient.

Effectiveness of the Small-Volume Nebulizer

A number of factors determine the effectiveness of SVNs, including dead volume, temperature and humidity, and nebulizer construction.

Dead volume, the amount of solution remaining in the nebulizer after the completion of a treatment, represents the solution adhering to the walls, cap, and patient connectors. Tapping the sides of the nebulizer during therapy causes droplets of solution adhering to the walls of the nebulizer to coalesce and renebulize, thus decreasing the dead volume. The dead volume depends on the volume of nebulizer solution, the nebulizer flow, and the temperature and humidity of the solution, the driving gas, and the entrained gas. Dead volume can be minimized with a solution volume of 4 mL at a nebulizer flow of 8 L/min. These higher flows decrease not only dead volume but also aerosol particle size.

The temperature and humidity of the nebulized solution and the driving and entrained gas also affect the particle size delivered by the SVN, as well as the concentration of the drug in the dead volume. Because of evaporation and adiabatic expansion of the driving gas, the

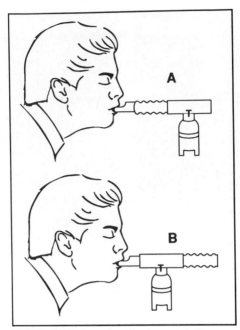

FIGURE 28–4: *A,* Small volume nebulizer with the reservoir in the inspiratory position. *B,* Small-volume nebulizer with the reservoir in the expiratory position. Placement of the reservoir in the expiratory position is preferred. (*A,* and *B,* From Pusit FM. Comparison of medication delivery by T-nebulizer with inspiratory and expiratory reservoir. Respir Care 34:985–988, 1989.)

temperature of aerosol solutions falls about 8 to 12°F below the ambient temperature. Ideally, the nebulizer should have a temperature between ambient temperature and body temperature; any entrained gas should be fully saturated with water vapor at room temperature. From a practical standpoint, temperature change in the nebulizer can be minimized by holding the SVN firmly in a closed hand.

The design of the nebulizer also affects the performance of the SVN. Differences exist not only between the performances of commercially available SVNs but between the SVNs of a particular manufacturer. One simple factor, an 50-mL expiratory reservoir, improves the performance of an SVN system (Fig. 28–4). Intermittent activation of the SVN (Fig. 28–5) during inspiration improves aerosol delivery because it minimizes the amount of aerosol lost during the patient's expiratory phase. However, this method is used infrequently because it is both time consuming and difficult for many patients.

Clinical Application

To minimize aerosol deposition in the nose and nasopharynx, the patient should inhale the aerosol through the mouth rather than the nose. However, when patients use a face mask and inspire through the mouth, no difference exists between the use of a mouthpiece and the use of a mask for aerosol delivery.

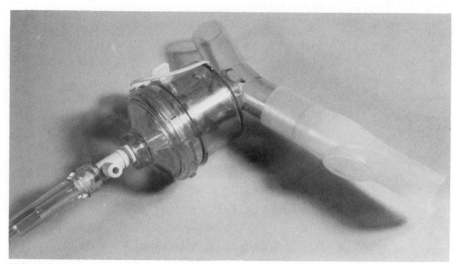

FIGURE 28–5: Small-volume nebulizer with a thumb port to allow intermittent nebulization.

Ventilatory patterns influence the deposition of SVN aerosols into the lower respiratory tract. A slow inspiratory flow (0.5 L/sec) at a normal tidal volume, with an occasional inspiration to total lung capacity and an inspiratory hold, is recommended. The specific technique for the use of an SVN is found in Table 28–1.

With spontaneously breathing patients, only about 10% of the aerosol from an SVN deposits in the lower respiratory tract (Fig. 28–6). However, considerable interindividual variability exists in pulmonary deposition with an SVN. During SVN use, the nebulizer retains a large fraction of the aerosol (dead volume), with some medication being wasted into the ambient environment during the patient's expiratory phase.

Techniques for using the SVN for continuous aerosol medication delivery have been described (Fig. 28–7). This therapy can deliver large amounts of aerosol and thus may be beneficial to patients with acute severe asthma. Although usually safe and effective, continuous nebulization requires more careful monitoring than the use of frequent SVN therapy by conventional means. With comparable doses, continuous aerosol therapy does not appear to be clearly superior to conventional intermittent aerosol therapy.

TABLE **28–1:** Technique for the Use of Small-Volume Nebulizers

Place the drug in the nebulizer
Use an appropriate volume of diluent to raise the total volume of the solution in the SVN
  to 4 mL
Set the driving gas flow at 8 L/min
Connect the patient to the SVN using a mouthpiece or mask
Instruct the patient to breathe through an open mouth if a mask is used or to close the
  lips around the mouthpiece
Grasp the nebulizer firmly in the hand to maintain its temperature during treatment
Have the patient slowly inhale normal tidal volumes
Have the patient occasionally inspire to total lung capacity and incorporate a 4- to 10-
  second breath hold
Tap the sides of the nebulizer periodically to minimize dead volume
Continue treatment until no aerosol is produced
Monitor the patient for the presence of side effects and beneficial effects

SVN, small-volume nebulizer.

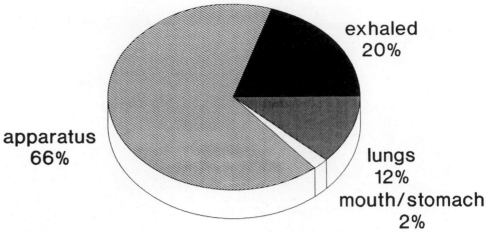

FIGURE 28–6: Deposition pattern of aerosol from a small-volume nebulizer.

For many years, the principal means of therapeutic aerosol administration by SVN was in conjunction with intermittent positive pressure breathing. Over the past 20 years, intermittent positive pressure breathing as a means of aerosol administration has been recognized as both unnecessary and undesirable. Intermittent positive pressure breathing may be indicated as a means of therapeutic aerosol administration in some acutely ill patients who are unable to spontaneously deep breathe. However, no benefit of intermittent positive pressure breathing exists over the use of an SVN or MDI in stable patients.

INHALERS

Technical Aspects

MDIs consist of the active drug in the form of micronized crystals, suspended with a surfactant in a mixture of two or three chlorofluorocar-

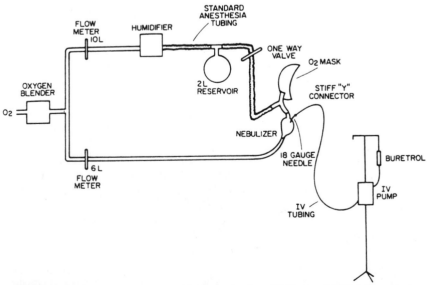

FIGURE 28–7: System for continuous aerosolization of beta-agonist. IV, intravenous. (From Moler FW, Hurwitz ME, Custer JR. Improvement in clinical asthma score and PaCO$_2$ in children with severe asthma treated with continuously nebulized terbutaline. J Allergy Clin Immunol 81:1101–1109, 1988.)

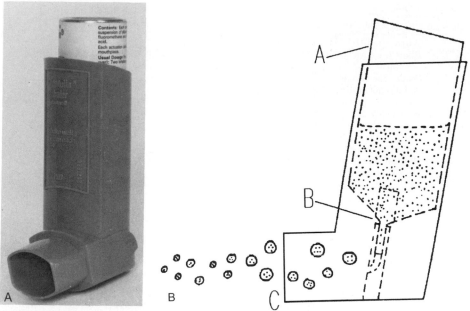

FIGURE 28–8: *A,* Typical metered dose inhaler. *B,* Schematic illustration of a metered dose inhaler. A, canister; B, metering chamber; C, mouthpiece.

bon propellants (Fig. 28–8). Activation by compression of the canister into the mouthpiece results in the release of a metered drug dose. With each activation, the MDI delivers 15 to 20 mL of gas. Because the canister is pressurized, the aerosol leaves the MDI rapidly and directionally. This results in deposition of the majority of the aerosol dose in the oropharynx (unless an auxiliary spacer device is used). As the aerosol particles move further from the MDI, their diameters decrease because of evaporation of the volatile chlorofluorocarbons. The cold propellant that leaves the MDI can be troublesome for some patients.

Effectiveness of Metered Dose Inhalers

Factors that determine the effectiveness of the MDI:

• Lung volume at actuation
• Inspiratory flow
• Breath hold
• MDI position relative to the mouth

Actuation of the MDI should occur near the beginning of a complete inhalation from functional residual capacity. Inspiration should be slow, with a 4- to 10-second end-inspiratory breath hold. Holding the MDI 4 cm from a wide open mouth during actuation is sometimes recommended. This may improve pulmonary deposition and decrease pharyngeal deposition; however, many patients find this method difficult and prefer to place the mouthpiece of the actuator between their lips. Although it is acceptable for patients to close their lips around the mouthpiece of the MDI, patients must be reminded to keep the tongue away from the outlet of the mouthpiece. Temperature also affects the particle size of the aerosol leaving the MDI. The MDI can be prewarmed to body temperature by rolling the canister between the hands before actuation and by carrying the MDI close to the body (i.e., in a pocket rather than in a purse).

The timing of actuation can also affect response, with some clinicians recommending a 3- to 10-minute period between actuations. Because this may not be practical for many patients, a 1-minute period before actuations is probably adequate.

TABLE **28–2:** Technique for the Use of Metered Dose Inhalers Without Auxiliary Spacer Devices

Warm the MDI to body temperature
Place the canister into the mouthpiece or actuator and remove the cap over the mouthpiece
Shake the canister
Exhale normally to functional residual capacity
Open the mouth and place the MDI mouthpiece at the mouth opening
Begin slow inspiration
Actuate the MDI
Continue to inspire to total lung capacity
Hold the breath for 4 to 10 seconds
Wait at least 1 minute before actuations
Rinse the mouth and pharynx if inhaling steroids
Monitor the patient for the presence of side effects and beneficial effects

MDI, metered dose inhaler.

Clinical Application of Metered Dose Inhalers

Many patients, especially the very young and the very old, have difficulty using an MDI correctly. Correct use of the MDI requires patient coordination and practice. A clinician (respiratory therapist, nurse, or physician) must teach the patient the correct method because most patients cannot learn to use an MDI correctly by reading the package insert. The proper technique for the use of the MDI is shown in Table 28–2. Although patients may benefit from the use of an MDI without a perfect technique, deviations from appropriate technique result in less aerosol deposition in the lungs. For patients with arthritic hands, a device called VentEase aids in activation of the MDI (Fig. 28–9).

Stable patients usually use the MDI three to four times per day at a dosage of two to three puffs per session. Acutely ill patients, particularly asthmatics, may need higher dosages. Although higher dosages may be necessary during acute exacerbations, patients should not increase their dosage without consultation with a physician. An increased bronchodilator requirement usually indicates a deterioration of lung function, which may require additional therapy such as corticosteroid administration.

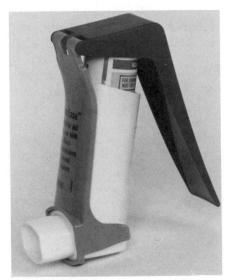

FIGURE 28–9: Metered dose inhaler with VentEase.

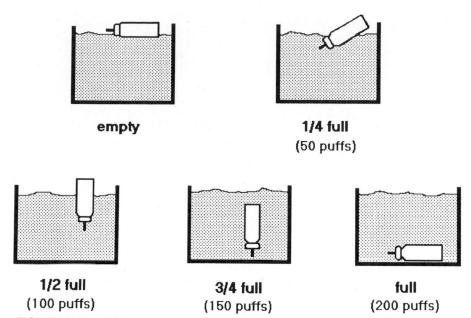

empty

1/4 full
(50 puffs)

1/2 full
(100 puffs)

3/4 full
(150 puffs)

full
(200 puffs)

FIGURE 28–10: Placing the metered dose inhaler canister into a pan of water can be used to estimate the amount of drug remaining. If the canister is full, it will sink to the bottom; if it is empty, it will float.

Increasing MDI usage without additional therapy may worsen the underlying pulmonary dysfunction. Clinicians must inform their patients of the dangers of increasing MDI use without medical direction. Just as patients should be warned of the dangers of overdosage from the MDI, they must also be reminded not to use the MDI at less than the prescribed dosage.

Nonhospitalized patients using an MDI can learn to estimate the amount of drug remaining in the canister (Fig. 28–10).

Metered Dose Inhalers With Auxiliary Spacing Devices

MDI auxiliary devices have been developed to overcome the problems of patient coordination and pharyngeal deposition. In the United States, the most commonly used of these include the InspirEase and the Aerochamber (Fig. 28–11). Auxiliary devices from other manufacturers have also recently become available. In each, the aerosol flows from the MDI into a holding chamber. The patient then inhales the aerosol from the holding chamber, rather than directly from the MDI. Thus, coordination between patient inhalation and MDI activation becomes less important. Further, large aerosol particles impact in the holding chamber rather than in the pharynx. These devices also provide auditory feedback to encourage a slow inspiratory flow. When inhaling steroids, the patient should always use an auxiliary device to minimize pharyngeal deposition. In patients who can use an MDI correctly, the use of an auxiliary device has little effect on pulmonary deposition. However, the use of an auxiliary device will increase pulmonary deposition in patients who have difficulty coordinating the use of an MDI alone; auxiliary devices should be used with such patients. The patient can use either MDI auxiliary device (the InspirEase, the Aerochamber, or another similar device) because no clear superiority of one device over another exists (Table 28–3).

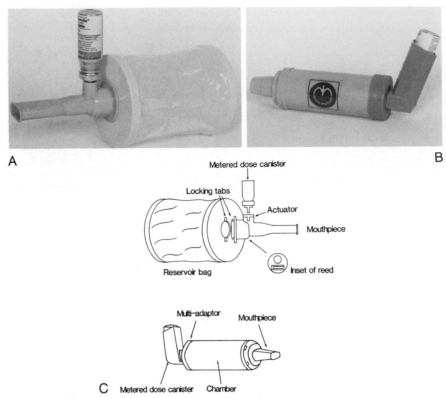

FIGURE 28–11: *A,* InspirEase metered dose inhaler auxiliary device. *B,* Aerochamber metered dose inhaler auxiliary device. *C,* Schematic illustrations of InspirEase (*top*) and Aerochamber (*bottom*). (*C,* From Newman SP. Aerosol generators and delivery systems. Respir Care 36:939–951, 1991.)

The technique for the use of an MDI with an auxiliary spacing device is listed in Table 28–4.

In spontaneously breathing patients using an MDI without an auxiliary device, about 10% of the aerosol deposits in the lower respiratory tract (Fig. 28–12). Considerable interindividual variability in deposition exists. With the MDI, a large fraction of the aerosol deposits in the upper airway unless an auxiliary device is used, in which case a large fraction of the aerosol deposits in the auxiliary device.

TABLE **28–3:** Characteristics of Metered Dose Inhaler Auxiliary Devices

	Aerochamber	**InspirEase**
Reservoir	Rigid	Collapsible
Volume	150 mL	700 mL
Valved	Yes	No
Less coordination (compared with an MDI)	Yes	Yes
Flow indicator	Yes	Yes
Pharyngeal deposition (compared with an MDI)	Less	Less
Increased bronchodilation (compared with an MDI)	Sometimes	Sometimes
Portable	Less than an MDI alone	Less than an MDI alone
Use with children	Yes	Older children but not preschoolers
Use with face mask	Yes	No

MDI, metered dose inhaler.

TABLE **28–4:** Technique for the Use of Metered Dose Inhalers With Auxiliary Spacer Devices

Warm the MDI to body temperature
Shake the canister
Actuate the MDI into the auxiliary spacer device
Exhale normally to functional residual capacity
Place the mouthpiece into the mouth and close the lips around the mouthpiece
Inspire slowly from the spacer
Continue to inspire to total lung capacity
Hold the breath for 4 to 10 seconds
Repeat the inspiration with breath hold if indicated by the spacer manufacturer
Wait at least 1 minute before actuations
Rinse the mouth and pharynx if inhaling steroids
Monitor the patient for the presence of side effects and beneficial effects

MDI, metered dose inhaler.

Dry Powder Inhalers

Advantages of the DPI:

- Breath activated
- Not dependent on ozone-depleting chlorofluorocarbons

Disadvantage of the DPI:

- Must be loaded with a drug capsule before each use; this may be inconvenient, particularly during acute exacerbations

The use of DPIs is less common in the United States than in Europe. The most commonly used DPIs in the United States include the Spinhaler (to administer cromolyn sodium) and the Rotahaler (to administer albuterol). Both the Spinhaler and the Rotahaler are single-dose devices (Fig. 28–13). A multidose DPI, the Turbohaler, is available in Europe and Canada for the administration of terbutaline and budesonide. With a DPI, unlike with an SVN or MDI, a high inspiratory flow must be used. With the DPI, an end-inspiratory breath hold is not needed. When the Rotahaler is used, care must be taken not to tilt the device after the capsule has been loaded and opened, which could result in loss of the drug. The technique for the use of the DPI is shown in Table 28–5. Pulmonary deposition patterns for the DPI are similar to those for the MDI.

CHOICE OF AEROSOL DELIVERY DEVICE IN ADULT AMBULATORY PATIENTS

When a therapeutic aerosol is prescribed, the clinician must decide which device to use: an SVN, an MDI, or a DPI. There are advantages and disadvantages to each (Table 28–6). Historically, the SVN has been the first choice, particularly in acutely ill patients. However, there has been a resurgence of interest in the use of MDIs in place of SVNs. Many studies have reported equal results with the SVN and the MDI in stable adult patients, acutely ill adult patients, adult patients with asthma,

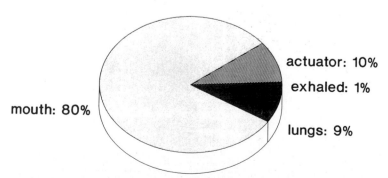

FIGURE 28–12: Deposition pattern of aerosol from a metered dose inhaler.

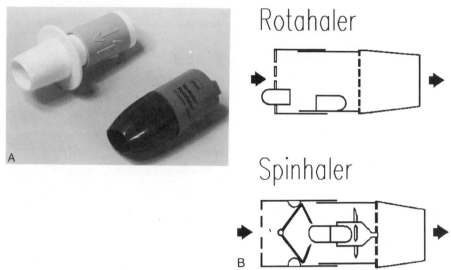

FIGURE 28–13: *A,* Spinhaler (*top*) and Rotahaler (*bottom*). *B,* Schematic illustration of Rotahaler and Spinhaler.

and adult patients with chronic obstructive pulmonary disease. For patients who can use the MDI correctly, an MDI costs less than an SVN. The MDI should now be considered the first choice of device for aerosol administration (Fig. 28–14). If the patient fails to use the MDI correctly or if the patient needs inhaled steroids, the patient should be given an MDI with an auxiliary device. If the patient is unable to use the MDI with an auxiliary device, an SVN should be used. The SVN may also be more convenient when the patient requires frequent or high dosages. If the patient cannot use the MDI with a spacer device, a DPI should be considered.

An interesting paradox emerges in a comparison of bronchodilator administration by SVN and MDI. The typical dose used with an SVN is approximately 10 times the dose used with an MDI. For example, a 0.3-mL dose of metaproterenol (5% solution) is equivalent to 15 mg, whereas a 2-puff dose of metaproterenol (0.65 mg each) is equivalent to 1.3 mg. The dose from the SVN may need to be greater to compensate for the volume of drug retained in the nebulizer and lost during the patient's expiratory phase. During acute exacerbations of obstructive lung disease, the standard SVN dose may actually deliver more drug to the patient's lungs than the standard MDI dose. This suggests that the SVN may be more beneficial than the MDI during acute exacerbations or when higher than usual MDI dosages must be used. The SVN may actually deliver more aerosol to lung receptors than the MDI, which may have clinical implications for some patients.

TABLE **28–5:** Technique for the Use of Dry Powder Inhalers

Assemble the apparatus
Open the capsule using a device-specific technique
Exhale normally to functional residual capacity
Place the inhaler mouthpiece into the mouth and seal the lips around the mouthpiece
Inhale rapidly through the device (a breath hold is not necessary)
Repeat the process until the capsule is empty
Rinse the mouth and pharynx if inhaling steroids
Monitor the patient for the presence of side effects and beneficial effects

TABLE **28–6:** Advantages and Disadvantages of the Use of Small-Volume Nebulizers, Metered Dose Inhalers, and Dry Powder Inhalers

Advantages	Disadvantages
Small-Volume Nebulizers	
Less patient coordination is required	Expensive
High doses are possible (even continuous)	Wasteful
No CFC release	Contamination is possible if the device is not carefully cleaned
	Not all medications are available
	A pressurized gas source is required
	More time is required
Metered Dose Inhalers	
Convenient	Patient coordination is required
Inexpensive	Patient activation is required
	Results in pharyngeal deposition
	Has the potential for abuse
	Difficult to deliver high doses
	Not all medications are available
	Dependent on ozone-depleting CFCs
Metered Dose Inhalers With Auxiliary Devices	
Less patient coordination is required	A more complex process for patients who can use an MDI alone
Results in less pharyngeal deposition	More expensive than MDI use alone
	Less portable than an MDI alone
Dry Powder Inhalers	
Less patient coordination is required	Requires a high inspiratory flow
A breath hold is not required	Most units are single dose
No CFCs are required	Can result in pharyngeal deposition
Breath activated	Cannot be used with intubated patients
	Not all medications are available
	Difficult to deliver high doses

CFC, chlorofluorocarbon; MDI, metered dose inhaler.

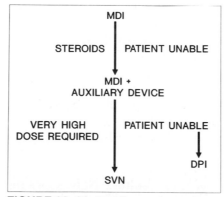

FIGURE 28–14: Decision tree to determine which aerosol delivery device should be used. MDI, metered dose inhaler; DPI, dry powder inhaler; SVN, small-volume nebulizer.

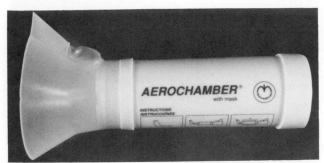

FIGURE 28–15: Aerochamber with mask for pediatric use.

AEROSOL ADMINISTRATION TO INFANTS AND CHILDREN

Therapeutic aerosols are used effectively in infants and children, especially those with asthma or bronchopulmonary dysplasia. Less information exists on aerosol delivery to pediatric patients, particularly infants, than on delivery to adults.

In infants and children, a physiologic response occurs even though aerosol deposition in the lower respiratory tract is as low as 1 to 2%. When an SVN is used, the dose must be tailored to each patient's individual response because the appropriate dose is unclear in small children.

Many children can effectively use an MDI. Patients younger than 10 years of age should use an auxiliary device because these patients have less ability to coordinate the use of an MDI. In very young children (those younger than 3 years of age), an auxiliary device with a mask can be used (Fig. 28–15). Because the delivery of aerosols to the lower respiratory tract is less efficient in children than in adults, the number of puffs from an MDI should not be reduced because of the patient's size. Children, like adults, need proper instruction in the use of the MDI. The clinician should periodically review the patient's technique and correct errors as necessary.

An SVN should be used to administer aerosols to intubated infants and children because no data exist on the use of MDIs in these patients. Effective aerosol therapy in intubated infants has been reported, despite very low pulmonary deposition fractions in this patient population.

AEROSOL DELIVERY DURING ADULT MECHANICAL VENTILATION

Intubated adult patients commonly receive aerosolized bronchodilators. Because the endotracheal tube presents a formidable barrier to the penetration of aerosols into the lower respiratory tract, higher dosages may be required for intubated patients than for ambulatory patients.

Use of Small-Volume Nebulizers in Intubated Patients

When an SVN is used with mechanically ventilated adult patients, only about 3% of the aerosol dose deposits in the lungs. When an SVN is used in a ventilator circuit, the SVN can be placed at the ventilator Y piece or at the circuit manifold, which is approximately midway between the ventilator and the Y piece. In addition, the nebulizer can be powered

Factors affecting aerosol delivery to pediatric patients:

- Patients' smaller airways
- Lack of cooperation
- Higher respiratory rates
- Shorter inspiratory times
- Decreased ability to breath hold

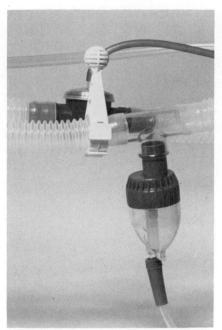

FIGURE 28–16: Small-volume nebulizer placed in the ventilator at the manifold, approximately midway between the ventilator and the patient.

continuously from an auxiliary gas flow (e.g., wall oxygen) or intermittently from the nebulizer drive line of the ventilator. The patient receives significantly more aerosol if the nebulizer is placed at the manifold (Fig. 28–16) and operated during inspiration only.

Several potential problems relate to the use of SVNs with mechanical ventilators. Contaminated nebulizers can be the source of bacterial aerosols in mechanical ventilator circuits. The continuous flow from an SVN increases the tidal volume (and associated pressure) delivered when volume ventilators are used. The continuous flow from an SVN introduces a bias flow, making it more difficult for the patient to generate the negative pressure required during assisted modes of ventilation, such as pressure supported and assist-control ventilation. The continuous flow of aerosol from the SVN can also damage the expiratory flow transducer of some ventilators. The recommended technique for the use of an SVN during mechanical ventilation is shown in Table 28–7.

TABLE **28–7:** Recommended Technique for the Use of Small-Volume Nebulizers During Mechanical Ventilation

Place the drug in the SVN
Dilute to a total solution volume of 4 mL
Insert the SVN into the inspiratory limb of the ventilator circuit at least 18 inches from the Y piece
Set the flow at 8 L/min, or use a ventilator nebulizer port
Set the ventilator rate at 4 to 8 per minute, or higher if not contraindicated
Set the tidal volume at 12 mL/kg, or greater if not contraindicated
Bypass the humidifier, or remove the artificial nose from the circuit
Tap the sides of the nebulizer to minimize dead volume
Continue treatment until no aerosol is produced
Remove the SVN from the ventilator circuit
Return the ventilator to pretreatment settings
Monitor the patient for the presence of side effects and beneficial effects

SVN, small-volume nebulizer.

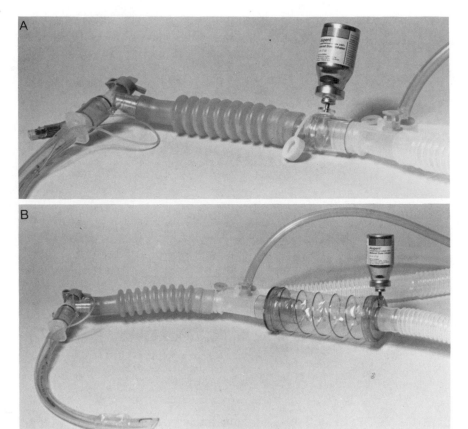

FIGURE 28–17: *A,* Instrumentation Industries metered dose inhaler adapter placed at the Y piece of the ventilator circuit. *B,* Monaghan AeroVent placed inline with the ventilator circuit. The AeroVent can be collapsed in the circuit between patient treatments.

Use of Metered Dose Inhalers in Intubated Patients

A number of adapters are commercially available to place the MDI in a ventilator circuit. Although various designs for these adapters are available (Fig. 28–17), insufficient evidence exists to indicate that one is superior to another. When an MDI is used with an intubated patient, about 3 to 6% of the aerosol penetrates the endotracheal tube. Although it is generally accepted that the use of an MDI and that of an SVN are virtually equivalent during mechanical ventilation, MDI use is recommended because this technique avoids the problems related to SVN use. In addition, an MDI is less expensive than an SVN. The recommended technique for the use of an MDI during mechanical ventilation is shown in Table 28–8.

AEROSOL DELIVERY FOR PARENCHYMAL LUNG DISEASE

Ribavirin and pentamidine are the principal therapeutic aerosols targeted to the lung periphery. Delivery of these agents requires specific equipment and procedures to protect the caregiver (e.g., respiratory therapists and nurses) from excessive environmental drug exposure.

TABLE **28–8:** Technique for the Use of Metered Dose Inhalers During Mechanical Ventilation

Place the MDI adapter into the ventilator circuit
Set the tidal volume at 12 mL/kg, or greater if not contraindicated
Warm the MDI to body temperature
Shake the MDI
Place the MDI in the circuit
Actuate the MDI immediately after the beginning of a mechanical breath; if a spacer is used, actuate 1 to 2 seconds before a mechanical breath or near end-exhalation, depending on the ventilator rate
Apply a 2- to 3-second inflation hold, if not contraindicated
Wait 1 minute before actuations
Return the ventilator to pretreatment settings
Monitor the patient for the presence of side effects and beneficial effects

MDI, metered dose inhaler.

Ribavirin

RSV—respiratory syncytial virus

Ribavirin is an antiviral agent used for the treatment of RSV infection in high-risk infants (e.g., those with congenital heart disease or bronchopulmonary dysplasia). Aerosolization of ribavirin is achieved with a small-particle aerosol generator (SPAG), which produces very small particles with an MMAD of 1.3 μm (Fig. 28–18). The SPAG, which is based on the Collison nebulizer design, includes three jets and a drying chamber into which dry air is metered to reduce particle size by evaporation. The inlet pressure of 40 to 60 psig decreases to 26 psig before the nebulizer jets and drying chamber are supplied. After the reservoir has been filled with 300 mL of ribavirin solution (20 mg/mL), the nebulizer flow and drying air flow are adjusted to achieve a total flow of 12 to 15 L/min. A usual course of ribavirin treatment involves a 3- to 7-day hospitalization, with administration of the aerosol for 12 to 18 hr/day.

Spontaneously breathing patients usually receive the ribavirin via hood, tent, or mask. Although the manufacturer does not recommend using ribavirin during mechanical ventilation because of concerns about crystallization in the ventilator circuit, techniques for its use with intubated mechanically ventilated patients have been described.

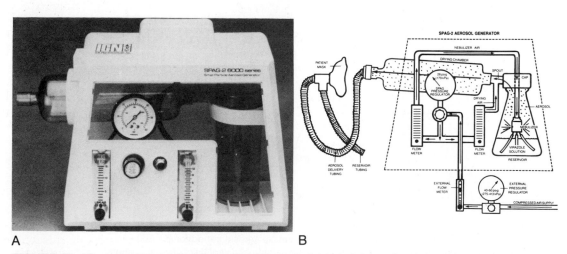

A   B

FIGURE 28–18: *A,* SPAG-2 small-particle aerosol generator for the administration of ribavirin. *B,* Schematic illustration of the SPAG-2 aerosol generator.

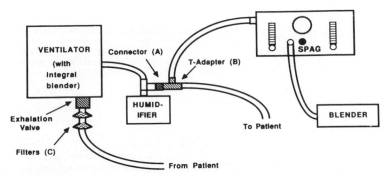

FIGURE 28–19: Use of a small-particle aerosol generator (SPAG) for ribavirin administration during pressure-controlled ventilation. (From Demers RR, Parker J, Frankel LR, Smith DW. Administration of ribavirin to neonatal and pediatric patients during mechanical ventilation. Respir Care 31:1188–1195, 1986.)

When the SPAG is used with a pressure-preset ventilator, the following are recommended (Fig. 28–19):

- Set the drying chamber flow on the SPAG to zero and the nebulizer flow to 4 to 6 L/min.
- Decrease the ventilator flow so that the sum of the SPAG flow and the ventilator flow equals the desired flow.
- Place two bacteria filters in series proximal to the exhalation valve of the ventilator.
- Replace the filters at intervals of 2 to 4 hours (this can be done by discarding the upstream filter, replacing it with the downstream filter, and placing a new filter at the downstream site).

When the SPAG is used with a volume-preset ventilator, the following are recommended (Fig. 28–20):

- Set the drying chamber flow on the SPAG to zero and the nebulizer flow to 4 to 6 L/min.

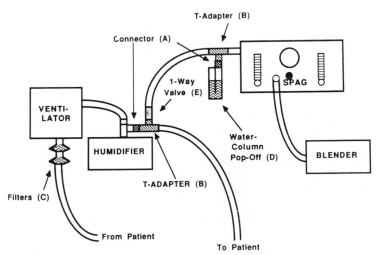

FIGURE 28–20: Use of a small-particle aerosol generator (SPAG) for ribavirin administration during volume-controlled ventilation. (From Demers RR, Parker J, Frankel LR, Smith DW. Administration of ribavirin to neonatal and pediatric patients during mechanical ventilation. Respir Care 31:1188–1195, 1986.)

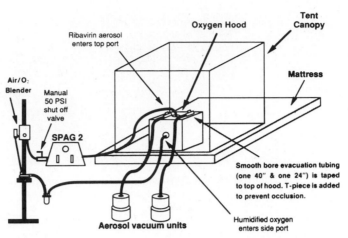

FIGURE 28–21: Scavenging system when ribavirin is used with a hood. (From Charney W, Corkery KJ, Kraemer R, Wugofski L. Engineering and administrative controls to contain aerosolized ribavirin: Results of simulation and application to one patient. Respir Care 35:1042–1048, 1990.)

- Place a one-way valve between the ventilator circuit and the SPAG.
- Place a pop-off valve between the SPAG and the ventilator circuit (optional).
- Place two bacteria filters in series proximal to the exhalation valve of the ventilator.
- Replace the filters at intervals of 2 to 4 hours (this can be done by discarding the upstream filter, replacing it with the downstream filter, and placing a new filter at the downstream site).

When ribavirin is used with mechanical ventilation, the ventilator circuit must be continuously monitored for signs of obstruction of the expiratory filters; this is best done by the use of a high positive end-expiratory pressure alarm proximal to the filters because expiratory obstruction should increase the positive end-expiratory pressure level. The circuit should be changed frequently because of the crystallization of ribavirin in the ventilator circuit.

Ribavirin has been shown to be teratogenic in some animal species, and for this reason there is concern about the exposure of health care personnel. Personnel should have limited exposure to ribavirin. Exposure is limited through the use of administrative controls (e.g., work assignments to avoid exposure to pregnant women), engineering controls (e.g., shutoff valves on the SPAG; scavenging systems; and appropriate venting of single-patient, negative pressure rooms), and protective devices (masks, gloves, gowns, and goggles). A scavenging system for ribavirin is shown in Figure 28–21. With this system, a hood is placed within a tent, and ribavirin is evacuated from the tent using two vacuum units equipped with high-efficiency particulate air filters. The SPAG is shut off when the tent is entered, with a parallel humidified oxygen source being used during these times.

Pentamidine

Aerosolized pentamidine is used for the prevention and treatment of *Pneumocystis carinii* infection in patients with acquired immunodefi-

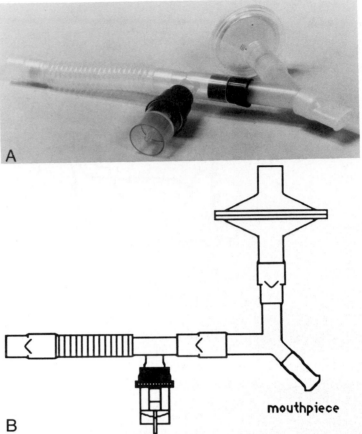

FIGURE 28–22: *A,* Respirgard II nebulizer for pentamidine administration. *B,* Schematic illustration of Respirgard II. (*B,* From Vinciguerra C, Smaldone G. Treatment time and patient tolerance for pentamidine delivery by Respirgard II and AeroTech II. Respir Care 35:1037–1041, 1990.)

ciency syndrome. Aerosolization of pentamidine is accomplished with nebulizers such as the Respirgard II (MMAD, 0.76 μm) (Fig. 28–22) and the AeroTech II (MMAD, 1.0 μm) (Fig. 28–23). Although there are differences in the performance of these nebulizers, either is acceptable. These nebulizer systems include one-way valves and filters to decrease environmental contamination with pentamidine and infectious organisms (e.g., *Mycobacterium tuberculosis*) from the patient's exhaled gases.

Although the mutagenic and teratogenic effects of pentamidine are unknown, there are concerns related to the occupational exposure of health care personnel to this agent, as well as concerns related to the exposure of health care personnel to tuberculosis-infected patients during treatment with pentamidine. As with ribavirin, the protection of personnel from exposure to pentamidine is prudent. This includes the use of engineering and administrative controls (e.g., high-efficiency particulate air filters, frequent air exchanges, and isolation rooms or treatment booths), protective devices (e.g., masks, goggles, gloves, and gowns), and rapid diagnosis and treatment of tuberculosis in patients with acquired immunodeficiency syndrome. Because pentamidine is irritating and frequently induces cough and bronchospasm, a beta-agonist should be administered (via an MDI) before pentamidine therapy.

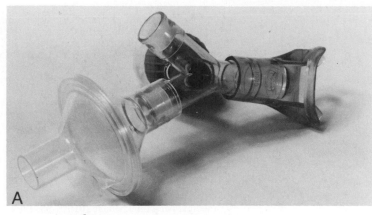

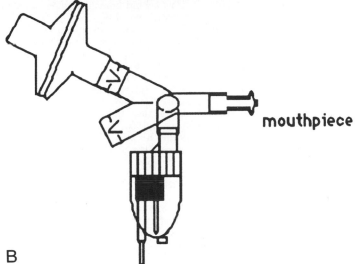

mouthpiece

FIGURE 28–23: *A*, AeroTech II nebulizer for pentamidine administration *B*, Schematic illustration of AeroTech II. (*B*, From Vinciguerra C, Smaldone G. Treatment time and patient tolerance for pentamidine delivery by Respirgard II and AeroTech II. Respir Care 35:1037–1041, 1990.)

SUMMARY

Aerosol therapy is commonly used in the treatment of patients with airway and parenchymal disease. Clinicians caring for respiratory patients have a responsibility to provide effective treatment at the lowest possible cost (e.g., an MDI versus an SVN). Clinicians also have a personal responsibility to protect themselves from a contaminated environment produced by therapeutic aerosols (e.g., ribavirin and pentamidine).

Suggested Readings

Alvine GF, Rodgers P, Fitzsimmons KM, Ahrens RC. Disposable jet nebulizers. How reliable are they? Chest 101:316–319, 1992.

Blake KV, Hoppe M, Harmon E, Hendeles L. Relative amount of albuterol delivered to lung receptors from a metered-dose inhaler and nebulizer solution. Bioassay by histamine bronchoprovocation. Chest 101:309–315, 1992.

Bowton DL, Goldsmith WM, Haponik EF. Substitution of metered-dose inhalers for hand-held nebulizers. Success and cost savings in a large, acute-care hospital. Chest 101:305–308, 1992.

Byron PR, Phillips EM, Kuhn R. Ribavirin administration by inhalation: Aerosol-generation factors controlling drug delivery to the lung. Respir Care 33:1011–1019, 1988.

Charney W, Corkery KJ, Kraemer R, Wugofski L. Engineering and administrative controls to contain aerosolized ribavirin: Results of simulation and application to one patient. Respir Care 35:1042–1048, 1990.

Colacdone A, Wolkove N, Stern E, et al. Continuous nebulization of albuterol (salbutamol) in acute asthma. Chest 97:693–697, 1990.

Demers RR, Parker J, Frankel LR, Smith DW. Administration of ribavirin to neonatal and pediatric patients during mechanical ventilation. Respir Care 31:1188–1195, 1986.

Dolovich M. Clinical aspects of aerosol physics. Respir Care 36:931–938, 1991.

Fallat RJ, Kandal K. Aerosol exhaust: Escape of aerosolized medication into the patient and caregiver's environment. Respir Care 36:1008–1016, 1991.

Fuller HD, Dolovitch MB, Posmituck G, et al. Pressurized aerosol versus jet aerosol delivery to mechanically ventilated patients: Comparison of dose to the lungs. Am Rev Respir Dis 141:440–444, 1990.

Guidry GG, Brown WD, Stogner SW, George RB. Incorrect use of metered dose inhalers by medical personnel. Chest 101:31–33, 1992.

Hess D. How should bronchodilators be administered to patients on ventilators? Respir Care 36:377–394, 1991.

Hess D, Daugherty A, Simmons M. The volume of gas emitted from metered dose inhalers (MDIs). Respir Care 37:444–447, 1992.

Hess D, Horney D, Snyder T. Medication-delivery performance of eight small-volume, hand-held nebulizers: Effects of diluent volume, gas flow rate, and nebulizer model. Respir Care 34:717–723, 1989.

Kacmarek RM. Ribavirin and pentamidine aerosols: Caregiver beware! [Editorial]. Respir Care 35:1034–1036, 1990.

Kacmarek RM, Hess D. The interface between patient and aerosol generator. Respir Care 36:952–976, 1991.

Kacmarek RM, Kratohvil J. Evaluation of a double-enclosure double-vacuum unit scavenging system for ribavirin administration. Respir Care 37:37–45, 1992.

Lewis RA, Fleming JS. Fractional deposition from a jet nebulizer: How it differs from a metered dose inhaler. Br J Dis Chest 79:361–367, 1985.

MacIntyre NR, Brougher P, Hess D, et al. Aerosol consensus statement—1991. Respir Care 36:916–921, 1991.

MacIntyre NR, Silver RM, Miller CW, et al. Aerosol delivery in intubated, mechanically ventilated patients. Crit Care Med 13:81–84, 1985.

Maguire GP, Newman T, DeLorenzo LJ, et al. Comparison of a hand-held nebulizer with a metered dose inhaler-spacer combination in acute obstructive pulmonary disease. Chest 100:1300–1305, 1991.

Moler FW, Hurwitz ME, Custer JR. Improvement in clinical asthma score and $PaCO_2$ in children with severe asthma treated with continuously nebulized terbutaline. J Allergy Clin Immunol 81:1101–1109, 1988.

Newman SP. Aerosol generators and delivery systems. Respir Care 36:939–951, 1991.

Sattler FR, Feinberg J. New developments in the treatment of Pneumocystis carinii pneumonia. Chest 101:451–457, 1992.

Sly RM. Aerosol therapy in children. Respir Care 36:994–1007, 1991.

Vinciguerra C, Smaldone G. Treatment time and patient tolerance for pentamidine delivery by Respirgard II and AeroTech II. Respir Care 35:1037–1041, 1990.

Waskin H. Toxicology of antimicrobial aerosols: A review of aerosolized ribavirin and pentamidine. Respir Care 36:1026–1036, 1991.

29

Airway Management

Michael S. Gorback, M.D.

Although the teeth usually provide a hindrance to laryngoscopy (especially in prognathic individuals), these structures play an important role in mask fit. Because it is often difficult to obtain a good mask fit in the edentulous patient, an oral airway can be inserted to compensate for this situation.

Macroglossia may hinder the performance of laryngoscopy.

Some authorities suggest that a high-arched palate in a long, narrow mouth is associated with difficult intubation.

Bilateral mandibular fractures can produce airway obstruction due to hypermobility of the tongue.

Several disorders, including degenerative, rheumatoid, and psoriatic arthritis and ankylosing spondylitis, may impair temporomandibular joint mobility.

To provide safe and effective airway control, the respiratory care practitioner must have a working knowledge of airway anatomy and know the application of basic and advanced management techniques. In addition, the practitioner must understand the physiologic responses to airway care, as well as how to avoid harming the patient while using management techniques. This chapter reviews the

- Basic anatomy of the upper and lower airways as it relates to airway management
- Basic information about establishing an airway
- Techniques for airway management
- Complications and hazards associated with airway care

AIRWAY ANATOMY (Figs. 29–1 and 29–2)

Upper Airway

Oral Cavity

The tongue is attached anteriorly to the mandible and the hyoid bone. Loss of muscle tone in the unconscious patient allows the tongue to fall posteriorly, obstructing the airway. Basic airway management maneuvers are aimed at relieving this obstruction. Anesthesia of the tongue is difficult to obtain with nerve blocks. Fortunately, topical anesthesia is easily provided.

The palate and the mandible provide the major bony framework of the oral cavity. The mandible serves as an anterior anchor for the tongue. The muscles of mastication insert on the ramus of the mandible. Motor block of these muscles is easily obtained by infiltration of the mandibular nerve in the pterygoid fossa, facilitating opening of the mouth without the use of parenteral muscle relaxants.

Nose

The nasal cavity borders on the base of the skull. In the presence of basilar skull fracture, nasotracheal or nasogastric tubes may accidentally pass into the cranial cavity. The nasal mucosa is highly vascular and easily damaged. Topical vasoconstrictors and generous lubrication decrease the likelihood of epistaxis during manipulation of this portion of the airway. When the nasal route is being used for intubation, several anatomic relationships must be kept in mind. The distance from the nares to the carina is 27 cm in the average adult woman and 32 cm in the average adult man. Because the meatus of the paranasal sinuses and lacrimal ducts open into the nasal cavity, prolonged intubation of the nose with nasogastric or nasotracheal tubes may cause sinus infections.

Nasogastric or nasotracheal tubes should be inserted perpendicular to the plane of the face because the floor of the nasal cavity runs parallel to the line of the teeth.

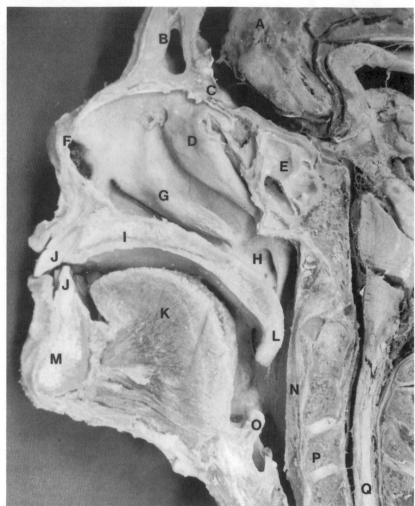

FIGURE 29–1: Sagittal section of the head. A, brain; B, frontal sinus; C, cribriform plate; D, superior concha; E, sphenoidal sinus; F, nostril; G, inferior concha; H, orifice of eustachian tube; I, hard palate; J, incisors; K, tongue; L, uvula; M, mandible; N, posterior pharyngeal wall; O, epiglottis; P, cervical spine; Q, spinal cord. (From Gorback MS. Emergency Airway Management. Philadelphia, BC Decker, 1990.)

Adenoids may block passage of a tube, become dislodged, or bleed during nasal intubation. The same may occur with nasopharyngeal tumors or abscesses. Enlargement of any of the pharyngeal structures may cause airway obstruction or complicate laryngoscopy.

The relative patency of each side of the nose should be checked to determine the presence of obstruction, such as a deviated septum.

Pharynx

The oral cavity and nasopharynx are continuous with the oropharynx, which contains the uvula, tonsils, and proximal epiglottis. The major structures of the nasopharynx are the adenoids. The laryngopharynx begins at the tip of the epiglottis.

Larynx

The adult larynx is located at the level of C4 to C5; in infants it is higher, at C3 to C4. The larynx passes anteriorly, extending to the level of the cricoid cartilage. Posteriorly, the pharynx joins the esophagus at the same level. Although this design may reflect a convenient economy on the part of evolution, it is disastrous for airway control: material intended for the posterior passage (e.g., a food bolus) may travel ante-

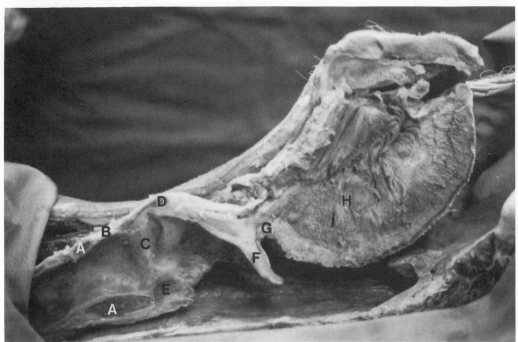

FIGURE 29–2: Detailed anatomy of the oral cavity and pharynx. A, cricoid cartilage; B, cricothyroid membrane; C, vocal cords; D, thyroid cartilage; E, arytenoid cartilage; F, epiglottis; G, vallecula; H, tongue. (From Gorback MS. Emergency Airway Management. Philadelphia, BC Decker, 1990.)

riorly into the larynx, and attempts to pass endotracheal tubes into the anterior passage may result in gastric insufflation.

As mentioned previously, the larynx ends at the cricotracheal junction. The only circumferentially complete laryngeal cartilage is the cricoid cartilage, located at C6. Cricoid pressure, part of Sellick's maneuver, compresses the proximal esophagus between the cricoid and the anterior cervical spine (Fig. 29–3). The narrowest part of the pediatric airway is the cricoid cartilage, whereas in the adult it is at the level of the vocal cords. The thyroid cartilage is a major anatomic landmark for both intubation and airway anesthesia. The superior laryngeal nerves can easily be blocked to provide supraglottic anesthesia. These nerves run past the superior horns of the thyroid cartilage as they enter the thyrohyoid membrane. The vocal cords are located inside the thyroid cartilage. The cricothyroid membrane is easily palpated between the thyroid and cricoid cartilages. This is the site of choice for emergency surgical access to the respiratory tract because of its relative avascularity and distance from the thyroid gland.

The epiglottis, a major landmark to look for during laryngoscopy, also impairs the view of the vocal cords. The upper part of the epiglottis is mobile, whereas the lower part attaches to the hyoid bone and the posterosuperior aspect of the thyroid cartilage.

Pressure on the thyroid cartilage during laryngoscopy will aid visualization by moving the larynx posteriorly.

Lower Airway

Trachea

The trachea is composed of 18 to 22 cartilaginous arches (approximately two rings per centimeter) joined by longitudinal elastic fibers,

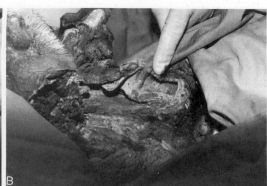

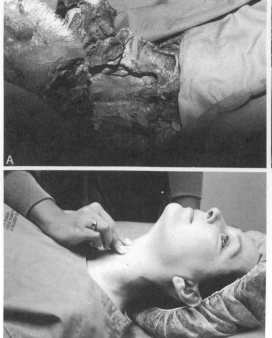

FIGURE 29–3: Cricoid pressure. *A,* The patent esophageal inlet is posterior to the cricoid cartilage. *B,* Pressure on the cricoid cartilage occludes the esophagus. *C,* Cricoid pressure is accomplished by placing the thumb and middle finger below and the index finger above the cricoid cartilage to form a stable tripod. (*A* to *C,* From Gorback MS. Emergency Airway Management. Philadelphia, BC Decker, 1990.)

allowing it to stretch and contract as the lungs move during the respiratory cycle. The posterior or membranous wall is closely applied to the esophagus throughout its length. The trachea is 10 to 13 cm long in the adult.

Bronchi, Conducting Airways, and Alveoli

The right mainstem bronchus is about 2 cm long before it divides into the right upper lobe bronchus and the bronchus intermedius. The left mainstem bronchus is about 5 cm long before it divides into the left upper and lower lobe bronchi. Therefore, there is a greater likelihood of obstructing the upper lobe with right endobronchial intubation.

AIRWAY MANAGEMENT

Simple Maneuvers to Relieve Airway Obstruction

The first step to relieve airway obstruction is to establish a patent airway. Foreign material should be removed from the mouth and the oropharynx, either manually (finger sweep) or with suction.

The presence of spontaneous respiration may dictate positioning. Apneic patients should be placed supine in anticipation of further airway support. An obtunded patient may alternatively be placed in the lateral decubitus position, with the head slightly down to prevent aspiration. Airway maneuvers such as the chin lift and jaw thrust are still possible in this position. A patient in respiratory distress will frequently prefer the sitting position, with the neck extended and the head moved anterior to the plane of the torso. This position, which is similar to the sniffing position used for laryngoscopy, aligns the major axes of the airway. The

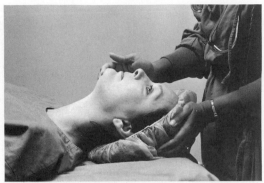

FIGURE 29–4: Chin lift maneuver. (From Gorback MS. Emergency Airway Management. Philadelphia, BC Decker, 1990.)

Any of the basic airway maneuvers may cause neurologic injury in patients with cervical spine instability.

sitting position removes the weight of the abdominal contents from the diaphragm. Forcing an awake dyspneic patient to lie flat may produce panic and struggling, as well as complicate management.

One of the simplest and most effective maneuvers to establish a patent airway is the chin lift. This maneuver is performed by placing the fingers under the chin and lifting upward to raise the chin while depressing the forehead with the other hand (Fig. 29–4). The thumb may be used to depress the lower lip or mandible, thus opening the mouth. The jaw thrust is another effective technique for opening the airway. The fingers are placed behind the angle of the mandible, lifting upward to displace it forward (Fig. 29–5). The thumbs may be used to hold the mouth open, to seal a mask on the face, or both. The chin lift and jaw thrust may be used together, with the thumbs employed to depress the mandible and open the mouth ("triple maneuver").

Artificial Airways

Nasal and oral airways are adjuncts to either mouth-to-mouth or mask ventilation. These devices establish a patent airway without intubation by overcoming soft tissue obstruction.

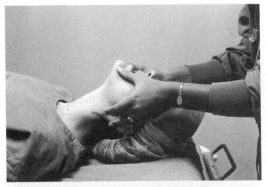

FIGURE 29–5: Jaw thrust maneuver (with depression of the mandible to open the mouth, the "triple maneuver"). (From Gorback MS. Emergency Airway Management. Philadelphia, BC Decker, 1990.)

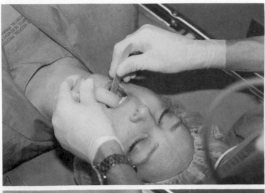
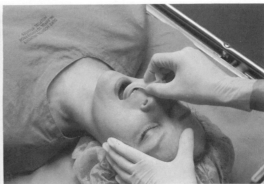
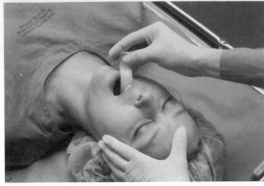

FIGURE 29–6: Insertion of an oral airway using a tongue blade *(A)*. The airway may be placed "upside down" *(B)* and rotated as it is advanced *(C)*. (*A* to *C*, From Gorback MS. Emergency Airway Management. Philadelphia, BC Decker, 1990.)

Oropharyngeal Airways

The primary function of the oropharyngeal airway is to establish airway patency. An airway that reaches from the corner of the mouth to the tragus of the ear when it is held next to the patient's face is most likely the proper size to use. There are two ways to insert an oral airway. With the use of a tongue blade or a finger to depress the tongue, the airway may be slid posteriorly (Fig. 29–6*A*). Alternatively, the airway may be inserted upside down (with the curvature facing the roof of the mouth) and rotated around into place (see Fig. 29–6*B* and *C*). This may require more mandibular excursion and may also dislodge loose teeth.

In a patient with intact gag reflexes, oral airway insertion is a very provocative stimulus. Prior topical application of local anesthetic may alleviate this response. It is possible to exacerbate obstruction with an oral airway. The airway must be seated posterior to the tongue (Fig. 29–7). If the airway is too small, the tip will be midway down the tongue, pushing it posteriorly against the back of the pharynx. Catching the tongue with the tip of the oral airway during insertion will push the tongue posteriorly against the pharyngeal wall, causing obstruction.

Nasopharyngeal Airways

Nasopharyngeal airways, which are better tolerated by the awake patient, can be inserted even if the patient is unable or unwilling to open the mouth. Generous lubrication will ease passage and prevent epistaxis. Topical vasoconstrictors may be used, but there is rarely time for their application. Topical anesthesia is not required, but coating the airway with lidocaine paste increases patient tolerance.

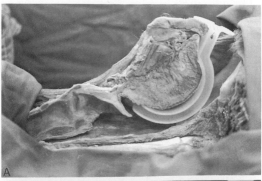
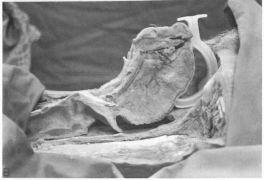

FIGURE 29–7: *A,* Correct placement of an oral airway, providing a stent between the tongue and the posterior pharyngeal wall. *B,* Incorrect placement and size. Too small an airway, or improper placement, will push the tongue down into the pharnyx. (*A* and *B,* From Gorback MS. Emergency Airway Management. Philadelphia, BC Decker, 1990.)

Intubation

Assessing the Patient for Intubation

A detailed evaluation must often be deferred in emergency situations (e.g., cardiac arrest). Unfortunately, management may be needlessly rushed when temporizing measures might have purchased a few extra moments for thought and preparation. For instance, a patient with impending respiratory failure may be assisted with a bag and mask while preparations are made for a more controlled, less stressful intubation. A small degree of preparation often tips the balance between an easy and a difficult procedure for both the intubator and the intubatee.

History

The practitioner must determine if the patient has any concurrent medical problems that could be exacerbated by the intubation procedure. The patient usually responds to intubation with hypertension and tachycardia. Occasionally, hypotension may ensue for a variety of reasons. The patient with respiratory failure may have high circulating levels of catecholamines in response to hypoxia or hypercarbia. Relief of the blood gas derangements may cause a drop in catecholamine levels and a fall in blood pressure. Manual hyperventilation following intubation is common; the resulting alkalosis may produce venodilatation, as well as decreased venous return due to positive pressure ventilation.

The practitioner must consider the impact of these responses on concurrent medical conditions. For example, patients with valvular disease, coronary artery disease, and congestive heart failure may respond poorly to increases in vasoconstriction or heart rate after intubation. Sudden elevations in arterial pressure may cause aneurysms to rupture. Patients with chronic hypertension often have a magnified pressor response to intubation. On the other hand, beta-receptor antagonists, vasodilators, or diuretics taken for chronic hypertension may blunt compensatory responses; in addition, profound hypotension may occur following the administration of sedatives, hypnotics, or muscle relaxants. Patients with reactive airway disease (asthma, bronchitis, or allergy) often respond to intubation with bronchoconstriction, which can be severe. Tracheal stenosis may be mistaken for asthma, with the diagnosis often missed in an emergency situation. Signs of prior tracheal trauma, such as tracheostomy, may indicate this condition.

Intubation usually increases intracranial pressure. Precautions should be taken before intubation to blunt this response. Care should be taken to avoid giving sedatives or other drugs that might produce hypotension in the presence of cerebrovascular insufficiency. Patients with carotid disease can develop bradycardia, cerebral ischemia, or both when the neck is extended for intubation.

Patients with myasthenia gravis have extreme sensitivity to nondepolarizing muscle relaxants. Anticholinesterase drugs taken for myasthenia prolong the half-life of drugs metabolized by plasma cholinesterases, such as succinylcholine. Ester-type local anesthetics may produce toxic side effects at lower doses in the presence of anticholinesterases.

The disposition of drugs given during airway management is affected by renal or hepatic impairment. Diminished drug excretion caused by renal or hepatic impairment may significantly delay neurologic assessment after intubation. For example, pancuronium excretion is greatly impaired in the presence of renal failure. The action of drugs whose primary route of elimination is hepatic (e.g., narcotics, vecuronium, and lidocaine) may be prolonged by hepatic disease. Chronic ethanol or other drug abuse may cause increased tolerance to central nervous system depressants.

Coagulopathy (e.g., due to thrombocytopenia, anticoagulant administration, or a clotting factor deficiency) may cause uncontrollable hemorrhage after airway instrumentation (especially with nasal intubation) or the performance of nerve blocks.

Most airway management maneuvers cause or require neck motion. Musculoskeletal disorders of the cervical spine have a profound impact on airway management. Patients with cervical spine instability (e.g., due to spinal trauma or rheumatoid arthritis) may suffer neurologic damage during airway manipulation (Fig. 29–8). Patients with ankylosing spondylitis may suffer neck fractures during neck manipulation.

Limited mobility of the head, neck, larynx, and temporomandibular joint may be caused by arthritis, ankylosing spondylitis, previous fusion, or placement in a halo. Infections such as epiglottitis or Ludwig's angina may precipitate airway embarrassment. Infections may complicate management if the infection is present at the site where a nerve block or tracheostomy is to be performed.

Aspiration risk factors include recent ingestion of food, gastric stasis (e.g., due to stress, anxiety, pain, gastric emptying disorders, or narcotic administration), gastroesophageal reflux, pregnancy, gastrointestinal obstruction, diminished level of consciousness (from any cause), and impaired protective reflexes (e.g., due to stroke).

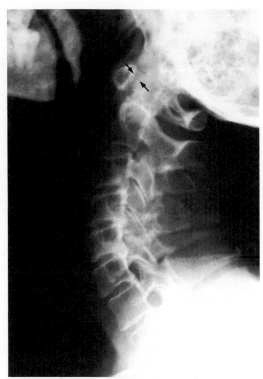

FIGURE 29–8: Cervical spine instability in rheumatoid arthritis. Many practitioners look for misalignment of the cervical vertebrae when they examine neck radiographs, but they fail to note atlantoaxial instability. Note the space that opens on extension between C1 and the dens *(arrows)*. (From Gorback MS. Emergency Airway Management. Philadelphia, BC Decker, 1990.)

Pregnancy produces changes in almost every major organ system. Mucosal capillary engorgement narrows air passages and increases the tendency for bleeding during manipulation. Precautions include the use of gentle technique during suctioning or intubation and the use of a smaller tube. As the pregnancy progresses, functional residual capacity diminishes, physiologic anemia worsens, and cardiac output increases, all of which contribute to rapid arterial oxygen desaturation during apnea. Preeclampsia further complicates management because of the cardiovascular, renal, and central nervous system derangements superimposed on the physiologic changes of pregnancy. Severe airway edema, intracranial pathology, and coagulopathy are common.

History of Previous Intubation Attempts

A great deal can be learned from records of previous intubations. Intubation procedure notes or anesthesia records often record the degree of difficulty encountered. In consideration of possible future intubations, the practitioner should document techniques and difficulties in the patient's record.

Physical Examination

Relative urgency can often be gauged with a brief determination of the patient's color, respiratory pattern, vital signs, level of distress, and level of consciousness. The autonomic stimulation of hypoxemia and hypercarbia produces hypertension, tachycardia, diaphoresis, and pallor. Hypotension and bradycardia are late signs. Drug overdose usually pro-

Subcutaneous air usually indicates airway disruption but is nonspecific as to location.

duces slow, deep, regular respiration. Metabolic acidosis accompanying diabetic ketoacidosis or renal failure (Kussmaul's breathing) may also produce this pattern.

Tachypnea is a nonspecific finding. Disorders of the conducting system (asthma), parenchyma (pulmonary edema), vasculature (pulmonary embolism), respiratory muscles (fatigue) or extrapulmonary diseases (e.g., salicylate toxicity, shock, or hyperventilation syndromes) can produce tachypnea.

Asymmetrical thoracic movement may reflect pneumothorax, major unilateral bronchial obstruction (e.g., foreign body aspiration), splinting due to injury, or atelectasis. These disorders may also be noted on chest percussion. Discoordinate movement is abnormal and suggests airway obstruction or respiratory muscle fatigue. The chest and abdomen should rise and fall together. Cheyne-Stokes, Biot's, or apneustic respiration often points to central disorders.

A prolonged inspiratory time with inspiratory stridor is characteristic of variable extrathoracic obstruction, whereas expiratory stridor, prolonged expiratory time, or wheezing suggests variable intrathoracic obstruction or bronchoconstriction. Fixed obstruction may affect one or both respiratory phases. Stridor indicates severe narrowing of the airway. Voice changes may result from vocal cord edema or palsy, dislocation or injury of laryngeal cartilages, or foreign bodies.

Airway Examination

If nasal intubation is anticipated, the practitioner should alternately compress each nostril as the patient breathes. This may provide a gross assessment of which passage is more patent. The patient may be able to indicate which nostril is the more patent. It is essential to assess temporomandibular joint mobility and mandibular morphology. In the normal adult, mandibular excursion is about 50 mm (2 inches, or three fingerbreadths). When excursion is reduced to half of that, or about 25 mm, difficulty with laryngoscopy may be anticipated. The distance from the symphysis of the mandible to the hyoid bone should also be about three fingerbreadths. Two fingerbreadths or less usually indicates a retrognathic mandible. According to one proposed scoring system, if the soft palate, fauces, and uvula are visible when the patient opens the mouth wide, the glottis should be visible at laryngoscopy. If only the soft palate and the uvular base are visible (or only the soft palate is visible), laryngoscopy may be difficult. The usefulness of this predictive technique has been questioned by at least one prospective investigation.

Examination of the mouth should include a search for loose or damaged teeth, dentures, and foreign bodies such as candy, chewing gum, tobacco, or food. Facial trauma can cause airway obstruction, complicate airway management, and accompany other, more serious injuries to the head and neck.

Goiters, abscesses, tumors, cysts, hematomas, or other neck masses may deviate or compress the airway. Neck mobility should be checked (provided that instability has been ruled out) because limited neck extension may hinder laryngoscopy. Patients with short, muscular ("bull") necks; morbid obesity; arthritis; radiation changes; or previous cervical fusion may have limited extension. Tracheostomy scars may indicate residual tracheal stenosis.

Chest radiography, arterial blood gas analysis, and pulmonary function tests are useful, time permitting. Electrocardiography, blood chemistry results, and hematologic profiles may be useful, but only tests used for evaluation for airway intervention are discussed here.

Arterial blood gas analysis findings must be interpreted in light of the clinical picture. An isolated oxygenation deficit may respond to O_2 supplementation without intubation. Compensated hypercarbia is not an indication for intubation. Narcotized patients may have moderate respiratory acidosis yet remain awake and stable. On the other hand, a normal Pa_{CO_2} at the expense of a respiratory rate of 60 breaths per minute is unacceptable.

Simple pulmonary function tests may be extremely useful, especially when they indicate a trend. A vital capacity of less than 10 to 12 mL/kg may indicate impending respiratory failure. The peak expiratory flow rate is sensitive to upper airway obstruction. If the ratio of FEV_1 (in milliliters) to peak expiratory flow rate (in liters per minute) is greater than 10, upper airway obstruction should be suspected.

Flow-volume loops are useful for evaluating airway obstruction. If the ratio of maximal expiratory flow to maximal inspiratory flow at midvital capacity is close to unity (i.e., the inspiratory and expiratory loops are equally diminished), there is probably a fixed obstruction. Variable intrathoracic lesions primarily distort the expiratory loop, with the ratio of maximal expiratory flow to maximal inspiratory flow at midvital capacity close to 0.3. Variable extrathoracic lesions behave in the opposite way, distorting the inspiratory loop. In this case, the ratio of maximal expiratory flow to maximal inspiratory flow at midvital capacity is close to 2.

When upper airway compromise is suspected, soft tissue films of the head, neck, and chest may be useful in revealing pathology not apparent on physical examination (Fig. 29–9). If airway obstruction is suspected,

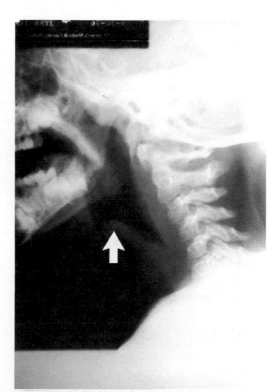

FIGURE 29–9: Epiglottitis. Swollen epiglottis and aryepiglottic folds *(arrow)*. (From Gorback MS. Emergency Airway Management. Philadelphia, BC Decker, 1990.)

this should be noted on the requisition; routine anteroposterior and lateral neck radiographs are usually optimized for bone. Overpenetrated chest films help to delineate the tracheobronchial tree, whereas expiratory chest radiographs are useful for demonstrating postobstructive emphysema distal to a radiolucent foreign body. Computed tomography is extremely useful but has inherent disadvantages:

* The patient must leave the care area.
* Patients who are unable to lie flat cannot be scanned.
* Some obese patients will not fit in the scanner.

Selecting Intubation Equipment

Laryngoscopes

Most laryngoscopes are either curved (e.g., the MacIntosh laryngoscope) or straight (e.g., the Miller or Wisconsin laryngoscope). The choice of blade is largely a personal one. The curved blade (Fig. 29–10) has a moderate curvature and a tapered flange along the left side. This blade elevates the epiglottis by stretching the hypoepiglottic ligament. Claimed advantages for the curved blade include

* Less dental trauma
* More room for passage of the tube
* Less chance of provocation of reflexes by pressing on the epiglottis

Straight blades (see Fig. 29–10), which come in a variety of configurations, are used in all age groups. The tip of a straight blade is used to lift the epiglottis directly to expose the vocal cords. Claimed advantages of this blade are greater exposure of the glottis and less need for a stylet.

Endotracheal Tubes

Contemporary high-volume, low-pressure, cuffed plastic endotracheal tubes have replaced low-compliance rubber tubes because the pressure required to obtain a good seal with the latter usually exceeds tracheal capillary pressure, thereby predisposing the patient to tracheal

> Curved blades are rarely used for infants: straight blades provide better control of the epiglottis in this age group.

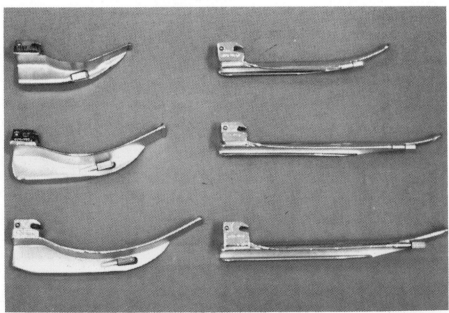

FIGURE 29–10: Laryngoscope blades. *Left,* Curved (MacIntosh). *Right,* Straight (Miller). (From Gorback MS. Emergency Airway Management. Philadelphia, BC Decker, 1990.)

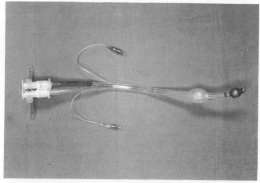

FIGURE 29–11: Endobronchial or double-lumen tube. Note the tracheal and bronchial cuffs above the respective lumens. (From Gorback MS. Emergency Airway Management. Philadelphia, BC Decker, 1990.)

injury. By convention, size is determined by the inner diameter of the tube (in millimeters).

The endotracheal tube has evolved in many specialized forms. Pediatric endotracheal tubes with an internal diameter of less than 4 mm are usually uncuffed. Flexible armored tubes are available if kinking or compression of the tube is of concern. Pulling on the ring of a "trigger" tube with a finger (or thumb) flexes the tube, maneuvering the tube tip. Double-lumen tubes (Fig. 29–11) isolate the two sides of the tracheobronchial tree to

- Prevent soiling of a healthy lung by pus or blood from the other
- Provide differential lung ventilation
- Perform lung lavage

Stylets and Guides

Stylets should be made of a malleable material (e.g., copper) and have a smooth surface, either of polished metal or plastic coated. After the lubricated stylet has been inserted into the tube, the tube is bent into the desired shape, usually a J or "hockey stick" configuration.

When the glottis cannot be seen, malleable plastic guides may be useful. The guide is shaped (usually into a J or hockey stick form, as with stylets) and slid under the epiglottis into the larynx. Flexible urethral sounds, nasogastric tubes, and suction catheters serve well. Dedicated bougies are also commercially available.

Fiberoptic Devices and Light Wands

The fiberoptic bronchoscope can be used for difficult or awake intubation. Light wands are malleable stylets with a light source on the end to aid intubation by transillumination of the airway. The Bullard laryngoscope, a rigid, curved fiberoptic device, is inserted like an oral airway, with the larynx being seen through its fiberoptic system. All three of these devices may be inserted orally in cases in which decreased mandibular excursion prevents conventional laryngoscopy. Flexible light wands are now available for the nasal route.

Monitoring Devices

Pulse oximetry allows continuous noninvasive assessment of oxygenation during airway management. Capnography allows early detection of failed intubation by revealing the absence of CO_2 in exhaled gas. Semiquantitative chemical sensors attach inline to the end of the endotracheal tube and change color with pH, thereby detecting the presence of CO_2. These devices may be included in an emergency bag for convenient determination of the end-tidal CO_2 at any clinical location.

Performing Intubation

Once the decision to intubate has been made, the practitioner must decide on the route of intubation and on whether to intubate the patient awake or under anesthesia.

Choice of Route

The two major routes for intubation are oral and nasal. The advantages of oral intubation include faster execution, the use of a larger tube, and a minimal risk of bacteremia. Oral intubation requires an open mouth (which dictates that the patient must be cooperative, paralyzed, or unconscious) and adequate mandibular excursion. Trauma to the teeth and lips is more likely with oral intubation. The patient can occlude the tube by biting down, but this can be prevented with the insertion of an oral airway or other bite block after intubation. Although it is frequently taught that oral intubation produces more laryngeal damage, this is true only in the short term.

Nasal intubation is feasible even if the patient cannot or will not open the mouth. There are no hard data to support the truism that nasal intubation is more comfortable once the tube is in place. Although occlusion by the teeth is not possible, kinking in the nasopharynx has been known to occur. Because the tube position is more stable, short-term laryngeal damage is decreased. Mouth care is easier without the impediment of an orotracheal tube.

Nasal intubation usually takes longer to perform. A longer and narrower tube must be used, and the increased respiratory workload may impede subsequent weaning attempts. Fiberoptic bronchoscopes or even suction catheters may be too large to pass through a narrower or kinked tube.

Injury is probably more common during nasal intubation. As opposed to the occasional tooth or lip damage seen with oral intubation, nasal mucosal and turbinate damage is common; the resultant epistaxis may be severe and difficult to control. Therefore, coagulopathy is a contraindication to nasal intubation. Nasopharyngeal tumors, adenoids, and abscesses may be disrupted. Submucosal tunneling or other injury to the posterior pharyngeal wall may occur during nasal intubation. The tube may be passed into the cranail cavity in the presence of basilar skull fracture. Pressure necrosis of the nasal septum or alae may occur.

Awake Versus Anesthetized

The advantages of awake intubation include maintenance of the airway, spontaneous respiration, and preservation of protective airway reflexes. If there is a question of central or peripheral nervous system derangement or damage, neurologic assessment is possible immediately after intubation. If sedation or local anesthesia is used, these advantages will be compromised to various degrees.

Awake intubation requires patient cooperation, especially for oral intubation. Nasal intubation can be performed in an uncooperative patient if active restraint by overwhelming force is used (also known as "brutane" anesthesia), but this is not recommended. Autonomic stress responses (e.g., hypertension, tachycardia, and elevated intracranial pressure) are practically guaranteed unless sedation and regional anesthesia are used.

Bacteremia during insertion, sinusitis, and otitis occur with significant frequency during nasal intubation. Therefore, immunocompromise should be considered a strong relative contraindication to nasal intubation.

Intubation under anesthesia or heavy sedation (e.g., using barbiturates, etomidate, ketamine, benzodiazepines, propofol, or narcotics) eliminates the requirement for patient cooperation. The stress response is usually less than with awake intubation. The major disadvantage of heavy sedation or general anesthesia is the production of apnea or profound respiratory depression. Such techniques should be used only by experienced personnel because the patient's life depends on the respiratory support skills of the operator. Anesthesia (whether general, regional, or topical) also obtunds or abolishes protective airway reflexes; in addition, postintubation neurologic assessment is impossible until the central nervous system depressants wear off.

Preparation for Intubation

Pharmacologic preparation of the patient is beyond the scope of this chapter. Detailed descriptions may be found in other sources.

In all but the most urgent cases, all necessary equipment should be set up and checked. A basic setup includes

- A laryngoscope and blade (or blades), with fresh batteries
- Endotracheal tubes of appropriate size, plus a few sizes larger or smaller
- A 5- or 10-mL cuff syringe
- An oxygen source capable of delivering 10 to 15 L/min, tubing, masks, and a bag-valve device
- Suction and suction catheter (Yankauer tip preferred)
- Stylets
- Intravenous access
- Emergency drugs
- A stethoscope

Oral Intubation

The occiput should be elevated about 5 cm. A folded blanket provides a firmer base than a pillow. The head is tilted back, aligning the axes of the larynx, pharynx, and mouth. Because this position mimics the posture of someone sniffing a flower, it is often called the sniffing position (Fig. 29–12). With the middle finger of the right hand placed on the

With the possible exception of ketamine, most central nervous system depressant drugs will cause variable degrees of cardiovascular depression.

Vital signs should be measured frequently, especially if sedatives or anesthetics are used. Electrocardiography, pulse oximetry, and capnography are highly recommended.

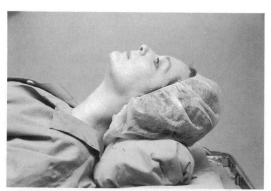

FIGURE 29–12: The sniffing position aligns the axes of the upper and lower airways. Some patients with respiratory distress prefer to sit in this position. (From Gorback MS. Emergency Airway Management. Philadelphia, BC Decker, 1990.)

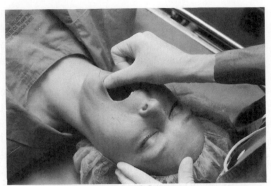

FIGURE 29–13: The scissors maneuver. (From Gorback MS. Emergency Airway Management. Philadelphia, BC Decker, 1990.)

upper teeth and the thumb on the lower teeth, the two are spread apart ("scissors maneuver," Fig. 29–13). The laryngoscope blade is inserted on the right side of the mouth, aiming for the right tonsillar pillar. The tongue is kept to the left of the flange. A common mistake is to place the blade down the middle of the tongue, which is a frequent cause of difficult intubation. The blade is slid into the pharynx until the epiglottis can be seen.

Up to this point, laryngoscopy is the same with either type of blade. If a curved blade is used, the tip of the blade is inserted into the space between the base of the tongue and the epiglottis (vallecula) as far as it will go. The blade is then lifted at a 45-degree angle in the direction of the axis of the handle. Tension on the hypoepiglottic ligament lifts the epiglottis (Fig. 29–14).

When a straight blade is used, the tip of the blade is inserted under (posterior to) the epiglottis, with the blade used to lift the epiglottis directly (see Fig. 29–14). Again, the practitioner lifts up on the handle: the laryngoscope should not be levered using the teeth as a fulcrum. With either type of blade, the tube is passed gently through the larynx until the cuff is seen to pass below the vocal cords.

Problems With Visualization

Poor technique is the most common cause of inadequate laryngoscopy. The two most common errors I have seen are improper positioning and failure to keep the tongue to the left of the blade. Sometimes the novice will insert the blade too far, neglecting to look for the epiglottis on the way in. On withdrawal of the blade from the esophagus, the epiglottis will fall into view. Displacing the glottis posteriorly toward the line of sight may be accomplished by pressure on the thyroid cartilage. The pressure should be applied such that the cartilage is not pinched, which will close the vocal cords. Suction should be used or the throat should be manually cleared of obstructing material. Magill forceps may be used to remove large pieces of solid material. Sometimes, using a different blade will make the difference between a successful and an unsuccessful intubation.

If the vocal cords still cannot be visualized but the epiglottis or the arytenoid cartilages can be seen, a malleable stylet is used to shape the tube into a J or hockey stick shape, and the practitioner tries to slide the tube along the underside of the epiglottis into the larynx (Fig. 29–15). When the tube can be felt to pass through the vocal cords, the stylet is removed and the tube is advanced into the trachea.

Unless laryngeal or cervical spine injury is suspected, there is no contraindication to pressing on the thyroid cartilage as a routine maneuver.

Many practitioners use a stylet for every emergency oral intubation.

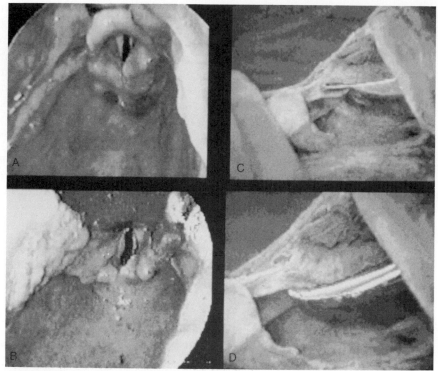

FIGURE 29–14: Laryngoscopy. *A*, View of the vocal cords with a MacIntosh No. 3 (curved) blade. Note that the epiglottis is visible below the blade. *B*, View of the vocal cords with a Miller (straight) blade. Note that the epiglottis is above the blade. *C* and *D*, Cadaver dissections showing placement of the curved and straight blades, respectively. (*C* and *D*, From Gorback MS. Emergency Airway Management. Philadelphia, BC Decker, 1990.)

The oral fiberoptic approach requires good topical anesthesia of the tongue. The use of a bite block or an intubating airway is highly recommended. The tongue should be displaced forward with an intubating airway, tongue traction, a jaw thrust maneuver, or a laryngoscope. An awake patient can be asked to protrude the tongue. Staying in the midline, the practitioner follows the tongue to the epiglottis.

Another approach in this situation is to intubate the larynx with a tube exchanger or another endotracheal guide and then to pass the en-

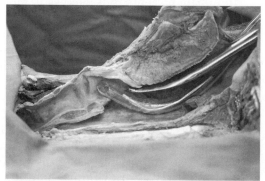

FIGURE 29–15: A "hockey stick" configuration is useful for guiding a tube into the larynx when only the epiglottis can be seen. (From Gorback MS. Emergency Airway Management. Philadelphia, BC Decker, 1990.)

dotracheal tube over it. Malleable urethral sounds, nasogastric tubes, and gum elastic bougies have all been used for this method.

The practitioner should not persist in an intubation attempt for more than 15 to 30 seconds unless continuous oxygen saturation monitoring (pulse oximetry) indicates that oxygenation is adequate. Cyanosis, a late sign of desaturation, should not be used as an end-point for an intubation attempt. Some practitioners have promulgated breath holding during intubation on the premise that when the intubator needs a breath so does the patient. However, the following points should be considered:

- Breath holding impairs concentration.
- The intubator's tolerance for apnea is likely to differ from the patient's.
- A dyspneic intubator is an impaired intubator.

Nasal Intubation

Anesthesia (either general or topical) and mucosal vasoconstriction are highly desirable. If nasal intubation will be performed under general anesthesia, topical anesthesia is not as necessary, but it will still help to blunt the response to intubation, allowing a lower dose of general anesthetic. Topical vasoconstrictors are recommended regardless of the choice of anesthetic.

The tube and the nasal passages should be lubricated generously. Insertion of a nasal airway lubricated with anesthetic paste (which also applies a final coat of lubrication and anesthetic) can help to determine patency as well. Through the insertion of successively larger nasal airways coated with anesthetic paste, the stimulus is gradually increased as more topical anesthesia is applied. Long cotton-tipped applicators can also be used to apply topical anesthesia and to explore the nasal passages. The tube is inserted with firm, steady pressure directed perpendicular to the face, not upward toward the forehead. Passage into the nasopharynx is usually accompanied by a sudden loss of resistance. The tube should not be forced if major resistance is encountered.

There are three general ways to perform nasal intubation:

- Blind
- Under direct vision
- With a fiberoptic scope

Blind nasal intubation requires no equipment other than the endotracheal tube itself. Contrary to popular belief, this technique often works in apneic patients, but success is more likely with spontaneous respiration. The practitioner advances the tube during inspiration while listening for breath sounds. If breath sounds are lost while the tube passes without resistance, esophageal placement is most likely. The tube should be withdrawn until breath sounds reappear. Extension of the neck will direct the tip of the tube anteriorly. If the tube has gone laterally or anteriorly, the loss of sounds will be accompanied by increased resistance. Rotating the tube will guide it laterally, and flexion of the neck will direct it posteriorly. A method of directing the tube anteriorly without neck manipulation is by inflation of the cuff. This technique may be used when the tube consistently passes posteriorly into the esophagus. The tube is withdrawn until breath sounds reappear, and then the cuff is inflated or overinflated. This displaces the tip of the tube away from the posterior wall of the pharynx. The tube is then advanced slightly. If it can be advanced past the point at which breath sounds were previously lost and if breath sounds continue to be present, the tip has probably

Continuing phonation by the patient is a sure sign that the tube is not translaryngeal. Coughing accompanied by loss of phonation indicates that the tube is in the trachea, whereas coughing with persistent phonation indicates that the tube is very close to the glottis. If the latter occurs, the position should be held until the cough is complete. During the subsequent forceful inspiration, the glottis is widely patent and the tube may be advanced at that moment.

entered the larynx. The cuff should be deflated and the tube advanced about 4 to 5 cm. This should place the tube below the vocal cords.

Nasal intubation may be performed under direct vision, but this requires laryngoscopy. Because this combines several of the disadvantages of both techniques, it is rarely a first choice for emergency intubation. It is useful for performing nasal intubation under controlled conditions, such as in changing an oral tube to a nasal one. Sometimes direct visualization is necessary when blind attempts fail but nasal intubation is the route of choice.

Nasal intubation with direct laryngoscopy is performed as for blind nasal intubation, except that the tube is advanced only into the pharynx. Laryngoscopy is then performed as described earlier for oral intubation, advancing the tube under direct vision. The manipulations described previously for blind intubation may be used to guide the tube into the larynx. Alternatively, the tube is grasped above the cuff with Magill forceps and is guided into the larynx while an assistant advances the tube slowly (Fig. 29–16). The cuff portion should not be grasped with the forceps because it may be torn.

Because the tongue is a major impediment to oral fiberoptic intubation, many prefer the nasal route. A disadvantage to the nasal route is that even slight amounts of blood impair visualization with the fiberoptic scope. Antisialagogues such as atropine or glycopyrrolate may be used to dry secretions in preparation for fiberoptic intubation. Elevation of the head helps to drain secretions and prevent posterior displacement of the tongue.

The dominant hand manipulates the controls while the nondominant hand controls the direction and depth of insertion. The scope must be rotated as a unit: it should be rotated by turning it with both hands. Body English should be avoided because this succeeds only in producing musculoskeletal reminders of the intubation in the operator.

As with other nasal intubations, anesthesia, vasoconstriction, and sedation are key elements to management. There are differences of opinion as to whether the tube or the scope should be passed first. If the scope is passed through the nose first, there will often be less epistaxis to obstruct vision. The major problem with this technique is that one may successfully pass the scope into the trachea only to find that the tube will not fit through the nose. Conversely, if the tube is passed through the nose first, patency is ensured, but the operating field is more likely to be obscured by blood. If the tube is inserted first, it should be

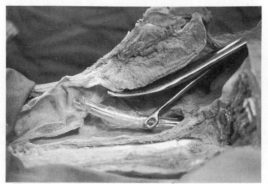

FIGURE 29–16: Use of the Magill forceps. (From Gorback MS. Emergency Airway Management. Philadelphia, BC Decker, 1990.)

passed just far enough to feel the "give" as the tube bends into the nasopharynx. If the tube is inserted in this way, the larynx will often be visible as the scope passes out of the end of the tube. If the tube is inserted too far initially, the first view from the end of the tube will be the esophagus. Having the patient breathe through the nose moves the soft palate anteriorly, which aids in nasal intubation. After the larynx has been visualized, the patient should pant, which will open the larynx and decrease the cough and gag reflexes.

Retrograde Intubation

Retrograde intubation kits are commercially available, but the components are simple and are easily assembled from equipment available in most clinical settings.

When standard approaches are not possible or fail, retrograde intubation (Fig. 29–17) may be attempted. The general principle is to introduce a slender, flexible guide through the cricothyroid membrane. Many variations on the technique have been reported, including the passage of epidural catheters through Tuohy needles, the passage of long central venous pressure catheters through introducer needles, and the passage of guidewires through intravenous catheters.

First, the intubator ensures that the flexible guide will pass through the selected introducer. This is ensured if a long central venous pressure catheter kit or an epidural tray is being used. A large-bore (No. 18 or larger) introducer needle or an intravenous catheter is inserted through the cricothyroid membrane until air is aspirated. The needle should be directed upward (cranially) toward the thyroid cartilage. A long, slender, flexible guide (e.g., a long central venous pressure catheter, an epidural catheter, or a guidewire) is threaded through the catheter and retrieved via the mouth or nose. A laryngoscope, a Magill forceps, or both may be

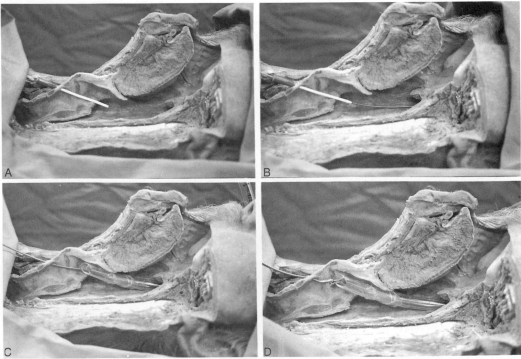

FIGURE 29–17: Insertion of an introducer through the cricothyroid membrane for retrograde intubation (A). A guide is passed through the introducer (B). The tube may be passed over the guide (C), or the guide may be tied to the tip of the tube (D). (A to D, From Gorback MS. Emergency Airway Management. Philadelphia, BC Decker, 1990.)

required. The guide can be tied to the endotracheal tube tip and the tube can be drawn into the larynx, or the tube may be passed over the guide. It is probably easier to pull the tube into the larynx than to thread it over a thin guide, but this leaves a knot on the end of the tube that could come loose in the trachea. The guide is cut at the skin level when the tube has entered the larynx, and the tube is inserted to the proper depth.

Tactile Orotracheal Intubation

The main danger with tactile orotracheal intubation is bitten fingers. This technique should be used only with paralyzed or deeply comatose patients or with the employment of a mouth prop or bite block. The tube is shaped into a J with a malleable stylet. Standing at the right side of the patient, the practitioner inserts the left hand into the right side of the mouth and into the pharynx. The epiglottis (the only firm mobile structure in the pharynx) is palpated with the middle finger, and the endotracheal tube is passed down the left side of the mouth. The tube is guided into the glottis with the middle and index fingers. The stylet is withdrawn before the tube is introduced more than a few centimeters past the cords.

Endobronchial Intubation

Indications for endobronchial intubation include

- Preventing contamination of a healthy lung by a contaminated one
- Bronchopleural fistula
- Giant lung cyst
- Tracheobronchial disruption
- Operations on the lung or esophagus
- Pulmonary lavage

Because double-lumen endotracheal tubes are rather bulky, only the oral route is available.

As described previously, the right upper lobe bronchus arises closer to the carina than the left upper lobe bronchus, so it is more likely to be occluded by the endobronchial cuff. Therefore, left-sided tubes are preferable.

Preparation for endobronchial intubation is similar to that for oral intubation with a single-lumen tube, with two major modifications:

1. Both cuffs (bronchial and tracheal) should be checked.

2. A stylet is inserted through the bronchial side of the catheter, giving it a slight curvature to the left toward the end of the tube (see Fig. 29–11).

With the airway adapters to the right, the distal part of the tube is inserted as if it were a single-lumen tube, and the stylet is withdrawn when the bronchial cuff passes through the vocal cords. The tube is rotated 90 degrees counterclockwise until the airway connectors are in the midline. This will direct the endobronchial side to the left. The tube is advanced until it is seated in the bronchus, and the laryngoscope is removed. The point at which the two lumina join should be at the level of the teeth. Placement and function are confirmed by inflating the tracheal cuff first and checking breath sounds during manual ventilation. If only one lung is ventilated, the tracheal cuff is probably in one of the mainstem bronchi; the cuff is deflated and the tube withdrawn slightly. This is repeated until bilateral breath sounds are heard, and the bronchial cuff is inflated using no more than 3 mL of air. The pilot balloon is palpated during inflation to ensure that excessive pressure is not applied. Breath sounds should still be bilateral after inflation of the bronchial cuff.

The tubing is clamped to the bronchial side. Breath sounds should disappear on the left and be present on the right. The process is repeated on the other side: the findings should reverse. If bilateral breath sounds are heard with either side clamped, the tube is not properly positioned. If the tube seems to be well seated and bilateral sounds persist with one side clamped, the bronchial cuff may be distal to a secondary bronchus. This is more likely to occur with a right-sided tube because of the early takeoff of the right upper lobe bronchus. The tube is pulled back 1 or 2 cm at a time, checking for proper function.

If both lumina are in one bronchus or if the tube is kinked, clamping one side abolishes breath sounds bilaterally. A remote possibility is occlusion of one of the ports. The intubator should try withdrawing the tube in 1- to 2-cm increments. If the tube has passed into the contralateral bronchus, ventilation will be absent on the right when the bronchial side is occluded. Positioning of the tube can be aided or confirmed by fiberoptic bronchoscopy. As viewed through the tracheal lumen, the right mainstem bronchus should be easily visible, whereas the endobronchial portion may be seen passing into the left mainstem bronchus. The tube may be withdrawn until the cuff is visible just distal to the carina, ensuring the proper position.

Light Wands

Lighted stylets (light wands) are used to intubate by transillumination of the airway in a dim room. The light wand stylet is lubricated and passed through an endotracheal tube. The tube is shaped into a J. The jaw is pulled forward, and the light wand is advanced into the pharynx until a bright area of light is seen below the cricoid cartilage, indicating that the tube is in the trachea. The stylet is removed and the tube is advanced to the desired depth.

Postintubation Procedures

The practitioner inflates the cuff while palpating the pilot balloon for excessive pressure. The cuff is slowly deflated until air can be heard escaping around it, and then just enough air is added to seal the leak. The following signs should be looked for:

- Bilateral chest movement during ventilation
- Condensation of moisture in the tube during exhalation
- Loss of phonation in an awake patient

Follow-up chest radiography is recommended to document satisfactory positioning of the tube.

Both lungs are auscultated, and the practitioner listens over the epigastrium to rule out esophageal intubation. The latter produces coarse flatulent sounds over the stomach. Esophageal intubation often produces a belching sound during ventilation. The depth of the tube is checked: it should be about 22 ± 2 cm at the level of the incisors (oral intubation) and 27 ± 2 cm at the level of the nares (nasal intubation) in the typical adult.

Because there is usually no CO_2 in the stomach, the presence of end-tidal CO_2 is a good indicator that the tube is placed correctly. If a functioning capnograph fails to detect CO_2, it is almost certain that the tube is not in the trachea. One notable exception to this rule is in cardiac arrest: if there is no circulation, no CO_2 will be delivered to the lungs, yielding a false-negative finding on capnography. Recent ingestion of

carbonated beverages or antacids may yield transient false-positive results after esophageal intubation. The end-tidal CO_2 should disappear
within a few breaths if this occurs. Hypoxemia (as indicated by pulse
oximetry or cyanosis) due to esophageal or endobronchial intubation is a
late sign. Tube placement may also be confirmed by bronchoscopy or
laryngoscopy.

Persistent air leaks are usually due to a leaky cuff or a malfunctioning pilot balloon valve. If an inordinate amount of air is required but the
cuff is not leaking (i.e., the pilot balloon does not lose pressure), the tube
may not be inserted far enough; the poor seal is due to the cuff's being
between or above the vocal cords.

Cricothyroidotomy

Cricothyroidotomy is performed when conventional intubation is impossible or contraindicated. Tracheostomy is technically more difficult
and time consuming, and its use as an emergency procedure is questionable unless laryngeal damage is present.

The cricothyroid membrane is palpable between the thyroid and
cricoid cartilages. A common error is to mistake the thyrohyoid space for
the cricothyroid space. The former is tucked up under the mandible,
whereas the latter is usually in the mid to lower neck. A good way to
identify the cricoid cartilage is to palpate in the suprasternal notch and
walk the finger up until the cricoid cartilage is encountered. This structure is much larger and firmer than the tracheal rings. If time permits,
the area is prepared and local anesthesia is administered. An incision is
made through the skin and the cricothyroid membrane. This incision
should not be too generous (perhaps 1.5 to 2 cm) because the carotid
arteries lie laterally. Some prefer to make the skin incision vertically,
allowing better palpation and identification of the cricothyroid membrane. The incision should be shallow so that the posterior larynx and
the esophagus are not injured. The incision can be opened by twisting
the scalpel handle in the incision, or a clamp may be used to spread the
margins of the incision. Any hollow stent may be used to maintain patency: it does not have to be a tracheostomy tube, although this is preferable.

Complications of emergency cricothyroidotomy include incorrect
placement (most commonly through the thyrohyoid membrane), false
passage, hemorrhage, thyroid cartilage fracture, subcutaneous emphysema, and laryngeal and esophageal laceration.

Needle Cricothyroidotomy

In the pediatric age group (patients younger than 12 years of age), needle cricothyroidotomy is the preferred treatment because of the possibility of cricoid damage.

Needle cricothyroidotomy is a temporizing measure to be used until
more definitive airway control is achieved. A large-bore catheter attached
to an oxygen source is inserted through the cricothyroid membrane (directed caudally). Intermittent occlusion of a Y connector or a side hole in
the tubing allows insufflation of oxygen. Some setups have a spring-
loaded valve that can be intermittently depressed. The practitioner in-
sufflates for 1 second and releases for 4 seconds.

The catheter can be connected to a conventional bag-valve setup.
The connector from a small endotracheal tube (approximately 3 mm in
diameter) will fit into the hub of an intravenous catheter. Alternatively,
a connector from a larger (7 to 8 mm in diameter) endotracheal tube will

fit the barrel of a 3-mL syringe. The syringe tip will fit into the intravenous catheter. It is very difficult to apply enough pressure to provide adequate ventilation, but it is better than nothing at all.

Changing Endotracheal Tubes

The nature of the procedure of changing endotracheal tubes implies that airway control has already been established. This allows the luxury of using sedation and paralysis to obtain optimal conditions. If possible, the stomach is emptied with an orogastric or a nasogastric tube to prevent aspiration during the exchange. The administration of 100% oxygen for several minutes before the procedure should provide an oxygen reserve unless a severe oxygenation deficit is present. When the same route will be used, a simple exchange over a guide is possible.

Direct visualization with either a laryngoscope or a fiberoptic bronchoscope allows the same or a different route to be chosen for the new endotracheal tube, but heavy sedation, anesthesia, and paralysis are often necessary to ensure good operating conditions and patient comfort. The larynx should be well visualized before the old tube is removed. One disadvantage to using the fiberoptic scope is that secretions dragged along when the old tube is removed may obscure vision. As a safety precaution, it is advisable to pass a tube exchanger down through the old tube first. Then, if airway control or visibility is lost before insertion of the new tube, a tube may be reinserted over the guide.

Tube exchanges can be performed by passing semirigid devices through an existing endotracheal tube. Some exchangers are hollow, allowing oxygen insufflation if difficulties arise in passing the new tube. An 18 Fr nasogastric tube with the suction ports cut off works very well. Some commercially available tube exchangers are very rigid and may cause tracheobronchial injury.

A tracheostomy tube that has been in place less than 7 days should not be changed unless absolutely necessary. If a fresh tracheostomy tube needs to be changed, a surgeon (preferably the surgeon who performed the tracheostomy) and equipment for emergency intubation should be available.

Exchange may be performed over a guide, as with other endotracheal tubes. The practitioner should always be prepared for oral or nasal intubation in case control of the airway is lost during the exchange. In some cases, it may be preferable to intubate the patient from above before the exchange, placing the tube proximal to the tracheostomy but below the vocal cords. The endotracheal tube can then be advanced past the stoma to ensure ventilation if the exchange is unsuccessful. Inadvertent decannulation of a fresh tracheostomy may not leave a clear track for reinsertion, and attempts to recannulate the trachea may result in blind passage into deep tissue layers. The patient may require intubation by the oral or nasal route, emergency surgical exploration, or both. Some surgeons place silk sutures into the walls of the tracheal stoma. In an emergency, pulling on the sutures will bring the tracheal stoma into approximation with the skin stoma.

Mature stomata do not require these special precautions.

SUMMARY

It is essential in providing state-of-the-art respiratory care for practitioners to understand basic principles of airway management. This first requires a fundamental understanding of the relationships of the oral cavity, nose, pharynx, larynx, trachea, and lower airways. Skilled clinicians should also know how to assess the need for airway care and be able to supply a patent airway noninvasively using proper positioning and masks. Tracheal intubation is an important skill that can be both lifesaving and life supporting. A number of techniques and types of equipment are available that sometimes must be used in conjunction with pharmacologic therapy to sedate and/or paralyze the patient. Complications of tracheal intubation are important to recognize and treat promptly.

Suggested Readings

1. Gorback MS. Emergency Airway Management. Philadelphia, BC Decker, 1990.
2. Block C, Brechner VL. Unusual problems in airway management II. The influence of the temporomandibular joint, the mandible, and associated structures on endotracheal intubation. Anesth Analg 50:114–123, 1971.
3. Grosfield O, Czarnecka B, Crecka-Kuzan K, et al. Clinical investigations of the temporomandibular joint in children and adolescents with rheumatoid arthritis. Scand J Rheumatol 2:145, 1973.
4. Jenkins LC, McGraw RW. Anesthetic management of the patient with rheumatoid arthritis. Can Anaesth Soc J 16:407–415, 1969.
5. Arens JF, Lejume FE, Webre DR. Maxillary sinusitis: A complication of nasal tracheal intubation. Anesthesiology 40:415–416, 1974.
6. Persico M, Barker GA, Mitchell DP. Purulent otitis media—A "silent" source of sepsis in the pediatric intensive care unit. Otolaryngol Head Neck Surg 93:330–334, 1985.
7. Seebacher J, Nozik D, Mathieu A. Inadvertent intracranial introduction of a nasogastric tube, a complication of severe maxillofacial trauma. Anesthesiology 42:100–102, 1975.
8. Fremstad JD, Martin SH. Lethal complication from insertion of nasogastric tube after severe basilar skull fracture. J Trauma 18:820–822, 1978.
9. Eckenhoff JE. Some anatomic considerations of the infant larynx influencing endotracheal anesthesia. Anesthesiology 12:401–410, 1951.
10. Gaskill JR, Gillies DR. Local anesthesia for peroral endoscopy. Arch Otolaryngol 81:654–657, 1966.
11. Benumof JL, Partridge BL, Salvatierra C, Keating J. Margin of safety in positioning modern double-lumen endotracheal tubes. Anesthesiology 67:729–738, 1987.
12. Knowlson GTG, Bassett HFM. The pressures exerted on the trachea by endotracheal tube cuffs. Br J Anaesth 42:834–837, 1970.
13. Murphy P. A fiberoptic endoscope used for nasal intubation. Anaesthesia 22:489, 1967.
14. Taylor PA, Toney RM. The broncho-fiberscope as an aid to endotracheal intubation. Anaesthesia 46:611, 1972.
15. Raj PP, Forestner J, Watson TD, et al. Techniques for fiberoptic laryngoscopy in anesthesia. Anesth Analg 53:708, 1974.
16. Ducrow M. Throwing light on blind intubation. Anaesthesia 33:827–829, 1978.
17. Ellis DG, Jakymec A, Kaplan RM, et al. Guided orotracheal intubation in the operating room using a lighted stylet: A comparison with direct laryngoscopic technique. Anesthesiology 64:823–826, 1986.
18. Stoelting RK. Circulatory changes during direct laryngoscopy and tracheal intubation: Influence of duration of laryngoscopy with or without prior lidocaine. Anesthesiology 47:381–384, 1977.
19. Hamill JF, Bedford RF, Weaver DC, et al. Lidocaine before endotracheal intubation: Intravenous or laryngotracheal. Anesthesiology 55:578–581, 1981.
20. Bishop MJ, Hornbein TF. Prolonged effect of succinylcholine after neostigmine and pyridostigmine administration in patients with renal failure. Anesthesiology 58:384–386, 1983.
21. Viby-Mogensen J. Cholinesterase and succinylcholine. Dan Med Bull 30:129–150, 1983.
22. Foldes FF, Davidson GM, Duncalf D, Kuwabara S. The intravenous toxicity of local anesthetic agents in man. Clin Pharmacol Ther 6:328–335, 1965.
23. Salathe M, Johr M. Unsuspected cervical fractures: A common problem in ankylosing spondylitis. Anesthesiology 70:869–870, 1989.
24. Sinclair JR, Mason RA. Ankylosing spondylitis. The case for awake intubation. Anaesthesia 39:3–11, 1984.
25. Lofgren RH, Montgomery WW. Incidence of laryngeal involvement in rheumatoid arthritics. N Engl J Med 267:193, 1962.
26. Heindel DJ. Deep neck abscesses in adults: Management of a difficult airway. Anesth Analg 66:774–776, 1987.

27. Crockett DM, Healy GB, McGill TJ, Friedman EM. Airway management of acute supraglottitis at the Children's Hospital, Boston: 1980–1985. Ann Otol Rhinol Laryngol 97:114–119, 1988.
28. Cheek TG, Gutsche BB. Maternal physiologic alterations during pregnancy. *In* Shnider SM, Levinson G (eds). Anesthesia for Obstetrics, 2nd ed. Baltimore, Williams & Wilkins, 1987, pp 3–13.
29. Heller PJ, Scheider EP, Marx GF. Pharyngolaryngeal edema as a presenting symptom in pre-eclampsia. Obstet Gynecol 62:523–527, 1983.
30. Porapakkham S. An epidemiologic study of eclampsia. Obstet Gynecol 54:26–30, 1979.
31. Bonnar J, Redman CWG, Denson KW. The role of coagulation and fibrinolysis in pre-eclampsia. *In* Lindheimer MD, Katz AI, Zuspan FP (eds). Hypertension in Pregnancy. New York, Wiley, 1976, pp 80–95.
32. Mallampati SR, Gatt SP, Gugino LD, et al. A clinical sign to predict difficult tracheal intubation. Can Anaesth Soc J 32:429–434, 1985.
33. Charters P, Perera S, Horton WH. Visibility of pharyngeal structures as a predictor of difficult intubation [Letter]. Anaesthesia 42:1115, 1987.
34. Brechner VL. Unusual problems in the management of airways: I. Flexion-extension mobility of the cervical vertebrae. Anesth Analg 47:362–373, 1968.
35. Empey DW. Assessment of upper airways obstruction. Br Med J 3:503–505, 1972.
36. Miller RD, Hyatt RE. Evaluation of obstructing lesions of the trachea and larynx by flow-volume loops. Am Rev Respir Dis 108:475–481, 1973.
37. Instructor's Manual for Basic Life Support. American Heart Association, Dallas, TX, 1987.
38. Guildner CW. Resuscitation—Opening the airway. A comparative study of techniques for opening an airway obstructed by the tongue. JACEP 5:588–590, 1986.
39. Berry FA, Blankenbaker WL, Ball CG. A comparison of bacteremia occurring with nasotracheal and orotracheal intubation. Anesth Analg 52:873–876, 1973.
40. Dubick MN, Wright BD. Comparison of laryngeal pathology following long-term oral and nasal endotracheal intubations. Anesth Analg 57:663–668, 1978.
41. Zwillich C, Peirson DJ. Nasal necrosis: A complication of nasotracheal intubation. Chest 64:376–377, 1973.
42. Gorback MS. Inflation of the endotracheal tube cuff as an aid to blind nasal intubation. Anesth Analg 66:913–922, 1987.
43. Latto IP, Rosen M (eds). Difficulties in Tracheal Intubation. London, Bailliere Tindall, 1984.
44. Benumof JL, Partridge BL, Salvatierra C, Keating J. Margin of safety in positioning modern double-lumen endotracheal tubes. Anesthesiology 67:729–738, 1987.
45. Ellis DG, Jakymec A, Kaplan RM, et al. Guided orotracheal intubation in the operating room using a lighted stylet: A comparison with direct laryngoscopic technique. Anesthesiology 64:823–826, 1986.
46. Flancbaum L, Wright J, Trooskin SZ, et al. Orotracheal intubation in suspected laryngeal injuries. Am J Emerg Med 4:167–169, 1986.
47. Flood LM, Astley B. Anaesthetic management of acute laryngeal trauma. Br J Anaesth 54:1339–1343, 1982.
48. Myers EM, Iko BO. The management of acute laryngeal trauma. J Trauma 27:448–452, 1987.
49. McGill J, Clinton JE, Ruiz E. Cricothyrotomy in the emergency department. Ann Emerg Med 11:361–364, 1982.
50. Weymuller EA, Pavlin EG, Paugh D, Cummings CW. Management of difficult airway problems with percutaneous transtracheal ventilation. Ann Otol Rhinol Laryngol 96:34–37, 1987.
51. Smith RB, Schaer WB, Pfaeffle H. Percutaneous transtracheal ventilation for anesthesia and resuscitation: A review and report of complications. Can Anaesth Soc J 22:607–612, 1975.
52. Stinson TW. A simple connector for transtracheal ventilation [Letter]. Anesthesiology 47:232, 1977.

Clinical Problems

30

Key Terms

Basal Metabolic Rate (BMR)

Calorie

Calorimetry

Carbohydrate

Fat

Indirect Calorimetry

Kwashiorkor

Marasmus

Protein

Nutrition

James R. Mault, M.D.

Nutrition is a study of basic economics: supply versus demand. To maintain normal physiology, healthy individuals must take in at least the number of calories, protein, and minerals expended over time. If supply consistently falls short of demand, malnutrition and physiologic illness are inevitable.

In hospitalized patients, the economics of nutrition is more complicated. Before admission, patients can be nutritionally depleted owing to anorexia, vomiting, diarrhea, cancer, or malabsorption, among many other causes. In addition, metabolic demands can be markedly elevated with fever, infection, surgery, or trauma. Lastly, alternative routes of delivery, such as enteral tube feeding or total parenteral nutrition, may be required to provide the necessary amounts of energy and protein substrates. Various formulations of these solutions exist for the management of specific illnesses. This chapter describes the principles of nutritional assessment and offers strategies for the administration of nutrition in the clinical setting.

NUTRITIONAL ASSESSMENT

Like any therapeutic modality, nutritional support should be based on objective data that can direct the type and amount of nutrition required. The first step is to determine the patient's baseline nutritional state. After this has been accomplished, the administration of nutritional support should be based on accurate measurements of calorie and protein requirements. These measurements can also be used to monitor the success of a chosen nutritional regimen.

General Survey of Baseline Nutritional State

In a state of normal health and nutrition, the human body maintains a reserve of energy in the form of glycogen, fat, and protein (Table 30–1). If dietary energy intake is less than energy expenditure, the deficit is compensated by utilization of these energy reserves. In a state of fasting, glycogen stores are exhausted within the first 24 hours. If calorie starvation persists, fat and protein stores are sufficient to sustain minimal bodily functions for an additional 30 to 60 days if adequate amounts of water are available. In hospitalized patients, in whom marasmus is usually secondary to an underlying illness, protein-calorie undernutrition for periods of only 2 to 3 days has been shown to cause measurable reductions in cardiac, renal, respiratory, and immune function, as well

The state of protein and calorie undernutrition is termed marasmus.

TABLE **30–1:** Energy Reserves of a Healthy 70-kg Man

Energy Substrate	Total Grams	Kilocalories
Glycogen	430	1720
Fat	6500	58,000
Protein	2400	9600

589

as impairment of wound healing. Therefore, a thorough evaluation of a patient's nutritional state at the time of hospital admission is an essential component of directed nutritional support.

The nutritional assessment of any patient begins with a thorough history taking and physical examination. Questioning should determine a patient's usual diet and reveal recent changes in appetite and weight, hair loss, weakness, or fatigue. A presenting history of nausea, vomiting, or diarrhea may indicate a nutritionally depleted state at the time of admission. Furthermore, chronic illnesses such as diabetes, peptic ulcer disease, renal or liver failure, carcinoma, and substance abuse should alert the interviewer to possible malnutrition. Information on the frequency and duration of any of these conditions is essential.

Physical findings suggestive of malnutrition include cachexia, muscle weakness, joint pain, ascites, signs of bleeding or bruising, and signs of dehydration, such as dry skin and mucous membranes. Height and weight must be measured accurately during this initial evaluation.

Several objective anthropometric and laboratory measurements have been shown to correlate with various degrees of malnutrition (Table 30–2). However, because of the influence of other factors on each of these measurements, no single test can reliably determine the baseline nutritional status of a patient. Therefore, some combination of objective parameters should be used for the assessment of malnutrition. These include anthropometric or body measurements, such as height, weight, midarm circumference, and triceps skinfold thickness. Objective laboratory measurements include serum albumin, transferrin, and prealbumin levels.

Anthropometric Measurements

If the general survey suggests malnutrition, a more quantitative evaluation is necessary to document the extent of depletion. Options include determination of the percentage of ideal body weight (IBW), midarm circumference, and triceps or subscapular skinfold thickness. These measurements guide the initial approach for support and serve as a baseline for later comparison as repletion is pursued.

Excluding changes in total body fluid, a net loss in body weight reflects inadequate caloric intake relative to caloric expenditure. With the use of insurance tables of IBW based on gender, height, and frame size, the percentage of IBW can be determined by dividing a patient's current weight by the IBW. If possible, these calculations should also be used to compare a patient's current weight with the patient's usual body weight. However, although comparisons with usual body weight will prevent errors in normally thin or obese patients, this information is often inaccurate if it is based only on the patient's memory. Previous medical records, if available, provide a more reliable account of usual body weight.

A weight of 80 to 90% of IBW is classified as mild marasmus; 70 to 79%, as moderate marasmus; and less than 70%, as severe marasmus.

TABLE **30–2:** Objective Parameters of Malnutrition

Parameter	Mild	Moderate	Severe
Ideal body weight (%)	80–90	70–79	<70
Usual weight (%)	90–95	80–89	<80
Triceps skinfold thickness (percentile)	40th–50th	30th–39th	<30th
Albumin (g/dL)	2.8–3.4	2.1–2.7	<2.1
Transferrin (mg/dL)	150–200	100–149	<100
Prealbumin (mg/dL)	10–15	5–9	<5

Midarm circumference is measured at the midpoint of the upper arm between the acromion process and the olecranon.

The midarm circumference value reflects changes in both muscle and adipose mass and accurately estimates degrees of marasmus-type malnutrition.

Triceps skinfold thickness is also measured at the midpoint of the right arm between the acromion process and the olecranon, where the skin and subcutaneous fat are gently pinched between Lange calipers for 3 seconds. This measurement quantifies changes in body adipose mass but does not indicate changes in muscle mass.

Laboratory Assessment of Nutritional Status

Direct measurements of certain visceral proteins have shown good correlations with protein-calorie malnutrition. Ideally, the protein of choice should have a short biologic half-life that allows a rapid response to a deficient diet. This deficiency should be reflected by decreased protein concentrations in the circulation. The total amount of free protein in the circulation should be small and should exhibit a rapid rate of synthesis and catabolism.

Changes in hydration or liver function can cause significant reductions in the serum albumin level independent of the patient's nutritional state.

Albumin, a water-soluble protein, is the classic parameter for monitoring a patient's nutritional state. With protein deprivation, the synthesis of albumin decreases, and its serum concentration correlates with the degree of malnutrition. Although albumin is a good indicator of general protein status, it has a long half-life of approximately 20 days and therefore is not a reliable indicator of acute changes in protein synthesis.

Transferrin, a beta-globulin that functions as a carrier protein of iron in the plasma, has a short half-life with a small body pool. Reduced serum transferrin levels accurately correlate with early protein malnutrition. Factors such as pregnancy, iron deficiency, and liver disease also influence transferrin production.

Prealbumin, also known as thyroxine-binding prealbumin, is a circulating glycoprotein synthesized in the liver. It has a very short half-life of 2 days and is a sensitive indicator of protein-calorie malnutrition. However, any sudden demand for new protein synthesis, such as occurs with trauma or acute infection, causes a rapid fall in prealbumin levels (see Table 30–2).

Measurement of Energy Metabolism

The original work of Harris and Benedict in 1919 first described the amount of energy required to maintain the most basic bodily functions.[1] This quantity of energy, expressed as kilocalories per day, is known as the basal metabolic rate (BMR). The BMR has a fixed relationship with gender, weight in kilograms, height in centimeters, and age in years. Although nomograms may accurately predict the energy requirements of normal, healthy subjects, the metabolic rates of hospitalized patients may be significantly different than those predicted by this calculation.[2-5] Energy metabolism has been shown to vary with injury, burns, sepsis, and surgery, in addition to the type and severity of disease. In these settings, actual measurement of energy requirements is preferred to any method of estimation because it may reduce morbidity, mortality, and hospital costs.

BMR (male) = 66.5 + (13.75 weight) + (5.00 height) − (6.78 age)

BMR (female) = 655.1 + (9.6 weight) + (1.85 height) − (4.68 age)

By definition, measurement of the energy loss of a substance or an individual is known as calorimetry.

Direct measurement of energy expenditure (direct calorimetry) is performed by placing a subject in a sealed, thermally insulated chamber. The heat liberated from the individual is then determined by measuring the change in the temperature of water circulated through the walls of the chamber. The use of direct calorimetry in the clinical setting is impractical for obvious reasons, and it is rarely performed even in research settings.

The most commonly applied technique for measuring energy requirements in the clinical setting is known as indirect calorimetry. Indirect calorimetry is based on the primary measurement of oxygen consumption ($\dot{V}_{O_2}$). At the time of measurement, $\dot{V}_{O_2}$ represents the actual rate of energy expenditure taking place for the measurement period.

Techniques of Indirect Calorimetry

Indirect calorimetry can be performed with one of several commercially available devices.[6] The complexity, capabilities, and cost of these devices range from simple and inexpensive with limited applications to extremely complex and expensive with broad applications (Table 30–3). These instruments accomplish measurement of $\dot{V}_{O_2}$ through one of three methods:

- Closed-circuit rebreathing spirometry
- Open-circuit mixed exhaled gas analysis
- Combined open- and closed-circuit technique

Determination of $\dot{V}_{O_2}$ may also be accomplished by calculation, through the Fick equation. The following section describes the basic working principles of each of these techniques.

Closed-circuit rebreathing spirometry uses an airtight breathing circuit and a volume spirometer filled with oxygen. With inspiration, volume is drawn from the spirometer to the subject, and a portion of oxygen is consumed. The unused oxygen and carbon dioxide produced are ex-

This technique allows accurate measurement of $\dot{V}_{O_2}$ and $\dot{V}_{CO_2}$ in both spontaneously breathing and mechanically ventilated patients at any inspired oxygen concentration and positive end-expiratory pressure. This system cannot be applied to patients with a bronchopleural fistula or a persistent cuff leak.

TABLE 30–3: Comparison of Gas Exchange Measurement Techniques

Method	Complexity	Cost	Advantages	Limitations
Closed circuit	+ +	+ +	Accuracy is independent of the $F_{I_{O_2}}$ Minimal calibration is needed Functional residual capacity measurement using helium	Errors due to circuit leaks Increased work of breathing Risk of CO_2 rebreathing
Open circuit	+ + +	+ + +	Minimal work of breathing Easy interface with ventilators Ideal for exercise measurements	Poor accuracy with $F_{I_{O_2}}$ > 60% Calibration drift Potential sampling errors
Combined open and closed circuit*	+	+	Accuracy is independent of the $F_{I_{O_2}}$ Minimal work of breathing Hand-held and portable	Measurement duration depends on the scrubber cartridge size Pneumotach accuracy is critical
Reverse Fick equation	+ +	+	Readily available in patients with pulmonary artery catheters	Potential error in cardiac output, hemoglobin, and saturation values

*Commercial device under development; advantages and disadvantages are theoretical.
+ = low; + + = moderate; + + + = high.

pired through a canister of sodium hydroxide crystals that chemically extract all of the carbon dioxide from the exhaled gas. The remaining gases return to the spirometer. Assuming that no air leak exists within the closed rebreathing circuit, the net volume loss from the system as recorded by the spirometer over time is the $\dot{V}_{O_2}$. Carbon dioxide production ($\dot{V}_{CO_2}$) can be measured in this system by performing capnometry on the exhaled gas before its removal by the sodium hydroxide crystals. Closed-circuit rebreathing spirometry can be applied to mechanically ventilated patients by adapting a bag-in-a-box bellows chamber to the breathing circuit (Fig. 30–1). With the patient's ventilator used for mechanical work, positive pressure is created within the chamber on the external surface of the bellows. As it collapses, the volume within the bellows is directed to the patient via one-way valves. After the compressible volume of the breathing circuit has been compensated for, this system delivers the same tidal volume, respiratory rate, and airway pressures as the baseline ventilator settings while maintaining a sealed breathing circuit to measure gas exchange.

Open-circuit, mixed-exhaled gas analysis is another method of measuring $\dot{V}_{O_2}$ and $\dot{V}_{CO_2}$. The simplest example of this approach is the Douglas bag technique, as illustrated in Figure 30–2. In this configuration, oxygen and carbon dioxide concentrations are measured in samples of inspired and expired gases. These concentrations can be determined very precisely by mass spectrometry, or more routinely by infrared carbon dioxide and paramagnetic or zirconium oxide oxygen analyzers. Accurate measurement of exhaled or inhaled minute volume is also required, usually by a precision volume pneumotach.

With data generated by these instruments, $\dot{V}_{O_2}$ is then determined by subtracting the volume of expired oxygen from the volume of inspired oxygen. Mixed exhaled gas analysis is a simple and accurate method of indirect calorimetry in relatively healthy subjects breathing room air.

$$\dot{V}_{O_2} = (1 - F_{E_{O_2}} - F_{E_{CO_2}}/[1 - F_{I_{O_2}}]) \times (F_{I_{O_2}} - F_{E_{O_2}}) \times \dot{V}_E$$

where $F_{E_{O_2}}$ is the expired oxygen concentration, $F_{E_{CO_2}}$ is the expired carbon dioxide concentration, $F_{I_{O_2}}$ is the inspired oxygen concentration, and $\dot{V}_E$ is the expired minute ventilation.

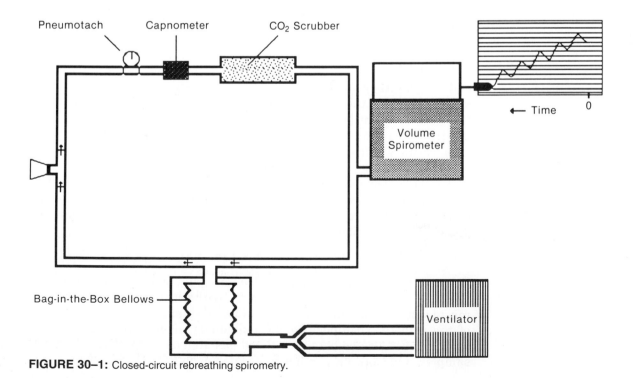

FIGURE 30–1: Closed-circuit rebreathing spirometry.

Pneumotach Capnometer CO_2 Scrubber

← Time   0

Volume Spirometer

Bag-in-the-Box Bellows

Ventilator

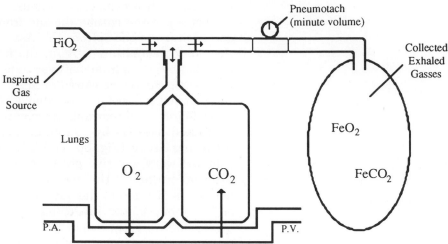

FIGURE 30–2: Open-circuit mixed-exhaled analysis: Douglas bag technique. PA, pulmonary artery; PV, pulmonary vein.

Carbon dioxide production is calculated as

$$\dot{V}_{CO_2} = F_{E_{CO_2}} \times \dot{V}_E$$

$\dot{V}_{O_2}$ is then calculated as follows:

$$\dot{V}_{O_2} = \dot{V}_I - \dot{V}_E - \dot{V}_{CO_2}$$

The standard Fick equation, as originally described by Fick in the 1880s, is as follows:

$$CO = \frac{\dot{V}_{O_2}}{C(a-v)_{O_2}}$$

where CO is cardiac output and $C(a-v)_{O_2}$ is the arteriovenous oxygen content difference.

However, the accuracy of this technique requires precise knowledge of the inspired oxygen content. With mechanical ventilation, the $F_{I_{O_2}}$ delivered to the patient varies by $\pm$ 1 to 2% oxygen per breath. Although this variation in $F_{I_{O_2}}$ has no clinical consequences for the patient, it significantly increases the standard error of the calculation. These problems are further compounded by compression of gasses being sampled by the analyzers. Therefore, this method of indirect calorimetry is generally limited to patients who are spontaneously breathing in room air and to those who are mechanically ventilated with an $F_{I_{O_2}}$ of less than 40%.

Combined open- and closed-circuit calorimetry is a new technique[7] that uses the closed-circuit measurement principle within an open-circuit architecture (Fig. 30–3). With a bidirectional, high-precision pneumotach, inspired volume ($\dot{V}_I$) is measured as the subject (or the mechanical ventilator) initiates a breath. Exhaled gases flow via one-way valves through a carbon dioxide scrubber (where all exhaled carbon dioxide is removed) and exit out via the pneumotach in the opposite direction ($\dot{V}_E - \dot{V}_{CO_2}$). $\dot{V}_{CO_2}$ and the respiratory quotient are easily determined by the addition of either a capnometer or a second pneumotach positioned immediately before the scrubber. This system is easily adapted into a positive pressure ventilator circuit, and $\dot{V}_{O_2}$ can be measured continuously (for the life of the carbon dioxide scrubber) without *any* change in ventilator settings. Although this device is still under commercial development, by design it will be hand-held, inexpensive, and simple to operate and will allow measurements of gas exchange at any $F_{I_{O_2}}$.

The Fick equation may also be applied for determining $\dot{V}_{O_2}$ and corresponding energy expenditure.[8] Simple manipulation of the equation allows the calculation of $\dot{V}_{O_2}$ as

$$\dot{V}_{O_2} = CO \times C(a-v)_{O_2}$$

To perform this calculation, an indwelling pulmonary artery catheter is required to determine cardiac output (by thermodilution) and obtain a mixed venous blood sample (which must be obtained from the distal port of the catheter positioned in the pulmonary artery). An arterial blood sample must also be obtained. Blood gas analysis is performed on both samples, and $C(a-v)_{O_2}$ is then calculated as follows:

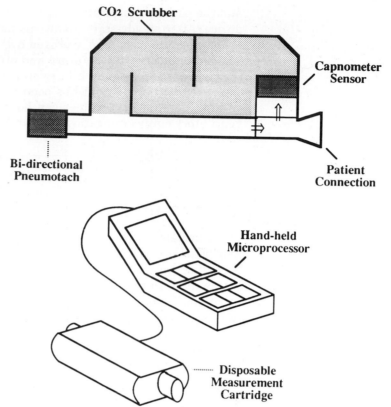

FIGURE 30–3: Combined open- and closed-circuit calorimetry.

$$C(a-v)O_2 = ([Sa_{O_2} - Sv_{O_2}] \times Hgb \times 1.36) + (0.0031 \times [Pa_{O_2} - Pv_{O_2}])$$

where S and P are the percentage saturations and partial pressures of oxygen of the respective arterial (a) and venous (v) blood samples and Hgb is the hemoglobin concentration in grams per deciliter.

Pulmonary artery catheterization is a valuable tool for the management of critically ill patients. The existence of these catheters in intensive care unit patients permits the Fick equation to be used for the calculation of $\dot{V}O_2$. However, the range of error of this calculation is significant when the individual errors of thermodilution cardiac output, blood gas determinations, hemoglobin measurement, and the estimation of the oxygen-carrying capacity of hemoglobin are added. Therefore, the Fick method for calculating $\dot{V}O_2$ and energy expenditure should be regarded as only an approximation of the metabolic rate. In addition, this method does not allow for measurement of $\dot{V}CO_2$ and the respiratory quotient (see Table 30–3).

Interpretation of Gas Exchange Measurements

When gas exchange measurements are conducted for the purpose of nutritional or hemodynamic management, every effort must be made to ensure that the conditions of the measurement are steady state.[9] Generally, during the measurement period, patients should be in a resting, recumbent state. If the patient is mechanically ventilated, appropriate adjustments should be made to duplicate the patient's usual oxygen concentration, minute ventilation, and airway pressure. If the patient is spontaneously breathing, measurements should be taken only after the patient has adjusted to breathing through the mouthpiece or face mask and the patient's respiratory effort is not influenced by the measurement device. After steady-state conditions have been confirmed, gas exchange measurements should be averaged over a period of at least 15 minutes. The patient's body temperature and other vital signs should be noted at the time of measurement as a reference for future studies.

After a measurement has been completed, the reliability of the resultant $\dot{V}O_2$ and $\dot{V}CO_2$ values can be verified through the calculation of ventilatory equivalent ratios, $\dot{V}e_{O_2}$ and $\dot{V}e_{CO_2}$, as follows:

$$\dot{V}e_{O_2} = \frac{\dot{V}E(L/min)}{\dot{V}O_2\ (dL/min)}\ (\text{normal range, 2.4 to 4.0})$$

$$\dot{V}e_{CO_2} = \frac{\dot{V}E(L/min)}{\dot{V}CO_2\ (dL/min)}\ (\text{normal range, 3.0 to 4.0})$$

Ventilatory equivalent values that fall below the normal ranges suggest that $\dot{V}O_2$ and $\dot{V}CO_2$ are falsely high relative to minute ventilation. Values above the normal ranges suggest that $\dot{V}O_2$ and $\dot{V}CO_2$ are falsely low relative to minute ventilation. In either case, technical errors such as tubing leaks, calibration errors, or non–steady-state conditions may have occurred during the measurement period. After these factors have been corrected, the gas exchange measurement should be repeated.

After the results of a gas exchange measurement have been confirmed, the corresponding energy expenditure can be calculated. Energy metabolism is divided into several categories of metabolic activity, as follows:

$$TEE = REE + AEE$$

where TEE is the total body energy expenditure, REE is the resting energy expenditure, and AEE is the energy expended by activity (exercise). REE is further defined by the following formula:

$$REE = BMR + SDA$$

where BMR is the basal metabolic rate (as defined earlier) and SDA is the specific dynamic action (energy expenditure due to the metabolic processing of dietary intake). In a hospital setting, patients are usually resting and recumbent, with minimal physical activity. Therefore, measurements of REE by indirect calorimetry accurately represent TEE for the purpose of guiding energy intake. If additional physical activity occurs, energy intake should be adjusted accordingly.

With the use of the stoichiometry of aerobic pathways, a caloric equivalent has been derived for each class of foodstuffs. The caloric equivalent of a given energy substrate is the amount of heat (in kilocalories) liberated when the substrate is burned in 1 L of oxygen. Similarly, each class of foodstuffs has a unique respiratory quotient (Table 30–4). The respiratory quotient is the ratio of carbon dioxide produced to oxygen consumed in the stoichiometric oxidation of a particular substrate.

TABLE **30–4:** Energy and Respiratory Values of Foodstuffs

Energy Substrate	Caloric Value (kcal/g)	Caloric Equivalent (kcal/L O_2)	Respiratory Quotient
Carbohydrate	4.1	5.05	1.00
Protein	4.1	4.46	0.82
Fat	9.3	4.74	0.71
Alcohol	7.1	4.86	0.60

By measuring $\dot{V}_{O_2}$, $\dot{V}_{CO_2}$, and urinary nitrogen excretion (Nu; in grams), it is possible to determine REE from the de Weir equation:[10]

$$REE \text{ (kcal)} = 3.581\ \dot{V}_{O_2} + 1.448\ \dot{V}_{CO_2} - 1.773\ Nu$$

where $\dot{V}_{O_2}$ and $\dot{V}_{CO_2}$ are in liters per minute. If the measurement of Nu or $\dot{V}_{CO_2}$ is unavailable, the REE can be accurately determined from $\dot{V}_{O_2}$ alone with the use of an estimated respiratory quotient of 0.85 (to generate a value for $\dot{V}_{CO_2}$) and an estimated Nu of 10 g. On the basis of comparisons with continuous 24-hour gas exchange measurements, extrapolation of single 15- to 30-minute measurements of $\dot{V}_{O_2}$ and $\dot{V}_{CO_2}$ to 24-hour values accurately describes daily energy requirements. Daily measurements are required because variability between days does occur.[11]

Measurement of Protein Metabolism

Protein, an essential component of most organs and bodily functions, is the basic material of metabolic enzymes, immunoglobulins, hormones, and support structures. Independent of caloric intake, when protein catabolism consistently exceeds protein intake, kwashiorkor is well known to result in impaired wound healing, immune function, coagulation function, and a host of other significant diseases and death. Therefore, the administration of nutritional support should be guided not only by knowledge of energy requirements but also by concurrent measurements of protein requirements.[12]

Because nitrogen exists only in proteins and amino acids, measurement of nitrogen excretion in the urine and other bodily fluids has provided a reliable means of determining protein requirements for the past 150 years. When protein is catabolized, liberated nitrogen is usually excreted via the urine as urea, but it may also be lost through feces, nasogastric suction, and wound drainage. With chemical luminescence techniques, analysis of total urinary nitrogen has become the gold standard for the accurate measurement of protein requirements in hospitalized patients.[13] The measurement of urinary urea nitrogen does not account for nonurea nitrogen losses but may be used reliably where total urinary nitrogen measurement is not yet available.

In contrast to the situation with gas exchange measurements, in which a single, brief gas exchange measurement is extrapolated to represent the energy requirements for an entire day, accurate measurements of net protein breakdown based on urinary nitrogen excretion must be performed over the entire 24-hour period. This is because of the large pool of urea nitrogen in the body and the large variability in nitrogen excretion from hour to hour.

After a 24-hour measurement of nitrogen excretion has been completed, the corresponding protein catabolic rate is calculated using a conversion factor of 6.25 g of protein per gram of nitrogen excreted.

STRATEGIES OF NUTRITIONAL MANAGEMENT

After the patient's baseline nutritional status has been assessed and the patient's energy and protein requirements have been measured, nutritional support should be initiated without delay. The type and route of nutritional support, however, depend on several factors. Once nutritional support has begun, efforts must be directed at repleting nutritional deficits and then achieving and maintaining a positive nutritional state.

Composition, Route, and Timing of Nutritional Support

The dietary habits of healthy humans are episodic, and their meals are variable in composition. In most circumstances, the type and amount of dietary intake are determined by appetite and the availability of foods. Regardless of the food eaten, digestion provides three types of substrates for human energy metabolism: carbohydrate, fat, and protein. With a stable weight, a regular diet, and normal activity, carbohydrate and fat intake is catabolized as energy for mechanical work and to carry out cellular functions. Protein intake is used to generate new cells and tissues, replacing enzymes, immunoglobulins, and so on.

In hospitalized patients, the mixture and amount of substrates provided are important. Excessive or deficient amounts or ratios of carbohydrate, fat, or protein intake can exacerbate illness. Therefore, careful attention must be directed at the type and amount of substrates provided. If the intake of energy substrates in the form of carbohydrate and fat is less than energy expenditure, dietary protein is catabolized as an energy source rather than used anabolically in the generation of new cells. If dietary protein is insufficient to supply the patient's energy requirements, protein from existing muscle cells and other tissues is cannibalized. Therefore, the goal of nutritional support in the hospitalized patient is to provide enough energy substrates, usually in the form of carbohydrate, fat, or both, to meet or exceed energy needs.

Carbohydrate is an essential component of nutrition for hospitalized patients. In particular, the brain and nervous tissue derive nearly all of their energy requirements from the oxidation of glucose and can account for 20% of the REE of adults (50% of the REE in neonates). After intestinal absorption, a portion of ingested carbohydrate is immediately hydrolyzed for energy needs, and the remaining portion is stored as glycogen in the liver and skeletal muscle. If glycogen stores are filled to capacity, additional carbohydrate intake is converted to fat.

Fat functions as the preferred source of energy for several organ systems (most notably the heart), but it is not an essential energy substrate. Certain types of fat, however, are critical components of all cell membranes. These essential fatty acids, linoleic acid and linolenic acid, cannot be synthesized de novo and must be provided as part of nutritional support. In addition to being needed for cell membrane generation, they are also required precursors for the production of prostaglandins, leukotrienes, and thromboxanes.

In general, because carbohydrate administration has been shown to cause significant sparing of nitrogen, in addition to other beneficial effects not provided by fat, it is recommended that the carbohydrate component of nutritional support equal 66 to 75% of REE, with fat comprising the remaining 25 to 33% of REE. The administered fat must include at least 5 to 10 g of omega-6 or omega-3 fatty acids.

Protein requirements for normal individuals are generally in the range of 1 g/kg/day. However, in critically ill hospitalized patients, protein requirements can exceed 3 g/kg/day. Large losses of protein can occur with wound drainage, ascites, peritoneal dialysis, bleeding, and infection. In these circumstances, nutritional support must provide the necessary amounts of complex proteins that contain both essential and nonessential amino acids. In addition, enhanced concentrations of branched-chain amino acids in parenteral nutrition have correlated with improved nitrogen balance. With enteral feeding, glutamine content may

The biochemical conversion of carbohydrate to fat causes liberation of carbon dioxide, which may exacerbate respiratory failure in patients with compromised respiratory function.[14, 15]

Excessive lipid intake via total parenteral nutrition may lead to the development of fatty liver disease.

In addition to providing sufficient amounts of energy substrates and protein, all nutritional support should include adequate amounts of vitamins, minerals, and trace elements.

play a critical role in the protection of normal gastrointestinal function and immune surveillance.

The route of nutritional support is strongly influenced by a patient's disease process or processes. Unconscious patients with normal gastrointestinal function can receive enteral nutrition via a feeding tube. In patients with absent gastrointestinal function, such as those with prolonged ileus, major gastrointestinal surgery, short bowel syndrome, or severe acute pancreatitis, total parenteral nutrition can fulfill all nutritional requirements for an indefinite period. Enteral nutrition is the most physiologic, the safest, and the most economic route for nutritional support. Total parenteral nutrition should be initiated only if enteral feeding is not possible by any means.

The timing of nutritional support is determined by two factors:

The risks of total parenteral nutrition are significant:

- Complications with central line placement
- Delayed catheter sepsis
- Cholestatic jaundice
- Impairment of gastric emptying

- The baseline nutritional state of the patient
- The estimated period that a normal, per os diet will not be adequate to supply energy and protein requirements

If on admission, a patient is clearly nutritionally depleted to any degree, some level of nutritional support should be initiated immediately. If a patient has little or no prospect of taking a normal diet for 3 days or longer, nutritional support, whether enteral or parenteral, should be initiated.

Balance of Nutrition

As emphasized in the beginning of this chapter, nutrition is a simple matter of supply and demand. After energy requirements have been determined through indirect calorimetry measurements, the daily and cumulative caloric balances should be tabulated. The daily caloric balance is calculated by subtracting the REE from the total energy (in kilocalories) administered per 24 hours. The cumulative caloric balance results from the addition of the consecutive daily balances (Fig. 30–4). The same format can (and should) be used to tabulate the daily and cumulative protein balances from measurements of total urinary nitrogen and protein intake. This approach to nutritional monitoring has shown significant value for the metabolic care of critically ill patients. Bartlett and coworkers performed indirect calorimetry, tabulated the daily and cumulative caloric balances, and related these findings to outcome in critically ill patients with multiple organ failure.[2] Of 57 patients studied in the surgical intensive care unit, 14 had a negative cumulative caloric balance of at least 10,000 kilocalories; 12 died (86%). Twenty-eight patients had a cumulative caloric balance of between 0 and −10,000 kcal; 11 died (39%). In contrast, of 15 patients who were discharged with a positive cumulative caloric balance, only four died (27%). The difference between these three groups was statistically significant ($P < .01$). Similar findings have more recently been demonstrated in a subgroup of critically ill multiple organ failure patients with acute renal failure.[16] Others have also shown benefit from the use of indirect calorimetry and protein balance measurements to guide nutritional support in critically ill patients.[17]

SUMMARY

As described previously, the metabolic needs of hospitalized patients are highly variable and cannot be predicted accurately from calculations

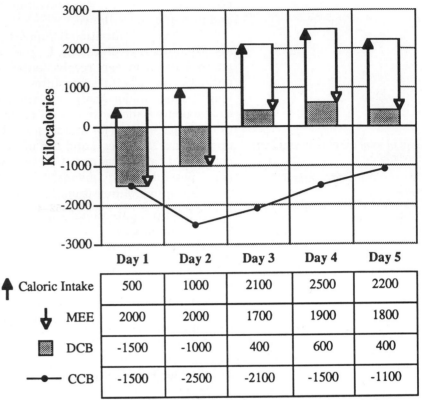

	Day 1	Day 2	Day 3	Day 4	Day 5
▲ Caloric Intake	500	1000	2100	2500	2200
▼ MEE	2000	2000	1700	1900	1800
▨ DCB	-1500	-1000	400	600	400
● CCB	-1500	-2500	-2100	-1500	-1100

FIGURE 30–4: Daily tabulation of energy balance. Routine metabolic monitoring can be charted in graphic or tabular form, as shown. After the measured energy expenditure (MEE) has been determined, the caloric intake is tabulated for the corresponding day. The daily caloric balance (DCB) is calculated by subtracting the MEE from the caloric intake. The cumulative caloric balance (CCB) is the running sum of each successive DCB. CCB values are listed as total kilocalories since admission, whereas all other values are kilocalories/24 hr.

or nomograms. Although the effects of underfeeding patients are well known, gross overfeeding of patients has also proved to be deleterious. These adverse effects can include hyperglycemia, fatty liver disease, hypervolemia, and exacerbation of respiratory failure through excess carbon dioxide production.[14, 18] In addition, overfeeding also results in unnecessary hospital costs. Interestingly, several publications have concluded that the use of indirect calorimetry and the subsequent custom-tailoring of nutritional support based on these measurements results in decreased length of stay and lower hospital costs.[17, 19, 20]

Indirect calorimetry is also used for nutritional assessment in other patient populations, including neonates and children,[21–24] cancer patients,[25–27] and patients with eating disorders such as obesity[28, 29] and anorexia nervosa.[30, 31] Indirect calorimetry is also helpful for measuring the work of breathing[32, 33] in patients with respiratory failure or chronic lung disease.[34]

In addition to having nutritional applications, $\dot{V}O_2$ is a primary value in hemodynamic monitoring. Because $\dot{V}O_2$ is one of the variables in the Fick equation, knowledge of this measurement may be useful in the assessment of the adequacy of oxygen delivery.[35] When $\dot{V}O_2$ measurements are combined with continuous mixed venous oximetry, the cardiac output can also be determined continuously.

References

1. Harris JA, Benedict FG. Biometric Studies of Basal Metabolism in Man. Washington, DC, Carnegie Institute, 1919. Publication 279.
2. Bartlett RH, Dechert RE, Mault JR, et al. Measurement of metabolism in multiple organ failure. Surgery 92:771–779, 1982.
3. Hunter DC, Jaksic T, Lewis D, et al. Resting energy expenditure in the critically ill: Estimations versus measurement. Br J Surg 75:875–878, 1988.
4. Roza AM, Shizgal HM. The Harris Benedict equation reevaluated: Resting energy requirements and the body cell mass. Am J Clin Nutr 40:168–182, 1984.
5. Weissman C, Kemper M, Askanazi J, et al. Resting metabolic rate of the critically ill patient: Measured versus predicted. Anesthesiology 64:673–679, 1986.
6. Branson RD. The measurement of energy expenditure: Instrumentation, practical considerations, and clinical applications. Respir Care 35:640–659, 1990.
7. Mault JR. Respiratory calorimeter with bidirectional flow monitor. United States Patent No. 5,179,958, 1993.
8. Cobean RA, Gentilello LM, Parker A, et al. Nutritional assessment using a pulmonary artery catheter. J Trauma 33:452–456, 1992.
9. McClave SA, Snider HL. Use of indirect calorimetry in clinical nutrition. Nutr Clin Pract 7:207–221, 1992.
10. de Weir JB. New methods for calculating metabolic rate with special reference to protein metabolism. J Physiol 109:1–9, 1949.
11. Vermeij CG, Feenstra BW, van Lanscot JJ, Bruining HA. Day-to-day variability of energy expenditure in critically ill surgical patients. Crit Care Med 17:623–626, 1989.
12. Konstantinides FN. Nitrogen balance studies in clinical nutrition. Nutr Clin Pract 7:231–238, 1992.
13. Dechert RE, Cerny JC, Bartlett RH. Measurement of elemental nitrogen by chemiluminescence: An evaluation of the Antek nitrogen analyzer system. JPEN J Parenter Enteral Nutr 14:195–197, 1990.
14. Askanazi J, Rosenbaum SH, Hyman AI, et al. Respiratory changes induced by the large glucose loads of total parenteral nutrition. JAMA 243:1444–1447, 1980.
15. Frayn KN. Calculation of substrate oxidation rates in vivo from gaseous exchange. J Appl Physiol 55:628–634, 1983.
16. Bartlett RH, Mault JR, Dechert RE, et al. Continuous arteriovenous hemofiltration: Improved survival in surgical acute renal failure? Surgery 100:400–408, 1986.
17. Foster GD, Knox LS, Dempsey DT, Mullen JL. Caloric requirements in total parenteral nutrition. J Am Coll Nutr 6:231–253, 1987.
18. Askanazi J, Weissman C, LaSala PA, et al. Effect of protein intake on ventilatory drive. Anesthesiology 60:106–110, 1984.
19. Schane J, Goede M, Silverstein P. Comparison of energy expenditure measurement techniques in severely burned patients. J Burn Care Rehabil 8:366–370, 1987.
20. Robinson G, Goldstein M, Levine GM. Impact of nutritional status on DRG length of stay. JPEN J Parenter Enteral Nutr 11:49–51, 1987.
21. Dechert RE, Wesley JR, Schafer LE, et al. A water-sealed indirect calorimeter for measurement of oxygen consumption (VO_2), carbon dioxide production (VCO_2), and energy expenditure in infants. JPEN J Parenter Enteral Nutr 12:256–259, 1988.
22. Schutz Y, Catzeflis C, Gudinchet F, et al. Energy expenditure and whole body protein synthesis in very low birth weight (VLBW) infants. Experientia 44(Suppl):45–56, 1983.
23. Forsyth JS, Crighton A. An indirect calorimetry system for ventilator dependent very low birthweight infants. Arch Dis Child 67:315–319, 1992.
24. Chwals WJ, Lally KP, Woolley MM. Indirect calorimetry in mechanically ventilated infants and children: Measurement accuracy with absence of audible airleak. Crit Care Med 20:768–770, 1992.
25. Koea JB, Shaw JH. The effect of tumor bulk on the metabolic response to cancer. Ann Surg 215:282–288, 1992.
26. Knox LS, Crosby LO, Feurer ID, et al. Energy expenditure in malnourished cancer patients. Ann Surg 197:152–162, 1983.
27. Hansell DT, Davies JW, Burns HJ. The effects on resting energy expenditure of different tumor types. Cancer 58:1739–1744, 1986.
28. Feurer ID, Crosby LO, Buzby GP, et al. Resting energy expenditure in morbid obesity. Ann Surg 197:17–21, 1983.
29. Tsoi CM, Westenskow DR, Moody FG. Weight loss and metabolic changes of morbidly obese patients after gastric partitioning operation. Surgery 96:545–549, 1984.
30. Vaisman N, Rossi MF, Goldberg E, et al. Energy expenditure and body composition in patients with anorexia nervosa. J Pediatr 113:919–924, 1988.
31. Dempsey DT, Crosby LO, Pertschuk MJ, et al. Weight gain and nutritional efficacy in anorexia nervosa. Am J Clin Nutr 39:236–242, 1984.
32. Lewis WD, Chwals W, Benotti PN, et al. Bedside assessment of the work of breathing. Crit Care Med 16:117–122, 1988.
33. Savino JA, Dawson JA, Agarwal N, et al. The metabolic cost of breathing in critical surgical patients. J Trauma 25:1126–1133, 1985.

34. Wilson DO, Donahoe M, Rogers RM, Pennock BE. Metabolic rate and weight loss in chronic obstructive lung disease. JPEN J Parenter Enteral Nutr 14:7–11, 1990.
35. Zwischenberger JB, Kirsh MM, Dechert RE, et al. Suppression of shivering decreases oxygen consumption and improves hemodynamic stability during postoperative rewarming. Ann Thorac Surg 43:428–431, 1987.

31

○

Myocardial Ischemia

James R. Bengston, M.D., M.P.H.,
J. Peter Longabaugh, M.D., and Mark Hamer, M.D.

Since the early 1980s, few other fields in medicine have experienced such tremendous advances in understanding of basic pathophysiology, diagnosis, and treatment as cardiology. Because of the close relationship among many respiratory and cardiovascular diseases, familiarity with these advances is often useful in managing patients with respiratory disease.

PATHOPHYSIOLOGY OF MYOCARDIAL ISCHEMIA

Myocardial ischemia occurs when oxygen supply is insufficient to meet oxygen demand. Because the heart maximally extracts oxygen from blood, the myocardial oxygen supply depends directly on coronary blood flow. Through autoregulation, increases in myocardial oxygen demand are normally met by coronary vasodilatation. The most common cause of reduced myocardial oxygen supply is atherosclerosis of the epicardial arteries. However, approximately 10 to 15% of patients who undergo cardiac catheterization to evaluate effort angina are found to have normal coronary arteries. In these patients, ischemia is probably due to reduced coronary flow reserve, which is in turn due to inappropriate dilatation of the small resistance vessels.

Progression from stable angina to unstable angina and other acute ischemia syndromes is initiated by the development of an ulcer or a fissure in the fibrous cap of the atheroma. The etiology of plaque fissuring is not well understood, but it is due at least in part to the action of shear forces of blood on the lesion. Platelet activation occurs almost immediately after plaque rupture. The magnitude of the platelet response depends on the extent of endothelial injury. When blood is exposed to the plaque, in particular to type I collagen, platelet adhesion occurs. Adhesion results from the bonding of exposed collagen to platelet receptor glycoprotein Ia, as well as from other endothelial ligand–platelet receptor interactions, including that of von Willebrand's factor with glycoprotein Ib, that of fibronectin with glycoprotein Ic, and that of thrombospondin with glycoprotein IV. Adhesion leads to further platelet activation and recruitment by the release of serotonin, adenosine diphosphate, arachidonic acid, and tissue thromboplastin. Intrinsic inhibitor systems are overwhelmed by massive platelet activation, leading to thrombus formation. The combination of the aggregating platelet-fibrin-thrombus matrix and vasospasm causes rapid narrowing of the arterial lumen, resulting in acute myocardial ischemia.

MYOCARDIAL ISCHEMIA SYNDROMES

Ischemia may be clinically "silent," but it is generally manifested by stable or unstable angina, myocardial infarction, or sudden death.

603

Stable Angina

The term *stable angina* typically describes the occurrence of midanterior chest discomfort brought on by exercise. The discomfort may radiate to the neck, jaw, or arms and may be associated with nausea, diaphoresis, dyspnea, or fatigue. Rest and sublingual nitroglycerin typically relieve the symptoms. A stable pattern implies that there is no chest pain at rest; that the frequency, severity, and duration of episodes are not increasing; and that relief is reliably achieved within approximately 15 minutes. A given level of exercise may or may not provoke angina at different times, depending on factors such as coronary artery smooth muscle tone, catecholamine levels, and peripheral vascular tone. The mechanism of stable angina is thought to be relatively fixed coronary artery stenosis that leads to ischemia only when the demand for perfusion exceeds the flow that can be achieved through the narrow coronary lumen.

Unstable Angina

The term *unstable angina* is commonly applied to a wide spectrum of presenting symptoms in patients with known or suspected coronary artery disease, encompassing crescendo angina, new-onset angina, angina at rest, and postinfarction angina. The angiographic appearance of coronary arteries in patients with unstable angina is also variable, although the majority of patients have eccentric lesions and visible thrombus. Coronary vasospasm and intermittent thrombosis are thought to be responsible for ischemia occurring in the absence of any increase in the demand for perfusion.

Myocardial Infarction

The diagnosis of myocardial infarction requires myocardial cell death, as evidenced by diagnostic electrocardiographic changes; elevated plasma creatine phosphokinase MB levels; or irreversible myocardial wall motion abnormalities, as noted with imaging techniques. Myocardial infarction is usually manifested by the typical chest discomfort and associated symptoms of angina, but it is more severe and prolonged. There is a wide variability of the level of pain experienced. In the Framingham study, 25% of myocardial infarctions were discovered only by routine electrocardiographic examination. The patients were presumably asymptomatic or experienced symptoms of infarction that were attributed to other causes (e.g., "indigestion"). The cause of myocardial infarction is usually thrombotic occlusion of a coronary artery segment, leading to a lack of distal perfusion and subsequent myocardial cell death. The occlusion may be transient, with factors other than thrombosis (e.g., coronary vasospasm, septic coronary emboli, and coronary arterial dissection) occasionally responsible for the occlusion.

APPROACH TO THE PATIENT WITH MYOCARDIAL ISCHEMIA

Patients with suspected acute ischemic syndromes require hospitalization. Initial therapy consists of pain relief, assurance of adequate oxygenation, stabilization of blood pressure, and control of dysrythmias. Potential precipitating factors, including anemia, hypertension, and congestive heart failure, should be treated. Pharmacologic therapy should be rapidly instituted to prevent further platelet aggregation and thrombus formation, decrease myocardial oxygen demand, and maximize myocardial oxygen supply.

Antiplatelet Agents

Inhibition of platelet aggregation with aspirin in dosages of 80 to 325 mg/day has been shown to have a beneficial effect in several large clinical trials. In the Veterans Administration study of unstable angina (Lewis et al.), for example, 1266 men were randomized to treatment with aspirin (324 mg/day) or placebo. The overall rate of myocardial infarction and death was 5% in the aspirin group, compared with 10.1% in the placebo group, after 12 weeks. Cairns and colleagues randomized 555 patients to aspirin (325 mg four times daily), sulfinpyrazone (200 mg four times daily), both, or neither. After a mean follow-up period of 19 months, the incidence of death and myocardial infarction was 8.6% in the aspirin-only patients, versus 17% in the other groups (Fig. 31–1).

Although clear evidence exists to support the use of aspirin in treating acute myocardial ischemia, the optimal dose continues to be controversial. Vejar and colleagues demonstrated that intravenous administration of 60 mg of aspirin for 24 hours, followed by 20 mg daily, was sufficient to reduce serum thromboxane B_2 to undetectable levels. However, 14 of 20 patients given this dose continued to have evidence of ischemia. The Research Group on Instability in Coronary Artery Disease conducted a trial in which 796 patients were randomized to treatment with aspirin (75 mg daily) or placebo. After 1 year, the aspirin-treated patients had a significant reduction in mortality, myocardial infarction, and severe angina necessitating referral to angiography (risk ratio, 0.65;

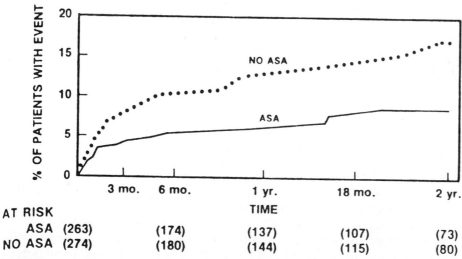

FIGURE 31–1: Kaplan-Meier curves showing the cumulative risk of cardiac death or nonfatal myocardial infarction in patients randomized to aspirin (ASA) or placebo. (From Cairns JA, Gent M, Singer J, et al. Aspirin, sulfinpyrazone, or both in unstable angina: Results of a Canadian multicenter trial. Reprinted, by permission, from the New England Journal of Medicine. 313:1373, 1985.)

confidence interval, 0.54 to 0.79). On the basis of these results and those of the randomized trials noted earlier, a daily aspirin dose of 75 to 325 mg should be administered.

Dipyridamole and sulfinpyrazone are poor substitutes for aspirin in treating patients with myocardial ischemia. Ticlopidine, an inhibitor of the adenosine diphosphate pathway of platelet aggregation, has been shown in a clinical trial (Balsano et al, 1990) to reduce morbidity among patients with unstable angina. However, this agent requires 3 days to achieve optimal efficacy. A monoclonal antibody to the platelet glycoprotein IIb/IIIa receptor blockers (7E3) has been shown to prevent thrombus formation in primates and is currently in clinical trials. The IIb/IIIa receptor can also be blocked by disintegrins, peptides with an arginine-glycine-aspartate recognition sequence; these peptides, derived from snake venoms, should soon be ready for clinical trials. Antagonists to thromboxane A_2 receptors and serotonin S_2 receptors have been found to delay reocclusion after thrombolysis in an animal model of coronary thrombosis and may prove to be effective in unstable angina. Prostacyclin and its analogues, iloprost and ciprostene, are potent vasodilators and platelet inhibitors. In small clinical trials (Lewis HD Jr), the inhibition of platelet function by these agents was confirmed, but no beneficial effects on the course of unstable angina were observed.

Antithrombotic Agents

Because patients with acute ischemic syndromes frequently have visible thrombus at the time of angiography, agents that prevent the extension or recurrence of thrombus are a logical component of therapy. The efficacy of heparin, a heterogeneous compound whose antithrombotic effect is mediated by antithrombin III and heparin cofactor II, has been extensively studied for the treatment of acute myocardial ischemia. Telford and Wilson, for example, conducted a double-blind study in which 214 patients with unstable angina were randomized to therapy with heparin, atenolol, both, or placebo. Patients treated with heparin had a reduced incidence of subsequent myocardial infarction—2%, versus 17% in those treated with placebo–after a mean follow-up of 8 weeks. In another study, 479 patients were randomized within 24 hours of hospitalization to treatment with heparin, aspirin, both, or neither. After a mean follow-up of 6 days, patients treated with heparin had significantly less refractory angina (8 versus 23%) and fewer myocardial infarctions (0.8 versus 11.9%) than patients who received placebo. No deaths occurred in the treated patients. Overall, those treated with heparin had somewhat better outcomes than those treated with aspirin. On the basis of the favorable results of these and other trials, intravenous heparin should be a standard component of therapy for patients with unstable angina, with dosing adjusted to maintain a partial thromboplastin time of 1.5 to 2 times control for 4 to 5 days.

Heparin is a relatively weak inhibitor of thrombin and is particularly ineffective for fibrin-bound clot. This fact has led to the development of a number of newer antithrombotic agents. Hirudin, a polypeptide found in the salivary glands of the leech *Hirudo medicinalis* and subsequently produced using recombinant techniques, is the most potent thrombin inhibitor known. A large clinical trial is currently in progress to study the safety and efficacy of hirudin in patients with unstable angina who have angiographically demonstrable thrombus. D-Phenylalanyl-L-prolyl-L-arginyl-chloromethyl ketone, a peptide that specifically inhibits the catalytic site of thrombin by irreversibly alkylating histidine, and argatroban, a synthetic N_2-substituted arginine derivative, have been studied in vitro and in experimental animals but not yet in clinical trials.

Nitrates

Nitrates, administered orally or intravenously, have several beneficial effects on ischemic myocardium:

- Decreased myocardial oxygen consumption through peripheral vasodilatation
- Increased oxygen supply through the dilatation of epicardial arteries
- Increased collateral flow
- Favorable redistribution of regional blood flow
- Inhibition of platelet aggregation

Intravenous nitroglycerin has been shown to be effective in relieving chest pain and to reduce mortality in acute myocardial infarction. Thus, nitrates should be considered a cornerstone of therapy in all acute myocardial ischemic syndromes unless significant hypotension exists.

Beta-Adrenergic Blockers

Beta-adrenergic blockers act primarily by reducing myocardial oxygen demand, as a result of decreasing the heart rate, arterial pressure, and inotropic force. Beta-blockers have been shown to be effective in decreasing effort angina. However, until recently, there was controversy about the use of beta-blockers in rest angina because of the theoretical risk of potentiating coronary vasoconstriction as a result of unopposed alpha-adrenergic tone. Several clinical trials have shown this concern to be unfounded. In the Holland Interuniversity Nifedipine/Metoprolol Trial of 515 patients with unstable angina, metoprolol (200 mg daily) reduced the incidence of recurrent ischemia and myocardial infarction during the 48-hour observation period. Propranolol, alone or in combination with nitrates and nifedipine, has also been shown to be effective in treating unstable angina. Esmolol, an ultrashort-acting beta-blocker (half-life, 8 minutes), was found in a placebo-controlled trial by Hohnloser and colleagues to reduce the incidence of myocardial infarction and the need for immediate revascularization. Thus, unless contraindications to their use exist, beta-blockers are important therapy for acute myocardial ischemic syndromes.

Calcium Channel Antagonists

The use of calcium channel antagonists in treating unstable angina is theoretically attractive because of the postulated involvement of dynamic coronary obstruction in the pathophysiology of the syndrome. Six clinical trials have randomized patients to treatment with oral calcium channel antagonists. In the largest of these trials (Holland Interuniversity), a trend toward more nonfatal myocardial infarctions in patients treated with nifedipine without concomitant metoprolol prompted early termination of the study. Taken together, these studies suggest that oral calcium channel antagonists are effective in relieving chest pain without concomitant therapy with nitrates or beta-blockers, but not in reducing adverse outcomes in unstable angina.

Thrombolytic Therapy

The frequent occurrence of refractory angina, myocardial infarction, and death after acute myocardial ischemia, together with evidence that coronary thrombosis plays an important role in unstable angina and acute myocardial infarction, has provided theoretical support for the use of thrombolytic therapy. Several randomized clinical trials have now clearly established the efficacy of such therapy for acute myocardial infarction.

Patients with subocclusive thrombus are most likely to benefit from thrombolytic therapy.

Despite a large number of clinical studies, comprising a total of approximately 188 treated patients, the role of thrombolytic therapy in the treatment of unstable angina remains controversial. Gold and colleagues treated 24 patients who had rest angina and ST segment changes with either a 12-hour infusion of recombinant tissue plasminogen activator (rt-PA) and heparin or heparin alone. Follow-up angiography demonstrated coronary thrombus in eight of the 11 patients who received placebo, versus none of the 11 patients treated with rt-PA. These impressive results were mitigated by bleeding in eight of the 12 rt-PA patients. In another placebo-controlled study, patients with angina refractory to conventional therapy were randomized to rt-PA or placebo. Patients treated with rt-PA had significantly less recurrent ischemia (Fig. 31–2). However, quantitative angiography did not reveal significant differences between the groups. Ongoing and future studies should help to define further which subgroups of patients with unstable angina are most likely to benefit from thrombolytic therapy.

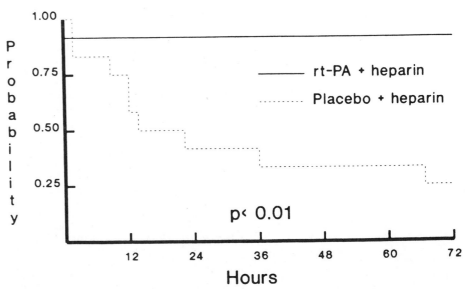

FIGURE 31–2: Kaplan-Meier curves comparing the probability of being ischemia-free as a function of recombinant tissue plasminogen activator (rt-PA) administration during a period of 72 hours in 24 patients whose conditions were refractory to conventional medical treatment. (From Ardissino D, Barberis P, De Servi S, et al. Recombinant tissue-type plasminogen activator followed by heparin compared with heparin alone for refractory unstable angina pectoris. Am J Cardiol 66:913, 1990.)

Cardiac Catheterization and Percutaneous Transluminal Coronary Angioplasty

Angiography should be performed urgently in patients whose conditions are not stabilized with pharmacologic therapy.

Because nearly 50% of patients with unstable angina have three-vessel or left main coronary artery disease, coronary angiography should be performed unless clear contraindications exist. On the basis of 15 reports of percutaneous transluminal coronary angioplasty published from 1981 to 1992, successful dilatation of the coronary arteries can be achieved in as many as 93% of patients, with an average success rate of 76%.

Coronary Artery Bypass Surgery

Compared with conventional medical therapy, surgical revascularization significantly reduces long-term mortality in patients with unstable angina who have left main disease, three-vessel disease, or specific types of two-vessel disease. The incidence of perioperative morbidity in large series has ranged from 6.1 to 16.7%, whereas perioperative mortality has ranged from 1.8 to 9%.

SUMMARY

Better understanding of the pathophysiology of myocardial ischemia, along with advances in diagnostic methods and therapies for ischemic syndromes, has been associated with improved survival of patients who have these syndromes. Nevertheless, morbidity and mortality remain substantial among patients with unstable angina and acute myocardial infarction. Although close monitoring and aggressive pharmacologic therapy are beneficial for relieving pain and reducing complications, invasive evaluation and revascularization are often warranted.

Suggested Readings

Ambrose JA, Winters SL, Stern A, et al. Angiographic morphology and the pathogenesis of unstable angina pectoris. J Am Coll Cardiol 5:609–616, 1985.

Ardissino D, Barberis P, De Servi S, et al. Recombinant tissue-type plasminogen activator followed by heparin compared with heparin alone for refractory unstable angina pectoris. Am J Cardiol 66:910–914, 1990.

Balsano F, Rizzow P, Violi F, et al. Antiplatelet treatment with ticlopidine in unstable angina. A controlled multicenter clinical trial. Circulation 82:17–26, 1990.

Bresnahan DR, Davis JL, Holmes DR Jr, Smith HC. Angiographic occurrence and clinical correlates of intraluminal coronary artery thrombus: Role of unstable angina. J Am Coll Cardiol 6:526–534, 1985.

Cairns JA, Gent M, Singer J, et al. Aspirin, sulfinpyrazone, or both in unstable angina: Results of a Canadian multicenter trial. N Engl J Med 313:1369–1375, 1985.

de Feyter PJ, Serruys PW, Arnold A, et al. Coronary angioplasty of the unstable angina related vessel in patients with multivessel disease. Eur Heart J 7:460–467, 1986.

Falk E. Unstable angina with fatal outcome: Dynamic coronary thrombosis leading to infarction and/or sudden death. Autopsy evidence of recurrent mural thrombosis with peripheral embolization culminating in total vascular occlusion. Circulation 71:699–708, 1985.

Fuster V, Chesebro JH. Mechanisms of unstable angina. N Engl J Med 315:1023–1025, 1986.

Gold HK, Johns JA, Leinbach RC, et al. A randomized, blinded, placebo-controlled trial of recombinant human tissue-type plasminogen activator in patients with unstable angina pectoris. Circulation 75:1192–1199, 1987.

Gruppo Italiano Per Lo Studio Della Streptochinasi Nell'Infarto Miocardico (GISSI). Effectiveness of intravenous thrombolytic treatment in acute myocardial infarction. Lancet 1:397–401, 1986.

Hohnloser S, Meinertz T, Kingenheben T, et al. Usefulness of esmolol in unstable angina pectoris. Am J Cardiol 67:1319–1323, 1991.

Holland Interuniversity Nifedipine/Metoprolol Trial Research Group. Early treatment of unstable angina in the coronary care unit: A randomized, double blind, placebo controlled comparison of recurrent ischaemia in patients treated with nifedipine or metoprolol or both. Br Heart J 56:400–413, 1986.

ISIS-2 (Second International Study of Infarct Survival) Collaborative Group. Randomized trial of intravenous streptokinase, oral aspirin, both, or neither among 17,187 cases of suspected acute myocardial infarction: ISIS-2. Lancet 2:349–360, 1988.

Kannel WB, Abbott RD. Incidence and prognosis of unrecognized myocardial infarction. An update in the Framingham study. N Engl J Med 311:1144, 1984.

Kemp HG, Vokonas PS, Cohn PF. The anginal syndrome associated with normal coronary arteriograms: Report of a six-year experience. Am J Med 54:735–742, 1973.

Kilton TC, Chaitman BR. The prognosis in stable and unstable angina. Cardiol Clin 9:27–38, 1991.

Lewis HD Jr. Which role for antiplatelet and anticoagulant drugs in unstable angina pectoris? Cardiovasc Drugs Ther 2:103–106, 1988.

Lewis HD, Davis JW, Archibald DG, et al. Protective effects of aspirin against acute myocardial infarction and death in men with unstable angina. Results of a Veterans Administration Cooperative Study. N Engl J Med 309:396–403, 1983.

Luchi RJ, Scott SM, Deupree RH. Comparison of medical and surgical treatment for unstable angina pectoris. Results of a Veterans Administration Cooperative Study. N Engl J Med 316:977–984, 1987.

Neri Serneri GG, Gensini GF, Poggesi L, et al. Effect of heparin, aspirin, or alteplase in reduction of myocardial ischaemia in refractory unstable angina. Lancet 335:615–618, 1990.

Rahimtoola SH, Nunley D, Grunkemeier G, et al. Ten-year survival after coronary bypass surgery for unstable angina. N Engl J Med 308:676–681, 1983.

Stuart RS, Baumgartner WA, Soule L, et al. Predictors of perioperative mortality in patients with unstable postinfarction angina. Circulation 78:I163–I165, 1988.

Telford AM, Wilson C. Trial of heparin versus atenolol in prevention of myocardial infarction in intermediate coronary syndrome. Lancet 1:1225–1228, 1981.

Theroux P, Latour J-G, Diodati J, et al. Hemodynamic, platelet and clinical responses to prostacyclin in unstable angina pectoris. Am J Cardiol 65:1084–1089, 1990.

Theroux P, Ouimet H, McCans J, et al. Aspirin, heparin, or both to treat acute unstable angina. N Engl J Med 319:1105–1111, 1988.

Vejar M, Hackett D, Brunelli C, et al. Comparison of low-dose aspirin and coronary vasodilators in acute unstable angina. Circulation 81(Suppl 1):I4–I11, 1990.

Wallentin LC, Research Group on Instability in Coronary Artery Disease in Southeast Sweden. Aspirin (75mg/day) after an episode of unstable coronary artery disease: Long term effects on the risk for myocardial infarction, occurrence of severe angina and the need for revascularization. J Am Coll Cardiol 18:1587–1593, 1991.

Williams DO, Kirby MG, McPherson K, Phear DN. Anticoagulant treatment of unstable angina. Br J Clin Pract 40:114–116, 1986.

32

○

Key Terms

Acute Renal Failure

Blood Urea Nitrogen (BUN)

Hemodialysis

Nephrotoxins

Nitrogenous Waste

Oliguria

Peritoneal Dialysis

Uremia

Nitrogenous waste materials—the breakdown products of ingested food and cellular metabolism.

Acute Renal Failure

John D. Wagner, M.D.

Beginning with an outline of normal renal function, this chapter reviews briefly the events that lead to renal failure in the hospitalized patient. This chapter defines the types of new-onset renal failure and the means of distinguishing them. The later sections of the chapter discuss basic principles of prevention and management and highlight some aspects of dialysis therapy.

Although therapeutic advances have had an impact on medical care, the prognosis for hospitalized patients with newly developed severe kidney failure has not changed much since the mid-1970s.[1-3] In the trauma or postoperative patient, severe kidney failure may be associated with a mortality rate of more than 50%.[4] Medical intensive care patients with multiorgan failure have a similarly poor prognosis when they also have severe renal failure. This is not to say that no progress has been made. With current management, most instances of renal failure developing in hospitalized patients are of a less severe nature than those seen previously.[5]

PHYSIOLOGY AND PATHOPHYSIOLOGY

The obvious role of the kidney is the excretion of salt, water, and waste material filtered from the blood.[6] Given the vagaries of the human diet, on any given day, ingested foodstuffs might impose a minimal burden of salt, water, and nutrients, followed on the next day by meals with large quantities of heavily salted food and beverages. On the day of minimal intake, the kidneys need to eliminate only relatively small amounts of salt, water, and nitrogenous waste materials. On the day of dietary surfeit, larger quantities of urine are excreted as the kidneys reject salt and water in excess of those quantities needed to maintain a normal intravascular fluid volume.

The kidneys regulate salt excretion independent of water excretion, allowing greater flexibility in adapting to particular dietary (or treatment-related) burdens of salt and water. Similarly, the mechanisms that alter salt and water excretion do not directly affect the elimination of nitrogenous wastes. In this way, patients can develop abnormalities of waste material accumulation without manifesting problems of salt or water imbalance.

The kidneys also produce important regulators of cell activity, some of which have systemic effects and some of which act locally. An example of the former is erythropoietin, a hormone produced in the kidney that stimulates the production of red blood cells in the bone marrow.[7] Erythropoietin serves to maintain the hematocrit. Intrarenal production of renin and angiotensin illustrates the latter point. Events in the kidney trigger kidney cells to release these substances in order to affect neighboring cells, thereby changing the renal excretory response.[8]

Urine is made by the transformation of blood in the kidneys into an ultrafiltrate of plasma, which is then further refined into the physiologically acceptable end-product. The kidneys are supplied by renal arteries, which deliver approximately 25% of the cardiac output to the renal tissue. These blood vessels divide into smaller branches, finally evolving into highly specialized capillaries called glomeruli (see Valtin for a synopsis of renal anatomy[6]). Each kidney has approximately 1 million such structures. Pre- and postcapillary muscular sphincters regulate the hydrostatic pressure within these glomeruli, and the cellular core changes shape to modify their volume. In this fashion, the circulating blood is forced against the semipermeable glomerular capillaries (Fig. 32–1), pushing salt, water, and its dissolved toxins through membrane pores, much like the water emanating from a sprinkler attached to a garden

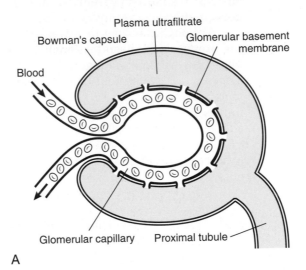

A

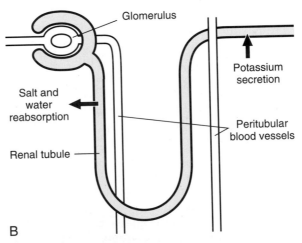

B

FIGURE 32–1: *A*, An idealized glomerular capillary enclosed by Bowman's capsule. This capsule delimits the urinary space. An ultrafiltrate of plasma escapes the blood contained within the glomerular capillary by traversing cells and the glomerular basement membrane on which the cells are anchored. The ultrafiltrate enters the urinary space and flows into the renal tubule. *B*, The anatomy of the renal tubule is such that different salt and water transport activities occur at different segments. The surrounding blood vessels carry the reabsorbed substances back into the bloodstream. The nature of the cells lining the tubules determines what transport activities may occur.

hose. In healthy glomeruli, blood cells and proteins are too large to pass through the pores; thus, they remain within the glomeruli (for a review of glomerular physiology, see Kanwar and coworkers[9]).

The plasma ultrafiltrate, which totals about 180 L/day (or more than four times the total body water of a 70-kg man), must be largely reabsorbed if the patient is to maintain fluid balance. The plasma ultrafiltrate exits from the glomerulus and enters the renal tubules, whose lining cells modify its composition, reabsorbing most of the salt, water, and some other constituents. Specialized transporting tubular cells directly transfer other substances, such as acids and potassium, from the blood surrounding the tubules in capillaries that course from the glomeruli. Chemical messengers and other signals may influence this transformation of ultrafiltrate into urine, so that the excretion of salt and water bears an appropriate relationship to what the patient's diet and metabolism require to be eliminated. Waste materials dissolved in the ultrafiltrate become constituents of urine as well (renal transport physiology is summarized in the textbook edited by Brenner and Rector[10-13]).

The urine exits the kidney via the collecting system, which consists initially of a sac called the renal pelvis attached to each kidney (Fig. 32–2). These two sacs narrow into two slender muscular tubes called ureters, which penetrate the bladder, from which urine is propelled ultimately into the outside environment via the urethra.

The most common measures of the kidney waste excretion function in clinical practice are the blood urea nitrogen (BUN) and serum creatinine levels.[14] Like other waste products of cellular metabolism, both substances are freely filtered by the glomerulus; patients therefore rely on glomerular filtration to rid themselves of them. Creatinine, a breakdown product of muscle metabolism, is relatively unaffected by the trans-

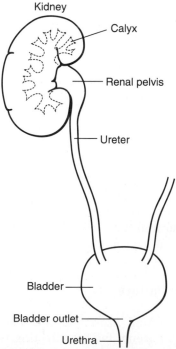

FIGURE 32–2: The gross anatomy of the urinary tract.

port processes of the renal tubules and consequently acts almost as an ideal marker of glomerular filtration.

A rise in the serum creatinine level reflects a fall in the glomerular filtration rate (GFR) because if the GFR falls, the ultrafiltration of creatinine will fall as well. With less ultrafiltration and with the production of creatinine continuing at the same rate, the blood level of this substance rises. Therefore, if one assumes that the production rate of creatinine has remained constant, a patient whose serum creatinine level rises must have had a fall in GFR.

Although termed BUN for historical reasons, the BUN test is typically performed on a serum sample. The BUN level also rises when the GFR falls, although the kidneys handle this substance a bit differently than they do creatinine. The liver makes urea as a byproduct of protein degradation. Unlike creatinine, the filtered urea undergoes reabsorption and secretion by the renal tubules. Hence, its level in serum may increase for reasons other than a diminution in the GFR. Furthermore, the production of BUN is not relatively fixed, as is that of creatinine; rather, it varies with diet, with the protein catabolic rate of the patient, and with the absorption of nondietary protein by the gastrointestinal tract (e.g., as in gastrointestinal bleeding). For these reasons, increases in the BUN level may be disproportionate to changes in the creatinine level.

Normal renal function encompasses the ability to balance salt and water output with intake, to excrete waste material, and to produce certain hormones and chemical messengers. Although a deficiency in renal performance in any of these areas might be construed as renal failure, this disorder is most commonly recognized when rising levels of BUN and serum creatinine indicate an impairment of the GFR and therefore an inability to excrete nitrogenous waste materials.[14]

In some cases of acute renal failure (ARF), a diminution in urine volume, salt excretion, or both may be perceived. As discussed previously, the renal regulation of the excretion of salt, water, and waste material occurs by diverse mechanisms, and a failure to excrete wastes does not necessarily also mean a failure to excrete salt and water. Occasionally, recognition of the diminution in urine output might prompt the discovery of the elevation in the BUN level, although monitoring of the BUN level tends to be routine. Patients with oliguric renal failure generally fare less well than nonoliguric patients (those with maintained urine outputs).[5] Patients who lose the ability to produce urine are called anuric.

ARF is further categorized as prerenal, intrinsic renal, or postrenal failure.[15] Factors external to the kidney that compromise renal blood flow can produce prerenal failure. Improvements in renal blood flow result in a rapid return of kidney function to normal. In contrast, intrinsic renal failure results from a process that directly damages kidney cells. The cells must recover from this damage in order for renal function to return toward normal. Postrenal failure results from the blockage of urine flow from the kidneys anywhere from the renal pelvis to the urethra.

Prerenal Failure

In prerenal azotemia, the disturbance in kidney function is due solely to nonrenal factors affecting renal blood flow. This renal hypoperfusion undermines the ability of the glomerulus to create an ultrafiltrate of the circulating blood, a process dependent on the amount of glomerular

It is useful to look at the levels of both BUN and creatinine in assessing renal function.

When the elevation of nitrogenous waste products in the blood occurs over a period of days, the renal failure is termed acute.

By definition, a daily urine volume of less than 400 mL denotes *oliguria*, a term that highlights the abnormality of such minimal urine formation.

blood flow as well as on the hydrostatic pressure generated in the glomerulus by that blood flow. The tubular cells and the glomeruli change their function in an attempt to adapt to a reduced renal perfusion, but this compensatory response can maintain glomerular filtration only to a limited extent, beyond which the filtration rate falls.

Table 32–1 provides examples of situations in which prerenal azotemia occurs. In all of them, the kidneys perceive a diminished effective arterial blood volume. In patients who develop shock, the renal hypoperfusion may occur suddenly. In other patients, it may evolve gradually following the deterioration of other body functions. For example, cardiac failure may cause renal hypoperfusion as the result of the loss of an effective blood pump. Bleeding tendencies or protracted vomiting and diarrhea can result in hypovolemia (low blood volume), with resultant low blood pressure and a shunting of blood away from the renal mass. Sepsis, hepatic failure, and malnutrition can result in a redistribution of the central blood volume to the extravascular space, again compromising renal blood flow.

In prerenal failure, the renal cells remain capable of normal function, despite the reduction in GFR. Indeed, this is why the disturbance in function is termed *pre*renal. Therefore, timely correction of the underlying problem (e.g., replacing fluid losses in a dehydrated patient) permits a rapid reversal of the elevated BUN level.[15] Associated oliguria should resolve as well, usually within 24 hours. Occasionally, patients at risk for prerenal azotemia do not develop prerenal failure until they receive a drug (e.g., a nonsteroidal anti-inflammatory agent such as ibuprofen) that interferes with a previously effective renal compensatory mechanism maintaining GFR.[16] Although such a drug disrupts renal function by a direct action on the kidney, it is the pre-existing renal hypoperfusion that makes the patient susceptible to the decrement in renal function. Cessation of the drug may allow a rapid return of function to normal.

Intrinsic Renal Failure

Table 32–2 lists examples of intrinsic renal failure, which refers to instances of kidney dysfunction related to problems within the kidney itself. Unlike prerenal failure, which may resolve within hours of correction of the abnormal prerenal factors, intrinsic ARF takes days to weeks

TABLE **32–1:** Prerenal Failure

Dehydration
  Vomiting
  Diarrhea
  Defective thirst mechanism or lack of access to fluids
  Diuretics
  Intra-abdominal redistribution of fluid into the extravascular
    space (related to gastrointestinal disease, surgery, or both)
Decreased effective arterial blood volume
  Congestive heart failure or pericardial disease
  Cirrhosis
  Nephrotic syndrome
  Sepsis
  Other low-albumin states
  Certain hypotensive drugs
Hemorrhage
Main renal artery stenosis or occlusion

TABLE **32–2:**   Intrinsic Renal Failure

Prerenal failure etiologies provoking acute tubular necrosis
  Sepsis
  Severe hemorrhage
  Severe volume depletion
  Drugs that interfere with intrarenal mechanisms maintaining
    glomerular filtration rate
  Surgical disruption of the renal blood supply (e.g., aortic cross-
    clamping)
Toxin-induced injury of tubular cells
  Aminoglycoside antibiotics
  Radiocontrast agents
  Rhabdomyolysis
  Hemolysis
Immunologically mediated renal disease
  Acute interstitial nephritis (from drugs, from infection, or
    idiopathic)
  Acute glomerulonephritis
Vascular insults
  Atheroemboli
  Thromboemboli
Intrarenal tubular obstruction
  Uric acid nephropathy
  High-dose methotrexate therapy

to reverse or may not reverse at all. Of all the forms of intrinsic renal failure, lowered blood flow with impaired oxygen delivery to the kidneys (termed ischemia) and exposure to agents (called nephrotoxins) that directly induce damage to kidney cells are the most common acute renal insults that occur in the hospitalized patient.[3]

As discussed earlier, renal hypoperfusion may cause a potentially reversible prerenal failure. However, prolonged or severe renal hypoperfusion may cause renal tubular cells to become nonviable,[17] leading to a form of intrinsic ARF sometimes known as acute tubular necrosis (ATN).[1] Such an outcome might eventuate from unremitting shock of any cause. Explanations for the reduction in GFR in ATN include blockage of the renal tubules by cellular debris and leakage of glomerular ultrafiltrate across a disrupted renal tubular lining back into the blood.

In ATN, as a type of intrinsic renal failure, the renal parenchyma is not normal by definition, although under the microscope the degree of discernible abnormality is highly variable.[18] For this reason, and on the basis of pathophysiologic insights gleaned from experimental animal models, some authors avoid the term *ATN*, preferring the more clinical diagnosis ARF instead. If the cause of ARF is ischemic injury, these authors would diagnose ischemic ARF rather than ATN.

Another frequent cause of intrinsic renal failure in hospitalized patients is the damage induced by drugs (nephrotoxicity).[19, 20] Toxin-induced ARF may appear clinically similar to the ATN of ischemia. Administration of the aminoglycoside antibiotics (e.g., gentamicin and amikacin), which are commonly used to treat serious gram-negative infections, can result in azotemia by poisoning renal tubular cells, although careful adjustment of the dosage according to serum drug levels may reduce the risk. Diuretics, another commonly administered class of drugs, may facilitate the toxicity of aminoglycosides.

Radiocontrast media given to enhance the appearance of vascular structures in various radiologic imaging formats (angiography, computed tomography, and pyelography) represent another potential source of renal injury to which hospitalized patients are exposed. The risk is particularly great in patients with underlying chronic renal disease, in diabetics, and in patients who are dehydrated.[19]

Although some drugs can cause a reversible deterioration in renal function by disrupting intrarenal mechanisms that serve to maintain the GFR (discussed previously), occasionally the renal failure induced by these agents runs a course more typical of ATN. For example, medications that lower blood pressure in severely hypertensive subjects may at times unpredictably lower the GFR.

However, in patients with atherosclerotic (or other) narrowing of the main renal arteries, antihypertensive drugs called angiotensin-converting enzyme inhibitors (e.g., captopril) may cause an abrupt, severe reduction in renal function.[21] Presumably, these drugs interfere with the intrarenal chemical signaling that permits maintenance of the GFR in the face of a subnormal renal blood flow. In some way, the disruption in the GFR induced by these drugs at times becomes sustained, outlasting the pharmacologic effects and therefore indicating that a more profound injury to the renal parenchyma has occurred.

Although ischemia or nephrotoxins account for most observed instances of intrinsic renal dysfunction in the hospitalized patient, drugs occasionally reduce the GFR by inducing an allergic reaction in the kidney.[22] The infiltration of immunologically reactive cells into the renal parenchyma prevents the normal functioning of tubular and glomerular transport processes. Although this reaction, termed acute interstitial nephritis, occurs rarely, commonly used drugs provoke it, such as antibiotics of the penicillin and cephalosporin classes.

Other less frequently observed causes of intrinsic renal dysfunction include various inflammatory renal diseases (called glomerulonephritis), which are sometimes seen in association with other organ system inflammatory disease. Examples of this include ARF associated with systemic lupus erythematosus, polyarteritis nodosa, and Wegener's granulomatosis.[23]

Acute intrinsic renal failure infrequently results from the occlusion of intrarenal blood vessels by cholesterol emboli.[24] Patients at risk are those with severe aortic atheromatous disease, particularly after aortic manipulation, such as might occur with angiography or vascular surgery. Atheroembolic renal disease may be associated with other organ system dysfunction, inasmuch as the emboli may lodge in mesenteric, intracranial, or extremity blood vessels in addition to those of the kidney.

Postrenal Failure

Postrenal failure is another broad pathophysiologic category.[25, 26] The blockage of urine flow may occur at the site where urine collects in the kidney after exiting from the tubules (the renal pelvis), in the ureter, at the bladder outlet, or in the urethra. Obstruction of the urinary tract must affect both kidneys or must affect the kidney that supplies the preponderance or totality of renal function in order to cause azotemia in a patient with previously normal renal function.

To understand this, one must realize that a healthy kidney is capable of an adaptive response to contralateral renal obstruction. The non-obstructed kidney is capable of increasing its GFR, mitigating the impact of unilateral obstruction on the overall GFR. In those uncommon patients who have congenital absence or atrophy of one kidney or in whom a kidney has been surgically removed, obstruction of the solitary "good" kidney would lead to a significant decrement in renal function. Bilateral obstruction leads to a similar decrement in renal function.

Typically, the process leading to obstruction occurs over a longer period than prerenal and intrinsic renal failure, but it may go unrecognized until a critical degree of obstruction has occurred, leading to symptomatic azotemia or obvious changes in urinary output. If this critical degree of obstruction occurs while the patient is hospitalized, ARF may result. For example, chronic narrowing of the bladder outlet from an enlarged prostate may progress to total occlusion in the postoperative or bedridden patient, preventing spontaneous voiding. In the absence of bladder emptying, renal obstruction results, accompanied by azotemia.

Table 32–3 summarizes selected etiologies of postrenal failure. Cancerous growths involving the bladder or the retroperitoneal space in which the ureters travel can block the flow of urine. Kidney stones or blood clots from urinary tract bleeding can lodge in the urinary tract and prevent urine flow. Sometimes the surgical correction of these problems leads to transient obstruction. Urinary catheters may become clogged. Fragmented stones can occlude the urinary tract before passing out of the patient.

DIAGNOSIS

History

A review of the fluid intake-and-output record and changes in body weight can shed light on a patient's volume status.

In ARF, as in many illnesses, the patient's history often suggests the etiology. Patients with congestive heart failure, liver disease accompanied by edema or ascites, or hypovolemia are at risk for prerenal azotemia.[15] Patients with profound circulatory disturbances, sepsis, or exposure to nephrotoxins are at risk for ATN.[1] In patients with known kidney stone disease, malignancy involving the retroperitoneum or the genitourinary tract, or bladder outlet obstructive symptoms, the possibility of postrenal failure exists. Especially in patients without any of these obvious historical clues, inflammatory renal disease (drug induced or otherwise) or vascular renal disease (e.g., that due to cholesterol emboli) must be considered.

TABLE **32–3:** Postrenal Failure

Bladder outlet or ureteral obstruction from malignancy
Prostate
Uroepithelial
Uterine
Cervical
Lymphoma
Bladder outlet obstruction from benign disease
Stones
Benign prostatic hypertrophy
Blood clots
Malfunctioning bladder catheter
Neurogenic bladder
Upper tract obstruction from benign disease
Stones
Strictures (congenital or related to trauma)
Retroperitoneal fibrosis
Blood clots
Papillary necrosis (sloughed tissue)

Physical Examination

The examination of the patient gives important clues. Low blood pressure and a rapid pulse suggest hypovolemia, severe heart failure, or the hemodynamic consequences of septic shock. Fever may indicate infection. Dryness of the skin and mouth cavity points to dehydration. Swelling of the legs or dependent tissues in a recumbent patient implies excessive total body hydration (although the intravascular volume might be low in such circumstances). Examination of the patient's lungs may provide evidence of circulatory overload. Tenderness in the flank or abdomen may suggest renal obstruction or inflammation. A large bladder above the symphysis pubis points to bladder outlet obstruction. Rectal or pelvic examination findings might suggest the presence of malignancy of the genitourinary tract.

Laboratory Testing

Laboratory data may provide diagnostically useful information. By definition, the BUN and creatinine levels are elevated, because ARF is recognized by azotemia and an abnormal creatinine level. Given the similar but not identical renal handling of BUN and creatinine, patients with intrinsic renal disease tend to have parallel rises in both, thereby maintaining the BUN-creatinine ratio of approximately 10:1.[27] Patients with prerenal azotemia may have a ratio of greater than 20:1, inasmuch as the mechanism of prerenal azotemia tends to influence urea clearance more than creatinine clearance.

The finding of a low total carbon dioxide level in a peripheral venous blood sample might indicate an accumulation of acid. An accumulation of acid and potassium out of proportion to the decrement in GFR might suggest renal obstruction.[26]

Microscopic and chemical analysis of the urine can suggest whether the intrinsic tubular function is intact (see later discussion). In prerenal azotemia, one would expect to find intact renal tubular function and the absence of features of intrinsic or postrenal failure.[15]

In intrinsic or postrenal failure, abnormal numbers of blood cells might point to the presence of malignancy, stones, or renal inflammation. The presence of renal tubular cells might indicate intrinsic kidney damage. Microscopic elements called casts provide further evidence of kidney cell damage. When excreted in the urine, they may be observed via the microscope. Red and white blood cell casts usually indicate inflammation. Muddy granular casts are suggestive of ATN. Detectable urinary protein might also suggest damage of the kidney cells (see Cadnapaphornchai and associates for a discussion[28]).

Additional, nonroutine tests often prove to be useful in distinguishing azotemia related to dehydration from actual injury to renal tubular cells. These tests include a determination of the sodium concentration in a randomly obtained urine specimen and an assessment of the urine osmolality.

The normal renal response to a patient's deficiency of salt and water (as might occur in prerenal azotemia) is to eliminate sodium from the urine and to reabsorb as much water as possible.[29] Renal conservation of sodium can result in a urine sodium concentration of less than 10 mEq/L. This is remarkable given that each of the 180 L of plasma filtered by the glomerulus each day contains approximately 140 mEq of sodium, for a

Casts—aggregated cells or proteinaceous debris that forms in and takes the shape of renal tubules.

620 Acute Renal Failure

total of more than 25,000 mEq of sodium filtered daily. Properly functioning renal tubular cells reabsorb more than 99% of this quantity in a volume of urine that may be less than 1 L.

The damaged renal tubular cells of ATN cannot achieve this high reabsorptive efficiency, resulting in a urine sodium concentration of greater than 40 mEq/L. Hence, the finding of a random (or "spot") urine sodium concentration of less than 20 mEq/L suggests that azotemia or oliguria relates to prerenal factors. A level of greater than 40 mEq/L (in a patient who is not receiving diuretics) does not confirm the normalcy of tubular function and lends support to a diagnosis of ATN.[30] However, the results of urinary chemistry studies from patients with prerenal versus intrinsic renal failure overlap in a small percentage of patients.[31]

The kidneys of volume-depleted subjects with prerenal azotemia might respond by maximally reabsorbing water. The urine specific gravity will rise to a level indicating an intact ability to concentrate (greater than 1.020). A more precise measure of urinary concentration than the specific gravity is the urine osmolality. Like the specific gravity, the urine osmolality rises when the urine is concentrated. Its value can be compared with serum osmolality as well.

Certain renal imaging tests can document the presence of two kidneys, assess the size of the renal parenchyma, and demonstrate renal obstruction if it is present.[32, 33] Ultrasonography most readily accomplishes these goals; bedside studies are possible. Computed tomography and magnetic resonance imaging performed without intravenous contrast can provide similar information without risk to renal function.

Imaging of the kidneys, ureters, and bladder and plain film radiography of the abdomen are traditional renal imaging tests that sometimes provide useful information pertinent to the evaluation of ARF. The outlines of the kidneys, the outline of the bladder, or both may be visible, thereby allowing determination of whether two kidneys are present and possibly assessment of renal size. Radiopaque stones might be visualizable. An enlarged bladder on a plain x-ray study might be a clue pointing to renal obstruction from bladder outlet disease. However, imaging of the kidneys, ureters, and bladder may not yield such information if the overlying intestinal contents obscure the genitourinary tract.

Intravenous pyelography is a radiographic procedure that uses intravenously administered radiocontrast to outline the kidneys and the collecting system.[32] Although this procedure defines the anatomy of the collecting system and shows obstruction if present, radiocontrast material may damage the kidneys in a patient who has an elevated BUN level. Therefore, avoiding intravenous pyelography in favor of other imaging studies is advisable. Occasionally, contrast is administered via a tube inserted into the bladder and then into the ureter under direct vision by the urologist. This retrograde pyelography does not expose the renal tissue to the risk of injury by radiocontrast material, but it is an invasive procedure.

Nuclear medicine techniques allow an assessment of renal function and renal blood flow without exposing the patient to the risk of radiocontrast. In the rare patient who has total renal artery occlusion, a nuclear renal flow scan might provide diagnostically useful information.[33]

Insertion of a bladder catheter can be diagnostically and therapeutically useful in patients with bladder outlet obstruction. In patients who cannot void spontaneously or who can void only incompletely, insertion of a bladder catheter might yield several hundred milliliters of urine, thereby suggesting the possibility that an overfilled bladder could be

A urine osmolality of more than 500 (compared with the normal serum value of 285) suggests that the renal cells are capable of normal function (a characteristic of prerenal failure). A low urine osmolality in an oliguric patient usually favors ATN over prerenal azotemia.

Abnormally small kidneys indicate pre-existing chronic renal disease.

The availability of noninvasive imaging studies limits the necessity to resort to retrograde studies.

blocking flow from the kidneys. It is then possible not only that bladder outlet obstruction may have caused renal failure but, if the diagnosis of obstruction is correct, that drainage of the bladder by a catheter may be followed by a return of renal function to normal.[15]

MANAGEMENT

General Approach

The development of ARF in the critically ill patient carries with it a less favorable prognosis and complicates management.[2, 34] The illnesses that make these patients so sick often predispose them to renal failure, either directly or through complications of necessary therapy. Whenever possible, the avoidance of renal injury assumes pre-eminent importance in the management of such patients. Treatment includes

- Maintaining adequate hydration and cardiac performance
- Aggressively treating infections
- Limiting or avoiding the use of drugs that might threaten renal function

After the diagnosis of ARF has been established, the therapeutic options become clear, although at times the diagnosis becomes clear only after a therapeutic trial (see Conger for a more extensive review[35]). Prerenal azotemia secondary to dehydration necessitates replacement of fluid losses. In prerenal azotemia from congestive heart failure, measures that improve cardiac output might benefit renal function. In patients with decreased effective arterial blood volume who have received drugs that interfere with intrarenal mechanisms helping to maintain GFR, cessation of those drugs may be necessary to counteract azotemia or prevent intrinsic renal failure. In septic patients, whose peripheral vascular dilatation may cause relative volume depletion by expanding the vascular volume, appropriate anti-infective therapy must be instituted.

No matter what the cause of renal failure, the staff must record daily weight changes and maintain intake-and-output records if they are not already available. Despite the information provided by the history, physical examination, and routine laboratory data, a clear picture of the patient's hydrational state sometimes remains elusive. In such cases, the right-sided intracardiac thermodilution catheter allows more precise monitoring of fluid requirements and permits insights into the effects of therapy aimed at improving cardiac performance.

If possible, attempts are made to treat the underlying process that has caused the renal failure in patients with intrinsic renal disease. In selected patients with glomerulonephritis or acute interstitial nephritis, anti-inflammatory drugs or other therapies may be given.[22, 23] Unfortunately, in the typical patient with nephrotoxic or ischemic ATN, no specific therapy expedites renal recovery, a process that may take weeks.[1] Therefore, the management of intrinsic renal failure often consists of attending to the complications of an acute disruption of renal salt, water, and waste handling.[3] Meticulous balancing of fluids corrects volume depletion and forestalls the development of overhydration. The latter becomes almost inevitable in the patient with minimal to no urine output unless significant extrarenal losses are present (e.g., gastrointestinal tract losses).

Abnormalities of plasma sodium, potassium, magnesium, calcium, and phosphorus concentrations may evolve, depending on the degree of renal damage, the patient's catabolic state, and the patient's intake of salts and fluids. Some restriction of dietary or medication-related sodium, potassium, fluid, magnesium, and phosphorus may therefore become necessary. In the critical care setting, the common use of parenteral alimentation or specialized enteral feeding solutions permits great flexibility in what nutrition the patient receives. However, the prescriber of these therapies must remember to tailor the choice of solutions to the particular needs of the patient. The standardized solutions employed successfully in the care of the nonrenal patient may contain dangerously inappropriate quantities of solutes.

Nondehydrated subjects without renal obstruction who have oliguria, even those with ATN, may respond to diuretic therapy. Therefore, a trial of diuretics to augment urine output in oliguric or fluid-overloaded patients is worth attempting.[1, 3] Successful conversion of a patient from an oliguric to a nonoliguric form of ARF facilitates fluid management.

Uremia

The accumulation of toxins normally excreted via the kidney ultimately produces symptoms, whether fluid overload or electrolyte imbalance is present or not. Although urea is not a toxic substance in and of itself, it serves as a surrogate marker for substances that are toxic. Therefore, uremia, the syndrome of poisoning by the accumulated circulating wastes of severe renal failure, is diagnosed at a time when the BUN level is high.[36] Clinical manifestations of uremia include

- Changes in the patient's level of alertness or other mental alterations
- Seizures
- Inflammation of the sac surrounding the heart (pericarditis)
- Nausea
- Vomiting
- Twitching
- Hiccuping

The actual BUN level at which these symptoms occur is quite variable, but they are more likely to be evident with a reduction in renal function to 10% or less of normal. Once these symptoms supervene, either improvement in renal function must occur or dialysis must be used to prevent the life-threatening complications of uremia.

Dietary protein restriction may defer the need for dialysis by restraining the accumulation of waste materials in the patient with renal failure. The BUN level of a protein-restricted patient is lower than that of a protein-loaded subject, and the previously described uremic symptoms tend not to appear as rapidly.[36] However, theoretical concerns about adequate nutrition in the critically ill patient may favor supplying adequate nutrition, including protein and calories, to meet the increased needs of catabolic patients with ARF.[3]

Dialysis

In the face of symptomatic volume overload unresponsive to diuretics, uremic manifestations of a serious nature (seizures, pericarditis, markedly altered mentation, and intractable nausea and vomiting), or life-threatening electrolyte abnormalities uncorrectable by dietary or pharmaceutical interventions, dialysis may be necessary. Dialytic therapies can be divided into those that require access to the patient's blood vessels (hemodialysis or some form of hemofiltration) and peritoneal dialysis. Dialytic therapy can be continuous or intermittent.

Hemodialysis

In hemodialysis, a specially designed catheter placed in a large vein (usually a femoral or subclavian vein) allows a blood pump to draw more than 200 mL/min into the central channels of thousands of hollow, hair-thin fibers of cellulosic or synthetic materials held within a cylinder called a dialyzer or an artificial kidney (less commonly, the dialyzer holds parallel plates instead of fibers). Surrounding the fibers is a dialysis solution (dialysate) containing a physiologically appropriate concentration of sodium, buffer (either bicarbonate or acetate), and other electrolytes. Fresh dialysate circulates through the dialyzer at a rate of 500 mL/min or greater[37] (Fig. 32–3).

Urea, which is not found in fresh dialysate, travels along its concentration gradient into the dialysate, thereby exiting the patient.[38]

The membranes of the dialyzer fibers are made of a material that is porous to small molecules, such as urea, salt, and water, but that prevents the transmembrane movement of protein and cells. Any difference between the concentration of a filterable substance on the blood side of the dialysis membrane and its concentration on the dialysate side favors movement of the substance from the higher-concentration side to the lower-concentration side. Therefore, the abnormally high blood waste concentrations cause shifts of these substances across the hollow-fiber membranes into the surrounding dialysate, which contains no wastes.

Because the dialyzer membrane is porous to water, hydrostatic forces applied across the membrane mimic what happens to blood flowing through the glomerulus. An ultrafiltrate of plasma traverses the dialyzer membrane, thereby relieving overhydration and affording additional clearance of the solutes dissolved in the ultrafiltrate.

The dialyzed blood then returns to the patient, either via a second catheter or via a second lumen in the catheter used to withdraw blood from the patient. To prevent the blood from clotting, the patient often receives heparin systemically throughout most of the dialysis treatment, although dialysis without anticoagulation or with nonsystemic anticoagulation is sometimes feasible.[38]

Treatments are typically rendered three or more times per week, for 3 hours or more for each dialysis, depending on patient requirements for fluid and uremic toxin removal.

The hemodialysis prescription includes

- Choosing a dialyzer with the desired permeability characteristics
- Setting the blood pump for a flow rate that the patient can tolerate hemodynamically
- Selecting a dialysate composition that meets the patient's needs
- Targeting fluid and urea removal (urea being the surrogate marker for waste removal) by ordering a specific duration of dialysis
- Adjusting the machine's transmembrane pressure to yield the desired fluid removal in that period

Hemofiltration

Continuous arteriovenous hemofiltration (CAVH) is another renal replacement therapy that uses a hollow-fiber artificial kidney connected

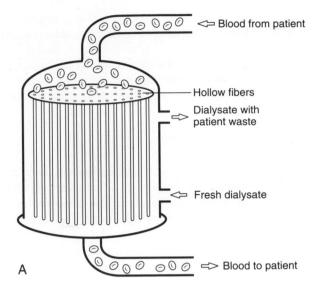

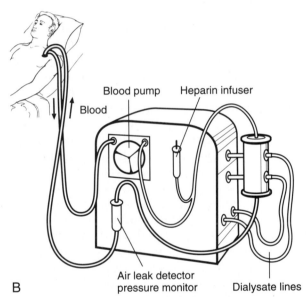

FIGURE 32–3: *A,* The hollow-fiber dialyzer. Blood enters the semipermeable hollow fibers, which allow movement of waste materials and excess salt and water from the blood side to the dialysate side. *B,* A hemodialysis machine. The machine incorporates a blood pump, a means of infusing anticoagulant, and monitoring devices to warn against excessive pressures within the dialysis circuit and against the development of air bubbles in the blood tubing. The machine also modifies the dialysate, adjusting its salt content and warming it to body temperature.

The CAVH artificial kidney, smaller than the hemodialysis kidney, is made of highly porous synthetic material.

to the patient's blood circulation[39] (Fig. 32–4). Unlike hemodialysis, CAVH avoids the use of a blood pump by employing a catheter in a large artery (usually the femoral). The patient's blood pressure rather than the blood pump then becomes the determining factor in the magnitude of the pressure exerted against the hollow-fiber membrane. Clearance from the blood of uremic toxins is the result of removing large volumes

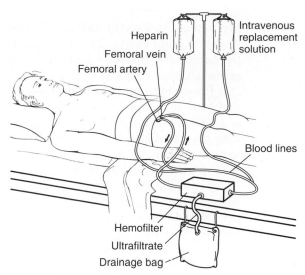

FIGURE 32–4: Continuous arteriovenous hemofiltration.

of ultrafiltrate (more than 500 mL/hr) and of replacing it intravenously with a physiologic solution (e.g., lactated Ringer's) that more closely resembles the salt content of nonuremic plasma.

The hemofilter operates continuously until it malfunctions or is removed; it requires no extra machinery. The patient receives heparin continuously (other anticoagulants are available) to prevent clotting in the tubing and dialyzer.

Variations on CAVH include continuous arteriovenous hemodialysis, in which dialysate infuses on the nonblood side of the dialyzer membrane at a rate of 1 L/h, somewhat increasing the efficiency at which uremic toxins escape the patient. Continuous venovenous hemofiltration spares the patient the potential trauma of cannulation of a large artery by using a venovenous circuit, accessing a large vein such as might be used for hemodialysis. However, to generate a suitable blood flow, continuous venovenous hemofiltration incorporates a blood pump into the circuit. This necessitates sensors and alarms not present in CAVH, making it a more complex procedure. Continuous venovenous hemodialysis further enhances this technique.[39]

Peritoneal Dialysis

Peritoneal dialysis uses the vascularized lining of the intestinal tract to serve as the membrane across which waste materials leave the blood.[40] In peritoneal dialysis, a sterile dialysate solution is instilled into the peritoneal (abdominal) cavity. Commercially available dialysate contains physiologically appropriate concentrations of salts and buffers. As in hemodialysis, salts move out of the blood compartment into the dialysate along their concentration gradients. The dialysate also contains a very high concentration of dextrose sugar. The high sugar content of the dialysate creates a concentration gradient favoring the formation of a large-volume plasma ultrafiltrate across the blood vessels of the peritoneum.

The dialysate is placed into the peritoneum via a semisoft catheter introduced into the abdominal cavity percutaneously. Alternatively, a soft catheter can be tunneled under the skin, with a cuff anchored to the peritoneum before the catheter is plunged through the peritoneum into the abdominal cavity. The dialysate exits from the abdominal cavity via the same catheter. Any amount drained in excess of that instilled represents net fluid removal from the patient (Fig. 32–5).

Prescribing peritoneal dialysis involves deciding how often to instill dialysate into and drain dialysate from the peritoneal cavity (each cycle of instillation and drainage constitutes an exchange), determining how long the instilled dialysate should remain in the abdomen before drainage (the dwell time), and choosing the right dextrose concentration so that neither too much nor too little fluid drains from the patient.

Typically, the critical care unit patient beginning peritoneal dialysis receives hourly exchanges of 2 L of dialysate. If this amount of dialysis proves to be in excess of patient needs, less frequent exchanges might suffice. Patients who have noncuffed, percutaneously placed dialysis catheters receive peritoneal dialysis for about 3 days. After 3 days, the catheter is removed to prevent the development of infection. If access to the abdominal cavity is via a subcutaneously tunneled catheter, dialysis need not be interrupted for catheter changes.

Choosing a Dialytic Therapy

The type of dialysis a patient receives depends on what fluid and electrolyte changes need to be effected and on technical considerations.[38] All the forms of renal replacement therapy described earlier correct fluid and electrolyte abnormalities and remove uremic toxins. However, the continuous therapies (CAVH, continuous venovenous hemofiltration, continuous arteriovenous hemodialysis, continuous venovenous hemodialysis, and peritoneal dialysis) allow daily adjustments of the dialysis prescriptions, which make them particularly advantageous in patients with large obligatory fluid intakes (e.g., those receiving parenteral nutrition) and in those who do not tolerate fluid overload well. On the other

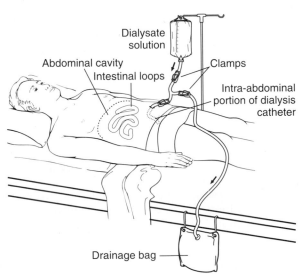

FIGURE 32–5: One type of peritoneal dialysis setup. The dialysis solution is directed into and out of the peritoneal cavity by setting the appropriate clamps.

hand, hemodialysis removes fluid and solute more efficiently than do the other therapies, making rapid relief of fluid overload or hyperkalemia (an elevated blood potassium level) a much more certain accomplishment in a limited period of time.

Therapies that rely on vascular access (hemodialysis, CAVH, and other forms of hemofiltration) typically require that the patient receive anticoagulants, a potential problem for patients with active bleeding or bleeding tendencies. Vascular access may be difficult to obtain or maintain in some patients, thereby eliminating the use of these therapies in a particular patient. Patients who are hemodynamically unstable may not tolerate the cardiovascular stresses engendered by hemodialysis, making this form of therapy hazardous to the patient. Patients receiving CAVH must have a blood pressure high enough to generate a sufficient pressure gradient across the hemofilter membrane such that filtration will proceed, which makes its use in patients in shock problematic.

Peritoneal dialysis avoids the problems of anticoagulation and perturbation of the cardiovascular system, but placement of the peritoneal dialysis catheter is an invasive procedure. In addition, the abdominal cavity must be suitable. Patients who have had recent abdominal surgery, who have intra-abdominal infection, or who have extensive adhesions from prior abdominal surgery may not be candidates for peritoneal dialysis. Even without obvious problems with the anatomy of the intra-abdominal cavity, the peritoneal dialysis procedure may not succeed.

Therefore, in patient whose cardiovascular status can be stabilized, who can receive some anticoagulation, and who have accessible large veins, hemodialysis usually offers the most certain avenue for rapid correction of the fluid, electrolyte, and uremic manifestations of ARF. The other forms of therapy might be useful when the patient's medical condition precludes hemodialysis for the reasons outlined or when continuous therapy manages the patient's problems more effectively.

Renal Recovery

In patients with reversible causes of ARF, dialysis supports the patient's well-being until the kidneys exhibit a return of function sufficient to maintain the patient's health without dialysis.[3] Evidence of this return of function may include an increase in urine output (most noticeable in the oliguric or anuric patient) and a fall in the predialysis peak BUN level. The high mortality rate of patients with ARF in the critical care setting generally stems from the severity of coexisting conditions, not from the renal failure itself.[2, 15] Whether ARF is a marker for the multiorgan failure or the postoperative patient's overall inability to survive or whether it predisposes the patient to continuing comorbid events (typically sepsis, gastrointestinal bleeding, or respiratory failure) from which the patient ultimately dies is unclear.

As mentioned previously, patients with ATN may not experience renal recovery for several weeks after the onset of therapy, at which point a rapid return toward premorbid renal function may occur over several days or a slower improvement may take place over weeks. In inflammatory renal disease, the GFR may return to normal gradually or suddenly, depending on the specific disease entity. Not all inflammatory renal disease benefits from or requires anti-inflammatory therapy. In those cases, spontaneous recovery can occur. In obstructive renal disease, renal recovery usually becomes evident within days of the relief of obstruction. In all forms of renal failure, incomplete recovery or no improvement of function may occur.

SUMMARY

ARF refers to a sudden lowering of the GFR that is clinically detectable by a rise in BUN and creatinine levels and by a variable change in urine output. ARF etiologically falls into one of three categories: prerenal azotemia, intrinsic renal failure, and postrenal failure. The context in which ARF occurs, a clinical assessment of the patient's volume status, microscopic and chemical testing of the urine, and renal imaging studies may contribute to a delineation of the cause of ARF in a given patient. Appropriate fluid replacement, dietary manipulation, and adjustment of medications may be all that is necessary to allow an uneventful recovery of renal function in patients whose renal failure is reversible. For patients with complications of renal failure that require more active intervention, several modalities of renal replacement therapy are available. Although dialysis can correct the life-threatening manifestations of renal failure in the critically ill patient, the likelihood of survival diminishes in patients who develop renal failure.

References

1. Lieberthal W, Levinsky NG. Treatment of acute tubular necrosis. Semin Nephrol 10:571–583, 1990.
2. Maher ER, Robinson KN, Scoble JE, et al. Prognosis of critically-ill patients with acute renal failure: APACHE II score and other predictive factors. Q J Med 72:857–866, 1989.
3. Nortman DF, Franklin SS. Acute renal failure in the critical care setting. Acute Care 13:127–156, 1987.
4. Stene JK. Renal failure in the trauma patient. Crit Care Clin 6:111–119, 1990.
5. Anderson RJ, Linas SL, Berns AS, et al. Nonoliguric acute renal failure. N Engl J Med 296:1134–1138, 1977.
6. Valtin H. Renal Function: Mechanisms Preserving Fluid and Solute Balance in Health. Boston, Little, Brown and Company, 1973.
7. Nimer SD. Molecular biology and hematology of erythropoietin. *In* Nissenson AR (moderator). Recombinant human erythropoietin and renal anemia: Molecular biology, clinical efficacy, and nervous system effects. Ann Intern Med 114:402–407, 1991.
8. Ingelfinger JR, Dzau VJ. Molecular biology of renal injury: Emphasis on the role of the renin-angiotensin system. J Am Soc Nephrol 2:S9–S20, 1991.
9. Kanwar YS, Liu ZZ, Kashihara N, Wallner EI. Current status of the structural and functional basis of glomerular filtration and proteinuria. Semin Nephrol 11:390–413, 1991.
10. Berry CA, Rector FC. Renal transport of glucose, amino acids, sodium, chloride, and water. *In* Brenner BM, Rector FC (eds). The Kidney, 4th ed. Philadelphia, WB Saunders, 1991, pp 245–282.
11. Giebisch G, Malnic G, Berliner RW. Renal transport and control of potassium excretion. *In* Brenner BM, Rector FC (eds). The Kidney, 4th ed. Philadelphia, WB Saunders, 1991, pp 283–317.
12. Alpern RJ, Stone DK, Rector FC. Renal acidification mechanisms. *In* Brenner BM, Rector FC (eds). The Kidney, 4th ed. Philadelphia, WB Saunders, 1991, pp 318–379.
13. Suki W, Rouse D. Renal transport of calcium, magnesium, and phosphorus. *In* Brenner BM, Rector FC (eds). The Kidney, 4th ed. Philadelphia, WB Saunders, 1991, pp 380–423.
14. Rudnick MR, Bastl CP, Elfenbein IB, Narins RG. The differential diagnosis of acute renal failure. *In* Brenner BM, Lazarus JM (eds). Acute Renal Failure, 2nd ed. New York, Churchill Livingstone, 1988, pp 177–232.
15. Conger JD, Briner VA, Schrier RW. Acute renal failure: Pathogenesis, diagnosis, and management. *In* Schrier RW (ed). Renal and Electrolyte Disorders, 4th ed. Boston, Little, Brown and Company, 1992, pp 495–537.
16. Stoff J, Clive DM. Role of arachidonic acid metabolites in acute renal failure. *In* Brenner BM, Lazarus JM (eds). Acute Renal Failure, 2nd ed. New York, Churchill Livingstone, 1988, pp 143–173.

17. Molitoris BA. New insights into the cell biology of ischemic acute renal failure. J Am Soc Nephrol 1:1263–1270, 1991.
18. Solez K, Morel-Maroger L, Sraer J-D. The morphology of "acute tubular necrosis" in man: Analysis of 57 renal biopsies and a comparison with the glycerol model. Medicine 58:362–376, 1979.
19. Coggins CH, Fang LS-T. Acute renal failure associated with antibiotics, anesthetic agents, and radiographic contrast agents. In Brenner BM, Lazarus JM (eds). Acute Renal Failure, 2nd ed. New York, Churchill Livingstone, 1988, pp 295–352.
20. Bennett WM, Plamp C, Porter GA. Drug-related syndromes in clinical nephrology. Ann Intern Med 87:582–590, 1977.
21. Eknoyan G, Suki WN. Renal consequences of antihypertensive therapy. Semin Nephrol 11:129–137, 1991.
22. Pusey CD, Saltissi D, Bloodworth L, et al. Drug associated acute interstitial nephritis: Clinical and pathological features and the response to high-dose steroid therapy. Q J Med 206:194–211, 1983.
23. Jennette JC, Falk RJ. Diagnosis and management of glomerulonephritis and vasculitis presenting as acute renal failure. Med Clin North Am 74:893–908, 1990.
24. Smith MC, Ghose MK, Henry AR. The clinical spectrum of renal cholesterol embolization. Am J Med 71:174–180, 1981.
25. Gillenwater JY. Clinical aspects of urinary tract obstruction. Semin Nephrol 2:46–54, 1982.
26. Klahr S. Obstructive uropathy. Pathophysiology and management. In Schrier RW (ed). Renal and Electrolyte Disorders, 4th ed. Boston, Little, Brown and Company, 1992, pp 581–633.
27. Levey AS, Madaio MP, Perrone RP. Laboratory assessment of renal disease: Clearance, urinalysis, and renal biopsy. In Brenner BM, Rector FC (eds). The Kidney, 4th ed. Philadelphia, WB Saunders, 1991, pp 919–968.
28. Cadnapaphornchai P, Dorman H, McDonald FD. Differential diagnosis of acute renal failure. In Jacobson HR, Striker GE, Klahr S (eds). The Principles and Practice of Nephrology. Philadelphia, BC Decker, 1991, pp 631–640.
29. Harrington JT, Cohen JJ. Measurement of urinary electrolytes—indications and limitations. N Engl J Med 293:1241–1243, 1975.
30. Pru C, Kjellstrand C. Urinary indices and chemistries in the differential diagnosis of prerenal failure and acute tubular necrosis. Semin Nephrol 5:224–233, 1985.
31. Miller TR, Anderson RJ, Linas SL, et al. Urinary diagnostic indices in acute renal failure. A prospective study. Ann Intern Med 89:47–50, 1978.
32. Kaye AD, Pollack IIM. Diagnostic imaging approach to the patient with obstructive uropathy. Semin Nephrol 2:55–73, 1982.
33. Fine EJ, Axelrod M, Blaufox MD. Physiologic aspects of diagnostic renal imaging. Semin Nephrol 5:188–207, 1985.
34. Schaefer J-H, Jochimsen F, Keller F, et al. Outcome prediction of acute renal failure in medical intensive care. Intensive Care Med 17:19–24, 1991.
35. Conger JD. Management of acute renal failure. In Jacobson HR, Striker GE, Klahr S (eds). The Principles and Practice of Nephrology. Philadelphia, BC Decker, 1991, pp 666–676.
36. Depner TA. Uremic toxins and dialysis. In Depner TA (ed). Prescribing Hemodialysis: A Guide to Urea Modeling. Boston, Kluwer Academic Publishers, 1991, pp 1–24.
37. Van Stone JC. Hemodialysis apparatus. In Daugirdas JT, Ing TS (eds). Handbook of Dialysis. Boston, Little, Brown and Company, 1988, pp 21–39.
38. Schetz M, Lauwers PM, Ferdinande P. Extracorporeal treatment of acute renal failure in the intensive care unit: A critical view. Intensive Care Med 15:349–357, 1989.
39. Dickson DM, Hillman KM. Continuous renal replacement in the critically ill. Anaesth Intensive Care 18:76–92, 1990.
40. Sorkin MI. Apparatus for peritoneal dialysis. In Daugirdas JT, Ing TS (eds). Handbook of Dialysis. Boston, Little, Brown and Company, 1988, pp 182–193.

33

◘

Trauma

Michael Rhodes, M.D., F.A.C.S., F.C.C.M.

This chapter reviews current principles of trauma management, with a specific emphasis on respiratory care of the injured patient. Because trauma care is a continuum, examining the epidemiology, prehospital care, resuscitation, surgery, critical care, specific injuries, and outcome is appropriate.

EPIDEMIOLOGY

Trauma is the fourth leading cause of death in the United States. More than 140,000 deaths and 340,000 permanent disabilities occur annually, with an estimated cost of $180 billion.[1, 2] Eighty per cent of injuries result from blunt mechanisms (e.g., motor vehicle accidents and falls), whereas 20% result from penetrating mechanisms, such as gunshot wounds and stabbings. In many major cities, penetrating trauma predominates as a result of increasing urban violence.[3, 4] Head injury, the leading cause of death from trauma (followed by hemorrhage and sepsis), is also the leading cause of disability, followed by injuries to the extremities, spine, and chest.[5, 6]

Trauma deaths occur in a trimodal distribution over time.[7] Immediate deaths occur from lethal head injury, transected major vessel injury, and high cervical cord injury. The only effective treatment for these injuries is taking preventive measures, such as using seat belts, airbags, and helmets; instituting gun control and drunk driving laws; and so forth. Early trauma deaths occurring within the first few hours of injury have been the primary focus for trauma system development. Treatable intracranial hematoma, tension pneumothorax, and intra-abdominal hemorrhage from visceral injury are examples of injuries leading to potentially preventable early deaths. Late deaths occur days to weeks after injury as a result of sepsis and multiple-organ dysfunction syndrome. Ironically, the advances in trauma systems, with rapid transport and early definitive care, have increased the number of patients in this latter category by preventing early deaths. Many patients who would have died within hours after injury 20 years ago are now surviving longer, only to develop organ failure later. As a result, increased effort has been placed into research and strategies to prevent these late deaths in the intensive care unit (ICU).[8]

Although the majority of traumatic injuries occur in persons between 15 and 45 years of age, 25% of traumatic injuries occur in patients older than 65 years of age, a group with twice the length of hospital stay and mortality of the younger group.[9] Furthermore, future projections suggest that the older group will increase dramatically over the next decade, a fact that will have a major impact on critical care units in the United States.[10]

PREHOSPITAL CARE

To identify patients who may require trauma center care, the American College of Surgeons' Committee on Trauma has published field triage criteria based on age, vital signs, anatomic findings, and mechanism of injury (Fig. 33–1).[11] Studies show that the use of these criteria results in an overtriage rate of 50% in order to maintain an undertriage rate of less than 10%.[12] Similar criteria have been developed for the interhospital transfer of patients to a trauma center.[11]

Most prehospital care is rendered by fire, rescue, and ambulance personnel, who provide basic life support skills. Basic life support training provides emergency medical technicians with the skills for noninva-

TRIAGE DECISION SCHEME

| Measure vital signs and level of consciousness |

Step I

Glascow Coma Score	< 13 or
Systolic Blood Pressure	< 90 or
Respiratory Rate	< 10 or > 29 or
Revised Trauma Score	< 11
Pediatric Trauma Score	< 9

YES → Take to trauma center

NO → Assess anatomy of injury

Step II

- All penetrating injuries to head, neck, torso, and extremities proximal to elbow and knee
- Flail chest
- Combination trauma with burns of 10% or inhalation injuries
- Two or more proximal long-bone fractures
- Pelvic fractures
- Limb paralysis
- Amputation proximal to wrist and ankle

YES → Take to trauma center

NO → Evaluate for evidence of mechanism of injury and high-energy impact

Step III

- Ejection from automobile
- Death in same passenger compartment
- Extrication time > 20 minutes
- Falls > 20 feet
- Roll-over

- High-speed auto crash
  - Initial speed > 40 mph
  - Velocity change > 20 mph
  - Major auto deformity > 20 inches
  - Intrusion into passenger compartment > 12 inches

- Auto-pedestrian injury with significant (>5 mph) impact
- Pedestrian thrown or run over
- Motorcycle crash > 20 mph or with separation of rider and bike

YES → Take to trauma center

NO →

Step IV

- Age < 5 to > 55 years
- Known cardiac disease; respiratory disease; or psychotics taking medication
- Diabetics taking insulin; cirrhosis; malignancy; obesity or coagulopathy

YES → Contact medical control and consider transport to trauma center

NO → Re-evaluate with medical control

WHEN IN DOUBT TAKE TO A TRAUMA CENTER

FIGURE 33–1: Field triage criteria for trauma patients. (Adapted from the Committee on Trauma, American College of Surgeons. Resources for Optimal Care of the Injured Patient. Chicago, American College of Surgeons, 1990.)

sive airway management, splinting, immobilization, external hemorrhage control, and oxygen therapy. Many areas in the United States have the advantage of advanced life support training in the prehospital environment. Advanced life support training provides paramedics with the skills for endotracheal intubation, intravenous fluid administration, and other therapeutic interventions. The ability to perform prehospital orotracheal and nasotracheal intubation has clearly had an impact on patient outcome, especially for head-injured patients.[13] The esophageal obturator airway has been largely abandoned in prehospital trauma care because of its ineffectiveness and high complication rate. However, if a patient arrives with an esophageal obturator airway in place, the patient should undergo orotracheal intubation before removal of the esophageal obturator airway to avoid profound aspiration. A modification of the esophageal obturator airway to limit these complications has been developed, but it has not been given wide clinical trial to date.

Prehospital intravenous fluid administration has been challenged as unnecessary and ineffective if the transport time is less than 20 minutes.[14] One study has suggested that intravenous therapy be withheld from victims of penetrating torso trauma until immediate definitive surgery is available.[15] This suggestion is based on the theory that intravenous volume will increase the blood pressure and exacerbate uncontrolled hemorrhage. However, if it does not delay transport, most field trauma protocols promote intravenous fluid therapy using a large-bore catheter (16 gauge or larger in adults) through which up to 2 L of crystalloid may be infused.

The pneumatic antishock garment (sometimes referred to as military antishock trousers), a compressive device, encircles the legs and abdomen for the purpose of combatting shock and hemorrhage. The pneumatic antishock garment has been the subject of much controversy because it has not been shown to alter outcome in patients with brief transport times.[16] In addition, the garment can potentially compromise pulmonary function in conditions such as a ruptured diaphragm, in which the intra-abdominal viscera may further herniate into the chest.[17] However, the garment still appears to have utility in victims of blunt trauma who have prolonged transport times, particularly in patients with pelvic or extremity fractures and shock.[18, 19]

Prehospital transtracheal ventilation, chest decompression, and chemical paralysis for patient control have been successfully used in some areas.[20–24] The use of transtracheal ventilation with a catheter is somewhat limited in the trauma patient because of the frequent presence of foreign bodies, vomitus, and blood and because of carbon dioxide retention. The use of pulse oximetry and carbon dioxide detectors has improved the monitoring of trauma patients in the field.[25–27]

The administration of solutions in the field, such as hypertonic saline and blood, is currently under trial.[28, 29] The main theoretical advantage of hypertonic saline administration in the field is to restore blood volume rapidly without worsening brain edema.[30, 31] The development of oxygen-carrying blood substitutes has been slow,[32] but this may become clinically feasible in the field within the next decade.

Aeromedical transport now plays a major role in trauma care. Throughout the United States, more than 50,000 trauma victims were transported by helicopter in 1989. Multiple studies demonstrate outcome advantages of air versus ground transport for certain patients; these advantages are mostly attributed to the skill of the flight crew, which may consist of physicians, paramedics, nurses, and respiratory therapists.[33, 34] Most investigators note that the skill of the flight crew is more important to patient outcome than the speed or size of the aircraft.[35]

A communication system must be in place to allow integration of the prehospital and in-hospital phases of trauma care. Field protocols and strong medical control are essential. A "trauma alert" system, used in many trauma centers, gathers the appropriate personnel as part of a resuscitation team before the patient's arrival. This prearrival notification allows for equipment checks (e.g., of airway equipment) and provides assignments to the appropriate personnel. The arrival of the trauma patient should be anticipated so that it is not perceived as disruptive to the hospital.

RESUSCITATION

Although early resuscitation starts in the field, formal resuscitation begins in the emergency department. Here, a team must be available that has the resources to provide life-saving measures using a well-rehearsed protocol. Even in nontrauma centers, a protocol should be in place that uses the principles developed by the American College of Surgeons' Committee on Trauma Advanced Trauma Life Support course for early stabilization and transport to a trauma center.

Airway

Early control of the airway remains the highest priority. In trauma patients, endotracheal intubation is indicated not only in patients who have airway obstruction and ventilatory failure but also in patients who do not follow commands or who have an obvious need for operative intervention (multiple open fractures, distended abdomen, or massive hemothorax).[36] It is no longer acceptable to delay intubation until ventilatory failure has become clinically obvious.

In order to provide appropriate airway management, adequate equipment must be available before the patient's arrival. Large-bore suction devices, adequate light, a pulse oximeter, carbon dioxide detectors, a volume-cycled ventilator, and protocols for intubation must be in place. The route of intubation depends on the preference of the person charged with the responsibility. In the breathing patient, the nasotracheal route is acceptable for airway management, especially for the less skilled intubator. This technique can usually be performed without neck extension, but on occasion it can be a traumatic event. Mild sedation, the use of local anesthetic spray, and lubrication are useful adjuncts for this route. The optimal route of intubation for trauma is the orotracheal route because it provides a larger, more permanent airway.

Emergent orotracheal intubation can be performed safely, even in the absence of normal findings on a lateral cervical spine x-ray study. An assistant must provide in-line cervical immobilization from below. Awake orotracheal intubation can be accomplished, but the preferred method is rapid-sequence induction using sedation and chemical paralysis. This technique is potentially useful in the combative head-injured patient because a struggling patient is at risk for exacerbating elevated intracranial pressure.

In essence, the patient in need of emergent intubation should be

The disadvantages of nasotracheal intubation include nasopharyngeal trauma and the placement of a small tube that may require subsequent change to a larger, orotracheal tube.

afforded all the resources available to the patient undergoing elective intubation. Chemical control of the patient allows a much smoother and efficient resuscitation.[37, 38] This requires a resuscitation area that is prepared with appropriate personnel and equipment before the patient's arrival. Appropriate knowledge of sedative and chemical paralyzing agents is essential.[39]

The use of a transtracheal needle catheter has been described for emergent airway management.[40] However, as noted previously, this technique may be of limited value in the trauma patient with vomitus and blood in the trachea. At best, this temporary catheter should be replaced with a definitive airway. Surgical cricothyroidotomy remains a valuable adjunct, especially in the patient with massive facial fractures, but it is infrequently required with modern intubation techniques.[41] A key to successful cricothyroidotomy is the availability of a scalpel and a 4- or 5-mm tracheostomy tube. A small endotracheal tube may be used as an alternative. Newer acute percutaneous techniques are available but have not been given wide clinical trial in the trauma patient.[42]

Checking the position of the endotracheal tube is paramount. Auscultation is important but not foolproof. The use of various portable carbon dioxide detectors now available should be part of the routine technique in emergent intubation for trauma. On occasion, the use of oral endotracheal intubation may promote the entrance of the endotracheal tube into the right mainstem bronchus, which mimics a left pneumothorax and prompts the placement of a tube into the left side of the chest. Because this is particularly true in children, this problem should be suspected in the almost total absence of left-sided breath sounds after intubation.

Other valuable adjuncts to airway control include frequent suctioning, jaw thrust, and oropharyngeal and nasopharyngeal airway placement. However, in the severely injured trauma patient, these temporizing procedures, with few exceptions, should be followed by endotracheal intubation.

> Cricothyroidotomy is contraindicated in small children: because of its small size and fragility, the trachea tends to tear, causing improper placement and permanent damage.

> When possible, all patients should receive preintubation oxygenation with a bag mask.

Ventilation

Clinical assessment of the chest after trauma is frequently rewarding. Observation for neck vein distention, splinting, flail, ecchymosis, and penetrating wounds should occur first. A flail may not be immediately visible in spontaneously breathing patients until there is a decrease in lung compliance from the underlying parenchymal contusion or adult respiratory distress syndrome. A flail is rarely visible in a mechanically ventilated patient. Anterior and lateral flails are much more apparent than posterior flail. Inspiratory stridor suggests upper airway obstruction (tongue, fractured mandible, neck hematoma, or foreign body), whereas expiratory stridor suggests lower airway compromise (chest wall injury, pneumothorax, pulmonary contusion, or ruptured diaphragm). Palpation for crepitus or pain can reveal rib fractures or pneumothorax. Auscultation can reveal decreased or absent breath sounds.

Patients requiring intubation should receive positive pressure ventilation, initially by bag and then by volume-cycled ventilator. In the patient with suspected head injury, early hyperventilation to a Pa_{CO_2} tube between 25 and 30 mm Hg may be helpful, although prolonged hyperventilation has not been shown to alter outcome.[43] In the hemodynamically stable patient without pulmonary injury causing increased dead space, capnometry may be used to titrate minute ventilation rapidly to a PET_{CO_2} of 22 to 26 mm Hg, assuming a normal Pa_{CO_2}-PET_{CO_2} gradient of 3 to 5 mm Hg. An FI_{O_2} of 100% and a positive end-expiratory pressure (PEEP) of 5 cm H_2O should be used empirically during early resuscitation in acutely traumatized patients. Further increases in PEEP may become necessary to oxygenate the patient with significant pulmonary contusion, which is frequently manifested by hypoxia and bloody endotracheal secretions. However, intravascular volume must be restored before PEEP is increased above 5 cm H_2O.

Ventilatory insufficiency may result from a decreased respiratory drive, as seen in severe head injury, or from mechanical failure, as seen in flail chest, pulmonary contusion, or pneumothorax. In addition to the provision of positive pressure ventilation, pleural decompression with a needle or chest tube may be required to remove air and blood.

In theory, a radiograph demonstrating a tension pneumothorax should rarely be seen because tension pneumothorax is usually a clinical diagnosis requiring immediate decompression without the need for a prior x-ray study. A patient presenting with hypotension, unilateral decreased breath sounds, and neck vein distention should have immediate needle chest decompression through the anterior second intercostal space, followed by the placement of a chest tube. A chest tube placed for the removal of either air, blood, or both should be large bore (36 or 40 Fr in the adult) and should be placed in the fifth intercostal space in the midaxillary line. Smaller tubes may clog and malfunction. The fifth intercostal space is used to avoid injuring the diaphragm or the abdominal viscera. The midaxillary line is used to facilitate dissection, avoiding the pectoralis and latissimus dorsi muscles. The pleural cavity can be inspected by the index finger before chest tube placement. A lacerated diaphragm may occasionally be detected with the finger. A sudden increase in peak airway pressures during resuscitation of the intubated trauma patient may signal the need for a chest tube if ventilator dysfunction and endotracheal tube dysfunction have been ruled out.

After a chest tube has been inserted, it should be placed to underwater seal and to suction at 20 cm H_2O. Thoracotomy may be indicated if more than 1 L of blood is suddenly evacuated or if, after the initial evacuation, bleeding continues at a rate of more than 200 mL/hr for 2 hours. However, 85% of chest injuries with hemothorax can be treated nonoperatively with placement of a large-bore chest tube. Most intrathoracic bleeding in trauma patients is from the parenchyma of the lung, which has a mean arterial pressure of 15 mm Hg. The 20-cm H_2O suction (equal to 15 mm Hg) causes tamponade of the bleeding lung by apposing the bleeding lung surface to the parietal pleura.

Chest tubes with trocars should be avoided in the acutely traumatized patient because of the potential for iatrogenic injury.

Circulation

To assess circulation, the pulse, blood pressure, skin color, level of consciousness, capillary refill, and evidence of external hemorrhage are measured. This may be helpful in predicting blood loss in the non–head-injured patient and in the nonelderly patient. However, normal assessment findings in the head-injured or elderly patient may be misleading, and an index of suspicion must be proportional to the mechanism of injury.

For adults, the placement of two large-bore (16- or 14-gauge) peripheral intravenous catheters, through which up to 2 L of warm crystalloid solution should be infused as a fluid challenge, is preferred. The speed of fluid administration is governed by Poiseuille's law (Fig. 33–2). This law of fluid flow through a cylinder suggests that warmed dilute fluid should be administered under pressure through a short, fat catheter. The radius of the catheter is the most important determinant of flow. Diluting packed red blood cells with warm saline will reduce viscosity and thereby increase flow.

Patients with hypotension whose conditions remain unstable may require blood replacement. For major hemorrhage, peripheral or central rapid-infusion catheters, together with a rapid-infusion pump device, can deliver warm fluid and blood at rates of up to 2 L/min.[44] The ultimate stability of the circulation may require exploratory laparotomy, pericardiocentesis, pelvic fixation, arterial embolization, thoracotomy, or correction of coagulopathy.

Overzealous fluid administration may precipitate acute pulmonary edema, high airway pressures, and frothy bloody secretions.

Monitoring

Ongoing assessment of the airway, ventilation, and circulation and of the effects of therapeutic intervention is essential in trauma management. A neurologic assessment can be performed by quantifying the patient's level of consciousness. A simplified technique is the AVPU method advocated in the Advanced Trauma Life Support course.[45] Subsequently, the more defined Glasgow Coma Scale is used for neurologic assessment.

Blood is sampled on admission for a complete blood count, determination of electrolyte and amylase levels, blood typing, and measurement of the alcohol level, if indicated. Continuous electrocardiographic monitoring and arterial blood gas analysis are performed. Pulse oximetry is a marvelous, noninvasive technology for measuring the oxygen saturation of arterial blood. This widely used tool is useful in virtually all phases of trauma care monitoring. Several precautions should be noted in the trauma patient. Because this technology is dependent on digital perfusion, any systemic or extremity hypoperfusion or traumatic ischemia to a limb will lead to false readings. This presents obvious limitations for its use in the patient in shock. In addition, dark skin, jaundice, and carboxyhemoglobin create artifactual readings. However, in most trauma situations, once the circulation has been restored, pulse oximetry is a valuable adjunct to trauma patient monitoring.

A nasogastric tube is placed unless the patient has severe midface

With the AVPU method, the patient is determined to be awake (A), responsive to verbal stimulation (V), responsive to painful stimulation (P), or unresponsive to pain (U).

$$Q = \pi\, r^4\, \frac{\Delta P}{8\eta L}, \text{ where}$$

Q = flow through a catheter

r = radius,

ΔP = change in pressure,

η = viscosity of fluid, and

L = length of catheter

FIGURE 33–2: Poiseuille's law governing the flow of liquid through a cylinder.

fractures, in which case the orogastric route is preferred. In the presence of midface fractures, a nasogastric tube may inadvertently be placed through fractured ethmoid sinuses into the brain. A method of preventing intracranial intubation in midface fracture is to first place a nasopharyngeal trumpet through which a nasogastric tube may be safely placed.[46] The placement of the nasogastric tube is checked by auscultation, and the tube is then irrigated to ensure patency. In the unstable patient, the nasogastric tube is placed after endotracheal intubation, using cricoid pressure against the esophageal opening (Sellick's maneuver) to avoid aspiration. Decompression of the stomach is particularly important in young children, who have a tendency to swallow large amounts of air, which results in abdominal distention.

A urinary catheter is placed unless gross blood presents at the urethra in the male patient. In this case, a urethrogram is necessary to rule out a ruptured urethra. If no gross blood is present at the urethra, a urethral catheter is placed, and urine is checked with a dipstick for the presence of blood. Urinalysis for blood is no longer necessary with clear urine.[47]

In the unstable patient, the placement of an arterial catheter for frequent sampling of arterial blood gases and continuous pressure monitoring helps in evaluating the patient. In the more stable patient, a noninvasive continuous blood pressure monitoring device (e.g., a Dinamap monitor) may be useful. Urinary output and central venous pressure measurements are of limited value in the first hour of resuscitation. However, the elderly patient may benefit from a pulmonary artery catheter early in resuscitation, as has been demonstrated in one study.[48]

Continuous electrocardiographic monitoring and pulse oximetry should continue during patient transfer to the operating room, ICU, or x-ray department. Patient transport ventilators are superior to manual bag ventilation, particularly in the management of acutely head-injured patients.[49]

DIAGNOSTIC IMAGING

Radiologic priorities in the patient with blunt trauma include lateral cervical spine, chest, and pelvic x-ray studies, although the need for the routine lateral cervical spine films has been questioned.[50, 51] The chest radiography technique is important. Most radiographs obtained with portable equipment are taken at a distance of 3 feet, with the patient in the supine position, and may result in an ill-defined or magnified mediastinum. This makes it difficult to rule out a torn thoracic aorta, especially in thick-chested large male patients. Providing a 5-foot distance from camera to cassette, either by using built-in x-ray equipment or by sitting the patient in the erect position, may help to define the mediastinum. In addition, the provision of a breath hold at end-inspiration by the respiratory therapist in the intubated patient may significantly reduce motion artifact.

After these priority films have been obtained, tests to determine occult intra-abdominal injury may be necessary, especially in the obtunded patient with unreliable physical examination findings. Controversy exists about the use of diagnostic peritoneal lavage versus abdominal computed tomography (CT) in detecting intra-abdominal injury.[52–55] Actually, these tests should be used in a complementary fashion (Fig. 33–3). Patients with unstable conditions and patients with obvious op-

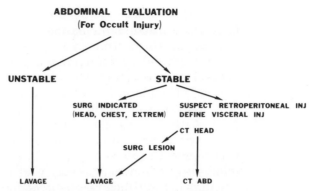

ABDOMINAL   EVALUATION
(For Occult Injury)

UNSTABLE

STABLE

SURG INDICATED
(HEAD, CHEST, EXTREM)

SUSPECT RETROPERITONEAL INJ
DEFINE VISCERAL INJ

CT HEAD

SURG LESION

LAVAGE

LAVAGE

CT ABD

FIGURE 33–3: Algorithm for detection of occult abdominal injury.

erative indications should have diagnostic peritoneal lavage and avoid CT. However, stable patients requiring head CT are ideal candidates for abdominal CT. The major concern with abdominal CT is the occasional missed hollow-viscus injury.[56, 57] Several centers successfully use ultrasonography for acute evaluation of the abdomen.[58–60] Laparoscopy for acute trauma is emerging.[61] After the abdominal evaluation, other imaging studies, such as extremity x-ray studies, CT head scans, and so forth, can be obtained.

SURGERY

The operating phase of trauma care requires that the resuscitation begun in the emergency department continue in the operating room. This is particularly important in the unstable patient. In many trauma centers, the respiratory therapist, as part of the resuscitation team, accompanies the patient into the operating room. In the seriously traumatized patient with pulmonary compromise, the ventilatory requirements of the patient may exceed the capabilities of most anesthesia machines, and a high-capacity ventilator may be needed through the operative phase. Intravenous narcotic anesthesia is frequently substituted for anesthetic gases in these patients.

Several aspects of operative trauma care deserve special comment. The unstable patient requiring massive blood and fluid transfusion may develop pulmonary edema, decreased pulmonary compliance, and high peak and mean airway pressures, especially if associated pulmonary contusions, coagulopathy, or both are present. Frequent suctioning and early application of PEEP may be required. Heating the ventilated air effectively prevents hypothermia, as does infusing warm fluids and covering the patient with insulating materials.

Performing arterial blood gas analysis as frequently as every 15 minutes may be necessary for the optimal assessment of ventilation, oxygenation, and control of acidosis in patients requiring massive resuscitation. The blood hematocrit, as well as the serum ionized calcium and potassium levels, should also be frequently measured. Portable tableside analyzers using small quantities of blood are now available for frequent measurements of hemoglobin, electrolyte, and blood gas levels, thereby eliminating the need for sending specimens to the laboratory.[62] Inline continuous measurement of these parameters is currently being introduced.[63, 64]

Another principle of operative trauma surgery is to correct as many problems as possible during the first surgery.[65, 66] Immediate and early fracture fixation exemplifies this principle. Significant reductions in morbidity, mortality, and hospital stay have been realized with immediate and early fixation of fractures.[67] In the polytraumatized patient, this may require up to 8 to 12 hours of surgery using several teams, with ongoing resuscitation and critical monitoring in the operating room.

Patients who require massive resuscitation as well as a laparotomy may develop massive tissue edema, particularly of the bowel and mesentery. Although this may prohibit closing of the abdomen, it is now not uncommon to leave the abdomen open and to perform closure at a later time.[68] This may be of great benefit in the ventilatory management of the noncompliant lung.

Certain trauma centers are bypassing the emergency department and admitting patients directly to the operating room for resuscitation. Studies have shown a reduction in mortality for certain types of patients.[69, 70] Respiratory therapists are part of the resuscitation team in most of these centers.

CRITICAL CARE

The critical care phase of trauma care is the most complex and resource consumptive.[71] In this phase, attention to providing optimal organ support is paramount. The goals of critical care management of the trauma victim are outlined in Table 33–1. This care must be provided by a team of professionals dedicated to the care of the critically ill, with constant attention at the bedside. Team members include physicians, nurses, respiratory therapists, nutritionists, clinical pharmacists, physical therapists, and psychologists.

Oxygen Transport

The major goal of critical care therapy is to provide optimal oxygen transport to the tissues. This means that oxygen delivery must be provided so that oxygen consumption is less than one third of the delivery and so that consumption does not rise when delivery increases (e.g., a non–flow-dependent oxygen consumption must be maintained) (Fig. 33–4). To reach this goal of optimal therapy, oxygen delivery may be augmented or oxygen consumption may be modified.[72]

Oxygen delivery may be increased by increasing any or all of three factors: arterial oxygen saturation, hemoglobin level, and cardiac output (Fig. 33–5). The hemoglobin level is optimal at approximately 10 g/dL unless the patient with a fixed cardiac output is stressed, such as the elderly trauma patient. In these patients, a hemoglobin level in the range

The arterial oxygen saturation should be maintained at greater than 90%, preferably at about 95%, by optimizing ventilatory management.

TABLE **33–1:** Goals of Critical Care Management

Optimize oxygen delivery
Prevent infection
Relieve pain, anxiety, and delirium
Provide adequate nutrition
Modify systemic inflammatory responses
Prevent complications
Promote cost-effective resource use

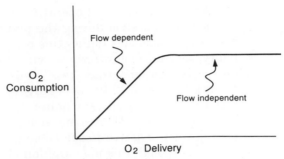

FIGURE 33–4: Conceptual oxygen consumption-delivery curve.

$S\bar{v}_{O_2}$ values of between 65 and 75% are considered normal but do not exclude abnormal oxygen transport.

of 12 to 13 g/dL may be necessary to maintain adequate oxygen delivery.[73] Cardiac output is usually optimized intrinsically in most trauma patients by virtue of the hormonal and endocrine response to trauma, whereby cardiac output improves through increases in stroke volume, rate, or both. However, in certain patients, such as septic or elderly patients with intrinsic coronary artery disease, this response is limited. In these situations, volume loading coupled with inotropic or vasodilatory support (or both) is used to optimize cardiac output.

Reducing an elevated oxygen consumption may be helpful in maintaining an adequate extraction ratio of less than 30% (Fig. 33–6). The most important step is to treat the underlying problem, such as sepsis, shock, or fever. Another approach is to reduce the metabolic demand through controlled ventilation using sedation, chemical paralysis, or both.

The presence of a pulmonary artery catheter is necessary to carry out this level of therapy because it allows frequent manipulation of both hemodynamic and oxygenation variables. The mixed venous oxygen saturation ($S\bar{v}_{O_2}$), which can be measured continuously by specific catheters, correlates with the oxygen extraction ratio, which is a useful indicator of global metabolic well-being in most circumstances (Fig. 33–7). However, because $S\bar{v}_{O_2}$ does not correlate with oxygen delivery or oxygen consumption, an abnormal $S\bar{v}_{O_2}$ requires measurement of these variables to diagnose and treat abnormal oxygen transport correctly. There is debate over the cost-effectiveness of continuous $S\bar{v}_{O_2}$ monitoring compared with fre-

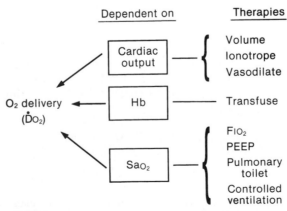

FIGURE 33–5: Determinants and therapies for oxygen delivery. Hb, hemoglobin.

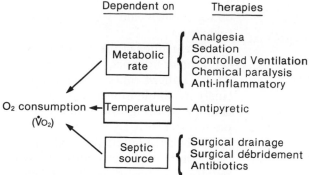

FIGURE 33–6: Determinants and therapies for oxygen consumption.

quent arterial blood gas measurement.[63, 74–76] Clinical judgment and unit protocols are necessary to use this resource appropriately.

Ventilatory Support

Ventilatory management of the trauma patient in the ICU requires precise tailoring to the patient and his or her injuries. A variety of modes are available, and clearly more than one method can be applied successfully. The hyperdynamic trauma patient or the patient with a severe head injury and suspected increased intracranial pressure usually requires controlled ventilatory support. This may reduce oxygen consumption while possibly alleviating the effects of motion and coughing on intracranial pressure. Controlled ventilation requires adequate sedation, chemical paralysis, or both, with absolute familiarity with these agents by the treating team. Good pulmonary toilet incorporating kinetic bed therapy may be necessary. Rigorous attention to ventilatory alarms and airway pressure monitors is crucial.

To avoid the use of high peak airway pressures (>40 cm H_2O), volume ventilation with high rates and low tidal volumes may be necessary. In addition, inverse ratio ventilation, with or without permissive hypercapnia, may also be a useful strategy. Less hyperdynamic trauma patients can be managed with assisted-controlled or synchronized intermittent mandatory ventilation mode ventilation. Weaning modes are numerous, and the use of pressure support ventilation and continuous positive airway pressure have gained popularity.[77] Weaning from ventilatory support should not be confused with extubation. Extubation of a trauma patient requires that the patient have a satisfactory cough, have

$$\text{Extraction ratio (ER)} = \frac{O_2 \text{ consumption } (\dot{V}O_2)}{O_2 \text{ delivery } (\dot{D}O_2)} = 25\%$$

$S\bar{v}_{O_2}$ correlates with ER

$S\bar{v}_{O_2}$ does not correlate with $\dot{V}O_2$ or $\dot{D}O_2$

FIGURE 33–7: Correlation of mixed venous oxygen saturation ($S\bar{v}_{O_2}$) with extraction ratio.

a patent airway, and be able to follow commands. A detailed discussion of ventilatory and weaning techniques is contained elsewhere in this text.

Techniques of precise pain, anxiety, and delirium management have been major advances in trauma patient ventilatory management (Table 33–2). Patient-controlled analgesia and epidural opioids should be routinely available in a trauma ICU. These techniques have facilitated ventilatory weaning and reduced the length of stay and the incidence of pneumonia in ICUs.[78]

Providing pulmonary toilet and pulmonary physiotherapy is of major importance in the traumatized patient. Incentive spirometry is also quite helpful in the unintubated patient. Intermittent positive pressure breathing is useful in delivering a bronchotherapeutic agent when the patient cannot take deep breaths on his or her own. The essence of promoting coughing and deep breathing is adequate analgesia and sedation. However, supplemental techniques to promote cough in the trauma patient also help, including the use of nasotracheal suctioning. This technique, sometimes referred to as "snaking," is performed by placing a soft catheter through the nose and intermittently entering the trachea, it is hoped with the patient's cooperation. Nasotracheal suctioning should not be used on a frequent basis because of discomfort and nasopharyngeal trauma to the patient. The placement of a well-lubricated nasopharyngeal trumpet through which the catheter is placed can sometimes reduce the soft tissue trauma.

Another technique for promoting coughing is placing a transtracheal catheter (cough tube) through which either saline or water can be instilled. A small catheter (e.g., an 18-gauge Intracath catheter), which is easily introduced through the cricothyroid membrane, is secured in place for 24 to 48 hours. In some patients, 1 to 3 mL of saline solution is effective, whereas sterile water may be more effective in promoting cough for others.

Postural drainage and percussion may effectively promote the drainage of secretions and assist in the coughing mechanism. Although the mechanical percussors are somewhat less labor intensive, the appropriately cupped hand in the well-trained percussionist is probably superior. These techniques are appropriate in a patient with either a normal airway or an artificial airway.

Flexible bronchoscopy in the ICU setting for traumatized patients is thought to be useful in the precise diagnosis of pneumonia; however, its utility in promoting bronchopulmonary toilet is controversial.[79] It is effective in diagnosing bronchial injuries and in clearing secretions to treat atelectasis. However, many trauma surgeons believe that this modality is overused to treat atelectasis because the techniques of snaking, cough

TABLE **33–2:** Techniques and Drugs for Relieving Pain, Anxiety, and Delirium

Reassurance	Morphine and fentanyl administration
Sedation	Intravenous bolus
Diazepam (Valium)	Intravenous continuous drip
Lorazepam (Ativan)	Patient controlled
Midazolam (Versed)	Transdermal
Propofol (Diprivan)	Epidural analgesia
Neurolepsis	Morphine
Haloperidol	Fentanyl
	Bolus
	Drip
	Intercostal nerve block

tube placement, postural drainage, and percussion, if used early and aggressively, could eliminate the need for most toilet bronchoscopies.

Tracheostomy Versus Prolonged Endotracheal Intubation

The complication rates from both tracheostomy and prolonged endotracheal intubation have been markedly reduced since 1975 because of the many advances in ventilatory management, particularly the development of high-volume, low-pressure cuffs. Therefore, most references to studies including patients treated before 1975 are irrelevant to today's critical care management. Secondly, patients with a tracheostomy can frequently be discharged from the ICU, whereas this is unlikely in patients with an endotracheal tube in place.[80, 81]

Evidence indicates that the patient with a rigid head injury (e.g., posturing of the upper or lower extremities) is a candidate for early tracheostomy.[82] Although patients can be managed by endotracheal tube for up to 3 weeks, studies have suggested that patients who are going to require a tracheostomy should have it done early when possible (i.e., within the first week).[83, 84] Nonemergent percutaneous tracheostomy has been shown to be a safe and effective bedside technique in the ICU.[85, 86] The respiratory therapist must constantly monitor airway pressure, tidal volume, and pulse oximetry during this procedure. End-tidal carbon dioxide monitoring is recommended to aid in the confirmation of proper placement.

Nutrition

The provision of adequate nutrition affects the respiratory aspects of trauma patient management (Table 33–3). Early nutritional support aids in ablating the hyperdynamic response of trauma and in speeding up the return of muscle function. Close monitoring helps to avoid overfeeding with carbohydrates. Carbohydrates may cause respiratory failure due to excess carbon dioxide production. Indirect calorimetry using a metabolic cart has been shown to be helpful in determining the respiratory quotient, oxygen consumption, and basal energy expenditure and in predicting a formula for more precise metabolic support.[87] A nutritional support team can be useful in calculating the daily requirements and in suggesting the appropriate formula.

Studies have suggested that postpyloric enteral feeding, especially when the feed is enriched with glutamine and arginine, results in lower morbidity than does total parenteral nutrition.[88, 89] In general, most clinicians believe that nasogastric tubes promote aspiration by interfering with gastroesophageal sphincter function and by providing a track for the migration of bacteria from the stomach to the pharynx, after which they may eventually find their way into the trachea. Smaller feeding tubes have been developed to obviate this risk.

TABLE **33–3:** Principles of Providing Adequate Nutrition

Early enteral feeding
Avoidance of overfeeding
Indirect calorimetry
Nutritional support team

Although feeding into the stomach is physiologically sound, this may increase the risk of regurgitation with aspiration, particularly in the supine patient receiving positive pressure ventilation. Therefore, placing the feeding tube beyond the pylorus by endoscopy or fluoroscopy has been advocated to reduce the risk of a full stomach. However, placing food in the duodenum, bypassing the stomach, may release hormones that lead to gastric stasis and hypoacidity with resultant bacterial overgrowth, theoretically increasing the risk of pneumonia from persistent microaspiration. Feeding into the proximal jejunum beyond the ligament of Treitz is probably the best option for the multiply injured supine patient on a ventilator, but this option usually requires a surgical procedure.

In the severely traumatized patient, especially the patient with a significant head injury, early oropharyngeal decontamination by removing tubes from the airway may be advantageous. Percutaneous endoscopic gastrostomy and percutaneous tracheostomy, which can be performed at the bedside, are effective techniques for removing these tubes from the oropharynx and for providing airway protection and nutritional support while reducing the incidence of sinusitis, pharyngeal ulceration, and pneumonia.[90] These techniques allow for more effective oral hygiene.

Additional Strategies

Efforts to prevent infection in the ICU are multifaceted (Table 33–4). Antibiotic therapy in a trauma patient is complex in the critical care unit. Strict protocol management is essential to prevent nosocomial pneumonia and antibiotic-associated diarrhea. Stress prophylaxis with sucralfate (which does not reduce gastric acid) to prevent stress ulceration of the stomach has been suggested to reduce the incidence of pneumonia compared with the use of H_2 blockers and antacids.[91, 92]

Renal function is best maintained by providing adequate urinary output (more than 50 mL/hr) and maintaining optimal oxygen transport. Avoidance of nephrotoxic drugs and dyes can reduce renal failure. Low-dose dopamine is thought to be useful in optimizing renal function in a compromised patient.[93]

Decreasing the incidence of deep venous thrombosis and pulmonary embolism has been accomplished by early patient mobilization and early use of sequential compression boots. Other therapeutic endeavors, such as the administration of low-dose heparin and low-dose warfarin, continue to be studied but thus far have not been definitely proved effective in trauma patients. Prophylactic vena caval filters for high-risk patients are currently under trial.

SPECIFIC INJURIES

Head Injury

The goals of early head injury management are early airway control, identification of a surgical lesion, and avoidance of worsening cerebral

TABLE **33–4:** Potential Strategies for Preventing Infection in the Trauma Patient

Hand washing	Stress prophylaxis
Dress code	Sucralfate
Clinical management protocols	Selective gut decontamination
Line changes	Early enteral feeding
Antibiotic use	

edema and intracranial pressure. Even transient hypoxia in these injuries may promote a "secondary brain injury," which may be more deleterious than the original trauma. Most patients suffering head injury have diffuse, nonsurgical lesions, and primary therapy is aimed at controlling intracranial pressure. In patients with severe head injury (Glasgow Coma Scale score of less than 8), controlled ventilation is required and is frequently combined with chemical paralysis, mannitol administration, hyperventilation, and on occasion, barbiturate coma. Intracranial pressure monitoring is now readily available by placing a catheter either in the subdural space or in the cerebral ventricle. An intracranial pressure of greater than 20 mm Hg usually requires treatment. A more precise measurement of brain perfusion is the calculated cerebral perfusion pressure, which is the mean arterial pressure minus the intracranial pressure. The calculated cerebral perfusion pressure should be greater than 60 mm Hg.

Cerebral perfusion pressures lower than 50 mm Hg are accompanied by a poor prognosis.

The traditional approach of hyperventilation to lower intracranial pressure has been shown to be effective. The classic range to strive for is a P_{CO_2} between 25 and 30 mm Hg. This causes cerebrovasoconstriction, reducing the cerebral blood volume and thereby lowering the intracranial pressure. Most investigators agree that this effect may not last beyond 24 to 48 hours. There is also concern that although the intracranial pressure may be lowered, the tradeoff of the vasoconstriction may actually cause ischemia to injured portions of the brain. Therefore, cerebral blood flow monitors, along with jugular bulb venous oxygen saturation catheters, are being used in some centers to help add precision to therapeutic modalities such as hyperventilation.[94]

After the acute stages of severe head injury management, the recovering head-injured patient presents continued challenges for the respiratory therapist. Restlessness, agitation, stupor, and a hypersympathetic metabolism can make secretion control, pulmonary toilet, and nutritional management extremely difficult. Weaning the head-injured patient from the ventilator requires patience and persistence. Extubation of the recovering head-injured patient who does not have a tracheostomy is one of the more confounding challenges in trauma care management. Determining whether the patient is restless and agitated from the presence of the endotracheal tube or from the underlying head injury process is frequently difficult before the extubation trial. A complete review of pulmonary mechanics, weaning spirometry, metabolic status, and so forth should be undertaken before restlessness, tachycardia, or hyperventilation is attributed to the patient's neurologic status. Premature extubation of the recovering head-injured patient who is either too stuporous to participate in pulmonary toilet or too agitated to be controlled without heavy sedation creates a difficult management problem. Experience, combined with the proper environment and the use of appropriate extubation protocols, can significantly facilitate this process.

Thoracic Injury

The chest wall and lungs are frequently injured together. After the evacuation of blood and air from the pleural space, attention is directed at pain management and ventilatory support until the pulmonary parenchyma can heal. It is not the presence of the flail chest but rather the underlying lung injury that determines the prognosis in pulmonary contusion with a flail chest.[95]

The elderly are particularly susceptible to respiratory failure after even one or two rib fractures. Early pain control with epidural opiates has proved to be extremely helpful in preventing or shortening the need for ventilatory support. Likewise, moderate pulmonary contusion may be managed without ventilatory support with careful fluid management, avoidance of fluid overload, precise analgesic control, and in some cases, the use of a continuous positive airway pressure mask.[95]

Most chest tubes placed for trauma should remain for 4 to 5 days, unless a persistent air leak and drainage of greater than 150 mL exists for 24 hours. In addition if the patient has a continued need for positive pressure ventilation, it is usually safe to remove the chest tubes after 7 days, unless the patient has a persistent air leak, more than 200 mL of drainage daily, or high peak airway pressures (peak inspiratory pressure of greater than 40 cm H_2O), or requires more than 5 cm H_2O of PEEP.

Abdominal Injury

It is more important to determine the presence of a surgical abdomen than to make a specific diagnosis in the early management of abdominal trauma. Some injuries to the liver and spleen diagnosed by CT are now safely managed with nonoperative therapy, especially in children.[96] This requires strict management protocols, including the immediate availability of an operating room. Patients who have multiple associated injuries are usually not candidates for a nonoperative approach. For example, the patient with rib fractures, pulmonary contusion, and a ruptured spleen may present a dilemma for the clinician trying to provide gentle management of the nonoperated fractured spleen as well as percussion and postural drainage to the left lower chest wall.

After exploratory laparotomy for massive trauma and hemorrhage, the abdominal wall may be difficult to close. Tight closure of the abdomen may cause elevated airway pressures, requiring a large minute ventilation for adequate ventilatory control. An alternative to tight closure of the abdomen is to leave the abdomen open for several days, with delayed closure performed later.[68]

Bladder injury is usually diagnosed with cystography and is frequently associated with pelvic fracture. Ureteral injuries, which almost always occur with penetrating trauma, are diagnosed with intravenous pyelography. Most renal injuries are diagnosed and staged by CT, and many can be managed nonoperatively.[97]

If a patient has had an intestinal anastomosis after abdominal trauma, care must be taken in using incentive spirometry and intermittent positive pressure breathing to avoid distending the gastrointestinal tract with air. A nasogastric tube may be necessary.

Pelvis and Extremities

A pelvic fracture associated with massive hemorrhage can be a life-threatening injury. Early fixation and, in some cases, arteriography with embolization may be necessary. Long bone extremity fractures may also be associated with blood loss. Early fixation of these fractures has been shown to reduce mortality and pulmonary complications with a reduction in pneumonia and fat embolism. Cast reduction and traction are rarely used in trauma patients, except in children. The technologic advances in external and internal skeletal fixation have been remarkable.

Fat embolism has been described in trauma patients suffering from long bone fractures, most commonly of the femur, tibia, and pelvis. Frequently, the signs and symptoms of fat embolism are hidden in the manifestations of the truly polytraumatized patient with associated chest and abdominal injuries. However, the diagnosis becomes more apparent in the patient with isolated extremity injuries who develops hypoxia, tachycardia, dyspnea, and fever 2 to 4 days after the injury. Ventilation-perfusion scan findings may be normal, but a chest x-ray study frequently displays the adult respiratory distress syndrome picture. In most instances, fat embolism responds well to supportive therapy. On occasion, the use of a continuous positive airway pressure mask or intubation with PEEP is necessary for severe cases. The origin of the fat in these cases remains subject to debate. Current thinking suggests that the fat droplets are formed de novo in the vascular system as a result of the rapid mobilization of free fatty acids as part of the endocrine and metabolic response to trauma. This helps to explain the finding of fat in the brain. However, the traditional thinking that the fat actually comes from the marrow of the fractured extremity has not been disproved. Thrombocytopenia and mucosal and upper chest wall petechiae are very common findings in this process. Fat droplets can be found in the urine but are not essential to make the diagnosis.

Spine

Spinal injury, with or without neurologic deficit, requires a team approach. Early fixation and immobilization have not markedly improved neurologic recovery, but they have reduced many of the associated complications, especially pulmonary complications.[98] The quadriplegic patient is a particular challenge because breathing may be only by virtue of the diaphragm. These patients may breathe adequately for several days, only to deteriorate from fatigue. Frequent measurement of respiratory mechanics is helpful in detecting early respiratory failure. Aggressive pulmonary care monitoring is essential to the recovering quadriplegic patient.

OUTCOME

Evidence continues to accumulate that organized trauma systems can reduce mortality and morbidity in seriously injured patients.[99–102] Studies have suggested that the outcome of trauma and critical care is reasonably optimistic, with the majority of survivors returning to meaningful lives.[103] However, patients may need up to 5 years after injury to reach their optimal recovery potential.

Several scoring systems have been described to predict outcome. The Trauma Score and the Revised Trauma Score are physiologic indicators measured on patient arrival. The Injury Severity Score is an anatomic measure of severity calculated at patient discharge. These scores have been combined with age in a formula weighted against a national database (major trauma outcome study) for the purposes of predicting expected outcome. This formula, known as TRISS,[104] is useful in predicting outcomes in trauma patient populations.

The Apache score (APACHE II and APACHE III) has been studied extensively as a measure for predicting outcome and resource utilization in critical care.[105] It has been validated in medical ICUs, but more recent studies of surgery and trauma patients have suggested that its use will be limited.[106] Clearly, there is a need to quantify the severity and treatment progress of critical care illness in trauma patients.

SUMMARY

Respiratory care of the trauma patient incorporates many of the principles described in detail in many of the accompanying chapters in this text. Factors unique to the trauma patient throughout the prehospital, resuscitative, operative, and critical care phases of treatment should be well understood by the respiratory specialist. The hyperdynamic metabolic response frequently encountered in the trauma patient requires special appreciation in order to provide optimal management. Exciting new therapies, such as manipulation of the mediator-driven hypermetabolic response, lie in the future. New technologies, such as inline blood gas and pH monitors, will allow a much more precise management of the injured patient. These developments will continue to expand the role of the respiratory therapist as a key member of the trauma team.

References

1. Rice DP, MacKenzie EJ, and associates. Cost of Injury in the United States: A Report to Congress. San Francisco, Institute for Health & Aging, University of California and Injury Prevention Center, The Johns Hopkins University, 1989.
2. Champion HR, Mabee MS. An American Crisis in Trauma Care Reimbursement. Emerg Care Q 6:65–87, 1990.
3. Magnuson E. Seven deadly days. Time, July 17, 1989, pp 30–61.
4. Morrissey TB, Byrd CR, Deitch EA. The incidence of recurrent penetrating trauma in an urban trauma center. J Trauma 31:1536–1538, 1991.
5. Gennarelli TA, Champion HR, Sacco WJ, et al. Mortality of patients with head injury and extracranial injury treated in trauma centers. J Trauma 29:1193–1202, 1989.
6. Committee on Trauma Research, Commission on Life Sciences, National Research Council and the Institute of Medicine. Injury in America: A Continuing Public Health Problem. Washington, DC, National Academy Press, 1985.
7. Trunkey DD. Trauma. Sci Am 249:28–35, 1983.
8. Baue A, Faist E. What's new in multiple system organ failure. In Maull KI, Cleveland HC, Feliciano DV, et al (eds). Advances in Trauma and Critical Care, vol 7. Chicago, CV Mosby, 1992, pp 1–21.
9. Finelli FC, Jonsson J, Champion HR, et al. A case control study for major trauma in geriatric patients. J Trauma 29:541–548, 1989.
10. Schneider EL, Guralnik JM. The aging of America: Impact on health care costs. JAMA 263:2335–2340, 1990.
11. Committee on Trauma, American College of Surgeons. Resources for Optimal Care of the Injured Patient. Chicago, American College of Surgeons, 1990.
12. Committee on Trauma, American College of Surgeons. Appendix F to the hospital resources document: Field triage categorization of trauma patients (field triage). Am Coll Surg Bull 71:21, 1986.
13. Baxt WG, Moody P. The impact of advanced prehospital emergency care on the mortality of severely brain-injured patients. J Trauma 27:365–369, 1987.
14. Lewis FR Jr. Prehospital intravenous fluid therapy: Physiologic computer modelling. J Trauma 26:804–811, 1986.
15. Martin RR, Bickell W, Mattox KL, et al. Prospective evaluation of preoperative volume resuscitation in hypotensive patients with penetrating truncal injuries—Preliminary report [Abstract]. J Trauma 31:1033, 1991.
16. Mattox KL, Bickell W, Pepe PE, et al. Prospective MAST study in 911 patients. J Trauma 29:1104–1112, 1989.
17. Riou B, Pansard JL, Lazard T, et al. Ventilatory effects of medical antishock trousers in healthy volunteers. J Trauma 31:1495–1502, 1991.

18. Rhodes M, Tinkoff G. Pneumatic anti-shock garment. *In* Cameron JL (ed). Current Surgical Therapy, 4th ed. St. Louis, Mosby–Year Book/BC Decker Imprint, 1992.
19. McSwain NE Jr. Pneumatic anti-shock garment: State of the art 1988. Ann Emerg Med 17:506–525, 1988.
20. MacLeod BA, Seaberg DC, Paris PM. Prehospital therapy past, present, and future. Emerg Med Clin North Am 8:57–74, 1990.
21. Xeropotamos NS, Coats TJ, Wilson AW. Prehospital surgical airway management: 1 year's experience from the Helicopter Emergency Medical Service. Injury 24:222–224, 1993.
22. Kern L, Komon H. An evaluation of mivacurium chloride: Can it be effective in the prehospital setting? Air Medical Journal September:344, 1993.
23. Syverud SA, Borron SW, Storer DL, et al. Prehospital use of neuromuscular blocking agents in a helicopter ambulance program. Ann Emerg Med 17:236–242, 1988.
24. Hedges JR, Dronen SC, Feero S, et al. Succinylcholine-assisted intubations in prehospital care. Ann Emerg Med 17:469–472, 1988.
25. Gabram SG, Jacobs LM, Schwartz RJ, Stohler SA. Airway intubation in injured patients at the scene of an accident. Conn Med 53:633–637, 1989.
26. McGuire TJ, Pointer JE. Evaluation of a pulse oximeter in the prehospital setting. Ann Emerg Med 17:1058–1062, 1988.
27. Melton JD, Heller M, Kaplan R. Occult hypoxia during aeromedical transport: Detection by pulse oximetry. Prehosp Disaster Med 4:115–120, 1989.
28. Mattox KL, Maningas PA, Moore EE, et al. Prehospital hypertonic saline/dextran infusion for post-traumatic hypotension. The USA Multicenter Trial. Ann Surg 213:482–491, 1991.
29. Vassar MJ, Perry CA, Gannaway WL, Holcroft JW. 7.5% sodium chloride/dextran for resuscitation of trauma patients undergoing helicopter transport. Arch Surg 126:1065–1072, 1991.
30. Battistella FD, Wisner DH. Combined hemorrhagic shock and head injury: Effects of hypertonic saline (7.5%) resuscitation. J Trauma 31:182–188, 1991.
31. Schmoker JD, Zhuang J, Shackford SR. Hypertonic fluid resuscitation improves cerebral oxygen delivery and reduces intracranial pressure after hemorrhagic shock. J Trauma 31:1607–1613, 1991.
32. Gould SA, Sehgal LR, Rosen AL, et al. The efficacy of polymerized pyridoxylated hemoglobin solution as an O_2 carrier. Ann Surg 211:394–398, 1990.
33. Boyd CR, Corse KM, Campbell RC. Emergency interhospital transport of the major trauma patient: Air versus ground. J Trauma 29:789–794, 1989.
34. Moylan JA, Fitzpatrick KT, Beyer AJ III, Georgiade GS. Factors improving survival in multisystem trauma patients. Ann Surg 207:679–685, 1988.
35. Moylan JA. Impact of helicopters on trauma care and clinical results. Ann Surg 208:673–678, 1988.
36. Rhodes M, Brader AH. Organization of a trauma resuscitation system. Adv Trauma 4:19–42, 1989.
37. Kuchinski J, Tinkoff G, Rhodes M, Becher JW Jr. Emergency intubation for paralysis of the uncooperative trauma patient. J Emerg Med 9:9–12, 1991.
38. Redan JA, Livingston DH, Tortella BJ, Rush BF Jr. The value of intubating and paralyzing patients with suspected head injury in the emergency department. J Trauma 31:371–375, 1991.
39. Durbin CG Jr. Neuromuscular blocking agents and sedative drugs: Clinical uses and toxic effects in the critical care unit. Crit Care Clin 7:489–506, 1991.
40. Committee on Trauma, American College of Surgeons. Advanced Trauma Life Support Program for Physicians: Instructor Manual. 5th Ed. Chicago, American College of Surgeons, 1993, pp 54–55.
41. Erlandson MJ, Clinton JE, Ruiz E, Cohen J. Cricothyrotomy in the emergency department revisited. J Emerg Med 7:115–118, 1989.
42. Ivatury R, Siegel JH, Stahl WM, et al. Percutaneous tracheostomy after trauma and critical illness. J Trauma 32:133–140, 1992.
43. Muizelaar JP, Marmarou A, Ward JD, et al. Adverse effects of prolonged hyperventilation in patients with severe head injury: A randomized clinical trial. J Neurosurg 75:731–739, 1991.
44. Satiani B, Fried SJ, Zeeb P, Falcone RE. Normothermic rapid volume replacement in traumatic hypovolemia. A prospective analysis using a new device. Arch Surg 122:1044–1047, 1987.
45. Committee on Trauma, American College of Surgeons. Advanced Trauma Life Support Program: Instructor Manual. Chicago, American College of Surgeons, 1989, p 15.
46. Bouzarth WF. Intracranial nasogastric tube insertion [Editorial]. J Trauma 18:818–819, 1978.
47. Kennedy TJ, McConnell JD, Thal ER. Urine dipstick vs. microscopic urinalysis in the evaluation of abdominal trauma. J Trauma 28:615–617, 1988.
48. Scalea TM, Simon HM, Duncan AO, et al. Geriatric blunt multiple trauma: Improved survival with early invasive monitoring. J Trauma 30:129–136, 1990.
49. Hurst JM, Davis K Jr, Branson RD, Johannigman JA. Comparison of blood gases during transport using two methods of ventilatory support. J Trauma 29:1637–1640, 1989.

50. Gbaanador GBM, Fruin AH, Taylon C. Role of routine emergency cervical radiography in head trauma. Am J Surg 152:643–648, 1986.
51. Diliberti T, Lindsey RW. Evaluation of the cervical spine in the emergency setting: Who does not need an x-ray? Orthopedics 15:179–183, 1992.
52. Fabian TC, Mangiante EC, White TJ, et al. A prospective study of 91 patients undergoing both computed tomography and peritoneal lavage following blunt abdominal trauma. J Trauma 26:602–608, 1986.
53. Marx JA, Moore EE, Jorden RC, Eule J Jr. Limitations of computed tomography in the evaluation of acute abdominal trauma: A prospective comparison with diagnostic peritoneal lavage. J Trauma 25:933–937, 1985.
54. Peitzman AB, Makaroun MS, Slasky BS, Ritter P. Prospective study of computed tomography in initial management of blunt abdominal trauma. J Trauma 28:585–592, 1986.
55. Davis RA, Shayne JP, Max MH, et al. The use of computerized axial tomography versus peritoneal lavage in the evaluation of blunt abdominal trauma: A prospective study. Surgery 98:845–850, 1985.
56. Fischer RP, Miller-Crotchett P, Reed RL II. Gastrointestinal disruption: The hazard of nonoperative management in adults with blunt abdominal injury. J Trauma 28:1445–1449, 1988.
57. Sherck JP, Oates DD. Intestinal injuries missed by computed tomography. J Trauma 30:1–7, 1990.
58. Thal ER, Meyer DM. The evaluation of blunt abdominal trauma: Computed tomography scan, lavage, or sonography? Adv Surg 24:201–228, 1991.
59. Gruessner R, Mentges B, Duber C, et al. Sonography versus peritoneal lavage in blunt abdominal trauma. J Trauma 29:242–244, 1989.
60. Tso P, Rodriguez A, Cooper C, et al. Sonography in blunt abdominal trauma: A preliminary progress report. J Trauma 33:39–44, 1992.
61. Fabian TC, Croce MA, Stewart RM, et al. A prospective analysis of diagnostic laparoscopy in trauma. Ann Surg 217:557–565, 1993.
62. Salem M, Chernow B, Burke R, et al. Bedside diagnostic blood testing. Its accuracy, rapidity, and utility in blood conservation. JAMA 266:382–389, 1991.
63. Shapiro BA, Cane RD. Blood gas monitoring: Yesterday, today, and tomorrow. Crit Care Med 17:573–581, 1989.
64. Chernow B. Blood conservation in critical care—The evidence accumulates [Editorial]. Crit Care Med 21:481–482, 1993.
65. Seibel R, LaDuca J, Hassett JM, et al. Blunt multiple trauma (ISS 36), femur traction, and the pulmonary failure-septic state. Ann Surg 202:283–295, 1985.
66. Border JR, Bone LB. Multiple trauma: Major extremity wounds; Their immediate management and its consequences. Adv Surg 21:263–291, 1988.
67. Bone LB, Johnson KD, Weigelt J, Scheinberg R. Early versus delayed stabilization of femoral fractures. A prospective randomized study. J Bone Joint Surg [Am] 71:336–340, 1989.
68. Smith PC, Tweddell JS, Bessey PQ. Alternative approaches to abdominal wound closure in severely injured patients with massive visceral edema. J Trauma 32:16–20, 1992.
69. Hoyt DB, Shackford SR, McGill T, et al. The impact of in-house surgeons and operating room resuscitation on outcome of traumatic injuries. Arch Surg 124:906–910, 1989.
70. Rhodes M, Brader A, Lucke J, Gillott A. Direct transport to the operating room for resuscitation of trauma patients. J Trauma 29:907–915, 1989.
71. Cullen DJ, Keene R, Waternaux C, et al. Results, charges, and benefits of intensive care for critically ill patients: Update 1983. Crit Care Med 12:102–106, 1984.
72. Moore FA, Haenel JB, Moore EE, Whitehill TA. Incommensurate oxygen consumption in response to maximal oxygen availability predicts postinjury multiple organ failure. J Trauma 33:58–67, 1992.
73. Shoemaker WC. A new approach to physiology, monitoring, and therapy of shock states. World J Surg 11:133–146, 1987.
74. Boutros AR, Lee C. Value of continuous monitoring of mixed venous blood oxygen saturation in the management of critically ill patients. Crit Care Med 14:132–135, 1986.
75. Vaughn S, Puri VK. Cardiac output changes and continuous mixed venous oxygen saturation measurement in the critically ill. Crit Care Med 16:495–498, 1988.
76. Norfleet EA, Watson CB. Continuous mixed venous oxygen saturation measurement: A significant advance in hemodynamic monitoring? J Clin Monit 1:245–258, 1985.
77. MacIntyre N, Nishimura M, Usada Y, et al. The Nagoya conference on system design and patient-ventilator interactions during pressure support ventilation. Chest 97:1463–1466, 1990.
78. Mackersie RC, Karagianes TG, Hoyt DB, Davis JW. Prospective evaluation of epidural and intravenous administration of fentanyl for pain control and restoration of ventilatory function following multiple rib fractures. J Trauma 31:443–451, 1991.
79. Dellinger RP, Bandi V. Fiberoptic bronchoscopy in the intensive care unit. Crit Care Clin 8:755–772, 1992.
80. Berlauk JF. Prolonged endotracheal intubation vs. tracheostomy. Crit Care Med 14:742–745, 1986.

81. Stauffer JL, Olson DE, Petty TL. Complications and consequences of endotracheal intubation and tracheotomy: A prospective study of 150 critically ill adult patients. Am J Med 70:65–76, 1981.

82. Dunham CM, LaMonica C. Prolonged tracheal intubation in the trauma patient. J Trauma 24:120–124, 1984.

83. Rodriguez JL, Steinberg SM, Luchetti FA, et al. Early tracheostomy for primary airway management in the surgical critical care setting. Surgery 108:655–659, 1990.

84. Astrachan DI, Kirchner JC, Goodwin WJ Jr. Prolonged intubation vs. tracheostomy: Complications, practical and psychological considerations. Laryngoscope 98:1165–1169, 1988.

85. Ciaglia P, Firsching R, Syniec C. Elective percutaneous dilatational tracheostomy: A new simple bedside procedure; Preliminary report. Chest 87:715–719, 1985.

86. Hazard PB, Garrett HE Jr, Adams JW, et al. Bedside percutaneous tracheostomy: Experience with 55 elective procedures. Ann Thorac Surg 46:63–67, 1988.

87. Makk LJK, McClave SA, Creech PW, et al. Clinical application of the metabolic cart to the delivery of total parenteral nutrition. Crit Care Med 18:1320–1327, 1990.

88. McAnena OJ, Moore FA, Moore EE, et al. Selective uptake of glutamine in the gastrointestinal tract: Confirmation in a human study. Br J Surg 78:480–482, 1991.

89. Pingleton SK. Enteral nutrition and infection in the intensive care unit. Semin Respir Infect 5:185–190, 1990.

90. Moore FA, Haenel JB, Moore EE, Read RA. Percutaneous tracheostomy/gastrostomy in brain-injured patients—A minimally invasive alternative. J Trauma 33:435–439, 1992.

91. McCarthy DM. Sucralfate. N Engl J Med 325:1017–1025, 1991.

92. Eddleston JM, Vohra A, Scott P, et al. A comparison of the frequency of stress ulceration and secondary pneumonia in sucralfate- or ranitidine-treated intensive care unit patients. Crit Care Med 19:1491–1496, 1991.

93. Parker S, Carlon GC, Isaacs M, et al. Dopamine administration in oliguria and oliguric renal failure. Crit Care Med 9:630–632, 1981.

94. Cruz J, Miner ME, Allen SJ, et al. Continuous monitoring of cerebral oxygenation in acute brain injury: Injection of mannitol during hyperventilation. J Neurosurg 73:725–730, 1990.

95. Richardson JD, Adams L, Flint LM. Selective management of flail chest and pulmonary contusion. Ann Surg 196:481–487, 1982.

96. Cywes S, Rode H, Millar AJW. Blunt liver trauma in children: Nonoperative management. J Pediatr Surg 20:14–18, 1985.

97. Herschorn S, Radomski SB, Shoskes DA, et al. Evaluation and treatment of blunt renal trauma. J Urol 146:274–277, 1991.

98. Schlegel JD. Timing of operative intervention in the management of acute spinal injuries. Submitted for publication.

99. West JG, Cales RH, Gazzaniga AB. Impact of regionalization: The Orange County experience. Arch Surg 118:740–744, 1983.

100. Cales RH. Trauma mortality in Orange County: The effect of implementation of a regional trauma system. Ann Emerg Med 13:1–10, 1984.

101. Shackford SR, Hollingworth-Fridlund P, Cooper GF, Eastman AB. The effect of regionalization upon the quality of trauma care as assessed by concurrent audit before and after institution of a trauma system: A preliminary report. J Trauma 26:812–820, 1986.

102. Clemmer TP, Orme JF Jr, Thomas FO, Brooks KA. Outcome of critically injured patients treated at level I trauma centers versus full-service community hospitals. Crit Care Med 13:861–863, 1985.

103. Rhodes M, Aronson J, Moerkirk G, Peterash E. Quality of life after the trauma center. J Trauma 28:931–938, 1988.

104. Boyd CR, Tolson MA, Copes WS. Evaluating trauma care: The TRISS method. Trauma Score and the Injury Severity Score. J Trauma 27:370–378, 1987.

105. Zimmerman JE (ed). Apache III study design: Analytic plan for evaluation of severity and outcome. Crit Care Med 17:S169–S221, 1989.

106. Civetta JM, Hudson-Civetta JA, Nelson LD. Evaluation of APACHE II for cost containment and quality assurance. Ann Surg 212:266–276, 1990.

34

■

Barotrauma in Mechanical Ventilation

Wayne M. Samuelson, M.D.,
David K. Handshoe, M.D., and
William J. Fulkerson, M.D.

Barotrauma, an unfortunately common and feared complication of mechanical ventilation, is a broad term for lung injury that may be manifested in a variety of ways. Some of the subtle signs of barotrauma may be missed, whereas others are obvious life-threatening emergencies. In some clinical series, the mortality rate from barotrauma has been reported to be as high as 13 to 35%. In addition to the mortality attributable to barotrauma, the morbidity induced by mechanical ventilation and its complications has also come under examination. Expanding critical care technology allows desperately ill patients to be supported for increasing lengths of time, thus compounding the features that may predispose to ventilator-associated injury.

BACKGROUND (Table 34–1)

In a landmark study of the mechanisms of barotrauma, Macklin and Macklin examined a number of recognized cases of pneumomediastinum. They found that many of these patients died of respiratory failure with stiff, overexpanded lungs that could not be collapsed by pressure at autopsy. Noting that these lungs also floated when placed in water, they discovered that this condition was secondary to ruptured alveoli and the dissection of air along vascular sheaths passing to the mediastinum and ultimately to the subcutaneous tissue and retroperitoneum. They termed this malignant interstitial emphysema. In an elegant series of experiments, they determined that the site of air escape was the alveolar base at the point at which it contacted the vascular sheath. Early studies demonstrated that high airway pressure alone was not the cause of alveolar rupture. In a canine model, air was insufflated into the lungs in large volumes, but expansion of the lungs was limited by thoracic binding. The marked elevation in intra-alveolar pressure was matched by the

TABLE **34–1:** Important Studies in Barotrauma

Study	Finding
Pollak and Adams	High insufflation pressure alone is not the cause of barotrauma
Macklin and Macklin	"Malignant interstitial emphysema"
Schaefer et al	Transpulmonic and transatrial pressure gradients
Lenaghan et al	Hemodynamic changes associated with lung rupture
Caldwell et al	Alveolar distention and pulmonary interstitial emphysema; role of the alveolar-arterial gradient

elevation in the supporting pressure on the outside of the chest, thus preventing a severe gradient between the intra-alveolar pressure and the external alveolar pressure. Under these conditions, the alveoli did not rupture. Macklin and Macklin determined that a gradient between the alveolus and the vascular sheath was necessary to produce alveolar rupture and interstitial emphysema. They hypothesized that the gradient could be produced either by alveolar overinflation without concomitant extension of the vascular lumen or by a reduction in the caliber of pulmonary vessels (as might occur in pulmonary embolization or states of decreased pulmonary flow). Table 34–2 summarizes the clinical conditions that may accentuate the alveolar gradient.

In 1970, Caldwell and coworkers conducted experiments in anesthetized rabbits to clarify the significance of the alveolar-arterial oxygen gradient in the development of pulmonary interstitial emphysema. Animals were instrumented after intubation and anesthesia. Both intrapulmonary pressures and intrapleural pressures were measured. Two groups of animals were studied. In one group, the animals were shaved and then wrapped tightly about the thorax and abdomen with adhesive tape in order to splint chest wall expansion. In both the bound and the unbound groups, the animals were divided into three subgroups according to pressure induced via a tracheal catheter. The frequency of induced lesions in the unbound animals correlated significantly with applied tracheal pressure. The frequency of induced lesions in the bound animals did not significantly correlate with induced pressure. Caldwell and coworkers concluded that airway pressure itself was not a primary cause of perivascular interstitial emphysema.

The influence of volumes on the occurrence of perivascular interstitial emphysema was also studied in bound and unbound animals. Again, the frequency of lesions was significantly lower in the bound animals than in the unbound animals. Caldwell and coworkers concluded that expansion of the lung is one of the primary factors in the development of perivascular interstitial emphysema. The alveolar-arterial oxygen gradient did not correlate with the occurrence of interstitial emphysema.

Lenaghan and associates examined hemodynamic changes associated with lung rupture. Lightly anesthetized dogs were instrumented such that intratracheal, pleural, central venous, and systemic arterial pressures could be monitored. Mediastinal pressures were recorded from an esophageal balloon and from a catheter in the anterior mediastinum. Lung rupture, produced by airflow into the trachea, was recognized by a steady stream of air bubbles from an intercostal drain. Insufflation continued until air leakage equaled input, which was believed to signify equilibration of pressures. Intratracheal and pleural pressures were then returned to normal.

Three groups of dogs were examined. In the first group, the intercostal tube was clamped in six of the 12 dogs. Nine of these dogs died. Each dog with a patent intercostal tube had air in the coronary arteries. In

TABLE **34–2:** Conditions That Accentuate the Alveolar Pressure Gradient

Cough
Airway obstruction with compensatory hyperinflation
Lobar atelectasis with compensatory hyperinflation
High peak ventilatory pressures
Rapid ascent from depth
Decreased pulmonary blood flow*

*Suspected, but not proven (see text).

these six, lung rupture occurred at a mean intratracheal pressure of 48.3 mm Hg. Intratracheal pressure reached equilibrium at an average of 104.8 mm Hg within a mean time of 44.2 seconds. The patency of the chest tube did not influence these readings. With insufflation, the intratracheal pressure initially increased slowly but later rose sharply. Lung rupture occurred with the abrupt change in the intratracheal pressure gradient. Circulatory arrest occurred within 90 seconds of the start of insufflation. Arterial pressure fell abruptly, whereas central venous pressure increased gradually. A pulse reappeared when pressure returned to normal, but blood pressure was not maintained. When the chest was opened, coronary artery air embolization and ventricular fibrillation were found. Air mixed with blood was found in both sides of the heart, in the pulmonary vessels, and in the proximal vena cava.

Monitoring catheters were placed via a median sternotomy into the right ventricles and pulmonary arteries of the next group of 18 dogs. The sternum was wired and the chest closed. At maximal intratracheal pressure, both the right ventricular and the pulmonary artery pressures were significantly elevated. When insufflation ceased, both pressures remained elevated. While the hypertension persisted, pulmonary circulation time was prolonged. With insufflation, the mean peripherally directed pulmonary artery gradient was reversed in direction. With this reversal in gradient, flow was reversed, resulting in radial expansion of the pulmonary artery and incompetence of the pulmonary valve. Tricuspid incompetence followed. After lung rupture, air entered the distal branches of the pulmonary artery and was seen to move centripetally in the right ventricle. Incompetence of the pulmonary valve resulted in an increase in mean right ventricular pressure. Tricuspid incompetence resulted in a fall in this mean pressure, followed by the appearance of right ventricular complexes on the central venous pressure tracing.

The third group of dogs was phlebotomized to a mean systemic arterial pressure of 40 mm Hg and maintained there for 1 hour. In these dogs, lung rupture and equilibrium occurred at much lower pressures than in normotensive dogs. All dogs in this group died of coronary artery emboli. In all dogs, acrylic casts of the bronchial tree confirmed that rupture occurred at a tissue level distal to the terminal bronchiole. These efforts became the foundation for clinically relevant studies. The advent of mechanical ventilation has made the consequences of barotrauma secondary to positive pressure ventilation much more pressing and important. The Macklins and their contemporaries were primarily concerned with the consequences of the slow accumulation of interstitial emphysema in spontaneously breathing patients. However, in ventilated patients, tension pneumothorax occurs with alarming frequency and may cause death if not rapidly treated. Thus, identifying the features that place a patient at high risk for barotrauma becomes increasingly important.

INCIDENCE OF BAROTRAUMA

Early reports of complications related to endotracheal insufflation came from the surgical and anesthesia literature. However, as mechanical ventilation has become a supportive therapy for critically ill patients for very prolonged periods, the incidence of complications has increased. Zwillich and colleagues prospectively studied 354 episodes of mechanical ventilation of longer than 24 hours in duration. Four hundred complications were discovered, including 15 episodes of pneumothorax and 39 cases of intubation of the right mainstem bronchus, leading to alveolar hyperventilation. Four of the 15 pneumothoraces occurred in patients with right mainstem bronchus intubation. However, pneumothorax did not correlate with decreased survival. A significant association between patient age and incidence of pneumothorax was discovered, with the complication being more frequent in patients younger than 30 years of age.

Fleming and colleagues reported a 15% incidence of pneumothorax in their ventilated patients, all of whom were treated in the 24th Evacuation Hospital in Vietnam. They followed up 128 patients requiring ventilatory support for more than 24 hours postoperatively. All patients had tracheostomies. Fifty-seven patients had chest injuries, and 23 (40%) had undergone thoracotomy. Pontoppidan noted that tension pneumothorax occurs with greater frequency in patients with chronic obstructive lung disease who are receiving mechanical ventilation. Steier and coworkers reported on a series of 544 patients who sustained pneumothorax between 1965 and 1972. Of these, 74 were patients receiving continuous ventilatory support. Steier and coworkers also noted that pneumothorax occurring during positive pressure breathing is highly dangerous; this situation demands immediate management. In their series, all 74 patients with pneumothorax on mechanical ventilation also developed subcutaneous emphysema.

ANATOMIC CONSIDERATIONS

The anatomic relationships of the chest, retroperitoneum, and neck divide the soft tissues of the chest into three compartments. The previsceral space, located anteriorly, extends superiorly to the mandible and inferiorly to the midsternum, merging laterally with the subcutaneous tissues of the neck. This compartment is separated from the visceral space by the pretracheal fascia. The fascia of the visceral space envelops the esophagus and trachea and follows these structures into the chest. This space, which is contiguous with the fascia surrounding the hilar vessels and major airways, terminates at the distal bronchovascular sheaths. The prevertebral space extends from the occiput to the upper thoracic spine. This space also extends laterally and communicates with the axillary sheath and the posterior triangle of the neck. The visceral space creates a conduit between the mediastinum and the neck that is most important in the movement of extra-alveolar air. The visceral space follows the esophagus through the diaphragmatic hiatus into the retroperitoneal space. The posterolateral portion of the retroperitoneal visceral compartment has anatomic continuity with the properitoneal fat, thus creating a means for extra-alveolar air entering this space to enter into the anterior abdominal wall. A similar conduit exists between the endothoracic fascia of the outer chest wall and the abdominal transverse fascia. This permits passage of gas to these soft tissue compartments as well.

FORMS OF BAROTRAUMA OTHER THAN PNEUMOTHORAX

Pneumothorax is not the only form of barotrauma that can be life threatening (Table 34–3). Pressure injury has been associated with hya-

Disruption of any of the fascial planes or soft tissue compartments by extra-alveolar air can readily result in the dissection of air into any other communicating compartment. Thus, the manifestations of pulmonary barotrauma can be diverse and far separated from the lung.

TABLE **34–3:** Forms of Barotrauma

Pneumothorax	Pneumoperitoneum
Pneumomediastinum	Pulmonary hyperinflation
Interstitial emphysema	Subpleural air cysts
Subcutaneous emphysema	Hyaline membranes*

*See text.

line membrane formation in children and adults (see Effects of Barotrauma at the Cellular Level, later). Hemodynamic alterations are also associated with mechanical ventilation, as is pulmonary overinflation. Although it is a less common complication in adults, air embolization can occur, with disastrous results. Marini and Culver described two critically ill patients who developed recurrent episodes of cerebral infarction, myocardial injury, and livedo reticularis while being supported by mechanical ventilation. In both cases, pre-existing extra-alveolar air collections had enlarged before the catastrophic clinical events took place. The pathophysiology of this event appears to be an extension of the extra-alveolar air, leading to interstitial emphysema and pneumothorax.

The most common initiating factor in the development of extra-alveolar air collections in the setting of mechanical ventilation is rupture of the alveolar wall with subsequent dissection of air along the bronchovascular sheaths, which is known as pulmonary interstitial emphysema. This condition is commonly recognized in neonates receiving mechanical ventilation and has also been noted in up to 15% of older children and adults receiving mechanical ventilation. The radiographic findings in this disorder reflect the underlying pathophysiology of barotrauma.

The earliest radiographic evidence of pulmonary interstitial emphysema is often an increase in tissue contrast within the consolidated lung, called parenchymal stippling. This renders a "salt-and-pepper" appearance to areas of the chest radiograph that were previously uniformly gray. This appearance is the result of air surrounding multiple small vessels viewed in cross section. Stippling is usually seen peripherally in the lung bases. The progression of air dissection leads to lucent mottling of the radiograph, reflecting the early development of air cysts. Perivascular dissection of air along the larger pulmonary vessels results in lucent streaking. This is most conspicuous in proximity to the hila. Lucent streaking may simulate air bronchograms, but it has a coarser appearance and a lack of distal tapering. As the process of dissection of extra-alveolar air continues, discrete airway cysts that resemble pneumatoceles may become evident in either the subpleural or the intraparenchymal regions of the lung.

Air cysts appear to be harbingers of tension pneumothorax.

Air cysts in the critically ill patient must be differentiated from emphysematous bullae, staphylococcal pneumatoceles, and abscesses secondary to necrotizing pneumonitis.

The development of subpleural air cysts is an underappreciated manifestation of barotrauma from mechanical ventilation. These thin-walled cavities, which are especially prominent at the lung bases, are generally 3 to 5 cm in size. They may expand rapidly and become quite large (Fig. 34–1). They may resolve spontaneously, or they may become secondarily infected and cause substantial morbidity. Air cysts may also simulate a loculated pneumothorax and may become large enough to develop tension and cause diaphragmatic inversion and mediastinal shift.

Subcutaneous emphysema, a very common sight in pulmonary barotrauma, may be present without detectable pneumothorax, but it often occurs in association with pneumothorax (Fig. 34–2). This condition develops from the dissection of air originating from ruptured alveoli into

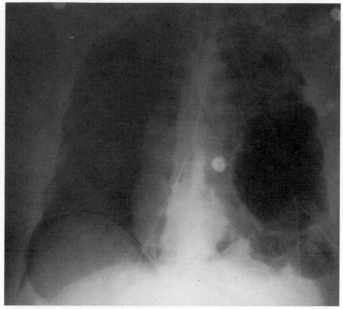

FIGURE 34–1: Large air cyst formed in association with pneumothorax.

subcutaneous tissue planes. It is usually most prominent in the head and neck, distending and distorting facial features and subcutaneous tissue (Fig. 34–3). Palpable subcutaneous emphysema can often be found even at very distal sites, such as the feet and abdomen (Fig. 34–4). Although this development is unsightly and is frequently upsetting to patients and their families, it rarely interferes with management and seldom poses a threat to the patient. However, it can complicate wound closure and may be associated with ischemic skin injury. Subcutaneous emphysema is not usually a life-threatening complication. However, its presence should be interpreted by the clinician to mean that more serious

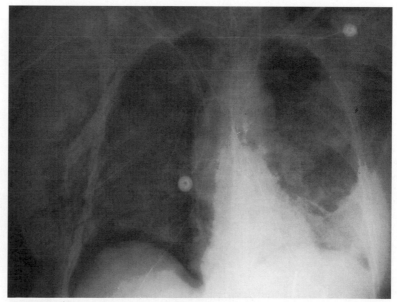

FIGURE 34–2: Subcutaneous emphysema with pneumothorax.

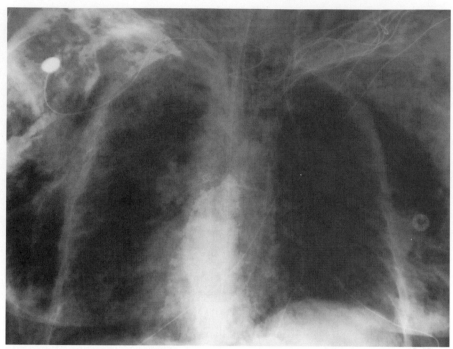

FIGURE 34–3: Widespread subcutaneous emphysema.

and potentially life-threatening complications are likely unless the course of events is reversed.

Pneumoperitoneum, which often follows pneumomediastinum, results from air dissecting into the retroperitoneum. The peritoneum itself may rupture (Fig. 34–5). This event, which can be painful, presents a diagnostic dilemma because it must be distinguished from the pain and the intra-abdominal air resulting from perforated viscus. Peritoneal lavage and even exploration may be necessary to rule out intra-abdominal pathology. Air under the diaphragm may interfere with effective venti-

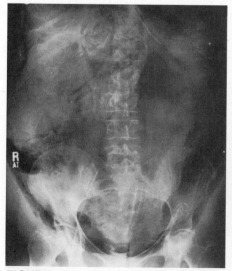

FIGURE 34–4: Subcutaneous emphysema spreading over the abdomen.

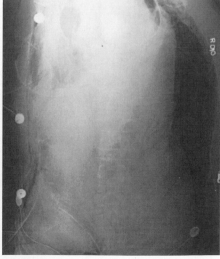

FIGURE 34–5: Pneumoperitoneum secondary to barotrauma mimicking perforated viscus.

lation. The evacuation of pneumoperitoneum is occasionally attempted, although it is often not successful. If pneumoperitoneum and pneumothorax exist concurrently, the placement of a chest tube may be definitive treatment for both conditions.

Pulmonary hyperinflation is another potentially serious complication of mechanical ventilation. This seems to be the result of ball-valve airway obstruction, small airway collapse, differential lung compliances, or a combination of these factors. Ball-valve airway obstruction is often caused by accumulated secretions that prevent the complete return of inspired volumes. When pulmonary injury or infiltration results in differential lung compliances, hyperinflation of the more compliant lung may be caused by attempts to ventilate diseased areas of low compliance. The patient usually presents with restlessness, respiratory distress, and intolerance of mechanical ventilation. Radiographs show

- Radiolucency of the affected areas
- Shift of the heart and mediastinum away from the involved side
- Widening of the intercostal spaces
- Depression and relative immobility of the ipsilateral diaphragm

The result of these events is worsening gas exchange secondary to a regional shift in lung perfusion, decreased alveolar ventilation, and compression effects on adjacent structures.

The treatment of pulmonary hyperinflation includes

- Decrease in or discontinuation of positive end-expiratory pressure (PEEP)
- Removal (if possible) of ball-valve mucus obstruction by bronchoscopy
- Judicious use of bronchodilators
- Avoidance of high peak inspiratory pressures

If triggering of assisted-supported mechanical breaths is hindered by the presence of diffuse hyperinflation from air trapping, applied PEEP may be beneficial (see Chapter 22).

Although an uncomplicated pneumothorax can be readily treated, the morbidity (and mortality) of more insidious lesions, such as hyaline membrane formation, is difficult to quantitate and more difficult to reverse. However, the most effective therapy for any of these complications is to correct the underlying disorder. Although caution should be exercised in the management of patients on mechanical ventilation, concern for potential complications should not override the clear indications for instituting and maintaining ventilatory support.

IDENTIFYING IMPENDING BAROTRAUMA (Table 34–4)

Most likely, the true incidence of pressure injury in mechanical ventilation is much higher than was originally thought.

Patients are at greater risk for developing complications of mechanical ventilation when ventilatory support is prolonged. Infiltrated paren-

TABLE **34–4:**   Conditions Predisposing to Barotrauma

High peak airway pressures
Bullous lung disease
High levels of positive end-expiratory pressure*
Necrotizing pneumonia
Aspiration of gastric acid
Adult respiratory distress syndrome*

*See text for discussion.

Pulmonary interstitial emphysema and pneumomediastinum are properly considered to be precursors of pneumothorax.

chyma may tether open vascular channels disrupted by inflammatory necrosis or shear stress, allowing the entry of gas leaking from ruptured alveoli into the interstitium. Pneumothorax is the most feared complication of barotrauma because it is potentially lethal. However, in the setting of mechanical ventilation, pneumothorax is rarely the initial manifestation of barotrauma. Once pulmonary interstitial emphysema and pneumomediastinum have been identified, a keen awareness of the subtle signs and symptoms of pneumothorax will aid the clinician in proper diagnosis and treatment. In a series reported on by Steier and coworkers, more than 60% of pneumothoraces were diagnosed on clinical grounds alone. Findings included hypotension, diminished breath sounds on the affected side, and tachycardia. Other signs and symptoms of pneumothorax may include hypoxemia, elevated peak airway pressure, tachypnea, and diaphoresis. An elevation in pulmonary artery pressures may suggest an occult pneumothorax, reflecting either the influence of increased pleural pressure on the pulmonary artery or hypoxemic vasoconstriction.

Recognition of air in the pleural space is difficult and challenging in the recumbent intensive care unit patient. The rate of misdiagnosis is reported to be as high as 30%. The classic findings are not always evident or may even be obscured by overlying support equipment. Air may accumulate in several different pleural recesses. Routine daily chest radiography is a standard practice in most intensive care units. Hall and associates, noting that a substantial number of radiographic findings were not anticipated by clinical evaluation, found that daily chest radiography led to a higher diagnostic and therapeutic efficiency. Additional radiographic views, including computed tomographic scans, should be obtained in any patient whose plain films are suggestive but not diagnostic of underlying barotrauma.

The anteromedial space is least dependent in the supine patient, so pleural air may collect there first. Air in the superior compartments yields sharp definition of the upper mediastinal contours, whereas an inferior anteromedial pneumothorax may create a deep anterior costophrenic sulcus or outline the medial diaphragm beneath the cardiac silhouette. The subpulmonic pneumothorax may be recognized by hyperlucency over the upper abdomen, a deep lateral costophrenic sulcus, and visualization of the inferior surface of the lung. The posteromedial pneumothorax, which appears as a lucent triangle whose base is outlined by the costovertebral sulcus, almost always occurs in association with lower lobe collapse or parenchymal disease. The lateral side of the triangle defines the medial edge of the collapsed or consolidated lobe, with the vertex pointing toward the hilum.

The presence of pulmonary interstitial gas on the chest radiograph is frequently difficult to recognize in adult patients. It is more often identified in the pediatric population. If seen in adults, it may be mistaken for an air bronchogram. Subpleural air cysts are also seen in the pediatric population. Although morbidity from these cysts is relatively low, their appearance should warrant identification and concern. Even when the cysts do not progress to pneumothorax, they may become secondarily infected and thus may increase patient morbidity and mortality.

Is there then a clear profile of the patient who is at risk for developing barotrauma? There are persuasive data suggesting that patients suffering from necrotizing pneumonia of any etiology are at increased risk for pneumothorax. Gastric acid aspiration may also increase the risk of pneumothorax. Gastric acid has been found to cause frank necrosis extending from the tracheobronchial tree to the periphery of the lungs. Pre-existing chronic obstructive lung disease also appears to predispose to barotrauma. Such patients, who generally have very little pulmonary reserve, may develop ventilatory failure after a fairly minor insult. If the lungs are not uniformly injured, positive pressure from the ventilator will be distributed to the more compliant areas of the lung, causing overdistention and probably barotrauma.

Asthmatic patients requiring intubation and mechanical ventilation are also at increased risk for pulmonary barotrauma. In one series, only one episode of mediastinal emphysema was observed in 48 episodes of assisted ventilation in 18 patients who had status asthmaticus. Another series reported five episodes of subcutaneous emphysema and seven episodes of pneumothorax during 21 courses of mechanical ventilation in 19 patients with status asthmaticus. The potential lethality of this complication is clear. Eight deaths occurred in 21 episodes of mechanical ventilation. Luksa and colleagues retrospectively evaluated 32 patients during 34 episodes of mechanical ventilation with intermittent positive pressure ventilation. Six episodes of pneumothorax were found. In all instances, pneumothorax was life threatening and was associated with hypotension and high ventilatory pressures. Another manifestation of barotrauma that may occur in patients with status asthmaticus is hyperinflation. A case has been described in which central airway plugging led to the creation of a one-way ball valve with air trapping beyond the inspissated mucus. Massive air trapping may be confused with tension pneumothorax, and a thoracostomy tube may be inadvertently placed into the affected side. Treatment consists of bronchoscopic removal of the mucous plug and possibly even bronchial lavage.

STRUCTURAL EVENTS IN THE DEVELOPMENT OF BAROTRAUMA

Macklin and Macklin defined a division in the bronchial tree of conducting and respiratory components. The respiratory element predominates in the periphery of the lung. However, expansion of the lung takes place throughout the whole lung during inspiration. The alveoli are of two types:

• Those whose bases lie against other alveoli (described as "partitional" by Macklin and Macklin)
• Those whose bases rest against some structure other than adjoining alveoli.

The latter group, whose bases are on bronchi, bronchial blood vessels, and connective tissue septa or pleura, are probably the source of the development of pulmonary interstitial emphysema. Pores exist between alveoli of the first type, so that the air can circulate from one alveolus to an adjoining one. However, when air escapes from the base of the second type of alveolus, it makes its way only into the underlying connective tissue. When air is drawn into the bronchial tree by enlargement of the thorax, the alveoli of the lung expand. As the alveoli abutting the bronchi and blood vessels open, the structures against which they rest must also change. The bronchial vessel elongates and at the same time expands in diameter. Pull of the expanding lung opens the vascular bed for increased blood flow during the inspiratory phase and opens the airway for greater inflow of air. The space between the alveolar bases and the bronchiolar vessel lumen stays constant in volume throughout the respiratory cycle because its interstices are filled with nonexpansile tissue fluid (Fig. 34–6).

If the alveoli are distended, and for whatever reason the vessel lumen is not correspondingly widened, a pressure gradient is created between the alveoli and the vascular sheath. Rupture of the bases takes place, and the air flows into the vascular sheath. Macklin and Macklin termed this factor overinflation factor A.

Macklin and Macklin also described factor B. In contrast to factor A, there is a second way in which a strong gradient between the alveolar base and the vascular sheath can be created: by a narrowing of the inner circle of vessel caliber without a corresponding diminution in the outer circle formed by the bases of surrounding alveoli. Although the features leading to the creation of factor A have been fairly widely accepted, the existence of the factor B conditions is largely undocumented.

After the introduction of air into the vascular sheath, continuation of the conditions that led to this rupture results in continued air leakage and accumulation of interstitial air. The accumulation of mediastinal air then leads to pneumothorax as the mediastinal pleura is ruptured. These conclusions have been fortified by various experimental data and autopsy studies, which appear to confirm the path of extra-alveolar air from the interstitium to the vascular sheath and finally to the mediastinum. In numerous radiologic series, pneumothorax was preceded first by the development of interstitial emphysema and pneumomediastinum.

Schaefer and colleagues examined mechanisms in the development of interstitial emphysema and air embolism on decompression from depth. Although they were primarily interested in decompression injuries and not in complications found in the intensive care unit, their clarification of the pathophysiology is important. Early studies had dem-

Pneumomediastinum results when sufficient interstitial air is accumulated and follows a path of least resistance toward the hilus.

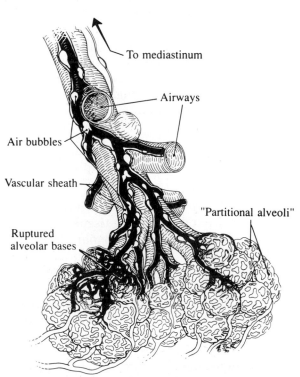

FIGURE 34–6: Development of interstitial emphysema. (Copyright 1990 by B. Smith.)

To mediastinum

Airways

Air bubbles

Vascular sheath

"Partitional alveoli"

Ruptured alveolar bases

onstrated that pulmonary rupture that occurs in dogs with an intratracheal pressure of 80 mm Hg can be prevented by controlling the distention of the abdomen and thorax with binders. Although control of distention could be the major benefit, the effects of binding on the circulation could not be discounted. Schaefer and colleagues examined the difference between intratracheal and intrapleural pressure (transpulmonic pressure), along with the difference between intratracheal and intra-atrial pressure (transatrial pressure). In experiments with instrumented dogs that were subjected to decompression from depth with tracheas open and closed, thoracoabdominal binding resulted in a significant rise in intrapleural, intra-atrial, pulmonary arterial, left atrial, and systemic venous pressures that was roughly parallel to the rise in intratracheal pressure. Thus, the effect of binding was to keep the transpulmonic and transatrial pressure gradients low. Without binding, systemic arterial pressure fell, and interstitial emphysema and air embolism developed. In their model, air embolism did not occur with transpulmonic gradients of less than 60 mm Hg or with transatrial gradients of less than 50 mm Hg, even when intratracheal pressure rose above 90 mm Hg. Necropsy findings supported Macklin and Macklin's data about the formation of interstitial air.

Immaturity may also be a risk factor in the development of barotrauma. Atkins and colleagues compared the effect of differing peak pressures (peak inspiratory pressures) in a group of 4- to 6-week-old rabbits with that in a group of adult rabbits. The young animals were exposed to 1 hour of peak airway pressure at 15, 30, and 45 cm H_2O, whereas the adult group received 1 hour at 15, 30, and 55 cm H_2O. The pulmonary capillary filtration coefficient was measured in an isolated lung perfusion system after the animals had been killed. This coefficient was significantly higher in the young rabbits than in the adult rabbits after ventilation with every level of peak inspiratory pressure. Pressure-volume loops demonstrated that immature rabbits had more compliant lungs and chest walls than adult rabbits. The increased coefficient was thought to indicate a higher baseline microvascular permeability. The immature animals were believed to be more susceptible to the development of ventilator-induced microvascular injury.

The site of injury, or the point at which pressure effects are most commonly seen, is usually the distal noncartilaginous airway. This is most clearly seen in immature infants with hyaline membrane disease, in whom the distal airways develop "ballooning" when the patient receives positive pressure ventilation. However, the distal airway, or alveolus, has been the apparent site of rupture in mature preparations as well.

EFFECTS OF BAROTRAUMA AT THE CELLULAR LEVEL

The importance of mechanical ventilation in the treatment of respiratory failure is undisputed. However, as with any therapy, the potential for side effects and complications is very real. The more clinically apparent complications of mechanical ventilation have been discussed. There are additional sequelae attributable to mechanical ventilation that are more subtle in their presentation. In many cases, these effects may not be distinguishable from the stigmata of the underlying disease process.

Treatment of the adult respiratory distress syndrome (ARDS) almost always includes mechanical ventilation. In patients from whom lung tissue is available for pathologic examination, the microscopic hallmark of early progressive ARDS is the presence of hyaline membrane. Some authors attribute hyaline membrane formation to oxygen therapy. Some evidence indicates that it is a manifestation of ventilator-induced injury.

Nilsson and coworkers induced hyaline membrane formation in the lungs of premature rabbits with mechanical ventilation for periods varying from 1 to 30 minutes. Fetuses were ventilated with a standardized tidal volume using no supplemental oxygen. Necrosis and desquamation of the bronchiolar epithelium was a constant finding in all fetuses that had been ventilated for 5 minutes or longer. The epithelial lesions seemed to reflect shear stress in the airway mucosa secondary to overdistention of preterminal conducting airways in a surfactant-deficient airway.

Dreyfus and associates used a murine model to show that mechanical ventilation with peak airway pressures (peak inspiratory pressures) of greater than 45 cm H_2O induced pulmonary edema. Four groups of animals were studied. Group 1 animals received mechanical ventilation with normal airway pressures of 7 cm H_2O for 30 minutes and served as a control group. Group 2 animals received mechanical ventilation with airway pressures of 45 cm H_2O for 5 minutes after 25 minutes of normal mechanical ventilation. Group 3 animals received peak airway pressures of 45 cm H_2O after 25 minutes of normal mechanical ventilation. Group 4 animals received mechanical ventilation for 20 minutes with peak airway pressures of 45 cm H_2O after 10 minutes of normal mechanical ventilation. At the completion of the study, physiologic data were collected, including extravascular lung water measurements. Some animals in each group were subsequently killed for anatomic studies, including electron microscopy. The findings in group 4 differed significantly from those in the other groups. In these animals, increased extravascular lung water and fractional albumin uptake per unit of sodium space were seen, reflecting increased extracellular water and increased transvascular protein flux. In group 4 rats, alveolar edema was diffuse, but it was markedly increased in the alveoli surrounding the bronchovascular space in subpleural areas. All animals in groups 2 to 4 were found to have damage of the blood-air interface at the ultrastructural level. Group 2 and 3 animals were found to have endothelial cell detachment. Group 4 animals had severe damage to type I cells, along with endothelial cell detachment and ultrastructural derangements. In a follow-up study in rats, these investigators showed a protective effect of PEEP during pulmonary edema experimentally induced by high-volume ventilation.

Kolobow and colleagues explored the effects of continued mechanical ventilation at peak airway pressures of 50 cm H_2O in healthy anesthetized adult sheep during a 48-hour period. The animals were divided into three groups. The control group of nine animals was ventilated with 40% oxygen and peak inspiratory pressures of 15 to 20 cm H_2O. In the second group, seven animals were ventilated with 40% oxygen and peak airway pressures of 50 cm H_2O with tidal volumes of 50 to 70 mL/kg. In the third group of animals, ventilatory parameters were identical to those in the second group, except that 3.8% carbon dioxide was added to the inspired gas to prevent transient pulmonary capillary alkalosis. During the first hours of the study, lung function remained excellent. Over the next 12 hours, however, a progressive decline in functional residual capacity, total lung compliance, and oxygenation was seen in all of the group 2 animals and in six of the nine animals in group 3. Severe atelectasis involving more than 50% of the lung was found at autopsy. Two animals in the second group and two animals in the third group developed pneumothorax. The authors concluded that mechanical ventilation with peak airway pressures in excess of 50 cm H_2O leads to progressive impairment in pulmonary mechanics and lung function.

Tsuno and associates, working with a piglet model, compared animals that were ventilated with peak airway pressures of 30 cm H_2O with a control group that had airway pressures maintained at less than 18 cm H_2O. Five piglets were killed for pathologic study after mechanical ventilation of 22 ± 11 hours. Light microscopy revealed alveolar hemorrhage, alveolar neutrophil infiltration, and type II cell proliferation. In addition, hyaline membranes were observed. These lesions were very similar to those seen in the early stages of ARDS. The control animals received mechanical ventilation for 3 to 6 days, with conventional respiratory care and appropriate ventilation. In addition to the lesions found in the earlier animals, a prominent alveolar exudate was found. These findings were indistinguishable from the chronic stage of ARDS. Six control animals ventilated with low peak airway pressures were found to have no change in lung function, gas exchange, or histopathologic findings. Parker and colleagues used an isolated, blood-perfused lung lobe model to explore the mechanism of this phenomenon. The left lower lobe of mongrel dogs was subjected to differing peak airway pressures ranging from 5 to 60 cm H_2O. The measured filtration coefficient was significantly increased in all models in which peak airway pressure exceeded 42 cm H_2O. The authors concluded that mechanical ventilation with airway pressures in excess of 42 cm H_2O was associated with a significant increase in microvascular permeability.

Schwieler and Robertson ventilated premature rabbits with air, oxygen, and oxygenated fluorocarbon. Histologic examination of the lungs from fetuses ventilated with air or oxygen revealed widespread necrosis and desquamation of the epithelium in conducting airways. Several preterminal airspaces were outlined with hyaline membranes containing remnants of necrotic epithelium. The animals exposed to fluorocarbon liquid had no hyaline membranes and little or no necrosis of bronchiolar epithelium. The results were thought to indicate that oxygen alone, without the trauma of ventilation (as provided by the fluorocarbon liquid), was not enough to cause damage to epithelium and the formation of hyaline membranes.

McAdams and coworkers examined the formation of hyaline membranes in premature rhesus monkeys. As with the experience in rabbits, epithelial damage and hyaline membrane formation were seen very early. Basement membrane and endothelial cells were not altered. Mechanical ventilation was essential for the production of epithelial necrosis, although the authors postulated that it played a facilitative rather than a primary role.

Presenti and colleagues compared premature lambs treated with apneic oxygenation (lung inflated to a constant intrapulmonary pressure) and extracorporeal carbon dioxide removal with a control group whose lungs were treated only with mechanical ventilation. Lambs whose lungs were at a constant apneic inflation and that were maintained by extracorporeal carbon dioxide removal rapidly improved and were soon maintained on normal ventilation. Lambs treated with mechanical ventilation alone did poorly. Five of seven so treated died within the first 24 hours of severe hyaline membrane disease.

Although these animal data tend to incriminate mechanical ventilation as the cause of hyaline membrane disease, a deficiency of surfactant may also play a role in the neonate. Lungs that have never been expanded or aerated may respond differently to injurious stimuli than do adult lungs.

Hayatdavoudi and associates studied lung injury in mature rats after oxygen exposure. While measuring the total lung capacity in intact animals, they observed that some oxygen-exposed animals developed pulmonary edema, whereas none of the control animals did. To explore the hypothesis that overdistention with large tidal volumes increased susceptibility to oxygen injury, animals were ventilated for 30 minutes at peak pressures of 30 and 40 cm H_2O. The lungs were then removed, and the ratio of wet weight to dry weight was determined. Animals exposed to 60% oxygen had normal lung weights and a normal lung wet weight–dry weight ratio if they were not subjected to mechanical ventilation or if they were ventilated at peak pressures of 30 cm H_2O. Control animals ventilated at 40 cm H_2O had a 50% greater lung wet weight. Animals exposed to 60% oxygen for 7 days and then ventilated at 40 cm H_2O had a 200% greater lung wet weight. The combination of repeated stretching of the pulmonary capillary bed along with the injury to the capillary bed induced by oxygen was believed to explain the greater degree of pulmonary edema in exposed animals.

An early study by Capers (1961) reported 37 cases of hyaline membrane formation in adults from a review of the autopsy files of the Dallas Veterans Administration Hospital. Among other features, it was noted that intermittent positive pressure breathing seemed to be "of some significance for the development of the membrane." This observation was also made by Barter and coworkers, who reported 10 cases of hyaline membrane formation in adults. Therapy with oxygen and intermittent positive pressure ventilation was believed to be a highly significant factor in the development of hyaline membranes.

Like all other therapies, mechanical ventilation has its risks. In the case of severe respiratory failure, the therapy may compound or at least prolong the lesion it is intended to treat. In the case of ARDS, it is difficult to determine the degree to which mechanical ventilation perpetuates the lesion. Patients who are hypoxemic and hypercarbic must be immediately treated with the therapy available despite the risk of compounding the underlying problems. Newer techniques have not yet proved to be superior to conventional ventilation. Several promising developments are currently under investigation.

It may eventually be possible to avoid the use of mechanical ventilation. Mortensen and colleagues described an intravascular device that, when placed in the inferior vena cava of laboratory animals, is capable of adding oxygen to and removing carbon dioxide from circulating blood. Such a device could sustain patients in respiratory failure. It could also be used in conjunction with mechanical ventilation, lowering the required level of support and therefore minimizing the risk of complications.

ADULT RESPIRATORY DISTRESS SYNDROME

Whether as a result of PEEP or of the disease process itself, ARDS is associated with a high incidence of barotrauma.

ARDS merits special attention. The syndrome was originally described by Ashbaugh and associates in 1967. They reported on 12 patients with the complex of severe dyspnea, tachypnea, and cyanosis that is refractory to oxygen therapy and is associated with diffuse alveolar infiltrates on chest x-ray studies and loss of lung compliance. They noted that the pathophysiology of this illness closely resembled that of the neonatal respiratory distress syndrome. They also reported that three of five patients with this syndrome who were treated with PEEP survived, whereas only two of seven patients survived who were not so treated. PEEP has long been advocated as the cornerstone of therapy for ARDS, although Ashbaugh and associates noted that it "merely buys time" until the underlying process is reversed.

The lesions seen on lung biopsy of patients with ARDS may vary, depending on the duration of ARDS before the time of biopsy. At the onset of disease, interstitial edema, often associated with fibrin thrombi in small vessels, is the major finding. Platelet and leukocyte aggregates are also seen, as are hyaline membranes. Hyaline membranes are the microscopic hallmark of early progressive ARDS. Marked capillary congestion and interstitial edema are also seen. The hyaline membrane is commonly found along alveoli making up the walls of the alveolar ducts. By electron microscopy, the membrane can be seen to be composed of fibrin, other proteins, and debris from necrotic cells (e.g., type 1 epithelium and macrophages).

Hyaline membranes, edema, and vascular congestion decrease with time. Alveolar epithelialization and interstitial fibrosis become progressively more prominent with time. The fibrosis involves primarily the alveolar ducts. This characteristic pattern allows the pathologist to recognize progressive ARDS on the basis of morphology alone.

Late-resolving ARDS is characterized by severe alveolar duct fibrosis, which apparently may resolve as the patient recovers. In one patient recovering from ARDS, bundles of loose fibrous tissue were noted within the alveolar ducts on microscopic examination, but the lungs appeared grossly normal. Macrophages were seen infiltrating these bundles, presumably lysing the collagen.

The etiology of these lesions is not clear, although both oxygen and barotrauma have been implicated. Kolobow and colleagues found that healthy sheep ventilated at peak airway pressures of 50 cm H_2O developed acute respiratory failure and alveolar cellular dysfunction. Pulmonary mechanics were also deranged. Sheep so ventilated died within 2 to 35 hours. All had highly abnormal lung parenchyma at autopsy.

Woodring reported on 15 consecutive patients with ARDS who were treated with mechanical ventilation. Pulmonary interstitial emphysema was seen in 13 of the 15 (87%). Ten of these patients also had pneumothorax. Half of the pneumothoraces appeared within 12 hours after the development of pulmonary interstitial emphysema was observed. The first radiographic evidence of pulmonary interstitial emphysema appeared at an average peak airway pressure of 45 cm H_2O (range, 18 to 59), a PEEP of 6 cm H_2O (range, 0 to 10), and a mean airway pressure of 14 cm H_2O (range, 4 to 28). There was no correlation between barotrauma and mean airway pressure or PEEP. In 12 of 13 patients, all manifestations of barotrauma occurred at or above a peak airway pressure of 40 cm H_2O.

Pratt and others have suggested that oxygen is the etiologic agent in the development of ARDS. Others have suggested that ARDS is a manifestation of barotrauma. The combination of high ventilatory pressures and oxygen is toxic to lung tissue.

POSITIVE END-EXPIRATORY PRESSURE

PEEP is commonly implicated as a cause of barotrauma. Its actual use dates back to 1938, when continuous positive pressure breathing was

The hyaline membrane is an eosinophilic layer found along the surface of the alveoli.

The association between the development of ARDS and pulmonary interstitial emphysema may rest on the effect of high peak pressures rather than on the use of PEEP. The alveolar duct may be the vulnerable site in ARDS, with the problem compounded by low compliance and other lung injury.

introduced by Barach and colleagues to treat acute pulmonary edema secondary to congestive heart failure. In the 1940s, it was studied as a means of preventing hypoxemia in pilots flying at high altitudes. However, the most common clinical use of PEEP was sparked by the experience of Ashbaugh and associates, who documented its efficacy in supporting oxygenation in patients with ARDS.

The most prominent benefit of PEEP therapy is an increased PaO_2, which permits a reduction in FIO_2 and reduces the risk of oxygen toxicity. The apparent mechanism for PaO_2 improvement is the prevention of airspace collapse and an increase in functional residual capacity. These effects seem to account for the decrease in pulmonary shunting that often results from the use of PEEP. Despite its utility, PEEP is not a panacea for ARDS. It has several deleterious effects on the cardiopulmonary system. Elevated airway pressure (and hence pleural pressure) is associated with decreased cardiac output. A variety of investigators have associated PEEP with an increased incidence of barotrauma.

PEEP may indirectly affect lung compliance. As PEEP is increased, the retrieval of collapsed alveoli improves compliance by increasing the functional residual capacity and raising the index inspiration point to a steeper portion of the pressure-volume curve. However, when alveoli become overdistended, they exhibit decreased compliance as the elastic properties of the lung are exceeded.

Radiographic changes after the institution of PEEP therapy may be quite striking. The most obvious manifestation is an increase in lung volume. The reversal of atelectasis and the shift of lung water from the alveoli may also contribute to radiographic improvement.

Complications of PEEP can be difficult to recognize. Whereas pneumothorax and pneumomediastinum are usually recognized on the chest radiograph, other manifestations of PEEP-induced barotrauma can be more subtle. Some complications may extend beyond the thorax. As previously described, air can be conducted to a wide variety of sites distal to the lung.

Monitoring PEEP therapy requires not only radiographic surveillance but careful attention to oxygen delivery, cardiac output, and lung compliance. Despite the concern about the predisposition to barotrauma, some studies suggest that PEEP is not a cause of injury and that very high levels of PEEP can be therapeutic and safe. Because the exact mechanism by which PEEP exerts its therapeutic benefit is still unknown, careful monitoring is indicated whenever it is used.

Monitoring PEEP and titrating therapy can be difficult. Various physiologic indices can be used, but the majority require invasive measurements and some degree of sophistication. Hemodynamic monitoring is important in avoiding deleterious effects on oxygen delivery. Monitoring of static compliance has been proposed as a method of monitoring PEEP and its effects. Although this is easily done, it may not be reliable.

Most discussions of PEEP in ARDS are conducted with the presumption that there is no PEEP unless it is instituted therapeutically. Broseghini and coworkers studied 14 consecutive patients with ARDS to determine respiratory resistance and compliance to assess the influence of "intrinsic" PEEP. They found that ARDS patients, like patients with chronic obstructive pulmonary disease, may have increased respiratory resistance with marked frequency dependence. They also noted that substantial added resistance is provided by the endotracheal tube, ventilation tubing, and attached devices. Intrinsic PEEP is not uncommon and

Although the alveolar-arterial oxygen gradient may narrow as PEEP is raised, oxygen delivery may actually fall as a result of decreased cardiac output.

Alveolar overdistention is thought to be a cause of the increased frequency of pneumothorax in patients receiving high levels of PEEP.

in these circumstances may lead to significant overestimation of static compliance.

THERAPY FOR PULMONARY BAROTRAUMA

With pulmonary barotrauma, as with most other medical conditions, the most effective treatment is prevention. Injuries secondary to mechanical ventilation range from the emergent to the subtle. Tension pneumothorax is probably the most frightening complication of barotrauma. Its immediate consequences are also the most readily treated. Chest tube thoracostomy is life saving and must be instituted immediately. In preparation for the insertion of a chest tube, the tension pneumothorax can be converted to an open pneumothorax by the insertion of a large-bore intravenous catheter into the intercostal space. This allows escape of the gas under tension, which usually results in the return of hemodynamic stability. Interstitial emphysema and pneumomediastinum are much more difficult to treat. Reports exist of improvement with the placement of mediastinal tubes. However, such insertion is difficult and hazardous. Once a chest tube is in place, it generally must remain throughout the course of mechanical ventilation.

Patients with ARDS present a particular therapeutic challenge. They require a high inspired oxygen tension but develop very noncompliant lungs, necessitating high peak inspiratory pressures and high levels of PEEP. Pressure control inverse ratio ventilation has been used effectively in patients with ARDS. The tidal volume in inverse ratio ventilation is generated at a constant pressure throughout the inspiratory time. Inspiratory flow decelerates once the peak inspiratory pressure has been reached. Peak inspiratory pressure is determined by the ventilator settings. Thus, peak inspiratory pressure, respiratory rate, and inspiratory time determine the minute ventilation delivered to each patient. This generally improves oxygenation, possibly from increased mean airway pressures and more even distribution of gas. A number of case reports and clinical series have suggested that this is an effective mode of ventilating patients with ARDS or severe bilateral pneumonia. However, it is not a comfortable mode of ventilation. Patients usually require heavy sedation, paralysis, or both for the technique to be effective (see Chapter 24).

Most conditions requiring mechanical ventilation are diffuse and bilateral. However, occasionally one lung will be more extensively involved than the other. Under these circumstances, ventilation and modalities such as PEEP are even more hazardous because of the tendency to deliver pressure preferentially to the less involved lung. Such conditions can be addressed by independent ventilation of each lung. Although the indications for such therapy are limited, it is possible to successfully ventilate lungs independently.

In the presence of established barotrauma, conventional ventilation may be less effective. In respiratory failure, convective gas distribution within the lung is generally abnormal. Adequate alveolar ventilation and arterial oxygenation can be maintained with ventilators that give tidal volumes substantially smaller than those of conventional ventilators. These devices operate at respiratory rates that are higher and sometimes substantially higher than more conventional respiratory rates (high-frequency ventilation). Adequate ventilation and oxygenation can usually be provided at lower peak inspiratory pressures. These modalities may

Chest tubes must be removed cautiously, usually after the acute illness has subsided.

If expiratory time is short enough, intrinsic PEEP may develop, which prevents alveoli from falling below their closing volume.

therefore be helpful in patients with significant **pre-existing** barotrauma or bronchopleural fistulas.

Despite the low tidal volumes generated by **high-frequency** ventilators, overdistention injury may occur. This can happen if there is insufficient time or space for jetted gas to be exhaled. Pressure builds in the tracheobronchial tree, and the point of rupture may not be close to the jet catheter. In cases in which only a small-bore jet catheter is placed, simple events such as the closure of vocal cords may result in overdistention. Migration or dislocation of the ventilator tube such that only a lobe or segment receives the full driving pressure also results in barotrauma. These problems may be prevented by the use of conventional endotracheal tubes that have a separate lumen for jet ventilation. This ensures adequate exhalation space and ease of securing the tube. In addition, the tube is less likely to migrate than a small-bore catheter (see Chapter 24 for further discussion of high-frequency ventilation).

Regardless of the methods used in the acute treatment of pulmonary barotrauma, the more obvious manifestations tend to resolve as the patient's underlying condition improves. Case reports suggest that interstitial emphysema, subcutaneous emphysema, pneumomediastinum, pneumoperitoneum, and pneumothorax all tend to resolve with improvement in the patient's overall condition. Few data exist to explain the course of recovery at the cellular level within the lung itself.

SUMMARY

Pneumothorax and its associated sequelae are the most obvious, but certainly not the only, manifestations of injury from mechanical ventilation. Barotrauma takes a variety of forms, and its initiation can be a very subtle event.

The occurrence of pneumothorax is not dependent on the rupture of peripheral airspaces. Rather, the initial injury seems to occur where alveoli abut the vascular bundle. Air then tracks along the vascular bundle toward the mediastinum. At this stage, the manifestations are usually limited to interstitial gas and can be very difficult to discern radiographically. As the process progresses, air accumulates in the mediastinum, where it often becomes more apparent. Sufficient pressure may accumulate to affect ventilation and circulation, or the mediastinal pleura may rupture, leading to pneumothorax.

The pressure gradient and thus the distention induced by insufflation are much more important in the development of pulmonary barotrauma than is the insufflation pressure itself. Animals whose abdominal and thoracic expansion is limited by external binding do not develop barotrauma even with very high insufflation pressures. Both animal studies and clinical experience suggest that peak inspiratory pressures in excess of 40 cm H_2O predispose to barotrauma. Several disease states, such as aspiration, pneumonia, and ARDS, are also associated with an increased incidence of barotrauma.

Mechanical ventilation induces other changes at the cellular level. There is evidence that ventilation itself causes epithelial injury that results in the formation of hyaline membranes. It also appears to potentiate the injury caused by high concentrations of inspired oxygen. The injudicious use of mechanical ventilation may, in fact, prolong the existence of the lesion it is intended to treat.

Avoiding barotrauma is far superior to responding to its occurrence. Alternative modes of mechanical ventilation may offer the ability to avoid dangerously high peak inspiratory pressures. This, in conjunction with tried and true methods of treating acute respiratory failure, should decrease the morbidity if not the mortality of the ventilated patient.

Suggested Readings

Ashbaugh D, Bigelow D, Petty T, Levine B. Acute respiratory distress in adults. Lancet 2:319–323, 1967.

Atkins WK, Hernandez LA, Coker PJ, et al. Age affects susceptibility to pulmonary barotrauma in rabbits. Crit Care Med 19:390–393, 1991.

Barter R, Finlay-Jones L, Walters N. Pulmonary hyaline membranes: Sites of formation in adult lungs after assisted respiration and inhalation of oxygen. J Pathol Bacteriol 95:481–488, 1968.

Broseghini C, Brandolese R, Poggi R, et al. Respiratory resistance and intrinsic positive end-expiratory pressure (PEEPi) in patients with the adult respiratory distress syndrome (ARDS). Eur Respir J 1:726–731, 1988.

Caldwell E, Powell R, Mullooly J. Interstitial emphysema: A study of physiologic factors involved in experimental induction of lesion. Am Rev Respir Dis 102:516–525, 1970.

Capers T. Pulmonary hyaline membrane formation in the adult. Am J Med 31:701–710, 1961.

Dreyfus B, Basset G, Soler P, Sammon G. Intermittent positive pressure hyperventilation with high inflation pressures produces pulmonary and microvascular injury in rats. Am Rev Respir Dis 132:880–884, 1985.

Fleming W, Bowen J, Hatcher C. Early complications of long-term respiratory support. J Thorac Cardiovasc Surg 64:729–738, 1972.

Hall JB, White SR, Karrison T. Efficacy of daily routine chest radiographs in intubated and mechanically ventilated patients. Crit Care Med 19:689–693, 1991.

Hayatdavoudi G, O'Neil J, Barry B, et al. Pulmonary injury in rats following continuous exposure to 60% O_2 for 7 days. J Appl Physiol 51:1220–1231, 1981.

Kolobow T, Moretti M, Fumagalli R, et al. Severe impairment in lung function induced by high peak airway pressure during mechanical ventilation. Am Rev Respir Dis 135:312–315, 1987.

Lenaghan R, Silva Y, Walt A. Hemodynamic alterations associated with expansion rupture of the lung. Arch Surg 99:339–343, 1969.

Luksa AR, Smith P, Coakley J, et al. Acute severe asthma treated by mechanical ventilation: Ten years' experience from a district general hospital. Thorax 41:459–463, 1986.

Macklin M, Macklin C. Malignant interstitial emphysema of the lungs and mediastinum as an important occult complication in many respiratory diseases and other conditions. Medicine 23:281–358, 1944.

Marini J, Culver B. Systemic gas embolism complicating mechanical ventilation in the adult respiratory distress syndrome. Ann Intern Med 110:699–703, 1989.

McAdams A, Coen R, Kleinman L, et al. The experimental production of hyaline membranes in premature rhesus monkey's. Am J Pathol 70:277–290, 1973.

Mortensen J, Berry G. Conceptual and design features of a practical, clinically effective intravenous mechanical blood oxygen/carbon dioxide exchange device (IVOX). Int J Artif Organs 12:384–389, 1989.

Nilsson R, Grossman G, Robertson B. Bronchiolar epithelial lesions induced in the premature rabbit neonate by short periods of artificial ventilation. Acta Pathol Microbiol Scand Sect 88:359–367, 1980.

Parker JC, Townsley MI, Rippe B, et al. Increased microvascular permeability in dog lungs due to high peak airway pressures. J Appl Physiol 57:1809–1816, 1984.

Pontoppidan H. Treatment of respiratory failure in nonthoracic trauma. J Trauma 8:938–951, 1968.

Pratt P. Pathology of adult respiratory distress syndrome: Implications regarding therapy. Semin Respir Med 4:79–85, 1982.

Presenti A, Kolobow T, Buckhold D, et al. Prevention of hyaline membrane disease in premature lambs by apneic oxygenation and extracorporeal carbon dioxide removal. Intensive Care Med 8:11–17, 1982.

Schaefer K, McNulty W, Carey C, Liebow A. Mechanisms in development of interstitial emphysema and air embolism on decompression from depth. J Appl Physiol 13:15–29, 1958.

Schwieler G, Robertson B. Liquid ventilation in immature newborn rabbits. Biol Neonate 29:343–353, 1976.

Steier M, Ching N, Roberts E, Nealon T. Pneumothorax complicating continuous ventilatory support. J Thorac Cardiovasc Surg 67:17–23, 1974.

Tsuno K, Miura K, Takeya M, et al. Histologic pulmonary changes from mechanical ventilation and high peak airway pressures. Am Rev Respir Dis 143:1115–1120, 1991.

Woodring J. Pulmonary interstitial emphysema in the adult respiratory distress syndrome. Crit Care Med 10:786–791, 1985.

Zwillich C, Pierson D, Creach C, et al. Complications of assisted ventilation. Am J Med 57:161–170, 1974.

Atelectasis

Continuous Positive Airway
Pressure (CPAP)

Incentive Spirometry (IS)

Intermittent Positive Pressure
Breathing (IPPB)

Laplace's Law

Sigh

Sustained Maximal
Inspiration (SMI)

35

Atelectasis: Pathophysiology and Treatment

Eric D. Bakow, M.A., R.T.T.

Atelectasis has long persisted as a clinical problem in many disease states and following surgery. In many ways, the field of respiratory care may trace much of its evolution to the pursuit of clinical interventions that prevent or treat this lung condition.

The incidence of atelectasis in the postsurgical patient varies and depends on many variables, including pre-existing patient risk factors and the surgical procedure performed. The incidence of clinically significant atelectasis may range from 6 to 75% in abdominal and thoracic surgery[1] and be as high as 61 to 84.5% after cardiopulmonary bypass.[2]

This chapter deals with

- The pathophysiology and clinical sequelae of atelectasis
- The efficacy of preoperative screening of patients
- Methods, old and new, in the treatment of "incomplete expansion" of the lung, with an emphasis on research methodologies in clinical studies that address these therapeutic modalities

PATHOPHYSIOLOGY

Some investigators describe the lung as a nonhomogeneous colloid of blood and air. Inherent in this notion is the image of millions of air-containing structures tethered to airways to form the parenchyma of the lung. Of course, gas transport is not the only physiologic function of the lung; however, this chapter focuses on this function. These air-containing structures are often depicted as round "air sacs" that fit nicely into physical laws defining spherical stability. Electron microscopy has demonstrated that alveoli are not round but may take on a variety of shapes, depending on their anatomic location and the body position of the lung.[3] Additionally, the transpulmonary pressure gradient (alveolar pressure–pleural pressure) that expands alveoli is not constant along the upright lung. This results in variations in the resting volume of the alveoli at functional residual capacity (FRC). Specifically, alveoli at the apex of the lung tend to be larger than those at the base of the lung. Gravity acts on the mass of lung tissue; this force tends to compress adjacent structures, also resulting in reduced alveolar volumes in "gravity-dependent" areas of the lung.

Alveolar volume and pressure are dynamic commodities that are in a constant state of flux. Surface tension results when molecules of different substances, gas and liquids, cause this interface to act like a stretched rubber membrane.[4] The end-result of this process is that a spherical structure tends to collapse with increases in surface tension. Surfactant, an acronym for surface-active agent, contains the substance

Laplace's law defines the mathematical model for such a system:

$$P = \frac{2T}{R}$$

where P is the pressure tending to collapse the alveolus, T is the surface tension, and R is the radius of the alveolar space.

dipalmitoyl lecithin, which acts to reduce the surface tension at the air-liquid emulsion of the alveolar lining. Reductions in this substance, for example by the immaturity of the type II cells that secrete this substance, result in the diffuse atelectasis common to infant respiratory distress syndrome. Although a more formal relationship can be used for nonspherical objects,[5] Laplace's law adequately describes the dynamic for our purposes. The collapsing tendency of the alveolar space is inversely related to its radius and directly proportional to the surface tension of the sphere. This explains why areas of lung that are underventilated relative to perfusion (i.e., areas with low $\dot{V}/\dot{Q}$ ratios) tend to become atelectatic: their reduced radius increases the pressure tending to collapse the airspace.

Of course, many factors may contribute to a reduction in alveolar ventilation. However, a monotonous tidal breathing pattern, devoid of intermittent deep breaths, seems to be the salient variable that leads to alveolar collapse. In their classic 1963 study, Bendixen and coworkers produced a 22% reduction in Pa_{O_2} and a 15% fall in compliance in 18 surgical patients who received general anesthesia with a ventilatory pattern that eliminated periodic deep breaths.[6] Figure 35–1 shows the data from this study. Note the rapid responses in both negative and positive changes in Pa_{O_2} and compliance. This initial study period, which averaged 76 minutes, was then followed by the reintroduction of mechanical sighs to the ventilatory pattern. This took the form of three successively deep breaths, spaced 4 or 5 minutes apart, that were sustained for

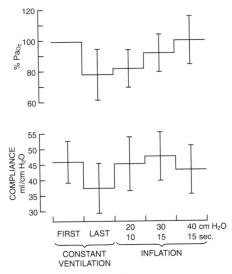

FIGURE 35–1: Average falls (with standard deviations) in oxygen tension and in total lung compliance as difference between first and last measurements during constant ventilation. Three successive inflations restore previous levels of compliance (with the first inflation) and oxygen tension (in steps). (From Bendixen H, Hedley-Whyte J, Laver MB. Impaired oxygenation in surgical patients during general anesthesia with controlled ventilation: A concept of atelectasis. Reprinted, by permission, from the New England Journal of Medicine 269[19]:991–996, 1963.)

several seconds. These sighs resulted in the return to baseline of both Pa_{O_2} and compliance within seconds of the deep breaths. The investigators concluded that "shallow tidal volumes lead to atelectasis and increased shunting," whereas "large tidal volumes appear to protect against falls in oxygen tension, presumably by providing continuous hyperinflation."[6]

Zikria and associates later established evidence that monotonous tidal breathing occurs in the postsurgical state in their study of 12 patients who were evenly divided between upper and lower abdominal surgery groups.[7] The investigators used spirometric tracings of the patients' breathing patterns 24 hours after surgery and found a 20% reduction in tidal volume and a 47% reduction in respiratory rate. Importantly, these authors also noted the complete elimination of sighing in the ventilatory pattern. These changes were found in patients who had upper abdominal surgery but were not present in those who had lower abdominal surgery. Narcotics and pain may eliminate the sigh mechanism and result in a pattern of monotonous tidal ventilation.[8] Other reasons for a reduction in alveolar ventilation include central nervous system depression, chronic obstructive pulmonary disease (COPD), thoracic pump abnormalities, and the presence of airway secretions. All of these factors could be important in reducing ventilation to the acinus such that alveolar volume and FRC are reduced. These variables produce a synergistic effect in that reductions in FRC lead to reductions in lung compliance, sputum retention, and hypoxemia. Figure 35–2 depicts this sequence of events that may eventually lead to infection, respiratory or ventilatory failure, or death. The introduction of deep breathing into the ventilatory pattern is needed to prevent or arrest this process at an early stage.

Absorption atelectasis describes the denitrogenation of the alveolar space with a subsequent loss of alveolar volume. Increased alveolar P_{O_2} levels have a resultant impact on the partial pressure of nitrogen in the alveolar space (P_{N_2}). This is due to Dalton's law of partial pressures, which states that the total gas pressure of a system must remain constant despite changes in the constituent gases of the system. So, while the alveolar P_{O_2} increases, there must be a concomitant decrease in the alveolar P_{N_2} to maintain a constant total alveolar pressure. Dale and Rahn described nitrogen as the "brake against atelectasis" because of this process.[9] However, the removal of nitrogen is not the only crucial variable. An additional defect, that of reduced alveolar ventilation, combines with denitrogenation of the alveolar space to produce lung collapse.[5] Airway closure, due to mucus plugging or an elevated closing volume, results in gas that is essentially "trapped" in the alveolar space. That is, this gas is not replenished with the next inspiratory phase of gas movement. In this scenario, alveolar volume, which is principally determined by the PA_{O_2} in the hyperoxygenated patient, is rapidly diminished as oxygen diffuses from the alveolar space into the capillary. This movement of oxygen is due to the lower total gas pressure of mixed venous blood compared with the total gas pressure in the alveolar space. The higher the $F_{I_{O_2}}$, the more rapidly this process can occur.[5, 9] Therefore, the combination of oxygen therapy and any one of several mechanisms of reduced alveolar ventilation (e.g., blunted drive to breathe, neuromuscular dysfunction, airway obstructive disease, or mucus plugging) predisposes the patient to absorption atelectasis.

Anesthesia presents a third major mechanism for the formation of atelectasis. A reduction in FRC by an average of 0.4 to 0.5 L has been

Nitrogen serves the important function of maintaining alveolar pressure and hence volume because this gas is not readily absorbed into the pulmonary capillary circulation.

Closing volume—the point in an expiratory maneuver in which collapse of the airways occurs

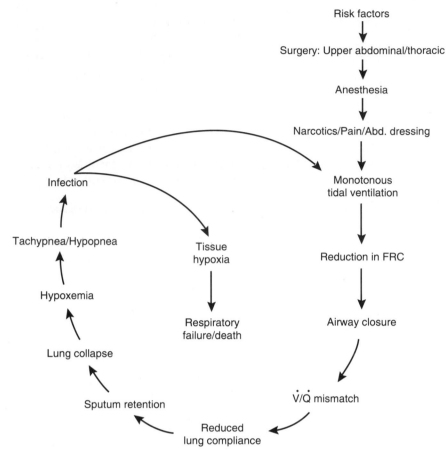

FIGURE 35–2: Pathogenetic mechanisms and sequelae of atelectasis. FRC, functional residual capacity.

measured during anesthesia.[10] Brismar and colleagues demonstrated a rapidly forming "crest-shaped" density detected by computed tomography (CT) in as little as 5 minutes after the induction of anesthesia.[11] This group postulated the cause of this density to be "compression atelectasis" that results from muscle paralysis. A possible mechanism may be that muscle relaxation causes an increase in the pleural pressure gradient surrounding the lung, thereby compressing and expelling gas from the airway.[11]

This notion is further supported by an apparent cephalad movement of the diaphragm with the use of general anesthesia. The ramifications of this change are important because Froese and Bryan noted a redistribution of inspired gas in supine patients who were paralyzed.[12] Specifically, they observed greater movement of *nondependent* lung zones with each mechanical inspiration. This was presumably due to the lower hydrostatic pressures placed on the diaphragm by the abdominal contents in this area (Figs. 35–3 and 35–4). Gravity-dependent areas of the lung, where the majority of blood flow occurs, were relatively hypoventilated, as demonstrated by little diaphragm excursion. Froese and Bryan also noted this same pattern when patients were placed in the left lateral decubitus position: the left lung responded as the posterior aspect in the earlier studies and received the majority of ventilation because of increased diaphragm displacement. It is interesting to note that this pattern was completely reversed in awake, spontaneously breathing pa-

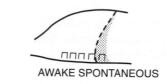

AWAKE SPONTANEOUS

ANESTHETIZED
SPONTANEOUS

PARALYZED

FIGURE 35–3: Diaphragm position and displacement during tidal breathing in a supine subject. Dashed lines indicate control functional residual capacity position of the diaphragm. Stippled areas represent diaphragmatic excursion during tidal breathing. (From Froese AB, Bryan AC. Effects of anesthesia in paralysis on diaphragmatic mechanics in man. Anesthesiology 41[3]:242–254, 1974.)

tients. Neither positive end-expiratory pressure nor large tidal breaths could restore ventilation to these areas. Although these data did not address atelectasis per se, they do illustrate the concept of reduced alveolar ventilation that may occur with anesthesia, which will set into motion progressive alveolar volume loss. It should be clear that this phenomenon applies to critically ill patients who are electively paralyzed, in addition to those patients in the operating room.

Additionally, other investigators have demonstrated a rapid onset of

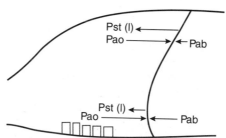

FIGURE 35–4: The balance of forces across the diaphragm in a dependent and a nondependent region during maintained positive airway pressure with the subject supine. The pressure relationships are shown for a lung volume large enough (e.g., greater than 60% of vital capacity) for transdiaphragmatic pressure to be zero in the relaxed subject. Therefore, Pst(l) = Pao − Pab in each region. Pao, airway pressure; Pst(l), elastic recoil pressure of the lung; Pab, abdominal pressure. (From Froese AB, Bryan AC. Effects of anesthesia in paralysis on diaphragmatic mechanics in man. Anesthesiology 41[3]:242–254, 1974.)

atelectasis with enflurane–nitrous oxide anesthesia that may be linked to the collapse of areas with low $\dot{V}/\dot{Q}$ ratios.[13] Klingstedt and coworkers also observed atelectasis formation with anesthesia induction and found the formation of collapse to be mainly distributed to gravity-dependent areas of the lung when patients were placed in lateral positions.[14] Using CT scans of the lung, they attributed these changes to alterations in lung geometry while patients were in the lateral position. Specifically, there were reductions in the transverse (lateral-lateral) diameter of the lung when the patient was turned from the supine to the lateral position. This positional change was associated with an almost doubling of the percentage of total atelectasis in the left lung when patients were placed in left lateral positions. The authors attributed these changes to atelectasis formation that was possibly due to mediastinal compression of lung tissue and a redistribution of blood volume.[14] Other related and important effects of anesthesia need to be highlighted here. Namely, general anesthesia has been known to produce a measurable increase in the ratio of dead space to tidal volume, an increase in shunt fraction, and a depression of mucociliary flow that may persist for 2 to 6 days.[15] If the effects of anesthesia are viewed collectively, it seems that general and prolonged anesthesia may contribute significantly to the formation of postoperative atelectasis.

Phrenic nerve damage also may lead to atelectasis. One recurring finding in patients who have had coronary artery bypass grafting (CABG) is left lower lobe collapse. Although the loss of volume may be bilateral, the persistent loss of volume on the left side has led investigators to hypothesize that the intraoperative use of a cold "slush" for topical cold cardioplegia may cause phrenic nerve damage and may therefore explain the left-sided atelectasis. In addition, Tulla and coworkers demonstrated that the rib cage contributed a greater proportion to tidal breathing in their study of 20 patients after CABG.[16] This implicates a reduced motion of the diaphragm in normal, quiet breathing. Wilcox and associates also examined the relationship of diaphragm function in the post-CABG patient and confirmed the preponderance of left-sided collapse in 57 patients following CABG.[17] Five patients in this study presented with "unequivocal" impairment in phrenic nerve conduction, with three of these patients having hemidiaphragm paralysis as confirmed by fluoroscopic examination. They also noted a reduction in phrenic nerve conduction (reduced amplitude in the latency to compound diaphragmatic action potentials) in 27 of these patients as compared with preoperative values. Because 90% of the patients in this study developed atelectasis of the left lower lobe, the authors concluded that factors other than phrenic nerve damage, such as the actual temperature of the cold slush and the duration of its application, may explain the incidence of left-sided lung collapse.

Spinal cord injury also is a major cause of phrenic nerve dysfunction that then progresses to atelectasis and infection. In fact, a summary of 20 years' experience in the treatment of cervical spine injuries by Bellamy and colleagues revealed a 40% incidence of death due to a pulmonary cause following spinal cord injury.[18] Fishburn and associates followed up 46 patients for the first 30 days after spinal cord injury and found that 53% of this population developed atelectasis and pneumonia in this period.[19] Interestingly, they found a large disparity in left versus right lung involvement, with 70% of the study patients developing left-sided pathology. No correlation was noted between the level of injury (a high level was involvement at C3, C4, or C5; a low level, involvement at

C6, C7, or C8) and the side of the lung involvement. The authors speculated that the predominance of left lung disease was due to the more acute angle of the left mainstem bronchus diverting from the trachea and the resultant adverse effect of that anatomy on the removal of secretions from the left lung.

RISK FACTORS

Atelectasis is one of the most common noninfectious pulmonary complications following surgery.[21]

Pre-existing patient conditions play an important role in predisposing the patient to the development of atelectasis. The two most important factors that predispose the patient to postoperative pulmonary complications (PPCs) are a history of smoking and the presence of obstructive lung disease.[20] In the context of this chapter, PPCs refer to increased cough and dyspnea, or atelectasis and pneumonia.

The time frame for smoking cessation in the avoidance of PPCs is an important variable. Cessation must occur approximately 8 weeks before surgery to achieve a statistically significant chance of reducing the incidence of PPCs.[22] Although smoking cessation that occurs in a more narrow window before surgery is certainly desirable, it may not result in a reduction in postoperative morbidity.

Pre-existing lung disease will predispose patients to an increased risk of developing PPCs.[23–25] Patients who present with a positive pulmonary history, a ratio of forced expiratory volume in 1 second to forced vital capacity (FVC) of less than 60%, a maximal ventilatory volume of 50%, and hypercapnia have been identified by Tisi as being at increased risk for PPCs.[21] Table 35–1 lists other risk factors that will influence the potential for atelectasis in patients who have had surgery. A multivariate study by Hall and associates found that fully 88% of patients who developed PPCs were identified by an age of older than 59 years and an American Society of Anesthesiology classification of greater than 1.[26]

Obviously, little can be done to positively influence the postoperative outcome of this patient population because the pre-existing disease is virtually not reversible in the short term preceding surgery. However, Celli emphasizes the need to begin postoperative care before surgery in an effort to optimize the patient's secretion status and therefore minimize postoperative morbidity.[20] A study by Stein and Cassara tested this strategy in 77 patients undergoing elective surgical procedures.[25] The majority of these patients had thoracic surgery (specific procedures were not reported) and abdominal surgery (again, specific procedures were not reported). The control group received traditional postoperative pulmo-

TABLE **35–1:** Risk Factors for the Development of Postoperative Pulmonary Complications

Age >59 yrs
ASA classification >2
Obesity
Chronic lung disease
Active or recent smoking
Duration of surgery
Surgical site
    Upper abdominal has more risk than thoracic
    Thoracic has more risk than lower abdominal
Surgical incision
    Lateral thoracic incision has more risk than median
    Subcostal incision has high risk

ASA, American Society of Anesthesiology.

nary care, whereas a second group received preoperative therapy that included smoking cessation, antibiotics as needed, deep breathing exercises, inhaled bronchodilators, and chest physiotherapy. This regimen was continued until the patient's condition was optimized, and for some it involved the delay of surgery until that condition was met. Twenty-one percent of the treatment group that received preoperative care developed PPCs, whereas 60% of the control group evidenced some form of PPCs. Additionally, the PPCs seen in the preoperative treatment group were clinically mild compared with those in the group that received postoperative care only. Patients were not randomized in this study design but were instead entered by members of the surgical service. This lack of randomization may imply a selection bias.

ROUTINE PREOPERATIVE SPIROMETRY

The value of routine preoperative spirometry to predict morbidity in the postoperative course is not clearly stated in the literature. At issue here is whether preoperative pulmonary function studies add any value to the management of postoperative patients that cannot already be perceived by a carefully constructed history and physical examination. A comprehensive review of existing studies that evaluated the role of routine preoperative spirometry was performed by Lawrence and coworkers.[27] They evaluated 135 clinical articles on this topic and concluded that serious methodologic flaws in the study designs precludes a definitive answer to the notion of spirometry as a value-added test in the postoperative course. Specifically, these authors identified the following flaws in 22 actual clinical studies (16% of the total of 135 papers reviewed) that assessed the predictive ability of spirometry:

1. Outcome assessments that were not blinded to the preoperative assessments of spirometry
2. The presence of selection bias in patient allocation to the study
3. Outcome measures that were poorly or incompletely defined
4. The presence of placebo or Hawthorne's effect (the patient's perception of well-being due to the use of medications or attention by medical staff that is unrelated to any actual therapeutic effect)

They concluded that the value of routine spirometry in predicting postoperative outcomes is unproved and that "generalizability from currently available studies to routine preoperative use of spirometry in patients undergoing abdominal surgery is limited." A similar conclusion regarding the efficacy of preoperative spirometry was reached by Zibrak and O'Donnell: available data do not support the contention that spirometry can reliably identify preoperative patients who will develop serious PPCs.[28] Interestingly, they do recommend the use of spirometry in patients who are currently cigarette smokers under the premise that this information may elicit a heightened "vigilance in the perioperative period and suggest helpful therapies." However, they cautiously note that even this assumption warrants further study.

CLINICAL FINDINGS

Atelectasis presents with various ausculatory findings that range from diminished or absent breath sounds to crackles and tubular sounds.

The general response to percussion is a dulled note with evidence of an elevated diaphragm over the affected area. With significant parenchymal involvement, the patient may evidence a tachypneic and hypopneic breathing pattern that also involves the use of accessory muscles. The need for supplemental oxygen is usually apparent at this point in the clinical course.

The radiographic findings of atelectasis include volume loss on the ipsilateral side with diaphragm elevation, mediastinal shift toward the affected side and displacement of the hilus, and fissures. The radiographic appearance of atelectasis is most often evidence of lobar involvement, although lung collapse may be difficult to distinguish from infiltrative disease or pleural fluid. There tends to be a recognizable pattern of radiographic changes as a function of the lobar anatomy that is involved.[29]

CLINICAL SEQUELAE

The insidious nature of this process should be underscored, because the development of alveolar collapse can be clinically undetected until a substantial amount of lung volume is involved. From the preceding discussion, it can be seen that as the process of alveolar collapse progresses, the stage is set for a "spiral effect" unless intervention occurs. Small reductions in alveolar volume result in reductions in the radius of the "sphere" (the acinus), which further increases the pressure tending to collapse the air sac (Laplace's law). The end-result of this progression is that the compliance of the lung unit is reduced, further impairing alveolar ventilation. This cycle self-perpetuates to complete collapse unless a significant intervention can reinflate the alveolus, restore alveolar compliance, and simultaneously reduce the pressure tending to collapse the airspace.

Because of the reduced lung compliance, a concomitant increase in the work of breathing is needed to maintain a physiologic alveolar minute volume. This may translate into a more energy-conserving breathing pattern that is characterized as both hypopneic (shallow tidal breathing) and tachypneic. Accessory muscle use and the complaint of shortness of breath are not uncommon at this point. Patients who present with respiratory muscle dysfunction are the first to manifest these signs and symptoms. Additionally, increases in both oxygen consumption and carbon dioxide production may result from the increased work of breathing that comes from these mechanical alterations.

Lindberg and coworkers compared traditional radiography and CT in 13 patients before and after anesthesia and for 4 days after abdominal surgery.[30] Using CT, this group found that six of the 13 patients demonstrated atelectasis while under anesthesia, and 11 (approximately 85%) evidenced atelectasis by 2 hours after surgery. This was associated with a doubling of the $P(A-a)O_2$. By the fourth postoperative day, 12 of 13 patients developed atelectasis on at least 1 day as determined by CT, whereas conventional radiography documented only one patient with atelectasis. These authors speculate that the more sensitive CT scan and the standard pulmonary x-ray study may be imaging lung collapse caused by different mechanisms: anesthesia-induced compression atelectasis that persists into the postoperative course may be seen on CT, and absorption atelectasis behind obstructed airways is possibly the pathology pictured on the routine radiographic images.[30] It is also interesting

Patients with lung collapse are also candidates for infection.

The process of lung infection may result in serious long-term effects, such as bronchiectasis, abscess formation, or parenchymal fibrosis.[32]

to note that only one patient developed fever in this study, and this patient had no findings of atelectasis on her radiograph. The one patient in this study who did evidence collapse on the chest x-ray film did not show any signs of infection and had minimal impairment of gas exchange or lung mechanics.

The study by Lindberg and coworkers is also interesting in that the authors were able to correlate atelectasis as per CT scan with other functional impairments: FVC and Pa_{O_2} (Figs. 35–5 and 35–6). It is worth noting that statistically significant correlations between the degree of lung collapse and the reduction in FVC or Pa_{O_2} existed for this patient population, despite the finding that only one of these patients presented with collapse by routine chest radiography. In addition, only one patient presented with fever but had normal chest x-ray findings. The authors found the majority of lung collapse to be in the dorsal and basal regions of the lungs and hypothesized airway closure as the pathogenetic mechanism.

Reductions in FRC as a result of lung collapse impair expiratory efforts to cough and inspiratory efforts to sigh and stretch (i.e., recruit) the lung parenchyma. This results in a patient who cannot clear secretions from the lung or maintain alveolar patency. Secretions then tend to become static, thereby favoring bacterial growth. Schlenker and Hubay noted that the lower airway is contaminated by oropharyngeal bacteria after surgery, but they were unable to demonstrate a correlation of this fact with the incidence of atelectasis, fever, or white blood cell elevation in an analysis of 151 patients who had abdominal surgery.[31] It is not surprising, then, that patients with lung collapse often develop a pulmonary infection.

TREATMENT

Many therapeutic approaches have come and gone over the years in the search for a truly effective way to treat atelectasis. One may recall blow bottles and carbon dioxide rebreathing techniques. Fortunately, these techniques have been shelved in favor of other approaches, but clearly no single intervention is as effective as one would like. The prin-

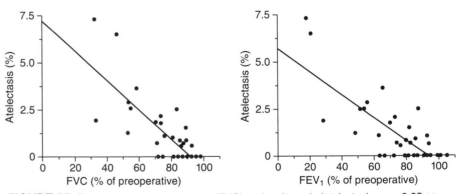

FIGURE 35–5: *Left,* Forced vital capacity (FVC) and atelectasis (atelectasis = $-0.08 \times$ FVC + 7.2, $r = -.78$, $P < .01$). *Right,* Forced expiratory volume in 1 second (FEV_1) and atelectasis (atelectasis = $-0.06 \times FEV_1 + 5.8$, $r = -.78$, $P < .01$). Postoperative data have been plotted (days 1, 2, and 4). (From Lindberg P, Gunnarsson L, Tokics L, et al. Atelectasis and lung function in the postoperative period. Acta Anaesthesiol Scand 36:546–553, 1992.)

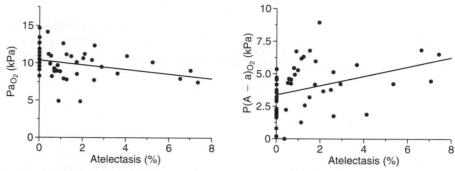

FIGURE 35–6: *Left*, Atelectasis and Pa_{O_2} ($Pa_{O_2} = -0.34 \times$ atelectasis $+ 10.4$, $r = -.33$, $P < .05$). *Right*, Atelectasis and $P(A - a)_{O_2}$ ($P(A - a)_{O_2} = 0.34 \times$ atelectasis $+ 3.4$, $r = .36$, $P < .01$). Postoperative data have been plotted (days 1, 2, and 4). (From Lindberg P, Gunnarsson L, Tokics L, et al. Atelectasis and lung function in the postoperative period. Acta Anaesthesiol Scand 36:546–553, 1992.)

ciples of atelectasis management, as outlined by Marini, are simple and straightforward: remove retained secretions from the airway and provide sufficient stretch to the lung tissue for the purpose of parenchymal re-expansion.[32]

Intraluminal secretions act to reduce alveolar ventilation, which can reduce lung volume and put into place the mechanisms that result in lung collapse. As many practitioners know, the removal of retained secretions can be most challenging in patients with existing lung disease. This task is difficult in a steady state, but when incisional pain, narcotics, binders, and wound dressings are added, the level of difficulty of this process elevates by an order of magnitude. Fortunately, the topic of bronchial hygiene is well covered in Chapter 21. Inhalation of beta-agonists, directed coughing, postural drainage therapy, positive expiratory pressure, and suctioning of the airway are all proven possibilities for the goal of sputum removal.

Perhaps less well defined is therapy to re-expand collapsed lung parenchyma. The ideal maneuver to recruit collapsed lung parenchyma is one in which a large transpulmonary pressure gradient and a large inflating volume are maintained for several seconds.[33] It is the transpulmonary pressure gradient that is responsible for "stretching" the lung and maintaining alveolar volume. Table 35–2 gives Bartlett and associates' original description of the ideal maneuver and a comparison of other therapies. Obviously, an inspiratory maneuver that can reliably reproduce these criteria will be useful in treating atelectasis. The current list of inspiratory maneuvers for this purpose now includes

- Sustained maximal inspiration, with or without incentive spirometry (IS)
- Intermittent positive pressure breathing (IPPB)
- Face mask continuous positive airway pressure (CPAP)
- Positive expiratory pressure (possibly)

Many studies have been published over the years to determine the relative value of IS and IPPB in preventing or treating PPCs. A careful review of the literature suggests that many of the studies are contradictory in their conclusions or contain distinct methodologic flaws that limit their interpretation. For example, a study by Oikkonen and colleagues randomly assigned 52 patients who had had CABG to treatment with IPPB or IS.[34] The authors found no difference in the incidence of atelec-

Transpulmonary pressure gradient—the difference between alveolar pressure and pleural pressure

TABLE **35–2:** Effects of Postoperative Respiratory Maneuvers

	Alveolar Inflating Pressure	Time for Alveolar Inflation	Inflating Volume
Ideal maneuver	High (40–60 cm H_2O—preferably negative intrathoracic)	Long (5–15 sec)	Largest possible (6–10 times tidal volume)
Expiratory maneuvers	Minimal (mostly deflating)	Minimal	Variable (not emphasized)
CO_2 hyperventilation	Moderate	Short (breathing deeper, but faster)	2–3 times tidal volume
Intermittent positive pressure breathing	Preset (usually 15–20 cm H_2O positive airway pressure)	Long (5–10 sec)	Unknown (2–3 times tidal volume)
Sustained maximal inspiration	Maximal (30–50 cm H_2O—negative intrathoracic pressure)	Long (5–10 sec)	Largest possible (2–6 times tidal volume)

From Bartlett RH, Gazzaniga AB, Geraghty TR. Respiratory maneuvers to prevent postoperative pulmonary complications: A critical review. JAMA 224(7):1017–1021, 1973. Copyright 1973, American Medical Association.

tasis in these two groups and concluded the study by considering "both devices equal in efficiency after coronary surgery."[34] However, it should be noted that these investigators excluded the following patients from the study: patients older than 70 years of age, those with a history of COPD, those who had had postoperative respirator treatment for longer than 20 hours, and those whose weight exceeded their ideal weight by more than 20%. Additionally, the IPPB treatments were delivered at 10 to 15 cm H_2O to "result in a sufficient widening of the thoracic cage," and physical therapists visited the patients at least once daily and "gave them conventional chest physiotherapy." It is not surprising that IPPB and IS may prove equally beneficial when one eliminates from the patient groups those who are elderly or obese, have COPD, and had difficulty in their ventilator course. One of the primary tenets of "modern" IPPB is that of a volume orientation to determine the inflating volume for each breath. Bartlett and associates alluded to inflating volume as being the most "critical measurement,"[33] but this idea was not incorporated into the design of the study. It is not specified what therapies constituted chest physiotherapy, which patients received the chest physiotherapy, or how often it was administered. It should be stated that this study does not stand alone in its design limitations.

Jung and associates compared the effect of IPPB, resistance breathing, and IS on the incidence of atelectasis and pneumonia in 126 patients after upper abdominal surgery.[35] They, too, concluded that IPPB was of no benefit in reducing the morbidity of these postoperative patients. However, the IPPB used in this study consisted of pressure-cycled ventilation with a pressure limit "arbitrarily set at 15 cm H_2O." Dohi and Gold also published a frequently referenced study that compared IS and IPPB in 64 patients who had abdominal surgery.[36] Here, "a registered respiratory therapist administered all treatments with IPPB. Flow, volume, and peak inspiratory pressures were adjusted maximally by the therapist for each treatment." No mention was made as to how the volume measurements were made or what inflating volumes were used. Interestingly, this technique, as just quoted, was referenced in Dohi and Gold's article to a letter to the editor that had appeared 2 years previously. In this letter, the reader is urged to use the IPPB device at flow rates that match the patient's inspiratory needs and at low cycling pressures.[37] Table 35–3, which lists several studies often cited in the literature, reveals the method of IPPB administration. Noting the dates of each study, one is not surprised at the uniform use of pressure-limited ventilation that, with few exceptions, is not concerned with the inspiratory volume being delivered to the patient.

   Could the literature have come to a premature conclusion regarding the merit of IPPB in treating postoperative patients? One is compelled to question the outcome of these studies had volume-oriented IPPB been used. The use of volume-oriented IPPB demonstrated reversal of atelectasis in four patients with roentgenographic evidence of lung collapse.[44] This uncontrolled trial used IPPB every 2 hours while patients were awake and at pressures of 35 to 45 cm H_2O, which increased patients' inspiratory capacities by an average of about 70%.

TABLE **35–3:** Clinical Studies Involving Intermittent Positive Pressure Breathing in Postoperative Pulmonary Complications and Their Methodology

Study	Technique	Conclusions	Comments
Calli et al[38]	All IPPB treatments were administered at 15 cm H_2O; no volume measurements were made. All treatments were qid.	IPPB, incentive spirometry, and DBE were compared in 200 patients after abdominal surgery; IPPB and IS were equally effective	Although not statistically significant, the clinical complication rate was 30% for IPPB, 32% incentive spirometry, 33% for DBE.
Gale and Sanders[39]	IPPB was delivered with the inspiratory pressure set at 20 cm H_2O; flow was set at 15 L/min and was then adjusted "according to patient's compliance." Incentive spirometry and IPPB treatments were given for 20 min qid.	In 109 patients who had had heart surgery, incentive spirometry was no better than IPPB in preventing atelectasis.	Incentive spirometry treatments were not defined.
Van De Water et al[40]	IPPB was given for 10 min qid at 20 cm H_2O.	IPPB was compared with incentive spirometry in 30 patients after adrenalectomy. No differences were noted in the incidence of postoperative pulmonary complications.	Incentive spirometry was unsupervised after instruction, and all patients could also receive chest physiotherapy, blow bottles, and breathing tubes. The frequency of use of these other therapies was not reported. The control group was retrospective, based on patients treated from 1961 to 1970.
Ali et al[41]	IPPB was given at 25 cm H_2O and 8–12 breaths per minute, which resulted in a tidal volume of 12–18 mL.	30 patients who had had cholecystectomy were studied; no difference in Pa_{O_2}, vital capacity, or functional residual capacity in the IPPB group compared with patients who received DBE, turning, and ambulation.	Patients with unusual cough, wheezing, shortness of breath, smoking history, and maximal breathing capacity less than 70% of predicted were excluded from the study.
Schuppiser et al[42]	IPPB was given at 15–20 cm H_2O tid for 10–15 min.	17 patients who had had upper abdominal surgery were studied. Neither IPPB nor the department's "standard chest physical therapy" was more effective than the other in preventing postoperative pulmonary complications.	Chest physiotherapy was "clearly preferred" because of potential hazards with IPPB. No complications of IPPB were reported in this group. No definition of the "department's standard chest physical therapy" was provided.
Anderson et al[43]	IPPB was administered at 20 cm H_2O for 15 min qid. Isoproterenol was also administered during the treatment.	19.5% of the control group (who received a "stirrup" regimen) experienced complications, and 2.5% of the IPPB group experienced pulmonary complications. It was concluded that all patients should receive IPPB with isoproterenol plus "stirrup" after thoracic or abdominal surgery.	160 patients comprised the control group, and 42 patients received IPPB. The IPPB group contained more patients older then 60 years of age and more patients with a maximal breathing capacity less than 60% of predicted.

DBE, deep breathing exercises; IPPB, intermittent positive pressure breathing; IS, incentive spirometry; qid, four times daily; tid, three times daily.

The previous statements are not a call for the widespread use of IPPB. This therapy is labor intensive and carries substantial risks for the patient. However, it could be correctly concluded that the role of volume-oriented IPPB in treating PPCs is not clearly defined. This approach therefore merits further investigation.

IS, the vehicle for sustained maximal inspiration, is regarded as the mainstay of therapy aimed at both treating and preventing atelectasis in the postsurgical patient. When performed correctly, this therapy fulfills Bartlett and associates' requirements of a large distending pressure and a large inflating volume that is held for several seconds, and it offers several advantages over IPPB. The use of a spontaneously deep breath avoids the problem of a pressurized thoracic compartment and the possible clinical problems associated with this phenomenon. IS is easier for the patient to perform: this facilitates closer adherence to the hourly time frame that seems to be important in the prevention of lung collapse.[33] Clinical studies have confirmed the utility of IS in treating PPCs.[45–47] Comparisons of IS with IPPB[34, 36, 39, 40] and with postural drainage therapy[48] have shown IS to be equally effective with these alternatives. One study documented a lack of therapeutic benefit with the use of IS in low-risk patients undergoing cholecystectomy.[49] The choice of volume- versus flow-oriented devices does not seem to alter patient outcomes,[50] but it seems to be a reasonable advantage to have accurate measurements of inspired volumes.

An interesting study of the need for supervision of IS was provided by Rau and associates. This evaluation included only CABG patients who evidenced a "freedom from disorientation or extreme lethargy and ability to cooperate."[51] Not surprisingly, no differences in outcomes (postoperative volumes, temperatures, productive cough, and days of hospitalization) were noted between the supervised and the unsupervised IS groups. It would be a mistake, however, to generalize these data to the world at large. The reality of routine care is that some patients *are* disoriented and uncooperative, and supervised IS is indicated for these patients until data to the contrary have been published.

The use of CPAP has a long history in the annals of pulmonary medicine. More recently, a substantive body of evidence has indicated a role for this therapy in the treatment of atelectasis. However, an elevated baseline of positive pressure during the entire respiratory cycle is a cause for concern regarding potential side effects. Table 35–4 lists commonly reported side effects, but it should be noted that few of these occur with great frequency.

The clinical benefit from face mask CPAP in treating PPCs lies in its ability to increase FRC and subsequently restore alveolar stability.[52, 53] A comparison of patients who developed PPCs with those who did not revealed a statistically significant reduction in FRC as early as 4 hours after surgery in patients who developed PPCs.[52] The process of FRC augmentation is a passive one from the perspective of patient effort; therefore, patient cooperation is not as essential for CPAP as it is for IPPB or IS.

TABLE **35–4:** Possible Side Effects Associated With the Use of Continuous Positive Airway Pressure

Hypotension	Nausea, vomiting, or aspiration
Pulmonary barotrauma	Tissue irritation at contact sites of mask
Gastric insufflation	Patient anxiety or discomfort

IS has been compared with mask CPAP, and significant improvements in the postoperative $P(A-a)O_2$ and in the incidence of atelectasis were noted with the use of CPAP.[54, 55] Ricksten and coworkers reported the simpler positive expiratory pressure system to be as effective as CPAP in their series of patients.[54] The statistical analysis of their data showed consistent differences supporting the superiority of CPAP over IS in a number of dependent variables (Pa_{O_2}, $P(A-a)O_2$, and FVC), but there were no such differences between CPAP and positive expiratory pressure. It is hoped that positive expiratory pressure will be more widely reported in future studies of PPCs.

The use of face mask CPAP postoperatively may be on an intermittent or a continuous basis.[56–58] The decision for either must be tempered by the severity of the pulmonary status and the patient's tolerance of the procedure. Although face mask CPAP offers putative advantages in the treatment of PPCs, it should be noted that the need for specialized masks, gas circuits, and properly trained personnel, as well as the potential for an array of complications, may limit the use of this therapy.

From the previous descriptions of IPPB, IS, and face mask CPAP, an attempt can now be made to synthesize these options into a coherent patient care approach. It must be emphasized that the clinical studies described earlier cannot be used as a template to establish a care plan for all patients. The obvious alternative is a rational approach to patient assessment, the identification of specific patient problems, and the individualized application of therapeutics for these problems. Each therapy should have an objective end-point that defines the effective use of therapy. Protocols for these therapies have been espoused, and considerable reductions in unnecessary care have been documented with their use.[59, 60]

At times, atelectasis can be especially severe, and the resultant patient condition may be critical. In cases of lobar or complete lung collapse, intubation and mechanical ventilation may be necessary to treat the patient successfully. More aggressive and invasive therapeutic interventions exist for these patients. The following paragraphs briefly describe therapeutic bronchoscopy, selective bronchial suctioning, and directed manual recruitment.

Therapeutic fiberoptic bronchoscopy is considered to be an effective approach to treating lobar atelectasis in critically ill patients when a central airway is obstructed by secretions.[32] Other causes of atelectasis, such as foreign bodies, tumors, and malposition of the endotracheal tube, are also responsive to this intervention. The principal mechanism of action for the effectiveness of this approach lies in the ability to remove secretions from the lumen of the airway, thereby restoring the channel for inflating volume and pressure to enter the acinus. Fiberoptic bronchoscopy also stimulates cough and may produce a localized "positive end-expiratory pressure effect" in the airway because of partial occlusion of the airway and increased airway pressure.[61]

However, considerable risks, such as significant arterial desaturation, have prompted providers to question the value of this approach compared with traditional respiratory therapy. Marini and coworkers investigated these two options in 31 patients with acute lobar atelectasis.[62] These authors randomly assigned patients to one of two groups: one group received bronchoscopy on detection of atelectasis, and the other group first received respiratory therapy and then had "delayed" bronchoscopy if they did not have at least a 50% radiographic resolution of the collapse. The respiratory therapy studied included deep breathing, bronchodilator administration, and chest physiotherapy. The investigators concluded that there were no differences in the resolution rate (i.e., the percentage of improvement in the original volume loss as detected by serial chest radiographs over 48 hours after treatment) of the lobar atelectasis between the two study groups. Additionally, the presence of an air bronchogram on chest radiography was associated with minimal improvements in volume resolution of the atelectatic area for both the bronchoscopy and the respiratory therapy treatment groups.

An interesting approach to the treatment of atelectasis is the use of directed manual recruitment of the lung. This technique involves the use of a hand bag resuscitator that provides large inflating volumes and pressures over 10 to 30 seconds. A pressure manometer is placed inline between the bag and the patient's artificial airway for precise monitoring of distending pressure. This technique is reported by Scholten and colleagues in a case report of four patients with radiographic evidence of atelectasis.[63] The authors placed these patients with the affected lung in the superior position and applied sustained airway pressures of up to 40 cm H_2O in an effort to re-expand the collapsed lung. They also elevated the patient's leg, used Trendelenburg positioning to maintain the patient's blood pressure; or did both. All four patients experienced significant improvement in their lung collapse, and no complications of this procedure were noted. The authors acknowledge the significant risk of barotrauma and cardiac compromise but urge the judicious use of this procedure in patients who would otherwise be candidates for invasive interventions such as bronchoscopy. From a theoretical perspective, this technique is compelling in that it satisfies the criteria of Bartlett and associates for an ideal maneuver (see earlier discussion), but this technique must be tested in a controlled trial for its role in the treatment of lung collapse to be fully appreciated.

SUMMARY

It should be clear that available information regarding therapies and diagnostic tests for postsurgical patients requires a healthy dose of critical scrutiny. It was observations concerning research methodology such as those stated previously that prompted O'Donohue to wonder aloud if postoperative atelectasis can or will be adequately studied.[64] Table 35–5 poses questions that must be addressed by all who are charged with reading and interpreting the clinical literature.

TABLE **35–5:**   Questions for Readers of Clinical Studies

What patient characteristics were *included* in this study? Which patients were *excluded* from the study design?

Was a concurrent (i.e., at the same time) control group employed? Or was a retrospective comparison used?

Were the control and treatment groups adequately matched for chronic obstructive pulmonary disease, other pre-existing diseases, and so forth?

How were the treatments performed? This area is typically lacking in detail. One should be able to identify important methodologic features of the procedure from the text; this information should not be inferred or assumed. How were volume and pressure measurements made, how often was therapy administered, was therapy supervised and by whom? One should be especially concerned with designs that include subjective interpretations, such as "adequate lung expansion" as an end-point that defines successful therapy.

Is a distinction made between clinically significant atelectasis and lung collapse that frequently resolves without any therapeutic intervention for the majority of patients?

Are various techniques of randomization, blindness, and statistical analysis adequately incorporated into the design?

The reader is referred to Chapter 62, which deals with these issues in a more complete fashion. However, it should be clear that the materials and methods section of a study must be carefully evaluated for completeness because the conclusions reached in any clinical study are only as good as the methods used to generate the information. The similarity of methodologic flaws in studies involving IPPB to those that evaluate routine spirometry is clear. At times, the past body of knowledge may not be as complete and reliable as one would like; future studies will need to provide more definitive answers to these problems. In view of the huge aggregate costs of these procedures, a scientific imperative must demand that these answers be determined.

References

1. Pontoppidan H. Mechanical aids to lung expansion. Am Rev Respir Dis 122(Suppl):109–111, 1980.
2. Gale GD, Teasdale SJ, Sanders DE, et al. Pulmonary atelectasis and other respiratory complications after cardiopulmonary bypass and investigation of aetiological factors. Can Anaesth Soc J 26(1):15–21, 1979.
3. Reifenrath R. The significance of alveolar geometry and surface tension in the respiratory mechanics of the lung. Respir Physiol 24:117–137, 1975.
4. Thomas CL (ed). Taber's Cyclopedic Medical Dictionary. Philadelphia, FA Davis, 1973, p S131.
5. Rigg JRA. Pulmonary atelectasis after anesthesia: Pathophysiology and management. Can Anaesth Soc J 28(4):305–313, 1981.
6. Bendixen H, Hedley-Whyte J, Laver MB. Impaired oxygenation in surgical patients during general anesthesia with controlled ventilation: A concept of atelectasis. N Engl J Med 269(19):991–996, 1963.
7. Zikria BA, Spencer JL, Kinner JM, Broell JR. Alterations in ventilatory function in breathing patterns following surgical trauma. Ann Surg 179(4):1–7, 1974.
8. Egbert LD. Effect of morphine on breathing pattern: A possible factor in atelectasis. JAMA 188:485–488, 1964.
9. Dale WA, Rahn H. Rate of gas absorption during atelectasis. Am J Physiol 70:606–615, 1952.
10. Rehder K, Sessler AD, Marsch HN. General anesthesia and the lung. *In* Mary JF (ed). Lung Disease: State of the Art. New York, American Lung Association, 1975–1976, pp 367–389.
11. Brismar B, Hedenstierna G, Lundquist H, et al. Pulmonary densities during anesthesia with muscular relaxation—A proposal of atelectasis. Anesthesiology 62(4):422–428, 1985.
12. Froese AB, Bryan AC. Effects of anesthesia in paralysis on diaphragmatic mechanics in man. Anesthesiology 41(3):242–254, 1974.
13. Gunnarsson L, Strandberg A, Brismar B, et al. Atelectasis and gas exchange impairment during enflurane-nitrous oxide anesthesia. Acta Anaesthesiol Scand 33:629–637, 1989.
14. Klingstedt C, Hedenstierna G, Lundquist H, et al. The influence of body position in differential ventilation on lung dimensions in atelectasis formation in anesthetized man. Acta Anaesthesiol Scand 34:315–322, 1990.
15. Sykes LA, Bowe EA. Cardiorespiratory effects of anesthesia. Clin Chest Med 114(2):211–226, 1993.
16. Tulla H, Alhava E, Takala J, et al. Respiratory changes after open heart surgery. Intensive Care Med 17:365–369, 1991.
17. Wilcox P, Baile EM, Hards J, et al. Phrenic nerve function and its relationship to atelectasis after coronary surgery. Chest 93(4):693–698, 1988.
18. Bellamy R, Pitts FW, Stauffer ES. Respiratory complications in traumatic quadriplegia. Analysis of 20 years' experience. J Neurosurg 39:596–600, 1973.
19. Fishburn MJ, Marino RJ, Ditunno JF. Atelectasis and pneumonia in acute spinal cord injury. Arch Phys Med Rehabil 71:197–200, 1990.
20. Celli BR. Perioperative respiratory care of the patient undergoing upper abdominal surgery. Clin Chest Med 14(2):235–261, 1993.
21. Tisi GM. Preoperative evaluation of pulmonary function validity, indications and benefits. Am Rev Respir Dis 119:293–310, 1979.
22. Warner MA, Divertie MB, Tinker JH. Preoperative cessation of smoking and pulmonary complications in coronary artery bypass patients. Anesthesiology 60:380–383, 1984.
23. Mittman C. Assessment of operative risk in thoracic surgery. Am Rev Respir Dis 84:197–207, 1961.

24. Gracey DR, Divertie MB, Didier EP. Pre-operative preparation of patients with chronic obstructive pulmonary disease. Chest 76:123–129, 1979.
25. Stein N, Cassara EL. Preoperative pulmonary evaluation and therapy for surgery patients. JAMA 211(5):787–793, 1970.
26. Hall JC, Tarala RA, Hall JL, Mander J. A multivariate analysis of the risk of pulmonary complication after a laparotomy. Chest 99(4):923–927, 1991.
27. Lawrence VA, Page CP, Harris GD. Preoperative spirometry before abdominal operations: A critical appraisal of its predictive value. Arch Intern Med 149:280–285, 1989.
28. Zibrak JD, O'Donnell CR. Indications for preoperative pulmonary function testing. Clin Chest Med 14(2):227–234, 1993.
29. Miller WT. Radiographic evaluation of the chest. *In* Fishman AP (ed). Pulmonary Diseases and Disorders. New York, McGraw-Hill Book Company, 1988, pp 479–527.
30. Lindberg P, Gunnarsson L, Tokics L, et al. Atelectasis and lung function in the post-operative period. Acta Anaesthesiol Scand 36:546–553, 1992.
31. Schlenker JD, Hubay CA. The pathogenesis of post operative atelectasis: A clinical study. Arch Surg 107:846–850, 1973.
32. Marini JJ. Post-operative atelectasis: Pathophysiology, clinical importance and principles of management. Respir Care 29(5):516–522, 1984.
33. Bartlett RH, Gazzaniga AB, Geraghty TR. Respiratory maneuvers to prevent postoperative pulmonary complications: A critical review. JAMA 224(7):1017–1021, 1973.
34. Oikkonen M, Karjalainen K, Kahara V, et al. Comparison of incentive spirometry and intermittent positive pressure breathing after coronary artery bypass graft. Chest 99(1):60–65, 1991.
35. Jung R, Wight J, Nusser R. Comparison of three methods of respiratory care following upper abdominal surgery. Chest 78:31–35, 1980.
36. Dohi S, Gold MI. Comparison of two methods of postoperative respiratory care. Chest 73(5):592–595, 1978.
37. Sheldon GP. IPPB: Yes or no [Letter]. Chest 69(1):133–134, 1976.
38. Celli BR, Rodriguez KS, Snider GL. A controlled trial of intermittent positive pressure breathing, incentive spirometry, and deep breathing exercises in preventing pulmonary complications after abdominal surgery. Am Rev Respir Dis 130:12–15, 1984.
39. Gale TD, Sanders DE. Incentive spirometry: Its value after cardiac surgery. Can Anaesth Soc J 27:475–480, 1980.
40. Van De Water JM, Watering WG, Linton LA. Prevention of postoperative pulmonary complications. Surg Gynecol Obstet 135:229–233, 1972.
41. Ali J, Serrette C, Wood LVH. Effective postoperative intermittent positive pressure breathing on lung function. Chest 85:192–196, 1984.
42. Schuppiser JP, Brandli O, Neili E. Postoperative intermittent positive pressure breathing vs. physiotherapy. Am J Surg 40:682–686, 1980.
43. Anderson WH, Dossett BE, Hamilton GL. Prevention of postoperative pulmonary complications: Use of isoproterenol and intermittent positive pressure breathing on respiration. JAMA 186:763–766, 1963.
44. O'Donohue WJ. Maximum volume IPPB for the management of pulmonary atelectasis. Chest 76(6):683–687, 1979.
45. Bartlett RH, Brennan ML, Gazzaniga AB, Hanson EL. Studies on the pathogenesis and prevention of postoperative complications. Surg Gynecol Obstet 137:1–9, 1973.
46. McConnell DH, Maloney JV, Duckberg GD. Postoperative intermittent positive pressure breathing treatments. J Thorac Cardiovasc Surg 68:944–948, 1984.
47. Craven JL, Evans GA, Davenport JC, Williams RHP. The evaluation of the incentive spirometer in the management of postoperative pulmonary complications. Br J Surg 61:793–797, 1974.
48. Hall JC, Tarala R, Harris J, et al. Incentive spirometry vs. routine chest physiology for prevention of pulmonary complications after upper abdominal surgery. Lancet 337:953–956, 1991.
49. Schwieger I, Gamulin Z, Forster A, et al. Absence of benefit of incentive spirometry in low risk patients undergoing elective cholecystectomy. Chest 89:5–8, 1986.
50. Lederer DH, Van de Water JM, Indeck RB. Which deep breathing device should the postoperative patient use? Chest 77:610–613, 1980.
51. Rau JL, Thomas L, Haynes RL. The effect of administering incentive spirometry on postoperative pulmonary complications in coronary artery bypass. Respir Care 33(9):771–778, 1988.
52. Linder KH, Lotz P, Ahnefeld FW. Continuous positive airway pressure effect on functional residual capacity: Vital capacity and its subdivisions. Chest 92(1):66–70, 1987.
53. Anderson JB, Olsen KP, Eikard E, et al. Periodic continuous positive airway pressure (CPAP) by mask and the treatment of atelectasis: A sequential analysis. Eur J Respir Dis 61:20–25, 1980.
54. Ricksten S, Bengtsson A, Soderberg C, et al. Effects of periodic positive airway pressure by mask on postoperative pulmonary function. Chest 89(6):774–781, 1986.
55. Stock MC, Downs JB, Gouer PK, et al. Prevention of postoperative pulmonary complications with CPAP, incentive spirometry and conservative therapy. Chest 87(2):151–157, 1985.
56. Smith RA, Kirby RR, Gooding JM, Sivetta JN. Continuous positive airway pressure (CPAP) by facemask. Crit Care Med 8:483–484, 1983.

57. Covelli HD, Weled BJ, Beekman JF. Efficiency of continuous positive airway pressure administered by facemask. Chest 81:147–150, 1982.
58. Wilson RS. Intermittent CPAP to prevent atelectasis in postoperative patients. Respir Care 28:71–73, 1983.
59. Torrington KG, Henderson CJ. Perioperative respiratory therapy (PORT): A program of preoperative risk assessment and individualized postoperative care. Chest 93(5):946–951, 1988.
60. Kester L, Stoller JK. Ordering respiratory care services for hospitalized patients: Practices of overuse and underuse. Cleve Clin J Med, November-December 1992, pp 581–585.
61. Marini JJ, Wheeler AP. Fiberoptic bronchoscopy in critical care. *In* Civetta JM, Taylor RN, Kirby RR (eds). Critical Care. Philadelphia, JB Lippincott, 1988, pp 425–436.
62. Marini JJ, Pierson DJ, Hudson LD. Acute lobar atelectasis: A prospective comparison of fiberoptic bronchoscopy and respiratory therapy. Am Rev Respir Dis 119:971–977, 1979.
63. Scholten DJ, Novak R, Snyder JV. Directive manual recruitment of collapsed lung in intubated and nonintubated patients. Am Surg 51:330–335, 1985.
64. O'Donohue WJ. Prevention and treatment of post operative atelectasis: Can it and will it be adequately studied. Chest 87(1):1–2, 1985.

36 Obstructive Lung Disease

David R. Dantzker, M.D.

Key Terms

Airflow Obstruction

Asthma

Bronchiectasis

Bronchoconstriction

Chronic Bronchitis

Chronic Obstructive Pulmonary Disease (COPD)

Cystic Fibrosis

Emphysema

Hyperinflation

Upper airway obstruction in general connotes disorders that affect the airway proximal to and including the mainstem bronchi.

Airflow obstruction occurs in a wide variety of acute and chronic disorders affecting the upper and lower airways as well as the lung parenchyma. This obstruction results in an increased work of breathing, dyspnea, disordered pulmonary gas exchange, and if it progresses sufficiently, respiratory failure. For discussion purposes, this chapter separates these disorders into upper and lower airway obstruction because the pathophysiologies and treatments are quite different. An upper airway obstruction is usually caused by an anatomic abnormality, such as a tumor or an inflammatory lesion. Neuromuscular abnormalities may cause anatomic obstruction of the upper airway, as with vocal cord paralysis, or functional obstruction, as is seen during obstructive sleep apnea. A more common clinical abnormality, obstruction of the lower airway is invariably due to a diffuse pulmonary process involving the airways, the pulmonary parenchyma, or both.

UPPER AIRWAY OBSTRUCTION

Acute or chronic obstruction of the upper airway is not uncommon because this is a complex passage with a variable cross-sectional area (see Chapter 1). Blockage sufficient to cause important clinical symptoms is more common in children than in adults. Table 36–1 lists a classification of conditions that lead to obstruction.

The symptoms of upper airway obstruction are generally nonspecific, consisting of dyspnea, cough, and if obstruction is severe enough, evidence of cor pulmonale. Stridor, a characteristic high-pitched musical sound that is heard with or without a stethoscope, localizes the problem to the upper airway. Occasionally, patients with upper airway obstruction present with the syndrome of sleep apnea (see Chapter 43). A fixed wheeze, recurrent infections, or roentgenographic evidence of atelectasis or volume loss may suggest bronchial obstruction.

TABLE **36–1:** Conditions Associated With Upper Airway Obstruction

Pharynx	Trachea
Enlarged tonsils	Tumor
Deep neck and pharyngeal abscess	Lymphadenopathy
Trauma	Aortic aneurysm
Foreign body	Mediastinal fibrosis
Sleep apnea	Thyromegaly
Larynx	Tracheomalacia
Foreign body	Trauma
Angioneurotic edema	
Intubation trauma	
External trauma	
Croup	
Epiglottitis	
Tumor	
Vocal cord paralysis	

The diagnosis of an upper airway lesions can be confirmed by direct visualization or radiographic studies. However, a severe obstruction may be suspected by the characteristic reduction in the peak inspiratory and expiratory flow rates, which is best appreciated on the maximal flow-volume curve (see Chapter 17).

Infections, which are probably the most important cause of acute upper airway obstruction because they involve the pharynx and larynx and especially the epiglottis, can rapidly progress to complete obstruction and death. Both bacterial (beta-hemolytic streptococci and *Haemophilus influenzae*) and viral pathogens (adenovirus, parainfluenza virus, coxsackie virus, and respiratory syncytial virus) are commonly found. More indolent infections, such as tuberculosis or fungal infections, occasionally involve the larynx and trachea; more often, they cause obstruction of the trachea or large bronchi by extrinsic compression owing to lymphadenopathy or mediastinal fibrosis.

Edema, another not infrequent problem in the upper airway, may be subsequent to trauma, either accidental or induced during attempts at intubation. Postintubation or post-tracheostomy edema and subsequent stenosis are unfortunately common. As many as 5% of intubated patients display stridor following extubation, with almost 2% requiring reintubation. The common site of involvement in intubated patients is the larynx, whereas the trachea, at the site of the cuff, is more commonly involved after tracheostomy.[2] Edema can also be seen after the inhalation of caustic materials or gases or after fires when thermal injury is a problem. Angioneurotic edema, which can rapidly lead to laryngeal obstruction, may occur secondary to external allergens or insect bites or spontaneously in patients with hereditary C1 esterase inhibitor deficiency.

Foreign bodies, which can lodge anywhere along the respiratory pathway, usually present as an acute onset of coughing and dyspnea. Chronic problems, such as progressive atelectasis or recurrent infections, may indicate an event forgotten by the patient.

Treatment

The treatment of upper airway obstruction should be directed at alleviation of the underlying problem. Infections of the epiglottis and occasionally of the larynx and pharynx can progress with frightening speed to upper airway obstruction. In adults, laryngitis is usually a viral illness, but in children, *Staphylococcus aureus* and *H. influenzae* infection can be seen. *H. influenzae* is the usual cause of acute epiglottis seen in children, but group A streptococci and *Haemophilus parainfluenzae* are also occasionally involved. Waiting for a culture of the organism is usually impractical; empiric therapy with a cephalosporin is recommended when impending obstruction is considered to be a possibility.

A number of nonspecific interventions should also be considered when obstruction is imminent, either from infectious or noninfectious causes. An inhaled alpha-adrenergic agent, most commonly racemic epinephrine, will reduce swelling. Although their onset of action is certainly slower, corticosteroids can provide anti-inflammatory action that may complement the vasoconstriction induced by the epinephrine. In patients in whom airway obstruction might develop, such as after a traumatic endotracheal intubation, expectant treatment with corticosteroids 2 to 6 hours before extubation may be useful.

The use of a mixture of oxygen and helium may be helpful in post-

Acute epiglottitis should always be considered a medical emergency.[3]

Helium, with a density of only about 15% that of nitrogen, will decrease the work of breathing through the obstruction.

poning the need for intubation in patients with upper airway obstruction. Bypassing the obstruction, the ultimate treatment, can usually be accomplished by intubation, although in situations in which there is marked edema, attempts at intubation may only worsen the situation and precipitate respiratory arrest. In these cases, the more conservative approach would be tracheostomy. In an emergency, oxygenation can be maintained through a large-bore needle placed through the cricothyroid membrane.

LOWER AIRWAY OBSTRUCTION

A reduction in expiratory flow rates is the distinguishing feature of a wide variety of pulmonary disorders (Table 36–2). These disorders constitute a significant cause of morbidity in the world. Asthma, which is thought to affect upwards of 5 to 10% of Americans, may be even more prevalent in underdeveloped countries. Chronic obstructive pulmonary disease (COPD) is one of the most significant causes of time lost from work in the United States and elsewhere. Where cigarette smoking is even more commonplace than in the United States, the impact is likely to be even greater. Cystic fibrosis is the most common significant hereditary disease found among whites in America. Although these diseases differ greatly in their etiologies and many of their manifestations, they also have much in common, in particular their pathophysiology and treatment. For this reason, they are treated as a group.

Pathophysiologic Principles

The determinants of airflow in the lungs are complex,[4] although for the sake of this clinical discussion, they can be simplified by the following equation:

$$\text{Airflow} = \text{driving pressure/airway resistance}$$

During most of a forced expiration, the driving pressure is the elastic recoil pressure of the lung. Thus, a reduction in lung elasticity (i.e., an increase in lung compliance) decreases expiratory flow. This is one of the prime mechanisms of the reduced flow seen in emphysema. Bronchoconstriction resulting from allergic or inflammatory stimuli or as a result of reflex mechanisms is a potent cause of increased airway resistance. Chronic inflammation in response to irritation by external pollutants (e.g., cigarette smoke) or infection or as a result of immunologic stimulation leads to goblet cell metaplasia, airway narrowing, and the production of excessive thick secretions. If inflammation is allowed to continue for a prolonged period, squamous metaplasia, loss of ciliated epithelium, and eventually peribronchial fibrosis will accentuate the problem.

Mild airway disease may result in a decrease in the flow rates only at low lung volumes, whereas a progressive illness eventually causes flow rates at all lung volumes to decline.

The important physiologic consequences of these anatomic and functional changes include an increase in the work of breathing and disordered pulmonary gas exchange.[5] The increased airway resistance requires a greater than normal amount of muscular effort for both

TABLE **36–2:** Conditions Associated With Lower Airway Obstruction

Asthma
Chronic obstructive pulmonary disease
Bronchiectasis

inspiration and expiration. It also leads to characteristic changes in pulmonary function (Table 36–3). The most prominent abnormality is a reduction in the expiratory flow rates, usually measured as a decreased 1-second forced expiratory volume or maximal midexpiratory flow rate.

The airway obstruction, as seen in asthma and COPD, also leads to distinctive changes in lung volumes. There is an increase in the residual volume and the functional residual capacity (FRC) and a normal or increased total lung capacity. The increasing residual volume encroaches on the vital capacity, which usually decreases. The mechanism of the increase in the residual volume and the FRC is not totally understood, but it is probably due to more than one factor, depending on the underlying disorder. In emphysema, the reduction in the elastic recoil of the lungs moves the FRC closer to the resting volume of the chest wall, which is normally about two thirds of the total lung capacity. Abnormal airways, particularly at the bases of the lungs, tend to collapse during expiration, trapping air beyond the closed airways. When airway resistance gets very high, there may not be sufficient time during expiration to allow for complete expiration, a phenomenon akin to the occurrence of "auto–positive end-expiratory pressure" in mechanically ventilated patients. Finally, patients with asthma have persistent inspiratory muscle activity during expiration, thereby actively maintaining an elevated FRC.

These changes in lung volume can have dramatic consequences for respiration. The pressure-volume curve of the lung is nonlinear, and breathing at high lung volumes requires a greater change in transpulmonary pressure than it does at a normal FRC. This increases the work of breathing. The work of breathing also may be increased by the need to overcome auto–positive end-expiratory pressure. The high lung volume also puts the respiratory muscles at a mechanical disadvantage because they are at a much shorter length at the beginning of a breath, reducing the force they can develop and predisposing them to fatigue (see Chapter 3). The hyperinflation does, however, have a beneficial effect. Because of the tethering effect of the alveoli on the airways, there is an inverse relationship between lung volume and airway resistance. Thus hyperinflation, by increasing the airway diameter, is one strategy immediately available to an individual to counter a sudden change in airway diameter, as might occur, for example, with the development of bronchospasm. Some investigators have noted persistent inspiratory activity in asthmatic subjects during expiration, as if they are invoking this compensatory mechanism.

Obstructive lung disease leads inevitably to abnormalities of pulmonary gas exchange. Airway obstruction, regardless of the cause, results in underventilation of some lung units and the creation of low ventilation-perfusion units (see Chapter 6). Emphysema results in the loss of

TABLE **36–3:** Pulmonary Function Changes in Obstructive Airway Disease

	COPD	Asthma	Bronchiectasis
Expiratory flow	D	D	D
Vital capacity	D	D	N or D
Total lung capacity	I	N	N or D
Residual volume/total lung capacity	I	I	I
Diffusing capacity	D	N or I	N or D
Arterial P_{O_2}	D, N	D, N	D or N
Arterial P_{CO_2}	D, N, or I	D, N, or I	D, N, or I

COPD, chronic obstructive pulmonary disease; D, decreased; I, increased; N, normal.

alveolar capillaries, causing a decrease in blood flow that is greater than the decrease in ventilation, thereby creating high ventilation-perfusion lung units. Both result in ventilation-perfusion inequality, which interferes with the transfer of both oxygen and carbon dioxide. As is characteristic of the arterial blood gas abnormalities seen with ventilation-perfusion inequality, hypoxemia is a more prominent problem than hypercapnia as long as patients are able to continue to increase their minute ventilation as the degree of lung disease worsens (see Chapter 6). However, because worsening disease is also accompanied by increasing work of breathing, a point may eventually be reached at which further increases in ventilation are no longer feasible, either because of the high energy costs or the impending onset of respiratory muscle fatigue. Any further increase in the degree of ventilation-perfusion inequality will then lead to hypercapnia. Allowing the Pa_{CO_2} to rise in this setting is actually energy efficient because the increased concentration of carbon dioxide in the alveolar gas permits elimination of the same amount of carbon dioxide per minute at a lower minute ventilation and thus reduced metabolic cost. However, the hypercapnia is also accompanied by the development of respiratory acidosis and a further worsening of hypoxemia. Acute exacerbations of any of the entities in this group of diseases invariably lead to a worsening of pulmonary gas exchange. During sleep, gas exchange also worsens as minute ventilation falls and respiratory drive diminishes.

Specific Entities

Despite the large amount of clinical and basic investigation focused on this group of conditions, a sizable measure of controversy and confusion remains with regard to the definition of the individual disorders falling under the rubric of obstructive lung disease. This exists to a great degree because of the considerable overlap of clinical and pathophysiologic features. By convention, emphysema and bronchiectasis have been defined by anatomic changes, and chronic bronchitis has been defined by its clinical presentation. A clear definition of asthma has never been agreed on. In an attempt to clarify the situation, other terms, such as COPD, were introduced but did little to help. Some people have suggested abandoning the traditional names and substituting groupings based on clinical symptoms. Such groups might include chronic mucus hypersecretion with or without airway obstruction or chronic reversible or nonreversible airway obstruction. However, because these are not in general use, this chapter attempts to define each of the diseases as presently understood and points out the controversies and overlaps that exist.

Asthma

Asthma is a disorder characterized by airway inflammation.[6] The inflammatory response consists of cellular infiltration, epithelial disruption, mucosal edema, and mucous plugging. Patients with asthma have episodic wheezing, cough, and shortness of breath, which are due to widespread narrowing of their airways, the severity of which varies over time. The narrowing is due to the inflammation, as well as to airway hyper-responsiveness and consequent bronchospasm. The stimulus to the bronchospasm may be immunologic in origin, as in the classic picture

In extrinsic asthma, airway mast cells, sensitized by IgE antibodies produced against various substances in the environment, degranulate after exposure to the proper antigen, releasing bronchoactive and inflammatory mediators.

of extrinsic asthma. Conversely, there may be no clear-cut immunologic overlay, with bronchospasm following exercise, cold exposure, or even emotional stress.

About half of the patients with asthma develop their first symptoms before the age of 5 years, with some becoming asymptomatic in their late teens. However, many of those who have an apparent resolution experience recurrences later in life. Even those who remain relatively symptom free can be shown to manifest bronchial hyper-reactivity and might even develop overt airway obstruction during episodes of infection or inhalation of irritants in the air. The remaining patients with asthma may manifest symptoms at any age.

Many categories of asthma have been defined (Table 36–4) based on the clinical presentation or the presumed inciting trigger. Because of the marked overlap in these groups, as well as the common approach to treatment, differentiation of these various forms is generally important only if there are clear-cut, easily identifiable, and avoidable extrinsic factors, such as drugs or industrial substances. A careful identification of all allergic factors is unnecessary because attempts at desensitization do not appear to alter the clinical course.

The diagnosis of asthma can be suspected from the symptoms of intermittent dyspnea and wheezing, especially if they are found in a patient who has a history of hay fever or eczema. On occasion, episodic cough will be the only presenting complaint. Pulmonary function studies, which are necessary to confirm the diagnosis, characteristically show decreased expiratory flows that correct fully or in part following acute bronchodilator administration. If a diagnosis of occupational asthma is suspected, a symptom diary with a record of peak flowmeter recordings can be valuable. Alternatively, the subject can be exposed to the suspected industrial substance in the laboratory, with flow rates measured before and after exposure.[7]

An exacerbation of asthma can vary in intensity from a mild increase in wheezing that is easily reversible with bronchodilator inhalation to an attack of increased severity that is unresponsive to acute treatment (status asthmaticus). The history of patients with status asthmaticus normally reveals a period of increased lability of expired flow rates unresponsive to gradually increasing amounts of medication. Occasionally, however, the attack may occur suddenly and without warning.

In addition to showing the obvious abnormalities of pulmonary mechanics, an acute asthmatic attack is accompanied by abnormal arterial blood gas values with a characteristic pattern of progression. Although arterial blood gas values may be normal in mild stable asthma, hypoxemia and hypocapnia are characteristic early in an attack. With increas-

As a general rule, the younger the onset of asthma, the more likely an allergic component will be found, whereas the older the onset, the more resistant the obstruction is to treatment.

If the patient is asymptomatic at the time of study, pulmonary function study results may be normal; the stimulation of bronchospasm with histamine, methacholine, or cold air may be necessary to confirm the diagnosis.

Although death from acute asthma is relatively rare, fatal episodes do occur, usually in a situation in which increasing symptoms are disregarded or correct therapy is not initiated.

In general, measurement of arterial blood gases is a less sensitive means of judging both the severity of disease and the response to therapy than is assessment of airway obstruction.

TABLE **36–4:** Types of Asthma

Type	Inciting Trigger
Extrinsic	IgE-mediated external allergens
Intrinsic	?
Adult onset	?
Aspirin sensitive (associated with nasal polyps)	Aspirin and other nonsteroidal anti-inflammatory drugs
Allergic bronchopulmonary aspergillosis	Hypersensitivity to *Aspergillus* species colonizing the airway
Exercise induced	Alteration in airway temperature and humidity
Occupational	Organic dusts; animal proteins; toluene diisocyanate

ing severity of the obstruction, the Pa_{O_2} falls further and the Pa_{CO_2} gradually returns toward normal as the combination of increasing ventilation-perfusion inequality and work of breathing progressively interferes with adequate alveolar ventilation. In cases of severe asthma, the hypoxemia may become profound, accompanied by a mixed respiratory and metabolic acidosis. The finding of hypercapnia is a worrisome feature that indicates the marked severity of the physiologic disturbance. It is not, by itself, an indication for intubation and mechanical ventilation because most of these patients have improvement with proper care.[8] However, these patients require very careful monitoring in an intensive care unit. Progressive and unresponsive hypercapnia plus acidosis is an indication for intubation.

Chronic Obstructive Pulmonary Disease

Normal subjects show a slow decrease in pulmonary function with increasing age, whereas patients with COPD show an exaggeration of this progression.[9] The steady increase in airway obstruction may be punctuated by exacerbations due to infections, poor compliance with prescribed medications, or the onset of heart failure. These exacerbations, which are distinguished by increasing dyspnea, cough, and sputum production, can occasionally precipitate respiratory failure. It used to be thought that acute respiratory failure in the setting of COPD was always associated with a poor prognosis; however, with the present understanding and management skills, even the requirement for intubation and mechanical ventilation need not significantly alter the natural progression of any individual's condition.

Patients with COPD, who are usually middle-aged or older, present to the physician with complaints of increasing shortness of breath and exercise limitation. Many of these patients have a long history of cough and sputum production before the point at which significant functional impairment causes them to seek medical help. The physical examination findings are nonspecific, showing the stigmata of airway obstruction: hyperinflation, decreased breath sounds, wheezes, and if the obstruction is severe enough, prominent use of the accessory respiratory muscles. Patients may vary in appearance from thin and almost cachectic to edematous with cyanosis and edema. These two clinical presentations, the "pink puffer" and the "blue bloater," were previously thought to represent the specific pathologic entities of emphysema and chronic bronchitis, respectively. However, clinicopathologic correlations have not supported this, demonstrating instead that emphysema is prominent in most patients with significant airway obstruction regardless of their clinical appearance.

In COPD, as in asthma, pulmonary function studies are necessary to confirm and quantitate the presence of airway obstruction. Although both disorders reveal reduced expiratory flow rates, patients with significant COPD are more likely to show marked overinflation. A reduced diffusing capacity is seen only in the presence of emphysema and never with asthma alone, where it is more likely to be increased. In patients with COPD, as in asthmatics, an improvement in flow rates in response to an acute trial of bronchodilators may be seen. However, the degree of improvement is usually modest, on the order of 15 to 25%.

Arterial hypoxemia is almost invariable in the patient with significant COPD, but hypercapnia is not usually seen until the degree of obstruction becomes very severe. Even with severe disease, the presence of hypercapnia is poorly correlated with airway function.[10] Patients with the same apparent degree of airway obstruction may vary from hypocapnia to hypercapnia (Fig. 36–1). Differences between patients may depend, in part, on the respiratory drive they had before the development of COPD. Patients with a high premorbid respiratory drive would maintain a normal or low Pa_{CO_2} (and thus a higher Pa_{O_2}) for any degree of airway obstruction, despite the marked increase in the work of breathing. In contrast, those with a lower drive would be satisfied with a higher Pa_{CO_2} but a lower Pa_{O_2}. The clinical consequences of these two patterns are important. The patients with the high respiratory drive would maintain better gas exchange but at the expense of a greater ventilatory effort and thus greater energy expenditure. This might in part explain the "pink puffer," who is thin and dyspneic with relatively well preserved arterial blood gas values. Conversely, the patient with the more sluggish respiratory drive would have the advantage of a lesser energy expenditure and greater ventilatory reserve but at the expense of more significant hypoxemia and as a result, pulmonary hypertension, heart failure, and reduced tissue oxygen delivery (i.e., the "blue bloater").

Patients with COPD are a clinically diverse group, dependent partially on the underlying lung disease. These diseases include emphysema, bronchitis, and small airway disease.[11] The clinical and physiologic pattern in any individual patient depends in part on the degree to which these are present.

Emphysema

Anatomically, emphysema is defined as an abnormal enlargement of the airspaces distal to the terminal bronchioles that is accompanied by changes in the alveolar walls. The pathologic type of emphysema has been further classified by the pattern of alveolar wall destruction (central lobular versus panlobular), but from a clinical standpoint, these have

> Gas exchange usually deteriorates during sleep, and patients with acceptable arterial blood gas values during the day may develop sufficient worsening during the night to develop cor pulmonale.

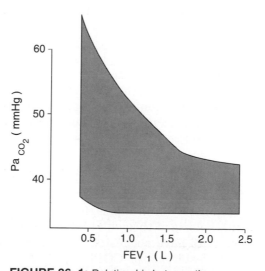

FIGURE 36–1: Relationship between the forced expiratory volume in 1 second (FEV₁) and the Pa_{CO_2} in chronic obstructive lung disease. The shaded area denotes the range of Pa_{CO_2} observed at any given level of obstruction. (From Anthonisen NR, Cherniack RM. Ventilatory controls in lung disease. *In* Hornbein TF [ed]. Regulation of Breathing. New York, Marcel Dekker, 1981.)

little functional importance. The diagnosis of emphysema is usually inferred from the clinical laboratory. These patients characteristically have a reduced elastic recoil pressure and a reduced diffusing capacity for carbon monoxide. Both findings correlate with the degree of anatomic emphysema. The degree of airway obstruction in patients with COPD correlates most closely with the severity of emphysema, and patients who have significant functional impairment usually have at least a moderate degree of emphysema.

The chest x-ray study shows nonspecific findings associated with hyperinflation, namely a depressed diaphragm, an increased anteroposterior diameter of the chest, and a widened retrosternal airspace. However, more specific features may be noted, such as the attenuation of pulmonary vessels and the presence of bullae. Computed tomography appears to be a sensitive method of quantitating the degree of emphysema.

The pathogenesis of emphysema is not known with certainty, but this condition may result from an imbalance in the lung between proteases and elastases, which can destroy tissues, and antiproteases and antielastases.[12] Cigarette smoking, the major factor in the production of emphysema, increases the number of alveolar macrophages and neutrophils in the lung and enhances their release of these tissue-destroying enzymes. In addition, cigarette smoke appears to impair the activity of the antiproteases and antielastases. However, other factors must also be involved, either directly or by increasing the lungs' susceptibility to these substances, because fewer than 10 to 15% of smokers develop emphysema and airway obstruction.

The clearest evidence of the theory of enzyme-antienzyme imbalance can be seen in patients who have an inherited deficiency of alpha$_1$-antiprotease (A1A).[13] The gene for the production of A1A has multiple alleles, with the commonest being M, S, and Z. Normal subjects have an MM phenotype and normal levels of A1A. Patients with the ZZ phenotype have very low levels of A1A and are at high risk for developing emphysema, especially if they also smoke. About 50% of people with ZZ A1A have an abnormally rapid fall in lung function with increasing age. Patients with other phenotypes have intermediate levels of A1A but no increased risk of emphysema. Replacement therapy for A1A is now available; patients with the ZZ phenotype who have demonstrated reduction in lung function are candidates for weekly infusions. Replacement therapy can replete the levels of A1A but there is no evidence to date that it will alter the rate of disease progression.

Small Airway Disease

A number of abnormalities have been identified in the small airways of patients with COPD. These include inflammation of the terminal and respiratory bronchioles, fibrosis and narrowing of the airway walls, and metaplasia of the goblet cells in the bronchiolar epithelium. Some investigators have suggested that these changes may represent the earliest manifestations of COPD.[14] Although these abnormalities undoubtedly contribute to the abnormal physiology of COPD, their relationship to airflow obstruction is much less clear than for emphysema. These lesions are probably due to long-term exposure to irritating and toxic inhalants, with cigarette smoke playing the most prominent role.

Chronic Bronchitis

Chronic bronchitis is perhaps the most common complaint of cigarette smokers, as well as of people regularly exposed to certain occupa-

Chronic bronchitis represents the overproduction of mucus with a chronic productive cough.

tional pollutants. The diagnosis requires exclusion of other causes of cough and sputum production, such as bronchiectasis. Pathologically, chronic bronchitis is recognized by hyperplasia of the mucous glands in the trachea and large bronchi.

The airway obstruction seen in chronic bronchitis does not, however, appear to be secondary to the hypersecretory lesion. Studies have failed to demonstrate any relationship between airflow obstruction and mucous gland hyperplasia.[15] When present, the reduction in flow rates in patients with chronic bronchitis is invariably due to the concomitant presence of emphysema, small airway disease, or bronchospasm. Perhaps more importantly, longitudinal studies have failed to demonstrate an independent effect of cough and sputum on the development of airflow obstruction. This means that although most patients with COPD at present have or previously had chronic bronchitis, most patients with chronic bronchitis never develop significant airway obstruction.

Bronchiectasis

Bronchiectasis is an abnormal and persistent dilatation of the airways due to destructive changes in the elastic and muscular layers of the airway wall.

Bronchiectasis, which may be a widespread process involving all lobes of the lung or may be localized to a single lung segment, is found as a consequence of various clinical disorders (Table 36–5).[16] In the past, bronchiectasis was often seen as a sequela of severe viral respiratory infections, such as measles and pertussis. As these diseases became less common, gram-negative necrotizing pneumonia became the leading post-infectious cause; immune deficiency states, which predispose to recurrent and severe pulmonary infections, are often associated with the development of bronchiectasis. Airway exposure to corrosive gases is an additional inflammatory injury that may lead to permanent airway damage, perhaps in association with superimposed infection. The anatomic changes of bronchiectasis can be seen after tuberculosis or fungal infection, but these patients rarely have the characteristic symptoms associated with this disease.

Interference with the normal pulmonary clearance of secretions also may result in chronic inflammation and eventually bronchiectasis. This may occur secondary to partial airway obstruction by tumor, lymph nodes, or scarring. More importantly, this causes bronchiectasis in patients with cystic fibrosis (see next section) and other congenital disorders. The immotile cilia syndrome (sometimes referred to as Kartagener's syndrome) results in decreased lung clearance due to a structural defect in the microtubular system of the cilia that paralyzes ciliary motion. This same defect in ciliary function has also been blamed for the other manifestations of this syndrome, namely sinusitis, situs inversus (or only dextrocardia), and infertility, although not all of these features must be present in each patient. The finding of obstructive azoospermia

TABLE **36–5:**   Clinical Disorders Associated With Bronchiectasis

Infection
Bronchial obstruction
Cystic fibrosis
Immotile cilia syndrome
Immunodeficiency
Allergic bronchopulmonary aspergillosis
Rare inherited and acquired disorders
   Young's syndrome
   Yellow nail syndrome
   Tracheobronchomegaly (Mounier-Kuhn syndrome)
   Unilateral hyperlucent lung (Swyer-James syndrome)

and chronic sinopulmonary infections (Young's syndrome), which occasionally leads to bronchiectasis, differs from immotile cilia syndrome because the cilia in these patients appear to be normal. In allergic bronchopulmonary aspergillosis, asthmatic patients develop an allergy to *Aspergillus* species that colonize their airways. Allergic bronchopulmonary aspergillosis is characterized by difficult-to-control bronchospasm, elevated IgE levels, and positive immediate and late (6- and 8-hour) skin test responses to aspergillum antigen. If this condition is not treated properly and vigorously with corticosteroids and bronchodilators, mucoid impactions occur and eventually bronchiectasis develops.

The diagnosis of bronchiectasis is suggested by historical evidence of long-standing cough and the production of large quantities of purulent, occasionally foul or bloody sputum along with the physical finding of persistent crackles over the affected lung zones.[17] With long-standing disease, clubbing and cor pulmonale can be seen. The definitive diagnosis is made roentgenographically. Early on, chest roentgenographic findings may be normal or may demonstrate only nonspecific features, such as increased markings and linear atelectasis. With time, thickening of the bronchial walls out to the periphery of the lungs and eventually even cystic lesions occur. Radiographic imaging of the airways by radiopaque substances (bronchography) is the gold standard for diagnosis but is rarely indicated. Computed tomography has been shown to demonstrate the dilated bronchi with a high degree of sensitivity.

Pulmonary function studies are not particularly helpful in differentiating bronchiectasis from other obstructive airway disorders. Most patients with bronchiectasis demonstrate a mild to moderate degree of airflow obstruction. However, as the disease progresses, lung volumes decrease; the combination of obstructive and restrictive lung disease may suggest the diagnosis.

Cystic Fibrosis

Cystic fibrosis, a generalized disorder of exocrine gland function, impairs the clearance of secretions from various organs in the body.[18] In the lung, it is manifested as thick, tenacious secretions and recurrent pulmonary infections leading to bronchial wall destruction (i.e., bronchiectasis). The basic pathophysiologic abnormality underlying cystic fibrosis is a defect of epithelial fluid and electrolyte exchange that is due to a faulty chloride channel.

The disease is usually first identified in childhood, often because of gastrointestinal disorders such as steatorrhea and bowel obstruction (Table 36–6). However, these abnormalities rarely prove to be fatal; the long-term morbidity is almost always associated with the pulmonary complications. The definitive diagnosis is based on the finding of an elevated concentration of sodium or chloride in the sweat. Although the

Cystic fibrosis, an autosomal recessive inherited disorder, occurs as frequently as one in every 200 white births. The gene for cystic fibrosis has been localized to chromosome 7.

Sweat sodium and chloride concentrations must be measured by experienced individuals using carefully standardized techniques. If this is done, levels above 60 mEq/L in children and 80 mEq/L in adults in the proper clinical setting are diagnostic.

TABLE **36–6:** Manifestations of Cystic Fibrosis

Pulmonary	Gastrointestinal
Cough and sputum productive	Meconium ileus
Recurrent infections	Chronic pancreatic insufficiency with malabsorption
Bronchospasm	Rectal prolapse
Pneumothorax	Hernias
Hemoptysis	Diabetes mellitus
Cor pulmonale	Cirrhosis and portal hypertension
Upper respiratory tract	Genitourinary
Nasal polyps	Sterility in men
Sinusitis	Low fertility in women

disease is usually diagnosed in childhood, and sometimes at birth, occasionally the pulmonary symptoms are mild enough that the diagnosis is not made until the patient is in the late teens or the early 20s. Many of these patients have had previous diagnoses of bronchitis or asthma, and the true diagnosis is made only when the lung disease worsens or some other manifestation, such as the discovery of infertility, suggests cystic fibrosis. Even older, only mildly symptomatic patients are now being recognized with the use of genetic analysis to make the diagnosis.

The gradual development of cor pulmonale and respiratory failure follows the natural history of cystic fibrosis.

Chronic and recurrent infections with *S. aureus* and various mucoid species of *Pseudomonas* are a consistent manifestation of cystic fibrosis. These infections are particularly difficult to treat because of the abnormally thick sputum and chronic colonization of the airways.[19] Although death from respiratory failure in early childhood used to be the rule, improvements in antibiotic therapy and general supportive care have markedly altered the outlook for these patients, whose median survival is now at more than 20 years of age. The introduction of lung transplantation promises to increase the longevity of selected patients. With the identification of the gene, it is hoped that further progress into the basic cellular defect will be made, allowing specific therapy to be finally developed.

Treatment

For the most part, the treatment of patients with all forms of obstructive lung disease is directed at correcting the physiologic consequences of the various disorders or at alleviating symptoms. Specific therapy aimed at correction of the underlying pathologic abnormalities is not yet possible, with the exception of A1A replacement in patients who have a homozygous deficiency of this important regulatory enzyme (see later discussion). For the majority of patients with obstructive lung disease, treatment is directed at reducing airway tone, combating inflammation, treating infection, improving the clearance of respiratory secretions, and correcting hypoxemia.

Bronchodilators

Three classes of bronchodilators are available at present: beta-adrenergic agonists, anticholinergics, and methylxanthines (Table 36–7).[20] Other drugs, such as calcium channel blockers, also have mild bronchodilating capabilities, but their clinical effectiveness is too small to make them effective therapeutic agents. Newer drugs that block putative mediators of bronchial smooth muscle constriction are being developed, but none is far enough along at this time to warrant discussion.

Beta-adrenergic agonists are the most potent and clinically useful

TABLE **36–7:** Drug Therapy for Airway Obstruction

Sympathomimetics	Anticholinergics
Beta$_2$-specific agents	Atropine
Metaproterenol	Ipratropium bromide
Terbutaline	Anti-inflammatory drugs
Albuterol	Corticosteroids
Epinephrine	Cromolyn sodium
Methylxanthines	
Theophylline	
Aminophylline	

For patients who are unable to coordinate the use of a metered dose inhaler, various spacer devices have been developed to improve the delivery of the drug.

bronchodilators. Agents such as isoproterenol are nonselective, stimulating both beta$_1$- and beta$_2$-receptors, and epinephrine has the additional undesirable effect of stimulating alpha-adrenergic receptors. The development of beta$_2$-selective drugs was a major advance, predominantly because these were noncatecholamine drugs (all but isoetharine). This protected them from being inactivated by the degradative enzymes of the body, increasing their duration of action (from 60 to 90 minutes for isoproterenol to greater than 4 hours) and allowing oral administration. In general, however, the preferred route for the administration of beta-agonists is by aerosolization because a lower dose is required with this route than with the oral route; thus, the incidence of side effects is minimalized. When used correctly, a metered dose inhaler is as effective as any nebulizer, and considerably more convenient.

Significant side effects of beta-agonists are rare. Tachycardia, palpitations, and muscle tremor are associated with excessive use, but tolerance to these symptoms usually develops with time. Importantly, tolerance to the bronchodilating ability of these agents does not appear to be clinically significant. Apparent failure of a bronchospastic patient to respond to a nebulized beta-adrenergic agonist is usually due to an insufficient dose or ineffective use of the metered dose inhaler or nebulizer.

Anticholinergic drugs were the first bronchodilators, probably used in one form or another for thousands of years. With the development of beta-agonists, their use declined, to a great degree because of mistaken concerns about their purported inhibition of lower airway secretions. As information on the importance of cholinergic mediation of airway tone has appeared, there has been a resurgence of interest in these agents.[21] The development of a new anticholinergic agent, ipratropium bromide, which unlike atropine is poorly absorbed into the circulation after aerosolization, has markedly reduced the extrapulmonary anticholinergic side effects (Table 36–8).

In asthmatic patients, anticholinergic agents are less potent bronchodilators than beta-adrenergic drugs. In some patients, however, the two types of drugs may have an additive effect and can be used together when a beta-agonist is insufficient. In patients with COPD, anticholinergic bronchodilators appear to be as effective as beta-agonists, and in some studies they have proved to be even more effective. In these patients, the two classes of drugs have also been shown to have an additive bronchodilating effect. As a general rule, anticholinergic bronchodilators have a slower onset of action than beta-agonists. For effective bronchodilatation and duration of action, a sufficient dose of the drug is necessary.

Methylxanthines, such as theophylline, are about 50% as potent a bronchodilator as the beta-agonists.[22] Their effectiveness depends on the blood level. The generally recommended blood level is in the range of 8 to 15 µg/mL, achievable in most patients at a dose of 10 to 12 mg/kg/day. The actual blood level attained for any dose of theophylline may vary widely, depending on factors that alter the metabolism of theophylline (Table 36–9). In some patients, continued improvement may be found at

TABLE **36–8:** Anticholinergic Side Effects

Dry mouth
Blurred vision
Urinary retention
Mydriasis
Central nervous system stimulation

TABLE **36–9:**   Factors Affecting Theophylline Clearance

Increase clearance	Decrease clearance
Cigarette smoking	Heart failure
Charcoal-broiled meat	Hepatic disease
Phenobarbital	Cimetidine
	Phenytoin
	Infection
	Erythromycin
	Propranolol
	Oral contraceptives

higher levels, but above 20 μg/mL, the toxicity becomes unacceptable (Table 36–10). The mechanism of action of theophylline is unknown but may relate to its mild anti-inflammatory action.

In relatively stable patients with COPD, it is often difficult to demonstrate an additional bronchodilating effect of theophylline above that achieved with optimal doses of a beta-agonist. However, many patients report symptomatic improvement after the addition of theophylline to the drug regimen, which may in part be due to the following nonbronchoactive effects of theophylline:

- Stimulates the respiratory center
- Has a mild inotropic effect on the heart
- Is purported to result in a small improvement in the strength and fatigue resistance of the respiratory muscles

In patients with asthma, theophylline is probably most useful as a means of reducing the increase in airway tone that occurs in the late night and early morning hours and that is presumably the cause of the common complaint of nocturnal wheezing. At present, theophylline is the only one of the three bronchodilators that can maintain a constant and therapeutic level with only twice-a-day dosing. The use of intravenous aminophylline in the acute exacerbation of COPD and asthma has been challenged because it adds little to the other drugs being administered (beta-agonists and corticosteroids) but significantly increases the likelihood of side effects.

Corticosteroids are not bronchodilators in the strict sense, but they are invaluable in the treatment of obstructive lung disease. The mechanism by which they reduce airflow obstruction results predominantly from their anti-inflammatory abilities. They also increase beta-adrenergic receptor responsiveness. Their ability to block the release of arachidonic acid metabolites or other bronchoactive mediators and their ability to prevent an increase in vascular permeability have been other suggested mechanisms of action.

The use of corticosteroids, early and in sufficient doses, in the treatment of the acute exacerbation of asthma has been shown to lessen the amount of airway obstruction and to reduce the time of hospitalization or even decrease the need for admission.[23] Evidence of a similar efficacy in acute exacerbations of COPD has also been claimed, but the data are less compelling. Inhaled corticosteroid is becoming the first-line drug for the treatment of chronic asthma. This approach emphasizes the under-

Long-term oral therapy with corticosteroids in patients with COPD should be used only as a last resort and only if there is clear-cut, objective evidence of efficacy. Toxicity-sparing approaches in the use of long-term corticosteroid therapy, such as every-other-day regimens, are often ineffective in bronchospastic diseases.

TABLE **36–10:**   Manifestations of Theophylline Toxicity

Headache	Restlessness
Nausea and vomiting	Cardiac arrhythmias
Abdominal pain	Seizures

TABLE **36–11:**   Complications of Steroid Use

Cutaneous	Gastrointestinal
Acne	Esophagitis and gastritis
Hirsutism	Pancreatitis
Poor wound healing	Endocrine
Petechiae and easy bruisability	Worsening of diabetes
Musculoskeletal	Menstrual disorders
Stunting of growth in children	Pituitary suppression
Osteoporosis	Ocular
Muscle weakness	Cataracts
Fractures	Immunologic
Abnormal fat deposition	Suppressed skin test hypersensitivity
Cardiovascular	Decreased response to infection
Edema	
Hypertension	

lying mechanism of the disease (i.e., inflammation).[24] Inhaled corticosteroids reduce the risk of complications associated with long-term oral corticosteroid use (Table 36–11). To be maximally effective, the inhaled corticosteroids often need to be used in doses two or even three times those at present recommended by the manufacturers. Aerosolized corticosteroids are also effective intranasally to treat allergic rhinitis. The use of inhaled corticosteroids in patients with COPD remains controversial because of the lack, to date, of sufficient long-term efficacy data.

Inhaled cromolyn sodium can be aerosolized to prevent bronchospasm in some patients with asthma.[25] It cannot be used to reverse an increase in airway tone and is thus of no use in the management of the acute asthma attack. No proven use exists in COPD. Cromolyn was initially thought to work entirely by stabilizing the mast cell membrane, preventing the mediator release that would otherwise follow exposure to an allergen in a sensitized individual. However, its effectiveness in some patients without atopic asthma suggests other mechanisms of action, probably a less specific anti-inflammatory effect. In patients with asthma that is difficult to control with inhaled corticosteroids and bronchodilators, cromolyn sodium should be tried before the patient is relegated to long-term oral corticosteroid use. The drug has a slow onset of clinically obvious action and should be used for 3 to 4 weeks before any conclusions are drawn as to its efficacy. It may also be used intranasally to relieve the symptoms of allergic rhinitis.

The appropriate use of single drugs and drug combinations to treat airway obstruction should be based on the underlying pathophysiology. Figure 36–2 outlines simplified treatment protocols.

Oxygen

Hypoxemia interferes with the normal delivery of oxygen to the tissues and may eventually lead to right-sided heart failure (cor pulmonale; see Chapter 47). Long-term supplemental oxygen therapy should be considered for patients with an oxygen saturation that is continuously less than 90%. Table 36–12 lists the generally accepted criteria for oxy-

TABLE **36–12:**   Indications for Long-Term Oxygen Therapy

Arterial $Po_2 < 55$ mm Hg
or
Arterial $Po_2 < 59$ mm Hg
and
Cor pulmonale or polycythemia

Outpatient Treatment of Stable Bronchospasm

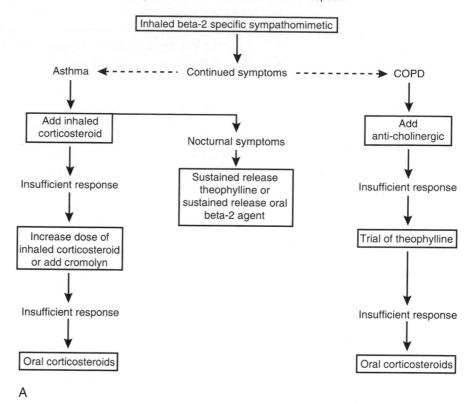

A

Emergency Room Treatment for Bronchospasm

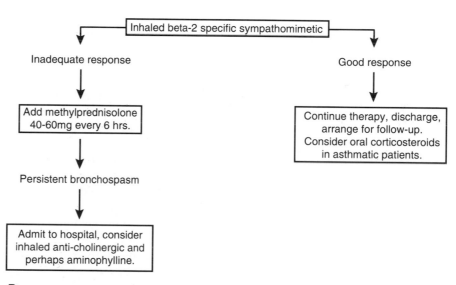

B

FIGURE 36–2: *A,* Outpatient treatment of stable bronchospasm. *B,* Emergency room treatment of bronchospasm. COPD, chronic obstructive pulmonary disease.

gen therapy in patients with COPD. Two large clinical trials have shown that patients meeting these criteria have an increased survival when long-term oxygen therapy is used.[26, 27] The degree of improvement appears to correlate with the amount of time the patient uses oxygen each day. In patients requiring long-term oxygen therapy, the goal should always be continuous use, or as close to this as possible. Usually, an adequate level of oxygen saturation can be achieved with very low flows (1 to 4 L/min). When oxygen flow rates higher than this are required, it becomes very difficult, expensive, or both to deliver. Some patients with COPD have an acceptable oxygen saturation at rest but desaturate during exercise or at night, when the normal respiratory drive diminishes (see Chapter 43). The usefulness of supplemental oxygen in these settings is not yet clearly defined. In the case of exercise-induced hypoxemia, the clinician should show that oxygen improves exercise tolerance before prescribing an expensive and potentially inhibiting form of therapy. In the case of nocturnal desaturation, perhaps some evidence of peripheral organ response to hypoxia, such as the presence of cor pulmonale or polycythemia, should be present before nocturnal oxygen therapy is recommended. Trials presently underway to study the incidence of pulmonary hypertension in patients who desaturate only at night should eventually provide more objective criteria.

Oxygen is often mistakenly prescribed to patients to be used intermittently as therapy for shortness of breath. Shortness of breath is an insensitive marker of hypoxemia because it is seen only with very low Pa_{O_2} levels (see Chapter 7). In addition, dyspnea in patients with obstructive airway disease due to the high work of breathing correlates poorly with the Pa_{O_2}. Breathing enriched oxygen mixtures may in fact reduce the sense of dyspnea in these patients even when they are significantly hypoxemic, probably by reducing the respiratory drive emanating from the carotid body. However, this is generally an expensive and misplaced use of oxygen therapy and may divert attention from the important goal of reducing the work of breathing.

Antibiotics

Patients with obstructive lung disease are prone to the development of pulmonary infections, which may contribute to an exacerbation of symptoms. This is most obvious in bronchiectasis and cystic fibrosis, in which *S. aureus* and mucoid *Pseudomonas* species are commonly isolated from the sputum. In these patients, therapy should begin early in the course of an exacerbation, before systemic signs of infection are present. Oral therapy is now available for both types of infection, but intravenous administration is often required. Aerosolization has also been suggested as a method of delivering antibiotics to the lower respiratory tract for bronchiectasis. The success of this form of therapy is not consistent from patient to patient; therefore, further study is necessary before it can be recommended for routine management. The use of prophylactic antibiotics in patients with bronchiectasis remains controversial. Although some investigators believe that this protocol decreases the chronic sputum production and the incidence of acute infections, most people choose to treat only when evidence of an acute infection is present.

In patients with COPD and asthma, *Streptococcus pneumoniae* and *H. influenzae* are the most commonly isolated bacterial pathogens. However, during most exacerbations, no bacterial pathogen is isolated. The relationship of the worsening of symptoms to the presence of infection is often unclear, especially in asthma; therefore, withholding antibiotics until there is clear-cut evidence of infection (a change in the quantity or quality of the sputum or the development of fever and leukocytosis) is justified.[28] In these cases, it is probably more cost-efficient to administer a broad-spectrum antibiotic, such as ampicillin, amoxicillin, erythromycin, or trimethoprim-sulfamethoxazole, than to waste time waiting for culture results, especially because cultures often fail to isolate the true pathogen. The prophylactic use of antibiotics has not been shown to be useful in preventing the onset of infection or in altering the natural history of disease.

Vaccines

Vaccines against specific strains of influenza have been shown to be effective in reducing morbidity and mortality during epidemic periods. Because these viruses mutate continuously, type-specific vaccine for the strain currently present in the environment must be used. The vaccine should be given to all patients with symptomatic lung disease. Unvaccinated patients can obtain variable protection from amantadine therapy if it is used prophylactically.

Pneumococcal vaccine has been proved effective in healthy subjects, but its ability to prevent debilitated patients from getting pneumonia is less certain. Although it is possible that many patients with chronic lung diseases obtain only a partial antibody response, pneumococcal vaccine is relatively safe (provided there is no egg allergy) and should be given.[29] Currently, only a single administration of the vaccine is recommended.

Mucolytics and Expectorants

Excessive and often difficult-to-clear mucus characterizes COPD, cystic fibrosis, and bronchiectasis and often complicates acute asthma. A number of agents allegedly have the ability to decrease the viscidness of these secretions, thereby improving clearance. Unfortunately, none of these agents worked effectively when studied during carefully controlled trials. A controlled trial of iodinated glycerol resulted in symptomatic improvement in patients with COPD, although there was no alleviation of functional abnormalities.[30] Proper use of beta-adrenergic agonists and corticosteroids improved sputum clearance, probably through these agents' ability to increase ciliary motion and reduce inflammation. It should be noted that although the use of anticholinergic agents may lead to drying of the upper respiratory tract, it does not substantially reduce secretions in the tracheobronchial tree. Although theoretically anticholinergic agents might reduce ciliary action, impaired clearance of secretions has not been described subsequent to their use.

Dehydration, which is often a problem in patients with exacerbations of airway obstruction, probably increases the viscidity of sputum. In this situation, rehydration is an important aid to clearing sputum. Overhydration, however, has no additional beneficial effects; in fact, overhydration may lead to the development of congestive heart failure, especially in older patients.[31]

Bland saline nebulization has also been shown to be ineffective as a means of mucolysis; in patients with airway hyperreactivity, it may lead to a worsening of the bronchospasm.

Alpha$_1$-antitrypsin Replacement

Alpha$_1$-antitrypsin (AAT) is now available as replacement for individuals with the AAT phenotypes associated with a high risk of lung disease. These include the ZZ, Znull, and nullnull variants. Weekly intravenous injections of AAT can significantly increase the serum and lung levels of AAT in these patients. Although AAT can now be replenished, it is not known whether this protects the lung against the development of emphysema.[13] In addition, the risk of emphysema development in these patients varies from 5 to 50%. In view of these two facts, and the major expense of AAT replacement (approximately $25,000 per year), treatment should be reserved for patients who, in addition to having the proper phenotype, have abnormal lung function as defined by spirometry.

Physical Therapy and Rehabilitation

Bronchial hygiene, namely postural drainage and chest percussion, is employed based on the assumption that it improves the ability to clear airway secretions.[32] Although this has never been rigorously proved, the general clinical impression is that for patients whose cough is ineffective and who have excessively viscid secretions, bronchial hygiene is a useful adjunct. Patients with bronchiectasis from any cause, hospitalized patients with respiratory failure, and patients who develop areas of atelectasis that do not rapidly clear are likely candidates for this form of therapy. Fiberoptic bronchoscopy is not any more effective than chest physiotherapy as a means of sputum removal.

The usefulness of exercise rehabilitation has been studied most carefully in patients with COPD. In carefully selected and highly motivated patients, regular exercise programs can increase exercise tolerance and efficiency, as well as improve the overall quality of life. Exercise rehabilitation does not, however, increase the maximal amount of exercise achievable, improve pulmonary function, or alter mortality or morbidity.[33]

Nutrition

Reduced body weight and poor nutritional status are commonplace in patients with cystic fibrosis because of the pancreatic insufficiency and the resultant intestinal malabsorption. Similar nutritional abnormalities appear in some patients with COPD. The etiology of the nutritional abnormalities in the COPD patients is unclear, although their presence correlates with reduced pulmonary function and increased mortality. Whether the nutritional abnormalities and weight loss are the cause of the reduced pulmonary function and increased mortality or whether body weight is falling because of the excessive ventilatory demands or because of some other factor common to both the nutritional changes and the deteriorating pulmonary function is unknown at this time.

The poor nutritional status of these patients is also reflected in abnormalities of the respiratory muscles, which have been shown to have a reduced bulk and in some settings a reduced strength and endurance as well. This may well predispose patients with constantly increased ventilatory demands to a greater risk of respiratory failure. In addition, malnutrition is associated with other systemic abnormalities, including depressed immunologic function. For all of these reasons, providing supplemental nutrition to debilitated patients with all forms of obstructive airway disease seems logical. In patients with cystic fibrosis, supplements should accompany pancreatic hormone replacement given to correct the malabsorption. No evidence exists that increasing weight by itself is beneficial; in fact, weight gain may be detrimental if it also increases metabolic oxygen demands and carbon dioxide production.

Smoking Cessation

Smoking probably worsens all forms of obstructive lung disease through its nonspecific irritative potential. In patients who are sensitive to cigarette smoke (about 10 to 15% of smokers), lung function declines faster when compared with that in nonsmokers. For example, the forced expiratory volume in 1 second declines about 30 mL/yr in the nonsmoker, compared with 80 mL/yr in the susceptible smoking patient with COPD (Fig. 36–3). If the smoking patient with COPD stops smoking, the rate

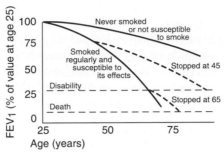

FIGURE 36–3: Pattern of decline in the forced expiratory volume in 1 second (FEV_1), with risk of morbidity and mortality from respiratory disease in a susceptible smoker compared with a normal subject or a nonsusceptible smoker. Although cessation of smoking does not replenish the lung function already lost in a susceptible smoker, it decreases the further rate of decline. (Adapted from Fletcher and Peto. Br Med J 1:1645, 1977.)

of decline falls over time to that of the nonsmoker. Thus, the sooner the COPD smoker stops, the less likely the patient with COPD is to develop respiratory failure.

Smoking cessation is very difficult to accomplish. Standard techniques, such as counseling, behavior modification, and adverse conditioning, have a success rate of 20 to 30%. The addition of pharmacologic intervention with a cutaneous nicotine patch may be useful for minimizing the physical effects of nicotine withdrawal. The role of more controversial approaches to smoking cessation, such as hypnosis, acupuncture, or the use of angiotensin-converting enzyme inhibitors, remains to be tested.

Lung Transplantation

In more recent years, lung transplantation and heart-lung transplantation have become feasible, and the role of this radical approach in the treatment of obstructive lung disease is now being defined. Heart-lung transplantation, and more recently double-lung transplantation, have been performed for a small number of cases of cystic fibrosis and emphysema.[34] Besides the usual technical problems of the surgery and the management of rejection, the number of such operations has been limited by organ availability. Single-lung transplantation, which is currently the operation of choice for transplantation in patients with pulmonary fibrosis and pulmonary hypertension, is a technically easier operation and should allow greater availability of organs. In cystic fibrosis, single-lung transplantation has not been favored because the continued presence of the remaining, chronically infected native lung would place the transplant in constant jeopardy. In emphysema, however, studies have shown that single-lung transplantation can be successful and may often be a viable option for carefully selected patients.

SUMMARY

Obstructive lung disease is a common cause of respiratory complaints and one of the most important reasons for hospitalization and time lost from work. The failure to diagnose and treat these patients correctly may result in respiratory failure and the development of right-sided heart failure. Proper diagnosis and treatment can alleviate the symptoms and physiologic abnormalities even in the setting of the lung destruction seen with emphysema. Future advances in the approach to the patient with obstructive lung disease will depend on a clearer understanding of the pathophysiology and will come in the area of prevention.

References

1. Miller RD, Hyatt RE. Evaluation of obstructing lesions of the trachea and larynx by flow-volume loops. Am Rev Respir Dis 108:475–481, 1973.
2. Stauffer JL, Olsen DE, Petty TL. Complications and consequences of endotracheal intubation and tracheotomy. A prospective study of 150 critically ill adult patients. Am J Med 70:65–76, 1981.
3. Hanallah R, Rosa JK. Acute epiglottitis: Current management and review. Can Anaesth Soc J 25:84–91, 1978.
4. Wilson TA, Hyatt RE, Rodarte JR. The mechanisms that limit expiratory flow. Lung 158:193–200, 1980.
5. Robins AG. Pathophysiology of emphysema. Clin Chest Med 4:413–420, 1983.
6. Busse WW. The role of inflammation in asthma: A new focus. J Respir Dis 10:72–80, 1989.
7. Guidelines for the Diagnosis and Management of Asthma. Washington, DC, US Department of Health and Human Services, 1991. Publication 91-3042.
8. Mountain RD, Sahn SA. Clinical features and outcome in patients with acute asthma presenting with hypercapnia. Am Rev Respir Dis 138:535–539, 1988.
9. Fletcher CM, Peto R, Tinker C, Speizer FE. The Natural History of Chronic Bronchitis and Emphysema. An Eight-Year History of Early Chronic Obstructive Lung Disease in Working Men in London. New York, Oxford University Press, 1976, p 272.
10. Anthonisen NR, Cherniack RM. Ventilatory controls in lung disease. *In* Horbein TF (ed). Regulation of Breathing. New York, Marcel Dekker, 1981, pp 965–987.
11. Nagai A, West WW, Thurlbeck WM. The National Institutes of Health. Intermittent Positive-Pressure Breathing Trial: Pathology studies II: Correlation between morphologic findings, clinical findings and evidence of expiratory-airflow obstruction. Am Rev Respir Dis 132:946–953, 1985.
12. Snider GL, Lucey EC, Stone PJ. Animal models of emphysema. Am Rev Respir Dis 133:149–169, 1986.
13. Crystal RG (ed). Symposium: Alpha-antitrypsin deficiency. Chest 95:181–208, 1989.
14. Niewoehner DE, Kleinerman J, Rice DB. Pathologic changes in the peripheral airways of young cigarette smokers. N Engl J Med 291:755–758, 1974.
15. Thurlbeck WM. Chronic airflow obstruction: Correlation of structure and function. *In* Petty T (ed). Chronic Obstructive Pulmonary Disease, 2nd ed. New York, Marcel Dekker, 1985, pp 129–203.
16. Barker AF, Bardana EJ. Bronchiectasis: Update of an orphan disease. Am Rev Respir Dis 137:969–978, 1988.
17. Stanford W, Galvin JR. The diagnosis of bronchiectasis. Clin Chest Med 9:691–699, 1988.
18. Davis PB, diSaint'Agnese PA. Diagnosis and treatment of cystic fibrosis: An update. Chest 85:802–809, 1984.
19. Hata JS, Fick RB. *Pseudomonas aeruginosa* and the airways disease of cystic fibrosis. Clin Chest Med 9:679–689, 1988.
20. Paterson JW, Woolcock AJ, Shenfield GM. State of the art: Bronchodilator drugs. Am Rev Respir Dis 120:1149–1188, 1979.
21. Gross NJ, Skorodin MS. State of the art: Anticholinergic, antimuscarinic bronchodilators. Am Rev Respir Dis 129:856–870, 1984.
22. Grant JA, Ellis EF. Update on theophylline: Symposium proceedings. J Allergy Clin Immunol 78:669–829, 1986.
23. Fanta CH, Rossing TH, McFadden ER. Glucocorticoids in acute asthma: A critical controlled trial. Am J Med 74:845–851, 1983.
24. Salmeron S, Guerin JC, Godard P, et al. High doses of inhaled corticosteroids in unstable chronic asthma. Am Rev Respir Dis 140:167–171, 1989.
25. Bernstein IL. Cromolyn sodium. Chest 87:685–735, 1985.
26. Nocturnal Oxygen Therapy Trial Group. Continuous O_2 nocturnal oxygen therapy in hypoxemic chronic obstructive lung disease: A clinical trial. Ann Intern Med 91:391–398, 1980.
27. Medical Research Council Working Party. Long-term domiciliary oxygen therapy in chronic hypoxic cor pulmonale complicating chronic bronchitis and emphysema. Lancet 1:681–686, 1981.

28. Anthonisen NR, Manfreda J, Warren CPW, et al. Antibiotic therapy in exacerbations of chronic obstructive pulmonary disease. Ann Intern Med 106:196–204, 1987.
29. Bolan G, Broome CV, Facklam RR, et al. Pneumococcal vaccine efficacy in selected populations in the United States. Ann Intern Med 104:1–6, 1986.
30. Petty TL. The National Mucolytic Study. Chest 97:75–83, 1990.
31. Shim C, King M, Williams MH. Lack of effect of hydration on sputum production in chronic bronchitis. Chest 92:679–682, 1987.
32. Kirilloff LH, Owens GR, Rogers MM, Mazzocco MC. Does chest physiotherapy work? Chest 88:436–444, 1985.
33. Hughes RL, Davison R. Limitations of exercise reconditioning in COPD. Chest 83:241–249, 1983.
34. Trulock EP, Cooper JD, Kaiser LR, et al. The Washington University–Barnes Hospital experience with lung transplantation. JAMA 266:1943–1946, 1991.

37

Congestive Heart Failure

Scott L. Roth, M.D.

Heart failure may be defined as the inability of the heart to pump an adequate amount of oxygenated blood to meet the metabolic demands of the tissues. Although this definition serves as an explanation of what may be happening at the cellular level, it is less useful in dealing with patients. Thus, in practice the clinical syndrome of congestive heart failure manifests as circulatory congestion. Congestion may be peripheral venous, pulmonary, or both. The syndrome may result from various causes of abnormal cardiac function, including malfunction of the heart muscle. This malfunction may be either primary, such as cardiomyopathy, or secondary, such as ischemic or valve disease.

The normal heart accepts a volume of blood (preload) and pumps the same volume against some degree of resistance (afterload). Normally functioning valves maintain one-way flow through the accepting chambers (the atria) and the pumping chambers (the ventricles). The atrial and ventricular septa normally separate the cardiac chambers into a right and a left side. The right side pumps blood to the lungs and receives venous return from the periphery. The left side pumps blood to the systemic circulation and receives pulmonary venous return from the lungs (Fig. 37–1).

COMPENSATORY MECHANISMS

The cardiovascular system, which is equipped with several adaptive or compensatory mechanisms, allows the heart to adapt to normal as well as abnormal changes in load. If cardiac overload persists over time (chronic heart failure), the compensatory mechanisms activate, accounting for much of the clinical syndrome observed.[1]

The first compensatory mechanism is the Frank-Starling relationship (Fig. 37–2). The performance of heart muscles relates to the length, or the amount of stretching, of the myocardial fibers. Thus, as the fibers stretch to a greater length, the force of contraction increases (within limits). Left ventricular diastolic volume can represent myocardial fiber length (Table 37–1). In the clinical setting, because volume is difficult to measure, the pulmonary artery diastolic or mean pulmonary capillary wedge pressure is usually substituted. Various measures of left ventricular performance, such as cardiac output and stroke volume, can represent myocardial fiber shortening.[2]

In Figure 37–2, the center curve represents the normal heart. Conditions that shift the curve upward and to the left represent states of enhanced pump function or contractility. This may occur with stimulation of the sympathetic nervous system, elevated circulating catecholamine levels, the use of inotropic drugs, or even increased heart rate. The curve shifted downward and to the right represents the failing myocardium, indicating a condition of reduced contractility. Patients with myocardial failure can increase their pump performance only at the expense

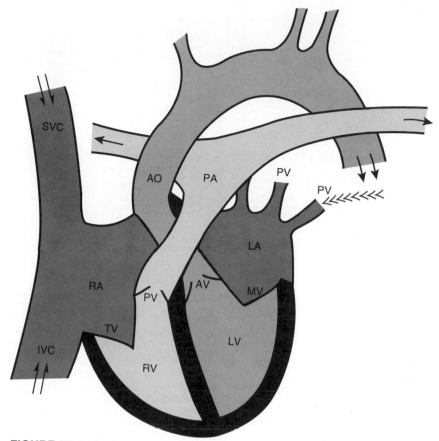

FIGURE 37–1: Cardiac anatomy. RA, LA, right and left atria; RV, LV, right and left ventricles; SVC, IVC, superior and inferior venae cavae; AO, aorta; PA, pulmonary artery; PVE, pulmonary vein; AV, aortic valve; TV, tricuspid valve; MV, mitral valve; PV, pulmonary valve.

Cardiac output = stroke volume × heart rate

of higher volume (dilatation), which leads to higher diastolic pressure, left atrial hypertension, and pulmonary congestion.

An increasing heart rate is a second compensatory mechanism to enhance left ventricular output. Cardiac output is a function of left ventricular stroke volume and heart rate. Stroke volume is the amount of blood pumped forward with each beat. Stroke volume is maximized in the failing heart by a dilated pumping chamber, as described earlier. An increasing heart rate will further enhance cardiac output. Patients in congestive heart failure due to reduced myocardial contractility are therefore usually tachycardic. In the patient with heart failure, the benefit derived from the increased heart rate is to some extent negated by the increase in cardiac work.

The activation of neurohormonal systems, an additional compensatory mechanism, includes sympathetic nervous system stimulation, elevated catecholamine levels, an activated renin-angiotensin system, and elevated atrial natriuretic peptide levels.[3] Although these mechanisms initially help to maintain blood pressure and perfusion in the face of failing pump function, the resulting salt and water retention worsen circulatory congestion.[4]

The myocardium adapts to chronic hemodynamic overload with its own intrinsic mechanisms. Various forms of valvular heart disease may

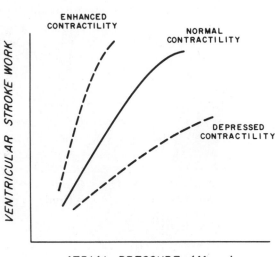

FIGURE 37–2: The Frank-Starling relationship. A family of ventricular function curves is diagrammed in which ventricular stroke work is plotted against the mean pressure in the corresponding atrium. In this model of ventricular function, enhanced contractility is defined as a shift of the function curve upward and to the left, and depressed contractility is defined as a shift of the function curve downward and to the right. (From Eagle K [ed]. The Practice of Cardiology. Boston, Little, Brown & Company, 1989, p 78.)

cause ventricular dilatation and hypertrophy. Once again, the initial effect of these responses to overload is to maintain pump performance, but as the condition persists, further myocardial dysfunction and circulatory congestion may ensue.[5]

PATHOPHYSIOLOGY

Congestive heart failure results when one or more of the previously described normal mechanisms is overloaded beyond the ability of the heart to adapt. This may occur from an excessive volume of blood return-

TABLE **37–1:**   Glossary of Terms

Systole	The period of time during which the heart chambers contract and eject blood
Diastole	The period of time during which the heart chambers dilate and fill with blood
Heart rate	The number of beats per minute
Cardiac output	The volume of blood delivered to the systemic circulation per unit of time (L/min)
Stroke volume	The volume of blood ejected from the pumping chamber (ventricle) with each beat
End-diastolic volume	The volume of blood contained in the ventricle at the end of filling, immediately before contraction
Contractility	The ability of muscle to shorten and develop tension
Ejection fraction	The ratio of stroke volume to end-diastolic volume *or* the percentage of blood volume that is ejected from the ventricle during systole

ing to the atria (preload), which may in turn result from valvular regurgitation or a shunt allowing blood to flow between the left and right sides of the heart. Overload can also occur when the ventricles must pump against a higher resistance (afterload), as in hypertension or outflow obstruction (e.g., aortic stenosis). If the heart muscle itself fails to generate sufficient force (poor contractility), the "normal" level of preload and afterload may be an excessive burden on the ventricles.[6] In addition, generalized hypervolemia (e.g., renal failure) may cause circulatory congestion in the setting of mild cardiac dysfunction.

Elevated pressures in the atria and the venous circulations cause edema in the presence of cardiac overload. However, this situation occurs only when the normal mechanisms for maintaining the integrity of the intravascular space have been overcome. The two forces that counteract the intravascular pressure (hydrostatic force) include the plasma oncotic pressure, which is created by proteins concentrated in the bloodstream, and the selective permeability of the capillary walls. These relationships are illustrated in Figure 37–3. A variety of noncardiac disorders may alter either the plasma oncotic pressure or the capillary permeability and thus cause interstitial edema (peripheral or pulmonary) in the absence of elevated atrial pressures. This accounts for the syndrome of noncardiogenic pulmonary edema.

Figure 37–4 illustrates the mechanism by which cardiac overload produces circulatory congestion. Right-sided heart overload produces el-

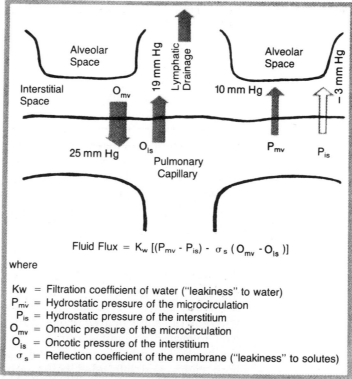

$$\text{Fluid Flux} = K_w \, [(P_{mv} - P_{is}) - \sigma_s \, (O_{mv} - O_{is})]$$

where

K_w = Filtration coefficient of water ("leakiness" to water)
P_{mv} = Hydrostatic pressure of the microcirculation
P_{is} = Hydrostatic pressure of the interstitium
O_{mv} = Oncotic pressure of the microcirculation
O_{is} = Oncotic pressure of the interstitium
σ_s = Reflection coefficient of the membrane ("leakiness" to solutes)

FIGURE 37–3: Factors affecting fluid filtration in the lung. The filtration is from the pulmonary microcirculation into the interstitium of the lung. Normally, excessive accumulation of fluid is prevented by the capacity of the lymphatics to drain it back into the systemic circulation. (From Roth SL. The adult respiratory distress syndrome and pulmonary critical care. *In* Andreoli TE, Bennett JC, Carpenter CCJ, et al [eds]. Cecil Essentials of Medicine, 3rd ed. Philadelphia, WB Saunders, 1993, p 161.)

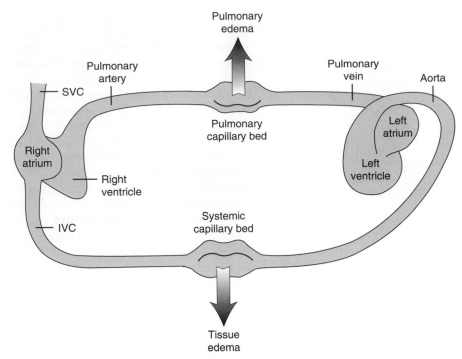

FIGURE 37–4: Left-sided heart overload causes elevated left ventricular end-diastolic pressure and therefore elevated left atrial pressure. This results in increased pressure in the pulmonary veins, which allows fluid to "leak out" of the pulmonary capillary system, causing interstitial pulmonary edema. Right-sided heart overload produces elevated right ventricular diastolic pressure and increased right atrial pressure. This results in high systemic venous pressure, which allows fluid to "leak out" of systemic capillaries, causing interstitial peripheral edema. SVC, IVC, superior and inferior venae cavae.

evated right ventricular diastolic and right atrial pressures. This causes high systemic venous pressure, which allows fluid to "leak" out of the systemic capillaries, causing peripheral edema. This may even lead to ascites and hepatic congestion if right atrial pressures become severely elevated for a prolonged period (severe right-sided heart failure). Left-sided heart overload produces elevated left ventricular diastolic and left atrial pressures. This causes high pulmonary venous pressure, which allows fluid to "leak" out of the pulmonary capillary system, causing interstitial pulmonary edema. If left atrial pressure becomes severely elevated, a larger amount of fluid leaks out, causing alveolar as well as interstitial edema (severe left-sided heart failure). This accounts for the syndrome of acute pulmonary edema, which is usually associated with a left atrial pressure of 25 mm Hg or greater. The level of atrial pressure at which pulmonary edema develops is a function of chronicity. Thus, moderate acute elevations in pressure may cause pulmonary edema, whereas the same degree of elevation, if it is present chronically, may be well tolerated without significant congestion. Because the two sides of the heart depend on each other for proper functioning, some degree of both right- and left-sided heart failure is frequently seen in a given patient: this is so-called biventricular failure.[7]

Some patients with dyspnea have preserved systolic function. Further study reveals that these patients have an elevated left ventricular diastolic pressure. Such patients have diastolic dysfunction, a disease that is due to myocardial hypertrophy and may be primary or secondary (e.g., due to systemic hypertension). The hypertrophy leads to a failure of the heart muscle to relax. Therefore, the left ventricle becomes stiff, which reduces its ability to fill with blood. This can lead to elevated diastolic pressures in the face of normal systolic function without significant volume overload.[8] The management of such patients is complex and is quite different from that of patients with heart failure and systolic dysfunction. Recognition of this syndrome is thus important because vasodilators and inotropic agents are of limited value.

The clinical syndrome of congestive heart failure may appear very similar in patients with vastly different disease etiologies. However, the diagnostic and therapeutic approach will be very different depending on the specific cause. Therefore, it is important to have a working knowledge of the various causes of heart failure (Table 37–2).

Usually, a single underlying cause exists for the syndrome in a given patient (e.g., myocardial failure and hemodynamic overload). However, many episodes of heart failure will be secondary to a precipitating cause, which can further interfere with the heart's ability to adapt to an underlying cardiovascular abnormality or stress. Recognition of both underlying and precipitating causes is necessary to institute effective therapy.

DIAGNOSTIC APPROACH

The first goal in evaluating the individual patient is to establish the presence of heart failure as the primary cause of the patient's signs and symptoms. The three major manifestations of the syndrome of circulatory congestion may be seen alone or in combination (Table 37–3). In the critical care setting, the clinician will most often encounter pulmonary congestion, the most common of the three manifestations. However, the other manifestations should be kept in mind because their presence will probably change the therapeutic approach to the patient.

When the clinician is confronted with a patient in acute respiratory distress, early recognition of acute pulmonary edema is crucial to rapid and effective management. A high level of suspicion is necessary because the condition of patients with acute pulmonary edema can deteriorate rapidly. Using the same logical, organized approach with every patient reduces the number of misdiagnoses and leads to effective treatment. Consider the following clinical situation:

TABLE **37–2:**   Causes of Heart Failure

Underlying causes
  Myocardial failure
    Loss of muscle cells with scarring (cardiomyopathy)
    Lack of oxygen delivery (ischemia)
    Acute myocardial infarction
    Diastolic dysfunction (ventricular hypertrophy)
  Hemodynamic overload
    Valvular stenosis or regurgitation
    Hypertension
    Congenital heart disease
Precipitating causes
  Increased salt intake
  Medication noncompliance
  Arrhythmia
  Infection (e.g., pneumonia)
  High-output state (anemia, hyperthyroidism, or pregnancy)
  Renal failure
  Myocardial depressant drugs (e.g., disopyramide)

TABLE **37-3:** Major Manifestations of Circulatory Congestion

Pulmonary congestion	Low-output state
Shortness of breath	Hypotension
Respiratory failure	Lethargy
Peripheral congestion	Low urine output
Jugular venous distention	
Enlarged liver	
Ascites	
Leg edema	

This case illustrates the cardinal features of acute cardiogenic pulmonary edema and demonstrates how the diagnosis may be suspected and confirmed with the history, physical examination, electrocardiogram (ECG), and chest x-ray study.

A 65-year-old man who had a myocardial infarction 6 months ago presents to the emergency department with the sudden onset of shortness of breath. He complains of having had progressive dyspnea on exertion for 1 month and of having had two-pillow orthopnea and paroxysmal nocturnal dyspnea for the past week. On initial evaluation, the patent is in severe respiratory distress sitting upright and is diaphoretic. His pulse is 120 beats per minute, and his blood pressure is 170/100 mm Hg. The physical examination reveals no apparent jugular venous distention, crackles and wheezes throughout both lung fields, a loud S_3 gallop, no significant murmur, and no hepatomegaly or peripheral edema. The skin is cool and clammy. The ECG reveals sinus tachycardia, left atrial enlargement, and Q waves from V_1 to V_6. The x-ray study reveals an enlarged cardiac silhouette, upper zone flow redistribution, and interstitial and alveolar edema with bilateral hilar "fluffiness." There is bilateral blunting of the costophrenic angles.

The history may have to be obtained from family members or emergency personnel because patients are often unable to provide adequate details. Establishing the presence of known potential causes of heart failure, such as prior heart attack, angina, or hypertension, raises the level of suspicion. A history of dyspnea on exertion, orthopnea, or paroxysmal nocturnal dyspnea suggests a cardiac etiology, but these features may be present with lung disease as well. An inquiry should be made about recent increases in salt intake or noncompliance with medications. The presence of palpitations, lightheadedness, or syncope may suggest arrhythmia as a precipitating factor. The recent onset of fever, cough, and sputum production should suggest the diagnosis of pneumonia, a common precipitating factor in elderly patients. Finally, the possibility of coexisting medical disorders that may exacerbate cardiac conditions, such as anemia, thyroid disease, and pregnancy, should be remembered.

The physical examination may or may not be helpful in differentiating cardiac from noncardiac causes of respiratory distress. The patient presented in the case study represents one end of the spectrum of left-sided heart failure. He has severe pulmonary congestion with bolt-upright posture, diaphoresis, tachycardia, hypertension, and crackles and wheezes (cardiac asthma) throughout the lung fields. Milder degrees of left-sided heart failure and pulmonary congestion may not be so obvious. Patients with mild to moderate pulmonary congestion usually have pulmonary crackles, perhaps only at the bases to the midlung fields. They are usually mildly tachycardic, and their blood pressure may be normal or slightly elevated. Pulsus alternans, a beat-to-beat variation in the systolic pressure, suggests the presence of significant left ventricular failure. Cardiogenic shock exists in the patient who exhibits a low systolic blood pressure, or hypotension, along with cardiogenic pulmonary edema. This dire situation, which has a high mortality rate, requires immediate and aggressive therapy. Pulmonary crackles may be absent in the early phase, with only expiratory rhonchi present. Similarly, upright posture, diaphoresis, tachycardia, and hypertension may be absent in patients with acute pulmonary edema.

Hypotension is a systolic blood pressure of less than 80 mm Hg.

On examination, an S_3 gallop or a prominent murmur, reflecting valvular dysfunction, helps to confirm the cardiac origin of pulmonary congestion. The specific findings may lead to a particular underlying cardiac etiology. Jugular venous distention, hepatomegaly, ascites, and peripheral edema should all be sought as signs of right-sided heart failure. These signs make the diagnosis of cardiogenic pulmonary edema more likely, in view of the fact that the most common cause of right-sided heart failure is left-sided heart failure. However, the absence of signs of right-sided heart failure does not exclude the presence of left-sided heart failure or pulmonary congestion. Specifically, patients with a sudden onset of acute pulmonary edema frequently do not have leg edema. Conversely, the presence of leg edema without other signs of heart failure does not imply a cardiac etiology for a patient's respiratory distress.

The ECG is helpful in detecting precipitating factors, such as the presence of ischemia (ST segment depression), acute myocardial infarction (ST segment elevation), prior myocardial infarction (Q waves), left atrial enlargement (seen with chronic congestive heart failure), and arrhythmias (especially atrial and ventricular tachyarrhythmias). The chest x-ray study provides important confirmatory evidence of pulmonary congestion. Because various lung disorders can cause pulmonary crackles on physical examination (e.g., pneumonia and chronic interstitial lung disease), the chest x-ray findings are often a decisive factor in clinical decision making. The most specific signs consistent with pulmonary congestion are upper zone flow redistribution and interstitial and alveolar edema. Bilateral pleural effusions may also be present, especially with severe left-sided heart failure. Cardiomegaly (a cardiothoracic ratio of greater than 0.5) usually helps to confirm only what is already known from the history, physical examination, and ECG. The absence of cardiomegaly does not exclude cardiogenic pulmonary edema.

The preceding discussion gives an overview of how the systematic application of the history, physical examination, ECG, and chest x-ray study can clarify the diagnosis of cardiogenic pulmonary edema. The information obtained up to this point suffices to begin therapy with general measures directed against pulmonary congestion (see the following section on management of acute pulmonary edema). However, many patients require further diagnostic testing to identify the specific underlying and precipitating causes of heart failure. These tests provide enough information to institute more directed, definitive therapy.[9]

Certainly, if the initial evaluation leaves the cause of respiratory distress unclear, further testing is required. For example, consider a patient without a cardiac history who has acute respiratory distress characterized by pulmonary crackles, normal cardiac examination findings, normal ECG results, and chest radiographic findings of diffuse bilateral alveolar edema. These findings suggest adult respiratory distress syndrome, or noncardiogenic pulmonary edema. The definitive diagnostic procedure is placement of a pulmonary artery catheter for precise measurement of the pulmonary capillary wedge pressure (PCWP), which provides an estimate of the left atrial pressure. A normal or low PCWP in this setting excludes the diagnosis of cardiogenic pulmonary edema. This also defines the syndrome of noncardiogenic pulmonary edema, the causes of which are listed in Table 37–4. A markedly elevated PCWP (i.e., greater than 20 mm Hg) confirms the diagnosis of cardiogenic pulmonary edema. Intermediate readings (13 to 19 mm Hg) need

A normal PCWP is 6 to 12 mm Hg.

TABLE **37–4:** Causes of Noncardiogenic Pulmonary Edema

Hypoalbuminemia (decreased plasma oncotic pressure)
  Renal or hepatic disease
  Malnutrition
  Protein-losing enteropathy
Adult respiratory distress syndrome (increased alveolar
    capillary permeability)
  Pneumonia
  Toxins (smoke inhalation)
  Uremia
Other causes
  Neurogenic
  High altitude
  Heroin overdose

to be evaluated in the context of other findings. The patient requires re-evaluation after a therapeutic trial.[10]

Thus, in the patient with physical examination and chest x-ray findings consistent with, but not diagnostic of, cardiogenic pulmonary edema, measurement of the PCWP can provide a definitive diagnosis. Additional valuable information can be obtained with the pulmonary artery catheter. For example, analysis of the waveform of the PCWP tracing may reveal prominent V waves, which are suggestive of significant mitral valve incompetence. Measurement of oxygen saturation of various levels in the right side of the heart may reveal a left-to-right shunt, diagnostic of ventricular septal rupture complicating acute myocardial infarction. These life-threatening causes of acute pulmonary edema may require urgent mechanical intervention.

Other diagnostic modalities that may be helpful at the bedside include noninvasive tests such as two-dimensional echocardiography and radionuclide angiography. Both of these tests, which are safe and easily performed in the critically ill patient, can directly assess left and right ventricular size and contractile function. Echocardiography can be applied in nearly all patients to assess chamber sizes and wall thickness, ventricular function, and valvular function. A small percentage of patients, particularly the obese, may be difficult to image. In these patients, radionuclide angiography can provide a quantitative assessment of right and left ventricular size and function.

MANAGEMENT OF ACUTE PULMONARY EDEMA

The initial therapeutic approach to acute cardiogenic pulmonary edema can be applied to all patients, regardless of the cause of the condition. The following general measures may be applied rapidly in conjunction with a continuing diagnostic evaluation.

Some patients with acute pulmonary edema are severely ill; the clinician must apply the ABCs (airway, breathing, and circulation) of resuscitation before any of the general measures can be instituted. In addition, all of the measures require an adequate blood pressure (greater than 95 mm Hg). Patients with pulmonary edema and systemic hypotension are considered to have cardiogenic shock, requiring intravenous pressor agents (to be described later).

The general goals of the initial management of acute pulmonary edema include

• Improve oxygenation

- Reduce anxiety
- Decrease venous return
- Decrease afterload
- Treat precipitating factors

The clinician evaluates and treats the patient by

- Placing the patient in the upright position
- Immediately administering oxygen by face mask or high-flow nasal cannula
- Securing an intravenous line, preferably a central or an antecubital line, if pressor agents are needed
- Monitoring vital signs frequently
- Obtaining a brief, directed history and performing a physical examination
- Sending blood samples for complete blood counts to reveal any anemia or an elevated white blood cell count as seen in infection; serum electrolyte levels should be measured
- Obtaining arterial blood gas measurements to assess oxygenation as well as ventilation and acid-base status; moderate acidosis, hypercarbia, and hypoxemia are frequently seen before effective therapy; blood gases may be repeatedly measured to determine the effectiveness of the general measures
- Performing a 12-lead ECG immediately, because the management differs in the presence of an acute myocardial infarction or ongoing ischemia; for example, if evidence of acute myocardial infarction exists, thrombolytic therapy must be considered; unstable angina without infarction may require intravenous nitroglycerin, as well as systemic anticoagulation with heparin; in addition, precipitating arrhythmias may be detected early

As long as the patient is adequately ventilated and has a reasonable systolic blood pressure (95 to 100 mm Hg), the following general measures should be instituted:

- Morphine sulfate should immediately be given intravenously, in doses of 3 to 5 mg, at 10- to 15-minute intervals.
- The patient should be monitored closely for lethargy, respiratory depression, and hypotension. Morphine increases venous capacitance, thus decreasing venous return and decreasing atrial pressure. It also decreases afterload somewhat. Anxiety will be reduced as well.[11]
- Nitrates also reduce venous return, because of their primary venodilating properties. They have a lesser effect on afterload, with a weaker arterial vasodilating effect. Nitroglycerin should be used immediately as long as blood pressure is maintained. Sublingual nitroglycerin has an onset of action of approximately 2 minutes. Nitropaste exerts its effect after several minutes, lasts for several hours, and may be removed if side effects develop. An intravenous nitroglycerin infusion provides an easily controllable route of administration. Dosing starts at 10 μg/min and may be increased by 5 to 10 μg/min every 5 minutes, titrating to systolic blood pressure.
- Intravenous diuretics should be used in nearly all patients. The rapidly acting loop diuretics, furosemide (Lasix) and bumetanide (Bumex), are used most commonly. Caution is needed in patients with low blood pressure and in those with suspected myocardial infarction or aortic stenosis, in whom hypotension must be avoided. Hypotension may occur with overdiuresis, especially with the use of nitrates and mor-

phine. Furosemide may be given initially as a 20- to 40-mg intravenous bolus; bumetanide may be started at 0.5 to 2 mg. Although the peak diuretic effect occurs in 15 to 30 minutes, furosemide appears to have some beneficial effects much sooner. This benefit is attributed to some vasodilatory properties of the drug. Electrolyte levels must be measured frequently when the loop diuretics are being used. Hypokalemia is particularly dangerous for patients with pulmonary edema and myocardial ischemia or infarction because a significant risk of ventricular arrhythmia exists.[12]

If acidosis and hypoxemia persist despite the reduction in venous return with the preceding measures, tracheal intubation with mechanical ventilation may be needed. The addition of positive end-expiratory pressure may be beneficial, despite its tendency to decrease cardiac output.

Most patients with acute pulmonary edema benefit from the reduction in venous return. In addition, a select group of patients may also require afterload reduction. These patients can be identified by using echocardiography to assess ventricular systolic and diastolic function. Afterload reduction is appropriate if systolic dysfunction is a major factor in the development of heart failure. Therapy with oral vasodilators should be instituted early.[13] The angiotensin-converting enzyme inhibitors are particularly useful in this regard. Captopril (Capoten) may be added to diuretics, starting with a test dose of 6.25 mg orally. The patient should be monitored carefully for the development of systemic hypotension, especially ½ to 1 hour after the initial dose. Subsequent dosing should be titrated to achieve a systolic blood pressure of approximately 100 mm Hg. Caution should be used in patients with renal insuffiency because these drugs may worsen renal function and cause hyperkalemia.[14] Parenteral vasodilators should be reserved for patients who do not respond to the previously mentioned therapy and for those with hypertensive crisis.

The methods of decreasing venous return and afterload should not be applied in patients with pulmonary edema and hypotension. These patients require intravenous catecholamine pressor agents to support systemic blood pressure and organ perfusion. With mild to moderate hypotension (80 to 100 mm Hg systolic pressure), dobutamine may be used alone. The starting dose is 5 to 10 μg/kg/min, with a positive inotropic effect. Invasive hemodynamic monitoring of the PCWP is usually required to assess the efficacy of treatment. Patients with more severe hypotension and signs of decreased tissue perfusion (lethargy, peripheral vasoconstriction, and decreased urine output) may require dopamine in as low a dose as possible (less than 10 μg/kg/min) to maintain renal and splanchnic perfusion. Sinus tachycardia and ventricular and atrial tachyarrhythmias may be precipitated. Norepinephrine, which has a greater alpha-adrenergic effect at low doses and a lower positive chronotropic effect, may be used as an alternative.

A small number of patients with acute myocardial infarction, ongoing ischemia, valvular disease (except aortic insufficiency), or ventricular septal rupture benefit from intra-aortic balloon counterpulsation. This mechanical technique provides superior afterload reduction and improves coronary perfusion. It may be used to stabilize the patient hemodynamically before cardiac catheterization and cardiac surgery.

Some patients with a history of systemic hypertension may develop acute pulmonary edema associated with a markedly elevated blood pres-

Dobutamine complications

- Ventricular arrhythmias
- Worsening of hypotension initially secondary to a vasodilator effect

sure. This constitutes a form of hypertensive crisis. These patients benefit from parenteral vasodilators. Intravenous nitroprusside, a powerful arterial vasodilator, is particularly efficacious in this setting. Its use is limited by the need for intensive blood pressure monitoring and by the possibility of toxicity with prolonged use (more than several days).

In addition to any or all of the previously mentioned measures, arrhythmia should always be sought as a precipitating factor, and specific therapy should be instituted. The supraventricular tachyarrhythmias commonly exacerbate pulmonary edema. Atrial fibrillation with rapid ventricular response leads to decreased diastolic filling. Slowing of the ventricular response with digitalis may lead to a dramatic improvement in selected patients. If the rhythm is associated with significant hypotension or ischemia, direct current cardioversion should be performed.

SUMMARY

Thus, the overall approach to managing acute pulmonary edema includes

- General measures (e.g., the use of oxygen, morphine, diuretics, and nitrates) that can be applied to most patients
- Specific measures applied to selected groups of patients, including afterload reduction for systolic dysfunction and the use of parenteral vasodilators for hypertensive crisis; more specific diagnostic information is required to apply the most definitive, selected therapeutic strategies

References

1. Weber KT, Janicki JS. Pathogenesis of heart failure. Cardiol Clin 7(1):11, 1989.
2. Braunwald E. Assessment of cardiac function. *In* Braunwald E (ed). Heart Disease: A Textbook of Cardiovascular Medicine, 4th ed. Philadelphia, WB Saunders, 1992, pp 419–443.
3. Just H. Peripheral adaptations in congestive heart failure: A review. Am J Med 90(5B):235, 1991.
4. Packer M. Neurohumoral interaction and adaptations in congestive heart failure. Circulation 77:721, 1988.
5. Opie LH. Compensation and overcompensation in congestive heart failure. Am Heart J 120(6 Pt. 2):1552, 1990.
6. Parmley WW. Pathophysiology and current therapy of congestive heart failure. J Am Coll Cardiol 13:771, 1989.
7. Braunwald E. Clinical aspects of heart failure. *In* Braunwald E (ed). Heart Disease: A Textbook of Cardiovascular Medicine, 4th ed. Philadelphia, WB Saunders, 1992, pp 444–463.
8. Yancy CW, Firth BG. Congestive heart failure. Dis Mon 34(8):465, 1988.
9. Smith TW, Braunwald E, Kelly RA. The management of heart failure. *In* Braunwald E (ed). Heart Disease: A Textbook of Cardiovascular Medicine, 4th ed. Philadelphia, WB Saunders, 1992, pp 464–519.
10. Forrester IS, Waters DD. Hospital treatment of congestive heart failure: Management according to hemodynamic profiles. Am J Med 65:173, 1978.
11. Stanley R. Drug therapy of heart failure. J Cardiovasc Nurs 4(3):17, 1990.
12. Cohn IN. Current therapy of the failing heart. Circulation 78:1099, 1988.
13. Katz AM. Changing strategies in the management of heart failure. J Am Coll Cardiol 13:513, 1989.
14. Thind GS. Angiotensin converting enzyme inhibitors: Comparative structure, pharmacokinetics, and pharmacodynamics. Cardiovasc Drugs Ther 4(1):199, 1990.

38

Respiratory Failure

David R. Dantzker, M.D.

◼

$$Pa_{CO_2} = \dot{V}_{CO_2} \times k/\dot{V}_A$$

where $\dot{V}_{CO_2}$ is CO_2 produced by the body each minute and k is a constant. $\dot{V}_A$ is the portion of the minute ventilation ($\dot{V}_E$) that actually partakes in gas exchange:

$$\dot{V}_A = \dot{V}_E - \dot{V}_D$$

where $\dot{V}_D$ represents ventilation of the dead space.

Respiratory failure, which causes marked interference with pulmonary gas exchange, is characterized by abnormal arterial blood gas values. Although the specific value of the arterial blood gases that defines respiratory failure is somewhat arbitrary, failure is usually said to be present when the Pa_{O_2} is less than 60 mm Hg or the Pa_{CO_2} is greater than 45 mm Hg in a person breathing room air at sea level. Respiratory failure may be caused by an abnormality of any of the components of the respiratory system and can be broadly categorized as being primarily due to ventilatory pump failure or to inefficient pulmonary gas exchange (Table 38–1). In many disorders, an overlap of these two broad mechanisms exists. Respiratory failure may progress slowly or occur acutely.

Ventilatory pump failure is the etiology of respiratory failure in patients with disorders of ventilatory control, in patients with neuromuscular and chest wall disease, and in the setting of respiratory muscle fatigue. Ventilatory pump failure, if allowed to progress, ultimately leads to hypoventilation and thus to the development of hypercapnia and hypoxemia (see Chapter 6). Hypoventilation as a mechanism of abnormal pulmonary gas exchange can be differentiated from other causes of respiratory failure by the presence of a normal alveolar-arterial gradient of O_2.

Inefficient gas exchange, the most common mechanism of both acute and chronic respiratory failure, is seen in patients with obstructive and restrictive lung diseases, in those with pneumonia, and in those with pulmonary edema. This inefficient exchange, which develops secondary to ventilation-perfusion ($\dot{V}/\dot{Q}$) inequality or shunt, is characterized by hypoxemia but often not by hypercapnia, as explained in Chapter 6.

In some patients, respiratory failure begins with inefficient gas exchange, but with progression of the underlying illness, there is a progressive requirement for increased ventilation in order to maintain a normal Pa_{CO_2}. Eventually, a point may be reached at which the respiratory pump either cannot continue to increase ventilation enough to keep up with the worsening degree of $\dot{V}/\dot{Q}$ inequality or may actually fail because of the excessive work of breathing or the development of respiratory muscle fatigue. This is commonly seen in patients with acute exacerbations of

TABLE **38–1:** Respiratory Failure

Ventilatory pump failure	Inefficient pulmonary gas exchange
Abnormal ventilatory control	Obstructive lung disease
Drug overdose	Restrictive lung disease
Cerebrovascular disease	Pneumonia
Sleep	Pulmonary edema
Neuromuscular disease	
Diaphragmatic paralysis	
Guillain-Barré syndrome	
Myasthenia gravis	
Muscular dystrophy	
Chest wall disease	
Scoliosis	
Ankylosing spondylitis	
Obesity	
Muscle fatigue	

chronic obstructive and restrictive lung disorders. Many of these patients maintain a normal or even a reduced arterial P_{CO_2} when their conditions are stable, but they become rapidly hypercapnic if the degree of the pulmonary abnormality worsens or an additional insult, such as infection, supervenes. Similarly, patients with ventilatory pump failure may develop an additional component of inefficient gas exchange due to complicating parenchymal lung disease.

VENTILATORY PUMP FAILURE

Alveolar gas equation:

$$PA_{O_2} = PI_{O_2} - PA_{CO_2}/R$$

where R is the respiratory exchange ratio.

In the otherwise normal lung, the Pa_{CO_2} directly depends on the alveolar ventilation ($\dot{V}A$). In the setting of ventilatory pump failure, $\dot{V}A$ falls because of inadequate $\dot{V}E$ (hypoventilation). In addition to hypercapnia, the reduction in $\dot{V}A$ leads to hypoxemia due to reduced alveolar P_{O_2} (see the alveolar gas equation).

This chapter cannot discuss each of the large number of disorders that result in failure of the ventilatory pump. However, some warrant emphasis because of their clinical importance.

Diaphragmatic Weakness and Paralysis

The diaphragm may be involved in a wide variety of neuromuscular disorders, including multiple sclerosis, poliomyelitis, and various neuropathies and myopathies. It may also be injured during trauma.[1] In patients undergoing open heart surgery, the phrenic nerve may be damaged by the ice used to cool the heart. The diaphragm may also function abnormally after upper abdominal surgery, although the mechanism is less clear. When only one side is involved, the patient may be relatively asymptomatic, but bilateral paralysis usually results in dyspnea and reduced exercise tolerance, as well as hypoxemia and hypercapnia. These abnormalities worsen when the patient is in the supine position because the flaccid diaphragm pushes up into the chest, further compromising respiratory function.

Spinal Cord Injury

Injuries to the spinal cord are, unfortunately, a common occurrence, especially as a result of motor vehicle accidents.[2] In addition to their effect on pulmonary function, they are associated with a myriad of other complications, including bowel and bladder dysfunction, recurrent infections, decubitus ulcers, and of course skeletal muscle paralysis. The pulmonary abnormalities depend on the level of the injury.

High cervical lesions, above the third cervical vertebra (C3), result in complete respiratory paralysis. These patients require continuous ventilatory assistance. Lesions at the mid and lower cervical regions usually leave sufficient accessory muscle function to permit reasonably good ventilatory function when the patient is awake, although hypoxemia may be present owing to basilar atelectasis. When sleeping, however, these patients often require complete or partial mechanical support to maintain adequate alveolar ventilation. Thoracic spine lesions compromise mainly expiratory muscle function and thus result in a weak, inefficient cough, which predisposes the patient to respiratory infections.

Guillain-Barré Syndrome

Guillain-Barré syndrome, a distinctive form of acute polyneuropathy in which a gradually progressive ascending paralysis occurs, usually follows a viral-like illness. Leg weakness is often greater than arm weakness, and full evolution of the paralysis usually occurs in 2 to 4 weeks. Progression to involve the respiratory muscles is common, with prolonged mechanical ventilation often necessary for 2 or more months. Studies have suggested that plasmapheresis[3] or intravenous immune globulin,[4] if used early in the course, will decrease the severity of Guillain-Barré syndrome.

Elective intubation and mechanical ventilation are recommended once the vital capacity falls below 1 L.

Myasthenia Gravis

Myasthenia gravis is a disease of the motor end-plate that is characterized by intermittent muscle weakness, especially after repeated muscular contraction. Although limb, ocular, and facial muscles are commonly involved, the respiratory muscles may also be affected, with resultant hypoventilation. Myasthenia gravis is often overlooked, sometimes with tragic consequences. Patients with acute myasthenic crises can often be helped by steroids or by plasmapheresis to remove autoantibodies to the acetylcholine receptor.[5] Respiratory failure due to myasthenia gravis must be differentiated from that due to a cholinergic crisis caused by too much cholinesterase inhibitor therapy.

The diagnosis of myasthenia gravis is made by giving patients a trial of a cholinesterase inhibitor such as edrophonium chloride (Tensilon), which causes an increase in muscle strength in patients with myasthenia gravis.

Kyphoscoliosis

Kyphoscoliosis is an excessive curvature of the thoracic spine both posteriorly and laterally. Its cause is unknown, but hereditary factors may play a role in most cases.[6] The spinal curvature, which leads to a progressive reduction in lung volumes, may eventually cause respiratory failure. The process usually progresses with age. Surgery to correct the skeletal disorder may be useful in children but not in adults.

Obesity

Individuals who are 150 to 200% or more of their ideal body weight suffer from a significant abnormality of pulmonary function.[7] There is a reduction in the compliance of the respiratory system, as well as an increased work of breathing. This is accompanied by a fall in lung volumes and hypoxemia due to poor or absent ventilation of the lung bases. The supine position aggravates all of these abnormalities. Obesity also increases the tendency to develop the obstructive sleep apnea syndrome, as described in Chapter 43.

Obstructive sleep apnea often leads to chronic hypercapnia and excessive daytime sleepiness, a constellation of symptoms and signs that when seen in obese people is classified as the obesity-hypoventilation syndrome or pickwickian syndrome.

MANAGEMENT OF VENTILATORY PUMP FAILURE

Diagnosis

The optimal management of ventilatory pump failure begins by making as specific a diagnosis of the underlying problem as possible.

Often, the diagnosis is obvious from the history or physical examination findings, such as with an overdose of sedatives or narcotics or an obvious neurologic or musculoskeletal disorder. On occasion, the realization that a patient has respiratory failure may be delayed until very late in the course of the illness. Individuals with chronic fatigue or decreased exercise tolerance as a result of early neuromuscular disease may initially be thought to be depressed. Paroxysmal arrhythmias, which are due to hypoxemia or respiratory acidosis, may lead to a cardiologic work-up. Morning headaches that are actually due to nocturnal hypercapnia may be ascribed to migraine.

When the suspicion of ventilatory pump failure is raised and the patient is stable enough to undergo a diagnostic work-up, pulmonary function testing is invaluable. The characteristic changes in lung volumes can often differentiate obstructive or restrictive lung disease from neuromuscular disease. Individuals with an isolated abnormality of ventilatory control usually have normal results on pulmonary function studies (Fig. 38–1). A measurement of maximal inspiratory and expiratory pressures should always be included (Table 38–2). Arterial blood gas measurements can differentiate pure hypoventilation (normal alveolar-arterial gradient for O_2) from disorders in which the lung is also involved. Patients with abnormal ventilatory control can often normalize their Pa_{CO_2} by voluntary hyperventilation. A discussion of the specific diagnostic approaches to the many causes of ventilatory pump failure is beyond the scope of this chapter.

Analysis of the P_{CO_2}-pH relationship suggests an acute versus a chronic problem. For an acute increase in the Pa_{CO_2}, there should be a decrease of 0.008 pH units/mm Hg P_{CO_2}. For chronic elevations, the change is 0.003 pH units/mm Hg P_{CO_2}.

Treatment

In patients with acute respiratory acidosis, the approach to treatment depends on the ability to reverse the underlying problem rapidly. Patients with an acute asthmatic attack can often be treated with aggressive bronchodilator and anti-inflammatory therapy, even after the onset of hypercapnia, without the need for intubation.[8] However, a patient with spinal cord trauma or drug overdose may require immediate intubation to stabilize the situation before an extensive diagnostic work-up can begin. Even in patients who do not require intubation, reversal of hypoxemia is a priority. In some cases, the administration of supplemental O_2 may lead to a further increase in P_{CO_2}, especially in patients with

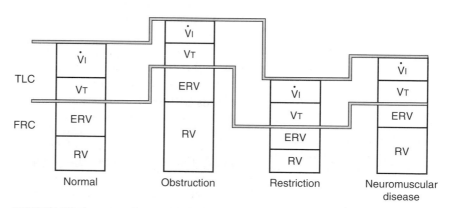

FIGURE 38–1: Lung volumes in various forms of respiratory failure. $\dot{V}I$, inspired volume; VT, tidal volume; ERV, expiratory reserve volume; RV, residual volume; TLC, total lung capacity; FRC, functional residual capacity.

TABLE **38–2:** Maximal Static Respiratory Pressure

	Men	**Women**
Maximal inspiratory pressure (mm Hg)*	− 130	− 100
Maximal expiratory pressure (mm Hg)†	240	180

*Residual volume.
†Total lung capacity.

pre-existing hypercapnia and marked hypoxemia. The cause of the increase in P_{CO_2} in this setting is multifactorial:

- A depression of respiratory drive
- An increase in ventilation-perfusion inequality
- A reduction in the affinity of hemoglobin for CO_2 (the Haldane effect)[9]

In many cases, the latter two mechanisms predominate. Small increases in P_{CO_2} are almost invariable when the $F_{I_{O_2}}$ of patients with previous chronic respiratory insufficiency is increased. This should not be a matter of immediate concern as long as the P_{CO_2} stabilizes and is not accompanied by central nervous system depression or marked acidosis. Sufficient but not excessive supplemental O_2 should be given to achieve an adequate O_2 saturation (about 90%); if progressive hypercapnia results, intubation may be necessary. It is often dangerous to treat the increasing hypercapnia by decreasing the inspired O_2 concentration because this may lead to the development of profound hypoxemia. It is important to remember that hypoxemia, not respiratory acidosis, is the serious immediate problem.

In patients with more chronic forms of ventilatory pump failure, the decision to resort to some form of assisted ventilation is often more difficult. In patients with progressive neuromuscular disorders or end-stage lung disease, the decision to treat acute respiratory failure with mechanical ventilation should be made only after discussion with the patient and family. Their understanding of the prognosis of the underlying disease and the likely benefits and complications of the treatment should be clear.

Sleep is often a particularly stressful time for patients with ventilatory pump failure. The supine position leads to a further reduction in functional residual capacity; at this lower lung volume, airway closure occurs and hypoxemia increases. In addition, respiratory drive is further reduced, and during certain phases of sleep, accessory muscle function is depressed (see Chapter 43). All of these factors may lead to an accentuation of the hypoxemia and hypercapnia, even in patients who are well compensated when awake. These repeated intermittent episodes of hypoxemia and hypercapnia may eventually result in the development of pulmonary hypertension and cor pulmonale. When right-sided heart failure develops in a patient in whom the awake blood gas values appear to be inappropriately normal, a sleep study should be performed.

In some cases, the problem of hypoventilation during sleep can be successfully treated with the use of nocturnal O_2 to correct the hypoxemia. However, some sort of ventilatory support is often necessary. Although this may require the placement of a tracheostomy, a number of ventilatory techniques exist that do not require direct access to the airway. These include the use of various types of negative pressure ventilators or rocking beds and more recently the use of nasal ventilation with a standard volume-limited positive pressure ventilator. These techniques are more fully described in Chapter 22.

INEFFICIENT PULMONARY GAS EXCHANGE

Inefficient pulmonary gas exchange, an almost invariable consequence of all lung disease, may be due to the development of ventilation-perfusion inequality, as seen in patients with obstructive and restrictive lung disease, or shunt, the cause of hypoxemia in pneumonia and pulmonary edema. For the most part, the characteristic abnormality of and the therapeutic approach to each of these are covered in the individual chapters devoted to the disorder. This section gives an overview of the most dramatic form of acute hypoxemic respiratory failure, commonly referred to as the adult respiratory distress syndrome (ARDS).

ARDS is characterized by severe hypoxemia, bilateral pulmonary infiltrates, and decreased lung compliance. Since the initial description of ARDS in 1967,[10] it has become increasingly clear that the pulmonary abnormalities are, in most cases, only the most obvious manifestations of a more diffuse process, often referred to as the syndrome of multiple-organ failure (MOF).[11] The etiology of MOF is uncertain and is likely to differ from patient to patient. The initiating event may be inflammatory or immunologic in origin and may involve damage to the microvascular bed, abnormal coagulation, mediator release, or cytokine activation. A clear exposition of the underlying mechanisms of injury will eventually be required before effective specific treatment protocols can be developed.

The incidence of ARDS has increased as improvements in the general care of the critically ill patient allow more of them to survive the initial phase of the catastrophic illness that acts as the stimulus. However, the mortality rate remains unacceptably high. More than 60% of patients with ARDS die; the prognosis worsens as the number of other failed organs increases.[12]

The pulmonary abnormalities seen in ARDS, regardless of the predisposing event, are caused by a flooding of the lung interstitium and the alveolar spaces by a proteinaceous and often hemorrhagic fluid.[13] This is due to damage to the vascular endothelium that leads to an increase in the permeability of the pulmonary vessels. Associated damage to the epithelial cells lining the alveoli is often present. This cause of increased extravascular lung water needs to be distinguished from other forms of pulmonary edema.

Early in the time course of the disease, fluid accumulates in the interstitial space, leading to an increased lung stiffness (i.e., a decrease in lung compliance) and the onset of dyspnea and tachypnea but with no significant changes in the arterial blood gas values. If the process continues, fluid begins to enter the alveoli, resulting in a further reduction in lung compliance and a fall in lung volume. The flooded alveoli can no longer be ventilated, converting their blood supply into intrapulmonary shunt, with the resultant onset of severe hypoxemia.

Diagnosis

ARDS is a clinically defined syndrome; thus, the diagnosis depends on finding the appropriate signs and symptoms (Table 38–3). Some clinical conditions are more commonly associated with the development of ARDS than others with the most important being sepsis (Table 38–4).

The clinical presentation of ARDS is dominated in the early stages by the underlying condition. However, within a short period, the patient develops dyspnea and has chest roentgenographic findings that show the appearance of a fine, diffuse reticular infiltrate. Unless the initiating

Cardiogenic pulmonary edema is due to an increase in the pressure in the pulmonary vessels. Fluid may also accumulate in the lung because of a low plasma oncotic pressure, as seen in patients with severe protein-losing states, such as nephrotic syndrome.

Most patients manifest the onset of respiratory failure within 24 hours of the onset of the predisposing event. Almost 90% of these patients will develop ARDS within 72 hours.[14]

TABLE **38–3:** Making the Diagnosis of Adult Respiratory Distress Syndrome

Proper clinical setting (see Table 38–4)
Exclusion of left ventricular failure
Diffuse pulmonary infiltrates on chest roentgenography
Pa_{O_2} of less than 50 mm Hg_{O_2} on an $F_{I_{O_2}}$ of greater than 0.60
Decreased respiratory compliance (less than 50 mL/cm H_2O)

condition is rapidly reversed, the picture quickly progresses to the full-blown syndrome, with the development of progressive bilateral pulmonary infiltrates and severe hypoxemia.

Treatment

The treatment of the patient with ARDS is mainly supportive and is directed at maintaining an adequate level of O_2 transport to the tissues while minimizing iatrogenic complications. Whenever possible, an attempt should be made to diagnose and treat the underlying condition because its continued presence prevents resolution of the ARDS. For example, in the setting of sepsis, the identification and successful treatment of the infection, particularly if it is localized as an abscess, can often lead to rapid clearing of the pulmonary edema.

Correction of the severe hypoxemia by increasing the $F_{I_{O_2}}$ can be accomplished early in the disease. As the percentage shunt increases, an increasingly higher $F_{I_{O_2}}$ is required (see Fig. 6–11). This high $F_{I_{O_2}}$ can by itself be toxic to the lung, resulting in many of the pathologic changes seen in ARDS.[15] The unknown threshold $F_{I_{O_2}}$ that produces O_2 toxicity to the lung in humans probably varies from individual to individual, depending on the duration of treatment and on the underlying condition of the lung.

When adequate oxygenation cannot be achieved at an acceptable $F_{I_{O_2}}$, mechanical ventilation is needed. Unlike in the case of ventilatory pump failure, in this setting mechanical ventilation is used primarily to oxygenate rather than to ventilate the patient because hypercapnia is unusual. The positive pressure generated by the ventilator increases mean airway pressure, which in turn increases lung volume. This results in the recruitment of collapsed and fluid-filled alveoli, a redistribution of some of the fluid into the interstitial space, and an improvement in pulmonary gas exchange. Mechanical ventilation also reduces the O_2 demands of the respiratory muscles as they attempt to cope with the increased work of breathing with stiff lungs. This permits more of the O_2 transport to be available to the critical visceral organs.

The many ways of delivering positive pressure ventilation are well covered in other chapters and are not discussed in detail here. It is sufficient to state that the goal of mechanical ventilation in the setting of ARDS, namely an increase in mean airway pressure, can be accomplished by any number of ventilatory modes with various tidal volumes

No specific $F_{I_{O_2}}$ can be guaranteed to be safe, although as a general rule, any $F_{I_{O_2}}$ can be tolerated for short periods (24 to 48 hours). Beyond this period, every effort should be made to lower the $F_{I_{O_2}}$ to below 0.6 to prevent further lung damage.

TABLE **38–4:** Clinical Conditions Commonly Associated With Adult Respiratory Distress Syndrome

Sepsis syndrome	Burns
Aspiration of gastric contents	Pulmonary contusion
Multiple transfusions	Pancreatitis
Pneumonia in the intensive care unit	Near-drowning
Disseminated intravascular coagulation	Caustic gas inhalation
Multiple bone fractures	

and levels of positive end-expiratory pressure. None of these techniques has been proved superior to any other, and each has the potential for significant complications, such as barotrauma and depression of cardiac output. In addition, animal studies have demonstrated that mechanical ventilation with large tidal volumes can, by itself, cause lung damage that is not different pathologically from that seen in ARDS.[16] Finally, no evidence exists that any particular technique of increasing lung volume with mechanical ventilation beneficially alters the primary pathologic condition or the healing process. For these reasons, mechanical ventilation should be used only to the degree that it helps to achieve a satisfactory O_2 saturation (about 90%) at a relatively nontoxic FI_{O_2} (less than 0.6) and a moderate tidal volume.

The improvement of arterial oxygenation is not by itself a sufficient guide to ventilatory therapy because an increase in airway pressure may cause a fall in cardiac output, thereby reducing O_2 transport at the same time that the Pa_{O_2} is rising. The mechanism for this fall in cardiac output is complex, but the major cause is a reduction in venous return to the heart due to the rise in intrathoracic pressure.[17] With small increases in intrathoracic pressure, such as may be seen with low levels of positive end-expiratory pressure, the reduction in cardiac output is minimal as long as intravascular volume remains normal. With higher levels of positive end-expiratory pressure (greater than 10 cm H_2O), cardiac output will almost certainly fall unless venous filling pressures are increased above normal in order to maintain the pressure gradient for venous return. Although this tactic will maintain cardiac output, the increased pressures are also reflected in the pulmonary microvessels, increasing the movement of fluid into the lungs and thus worsening the gas exchange abnormalities. Mechanical ventilation has also been shown to reduce cardiac output by altering left ventricular compliance or by reducing ventricular filling volume owing to direct compression of the heart by the surrounding lungs. These are also corrected, to some degree, by an increase in intravascular volume.

In order to monitor this complex interplay of pulmonary and cardiac function, it is often necessary to follow changes in intravascular pressures and cardiac output with a flow-directed pulmonary artery catheter. With the use of this invasive monitoring, both pulmonary artery and pulmonary artery occlusion pressure (an estimate of left atrial pressure), as well as cardiac output, can be followed. The catheter is useful to help differentiate between ARDS and congestive heart failure, a distinction that is often difficult to make by the history and physical examination in many sick patients.

The most difficult task in patients with ARDS, especially if it is accompanied by MOF, is to monitor the adequacy of tissue O_2 delivery and utilization. Despite our ability to measure many of the parameters of O_2 transport, this remains an as yet unsolved problem. A complete discussion of tissue O_2 transport is found in Chapter 9.

The correct use of antibiotics is key to the successful management of ARDS. The prompt treatment of infection may be life saving, whereas a failure to recognize and treat it may result in the continuation of the capillary leak. Empiric therapy is usually required while the culture results are awaited. Persistent bacteremia in the face of apparently adequate antibiotic administration should raise the spector of abscess formation and should lead to a vigorous diagnostic search. The lungs and abdomen are the most common sites of undiagnosed infection.

Care must be taken in the insertion and maintenance of pulmonary artery catheters because a number of significant complications associated with their use can occur:

- Pneumothorax
- Myocardial and vascular perforation
- Bleeding
- Air embolism
- Arrhythmias
- Valve trauma
- Endocarditis
- Sepsis
- Pulmonary embolism and infarction.[18]

SUMMARY

To date, no therapy is available to prevent or treat ARDS or MOF. High doses of corticosteroids have now been shown to be of no efficacy in treating or preventing either ARDS or sepsis.[19] Prostaglandin inhibitors affect the course of experimental ARDS but are as yet unproven in humans. Monoclonal antibodies against endotoxin once thought to reduce the mortality from sepsis have been shown to be ineffective in most patients. Other monoclonal antibodies and receptor blockers directed at cytokines, such as tumor necrosis factor and the interleukins, are being studied, but none have yet been shown to be effective.

Patients who survive an episode of ARDS can usually be assured of a slow normalization of pulmonary function.[20] A small percentage may be left with some residual lung pathology characterized by mild restrictive lung disease and hypoxemia. Some patients may develop obstruction and even hyperactive airway disease, although this is very uncommon. The long-term prognosis for survivors depends, for the most part, on the presence or absence of other underlying disorders.

References

1. Belman MJ. Respiratory muscles: Function in health and disease. Clin Chest Med 9:441–691, 1988.
2. Albin MS. Acute spinal cord injury. Crit Care Clin 3:441–691, 1987.
3. Guillain-Barré Syndrome Study Group. Plasmapheresis and acute Guillain-Barré syndrome. Neurology 35:1096–1104, 1985.
4. Van der Meche FGA, Schmitz PIM, and the Dutch Guillain-Barré Study Group. A randomized trial comparing intravenous immune globulin and plasma exchange in Guillain-Barré syndrome. N Engl J Med 326:1123–1129, 1992.
5. Drachman DB. Myasthenia gravis. N Engl J Med 298:136–142, 186–193, 1978.
6. Bergofsky EH. Respiratory failure in disorders of the thoracic cage. Am Rev Respir Dis 119:643–669, 1979.
7. Sharp J, Barrocas M, Chokcovertz S. The cardiorespiratory effects of obesity. Clin Chest Med 1:103–118, 1980.
8. Mountain RD, Sahn SA. Clinical features and outcome in patients with acute asthma presenting with hypercapnia. Am Rev Respir Dis 138:535–539, 1988.
9. Aubier M, Marviano D, Milic-Emil J, et al. Effects of the administration of O_2 on ventilation and blood gases in patients with chronic obstructive pulmonary disease during acute respiratory failure. Am Rev Respir Dis 122:747–754, 1980.
10. Ashbaugh DG, Bigelow DB, Petty TL, Levine BE. Acute respiratory distress in adults. Lancet 2:319–323, 1967.
11. Montgomery AB, Stager MA, Carrico J, Hudson CD. Causes of mortality in patients with the adult respiratory distress syndrome. Am Rev Respir Dis 132:485–489, 1985.
12. Bell RC, Coalson JJ, Smith JD, Johanson WG. Multiple organ system failure and infection in adult respiratory distress syndrome. Ann Intern Med 99:293–298, 1983.
13. Meyrick B. Pathology of the adult respiratory distress syndrome. Crit Care Clin 2:405–428, 1986.
14. Pepe PE, Potkin RT, Reus DH, et al. Clinical predictors of the adult respiratory distress syndrome. Am J Surg 144:124–130, 1984.
15. Barber RE, Lee J, Hamilton WK. Oxygen toxicity in man: A prospective study in patients with irreversible brain damage. N Engl J Med 283:1478–1485, 1970.
16. Dreyfuss D, Soler P, Basset G, Sauman G. High inflation pressure pulmonary edema. Am Rev Respir Dis 137:1159–1164, 1988.
17. Biondi JW, Schulman DS, Matthay RA. Effects of mechanical ventilation on right and left ventricular function. Clin Chest Med 9:55–72, 1988.
18. O'Quin R, Marini JJ. Pulmonary artery occlusion pressure: Clinical physiology, measurement and interpretation. Am Rev Respir Dis 128:319–326, 1983.
19. Bone RC, Fisher CJ, Clemmer TP, et al. Early methylprednisolone treatment for septic syndrome and adult respiratory distress syndrome. Chest 92:1032–1035, 1987.
20. Ingbar DH, Matthay RA. Pulmonary sequelae and lung repair in survivors of the adult respiratory distress syndrome. Crit Care Clin 2:629–665, 1988.

39

Weaning Mechanical Ventilatory Support

Neil R. MacIntyre, M.D.

Weaning is the process of gradually withdrawing mechanical ventilatory support. Weaning can also refer to the process of gradually withdrawing oxygenation support (i.e., FI_{O_2} or positive end-expiratory pressure). However, in this discussion, weaning means the gradual return of the work of breathing back to the patient. Extubation, the final step in the weaning process, takes place when the patient can once again tolerate the total work of breathing indefinitely. Indications of a high likelihood of a successful extubation (Table 39–1) are frequently referred to as weaning criteria. These criteria, however, should more properly be referred to as extubation criteria.

WHO NEEDS WEANING?

Early approaches to mechanical ventilatory support involved total mechanical ventilatory support until the patient was extubated. Weaning, or the use of a gradual reduction in partial support, was not usually done. There are, however, reasons why gradual support reduction might be a better approach in the patient with a prolonged need for ventilatory support:

• Partial support involves less of a need for positive pressure in the thorax, thereby reducing the risk of barotrauma and cardiac depression.
• Partial support requires that ventilatory muscles be active, reducing the risk of disuse atrophy. If muscle loads are appropriate, this activity may also result in a conditioning effect.

Weaning is indicated in the patient who no longer requires total mechanical ventilatory support but who is unable to sustain adequate ventilation on his or her own. Patients fitting this description are actually a minority of patients receiving mechanical ventilatory support. In fact, in my institution, two thirds of patients receiving ventilatory support can be extubated in less than 24 hours, and almost 80% can be extubated in less than 72 hours. Weaning techniques are thus really of importance only in the fewer than 20% of patients who remain in need of ventilatory support beyond the 72-hour mark.

The causes of ventilator dependence beyond 72 hours influence the rate at which weaning can start and progress. Three broad physiologic derangements can be used to classify ventilator dependence:

• Neurologic dysfunction (i.e., inability to generate a stable respiratory pattern)
• Oxygenation failure (i.e., inability to maintain a satisfactory Pa_{O_2} without potentially toxic levels of FI_{O_2} or the need for positive end-expiratory pressure)
• Muscle overload (i.e., ventilatory muscle loads imposed by compliance,

735

TABLE **39–1:** Commonly Used Criteria to Assess the Likelihood of Successful Ventilator Withdrawal

Minute ventilation	≤ 10 L
Maximal voluntary ventilation	$2 \times$ minute ventilation
Vital capacity	≥ 10–15 mL/kg
Unassisted breathing rate	≤ 25 breaths per minute
Maximal inspiratory pressure	≤ -25 cm H_2O
Rapid shallow breathing index (f/V$_T$)	< 105

resistance, and ventilation demands that exceed ventilatory muscle capabilities)

The distribution of these causes in the medical intensive care unit at Duke University Medical Center is given in Table 39–2. Note that combinations are frequent but that muscle overload factors were present in 75% of ventilator-dependent patients. Although weaning involves the muscle-reloading process in these patients, weaning cannot progress any faster than the resolution rate of *all* of the factors involved.

CURRENTLY AVAILABLE PARTIAL SUPPORT MODES (WEANING MODES)

Weaning modes are partial support modes designed to shift ventilation loads gradually from the ventilator to the patient. This reloading process can be characterized by three factors:

- Amount of load placed on the patient (quantitated by work or pressure-time indices): In general, the greater the load applied to the ventilatory muscles, the more energy and O_2 demands are placed on the muscle.
- Pressure-volume (P-V) characteristics of the load: In general, the more normal the P-V relationships, the more efficient is the muscle (i.e., work/muscle O_2) and the greater is the emphasis placed on endurance (as opposed to strength) conditioning.
- Regularity of the load: In general, the more consistent the stretch and tension in the thorax with every breath, the more likely the spontaneous ventilatory drive is to synchronize with the remaining ventilatory support.

Each of the specific techniques described in the following sections should be assessed in view of these reloading characteristics (Fig. 39–1 and Table 39–3).

Spontaneous Breathing Trials Alternating With Total Support (T Tube Weaning)

T tube weaning

T tube weaning (see Fig. 39–1A) is the oldest approach to weaning. Ventilatory muscle reloading occurs through periods of spontaneous breathing. Muscles rest with total support between these periods. The longer the spontaneous breathing period, the more reloading takes place and the more weaning progresses. Muscle reloading is regular during the spontaneous breathing trials. However, the P-V configuration of the load is fixed in a high P-V relationship because of disease-imposed ventilatory system impedances (i.e., respiratory system compliance and airway resistance) and the high-resistance endotracheal tube.

TABLE **39–2:** Physiologic Causes of Ventilator Dependence Beyond 72 Hours in 81 Medical Intensive Care Unit Patients

	Alone	In Combination With Other Factors	Total
Neurologic factors (%)	10	21	31
Oxygenation factors (%)	10	35	45
Mechanical overload (%)	29	46	75

Intermittent Mandatory Ventilation

IMV—intermittent mandatory ventilation

IMV (see Fig. 39–1B) allows spontaneous breaths to be interspersed with ventilator-assisted or -controlled breaths. The number of spontaneous breaths that the patient is allowed to take determines the amount of muscle reloading. As with T tube trials, the P-V characteristics are fixed in a high P-V configuration. Reloading is also irregular because of the intermittent provision of the ventilator breaths.

With IMV using volume-assist breaths, the issue of patient-ventilator synchrony must also be considered. As noted in Chapter 22, synchrony refers to the process of matching a ventilator's delivered flow and volume to the flow and volume demands of the patient's ventilatory effort. Dyssynchrony can produce a significant imposed load on the ventilatory muscles, resulting in significant muscle oxygen demand with a consequent tendency to fatigue. Volume-assist dyssynchrony worsens as the ventilatory drive increases; thus, it may worsen with aggressive reloading (i.e., weaning is done too rapidly). Volume-assist synchrony can be improved with manipulations of the assisted flow or volume, but it may require sedation or a change of mode (i.e., using pressure assist-control breaths with IMV or using pressure support).

Dyssynchrony—the mismatch of delivered and demanded breath patterns

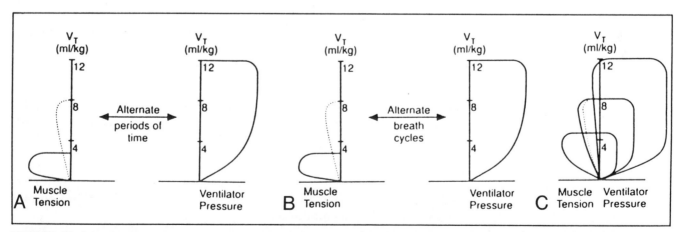

FIGURE 39–1: Quantity and characteristics of the patient's and the ventilator's contributions to the work of breathing during various modes of mechanical ventilatory support. Work per tidal breath is the area inscribed by the pressure-volume relationship during that breath. Spontaneous breaths are depicted with leftward-directed muscle tension; ventilator breaths are depicted with rightward-directed airway pressure. The dashed line represents a normal pressure-volume relationship. *A*, Assist-control T tube ventilation. This approach enables patients to work only during T tube trials. Patient work quantity is controlled by the duration of the T tube trial, whereas work characteristics are fixed as a higher than normal pressure-volume configuration reflecting abnormal impedances imposed by disease. *B*, Intermittent mandatory ventilation. This approach allows patients to work between mandatory ventilator breaths. Patient work quantity is thus controlled by the number of mandatory breaths given. Work characteristics are again fixed in a higher than normal pressure-volume configuration. *C*, Pressure-support ventilation. Patient work quantity is controlled by the level of pressure applied with every breath. With pressure support, unlike with volume-cycled ventilator modes, work characteristics are changed to a more normal configuration. (Reprinted from MacIntyre NR. Pressure support ventilation. *In* Banner MJ [ed]. Problems in Critical Care. Philadelphia, JB Lippincott, 1990, p 227.)

TABLE **39–3:** Muscle Reloading Characteristics of Three Commonly Used Weaning Modes

	Assist-Control Ventilation–T Tube Weaning	Intermittent Mandatory Ventilation	Pressure-Support Ventilation
Load quantity	Set by length of T tube breathing (guide by load tolerance)	Set by number of mandatory breaths (guide by load tolerance)	Set by level of inspiratory pressure (guide by load tolerance)
Load P-V characteristics	Fixed high P-V relationship by respiratory system and endotracheal tube	Fixed high P-V relationship by respiratory system and endotracheal tube	P-V relationship more normal depending on level of inspiratory pressure
Load regularity	Regular	Irregular	Regular
Synchrony	Volume assist has fixed clinician-set $\dot{V}$ and V_T	Volume assist has fixed clinician-set $\dot{V}$ and V_T	Inspiratory pressure support gives patient input on $\dot{V}$ and V_T
Minute ventilation guarantee	All or none	Minimum guaranteed by mandatory rate	None guaranteed*; minute ventilation depends on patient drive and respiratory system impedances

*Newer systems are being designed to provide a volume "guarantee" to the pressure-supported breath.
P-V, pressure-volume.

Pressure-Support Ventilation

PSV—pressure-support ventilation

PSV (see Fig. 39–1*C*) delivers a set amount of inspiratory pressure with each spontaneous effort. In contrast to volume assist-control ventilation, PSV supplies only a guaranteed pressure. The patient's interaction with this pressure determines the flow and volume. With pressure support, reloading occurs with every breath, adjusted by the level of inspiratory pressure given (i.e., the more inspiratory pressure given, the lower the load placed on the patient). In fact, levels of pressure support that result in a tidal volume of 10 mL/kg usually result in virtual total ventilatory support (i.e., no load on the patient's muscles). PSV weaning is accomplished with set pressures gradually reduced below this level.

The conceptual benefits of this approach to reloading are two-fold:

- Muscle reloading is done with a more normal P-V configuration. This should result in better muscle efficiency and may be a more appropriate conditioning stimulus.
- Because loads are regular and flow responds to patient demand, a high level of patient-ventilator synchrony should be expected. Indeed, patient comfort is a commonly reported feature of PSV weaning.

The disadvantage of a stand-alone pressure-support approach is that because delivered volume depends on the patient's ventilatory drive and ventilatory system impedances, unstable ventilatory support can occur in patients with unreliable ventilatory drives or a rapidly changing respiratory system compliance or airway resistance. Newer ventilator designs that offer a volume "guarantee" to a pressure-support breath may help to address this limitation.

Spontaneous Breathing During Pressure-Controlled Inverse Ratio Ventilation

APRV—airway pressure release ventilation

This relatively new approach to partial ventilatory support can be used as a weaning technique. In essence, long periods of moderately high airway pressures are interspersed with short deflation periods. The mode is considered to be a partial support mode because the ventilatory effects of the periodic short deflations are not sufficient to provide all the required ventilatory needs. Spontaneous unassisted breathing during both the high and low airway pressure periods is thus required to maintain adequate ventilation.

The advantage of this approach is that progressively lower peak airway pressures are required as weaning progresses, in marked contrast to volume assist-control ventilation with T tube trials or IMV. Pressure reductions, however, may be similar to those used during PSV weaning. With airway pressure release ventilation, the muscle loads have a high P-V configuration. This, along with the periodic inflation-deflation cycle, has the potential to produce an uncomfortable imposed load.

Comparing Approaches

Although each of these approaches has conceptual advantages and disadvantages, no clinical trial has conclusively demonstrated that any one is superior in terms of patient outcome. The choice of weaning mode must therefore be based on other factors (e.g., device availability, operator expertise, physiologic principles, and clinical assessment of patient tolerance).

INITIATING AND MONITORING WEANING

As noted previously, weaning is defined as the process of withdrawing ventilatory support and the consequent shifting of loads from the ventilator to the patient. This implies that the other two causes of ventilator dependence listed in Table 39–2 (neurologic dysfunction and oxygenation impairment) are resolved enough to allow the ventilatory muscles to be reloaded. Once the decision to begin reloading has been made, the clinician must remember that regardless of the techniques used, this process can progress only as fast as patient tolerance of the load permits. Resolution of the underlying process or processes that precipitated the overload condition is usually the rate-limiting step to weaning. On the other hand, a delay in clinician recognition of patient changes can result in unnecessary weaning delays (if patient recovery is rapid) or unnecessary fatigue (if reloading is too rapid). Proper monitoring is thus crucial to appropriate weaning.

Monitoring of the weaning process should focus on patient tolerance of the returned load. A number of possible load-monitoring techniques have been proposed (Table 39–4). Direct load calculations may be helpful, but blood gas monitoring can be quite insensitive to overload (e.g., gas exchange parameters often lag hours behind the development of muscle fatigue). The patient's own load sensors (i.e., stretch receptors) in the central nervous system (see Fig. 22–3) may be the most useful in that they produce characteristic reflex ventilatory pattern changes in response to excessive muscle loading. These changes, as listed in Table 39–5, should be used as the primary monitors of muscle reloading during

TABLE **39–4:** Load Tolerance Monitors

Load calculations (minute ventilation, work, pressure-time index)
Muscle capabilities (maximal inspiratory pressure, electromyography)
Load-muscle relationship (inspiratory pressure–maximal force ratio)
Arterial blood measurements
Ventilatory pattern

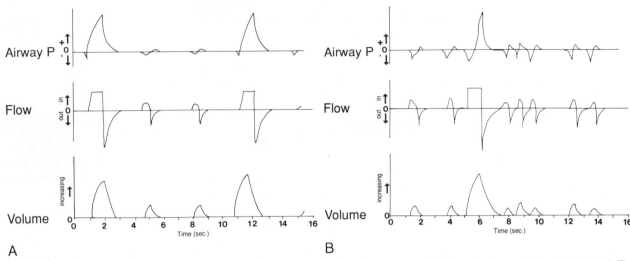

A   B

FIGURE 39–2: Airway pressure (P), flow, and volume over time during partial support with intermittent mandatory ventilation. *A,* The intermittent mandatory ventilation rate is 7 breaths per minutes and the total breathing frequency is 20 breaths per minute and regular. In addition, the assisted breath appears synchronous with patient effort (smooth convex upward airway pressure tracing). These all reflect patient tolerance of the loads being placed on the muscles and thus a weaning process that has been successful to this point. *B,* The intermittent mandatory ventilation rate is 4 breaths per minute and the total breathing frequency is rapid and irregular. In addition, the assisted breath is dyssynchronous with patient effort (concave downward airway pressure tracing). These all reflect patient intolerance of the loads being placed on the muscles and thus a weaning process that has been pushed too far.

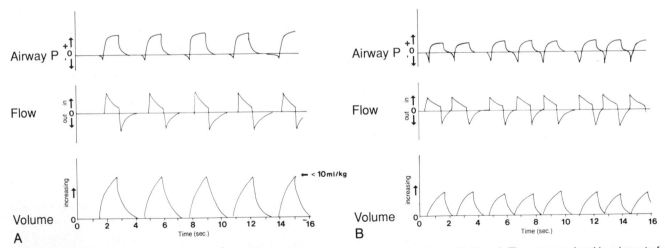

A   B

FIGURE 39–3: Airway pressure (P), flow, and volume over time during pressure-support ventilation. *A,* The pressure level is adequate for a V_T of 10 mL/kg. The breathing frequency is 20 breaths per minute and regular. In addition, the pressure-support breaths are synchronous with patient efforts. These all reflect patient tolerance of the very small loads being placed on the muscles with this high level of pressure support ventilation. *B,* The pressure level is much lower and the resulting breathing pattern is rapid and irregular. These reflect patient intolerance of the loads being placed on the muscles and thus a weaning process that has been pushed too far.

TABLE **39–5:** Ventilatory Pattern Changes Associated With Intolerable Loads

Tachypnea	Accessory muscle activity
Increased inspiratory effort (i.e., $P_{0.1}$)	Abdominal paradox

the weaning process, regardless of the technique used. Examples of ventilatory patterns during weaning are given in Figures 39–2 and 39–3.

SUMMARY

Weaning, or the gradual reduction in partial ventilatory support, is required in only a minority of patients receiving mechanical ventilatory support (i.e., those who need prolonged ventilatory support, generally for more than 72 hours). Weaning techniques involve muscle reloading and generally require intact ventilatory drives and reasonable oxygenation before they can be initiated. Weaning is best monitored by determining load tolerance, which is best accomplished by assessing the ventilatory pattern. Reloading techniques usually involve either allowing spontaneous unassisted breaths (as T tube trials, as breaths interspersed with intermittent volume-assist breaths, or as breaths superimposed on prolonged periods of lung inflation alternating with short deflations) or providing partial support of every spontaneous effort through a delivered inspiratory pressure-assist or support. Different effects on load characteristics and ventilator synchrony can be seen with different modes. Although these effects may have an impact on outcome, it is important to remember that disease resolution is generally the rate-limiting step in weaning.

Suggested Readings

Brochard L, Harf A, Lorino H, et al. Pressure support prevents diaphragmatic failure during weaning from mechanical ventilation. Am Rev Respir Dis 139:513–521, 1989.

Cohen CA, Zagelbaum G, Gross D, et al. Clinical manifestations of inspiratory muscle fatigue. Am J Med 73:308–316, 1982.

Downs JB, Klein EF, Desautels D, et al. Intermittent mandatory ventilation: A new approach to weaning patients from mechanical ventilation. Chest 64:331–341, 1973.

Garner W, Downs JB, Stock MC, et al. Airway pressure release ventilation (APRV). Chest 94:779–781, 1988.

Gillespie DJ, Marsh HMM, Divertie MB, et al. Clinical outcome of respiratory failure in patients requiring prolonged (> 24 hours) mechanical ventilation. Chest 90:364–369, 1986.

Leith DE, Bradley M. Ventilatory muscle strength and endurance training. J Appl Physiol 41:508–516, 1976.

MacIntyre NR. Weaning from mechanical ventilatory support: Volume-assisting intermittent breaths versus pressure-assisting every breath. Respir Care 33:121–125, 1988.

MacIntyre NR, Leatherman NE. Ventilatory muscle loads and the frequency-tidal volume pattern during inspiratory pressure-assisted (pressure-supported) ventilation. Am Rev Respir Dis 141:327–331, 1990.

MacIntyre NR, Leatherman NE. Mechanical loads on the ventilatory muscles: A theoretical analysis. Am Rev Respir Dis 139:968–973, 1989.

Marini JJ. Exertion during ventilator support: How much and how important? Respir Care 31:385–387, 1986.

Marini JJ. The physiologic determinants of ventilator dependence. Respir Care 31:271–282, 1986.

Marini JJ, Smith TC, Lamb VJ. External work output and force generation during synchronized intermittent mechanical ventilation: Effect of machine assistance on breathing effort. Am Rev Respir Dis 138:1169–1179, 1988.

Montgomery AB, Holle RHO, Neagley SR, et al. Prediction of successful ventilator weaning using airway occlusion pressure and hypercapnic challenge. Chest 91:496–499, 1987.

Morganroth ML, Morganroth JL, Nett LM, et al. Criteria for weaning from prolonged mechanical ventilation. Arch Intern Med 144:1012–1016, 1984.

Sahn SA, Lakschminarayan MB. Bedside criteria for the discontinuation of mechanical ventilation. Chest 63:1002–1005, 1973.

Tobin MJ, Perez W, Guenther SM, et al. The pattern of breathing during successful and unsuccessful trials of weaning from mechanical ventilation. Am Rev Respir Dis 134:1111–1118, 1986.

Tokioka H, Saito L, Kosaka F. Comparison of pressure support ventilation and assist control ventilation in 20 patients with acute respiratory failure. Intensive Care Med 15:364–367, 1989.

40
Gastrointestinal Emergencies in the Intensive Care Unit

Isaac Raijman, M.D., and Larry D. Scott, M.D.

The challenges a physician confronts when evaluating a patient in the intensive care unit who has an acute gastrointestinal event are vast. The physician's awareness and expertise in obtaining a careful history and in performing a careful physical examination, along with laboratory and radiologic data, may abort a potential catastrophe. The following discussion focuses first on gastrointestinal and pancreatobiliary syndromes in acutely ill patients. These syndromes include acute abdominal pain, jaundice, nausea and vomiting, abdominal distention, gastrointestinal bleeding, and diarrhea. An overview of specific digestive diseases follows. Although this is not intended to provide encyclopedic coverage of gastrointestinal emergencies, it is hoped that the chapter will provide important information necessary to make the proper diagnostic and therapeutic decisions when the physician confronts an acutely ill patient.

ACUTE ABDOMINAL PAIN

A broad spectrum of intra- and extra-abdominal disorders may present with acute abdominal pain and symptoms and similar physical findings. Several factors are important in determining the cause of the pain,[1] including:

- The site and time of onset
- Radiation characteristics
- Aggravating and relieving factors
- A history of similar episodes
- Associated symptoms
- Concomitant diseases
- Prior operations
- Medications

Visceral pain is poorly localized, diffuse, and dull, whereas somatic pain is well localized and sharp, as with pain at the site of peritoneal irritation.[2]

When taking the clinical history, the physician should try to determine if the pain is visceral or somatic in origin. In the intensive care unit, where a detailed history may be difficult to obtain, a physician must rely on his or her ability to perform a thorough physical examination. In examining the abdomen, important signs to look for include skin discoloration, scars, distention, visible peristaltic waves, fluid wave, visceral borders, tympanism, shifting dullness, abdominal bowel sounds, and bruits. Abdominal tenderness, the physical finding that correlates with the subjective complaint of pain, may localize the abnormality, particularly if peritoneal irritation is present. Associated muscular rigidity indicates peritonitis. Because movement aggravates the pain, such patients tend to stay immobile. In any patient, acute abdominal pain may

743

TABLE **40–1:**   Acute Abdominal Pain: Most Common Causes*

Cause	Patients (%)
Unknown	41.3
Gastroenteritis	6.9
Pelvic inflammatory disease	6.7
Urinary tract infection	5.2
Ureteral stone	4.3
Appendicitis	4.3
Acute cholecystitis	2.5
Intestinal obstruction	2.5
Constipation	2.3
Duodenal ulcer	2.0
Dysmenorrhea	1.8
Pregnancy	1.8
Pyelonephritis	1.7
Gastritis	1.4
Chronic cholecystitis	1.2
Ovarian cyst	1.0
Incomplete abortion	1.0
Pancreatitis	0.9
Abdominal aneurysm	0.7
Epididymitis	0.7

Adapted from Brewer RJ, Golden GT, Hitch DC, et al. Abdominal pain: An analysis of 1000 cases in a university hospital emergency room. Am J Surg 131:219, 1976.

*The 20 most common causes of acute abdominal pain in a group of 1000 patients in a university hospital emergency room.

evolve into an acute abdominal catastrophe, which if not recognized early may result in significant morbidity and death.[3] The presence of peritonitis implies that the peritoneal cavity has already been contaminated with either gastrointestinal contents, body fluids, or septic material. Intense pain accompanies peritonitis because the peritoneum lining the anterior wall is richly innervated.[2] On occasion, major disorders that require immediate intervention may have completely normal abdominal examination results; mesenteric ischemia is a good example.[4] Table 40–1 lists the 20 most common causes of abdominal pain,[5] and Table 40–2 lists extraintestinal conditions simulating an acute abdomen. Anatomic and pathophysiologic considerations help the physician to arrive at a differential diagnosis.[6]

Useful objective information includes the results of laboratory (Table 40–3) and radiologic studies.[7–10] A plain film of the abdomen, which may be very helpful in evaluating a patient with abdominal pain, will show bowel gas patterns and the presence or absence of extraintestinal gas (in the peritoneum, urinary tract, biliary tract, abdominal wall, or portal and mesenteric veins). Calcifications and foreign material may be noted, along with information about bone structures and lung bases.[10] When

TABLE **40–2:**   Acute Abdominal Pain: Extra-abdominal Conditions Simulating an Acute Abdomen

Cause	Examples
Cardiac	Acute myocardial infarction, pericarditis
Drugs or toxins	Lead, arsenic, mushroom poisoning
Endocrine	Diabetic ketoacidosis, addisonian crisis
Functional	Somatization, Münchausen's syndrome
Familial	Acute intermittent porphyria, familial Mediterranean fever
Hematologic	Sickle cell disease, acute leukemia
Infectious	Rocky Mountain spotted fever, malaria
Neurologic	Tabes dorsalis, thoracic neuropathy
Pulmonary	Pneumonia, pulmonary embolus

TABLE **40–3:** Acute Abdominal Pain: Useful Laboratory Data

Test	Information
Complete blood count with cell differential	Infection, blood loss
Serum electrolytes	Deficiencies, calculate anion gap
Blood glucose	Diabetic ketoacidosis, prognostic factor in pancreatitis
Blood urea nitrogen	Gastrointestinal bleeding, intravascular volume contraction
Serum amylase	Pancreatitis
Arterial blood gases	Acid-base analysis
Urinalysis	Renal function, hematuria, pyuria
Pregnancy test	Ectopic pregnancy

Pain of less than 2 days in duration, patient age older than 65 years, and pain followed by vomiting point to a possible surgical disorder.[5]

the plain film findings are normal, with no evidence of peritonitis, ultrasonography may be useful, although obesity and abdominal distention due to intestinal gas will adversely affect its resolution. Computed tomography has proved to be of great value in confusing cases, complementing ultrasonography and plain radiography. All these tests should be considered complementary and should be used according to the clinical data obtained. In evaluating a patient with acute abdominal pain, the goal is to determine whether the patient needs surgery; laboratory and radiologic evaluations should not delay surgical intervention when the diagnosis is strongly suspected on the basis of clinical data. About 75% of patients with acute abdominal pain require surgical intervention.[5]

Immunocompromised patients, including those with the acquired immunodeficiency syndrome, those receiving chemotherapeutic agents or corticosteroids, those who have had transplantation, and those with underlying malignancies, should be considered separately.[11, 12] Such patients may harbor an acute life-threatening disorder but have a paucity of clinical manifestations. In addition, the underlying disease may suggest a specific set of diagnostic possibilities. For example, splenic rupture needs to be considered in a patient with acute leukemia, hypotension, and acute abdomen.[13] Abdominal films showing subserosal gas parallel to the intestinal lumen suggest pneumatosis cystoides intestinalis occurring in a patient with vasculitis.[14] A systemic process causing hepatitis, pancreatitis, and interstitial pneumonia should alert the clinician to the possibility of cytomegalovirus infection, which may be accompanied by mucosal ulceration.[15] Other entities causing pain in this group of patients include necrotizing enterocolitis, especially in patients with hematologic disorders;[16] splenic and liver abscesses due to candidal infection;[17] and acute graft-versus-host disease in bone marrow recipients.[18]

JAUNDICE

Although mechanical biliary obstruction leading to jaundice can be accurately diagnosed in the vast majority of patients,[19] the differential diagnosis of jaundice remains a clinical challenge. The most common cause of jaundice is cholestasis, or impaired bile flow, of either an intra- or an extrahepatic etiology. A carefully obtained clinical history, including information on contacts, drug exposure, medications, alcohol use, blood transfusions, sexual preference, recent travel, and constitutional symptoms, along with a thorough physical examination, should lead the physician to a possible etiology that may later be more precisely defined

TABLE **40–4:** Clinical Differentiation of Cholestatic and Hepatocellular Jaundice

Clinical or Laboratory Finding	Cholestatic	Hepatocellular
Drugs or medications	+	+
Alcohol	+	+
Blood transfusions	−	+
Acute onset	−	+
Prolonged course	+	−
Pruritus	+	−
Light-colored stools	+	+
Dark urine	+	+
Systemic symptoms	−	+
Hepatomegaly	+	+
Elevated bilirubin level	+ +	+
Elevated alkaline phosphatase level	+ +	+
Elevated aspartate aminotransferase and alanine aminotransferase levels	+	+ +

−, Generally absent; +, generally present; + +, almost always present.

by laboratory and radiologic tests (Table 40–4).[20] In general, patients with obstructive jaundice have a more prolonged course and are often otherwise asymptomatic, whereas patients with jaundice secondary to a hepatocellular process are symptomatic and seek medical attention shortly after the initiation of symptoms.[21] Pruritus, dark urine, and light stools suggest cholestasis, whereas the patient with hepatocellular disease has constitutional symptoms such as fever, malaise, and anorexia. Jaundice developing in a patient who is already hospitalized suggests a different set of possibilities. Conditions and situations that may produce jaundice in an acutely ill patient include hepatic congestion, the use of total parenteral nutrition, the administration of medications, acute calculous and acalculous cholecystitis, acute biliary obstruction, sepsis, and intravascular hemolysis (Table 40–5).

Jaundice is detectable on physical examination when the bilirubin level exceeds 3.5 mg/dL (normal, less than 1.2). The breakdown product of hemoglobin, bilirubin, is normally transported on albumin from the reticuloendothelial system to the liver, where it is conjugated with glucuronic acid before secretion into the bile. Thus, an excess production of bilirubin, as in hemolysis, can produce jaundice. Alternatively, any disorder of the liver cell can impair the conjugation and secretion of bilirubin and lead to jaundice. Lastly, obstruction to the flow of bile can cause jaundice. Measurement of the bilirubin concentration in blood and of the fractions conjugated (direct bilirubin) and unconjugated (indirect bilirubin) can be useful in determining the possible cause of jaundice. If liver enzyme abnormalities are present, a distinction between hepatocellular damage and cholestasis may be made. In hepatocellular damage, serum aminotransferase levels (aspartate and alkaline aminotransferase) are expected to be elevated out of proportion to the level of alkaline phosphatase, whereas in obstructive jaundice, the inverse should hold true. An easy distinction cannot always be made because patients may have a combination of both. In these patients, abdominal ultrasonography, com-

TABLE **40–5:** Causes of Jaundice in Critically Ill Patients

Cause	Examples
Hepatocellular injury	Acute hepatitis, drugs, sepsis
Cholestasis	Biliary tract obstruction, drugs, sepsis
Hemolysis	Thrombotic thrombocytopenic purpura

puted tomography, percutaneous transhepatic cholangiography, endo-scopic retrograde cholangiopancreatography (ERCP), or radionuclide studies may play an important diagnostic role. If extrahepatic obstruction is suspected, the next step is to visualize the biliary tree, either by percutaneous transhepatic cholangiography or by ERCP,[22] both of which not only help establish the presence or absence of obstruction but also provide information about the location and nature of the obstruction that will help treatment.[19] Therapeutic options to relieve biliary obstruction, which may be surgical, endoscopic, or radiologic, depend on the diagnosis and the clinical status of the patient.

NAUSEA AND VOMITING

Nausea and vomiting, manifestations not always specific to the gas-trointestinal tract, can be caused by a large number of conditions.[23, 24] However, the potential complications of vomiting, which include esopha-geal rupture and tear of the esophageal mucosa with associated bleeding (Mallory-Weiss syndrome), can be life threatening. Other complications are aspiration pneumonitis, asthma, acid-base disturbance, electrolyte imbalance, and malnutrition.

Patients in the intensive care unit are often taking many drugs, any one of which may have nausea and vomiting as side effects. The most commonly involved agents include nonsteroidal anti-inflammatory drugs, bromocriptine, levodopa, opiate analgesics, digitalis, and cancer chemo-therapeutic agents.[23] It is also very common for acutely ill patients with underlying systemic disorders to experience vomiting. Gastrointestinal conditions complicated by vomiting include those that mechanically ob-struct (by either an intraluminal, a mural, or an extrinsic process) and nonobstructive inflammatory conditions, such as pancreatobiliary dis-eases.

In the initial evaluation of the acute (less than 24 hours) onset of vomiting, the clinical history, physical examination, initial laboratory screen (including a complete blood cell count, measurement of electrolyte levels, serum chemistries, amylase, and assessment of renal parame-ters), and plain radiography of the abdomen are all important. Once they have been completed, the next step is to screen for metabolic disorders, infections, drugs, and intoxication as possible causes. At this point, dis-tinguishing between intrinsic gastrointestinal disease and systemic or metabolic causes may be possible. For example, large-volume emesis, abdominal distention, hyperactive bowel sounds, and distended small bowel loops on x-ray studies point to mechanical intestinal obstruction. On the other hand, generalized malaise, hypotension, hyperkalemia, and hypoglycemia suggest adrenal insufficiency.

Therapy for vomiting includes (1) treating the underlying cause when it has been identified and (2) providing relief to the patient while preventing the complications noted previously. If mechanical obstruction is unlikely, symptomatic treatment with drugs such as metoclopramide or phenothiazines (chlorpromazine and prochlorperazine) may be useful.

ABDOMINAL DISTENTION

In general, abdominal distention can be caused by

* Distention of gas-containing viscera

Vomiting may be seen in uremia, diabetes, diabetic ketoacidosis, adrenal insufficiency, hypothyroidism, hyperthyroidism, myocardial ischemia, electrolyte imbalances, and other metabolic derangements.

Metoclopramide is a dopamine antagonist with cholinomimetic activity that helps the coordination of gastric, pyloric, and duodenal motor activity to propulse intraluminal contents aborally.[25] This is supplemented by its central antiemetic effect. In up to 20% of patients, however, side effects, including drowsiness, anxiety, motor restlessness, and rarely extrapyramidal manifestations and hypertensive crises, may be encountered.

- Intraperitoneal fluid (ascites)
- Urinary bladder distention
- Tumors, especially those containing mucinous material

The following discussion focuses on the former two as the most likely conditions encountered.

Intestinal Distention

Gaseous distention of small or large bowel may result from mechanical or nonmechanical causes. The most common causes of mechanical small bowel obstruction (SBO) are adhesions, which are usually due to previous abdominal or pelvic surgery; neoplasms; and hernias.[26-29] Large bowel obstruction (LBO) may complicate carcinoma, volvulus, and diverticulitis.[26, 27, 29]

During mechanical obstruction, the intraluminal contents accumulate, producing distention, which promotes intestinal secretion of water and electrolytes. The stagnation of intestinal contents in the obstructed bowel facilitates the growth of bacteria, both aerobic and anaerobic, with the further production of gas. Retrograde peristalsis may then ensue, leading to vomiting. Usually, in proximal SBO, vomiting is prominent but not foul smelling, whereas in distal SBO, vomiting, when present, may be large in volume (greater than 500 mL) and have a feculent odor. Vomiting, along with third-space losses of fluid, produces severe water and electrolyte imbalance that may lead to dehydration, hemoconcentration, oliguria and azotemia, systemic hypotension, hypokalemia, and metabolic alkalosis. The presence of metabolic acidosis is an ominous sign, suggesting severe tissue underperfusion, sepsis, or necrotic bowel. This usually occurs with strangulation obstruction, which is more frequently seen in obstruction secondary to volvulus, hernia, or adhesions; it is uncommon in colonic obstructions due to carcinoma or diverticular disease.[26]

The diagnosis of bowel obstruction is made on clinical grounds, complemented by plain films of the abdomen.[26-29] Low-grade fever and leukocytosis may be seen, although peritoneal signs, severe pain, high fever, and marked leukocytosis are present in patients with strangulation obstruction. Plain radiography of the abdomen is helpful in distinguishing SBO from LBO. In the former, distended bowel loops have a central location, and valvulae conniventes can be seen (Fig. 40–1). In LBO, the distended bowel is more peripheral, and the colonic haustrations do not completely transverse the width of the gas-filled loop. The more distal the obstruction, the greater the abdominal distention is and the more air-fluid levels are likely to be visible. In distal colonic obstruction, however, small bowel dilatation may not be present in the presence of a competent ileocecal valve.

The initial assessment dictates the therapeutic approach in most patients. Intravenous fluids, supplementation of electrolyte deficiencies, and nasogastric decompression may be indicated in all patients with obstruction, regardless of the cause. Many patients with SBO require exploratory laparotomy. In as many as 20% of these patients with prior laparotomy, SBO resolves spontaneously with medical management alone. If after the initial 24 to 48 hours of decompression the patient has pain, fever, leukocytosis, or metabolic acidosis, the likelihood of spontaneous resolution is remote, and surgery is indicated.[26, 29] It is critically

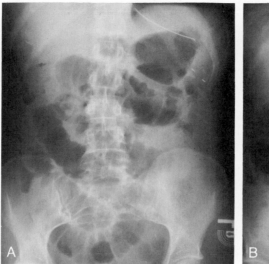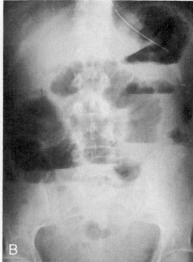

FIGURE 40–1: Flat *(A)* and upright *(B)* views of the abdomen in a patient with mechanical small bowel obstruction. The gas-filled loops of small intestine display prominent valvulae conniventes with uneven air-fluid levels on the upright view. No colonic gas is present. The tip of a nasogastric tube is visible in the stomach.

The mortality from elective surgery is two to four times lower than that from emergency colonic operations.[31]

important to distinguish radiographically between partial and complete SBO, which can be predicted in 82% by the initial abdominal films, because as many as 75% of patients with partial obstruction respond to medical management.[30] Like SBO, LBO is treated nonoperatively only when the obstruction is incomplete. In view of the common causes of colonic obstruction, it is often possible to prepare the patient for an elective operation. Colonoscopy or sigmoidoscopy and the placement of a decompression colonic tube may help to reverse cecal and sigmoidal volvulus and may be useful in the decompression of nonobstructive colonic distention. In a patient with a competent ileocecal valve, distention of the colon may be dramatic, with a risk of perforation if the cecal diameter is more than 10 cm. Rapid decompression is of importance in preventing cecal gangrene or perforation. Nonmechanical distention of the intestine, or ileus, may occur in any intra-abdominal inflammatory process, such as appendicitis, pancreatitis, and so forth. A similar picture may also complicate electrolyte disorders (e.g., hypokalemia) and the administration of drugs, such as narcotic analgesics. Table 40–6 lists these conditions.

Ascites—the accumulation of fluid within the peritoneal cavity, which when excessive can cause abdominal distention

Ascites

The majority of patients with ascites have underlying hepatic disease, usually cirrhosis. Table 40–7 lists other causes of ascites. When

TABLE **40–6:** Causes of Ileus in Critically Ill Patients

Gram-negative sepsis	Spinal or pelvic fractures
Postsurgical	Pneumonia
Abdominal trauma	Peritonitis
Acute myocardial infarction	Pancreatitis
Drugs (e.g., narcotics)	Electrolyte disorders (e.g., hypokalemia)
Mesenteric ischemia	

TABLE **40–7:** Causes of Ascites in Critically Ill Patients

Cirrhosis	Pancreatitis
Constrictive pericarditis	Cardiac failure
Inferior vena cava obstruction	Cardiac tamponade
Budd-Chiari syndrome	Hypoalbuminemia
Portal vein occlusion	

due to hepatic disease, the formation of ascitic fluid is determined by several factors:

- Increased hydrostatic pressure due to portal hypertension
- Decreased oncotic pressure due to hypoalbuminemia
- Extravasation of lymph due to abnormalities in the hepatic sinusoidal endothelium
- Renal sodium retention with an inability to excrete a water load

Ascites developing in the hospital may be seen in a patient with marginally compensated liver disease who received sodium-containing fluids. Clinically, patients with ascites complain of abdominal distention and fullness. As the amount of fluid increases, complaints of dyspnea, nausea, anorexia, heartburn, or pain may appear. In the majority of patients, the underlying cause of the ascites is manifest clinically. For example, the patient may also have jaundice and stigmata of chronic liver disease, suggesting cirrhosis. The physical examination is insensitive in diagnosing ascites unless large amounts of fluid are present (usually more than 1.5 L), demonstrable by bulging flanks, shifting dullness, and fluid wave.[32] Umbilical herniation, penile or scrotal edema, and pleural effusions may also be present. The abdominal plain film may show separation of bowel loops, abdominal haziness, visualization of the liver edge, and erasure of the psoas shadows. Abdominal ultrasonography is a highly sensitive test that is able to detect as little as 100 mL of fluid and is also able to differentiate between loculated and free fluid; clues to the underlying disease process might also be noted.[33]

Abdominal paracentesis and ascitic fluid analysis are essential in evaluating a patient with ascites because they may provide invaluable information with a very low risk.[34] Analysis of the ascitic fluid total protein, glucose, lactate dehydrogenase, and albumin levels; a cell count; Gram's stain; and culture should be performed, with simultaneous measurement of the serum albumin, glucose, and lactate dehydrogenase levels. Amylase measurements may also be useful. Distinguishing between a transudate and an exudate may be helpful in suggesting a diagnosis, although overlap exists.

The management of patients with cirrhosis and ascites includes bed rest, sodium restriction, and the administration of diuretics such as spironolactone and furosemide.[36] Large-volume paracentesis can be performed safely if appropriate colloid replacement, such as albumin, is given intravenously.[37] All in all, large-volume paracentesis is a safe procedure that can reduce a patient's discomfort, improve cardiorespiratory function, shorten the hospital stay, and decrease hospital costs.[38] Patients with moderate ascites who have few or no symptoms can usually be treated with paracentesis. The development of ascites in cirrhotic patients conveys a poor prognosis, with only 59% surviving the first year.[36] Complications of cirrhotic ascites include spontaneous bacterial peritonitis in 10%, pleural effusions in 6%, umbilical herniations in 20%, atelectasis, dyspnea, and poor nutrition due to anorexia and nausea.[39]

Computed tomography is very sensitive for small amounts of ascites but is rarely needed to confirm a clinical diagnosis.

The serum–ascitic fluid albumin gradient may be the most sensitive test in separating transudates (greater than 1.1) and exudates (less than 1.1), although this has been shown mainly in patients with alcohol-induced liver disease.[35]

GASTROINTESTINAL BLEEDING

Despite technical advances in controlling bleeding and the availability of a large array of drugs, gastrointestinal hemorrhage remains a common and considerable problem. Fortunately, in most patients, gastrointestinal bleeding stops spontaneously. The 15% of patients with continued bleeding who require more aggressive therapeutic intervention have a much higher mortality rate.[40] Physicians who care for acutely ill patients, especially in intensive care units, confront two different clinical situations with regard to gastrointestinal hemorrhage. The first is the patient who is already bleeding at the time of admission. The second, and frequently the more severely ill, type of patient develops gastrointestinal bleeding as a complication of the underlying disease or the management.

The evaluation of a patient with active gastrointestinal bleeding consists of a rapid assessment of the presenting manifestations and an evaluation of the patient's hemodynamic status. This initial assessment, which determines the severity of the episode, dictates the management. Needless to say, before any diagnostic procedure is attempted, resuscitative measures should be the first priority in managing the hemodynamically unstable patient.

Hematemesis and melena suggest an upper gastrointestinal source, whereas hematochezia occurs more commonly with lower gastrointestinal bleeding. The most important aspect of the physical examination is measurement of the blood pressure and heart rate. In patients in whom tachycardia and peripheral vasoconstriction are found, postural hypotension may be the only finding of hemodynamic instability early after the onset of bleeding. However, if the bleeding is not corrected, circulatory collapse and shock may result. Individual variations to this sequence of events depend on the patient's cardiac and neural integrity, as well as on the patient's intravascular volume status before the bleeding episode. On examination of the abdomen, the presence of hyperactive bowel sounds favors a proximal source of bleeding.[41]

This initial evaluation can be conducted rapidly. Venous access, usually with one or two large-bore catheters, should be established in the patient with active bleeding. At the same time, blood can be collected and sent to the laboratory for a complete blood cell count, coagulation studies, assessment of electrolyte levels, and typing and cross-matching. In addition, physical findings may indicate underlying disease, which may have bleeding as a complication. For example, the findings of jaundice, palmar erythema, and spider angiomas suggest chronic liver disease and thus the possibility of bleeding esophageal varices.

In addition to the history and physical examination, lavage of the stomach through a nasogastric tube may help to localize the site the bleeding. The presence of blood confirms a proximal source, whereas its absence usually favors a lower source. However, an inactive or intermittently active upper gastrointestinal bleeding source or a duodenal ulcer may have negative lavage findings.[42] In addition to its diagnostic value, the placement of a nasogastric tube helps in the initial management of upper gastrointestinal bleeding by permitting gastric lavage with room temperature tap water to prepare the stomach for endoscopy and to assess the rate of bleeding.

Once the patient has been hemodynamically stabilized, a diagnostic work-up can be started. Table 40–8 outlines the many causes of acute gastrointestinal bleeding. Upper gastrointestinal bleeding developing in

A laboratory clue to gastrointestinal bleeding is an elevated serum blood urea nitrogen level that is out of proportion to the serum creatinine level, reflecting depleted intravascular volume plus absorbed proteins.[43]

TABLE **40–8:** Causes of Acute Gastrointestinal Bleeding in Critically Ill Patients

Upper	Upper or Lower
Esophageal varices	Enterovascular fistulas
Mallory-Weiss syndrome	Arteriovenous malformations
Stress-related ulcers	Angiodysplasia
Gastric varices	Vasculitis
Gastric ulcer	**Lower**
Acute gastritis	Diverticulosis
Duodenal ulcer	Ischemic bowel disease
	Inflammatory bowel disease

Both the injection catheter and the bipolar electrode or thermal probe are small-diameter devices that can easily be passed down the biopsy channel of the endoscope, allowing direct application to the bleeding site.

the patient in the critical care unit is often due to stress ulcer or stress-related mucosal damage. Investigation is best carried out with endoscopy, which not only is more sensitive than radiologic contrast studies but also can visualize an active site of bleeding, provide prognostic information, characterize the lesion or lesions, be used to obtain biopsy samples, and be used to intervene therapeutically if necessary.[44] In patients with lower gastrointestinal bleeding, the value of early colonoscopy may be limited. However, studies have suggested that when colonoscopy is performed within 24 hours and after an oral purge, it may identify or exclude a colonic source 70 to 77% of the time.[45-47]

Therapy for gastrointestinal bleeding involves both general measures designed to replace loss and stabilize the patient hemodynamically and specific intervention directed at the bleeding site. With respect to the latter, both injection and coagulation methods are available through the endoscope. A bleeding varix in the esophagus can be injected with a sclerosing agent or banded, or the base of a bleeding ulcer can be injected with a vasoconstrictor such as epinephrine. Alternatively, a bipolar electrocoagulator or a thermal probe can be applied directly to a bleeding vessel for control of hemorrhage. Overall, endoscopic therapy has reduced mortality, transfusion requirements, the need for emergency surgical intervention, and cost (by reducing the duration of the hospital stay). In addition to the previously mentioned therapies, antisecretory drugs, mucosal protectants, and antacids are often given in managing patients with bleeding ulcers, although their benefit is limited in the presence of active bleeding.

Special attention has been given to what physicians can do to prevent the development of gastrointestinal hemorrhage due to a stress ulcer in patients who are critically ill. When prospectively evaluated, patients admitted to an intensive care unit who are at high risk for developing gastrointestinal bleeding are those with multiple trauma, burns, sepsis, or multiorgan failure and those requiring mechanical ventilation. The incidence of gastrointestinal bleeding in such patients is between 6 and 14%, depending on the criteria used to define gastrointestinal bleeding.[48] A large number of trials have assessed the efficacy of decreasing or neutralizing gastric acidity in order to prevent gastrointestinal bleeding. Both antacids and H_2 receptor antagonists have been shown to reduce the frequency of bleeding in this population. More recently, major emphasis has been placed on the rate of complications these prophylactic measures may convey, especially in mechanically ventilated patients. Alkalinization of the gastric environment by antacids or H_2 antagonists may increase the risk of bacterial overgrowth in the respiratory tract by retrograde colonization, putting the patient at risk for pulmonary infections, especially secondary to gram-negative bacilli.[49-51] This respiratory tract colonization has been correlated with a gastric pH of greater than 4.0. Sucralfate, a complex of sulfated sucrose and aluminum hydroxide that works as a mucosal protectant, has been shown to be as effective as antacids in the prevention of gastrointestinal bleeding without neutralizing acid. The use of this agent may therefore be associated with a reduced incidence of nosocomial pneumonia in mechanically ventilated patients being treated with a stress ulcer prophylactic regimen.[49–50]

DIARRHEA

Diarrhea developing in hospitalized patients, especially in the intensive care unit setting, is a common complication in critically ill patients, afflicting as many as 41%.[52] Potential causes include nasogastric tube feedings, dietary changes, drug administration, infections, and multiorgan failure. More often, diarrhea is a side effect of treatment.[53]

Diarrhea related to nasogastric tube feeding, which has long been recognized, has been estimated to affect as many as 68% of patients.[52] This may be related to the high osmolality of the solutions used, to patient lactose intolerance due to disaccharidase deficiency, or to bacterial contamination. Although diarrhea usually develops in patients who have predisposing conditions, as many as 36% of patients have diarrhea without a predisposing factor.[54] Because nutritional support is of tremendous importance and the enteral route is the preferred choice whenever possible, various attempts have been made to decrease diarrhea as a complication. These include the use of low-fat, lactose-free, less concentrated solutions; slower rates of delivery; continuous infusion as opposed to intermittent boluses; and the addition of bulk-forming agents. Adding fecal bulking agents appears to be one of the most useful.[55]

Drug-induced diarrhea is one of the commonest causes of diarrhea in hospitalized patients. Antacids, magnesium sulfate, sodium phosphate, sodium citrate, lactulose, laxatives, H_2 receptor antagonists, and antibiotics are the most frequently involved.[56] The produced diarrhea may be secondary to increased intraluminal osmolality; to bacterial colonization, including by *Clostridium difficile*; and to increased intestinal secretion.

Infection-related diarrhea in hospitalized adult patients is almost always related to the development of *C. difficile* infection complicating antibiotic administration. Other predisposing factors include chemotherapy, underlying malignancies, the use of enemas, inflammatory bowel disease, and severe immunocompromised states. Transmission of the organisms has been documented in hospitalized patients.[58] The diagnosis is confirmed by the presence of *C. difficile* toxin in stool.[59] Pseudomembranous colitis encompasses the presence of colitis, positive culture findings, and pseudomembranes seen on endoscopy, occurring in about 33% of the patients.[60] The endoscopic picture is that of diffuse ulcerations with multiple raised yellow-white plaques and normal intervening mucosa. Although the majority of cases are diagnosed during flexible sigmoidoscopy, local colonic pseudomembranes have been found on colonoscopy in patients with negative proctosigmoidoscopic findings.[61]

Symptomatic patients should be treated, whereas asymptomatic patients should not. Discontinuing antibiotics alone may correct diarrhea in 23% of the patients.[60] Metronidazole and oral vancomycin have been the mainstays of antibiotic therapy directed against *C. difficile* infection. They have similar efficacies (95%) and relapse rates (5 to 15%), but metronidazole is considerably cheaper.[60] Bacitracin and toxin-binding

C. difficile organisms produce a wide spectrum of gastrointestinal disorders, ranging from asymptomatic carrier to antibiotic-associated diarrhea to states of fulminant toxic megacolon. It is the most commonly isolated organism in adult patients who develop diarrhea while hospitalized,[57] and the immense majority of cases are related to the use of antibiotics.

Other intestinal pathogens, such as *Salmonella, Shigella,* and *Campylobacter* species, are very uncommonly isolated.[52, 53, 62]

drugs such as cholestyramine may be an effective alternative therapy. Cholestyramine binds vancomycin; therefore, their concomitant use is contraindicated.

Diarrhea can also be a manifestation of multiorgan failure.[63] In these patients, diarrhea develops with or without enteral feedings. Hypoalbuminemia has been found to be present in many critically ill patients with diarrhea.[64] This association has been found to be as high as 34%, especially in patients in whom no other explanation for the diarrhea exists. The majority of patients have had a serum albumin level of less than 2.5 g/dL. It is likely that diarrhea developing in patients with multiorgan failure is multifactorial in origin because most are also receiving antacids, H_2 antagonists, enteral feedings, antibiotics, and other drugs associated with this adverse reaction.

The importance of diarrhea developing in these patients relates not only to the possibility of inducing water and electrolyte imbalance but also to nutritional deficiency, skin breakdown with subsequent ulceration, changes in intestinal structure, increased cost and nursing time, and a great deal of discomfort for both patients and their relatives.

Management is directed at the precipitating factor. All unnecessary medications should be stopped. Changes in enteral feedings, as mentioned earlier, should be tried. Toxin assay and cultures for *C. difficile* are indicated. Other cultures for enteropathogens and parasites are indicated only if suggested by the clinical evaluation. Adequate replacement of water and electrolytes is mandatory. Continuous positional changing and cleansing are necessary to avoid skin breakdown. In patients with continuous fecal flow or in those in whom continuous turning is not possible, a soft-walled rectal tube can be used. Therapeutically, medications such as methylcellulose and kaolin pectate can be tried. Antidiarrheals such as diphenoxylate with atropine, loperamide, and opiates should be avoided as much as possible because of their side effects and potential complications.

ESOPHAGEAL PERFORATIONS

Perforation of the esophagus is an unusual event, but when present, it is life threatening. The majority of cases (64%) are iatrogenic: that is, perforation is a complication of medical instrumentation, such as esophageal dilatation.[65] Because perforation occurs shortly after the procedure, the diagnosis is often self-evident. The patient may complain of worsening chest pain, often pleuritic in nature; a low-grade fever may be noted. Subcutaneous emphysema may be present on physical examination, along with a mediastinal "crunch," a crackling sound audible over the anterior chest wall, usually in concert with cardiac systole. A more difficult diagnosis may be spontaneous esophageal perforation, also called Boerhaave's syndrome. Typically, this patient, after a heavy meal and often a large alcohol intake, presents with chest pain, dyspnea, and vascular collapse.[66] Abdominal pain, pneumothorax, pleural effusions, and pneumomediastinum are frequent complications.

The diagnosis of suspected esophageal perforation may be suggested by the finding of air in the mediastinum on plain radiography of the chest; pleural effusion may also be present. The diagnosis is confirmed by the finding of extravasation of water-soluble contrast administered orally.

Although there is precedent for nonoperative management with nasogastric suction, antibiotics, and parenteral nutrition,[67] this is successful only when initiated early. In addition, no evidence of shock or hemorrhage or of communication between the perforation and the pleura or peritoneal cavity should be present, and the perforation cavity should be in free communication with the esophageal lumen. A more aggressive but probably more conservative approach is surgical treatment. Mortality is influenced by factors such as the patient's age, the patient's overall clinical status, the presence of sepsis, the time of the initiation of treatment (less than 24 hours after perforation), and the location of the perforation (with intrathoracic perforations carrying the highest mortality).

PEPTIC ULCER DISEASE

Hemorrhage and perforation are the major complications of peptic ulcer disease for which critical care may be required. Although the incidence of peptic ulcer disease in the United States has declined over the last three decades, the number of patients with perforated and bleeding ulcers has remained constant.[68, 69] The problem of upper gastrointestinal bleeding was discussed earlier. Perforated ulcer diseases account for 10% of all hospital admissions related to peptic ulcer disease,[68–70] remaining a more common problem among male patients, with a peak in the fifth decade. The use of anti-inflammatory drugs, especially nonsteroidal agents and particularly among elderly women, is an important factor in the development of peptic ulcer and perforation, including both gastric and duodenal ulcers.[71] Although nonsteroidal anti-inflammatory drugs may differ in their propensity to produce acute injury, no differences are seen with respect to ulcer complications, including perforation. The use of antiulcer drugs such as H_2 blockers has not prevented this complication.[72]

The most frequent mode of presentation is that of sudden, severe epigastric pain with signs of peritoneal irritation, such as rigidity and rebound tenderness on physical examination. Maximal tenderness may be in the epigastric area.[68] As discussed in the section on abdominal pain, the elderly may have a paucity of manifestations, which may delay recognition and treatment. The major laboratory abnormality early in the course is leukocytosis. Radiographic evaluation shows free intra-abdominal air in 60 to 85% of cases; with this finding in a typical clinical setting, no further diagnostic tests are needed. If the picture is confusing, however, peritoneal lavage may be helpful.[68] Rarely is a contrast x-ray study required to confirm the diagnosis. The mortality rate from perforated gastric ulcer is 10 to 40%, whereas that from perforated duodenal ulcer is 0 to 10%.[68] Treatment should ideally be surgical, although nonoperative management has been advocated for selected cases.[73] Although this approach may be useful in young patients who have spontaneously sealed perforated ulcers or in patients presenting an excessive surgical risk, most authors agree that operative intervention is the therapeutic method of choice. The primary surgical goal is closure or oversewing of the perforation and irrigation plus drainage of the peritoneal cavity. The decision to proceed simultaneously with definitive ulcer surgery depends largely on the presence or absence of associated risk factors.[68]

Gastric ulcers most commonly perforate along the anterior wall of the antrum between the pylorus and the incisura near the lesser curvature, whereas duodenal ulcers more commonly perforate through the anterior wall of the duodenal bulb.[68]

DISORDERS OF THE BILIARY TRACT AND PANCREAS

The most commonly encountered complications of biliary tract disease are those causing obstruction, leading to jaundice and sepsis due to secondary bacterial infection (cholangitis). Hemobilia, bleeding into the biliary tract, is a rare but potentially life-threatening disease if major gastrointestinal hemorrhage results. Acute pancreatitis is the major pancreatic disorder seen in the intensive care unit. Complications of chronic pancreatitis, such as pseudocyst, abscess, and so forth, may also present as an acute illness, although this is unusual. The diagnosis and treatment of both acute biliary and pancreatic diseases have been dramatically influenced by endoscopy, specifically ERCP, which not only can facilitate the diagnosis when noninvasive modalities are unsuccessful but also can provide definite therapy, as is discussed later. A newly developed interest in percutaneous cholecystostomy in the treatment of acute cholecystitis, especially in high operative risk patients, has added a valuable tool to the therapeutic armamentarium of this common disorder.

Acute Cholecystitis

The vast majority of cases of acute cholecystitis occur in association with gallstones, although as many as 10% occur in the absence of stones.[74] The key pathogenetic event is occlusion of the cystic duct, in most cases by a stone. Early in the course of the disease, the gallbladder contents may be sterile, but with time, secondary infection may result, particularly with organisms such as *Escherichia coli,* group D streptococci, *Staphylococcus* species, and *Klebsiella* species.[75] The most common clinical presentation is that of epigastric pain of sudden onset, constant, with radiation to the right upper quadrant and occasionally to the back and shoulder, which persists in contrast to biliary colic; in the latter, an inflammatory process does not develop and pain gradually resolves over the next 2 to 6 hours. Often, nausea, vomiting, and fever are present. Physical findings include fever and a tender right upper quadrant. Jaundice is found infrequently. Laboratory data show moderate leukocytosis with left shift. Elevated bilirubin and alkaline phosphatase levels may be found, although in the absence of common duct stones, the degree of elevation is usually minor. Plain radiography of the abdomen may demonstrate stones in only 15% of cases because most stones are predominantly cholesterol in composition and thus are radiolucent.[75] Abdominal ultrasonography, however, has a sensitivity of 90% and a specificity of 95% in detecting gallstones.[76] Sonographic criteria for acute cholecystitis include pericholecystic edema and thickening of the gallbladder wall. Nuclear hepatobiliary imaging (cholescintigraphy), by assessing the patency of the cystic duct, may be very useful in confirming a suspected diagnosis. Positive cholescintigraphic findings indicate obstruction of the cystic duct, as evidenced by radionuclide in the common bile duct but no uptake in the gallbladder. The initial therapy for acute calculous cholecystitis is conservative in most cases; it includes the administration of intravenous fluids, antibiotics, and analgesics and surgical consultation. An operation is indicated for patients suspected of having a perforation, for those not responding to medical therapy, and for those with suppurative cholangitis. In high-risk surgical patients, percutaneous cholecystostomy, which produces favorable results, can be performed by an interventional radiologist under ultrasonographic or computed tomographic guidance with local anesthesia.[77, 78]

Acute acalculous cholecystitis is an uncommon entity that occurs in fewer than 10% of all cases of acute cholecystitis. However, it is an important diagnosis to be aware of because it typically occurs clinically in the critical care unit. The majority of cases are found in critically ill patients who have sepsis or burns or have had major trauma or who are receiving nasogastric suctioning or narcotics.[79, 80] The onset of acalculous cholecystitis may manifest as unexplained fever or deterioration; many such patients may be unable to voice complaints. The diagnostic approach is similar to that used with calculous cholecystitis, with ultrasonography and hepatobiliary imaging; even in the absence of stones, thickening of the gallbladder wall and cystic duct obstruction suggest the diagnosis. The physician's knowledge and awareness of this complication are crucial to making a prompt diagnosis. Treatment is generally surgical, but percutaneous cholecystostomy or endoscopic placement of a gallbladder stent, described earlier, appears to be a good alternative.[77, 78]

Acute Suppurative Cholangitis

Obstruction of the common bile duct with bile stasis may, on occasion, be complicated by secondary infection, which in turn results in a clinical syndrome called ascending cholangitis. Patients with this condition are acutely ill, febrile, jaundiced, and hypotensive, with right upper quadrant pain and tenderness. Gallstones account for almost all cases, followed rarely by neoplastic obstruction. The majority of patients have positive bile culture results; in most cases, gram-negative microorganisms are found, including *E. coli, Proteus* species, *Klebsiella* species, and *Pseudomonas* species. Group D streptococci and gram-positive bacteria have also been reported. Approximately 25 to 40% have positive blood culture findings.[81] Although abdominal ultrasonography may reveal evidence of obstruction (usually a dilated biliary system), close to 10% of patients have obstruction with normal sonographic findings.[82] Thus, a high index of suspicion is needed in order to avoid overlooking this diagnosis because rapid intervention is required. In view of the high accuracy of ERCP in detecting and localizing the site of obstruction and because of the possibility of intervening therapeutically with it,[19] ERCP is the first choice if experienced personnel are available. Percutaneous transhepatic cholangiography could also provide access to the biliary tree and drainage of a suppurative process.

Therapy is aimed at controlling the infection with drainage and antibiotics and at stabilizing the patient hemodynamically with intravenous fluids. Although logic suggests that immediate decompression is indicated, emergent operative drainage is associated with a high mortality of up to 40%, which can be reduced dramatically if the infection can be controlled and surgery can be performed electively.[83] It is here that biliary decompression by either endoscopy (ERCP) or percutaneous techniques (percutaneous transhepatic cholangiography) can play a major role. Morbidity and mortality rates are lower with ERCP than with surgery, and endoscopic sphincterotomy and stone extraction may provide definitive therapy.

Acute Pancreatitis

Most episodes of acute pancreatitis resolve spontaneously, with the condition of no more than 5% of patients progressing to a more devastating and life-threatening illness.[84]

Acute pancreatitis is a common disorder. Although many etiologic factors are associated with the development of acute pancreatitis, chronic alcohol ingestion and biliary lithiasis account for up to 70% of all in-

Most alcoholic patients have sustained permanent pancreatic damage before their first attack of pancreatitis, which usually occurs after 10 to 20 years of alcohol ingestion.

stances; however, idiopathic pancreatitis is also common, comprising 20% of reported cases.[84, 85] Other causes include trauma, drugs, viral infections, anatomic abnormalities, previous surgery, and hyperlipidemic syndromes. The highest mortality occurs in postoperative pancreatitis, although these patients are often ill with other problems. The pathogenesis of pancreatitis due to gallstone disease has not been elucidated, although most cases are associated with passage of a stone through the ampulla of Vater.[86] The association of acute pancreatitis and alcohol intake is well established, but its pathogenesis also remains obscure. Regardless of the cause, once pancreatic enzymes have been activated, an autodigestive process begins; the balance between activated proteases and protease inhibitors determines the subsequent course of acute pancreatitis.[87] Both exocrine and endocrine functions are impaired to a variable extent and for a variable duration. Only rarely does acute pancreatitis lead to chronic pancreatitis.

Acute pancreatitis is characterized by acute abdominal pain accompanied by increased levels of pancreatic enzymes in blood, urine, or both. The pain is usually severe, is located in the epigastric region, and is sometimes accompanied by fever, nausea, vomiting, and intravascular volume contraction. A soft abdomen may be found, presumably due to the retroperitoneal location of the organ, but it may progress to an acute abdomen based on the severity of the pancreatic injury.[84, 85, 87] The pain is usually worse in the supine position. Emesis may alleviate the pain. Fewer than 2% of patients have painless pancreatitis, but their prognosis is worse because they present in shock.

Once the diagnosis of acute pancreatitis has been established, an accurate assessment of the severity of the pancreatitis provides important information for optimal patient care. Mortality is directly related to the number of clinical and laboratory characteristics that are present at the time of diagnosis or that develop during the first 48 hours after diagnosis (Table 40–9).[88] Mortality is higher in the presence of three or more of these signs. When acute pancreatitis is mild, the inflammatory process is characterized primarily by interstitial edema, and the patient usually recovers after fluid replacement. In contrast, when the inflammatory process is severe, life-threatening complications may ensue. Systemic hypotension, tachycardia, decreased urine output, altered sensorium, and hemoconcentration indicate intravascular volume contraction and a more severe attack. Hypocalcemia producing tetany is extremely rare but indicates a poor prognosis. When fewer than three signs in Ranson's criteria are positive, virtually all patients survive, although there are exceptions. Somewhat paradoxically, Ranson and coworkers have also shown that patients with a poor prognosis had fewer or no preceding attacks and that they had lower serum amylase levels on admission than did patients with a benign course.[88] The major use of

TABLE **40–9:** Ranson's Criteria in Acute Pancreatitis

At Admission or Diagnosis	During Initial 48 Hours
Age > 55 yr	Decreased hematocrit $> 10\%$
White blood cell count $> 16,000/mm^3$	Increased blood urea nitrogen level > 5 mg/100 mL
Blood glucose level > 200 mg/100 mL	Serum calcium level < 8 mg/100 mL
Serum lactate dehydrogenase level > 350 IU/L	Arterial $Po_2 < 60$ mm Hg
Serum aspartate aminotransferase level > 250 IU/L	Base deficit > 4 mEq/L
	Fluid loss > 6 L

From Soergel KH. Acute pancreatitis. *In* Sleisinger MH, Fordtran JF (eds). Gastrointestinal Disease: Pathophysiology, Diagnosis, and Management, 4th ed. Philadelphia, WB Saunders, 1989, p 1825.

prognostic signs is in trying to identify patients who are at risk for a complicated course and who require more specialized care.[89]

Abdominal ultrasonography, abdominal computed tomography, or both, help to determine the presence of pancreatitis, to assess the severity of pancreatitis and the development of local complications, and to evaluate the biliary tract for the presence of stones or ductal dilatation.[87] Computed tomography is considered to be the imaging method of choice for any pancreatic disease when a complication is suspected. In mild pancreatitis, ultrasonography alone is sufficient.

After the first 48 hours from admission, the patient should continue to be carefully monitored. Most deaths within the first week are related to refractory shock, respiratory failure, intra-abdominal hemorrhage, acute renal failure, and complicating septic cholangitis.[87] Septic complications, including pneumonia and pancreatic abscess, account for late mortality, usually after the first week. At present, pancreatic infection is the most common cause of death.[90]

Complications of acute pancreatitis are categorized in two different groups (Table 40–10).

During the first several days of illness, therapeutic efforts are directed at fluid resuscitation and the prevention of end-organ damage.[87] At this point, no specific therapy will abort the autodigestive process, but in most cases the illness is self-limited. Prophylactic antibiotics have been of no value. The replacement of fluid losses with crystalloids, or colloids if necessary; the use of analgesics; nasogastric suctioning if ileus or persistent vomiting is present; withholding oral intake; close monitoring of vital signs; and physical examination are the mainstays of the treatment of mild pancreatitis. In severe pancreatitis, the same principles of therapy apply, but the patient often needs to be admitted to an intensive care unit with hemodynamic monitoring. Identification and treatment of complications are necessary in conjunction with a surgical consultation, although fewer than 5% of patients require surgery.[85] Nutritional support is also of crucial importance in severe acute pancreatitis. Patients with mild pancreatitis usually tolerate oral feeding without difficulty once the acute inflammatory process has resolved.

HEPATIC FAILURE

The patient with advanced chronic liver disease is at risk for several complications, including upper gastrointestinal bleeding from varices, ascites, coagulopathy, encephalopathy, infection, and renal failure. Some of these have been discussed earlier. Hepatic encephalopathy, or hepatic coma, results from exposure of the brain to neurotoxic substances that have bypassed the liver because of the development of shunts from the portal to the systemic circulation. These products are for the most part

TABLE **40–10:** Complications of Acute Pancreatitis

Local	Systemic
Abscess	Adult respiratory distress syndrome
Pseudocyst	Pleural effusion
Phlegmon	Decreased cardiac output
Ascites	Disseminated intravascular coagulation
Jaundice	Acute renal failure
Ileus	Hypocalcemia, hyperglycemia
	Encephalopathy, psychosis

nitrogenous, originating in the gut. Among the putative toxins, ammonia has received the most attention. Other important mechanisms include enhanced permeability of the blood-brain barrier, abnormal cerebral metabolism, and the presence of false neurotransmitters.[91] A precipitant factor can usually be found to explain the hepatic encephalopathy. Such factors include increased dietary protein intake, the use of sedatives and analgesics, metabolic changes including hypokalemia, coexistent infections, and gastrointestinal bleeding.[92]

Clinically, patients may exhibit only subtle behavioral changes in mild cases but can progress to frank coma in stage 4 encephalopathy. Little correlation exists between the blood ammonia level and the extent of hepatic encephalopathy,[93] and this is therefore not a useful diagnostic test. The diagnosis is largely clinical by noting the appearance of mental or behavioral changes in a patient with liver disease. As with encephalopathy of any metabolic cause, patients may demonstrate a flapping tremor of the outstretched hands called asterixis. Early recognition and treatment are of great importance because in its early stages the encephalopathy may be fully reversible. Therapy is aimed at treating the precipitating factor and diminishing the load of toxic metabolites absorbed from the gastrointestinal tract into the systemic circulation. Dietary protein restriction is necessary during the acute phase, and protein is gradually reintroduced in small increments if improvement has occurred. Lactulose, which has been used extensively, is a disaccharide that passes unchanged to the lower intestine, where it is metabolized by bacteria, reducing the pH of the colonic contents. This traps ammonia in the colon, promoting its excretion. Other mechanisms may also contribute to its efficacy.[94] Lactulose is usually administered orally, but it can be given as a retention enema, particularly in patients who are comatose. Neomycin is an antibiotic with very poor gastrointestinal absorption that lowers the production of ammonia by inhibiting urea-splitting bacteria. It is recommended in patients who do not respond to lactulose. Other supportive measures include the correction of electrolyte imbalance and the replacement of deficient minerals and vitamins. Potentiating drugs should also be discontinued. Other forms of therapy have been proposed but provide no advantage over conventional therapy, such as lactulose.

Another problem in patients with advanced liver disease and ascites is primary infection of the peritoneal space, which is called spontaneous bacterial peritonitis to distinguish it from peritonitis that is secondary to another process, such as perforated viscus. In the laboratory, it is defined as positive ascitic fluid culture findings and a cell count showing more than 250 polymorphonuclear leukocytes/mm^3 in the absence of an intra-abdominal source of infection. As mentioned earlier, it complicates the conditions of 12 to 15% of cirrhotic patients. The most commonly isolated organisms are *E. coli,* streptococci, and *Klebsiella* species. Anaerobes cause spontaneous bacterial peritonitis in 6% of cases. The diagnosis should be suspected in the cirrhotic patient with ascites who is showing deterioration, such as worsening of the encephalopathy or unexplained fever. Abdominal pain may or may not be present, and physical findings of peritoneal irritation (e.g., rigidity or rebound) are seldom noted. The diagnosis is established with paracentesis and analysis of the ascitic fluid demonstrating a polymorphonuclear leukocyte count of greater than 250 cells/mm^3 and positive culture results. If the clinical suspicion of spontaneous bacterial peritonitis is strong, treatment should be initiated, preferably with a third-generation cephalosporin,[95] and should be adjusted later according to the susceptibility of the isolated organism. With appropriate therapy, the absolute polymorphonuclear leukocyte count should decrease by 50% after 48 hours of treatment.[96] Unfortunately, despite treatment, mortality remains very high.

HEPATORENAL SYNDROME

The hepatorenal syndrome is also called functional renal failure because in this situation the kidney is anatomically normal. Renal insufficiency results from a shift of renal blood flow from the cortical to the medullary region of the kidney, probably due to vasoactive substances, such as prostaglandins. This syndrome continues to have a devastating outcome with a high mortality.[97] Thus, it needs to be differentiated from other forms of renal dysfunction in patients with hepatic disease because treatment and prognosis differ markedly. Most patients have alcoholic cirrhosis, but it has also been documented in other forms of hepatic disease. The majority have evidence of advanced hepatic disease manifested by hypoalbuminemia, jaundice, portal hypertension, and ascites. Hepatorenal syndrome is often precipitated by abrupt disturbances in intravascular volume of any etiology, including bleeding, the use of diuretics, and diarrhea. The use of prostaglandin inhibitors, such as nonsteroidal anti-inflammatory drugs, may precipitate this syndrome. The diagnosis is suggested when in the absence of other causes, oliguria and azotemia develop in a patient with hepatic dysfunction; the urinalysis results are usually normal, and no improvement is seen in renal function after volume expansion. Typically, the urinary sodium concentration is less than 10 mmol/L, reflecting normal tubular function. It is important not to assume that all patients with hepatic dysfunction and renal failure have hepatorenal syndrome. If known precipitants of renal failure are excluded, fluid challenge with central venous pressure monitoring is helpful to exclude prerenal azotemia because the latter benefits from volume expansion. The mortality associated with this syndrome remains very high, with most patients dying of encephalopathy and not of uremia. The best treatment is prevention because no medical therapy has been predictably successful.

ACUTE COLONIC DIVERTICULITIS

The incidence of diverticular colon disease, both diverticulosis and diverticulitis, increases with advancing age. Only 5% or fewer of patients admitted for diverticular disease are younger than 40 years of age.[98] The disease is most common in the sigmoid colon. One explanation for this is that diverticular disease is more common in bowel with a narrow lumen and a thick wall because a higher intraluminal pressure is generated. This increased pressure causes mucosal herniation through a weakened portion of the bowel wall, presumably where nutrient vessels penetrate. In 80% of cases, colonic diverticulosis is asymptomatic. When symptomatic, it manifests clinically as rectal bleeding (discussed earlier) or as diverticulitis, with the latter being the most common complication of diverticulosis.

Acute diverticulitis complicates approximately 20% of known cases of diverticular disease.[99] Commonly, only one diverticulum is involved, and most of the time it is located in the sigmoid colon. The process is thought to be initiated by a microperforation leading to a pericolic inflammatory reaction or pericolitis. The diagnosis of acute diverticulitis is based primarily on clinical judgment. Fever, abdominal pain localized to the left lower quadrant, and abdominal distention suggest the diagnosis. The patient may also complain of diarrhea or constipation. Urinary symptoms may occur and suggest bladder involvement. An associated ileus may be found, producing more abdominal distention, nausea, and vomiting. Because of the inflammatory process, a mass may be palpated. Rectal examination may disclose a mass, mucosal tenderness, and induration.[100] Leukocytosis is often present, but the white blood cell count may be normal even in the presence of complicated diverticulitis.[101] Plain radiography of the abdomen may show bowel obstruction or ileus. Occasionally, a soft tissue mass may be noted in the pelvis. Computed tomography may provide more detailed evidence of inflammation by demonstrating localized thickening of the colonic wall and increased density in the pericolic fat or by showing related abscesses and fistulas. Barium enema should generally be avoided during the acute illness, but if a contrast study is deemed necessary, a water-soluble contrast agent may be used. The presence of fistula, pericolic mass, extravasation of the contrast agent, or an intramural abscess favors the diagnosis of acute diverticulitis. Endoscopic evaluation is rarely needed or indeed useful in making a diagnosis, but it may be used during the acute phase if it is performed gently, with minimal bowel preparation and air insufflation.[100] The major complications of acute diverticulitis, which occur in as many as 38% of patients, include intra-abdominal abscesses, fistula formation, perforation, and obstruction.

The management of acute diverticulitis is initially supportive, with the use of intravenous fluids, bowel rest, intravenous broad-spectrum antibiotics, nasogastric suction if bowel obstruction or ileus is present, and analgesics. It is best to use morphine derivatives such as meperidine because morphine itself may increase intracolonic pressure and, at least theoretically, adversely affect the course of the illness.[102] Approximately 85% of patients respond to medical therapy. Right colon diverticulitis is rare but may be a more aggressive form of the disease, with almost 90% of patients requiring surgical intervention.[98] Surgical intervention is indicated when there is evidence of perforation, high-grade bowel obstruction, symptomatic fistula, or no response to appropriate medical therapy. An abscess requiring drainage may be treated nonoperatively by percutaneous drainage and catheter placement under sonographic or computed tomographic guidance, allowing the patient to recover for a later elective surgery, if required. Complete obstruction is treated with diverting colostomy. Eventually, many such patients require resection of the involved segment of the colon.

MESENTERIC ISCHEMIA

Blood nourishment to the intra-abdominal viscera is supplied by three major vessels arising from the abdominal aorta: the celiac axis, the superior mesenteric artery, and the inferior mesenteric artery.[103] The celiac axis gives rise to the splenic, left gastric, and hepatic arteries. Other arteries that originate from these vessels supply blood to the duodenum and pancreas. The superior mesenteric artery nourishes the jejunum, the ileum, the cecum, the ascending colon, and the proximal portion of the transverse colon. The inferior mesenteric artery carries blood to the distal part of the transverse colon, the descending colon, the sigmoid, and proximal portions of the rectum, whereas the distal portion is supplied by arteries derived from the hypogastric artery. Although the blood supply to the intra-abdominal organs may be perceived as vast, major areas of ischemia and necrosis may occur in the absence of collaterals or in other potentially vulnerable areas, defined as watershed areas (the splenic flexure and the junction of the superior and middle portions of the rectum). Regulators of mesenteric blood flow include the autonomic nervous system, cardiac output, systemic arterial blood pressure, the volume and viscosity of blood, circulating vasoactive peptides, and intrinsic vascular properties.

Causes of vascular insufficiency are included in two major categories occlusive and nonocclusive. In the latter, abnormalities arise that lead to low-flow states. Data have indicated that the most common cause of acute mesenteric ischemia is superior mesenteric artery embolus (50%), followed by nonocclusive ischemia (25%).

Acute mesenteric ischemia, either occlusive (due to embolus) or nonocclusive, is often precipitated by a cardiac disorder such as a myocardial infarction, an arrhythmia, or bacterial endocarditis or in the setting of a prosthetic valve. The patient appears acutely ill, with abdominal pain out of proportion to the physical findings. As the disease progresses, the abdomen becomes distended and tender, bowel sounds are hypoactive, and peritoneal signs become obvious. Systemic manifestations such as fever, hypotension, and tachycardia are common. The laboratory results show hemoconcentration, leukocytosis, uremia, and metabolic acidosis. Plain x-ray films of the abdomen may show ileus, gas in the intestinal wall, or thumbprinting (Fig. 40–2). If angiography is performed, the site of occlusion may be seen, or only splanchnic vasoconstriction may be noted. However, normal study findings do not rule out ischemia. Angiography not only helps to make the diagnosis but also helps in the treatment because vasodilators such as papaverine may be given (see later).

Thumbprinting—a scalloped appearance of the intestinal wall secondary to submocosal edema and hemorrhage

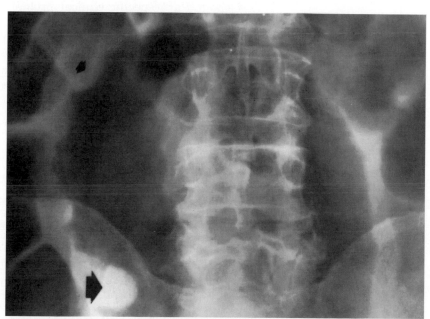

FIGURE 40–2: Plain film of the abdomen in a patient with acute mesenteric ischemia. The scalloped soft tissue contour of the walls of the gas-containing loops of intestine represents submucosal hemorrhage, often referred to as "thumbprinting" *(arrows)*. (Courtesy of E. T. Stewart, M.D., Milwaukee, WI.)

The overall mortality associated with mesenteric infarction is about 80%.[104] This mortality directly relates to the presence of advanced atherosclerosis and to the physiologic adaptation to the low-flow state.

Therapy involves general supportive measures such as volume repletion, central pressure monitoring, nasogastric suction, and the use of broad-spectrum antibiotics. The use of arterial vasodilators (e.g., papaverine) administered at the time of angiography has been advocated. Surgery is often necessary in a deteriorating course if the patient's general condition allows it. A "second-look" operation 12 to 36 hours after the first intervention is sometimes advocated to determine residual intestinal viability.

SUMMARY

A variety of gastrointestinal and hepatobiliary problems may be sufficiently severe that their management in a critical care setting is required. Furthermore, such problems may complicate the course of a patient who is admitted to the intensive care unit for other reasons and, in so doing, may contribute directly to morbidity and mortality. Acute abdominal pain may reflect extra-abdominal as well as intra-abdominal pathology. Jaundice may be hepatocellular or cholestatic in origin, reflecting both intrahepatic and extrahepatic processes. In most cases abdominal distention is caused by intraperitoneal fluid accumulation (ascites) or gaseous distention of the bowel. Gastrointestinal bleeding may arise from anywhere in the gastrointestinal tract; when it develops after the patient is admitted to the intensive care unit, it is often caused by stress-related gastric mucosal injury. Hospital-acquired diarrhea is commonly due to *Clostridium difficile* colitis associated with antibiotic use, adverse effects of medications, or tube feedings. Esophageal rupture, perforated peptic ulcer, acute cholecystitis (calculous and acalculous), acute pancreatitis, hepatic failure, acute diverticulitis, and mesenteric ischemia are specific clinical problems that present unique diagnostic and management issues. When such problems develop in the hospital setting, many are as likely to be complications of disease management as of the underlying disease. As with most clinical challenges, appropriate use of data from the medical history, physical examination, laboratory, and radiologic resources is instrumental in achieving a favorable outcome.

References

1. Hickey MS, Kiernan GJ, Weaver KE. Evaluation of abdominal pain. Emerg Med Clin North Am 7:437, 1989.
2. Jung PJ, Merrell RC. Acute abdomen. Emerg Med Clin North Am 7:227, 1989.
3. Young GP. Abdominal catastrophes. Emerg Med Clin North Am 7:699, 1989.
4. Brandt LJ, Boley SJ. Nonocclusive mesenteric ischemia. Annu Rev Med 42:107, 1991.
5. Brewer RJ, Golden GT, Hitch DC, et al. Abdominal pain: An analysis of 1,000 cases in a university hospital emergency room. Am J Surg 131:219, 1976.
6. Purcell TB. Nonsurgical and extraperitoneal causes of abdominal pain. Emerg Med Clin North Am 7:721, 1989.
7. Field S. Plain films: The acute abdomen. Clin Gastroenterol 13:3, 1984.
8. Shaff MI, Tarr RW, Partain CL, James AE Jr. Computed tomography and magnetic resonance imaging of the acute abdomen. Surg Clin North Am 68:233, 1988.
9. Levine MS. Plain films of the acute abdomen. Emerg Med Clin North Am 3:541, 1985.
10. Preger L, Gronner AT, Glazer H, et al. Imaging of the nontraumatic acute abdomen. Emerg Med Clin North Am 7:453, 1989.
11. Nylander WA. The acute abdomen in the immunocompromised host. Surg Clin North Am 68:457, 1988.

12. Sievert W, Merrell RC. Gastrointestinal emergencies in the acquired immunodeficiency syndrome. Gastroenterol Clin North Am 17:409, 1988.
13. Bower TW, Haskins GE, Armitage JO. Splenic rupture in patients with hematologic malignancies. Cancer 48:2729, 1981.
14. Karp DR, Kantor OS, Halverson JD, Atkinson JP. Successful management of catastrophic gastrointestinal involvement in polyarteritis nodosa. Arthritis Rheum 31:683, 1988.
15. Cohen EB, Kamarowski RA, Kauffmann HM, et al. Unexpectedly high incidence of cytomegalovirus infection in apparent peptic ulcers in renal transplant recipients. Surgery 97:606, 1985.
16. Hawkins JA, Mower WR, Nelson EW. Acute abdominal conditions in patients with leukemia. Am J Surg 150:739, 1985.
17. Helton WS, Carrico CJ, Zaveruha PA, et al. Diagnosis and treatment of splenic fungal abscesses in the immunosuppressed patient. Arch Surg 121:580, 1986.
18. McDonald GB, Shulman HM, Sullivan KM, et al. Intestinal and hepatic complications of human bone marrow transplantation. Gastroenterology 90:460, 1986.
19. Frank BB, Members of the Patient Care Committee of the American Gastroenterological Association. Clinical evaluation of jaundice: Guidelines of the Patient Care Committee of the American Gastroenterological Association. JAMA 262:3031, 1989.
20. O'Connor KW, Snodgrass PJ, Swonder JE, et al. A blinded prospective study comparing four current noninvasive approaches in the differential diagnosis of medical versus surgical jaundice. Gastroenterology 84:1498, 1983.
21. Marin GA. Differential diagnosis of jaundice. Postgrad Med 81:178, 1987.
22. Olen R, Pickleman J, Freeark RJ. Less is better: The diagnostic workup of the patient with obstructive jaundice. Arch Surg 124:791, 1989.
23. Feldman M. Nausea and vomiting. *In* Sleisinger MH, Fordtran JS (eds). Gastrointestinal Disease: Pathophysiology, Diagnosis and Management, 4th ed. Philadelphia, WB Saunders, 1989, pp 222–237.
24. Hanson JS, McCallum RW. The diagnosis and management of nausea and vomiting: A review. Am J Gastroenterol 80:210, 1985.
25. Albibi R, McCallum RW. Metoclopramide: Pharmacology and clinical application. Ann Intern Med 98:86, 1983.
26. Holder WD. Intestinal obstruction. Gastroenterol Clin North Am 17:317, 1988.
27. Richards WO, Williams LF Jr. Obstruction of the large and small intestine. Surg Clin North Am 68:355, 1988.
28. Mucha P. Small intestinal obstruction. Surg Clin North Am 67:597, 1987.
29. Jones RS, Schirmer BD. Intestinal obstruction, pseudo-obstruction, and ileus. *In* Sleisinger MH, Fordtran JS (eds). Gastrointestinal Disease: Pathophysiology, Diagnosis and Management, 4th ed. Philadelphia, WB Saunders, 1989, pp 369–380.
30. Brolin R, Crasna M, Mast R. Use of tubes and radiographs in the management of small bowel obstruction. Ann Surg 206:126, 1987.
31. Irvin GL III, Horseley JS III, Caruana JA Jr. The morbidity and mortality of emergent operations for colorectal disease. Ann Surg 199:598, 1984.
32. Cummings S, Papadakis M, Melnick J, et al. The predictive value of physical examination for ascites. West J Med 142:633, 1985.
33. Black M, Friedman AC. Ultrasound examination in the patient with ascites. Ann Intern Med 110:253, 1989.
34. Runyon BA. Paracentesis of ascitic fluid; A safe procedure. Arch Intern Med 146:2259, 1986.
35. Rector WG Jr, Reynolds TB. Superiority of the serum-ascites albumin difference over the ascites total protein concentration in separation of transudative and exudative ascites. Am J Med 77:83, 1984.
36. Herrera JL. Current medical management of cirrhotic ascites. Am J Med Sci 302:31, 1991.
37. Gines P, Arroyo V, Quintero E, et al. Comparison of paracentesis and diuretics in the treatment of cirrhotics with tense ascites: Results of a randomized study. Gastroenterology 93:234, 1987.
38. Simon DM, McCain RJ, Bonkovsky HL, et al. Effects of therapeutic paracentesis on systemic and hepatic hemodynamics and on renal and hormonal function. Hepatology 7:423, 1987.
39. Bender MD, Ockner RK. Ascites. *In* Sleisinger MH, Fordtran JS (eds). Gastrointestinal Disease: Pathophysiology, Diagnosis and Management, 4th ed. Philadelphia, WB Saunders, 1989, pp 428–454.
40. Gostout CJ. Acute gastrointestinal bleeding—A common problem revisited. Mayo Clin Proc 63:596, 1988.
41. Peterson WL. Gastrointestinal bleeding. *In* Sleisinger MH, Fordtran JS (eds). Gastrointestinal Disease: Pathophysiology, Diagnosis and Management, 4th ed. Philadelphia, WB Saunders, 1989, pp 397–427.
42. Cuellar RE, Gavaler JS, Alexander JA, et al. Gastrointestinal tract hemorrhage: The value of nasogastric aspirate. Arch Intern Med 150:1381, 1990.
43. Olsen LH, Andreassen KH. Stools containing altered blood-plasma urea: Creatinine ratio as a simple test for the source of bleeding. Br J Surg 78:71, 1991.
44. Marshall JB. Acute gastrointestinal bleeding, a logical approach to management. Postgrad Med 87:63, 1990.

45. Potter GD, Sellin JH. Lower gastrointestinal bleeding. Gastroenterol Clin North Am 17:341, 1988.
46. Caos A, Benner KG, Manier J, et al. Colonoscopy after Golytely preparation in acute rectal bleeding. J Clin Gastroenterol 8:46, 1986.
47. Jensen DM, Machichado GA. Diagnosis and treatment of severe hematochezia. Gastroenterology 95:1569, 1988.
48. Derrida S, Nury B, Slama R, et al. Occult gastrointestinal bleeding in high risk intensive care unit patients receiving antacid prophylaxis: Frequency and significance. Crit Care Med 17:122, 1989.
49. Driks MR, Craven DE, Celli BR, et al. Nosocomial pneumonia in intubated patients given sucralfate as compared with antacids or histamine type 2 blockers. N Engl J Med 317:1376, 1987.
50. Cook DH, With LG, Cook RJ, Guyat GH. Stress ulcer prophylaxis in the critically-ill: A meta-analysis. Am J Med 91:519, 1991.
51. Tryba M. Prophylaxis of stress ulcer bleeding. A meta-analysis. J Clin Gastroenterol 13(Suppl 2):S44, 1991.
52. Kelly WJ, Patrick MR, Hillman KM. Study of diarrhea in critically ill patients. Crit Care Med 11:7, 1983.
53. Dobb GJ. Diarrhea in the critically ill. Intensive Care Med 12:113, 1986.
54. Pesola GE, Hogg JE, Yonnios T, et al. Isotonic nasogastric tube feedings: Do they cause diarrhea? Crit Care Med 17:1151, 1989.
55. Broom J, Jones K. Causes and prevention of diarrhea in patients receiving enteral nutritional support. J Hum Nutr 35:123, 1981.
56. Fine KD, Krejs GJ, Fordtran JS. Diarrhea. *In* Sleisinger MH, Fordtran JS (eds). Gastrointestinal Disease: Pathophysiology, Diagnosis and Management, 4th ed. Philadelphia, WB Saunders, 1989, pp 290–316.
57. Gilligan PH, McCarthy LR, Genta VM. Relative frequency of *Clostridium difficile* in patients with diarrheal disease. J Clin Microbiol 14:26, 1981.
58. Delmee M, Michaux JL. Prevention of *Clostridium difficile* outbreaks in hospitals. Lancet 2:350, 1986.
59. Lashner BA, Todorczuk J, Salm DF, Hanauer SB. *Clostridium difficile* culture-positive toxin-negative diarrhea. Am J Gastroenterol 81:940, 1986.
60. Teasley DG, Gerding DN, Olson MM, et al. Prospective randomized trial of metronidazole versus vancomycin for *Clostridium difficile*–associated diarrhea and colitis. Lancet 2:1043, 1983.
61. Tedesco FJ. Antibiotic associated pseudomembranous colitis with negative proctosigmoidoscopic examination. Gastroenterology 77:295, 1979.
62. Gilligan PH. Diarrheal disease in the hospitalized patient. Infect Control 7:607, 1986.
63. Dark DS, Pingleton SK. Nonhemorrhagic gastrointestinal complications in acute respiratory failure. Crit Care Med 17:755, 1989.
64. Brinson R, Guild R, Kolts B. Hypoalbuminemia as an indicator of diarrheal incidence in critically ill patients. Crit Care Med 15:506, 1987.
65. Goldstein LA, Thompson WR. Esophageal perforations: A 15 year experience. Am J Surg 143:495, 1982.
66. Jaworski A, Fischer R, Lippmann M. Boerhaave's syndrome. Computed tomographic findings and diagnostic considerations. Arch Intern Med 148:223, 1988.
67. Swedlund A, Traube M, Sisking BN, McCallum RW. Non-surgical management of esophageal perforation from pneumatic dilation in achalasia. Dig Dis Sci 34:379, 1989.
68. Jordan PH, Morrow CH. Perforated peptic ulcer. Surg Clin North Am 68:315, 1988.
69. Elashoff JD, Grossman MI. Trends in hospital admissions and death rates for peptic ulcer in the United States from 1970–1978. Gastroenterology 78:280, 1980.
70. Miller TA. Emergencies in acid peptic disease. Gastroenterol Clin North Am 17:303, 1988.
71. Smedley FH, Hickish T. Non-steroidal anti-inflammatory drugs and peptic ulcer perforation. Gut 27:114, 1986.
72. Sherlock DJ, Holl-Allen RTJ. Duodenal ulcer perforation whilst on cimetidine therapy. Br J Surg 71:586, 1984.
73. Sachdeva AK, Zaren HA, Sigel B. Surgical treatment of peptic ulcer disease. Med Clin North Am 75:999, 1991.
74. Sievert W, Vakil NB. Emergencies of the biliary tract. Gastroenterol Clin North Am 17:245, 1988.
75. Young M. Acute diseases of the pancreas and biliary tract. Emerg Med Clin North Am 7:555, 1989.
76. Marton KI, Doubilet P. How to image the gallbladder in suspected cholecystitis. Ann Intern Med 109:722, 1988.
77. Werbel GB, Nahrwold DL, Joehl RJ, et al. Percutaneous cholecystostomy in the diagnosis and treatment of acute cholecystitis in the high-risk patient. Arch Surg 124:782, 1989.
78. Klimberg S, Hawkins I, Vogel SB. Percutaneous cholecystostomy for acute cholecystitis in high risk patients. Am J Surg 153:125, 1987.
79. Frazee RC, Nagorney DM, Mucha P Jr. Acute acalculous cholecystitis. Mayo Clin Proc 64:163, 1989.
80. Orlando R, Gleason E, Drezner AD. Acute acalculous cholecystitis in the critically ill patient. Am J Surg 145:472, 1983.

81. Thompson JE, Tompkins RD, Longmire WP. Factors in management of acute cholangitis. Ann Surg 195:137, 1983.
82. Beinart C, Efremidis S, Cohen B, et al. Obstruction without dilation: Importance in evaluating jaundice. JAMA 245:353, 1981.
83. Lipsett PA, Pitt HA. Acute cholangitis. Surg Clin North Am 70:1297, 1990.
84. Moody FG. Pancreatitis as a medical emergency. Gastroenterol Clin North Am 17:433, 1988.
85. Potts JR. Acute pancreatitis. Surg Clin North Am 68:281, 1988.
86. Winslet MC, Imray C, Neoptolemos JP. Biliary acute pancreatitis. Hepatogastroenterology 38:120, 1991.
87. Soergel KH. Acute pancreatitis. *In* Sleisinger MH, Fordtran JF (eds). Gastrointestinal Disease: Pathophysiology, Diagnosis and Management, 4th ed. Philadelphia, WB Saunders, 1989, pp 1814–1841.
88. Ranson JHC, Rifkind KM, Turner JW. Prognostic signs and nonoperative peritoneal lavage in acute pancreatitis. Surg Gynecol Obstet 143:209, 1976.
89. Buchler M. Objectification of the severity of acute pancreatitis. Hepatogastroenterology 38:101, 1991.
90. Beger HG, Bittner RG, Block S, et al. Bacterial contamination of pancreatic necrosis. Gastroenterology 91:433, 1986.
91. Fraser CL, Arieff AI. Hepatic encephalopathy. N Engl J Med 313:865, 1985.
92. Schafer DF, Jones AE. Hepatic encephalopathy. *In* Zakim D, Boyer TD (eds). Hepatology: A Textbook of Liver Disease, 2nd ed. Philadelphia, WB Saunders, 1990, pp 447–459.
93. Munoz SJ, Maddrey WC. Major complications of acute and chronic liver disease. Gastroenterol Clin North Am 17:265, 1988.
94. Mortensen PB, Rasmussen HS, Holtug K. Lactulose detoxifies in vitro short-chain fatty acid production in colonic contents induced by blood: Implication of hepatic coma. Gastroenterology 94:750, 1988.
95. Felisart J, Rimola A, Arroyo V, et al. Randomized comparative study of efficacy and nephrotoxicity of ampicillin plus tobramycin versus cefotaxime in cirrhotics with severe infections. Hepatology 5:457, 1985.
96. Akriviadis EA, Runyon BA. When should paracentesis be repeated to assess the response of infected ascites to antimicrobial therapy? Hepatology 7:1030, 1987.
97. Ullian ME, Berl T. The hepatorenal syndrome: Recognition, management and prevention. J Crit Illness 1:67, 1986.
98. Freischlag J, Bennion RS, Thompson JE. Complications of diverticular disease of the colon in young people. Dis Colon Rectum 29:639, 1986.
99. Almy TP, Howell DA. Diverticular disease of the colon. N Engl J Med 302:324, 1980.
100. Naitove A, Almy TP. Diverticular disease of the colon. *In* Sleisinger MH, Fordtran JS (eds). Gastrointestinal Disease: Pathophysiology, Diagnosis and Management, 4th ed. Philadelphia, WB Saunders, 1989, pp 1419–1434.
101. Hackford AW, Schoetz DJ, Coller JA, et al. Surgical management of complicated diverticulitis. Dis Colon Rectum 28:317, 1985.
102. Painter NS, Truelove SC, Ardran GM, et al. Effect of morphine, Prostigmin, pethidine, and Pro-Banthine on the human colon in diverticulosis studied by intraluminal pressure recording and cineradiography. Gut 6:57, 1965.
103. Grendell JH, Ockner RA. Vascular diseases of the bowel. *In* Sleisinger MH, Fordtran JS (eds). Gastrointestinal Disease: Pathophysiology, Diagnosis and Management, 4th ed. Philadelphia, WB Saunders, 1989.
104. Sitges-Serra A, Mas X, Roqueta F, et al. Mesenteric infarction: An analysis of 83 patients with prognostic studies in 44 cases undergoing a massive small bowel resection. Br J Surg 75:544, 1988.

41

General Management Principles of Poisoning and Overdose

R. Phillip Dellinger, M.D.

Key Terms

Cathartics

Lavage

Miosis

Mydriasis

Poisoning and overdose continue to be major medical problems in the United States, consuming significant health care resources. The health care professional managing such patients should possess the ability to predict complications of known overdoses, as well as be able to offer a differential diagnosis for suspected overdose in which the toxic substance is not known. This chapter presents the general management principles pertinent to poisoning, overdose, and substance abuse, as well as management tips for specific overdoses that might be encountered.

TOXICITIES

Although minor toxicities from poisoning and overdose are numerous, the primary life-threatening toxicities are respiratory depression, cardiac dysrhythmias, hypotension and hypertension, metabolic acidosis, coma, seizures, and hypoxemia. The ability to classify unknown poisonings on the basis of clinical presentation may be helpful. Table 41–1 presents various toxidromes and their possible causative agents.

DIFFERENTIAL DIAGNOSIS

Drugs and conditions that may be associated with toxic psychosis or delirium are as follows:

Many prescription medications and substances of abuse are associated with toxic psychosis and delirium, as are some acute psychiatric

TABLE **41–1:** Examples of Using Toxidromes to Predict Potential Poisonings

Hyperadrenergic states (tachycardia, hypertension, anxiety)	Cocaine, amphetamines, decongestants
Sedation, respiratory depression	Opioids, barbiturates, antidepressants, benzodiazepines and ethanol (less likely to cause respiratory depression)
Depressed level of consciousness with metabolic acidosis	Carbon monoxide, cyanide, methanol, ethylene glycol
Seizures	Antidepressants, theophylline, cocaine, amphetamines, phenothiazines
Hypotension and bradycardia	Beta-blockers, calcium channel blockers
Hyperthermia	Cocaine, amphetamines, salicylates, phenothiazines
Hypothermia	Barbiturates

Conditions confused with poisoning and overdose:

- Psychosis
- CNS infection
- Hypoxia
- Sepsis
- Hypoglycemia
- Postictal state
- Hyponatremia
- Hyperthermia
- Hypercarbia
- Intracranial mass lesion (particularly subdural hematoma)

Drugs potentially producing toxic psychosis and delirium:

- Lysergic acid diethylamide
- Anticholinergics
- Phencyclidine
- Ethanol
- Marijuana
- Amphetamines
- Hashish
- Opioids (particularly oxycodone)
- Cocaine

Glycogen depletion:

- Acute or chronic ethyl alcohol abuse
- Fad dieting
- Liver disease
- Known poor nutrition
- Fasting in pediatric patients

Hypothermia: phenobarbital
Hyperthermia: cocaine

disorders. More important, however, is knowledge of the spectrum of metabolic or electrolyte, organic, infectious, and structural disorders associated with altered mental status. The clinician must be particularly alert to the possibility of hypoglycemia, central nervous system (CNS) infection, and intracranial mass lesions in patients suspected of having poisoning or overdose, or of being substance abusers.

CLINICAL PRESENTATION

Minimal time and effort are required when patients present with suspected poisoning or overdose to ascertain the presence of potentially life-threatening problems. The physical examination will reveal severe respiratory depression, whereas occult increases in Pa_{CO_2} may require arterial blood gas (ABG) measurement. Cardiac monitoring and electrocardiography (ECG) should reliably reveal the presence of dysrhythmias. Assessment of the vital signs will determine hypotension or hypertension. Metabolic acidosis may not be suspected and is another reason for early ABG measurement in the poisoned patient. Hypoxemia may be evident clinically or may be occult, diagnosed only with ABG measurement or pulse oximetry. Seizures are self-evident.

INITIAL MANAGEMENT

The ABCs (airway, breathing, and circulation) are paramount. Normal saline is the preferred intravenous fluid because hypotension is more likely than hypertension and seizures may require phenytoin therapy (phenytoin infusion requires solutions that do not contain dextrose). Naloxone (2 mg intravenously initially) and glucose (25 to 50 g of 50% dextrose) should be given to all patients who present with altered mental status or a depressed level of consciousness unless the bedside glucose determination is elevated or stroke is suspected. If glycogen depletion is a possibility, the addition of thiamine (a 100-mg intravenous bolus) with glucose administration is desirable to prevent the development of acute Wernicke's syndrome. As a practical rule, thiamine should be administered with glucose in all patients. The initial finger stick glucose determination is important, as is the laboratory blood glucose determination performed on a sample drawn before the administration of glucose (for retrospective documentation of the baseline blood glucose level). However, the clinician should not rely on a midrange finger stick glucose determination to negate empiric glucose administration. To avoid later diagnostic confusion, blood for the laboratory glucose determination should be obtained before glucose administration.

The patient's cardiac rhythm should be monitored, and the patient's vital signs should be assessed frequently. Hypo- and hyperthermia may be manifestations of specific poisonings. Early ABG measurements are very important, with oxygen therapy administered for possible hypoxemia.

After the stabilization of vital signs, the next consideration is the elimination of orally consumed toxins from the gastrointestinal (GI) tract. Gastric lavage and emesis induced with ipecac have been traditionally used. This area has been the subject of much controversy and changing opinion over the last several years. Ipecac has few indications, with the current consensus indicating that it is not recommended for use in

770 General Management Principles of Poisoning and Overdose

Charcoal does not absorb iron, lithium, hydrocarbons, or alcohols.

Cathartics that have been used:

- Sodium sulfate
- Magnesium citrate
- Magnesium sulfate
- Sorbitol

the hospital in adult patients. Induced emesis, which is not clinically more effective than lavage, has numerous shortcomings, such as delaying charcoal administration and causing possible aspiration in a patient who subsequently develops seizures or altered mental status. If ipecac is used, the patient should be alert and the overdose substance must not be caustic or associated with the potential for seizures or a sudden depression of the level of consciousness. The more important issue is that no method of GI elimination removes more than 50% of ingested toxin from the upper GI tract. This emphasizes the importance of the early administration of charcoal, which absorbs most poisons. Charcoal does not bind lithium or iron. In view of recent study findings, it could be argued that with the exception of ingestions that have occurred within 1 hour in patients with unstable vital signs or a depressed level of consciousness, charcoal alone may be as effective as lavage followed by charcoal. If the patient has a potentially life-threatening overdose or has unstable vital signs or if a gastric tube would have to be placed to deliver charcoal, then orogastric lavage with a 30 to 42 Fr tube should be performed before the administration of charcoal. The use of indiscriminant gastric lavage may increase morbidity because gastric lavage may be associated with aspiration, hypoxia, or esophageal injury. Patients who are unconscious or have an absent gag reflex should have an endotracheal tube placed before lavage. Lavage with bicarbonate solution may decrease absorption in iron overdose by converting the ferrous cation to the less absorbable ferric form. With few exceptions, charcoal should be used in all patients. Because charcoal partially binds N-acetylcysteine, consideration should be given to increasing the dosage of N-acetylcysteine (to approximately 1.5 times the calculated dose) if this agent is given in the presence of charcoal. Repetitive charcoal dosing may be useful with toxic substances that have well-identified enterogastric, enterohepatic, or enteroenteric circulations (e.g., phenobarbital or theophylline).

The use of cathartics is controversial. No prospective controlled studies have shown that cathartics decrease morbidity or mortality. They should be used with caution in the very young and the very old because of a predisposition for dehydration and electrolyte disturbances. The magnesium-containing cathartics may be associated with hypermagnesemia in patients who receive repetitive charcoal dosing combined with a cathartic.

Whole bowel irrigation with polyethylene glycol electrolyte solution has been used in experimental overdoses, with mixed reviews. It might be useful in patients with potentially life-threatening overdoses of substances that do not bind to charcoal (iron and lithium) or have already moved past the proximal GI tract. It has been used anecdotally in a cocaine body packer to facilitate the passage of cocaine packets.

Forced diuresis plus alkalinization of the urine may increase the clearance of some toxic substances (salicylates and phenobarbital). The possibility of volume overload and alkalemia should be considered and monitored closely. Acidification of the urine is much more controversial. Although substances such as amphetamine and phencyclidine do have increased renal clearance with urine acidification, blood acidemia (which is not desirable) must usually be achieved to obtain urine acidity. In addition, because the substances of abuse mentioned previously are associated with rhabdomyolysis, acidification of the urine may increase myoglobin toxicity to the renal tubules and is probably not indicated. Hemodialysis and hemoperfusion may be useful in some life-threatening

TABLE **41–2:** Poisoning and Overdose Substances With Potentially Efficacious Antidotes

Substance	Antidote
Acetaminophen	*N*-Acetylcysteine
Benzodiazepines	Flumazenil
Carbon monoxide	Oxygen (consider hyperbaric)
Cyanide	Nitrites, thiosulfate
Isoniazid	Pyridoxine
Lead, mercury, arsenic	Chelator therapy
Methanol, ethylene glycol	Ethanol
Nitrites	Methylene blue
Opioids	Naloxone
Organophosphates	Atropine, pralidoxime

overdoses, such as theophylline and methanol overdoses. It may also be useful in life-threatening lithium intoxication.

CLINICAL PEARLS

It is important to know specific antidotes that exist for some substances with potentially life-threatening toxicity. Table 41–2 lists the limited number of antidotes available.

Some overdoses are associated with a significant anion gap acidosis. Table 41–3 lists a mnemonic for etiologies of anion gap acidosis.

The osmolal gap may be useful in supporting the presence of some poisonings. The osmolal gap is the calculated osmolality ($2 \times$ sodium + glucose/18 + blood urea nitrogen/2.8) subtracted from the laboratory-measured osmolality. The normal osmolal gap is 10. Overdose substances associated with a high osmolal gap, in order of prominence, are methanol, ethanol, ethylene glycol, acetone, and isopropyl alcohol. Of this group, only isopropyl alcohol is not associated with an anion gap metabolic acidosis.

Many patients have mixed poisonings, making pupillary findings unreliable. If a single substance is taken, examination of the pupils may be helpful. Listed to the left are overdose substances that, if taken alone, are likely to produce miosis and those that are likely to produce mydriasis. Remember that mixed overdoses may negate the value of pupillary findings.

The capability to screen for poisoning and overdose substances and to order specific quantitative serum levels when appropriate is needed to manage poisoning and overdose patients optimally.

Table 41–4 lists a recommended urine screen (qualitative) and quantitative blood assays that should be available in most large-volume emergency departments to screen for potential toxins. New bedside, rapid-

Miosis (small pupils):

Opioids (except meperidine)
Pilocarpine
Organophosphates
Barbiturates
Clonidine
Parasympathomimetics

Mydriasis:

Amphetamines
Lysergic acid diethylamide
Cocaine
Marijuana
Anticholinergics
Ethanol
Meperidine
Sympathomimetics

TABLE **41–3:** Possible Causes of Anion Gap Metabolic Acidosis

M	*Methanol**
U	Uremia
D	Diabetic ketoacidosis
P	Paraldehyde (no longer available)
I	*Iron, isoniazid, inhalants*
L	Lactate
E	Ethanol, *ethylene glycol*
S	Shock, sepsis, *salicylates, solvents,* starvation ketosis

*The italicized causes are those associated with poisoning or overdose.

TABLE **41–4:** Typical Urine Screen and Blood Assays Available for the Diagnosis and Estimation of Potential Toxicity

Urine Screen—Qualitative	Blood Assays—Quantitative
Amphetamines	Acetaminophen
Barbiturates	Antidepressants
Benzodiazepines	Barbiturates
Cocaine	Carboxyhemoglobin
Ethanol	Ethanol
Lysergic acid diethylamide	Methanol
Marijuana	Salicylate
Opioids	Theophylline
Phencyclidine	

turnaround, monoclonal antibody, single-use urine toxicology screens may facilitate prompt management of some overdoses.

SPECIFIC POISONING AND OVERDOSE PROBLEMS

Cocaine

A 35-year-old man, a known cocaine abuser, is admitted to the intensive care unit (ICU) with a depressed level of consciousness and a blood pressure of 140/96 mm Hg. An unenhanced computed tomographic scan of the head showed an intracerebral hemorrhage. He does not respond to glucose or naloxone. His reflexes are increased.

A 26-year-old man is admitted to the ICU for hyperthermia and a depressed level of consciousness after intravenous cocaine abuse. His temperature is 104.8°F. A thorough evaluation for any evidence of associated infection yields negative results. The initial creatine phosphokinase level was 2000 U/L, and the repeated creatine phosphokinase level after 6 hours is 13,400 U/L. The patient's urine output is currently 50 mL/hr. The blood urea nitrogen and creatinine levels were initially 28 mg/dl and 1.2 mg/dl and are now 40 mg/dl and 1.6 mg/dl. The prothrombin time, partial thromboplastin time, and platelet count are normal. His blood pressure is 160/100 mm Hg and his pulse is 120/min. The lungs are clear to auscultation. Cocaine-induced hyperthermia with rhabdomyolysis is diagnosed.

These cases demonstrate cocaine's cerebrovascular and muscle toxicity, respectively. Cocaine is potentially lethal by all routes, including nasal insufflation and the intravenous, smoking, and oral routes. Although it is absorbed less rapidly and is not usually abused by this route, cocaine by mouth can, however, be very toxic if large quantities are consumed or if packages containing uncut cocaine rupture within the GI tract (body packing, used for illicit transport). Smoked cocaine rapidly absorbs across the alveolar-endothelial surface and readily crosses the blood-brain barrier. This produces a rapid but nonsustained euphoria that leads to repetitive use and associated morbidity.

Cerebrovascular accidents associated with cocaine abuse are a catastrophic event seen with increasing frequency. Both intracerebral and subarachnoid hemorrhage are seen. Strokes possibly due to thrombosis or vasculitis may also be linked to cocaine abuse. Cocaine-induced chest pain may be associated with myocardial infarction, as well as with ECG abnormalities without infarction. Recurrent chest pain with normal coronary arteries and persistent ECG abnormalities has also been reported. This may be related to abnormalities in small penetrating intramyocardial arteries. Seizures may be induced in patients with or without a history of seizures. Cocaine-induced rhabdomyolysis with or without hyperthermia has significant morbidity and mortality. Table 41–5 displays cocaine toxicities and the recommended management. Alveolar hemorrhage and hypersensitivity pneumonitis occur in cocaine smokers, as does barotrauma with efforts to accentuate pulmonary absorption.

Carbon Monoxide

A 25-year-old man is found in a parked car. The engine is not running. The patient is unconscious, plethoric, and known to be taking a tricyclic antidepressant and seizure medication. He is intubated in the emergency center for airway protection and is admitted to the ICU. His ABG values before intubation are as follows: Pa_{O_2}, 98 mm Hg; Pa_{CO_2}, 30 mm Hg; and pH, 7.24. Carboxyhemoglobin level is 50%.

Smokers may have low levels of carboxyhemoglobin in the blood.

This case indicates intentional carbon monoxide poisoning with diversion of carbon monoxide from the exhaust system to the inside of the car. The car had run out of gas. The patient eventually died. The unconscious state was predominantly due to cellular hypoxia. Because hemoglobin has 210 times the affinity for carbon monoxide as for oxygen, significant carboxyhemoglobin is produced when small concentrations of carbon monoxide are inhaled. The diagnosis is made by demonstrating an elevated level of carboxyhemoglobin in the blood. Remember, in the absence of smoke inhalation, induced lower airway injury carbon monoxide poisoning does not decrease Pa_{O_2}. Not only is the oxygen-carrying capacity of hemoglobin decreased by carboxyhemoglobin, but also the oxyhemoglobin saturation curve is shifted to the left, producing decreased off-loading. Perhaps most importantly, carbon monoxide exerts a direct cellular toxic effect. A sign of severe carbon monoxide poisoning

TABLE **41–5:** Problem-Oriented Cocaine Toxicity Management

Problem	Treatment
Anxiety or psychosis	Diazepam or haloperidol, respectively
Supraventricular tachycardias	Esmolol,* cardioversion if unstable
Ventricular tachycardia	Lidocaine, esmolol,* cardioversion if sustained and unstable
Severe hypertension (unlikely to occur in patients without a history of hypertension)	Rule out end-organ damage, diazepam, labetalol for a hypertensive emergency
Severe headache	Computed tomography of the head
Seizures	Diazepam and phenytoin for persistent seizures, computed tomography of the head if there is a decreased level of consciousness or a lateralizing defect on neurologic examination
Myocardial ischemia	Nitrates, calcium channel blocker, beta-blockers,* rule out myocardial infarction if appropriate
Cerebrovascular accident	Supportive, treatment of blood pressure if markedly elevated (diastolic > 120 mm Hg), possible surgery for berry aneurysm
Rhabdomyolysis (usually associated with hyperthermia)	Standard therapy to include volume therapy to maintain a high urine output (alkalinization of the urine and mannitol are controversial)
Barotrauma	Observation for pneumomediastinum, consider chest tube for pneumothorax

*Some concern has been raised about the possible iatrogenic induction of systemic hypertension by administering a beta-blocker in the presence of cocaine, because an unopposed peripheral alpha-effect may be unmasked by blocking peripheral beta-receptors. Labetalol, a combined alpha- and beta-blocker, may be considered in response to this concern.

may be metabolic acidosis, implying inadequate availability of oxygen utilization at the tissue level. The cellular toxic effect may not correlate directly with the carboxyhemoglobin level. Although the diagnosis of significant carbon monoxide poisoning should be based on elevated carboxyhemoglobin levels, decisions for aggressive therapy (100% oxygen with intubation or hyperbaric oxygen) should be based primarily on abnormal neurologic examination findings. All patients with suspected carbon monoxide poisoning should receive high-flow supplemental oxygen. Patients considered for aggressive therapy include any patient with a depressed level of consciousness or an objective abnormality on neurologic examination. Headache as an isolated single variable probably does not mandate aggressive therapy. Most clinicians would aggressively treat very high carboxyhemoglobin levels (40% or greater) as potentially morbid even in the absence of neurologic findings.

Antidepressants

A 28-year-old woman is admitted to the ICU in an unconscious state with poor respiratory effort. She is unresponsive to pain and has dry skin and dilated pupils. After lavage and the insertion of 50 g of charcoal into the stomach, the patient was intubated for airway protection. The current mental status examination reveals a localizing response to pain only. ECG reveals sinus tachycardia with a QRS of 0.09 millisecond. The cardiac rhythm subsequently changes from sinus tachycardia to a wide QRS rhythm with complete heart block. The patient's blood pressure decreases from 130/100 to 70/50 mm Hg. An empty bottle of antidepressants and a suicide note are found in the patient's home.

Primary toxicity from antidepressant poisoning includes seizures, dysrhythmias, hypoventilation, a depressed level of consciousness, and hypotension. Contrary to earlier literature reports, the current consensus is that the onset of antidepressant morbidity occurs within the first 24 hours after ingestion. Therapy is primarily supportive, with standard therapy directed at the particular toxic manifestation. The exception is the use of bicarbonate, which may be effective in decreasing acute toxicity. Alkalinization of the blood to a pH of 7.50 to 7.55 increases the protein binding of the antidepressant, decreasing free drug levels and toxicity. Metabolic alkalinization may be more effective than hyperventilation. Predicting the development of toxicity is difficult. Many studies have attempted to identify variables that can be used. Antidepressant levels are probably not helpful in predicting toxicity but are needed for the documentation of overdose. A QRS of 0.10 to 0.15 millisecond correlates with increased risk for seizures, whereas a QRS of 0.16 millisecond or greater puts the patient at risk for both seizures and dysrhythmias. A QRS of less than 0.10 millisecond does not, however, rule out the possibility of developing significant cardiac or noncardiac toxicity. Seizures may occur in the absence of signs of cardiac toxicity. The level of consciousness seems to be a good predictor of toxicity.

Physostigmine, although of potential benefit in reversing a depressed level of consciousness and in treating refractory ventricular dysrhythmias, should probably be avoided because it may produce seizures and asystole. It is contraindicated in the presence of bradycardia. Ventricular dysrhythmias are best treated with alkalinization and the standard advanced life support protocol. Phenytoin might be considered in refractory dysrhythmias. Other considerations are based on the known adrenergic effects of antidepressants. Beta-blockers for refractory ventricular dysrhythmia should be used with caution because hypotension is a potential consequence. Phenytoin may offer utility in refractory ventricular dysrhythmias. If vasopressors are used, norepinephrine or phenylephrine is recommended over dopamine. Dopamine requires the release of norepinephrine, and antidepressants deplete norepinephrine stores.

Opioids

A 35-year-old man who is a known intravenous heroin abuser presents to the emergency center unconscious, with shallow respirations and small pupils. The patient is intubated for respiratory depression, has a subsequent positive response to naloxone, and is admitted to the ICU.

Potential respiratory depressants:

Heroin
Pentazocine
Methadone
Morphine
Oxycodone
Diphenoxylate
Meperidine
Hydromorphone
Butorphanol
Codeine
Propoxyphene
Nalbuphine

The classic triad of opioid toxicity is miosis, respiratory depression, and a depressed level of consciousness. Respiratory depression, loss of airway protection secondary to a depressed level of consciousness, and hypotension are the primary morbidity-producing events. Naloxone (2 mg initially) should be given to reverse respiratory depression. Alternative routes of administration include via endotracheal tube (the best route if an intravenous line is not in place) and sublingual injection. Intramuscular and subcutaneous injection are less effective. Naloxone reliably reverses respiratory depression in most cases of overdose with semisynthetic, synthetic, and naturally occurring opioids.

More than 2 mg of naloxone (10 to 20 mg) may be required to reverse the respiratory depressant effects of pentazocine, propoxyphene, codeine, and methadone. Essentially all opioids have longer half-lives than naloxone, and repeated dosing or continuous infusion of naloxone may be necessary.

Beta-Adrenergic Blockers

A 47-year-old woman is admitted to the ICU hypotensive, with a pulse of 34/min. Her blood pressure in the emergency center was 70/40 mm Hg. After treatment with volume, atropine, and dopamine (10 μg/kg/min), her blood pressure remains at 90/60 mm Hg. Her pulse is 44/min. She admits to taking a full bottle of propranolol in a suicide attempt.

Beta-adrenergic blockers produce toxicity through bradycardia and depression of cardiac contractility (decreased inotropy). Although increasing the pulse rate is desirable and atropine is indicated in the presence of bradycardia, treatment is oriented toward reversing the negative inotropy that is the primary cause of the hypotension. Although epinephrine, atropine, isoproterenol, and dopamine may be variably effective in reversing life-threatening beta-blocker toxicity, glucagon is considered to be the initial drug of choice because it boosts inotropy and does not compete with the beta-blocker at the beta-receptor. In life-threatening hypotension from beta-blocker overdose, 3 mg of glucagon may be given initially intravenously. A glucagon drip may subsequently be necessary to maintain adequate blood pressure. Failure to achieve an immediate satisfactory response with glucagon warrants the administration of adrenergic therapy by continuous infusion.

Calcium Channel Blockers

A 15-year-old boy presents to the emergency center at 9:00 A.M. following the consumption of his parents' prescription medications at 2:00 A.M. in a suicide attempt. The patient is diaphoretic and pale but oriented. His blood pressure is 60 mm Hg systolic, and his pulse rate is between 30 and 40/min.

This patient had consumed a significant quantity of a long-acting calcium channel blocker. Guidance for the treatment of calcium channel blocker overdose comes primarily from anecdotal case reports, retrospective collective studies, and animal studies. Intravenous calcium chloride has been recommended and was used in this case without significant effect. The patient also received glucagon, which has been recommended in a dose of 2 to 4 mg in a slow intravenous push for life-threatening calcium channel blocker overdose. This was accomplished without effect. A glucagon drip of 2 mg/hr was also initiated (infusion rates of 2 to 4 mg/hr are recommended in adults). A noninvasive pacer was used that initially captured and brought the systolic blood pressure to 100 mm Hg. Subsequently, the noninvasive pacer failed, and the patient was started on an isoproterenol infusion and transferred to the cardiac catheterization laboratory, where a temporary transvenous pacer was inserted. This case demonstrates the use of most of the medications and interventions that have been recommended to treat calcium channel blocker overdose. Variable success may be encountered, as was seen in this particular case.

Hydrocarbons

A 28-year-old man is evaluated in the emergency center after the intentional ingestion of 1 cup of gasoline. The patient is in no acute distress.

Group 1 hydrocarbons
- Greases—nontoxic

Group 2 hydrocarbons
- Kerosene, gasoline—toxic, primarily by aspiration pneumonitis; potential systemic toxicity with large quantities (more than 1 mL/kg)

Group 3 hydrocarbons
- Ring hydrocarbons (benzene)—very systemically toxic

Group 4 hydrocarbons
- Chlorinated hydrocarbons (carbon tetrachloride)—very systemically toxic

Hydrocarbon toxicity from group 2 hydrocarbons comes primarily from aspiration and resultant pneumonitis at the time of swallowing. GI elimination is therefore not indicated because pulmonary toxicity may be increased. With the ingestion of large quantities of grade 2 hydrocarbons (more than 1 mL/kg), systemic absorption may occur and may result in cardiac toxicity, CNS toxicity, or GI toxicity. Group 3 and 4 hydrocarbons are always considered to be potentially life threatening, and GI elimination is indicated. Potential toxicities of the various hydrocarbon groups are detailed in the margin.

Phencyclidine

A 26-year-old man is admitted to the ICU in four-point leather restraints. The patient had presented to the emergency center with alternating periods of "almost catatonia" with a blank stare followed by violent periods of uncontrollable aggressive behavior. During the periods of violent behavior, no communication could be established with the patient. The patient's laboratory results reveal a creatine phosphokinase level of 6000 U/L. Urine toxic screen reveals phencyclidine.

The hallmark of phencyclidine toxicity is violent or bizarre behavior. The patient may exhibit any of the following:

- Intermittent blank stare
- Intermittent facial grimacing

- Intermittent abnormal posturing
- Irregular respiratory pattern
- Visual hallucinations
- Nystagmus

The primary toxicity associated with phencyclidine is self-induced injury, but hypertension, seizures, and severe rhabdomyolysis may occasionally be manifest. Treatment is usually supportive. A calm environment is ideal. If the patient needs to be chemically calmed, diazepam (for anxiety) and haloperidol (for frank psychosis) are the drugs of choice. The patient's urine should be screened for myoglobin because rhabdomyolysis may occur. Physical restraints may prevent self-injury but increase the severity of rhabdomyolysis.

Theophylline

A 19-year-old woman with a history of suicide gestures is admitted to the ICU with persistent seizures. Her family relates that she had severe nausea and vomiting before the onset of the seizures. She has a sinus tachycardia (rate, 150/min), and her blood pressure is 140/100 mm Hg. Her serum theophylline level is 50 mg/dl.

A 64-year-old woman with chronic obstructive pulmonary disease has increased her dosage of sustained-release theophylline on subsequent days from (1) 200 mg twice daily to (2) 300 mg twice daily to (3) 300 mg three times a day to (4) 300 mg four times a day. The patient presents to a small hospital emergency center with complaints of being jittery and having nausea and palpitations. ECG reveals no premature ventricular contractions, and the theophylline level is 48.6 mg/L. During transfer to a tertiary care center, multiple runs of ventricular tachycardia are noted.

Toxicity begins at a concentration of 20 mg/L. Life-threatening toxicity is unusual with levels of less than 50 to 60 mg/L in acute ingestion.

Theophylline toxicity is characterized by nausea, vomiting, and agitation. More serious complications include ventricular dysrhythmias and seizures. A chronic user may have a life-threatening toxicity with levels of less than 50 to 60 mg/L (the second of the previous two cases). With the same blood level of theophylline, toxicity is more likely to occur in a patient receiving long-term theophylline therapy than in a person not receiving theophylline who takes an intentional overdose. Levels of greater than 30 mg/L are concerning in this group. Hypokalemia may exacerbate dysrhythmias. Seizures may be poorly responsive to phenytoin but should respond to benzodiazepines (as is true for most seizures due to drug or medication toxicity). In addition to standard supportive therapy and GI elimination, repetitive charcoal administration may be effective. Any patient with a life-threatening complication, such as seizure, and a level of 60 mg/L or greater and rising should be considered for hemoperfusion.

Organophosphates

A 32-year-old woman is admitted to the ICU following the ingestion of insecticide. The patient has small pupils and is drooling from the corners of the mouth. The patient has abdominal cramps and diarrhea. Her pulse is 90/min, and her blood pressure is within normal limits. Auscultation of the lungs reveals diffuse wheezing with evidence of increased upper airway secretions.

Organophosphate poisoning exerts potential deleterious effects on three body systems:

- Muscarinic (parasympathetic) system—inducing bronchorrhea, bradycardia, and SLUDGE (salivation, lacrimation, urination, defecation, GI pain, and emesis)
- Nicotinic autonomic system—resulting in muscle weakness
- CNS—less commonly a problem, but effects may include confusion, slurred speech, and respiratory depression

Muscarinic poisoning is most likely to produce morbidity and mortality, followed by nicotinic and finally by CNS effects. Pulmonary toxicity (bronchorrhea, bronchospasm, and respiratory depression) are the primary concerns. Cholinesterase levels may be measured. Pseudocholinesterase can be measured in the plasma (easier measurement), and true cholinesterase (acetylcholinesterase) can be measured in the red blood cells. The latter is a better measurement of actual cholinesterase activity. Unfortunately, the availability of these tests makes them unlikely to be of benefit in clinical decision making. Both intravenous atropine and pralidoxime are indicated. Atropine does not reverse nicotinic manifestations; therefore, patients with significant respiratory muscle weakness will not have improvement. Pralidoxime does reverse the nicotinic effect but does not exert an effect for approximately 15 to 20 minutes. The initial therapy with atropine is 2 to 4 mg, repeated every 5 minutes until atropinization has occurred. Large amounts may be required. Atropinization is best assessed by dryness of the oral secretions, not by pupillary size.

Barbiturates

A 52-year-old woman is admitted to the ICU with a depressed level of consciousness following a barbiturate overdose. The patient had been intubated in the emergency center for airway protection. Her reflexes are depressed diffusely. After transfer to the ICU, the patient's blood pressure is noted to have decreased from 120/70 to 90/50 mm Hg.

Barbiturate toxicity is characterized by respiratory depression, hypotension, and a depressed level of consciousness. Standard therapy for barbiturate overdose is GI elimination and supportive therapy. Forced diuresis, alkalinization of the urine, and repetitive charcoal administration may all increase clearance. Hypotension is primarily due to an increase in venous capacitance and should be treated initially with volume therapy.

Methanol and Ethylene Glycol

A 42-year-old alcoholic admitted to the ICU is lethargic, with a profound anion gap metabolic acidosis. A large osmolal gap is present. His breath smells of antifreeze.

The patient's breath odor may support alcohol substitute poisoning (wood alcohol for methanol, antifreeze for ethylene glycol). Anion gap metabolic acidosis is usually present with significant overdoses. An osmolal gap should be present. With ethylene glycol toxicity, urinalysis demonstrates oxalate crystals in fewer than one third of cases. Visual problems are a primary and often permanent manifestation of methanol toxicity (because of optic nerve injury). The urine of a patient who overdoses on antifreeze may fluoresce with a Wood light because of the fluorescent material added to assist mechanics in diagnosing leaks in auto cooling systems. Treatment for life-threatening poisonings includes the use of intravenous ethanol. The hepatic alcohol dehydrogenase system preferentially metabolizes ethanol over methanol and ethylene glycol. The toxic products of methanol and ethylene glycol metabolism are therefore decreased by the infusion of ethanol. The metabolic acidosis is treated with sodium bicarbonate.

Acetaminophen

A patient admitted to the ICU with a significantly depressed level of consciousness has been prophylactically intubated for airway protection. The patient had consumed a large quantity of multiple medications from the home medicine cabinet (polypharmacy overdose). The urine toxic screen results are pending.

In patients who consume multiple medications for which the identity is not known, it is important to screen for acetaminophen because there may be few or no acute toxic manifestations. Knowledge of how to treat these patients is important. Normally, only 4% of medicinal acetaminophen is metabolized by the cytochrome P-450 system. Cytochrome P-450 system byproducts are thought to produce the liver toxicity seen with acetaminophen overdose. Glutathione metabolizes the toxic byproducts of acetaminophen metabolism. Patients who take large quantities of acetaminophen overwhelm the normal metabolic pathway, and an increasing percentage of acetaminophen is then metabolized by cytochrome P-450, with a marked increase in toxicity. Glutathione stores are rapidly depleted, especially in people with pre-existing liver disease. A latent period for the manifestation of hepatic damage exists (12 hours to 3 days). Life-threatening toxicity may therefore be present with no initial symptoms. Acetaminophen levels should probably be measured in all potential polypharmacy suicide gestures or attempts. Acetaminophen levels are measured 4 hours or more after ingestion and are plotted on the Rumack-Matthew nomogram for decisions on N-acetylcysteine therapy. N-Acetylcysteine as an antidote is most effective when given within the first 8 to 12 hours after acetaminophen overdose, and it is still used with some hope for benefit up to 24 hours. Lavage is preferred over ipecac because the patient is more tolerant of the noxious-smelling N-acetylcysteine if it is delivered by gastric tube. Charcoal binds N-acetylcysteine to some degree, and this fact should be considered in management decisions, as discussed earlier.

Salicylates

A 68-year-old woman is admitted to the ICU with altered mental status, metabolic acidosis, and diffuse infiltrates with hypoxemia. Head computed tomographic findings are within normal limits. The patient's blood pressure is 130/100 mm Hg, and her pulse is 118/min. A pulmonary artery catheter is inserted, and the pulmonary artery occlusive pressure is normal. The patient is afebrile. Her sister reports she has had heavy aspirin use in the previous week.

Examples of over-the-counter preparations containing salicylates:

Anacin
Alka-Seltzer
Bufferin
Dristan
Empirin
Excedrin
Midol

Salicylates are found in many over-the-counter preparations, as well as in prescription medications (Fiorinal and Percodan). There is a decreasing rate of absorption with aqueous, tablet, and enteric-coated compounds, in that order. The most highly concentrated salicylate preparation is methyl salicylate (oil of wintergreen). Symptoms of salicylate poisoning include tinnitus, nausea and vomiting, and in severe cases, a depressed level of consciousness. Noncardiac pulmonary edema and metabolic acidosis may be present. The Done nomogram with a blood salicylate level plotted 6 hours or more after acute intake is helpful in decision making with regard to the need for admission and for treatment, observation, or support (usually including diuresis and alkalinization of the urine). Measurement of salicylate levels is not helpful in enteric-coated overdose or chronic salicylate intoxication. The Done nomogram assumes a normal pH. Nomogram toxicity may be underestimated in the case of a low pH. In the case of a normal pH and acute ingestion of non–enteric-coated salicylates, moderate to severe toxicity may be overestimated by the nomogram. Empiric therapy may be indicated in cases of chronic salicylate toxicity based on the clinical scenario.

The clinician should beware of unrecognized salicylate toxicity (particularly chronic toxicity in elderly patients presenting with a depressed level of consciousness and metabolic acidosis). Salicylate toxicity may be associated with both centrally mediated respiratory alkalosis and metabolic acidosis. Although children usually present with respiratory alkalosis followed by the development of metabolic acidosis, adults with clinically significant salicylate toxicity usually present with the combined acid-base disorder. Bicarbonate therapy cannot be initiated during the early phases of toxicity, when the respiratory component may predominate.

Toluene

A 27-year-old man presents to the emergency department (brought by family) with complaints of severe weakness. The physical examination reveals a marked decrease in motor strength in both the upper and the lower extremities. The patient's respirations are rapid and shallow. His blood pressure is 150/100 mm Hg, and his pulse is 135/min. The ABG values on high-flow oxygen are as follows: pH, 7.18; Pa_{CO_2}, 50 mm Hg; and Pa_{O_2}, 150 mm Hg. Electrolyte assessment reveals a potassium of 1.6 mEq/L and the absence of an anion gap. Friends report frequent inhalation of metal spray paint fumes.

Toluene, found in model cement and spray paints, is abused by the inhalant route for its mood-altering properties. Toluene may acutely produce a lactate acidosis, cardiac dysrhythmias (primarily bradydysrhythmias), and altered mental status. Chronically, it produces cerebral atrophy, loss of cognitive function, peripheral neurologic abnormalities, and renal tubular acidosis. The renal tubular acidosis may be the reason for ICU admission because of severe hypokalemia with a nonanion gap metabolic acidosis. Correcting the pH in the preceding case without first initiating potassium replacement could be catastrophic.

Amphetamines

A 28-year-old man presents to the emergency department with acute psychosis. The patient's behavior is somewhat paranoid. He is tachycardic and minimally hypertensive. Diaphoresis is present, and needle marks are noticed on both arms. Friends report that he "does speed."

Amphetamine toxicity is similar to cocaine toxicity. The symptoms include tachycardia, mydriasis, and diaphoresis. The toxic effects are primarily hypertension, hyperthermia, rhabdomyolysis, seizures, and dysrhythmias. Treatment is supportive and is directed toward specific organ toxicity. Diazepam is the nonspecific drug of choice to combat the hypersympathetic state.

Benzodiazepines

A 24-year-old man presents to the emergency department responsive to pain only. The neurologic examination results are nonfocal, and the breath does not smell of ethanol. He is found to have many pills for "nerves."

Benzodiazepines are unlikely to produce life-threatening toxicity as a single overdose. However, they produce a differential diagnosis for substances that may later manifest with more severe toxicity, such as barbiturates, antidepressants, and so forth. They are likely to be a problem through additive respiratory depression when they are combined with other potential respiratory depressants. Loss of airway protection with resultant aspiration is perhaps the greatest concern. The primary manifestation is somnolence. Occasionally, a primary respiratory depression may be seen in young, healthy patients, although this is more likely to occur in older patients or in patients with severe chronic lung disease. Treatment has traditionally been supportive. Flumazenil, a benzodiazepine antagonist, has become available and may be effective in reversing the depressed level of consciousness. The dosage for intentional overdose is an initial 0.2 mg intravenously over 30 seconds. If the desired level of consciousness is not obtained in 30 seconds, an additional intravenous dose of 0.2 mg can be given. If the desired response is not realized, additional intravenous doses of 0.5 mg over 30 seconds, every 1 minute to a total of 3 mg, may be given. Occasionally, a total of 5 mg may be required. Resedation is common because the half-life of flumazenil is shorter than that of most benzodiazepines. The use of flumazenil is not a substitute for other supportive care, including airway management and ventilation when necessary. Flumazenil should not be administered to patients with known or suspected antidepressant overdose or to those in whom benzodiazepines are needed for seizure control because of the possibility of lowering the seizure threshold.

Warfarin Compounds

A 28-year-old man who is depressed presents to the emergency department with hematuria and a swollen submandibular area. The patient also relates a history of intermittent hematemesis. His vital signs are as follows: blood pressure, 150/80 mm Hg supine and 130/90 mm Hg standing; pulse, 100/min supine and 90/min standing; afebrile. His platelet count is 330,000/cu mm, and his hematocrit is 30%. The patient's prothrombin time is 91.8 seconds, and his partial thromboplastin time is 71 seconds. He admits to ingestion of rat poison.

This example is that of poisoning with a long-acting warfarin compound called superwarfarin (brodifacoum). All warfarin compounds are potentially lethal because of the possibility of severe hemorrhage. Both the prothrombin time and the partial thromboplastin time are prolonged. Treatment includes the use of fresh frozen plasma and vitamin K if acute hemorrhage is present and observation and the institution of vitamin K therapy only if hemorrhage is absent. For superwarfarins, the half-life is long and the elevation in clotting parameters may persist for weeks to months. Repetitive vitamin K therapy is necessary in this circumstance. Some investigators have noted the theoretical benefit of phenobarbital in inducing the liver metabolism of warfarins, but this has not been proved.

SUMMARY

The health care professional should have an understanding of the diagnosis and treatment of poisonings. A knowledge of initial stabilization techniques and GI elimination procedures is essential. Availability and proper knowledge of effective antidotes are needed. It is essential to be able to use presenting findings in the patient with known or suspected poisoning or overdose to:

- Support the diagnosis of the type of poison likely to be involved
- Initiate diagnostic tests
- Make rational decisions for empiric and definitive therapy

Acknowledgment

I wish to thank Dr. Janice L. Zimmerman, Ben Taub General Hospital, Baylor College of Medicine, for her input and critique of this manuscript.

Suggested Readings

Brody SL, Wrenn KD, Wilber MM, et al. Predicting the severity of cocaine-associated rhabdomyolysis. Ann Emerg Med 19:1137–1143, 1990.

Bryson PD. Comprehensive Review in Toxicology. Rockville, MD, Aspen Publication, 1986.

DeBroe ME, Bismuth C, DeGroot G, et al. Haemoperfusion: A useful therapy for a severely poisoned patient? Hum Toxicol 5:11–14, 1986.

Dice WH, Ward G, Kelley J, et al. Pulmonary toxicity following gastrointestinal ingestion of kerosene. Ann Emerg Med 11(3):128–132, 1982.

Frommer DA, Kulig KW, Marx JA, et al. Tricyclic antidepressant overdose: A review. JAMA 257:521–525, 1987.

Gold MS. Cocaine: Helping patients avoid the end of the line. Emerg Med Rep 6:17, 1985.

Goldberg MJ, Spector R, Park GD, et al. An approach to the management of the poisoned patient. Arch Intern Med 146:1381–1385, 1986.

Goldfrank LR. Toxicologic emergencies. In Goldfrank LR, Flomenbaum NE, Lewin NA, et al (eds). 3rd ed. Norwalk, CT, Appleton-Century-Crofts, 1986.

Henry JA. Specific problems of drug intoxication. Br J Anaesth 58:223–233, 1986.

Ilano AL, Raffin TA. Management of carbon monoxide poisoning. Chest 97:165–169, 1990.

Jones J, McMullen MJ, Dougherty J, et al. Repetitive doses of activated charcoal in the treatment of poisoning. Am J Emerg Med 5:305–310, 1987.

Katona B, Wason S. Superwarfarin poisoning. J Emerg Med 7:627–631, 1989.

Kellermann AL, Fihn SD, LoGerfo JP, et al. Impact of drug screening in suspected overdose. Ann Emerg Med 16(11):1206–1216, 1987.

Kulig K, Duffy JP, Linden CH, et al. Toxic effects of methanol, ethylene glycol, and isopropyl alcohol. Top Emerg Med 6:14, 1984.

Levine SR, Brust JCM, Futrell N, et al. Cerebrovascular complications of the use of the "crack" form of alkaloidal cocaine. N Engl J Med 323:699–704, 1990.

Mitchell JR. Acetaminophen toxicity. N Engl J Med 319(24):1601–1602, 1988.

Nejman G, Hoekstra J, Kelly M. Gastric emptying in the poisoned patient. Am J Emerg Med 8:265–269, 1990.

Olson KR. Is gut emptying all washed up? Am J Emerg Med 8(6):560–561, 1990.

Paloucek FP, Rodvoid KA. Evaluation of theophylline overdoses and toxicities. Ann Emerg Med 17:135–144, 1988.

Ramoska EA, Spiller HA, Myers A. Calcium channel blocker toxicity. Ann Emerg Med 19:649–653, 1990.

Renzi FP, Donovan JW, Martin TG, et al. Concomitant use of activated charcoal and *N*-acetylcysteine. Ann Emerg Med 14(6):568–572, 1985.

Shannon M, Fish SS, Lovejoy FH. Cathartics and laxatives: Do they still have a place in management of the poisoned patient? Med Toxicol 1:247–252, 1986.

Snyder JW, Vlasses PH. Role of the laboratory in treatment of the poisoned patient. Arch Intern Med 148:279–280, 1988.

Sullivan JB. Planning an effective therapeutic strategy in salicylate poisoning. Emerg Med Rep 7(12):1–10, 1986.

Tafuri J, Roberts J. Organophosphate poisoning. Ann Emerg Med 16:193–197, 1987.

Tenenbein M, Cohen S, Sitar DS. Whole bowel irrigation as a decontamination procedure after acute drug overdose. Arch Intern Med 147:905–907, 1987.

Votey SR, Bosse GM, Bayer MJ. Flumazenil: A new benzodiazepine antagonist. Ann Emerg Med 20(2):181–188, 1991.

Weinstein RS. Recognition and management of poisoning with beta-adrenergic blocking agents. Ann Emerg Med 13(12):1123–1131, 1984.

Zimmerman JL, Dellinger RP, Majid P. Cocaine-associated chest pain. Ann Emerg Med 20(6):611–615, 1991.

42

■

Pulmonary Thromboembolic Disease

Gilbert E. D'Alonzo, D.O.

Venous thrombosis, along with its sequela pulmonary embolism, is a serious and at times fatal disease that often complicates the course of chronically ill patients and occasionally affects otherwise healthy individuals. Nearly 5 million episodes of deep venous thrombosis occur and upward of 600,000 people suffer from pulmonary thromboemboli each year in the United States;[1] most alarmingly, however, it may be responsible for up to 200,000 deaths. More than half of these deaths occur in patients in whom the diagnosis of pulmonary embolism is not made and to whom therapy is never given. Approximately 60,000 to 90,000 patients with pulmonary emboli die within the first few hours of the acute event, with nearly 10,000 dying subsequently despite a correct early diagnosis and the initiation of therapy. The mortality rate is four- to six-fold greater in patients in whom the diagnosis is missed and appropriate therapy is not instituted. This information stresses not only the importance of early disease recognition and the institution of therapy but also the necessity of preventing deep venous thrombosis from developing in the first place.

Because of the relative lack of specificity of the tests used to demonstrate emboli or their progenitor deep venous thrombosis, the condition has the potential for being overdiagnosed. No single component of the history, physical examination, or routine laboratory work-up is specific. Diagnostic difficulties are often confounded by the patient's having another disease that when exacerbated has many of the clinical features of pulmonary embolism. A review of the literature suggests that unless the diagnosis of pulmonary embolism is vigorously pursued, it may well be overdiagnosed in the healthy ambulatory population, in which it is often confused with other, less serious causes of nonspecific chest pain. However, pulmonary embolism is frequently missed in high-risk hospitalized patients, in whom it continues to be a significant cause of both morbidity and mortality.

This chapter

- Focuses on the challenging problem of pulmonary thromboembolism
- Presents a pathophysiologic and clinical review
- Develops a logical approach to diagnosis
- Addresses accepted forms of treatment

Substances other than venous thrombi can also embolize to the lung. The clinical syndromes associated with air, tumor, fat, and foreign body emboli are quite different from that associated with intrinsic thromboemboli. Finally, a brief discussion of these conditions touches on their expressive clinical differences from pulmonary thromboembolism.

DEEP VENOUS THROMBOSIS

Injury to the pelvis or the lower extremities, surgery involving the lower extremities, all surgical procedures requiring prolonged general anesthesia, burns, pregnancy and particularly the postpartum state, prior venous thrombosis with residual venous obstruction, congestive heart failure, cancer, and any medical condition that is associated with bed rest for a prolonged period have all been implicated.

Because venous thrombosis is a precursor of pulmonary embolism, an understanding of its pathophysiology, diagnosis, and prevention is necessary. A number of clinical conditions, diseases, and laboratory findings have been associated with an apparent predisposition to the development of deep venous thrombosis (Table 42–1). Many of these so-called risk factors have been found to be associated with one or more of the thrombogenic alterations responsible for the development of a hypercoagulable state. In most patients, some clinical state associated with venostasis, vascular intimal injury, or both increases the risk of pulmonary embolism from deep venous thrombosis. Additionally, a number of relatively uncommon disorders are associated with venous thromboembolism, including systemic lupus erythematosus[2] and polycythemia vera.[3] Other risk factors are older age (particularly older than 65 years), obesity, and the use of estrogen-containing medications. Risk factors are cumulative in their effect, and generally more than one factor is present in patients with deep venous thrombosis.[4] A number of laboratory abnormalities correlate with an increased incidence of thrombosis. These abnormalities are due to inherited or acquired diseases that seriously alter the coagulation system.[5] Such disorders include deficiencies in antithrombin III, protein C, protein S, and various plasminogen activators. For example, low antithrombin III levels can be acquired with liver disease, with oral contraceptive use and heparin therapy, and during the course of consumptive coagulopathy.

Clinically detectable pulmonary emboli arise chiefly from thrombosis of the deep veins of the leg. Autopsy studies have shown that approximately 80 to 95% of pulmonary emboli that achieve clinical importance arise from venous thrombosis in the veins of the lower extremities.[5, 6] The likelihood of embolization seems to be heavily dependent on the location of thrombi in the veins of the lower extremity. Thrombi found in the popliteal and other more proximal veins have a high risk of embolization. In contrast, calf vein thrombosis seems to be less associated with pulmonary embolization, unless the thrombosis propagates proximally. Probably 10 to 15% of emboli come from the pelvic veins, the right side of the heart, and the upper extremity veins. Indeed, with the increasing use of subclavian and internal jugular venous access, more cases of sub-

TABLE **42–1:** Individuals at Increased Risk for Venous Thromboembolism

Surgical Patients
Orthopedic surgery and lower extremity fractures
Major surgical procedures (general anesthesia > 30 min)
Urologic, gynecologic, and neurosurgical procedures
Medical Patients
Cancer
Stroke
Myocardial infarction
Congestive heart failure
Sepsis
Acquired Risks
Lupus anticoagulant
Nephrotic syndrome
Paroxysmal nocturnal hemoglobinuria
Polycythemia vera
Inherited Risks
Antithrombin III, protein S, and protein C deficiency
Dysfibrinogenemia
Plasminogen and plasminogen activation disorders

clavian, axillary, and internal jugular venous thromboembolism are being diagnosed. However, in the absence of right ventricular failure or indwelling catheters, emboli from the upper extremity veins or the right cardiac chamber are probably quite rare. Available evidence obtained from an analytic review of 20 relevant studies suggests that calf deep vein thrombosis propagates to the thigh in up to 20% of cases and that propagation invariably occurs before embolization.[7]

The clinical diagnosis of venous thrombosis is both insensitive and nonspecific. It is insensitive because often thrombosis is present but clinical manifestations are absent. This may be because phlebitis is not present or is only minimal or because venous blood flow is not completely obstructed. Thus, dangerous venous thrombosis can be present in patients with no or only minor signs and symptoms. The clinical diagnosis is nonspecific because the classic symptoms of pain, erythema, and swelling, when present, may not be due to venous thrombosis. In fact, only about 50% of patients suspected of having venous thrombosis are diagnosed with this condition by venography.[8] The eventual diagnoses in patients who did not have thrombosis included disorders of subcutaneous tissue, lymphatics, muscles, nerves, bones, and joints. In the group that had thrombosis, two thirds had distal involvement only. From these observations, it becomes obvious that a clinically suspected diagnosis must be confirmed by a reliable test and that early detection of thrombosis in high-risk patients requires a monitoring process.

PATHOPHYSIOLOGY OF PULMONARY EMBOLISM

Embolic obstruction of the pulmonary arteries affects lung tissue, the pulmonary circulation, and the function of the right and left sides of the heart. Generally, the degree of compromise depends on the extent of embolic obstruction and the degree of pre-existing cardiopulmonary disease. Hemodynamic alterations that occur with acute pulmonary embolism correlate with the degree of vascular obstruction in patients without previous cardiopulmonary disease. However, in patients with underlying heart or lung disease, severe hemodynamic instability and collapse can occur even with submassive (less than 50% of the pulmonary vasculature) occlusion.[9] The initial hemodynamic consequence of embolization is an acute reduction in pulmonary vascular cross-sectional area, with a subsequent increase in the resistance to blood flow through the lungs. If the cardiac output is to remain adequate, the pulmonary arterial pressure must rise. The maintenance of flow then depends on the ability of the right ventricle to pump against the added pressure afterload. If it cannot, right-sided heart failure ensues. In previously normal patients, significant pulmonary hypertension and right-sided heart dysfunction do not usually occur until approximately 50% of the pulmonary vascular bed is occluded.[10] The normal right ventricle is unable to develop high pressures acutely and to perform high-intensity work for extended durations. Thus, there are limits to the ability of the right ventricle to compensate for embolic occlusion. In patients without previous cardiopulmonary disease, the maximal mean pulmonary arterial pressure that can be generated and maintained is approximately 40 mm Hg. If this load is exceeded, right ventricular failure generally develops.

If cardiac or pulmonary disease exists and impairs the pulmonary vascular reserve capacity or results in right ventricular hypertrophy, then a relatively smaller degree of vascular occlusion will result in a greater amount of pulmonary arterial hypertension and more serious right ventricular dysfunction.[10] When compared with patients who were healthy before the embolic event, patients with prior cardiopulmonary disease showed a level of pulmonary hypertension that was disproportionate to the extent of embolic obstruction.

Abnormalities of pulmonary gas exchange are an inevitable consequence of pulmonary embolization.[11] The etiology of the gas exchange abnormality, which is likely to be complex and multifactorial, can differ from patient to patient. The degree of abnormal gas exchange is influenced by

- The size of the embolized vessels
- The character of the embolized material
- The completeness of the occlusion
- The presence or absence of underlying cardiopulmonary disease
- The time that has elapsed since embolization

An increase in physiologic dead space (nonperfused but aerated alveoli) is an inevitable consequence of pulmonary embolism. Right-to-left shunting, ventilation-perfusion inequality, and in certain patients, a fall in the oxygen tension of the mixed venous blood have all been shown to play a role in the development of hypoxemia subsequent to pulmonary embolism.

Pulmonary infarction, an uncommon consequence of embolism, occurs after the ischemic death of lung tissue.[12] The lung receives its oxygen from the bronchial circulation, the pulmonary arterial circulation, and alveolar gas. Because of multiple oxygen supply sources, impairment of the pulmonary arterial flow does not generally produce parenchymal ischemia. However, if ischemia or infarction is going to occur, it will most likely develop in the periphery of the lung, where the bronchial circulation is minimal and postembolic bronchoconstriction is likely to occur. This probably explains why infarctions are more likely to occur with small peripheral emboli than with large central clots. Infarction is also more likely to occur in patients with underlying left ventricular failure or chronic obstructive lung disease, two clinical situations in which the two sources of oxygen supply to the lung tissue besides the pulmonary artery may be impaired.

DIAGNOSIS OF PULMONARY EMBOLISM

A high index of suspicion is paramount for the diagnosis of pulmonary emboli in the majority of patients.

Many different diseases can produce manifestations similar to pulmonary embolism. Often, pulmonary emboli are clinically silent. Thromboembolism should be considered in any patient who is at significant risk for the development of deep venous thrombosis and who has a compatible clinical picture.

Signs and Symptoms

The signs and symptoms of pulmonary embolism are nonspecific and are typical of many cardiopulmonary diseases.[13] The frequencies of the many symptoms observed in patients with pulmonary emboli are shown in Table 42–2. As mentioned, two factors play an important role in determining the clinical presentation of pulmonary embolism in a given patient: the pre-embolic cardiopulmonary status and the extent of embo-

TABLE **42–2:** Symptoms Observed in 327 Patients With Angiographically Proven Acute Pulmonary Emboli

	Patients (%)		
Symptom	Total (n = 327)	With Massive Embolism (n = 197)	With Submassive Embolism (n = 130)
Chest pain	88	85	89
Pleuritic	74	64	85
Nonpleuritic	14	6	8
Dyspnea	85	85	82
Apprehension	59	65	50
Cough	53	53	52
Hemoptysis	30	23	40
Syncope	13	20	6

Adapted from Bell WR, Simon TL, DeMets DL. The clinical features of submassive and massive pulmonary emboli. Am J Med 62:355–360, 1977.

lization. Generally, dyspnea and chest discomfort are the most common signs, with more than half of patients complaining of apprehension and cough. Dyspnea varies in intensity and duration, and in many patients, it lasts only a brief period. The duration and intensity of dyspnea are most likely related to the extent of embolization. Pleuritic chest pain is most commonly found after submassive embolic events, especially when an infarction or congestive atelectasis has occurred. Occasionally, especially after an acute massive embolic event, a dull, substernal heaviness or tightness is noted. Syncope is rare, but when it occurs, it generally implies that a massive embolic event has taken place, with a serious reduction in cardiac output and cerebral blood flow. Like pleuritic chest pain, hemoptysis is more likely to occur after a submassive embolic event.

Tachypnea is the only consistent physical finding after pulmonary embolism (Table 42–3).[13] Other physical findings typical of cardiopulmonary disease, such as tachycardia, an accentuated second heart sound, and crackles on auscultation, are found in fewer than 50% of cases. Low-grade fever is common, but a sustained temperature elevation, which is uncommon, points more to an infectious process, especially if it is accompanied by an elevated white blood cell count. Wheezing is uncommon. Hypotension leading to shock occurs in about 10% of patients and is almost always associated with a massive embolic event. If a patient does not complain of shortness of breath or chest pain and does not have tachypnea, then the diagnosis of pulmonary embolism is very unlikely.

The measurement of arterial blood gases provides minimal diagnostic help.[11]

The degree of hypoxemia, when present, is usually moderate, although approximately 25% of patients have a Pa_{O_2} of less than 60 mm Hg, which is usually associated with a high degree of embolic vascular occlusion and low cardiac output or pre-existing pulmonary disease.

Arterial Blood Gas Measurement

Routine laboratory studies play no role in the diagnosis of acute pulmonary embolism. Hypoxemia is a common but not inevitable finding in patients with pulmonary embolism. Approximately 13% of patients have an arterial partial pressure of oxygen (Pa_{O_2}) of greater than 80 mm Hg. Because of the hyperventilation that accompanies pulmonary embolism, arterial hypocapnia is common. In patients who do not have substantial hypoxemia, the alveolar-arterial oxygen gradient is often, but not always, elevated.[14]

TABLE **42–3:** Signs Found in 327 Patients With Angiographically Proven Acute Pulmonary Emboli

	Patients (%)		
Symptom	Total (n = 327)	With Massive Embolism (n = 197)	With Submassive Embolism (n = 130)
Respiration > 20/min	92	95	87
Rales	58	57	60
Increased S$_2$P*	53	58	45
Pulse > 100/min	44	48	38
Temperature > 37.8°C	43	43	42
Diaphoresis	36	42	27
Gallop	34	39	25
Phlebitis	32	36	26
Edema	24	28	28
Cyanosis	19	25	9

Adapted from Bell WR, Simon TL, DeMets DL. The clinical features of submassive and massive pulmonary emboli. Am J Med 62:355–360, 1977.
*S$_2$P is the intensity of the pulmonic component of the second heart sound.

Chest Radiography

The chest radiographic findings are frequently abnormal, but once again, the findings are too nonspecific to be useful.[15] Lung parenchymal abnormalities, including consolidation and atelectasis, are common. Occasionally, the infiltrates are pleural based and more commonly found in the lower and midlung fields. Elevation of a hemidiaphragm is also common. More subtle roentgenographic signs involve changes associated with the pulmonary vessels. Two such findings are areas of absent vascular markings or oligemia and unilateral distention of a proximal pulmonary artery. The chest x-ray film can be most useful in providing evidence of another diagnosis that may emulate pulmonary embolism, such as pneumothorax, congestive heart failure, or pneumonia.

Electrocardiography

In the majority of patients with pulmonary embolism, electrocardiography shows nonspecific alterations, which are difficult to separate from abnormalities caused by pre-existing cardiopulmonary disease.[15] Changes in the ST segment and T wave inversion are common. Other observed electrocardiographic changes are low QRS voltage in the frontal plane, complete right bundle branch block, left axis deviation, and premature ventricular contractions. P pulmonale, right axis deviation, and atrial fibrillation are uncommon, occurring in 5% or fewer of patients.

Ventilation-Perfusion Lung Scanning

The key to the diagnosis of acute pulmonary embolism is the ventilation-perfusion ($\dot{V}/\dot{Q}$) lung scan. A high-probability scan, defined as perfusion defects that are segmental or larger, combined with normal ventilation in the correct clinical situation is sufficient to make the diagnosis.[16] Patients for whom routine anticoagulation is contemplated and who have no contraindication to anticoagulation may be treated on the basis of a high-probability $\dot{V}/\dot{Q}$ scan. All other combinations of abnormalities should be considered as indeterminate, with the risk of throm-

Electrocardiographic findings are frequently normal or show only sinus tachycardia.

Like chest radiography, electrocardiography may be most useful in ruling out cardiac conditions that mimic pulmonary embolism, such as acute myocardial infarction and pericarditis.

A normal lung scan result effectively rules out the diagnosis.

boembolic disease ranging from 10 to 50%.[16-18] In these patients, other studies are necessary to confirm or exclude the diagnosis of thromboembolic disease.

Detection of Lower Extremity Venous Thrombosis

The diagnostic tests for deep venous thrombosis can be divided into invasive and noninvasive studies (Table 42–4). Each has advantages and disadvantages, and the specific test chosen depends on patient-related factors, the availability of equipment, technical and interpretive experience, and the question being addressed. The gold standard for the diagnosis of deep venous thrombosis is contrast venography, a difficult invasive procedure that requires considerable experience not only to execute but to interpret properly. At times, the venous system is not satisfactorily visualized, raising questions about whether nonvisualization indicates thrombosis or is merely the result of technical problems. Venography has been reported to be 90% accurate for deep venous thrombosis. It is associated with adverse side effects ranging from pain to hypersensitivity reactions, and finally, it is expensive.

Because of these problems, noninvasive standardized tests have been sought. One of these tests is impedance plethysmography (IPG). The sensitivity and specificity of IPG for the diagnosis of venous obstruction of the iliofemoral system have been reported to be in the 90% range.[19] A normal test finding essentially excludes the presence of a proximal but not distal leg venous thrombus, although a false-negative IPG finding can occur when the thrombus is small and nonocclusive. IPG is not very sensitive in the detection of calf vein thrombosis. Fortunately, this limitation is not clinically important because treatment of calf vein thrombosis is required only if it extends into the proximal leg deep venous system. If popliteal extension of calf vein thrombosis is going to develop, it generally occurs during the first 7 days of presentation, and it can be detected by performing serial IPG tests.[17, 20, 21] IPG loses its specificity for iliofemoral thombosis in the presence of other conditions that impede venous flow from the legs. These include pregnancy, congestive heart failure, and ascites. A false-positive IPG result can also be caused by related, unrecognized leg muscle contraction, by the improper positioning and fitting of electrodes and cuff, and by reduced arterial filling.

Like IPG, Doppler ultrasound examination is sensitive and specific

TABLE **42–4:** Diagnostic Tests for Venous Thrombosis of the Lower Extremities

Test	Comments
Venography	Reference standard, but the most invasive of all tests; painful; contrast material may cause an allergic reaction or induce phlebitis
Radionuclide venography	Sensitive for inferior vena cava and proximal vein thrombosis, especially in patients with a known history of contrast media allergy; high incidence of false-positive results
Impedance venography	Sensitive and specific for proximal vein thrombosis; generally considered to be the procedure of choice for the diagnosis of deep venous thrombosis
Real-time ultrasonography	Sensitive and specific for proximal vein thrombosis; not reliable for iliac vein thrombosis; requires skill and experience to perform reliably

for proximal venous thrombosis, but the test is highly dependent on the subjective interpretation of variations in sound that represent changes in venous blood flow characteristics. This requires skill and experience, but when the technician or physician who performs the test has these attributes, the test becomes almost as sensitive as IPG. Like IPG, the Doppler technique is less sensitive to nonocclusive proximal thrombosis and to calf vein thrombosis. Real-time ultrasonic imaging has been used to diagnose deep venous thrombosis. This technique uses B-mode scanning to visualize the deep venous system of the lower extremities noninvasively for patency, blood flow, and the presence of thrombosis. Thrombi are identified by their noncompressibility and by absent or altered flow sounds. This form of ultrasonic testing is an accurate and noninvasive test for femoral and popliteal clots,[22] but because of certain technical limitations, the test is not useful for calf or iliac thrombi.

The other commonly used technique, radionuclide venography, like many other radionuclide techniques, is most useful if findings are normal because there is a high incidence of false-positive studies. To its advantage, it has a lower incidence of complications than venography and can be performed at the time of lung scanning. It might be considered if the patient has an absolute contraindication to the use of radiographic contrast media, such as a history of contrast dye hypersensitivity.

Pulmonary Angiography

The risks of angiography include cardiopulmonary arrest, heart and pulmonary artery perforation, serious life-threatening arrhythmias, vascular intimal injection, and contrast allergy.

Pulmonary angiography, although the most invasive of all diagnostic studies for pulmonary embolism, is considered to be the most definitive test available. When properly performed and interpreted, pulmonary angiography should be considered the gold standard. In experienced hands, pulmonary angiography is safe, even in the patient with an unstable condition, and it is preferable to empiric treatment with a potentially dangerous drug for a condition that may not be present. The vast majority of fatalities occur in patients who are critically ill or who have pulmonary hypertension. Other drawbacks include the need for sophisticated equipment, the discomfort, and the cost. Therefore, angiography should be performed only when less invasive procedures do not confirm or exclude the diagnosis.

Diagnostic Work-Up

A high index of suspicion is key to the diagnosis of pulmonary embolism. As stated previously, the clinical findings are often subtle; therefore, knowing who is at risk for the development of pulmonary embolism is essential (see Table 42–1). Once a clinical suspicion has been raised, the course and extent of the diagnostic evaluation for pulmonary embolism must be tailored to the individual patient, with consideration given to the stability of the patient's condition and to the risk of the planned therapeutic interventions. Additionally, certain diagnostic decisions depend on local expertise and equipment availability. For most patients, respiratory gas exchange and hemodynamic stability allow time for a systematic diagnostic approach, as shown in Figure 42–1. If chest x-ray findings are markedly abnormal, then pulmonary angiography should be considered. Otherwise, lung scanning should be the first diagnostic test employed. Some clinicians may be tempted to bypass the lung scan in

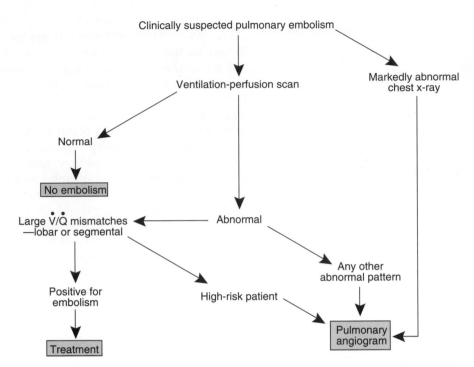

FIGURE 42–1: Practical approach to the diagnosis of pulmonary embolism in patients with clinical stability.

patients with marked airway obstruction that is due to either asthma or chronic obstructive lung disease, on the assumption that the abnormal ventilation is bound to lead to abnormal perfusion secondary to hypoxic vasoconstriction. However, many of these patients with normal chest x-ray findings and no pulmonary emboli have normal perfusion lung scan results despite the abnormalities of ventilation, making angiography unnecessary.

Another modification of the scheme may be reasonable in patients with an indeterminate lung scan result. Finding a source of the clot in these patients would be as useful in clinical decision making as seeing the embolus itself, and this process could thus be substituted for pulmonary angiography. Because the overwhelming majority of pulmonary emboli come from the deep veins of the leg, an alternative approach would be to replace pulmonary angiography in patients who do not have a diagnostic lung scan with a study that demonstrates the presence of deep venous disease. Figure 42–2 shows a practical approach that relies chiefly on IPG or Doppler ultrasound evaluation. The absence of an obvious clot cannot be used to rule out pulmonary embolism because the entire lower extremity thrombus may have already embolized. As many as 40% of patients with proven pulmonary emboli have negative findings on lower extremity studies. In these patients, a repeated noninvasive lower extremity study may be performed in a serial fashion in an attempt to identify patients who redevelop deep venous thrombosis.

Remember, anticoagulants are meant to prevent the development of the next thrombus, not to treat the embolism that has already occurred.

PREVENTION AND TREATMENT OF VENOUS THROMBOEMBOLISM

The prevention of pulmonary embolism is its best treatment. Appropriate prophylaxis in the high-risk patient will significantly reduce the

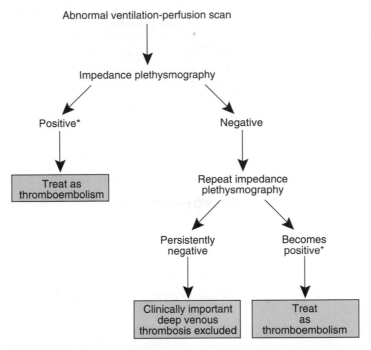

Abnormal ventilation-perfusion scan

Impedance plethysmography

Positive*

Negative

Treat as
thromboembolism

Repeat impedance
plethysmography

Persistently
negative

Becomes
positive*

Clinically important
deep venous
thrombosis excluded

Treat
as
thromboembolism

FIGURE 42–2: Alternative diagnostic approach to pulmonary embolism in patients whose ventilation-perfusion scan findings are other than normal or high probability (multilobar or segmental perfusion defects with normal ventilation scan and chest x-ray film findings). An asterisk indicates that the test results were determined to be positive in the absence of conditions that produce a false-positive result.

Therapy must be tailored individually to enhance efficacy and to reduce disease- and treatment-related complications.

incidence of this potentially lethal consequence of venous thrombosis. Table 42–5 presents a strategy for the prevention of deep venous thrombosis according to risk category. Recommended modalities range from the use of simple graduated compression stockings to the use of anticoagulation therapy. In certain very high risk patients (patients requiring knee and hip surgery), prophylactic doses of heparin may not be sufficiently protective. In these individuals, the use of adjusted-dose heparin therapy subcutaneously or low doses of warfarin, with or without the concomitant use of intermittent pneumatic compression devices, has improved the ability to prevent the development of venous thrombosis.[23, 24]

Supportive care continues to be the first step in the management of patients who have suffered an acute pulmonary embolism. Oxygen should be used to reverse hypoxemia, and intravenous fluids should be given to support right ventricular output. Vasopressors, inotropic agents, and antiarrhythmics may be indicated for the most unstable patients. Unless there is a contraindication, anticoagulant therapy should be initiated based on the suspicion of pulmonary embolism before definitive studies, with the realization that the decision to continue therapy will be predicated on the outcome of the diagnostic work-up. The most important goal of treatment is to prevent the continued propagation of clotting. The treatment of deep venous thrombosis in pulmonary embolism involves multiple options, including a variety of pharmacologic and surgical interventions (Fig. 42–3).

In patients with thromboembolic disease, an adequate course of therapy almost always involves the initial use of heparin and then the use of warfarin. The coagulation status of the patient should be checked at

TABLE **42–5:** A Strategy for the Prevention of Deep Venous Thrombosis

Risk Category	Recommended Modalities
Low Risk	
< 6% incidence of DVT	GCS and early ambulation
Under 40 years of age	
Minor surgery	
Bedridden patients with uncomplicated medical conditions	
Intermediate Risk	
6–40% incidence of DVT	LDH or dextran or IPC* of the legs and early ambulation
Over 40 years of age or obese	
Abdominal, pelvic, or thoracic surgery	GCS and IPC or LDH and early ambulation
Uncomplicated myocardial infarction	
High Risk	
> 40% incidence of DVT	Combined methods (IPC with GCS and LDH and early ambulation)
Elderly	
Extensive abdominal, pelvic, or thoracic surgery	For elective hip and major knee surgery, low-dose warfarin or dextran or adjusted-dose heparin and IPC; early mobilization and elevation of the foot of the bed or the involved limb are also recommended
Hip and major knee surgery	
Fractured hip	
Malignancy	
History of DVT	

*IPC is the method of choice in neurosurgery, ophthalmologic surgery, urologic procedures, or when the risk of hemorrhage is judged to be high.

DVT, deep venous thrombosis; GCS, graduated compression stockings; IPC, intermittent pneumatic compression; LDH, low-dose heparin.

baseline by determining the activated partial thromboplastin time, the prothrombin time, and the platelet count. In all clinically stable patients, heparin should be given as an initial loading dose of at least 5000 U followed by a continuous infusion at a rate sufficient to maintain the activated partial thromboplastin time at 1.5 to 2.0 times the control value.[25] Alternatively, heparin could be given by intermittent boluses or by adjusted-dose subcutaneous dosing[26] to achieve the same prolongation

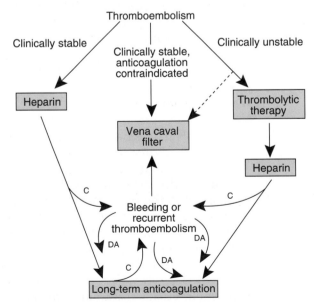

FIGURE 42–3: Management of documented pulmonary embolism. C, complication; DA, dosage adjustment.

of the activated partial thromboplastin time. Heparin requirements are usually greater during the first few days after a thromboembolic event; therapy should therefore be monitored very closely during this time. It is also important to monitor the platelet count every 2 to 3 days when heparin is being administered because the drug can induce thrombocytopenia and bring about paradoxical arterial thrombosis.

Heparin is usually continued for the first 5 to 10 days, but after the first 48 to 72 hours of heparin therapy, oral anticoagulant therapy can be concomitantly initiated, with a 5- to 7-day overlap of the two medications. This allows sufficient time for inhibition of the hepatic syntheses of vitamin K–dependent clotting factors and fibrin formation. Warfarin should be given in doses sufficient to maintain the prothrombin time at 1.3 to 1.5 times the control value.[25] Increasing the prothrombin time above 1.5 times the control value increases the incidence of hemorrhagic side effects. An alternative to warfarin therapy for the long-term maintenance of anticoagulation is the use of subcutaneous adjusted-dose heparin in a dose that prolongs the activated partial thromboplastin time to 1.3 to 1.5 times the control measured at the middose time.[27] Like intravenous heparin therapy, subcutaneous adjusted-dose therapy can induce thrombocytopenia, and after prolonged use, osteoporosis. Recommendations as to the total duration of anticoagulation are somewhat controversial because there are few control trials to provide guidance. The total duration of long-term anticoagulation therapy should be based on the continued presence of predisposing factors for venous thrombosis. Anywhere from 3 to 6 months has been recommended for most patients.

For many years, anticoagulation was the only form of therapy available for venous thrombosis and pulmonary embolism. Although anticoagulation markedly reduces the likelihood of recurrent embolism, it does not lyse the clot and thus does not treat the morbid consequences of the existing thrombi. It also fails to eliminate the potential source of subsequent embolization or the vascular disturbances associated with this occlusive process. For these reasons, thrombolytic therapy has been proposed as the treatment of choice in selected patients with venous thromboembolic disease. The Urokinase Pulmonary Embolism Trial[15] compared the use of heparin alone with the use of an initial infusion of urokinase followed by heparin. The use of urokinase led to a more rapid resolution of the pulmonary embolism at 24 hours, but no significant differences were found between the groups in terms of short- and long-term survival. Significant bleeding occurred in 27% of the heparin group and in 45% of the urokinase plus heparin patients. On the basis of these data, it appears prudent to reserve thrombolytic therapy for patients with markedly unstable hemodynamics and pulmonary gas exchange in whom more rapid resolution over the first 24 hours may be life saving.

Thrombolytic therapy has been compared with heparin alone in the treatment of acute deep venous thrombosis.[28, 29] Although the results of these trials have been questioned,[30] they appear to indicate that the improvement was significantly greater with thrombolytic therapy. Patients with acute symptoms of less than 3 days' duration showed more improvement than those with chronic symptoms. Extensive lower extremity proximal vein thrombosis responded better than isolated calf vein thrombosis. Rapid clot lysis in the deep venous system of the lower extremity is thought to preserve valve cusp anatomy and function, whereas a slow resolution with heparin therapy may not prevent valve distortion. Patients who are asymptomatic after thrombolysis are more likely to have normal valve function and normal venographic findings,

Adjusted-dose subcutaneous heparin therapy is the long-term regimen of choice in pregnancy and in patients in whom careful monitoring is not practical.

whereas patients with persistent venous abnormalities usually have symptoms of chronic venous insufficiency.[31]

Newer thrombolytic agents for the treatment of pulmonary embolism are now being considered. Both intravenous and intrapulmonary infusions of tissue plasminogen activator have been used to treat acute massive pulmonary embolism.[32] Compared with urokinase, tissue plasminogen activator may be safer and may act more rapidly and completely at lysing clot.[33]

Many contraindications to thrombolytic therapy exist. Because they are often present in patients with massive pulmonary embolism, the actual number of embolic patients in whom thrombolytic therapy might be appropriate is likely to be small. An increased likelihood of bleeding prohibits thrombolytic therapy in patients who have active internal bleeding or who have had a cerebrovascular accident within 2 months of the consideration to use thrombolytic therapy. Relative contraindications include

- Diastolic hypertension above 100 mm Hg
- Trauma
- Closed biopsy or surgery within 10 days
- Recent closed-chest cardiopulmonary resuscitation

A recent puncture of a noncompressible vessel, whether arterial or venous, may also be a contraindication to therapy.

The need for vena caval interruption in patients with pulmonary embolism has decreased because of the improved use of anticoagulation therapy. However, it should be considered in the following patients:

- The patient who has an active pulmonary embolism and a major contraindication to anticoagulation therapy
- The unusual patient who has documented recurrent pulmonary embolism despite adequate anticoagulation
- The rare patient who requires a surgical embolectomy, because anticoagulation will be contraindicated postsurgically
- The patient who has sustained a massive embolism and who is at risk for developing a recurrence, with an increased likelihood of death occurring
- The patient who has septic emboli from the pelvis or lower extremities
- The patient who has paradoxical emboli to the arterial circuit via a patent foramen ovale

Vena caval interruption is best accomplished by the insertion of a transvenous intracaval device.[34] At present, the most commonly used device is the Greenfield filter; however, the bird's nest filter is increasingly being placed.[35]

Percutaneous transvenous embolectomy and open-chest pulmonary embolectomy while the patient is on cardiopulmonary bypass are alternative treatments for a select group of patients. These interventions should be considered only in patients with acute massive pulmonary embolism documented by angiography who have persistent hemodynamic instability despite optimal medical therapy or who have an absolute contraindication to anticoagulation. Acute embolectomy should not be confused with the open-chest pulmonary endarterectomy used for the surgical treatment of chronic recurrent thromboembolic pulmonary hypertension and cor pulmonale.[36] This intervention can produce remarkable symptomatic relief and hemodynamic improvement in carefully selected patients without the high mortality that is seen in the acute setting.

COMPLICATIONS OF ACUTE THROMBOEMBOLIC DISEASE

The complications of acute thromboembolic disease can be divided into those that are due to the disease and those that result from the therapy. As mentioned previously, the major complication of treatment is bleeding, which can be minimized by maintaining the degree of anticoagulation carefully within the guidelines already discussed. Complications other than hemorrhage include thrombocytopenia and paradoxical arterial thrombosis when heparin therapy is used, and vascular purpura when warfarin is employed.

The natural history of recurrent deep venous thrombosis and postphlebitic syndrome is poorly understood. Postphlebitic syndrome occurs when the destruction of valves results in the redirection of venous flow into the superficial veins of the legs, with induced swelling, inflammation, and pain. Eventually, ulceration of the overlying skin occurs, and a secondary infection develops that is extremely resistant to therapeutic intervention.

An uncommon complication of acute pulmonary embolism is chronic embolic pulmonary hypertension, which is thought to occur because of recurrent episodes of subclinical embolization.[37] Unfortunately, this complication is usually not diagnosed until symptoms of pulmonary hypertension and cor pulmonale develop. Often, no clear history of acute pulmonary embolism precedes the diagnosis. It is important that this condition be differentiated from other disorders causing chronic pulmonary hypertension, such as primary pulmonary hypertension.[38] As mentioned previously, in carefully selected patients with chronic embolic pulmonary hypertension in whom the clots are predominately central in location, surgical removal can be performed during cardiopulmonary bypass. This procedure has had its greatest success by surgeons at institutions that have a particular interest in this form of surgical intervention. Occasionally, vasodilator therapy improves hemodynamic performance,[39] but the effect of this form of therapy on functional performance and survival is unclear. In patients who are candidates for neither form of therapy, the prognosis is poor and is likely to be similar to that seen in primary pulmonary hypertension.

OTHER FORMS OF PULMONARY EMBOLISM

Because the lung receives all the blood flow returned from the venous system, the pulmonary vascular bed serves as a filter for all particulate matter entering the venous blood, both intrinsic debris and extrinsic intravenously injected substances.

Venous Air Embolism

The incidence of venous air embolism is unknown. This condition is associated with

- A wide variety of invasive surgical and medical procedures

Most deaths from pulmonary embolism are seen in patients in whom the diagnosis is not made and treatment is not initiated promptly. In patients in whom the diagnosis is made and treatment is appropriately instituted, embolic recurrences are avoided, and the mortality rate is less than 10%.

- Various types of trauma, particularly penetrating lung injury
- The use of indwelling venous catheters[40]
- Positive pressure mechanical ventilation
- Tension pneumothorax
- Hemodialysis
- Insufflation of the genitourinary tract
- Both uncomplicated and complicated labor and delivery[41]

Air embolism is commonly reported in surgical patients, especially during craniotomy performed in the sitting position. Accidental intravenous injections of air have been reported to be fatal in humans. This is a particular risk if the site of infusion is above the heart, particularly from the jugular or subclavian vein, and the patient generates large negative intrathoracic pressure swings. Air bubbles enter the pulmonary capillary bed and diffusely distribute throughout the body. It is estimated that during a 1-second period, approximately 100 mL of air can flow through a 14-gauge needle with a 5-cm H_2O pressure drop across it.

The clinical presentation of injury in venous air embolism, which is nonspecific and difficult to recognize, depends on the rate and the amount of air infusion and on the underlying disease of the patient. A mill wheel murmur, although specific for air embolism, is infrequently heard. Large air emboli cause acute pulmonary hypertension, precipitate right-sided heart failure and sudden systemic hypotension, and may lead to death. The increase in right-sided heart pressure associated with large air emboli may facilitate the opening of the foramen ovale and lead to systemic embolization (paradoxical emboli). Pulmonary edema secondary to microvascular permeability may develop. In extremely large embolic episodes, air can escape through the lung vascular bed and into the systemic arterial circulation, even in the absence of a foramen ovale. The formation of platelet aggregates on air bubbles creates diffuse platelet microthrombi, which can lead to thrombocytopenia.[42] Therefore, the clinical picture can include confusion, seizure, coma, tachypnea, dyspnea, cough, tachycardia, and diaphoresis.

The administration of 100% oxygen decreases the size of the air emboli by causing reabsorption of the nitrogen component in air. Some medical institutions have access to a hyperbaric chamber, and rapid decompressive therapy may be of benefit.[43]

The best approach to air embolism is prevention, and if this fails, early detection. Measures to prevent the development of air embolism during central venous cannulization include placing the patient in the Trendelenburg position, having the patient breath hold or perform a Valsalva maneuver when the catheter is being quickly inserted into the needle or introducer, and at the same time occluding the hub as much as possible with the operator's finger. During high-risk surgical procedures, such as procedures performed in open heart, lung, and neurologic surgery, a Doppler ultrasound device placed over the right side of the heart can promptly detect air entry into the circulation. If air embolism is suspected, the patient should be placed in the left lateral decubitus position, which facilitates air bubble flow to the apex of the right ventricle and reduces bubble transgression into the pulmonary vascular bed. Aspiration of the air from the right side of the heart and the pulmonary artery via a pulmonary artery catheter may be efficacious.

Fat Embolism

The incidence of fat embolism increases with the number of fractures.[44]

The nonthrombotic embolic condition, fat embolism, refers to a clinical presentation of neurologic, hematologic, and respiratory abnormalities that occurs from as early as 3 to as late as 72 hours after traumatic fracture of the pelvis or a long bone. Trauma to other fat-laden tissue, such as a fatty liver, has also been associated with this syndrome.[45] Although the cause of the fat embolism syndrome is not entirely clear, it does seem to be associated with the release of neutral fat from bone marrow after bone injury. Initially, these fat globules cause mechanical obstruction of portions of the end-organ tissue to which they embolize, but after a latent period, lipase hydrolyses the neutral fat into fatty acids, which cause inflammation and local tissue damage.

The patient often develops fever, tachycardia, respiratory distress, mental confusion, and a petechial rash associated with thrombocytopenia. The chest x-ray film usually remains clear for 12 to 24 hours and then often displays diffuse infiltrates. The petechial rash, which generally develops after 24 hours, is distributed across the upper thorax, including the axillae, flanks, and conjunctivae. Occasionally, retinal exudates and hemorrhages are found.

Certain laboratory tests provide additional information but cannot be considered diagnostic of the fat embolism syndrome. High concentrations of lipase in serum may be useful as confirmatory evidence. Fat globules may be found in the blood, urine, and sputum, but again these findings are neither sensitive nor specific for the syndrome.

Management consists of supportive care, including mechanical ventilation when necessary.[47] Attention should be quickly given to orthopedic issues such as proper traction and immobilization of fractured extremities. Survival is the rule with meticulous supportive care. In high-risk patients, corticosteroid prophylaxis appears to be useful.[48] Methylprednisolone at a dose of 7.5 mg/kg every 6 hours for 4 days was found to markedly decrease the incidence of the syndrome. Convincing evidence to support the use of corticosteroids once the syndrome has developed is lacking. The use of ethanol infusion, low molecular weight dextran, or heparin has not altered the clinical course of this syndrome.

Amniotic Fluid Embolism

Amniotic fluid embolism is an uncommon but catastrophic obstetric complication that occurs during or after delivery when amniotic fluid and debris enter the uterine venous channels and embolize to the pulmonary and systemic circulations.[49] This disorder nearly always accompanies labor, although cases have been reported preterm or without apparent uterine manipulation. Predisposing factors for amniotic fluid embolism include older age, multiparity, amniotomy, cesarean section, premature placental separation, and the use of intrauterine monitoring devices. Tumultuous labor, large fetal size, and intrauterine fetal death are of questionable predisposing risk significance.

Patients with amniotic fluid embolism typically present with sudden, severe dyspnea, pulmonary edema, and vascular collapse. Seizures and bleeding diathesis may also be found. Nearly half of the patients die within the first hour of presentation. The pulmonary edema that develops may be both hydrostatic and nonhydrostatic in origin.[51] The coagulopathy that develops may result from the thromboplastin-like effect of amniotic fluid and its ability to activate the complement cascade. This activity leads to extensive fibrin deposition in the vasculature of the lung and other organs; a severe consumptive coagulopathy develops with its accompanying hypofibrinogenemia. Subsequent multisystem organ failure often develops in patients who survive more than a few days.

The earlier the patient presents with the fat embolism syndrome, the more likely is the development of severe cardiopulmonary impairment.

Arterial hypoxemia occurs almost invariably in fat embolism.

Bronchoalveolar lavage has been described as a method for the rapid diagnosis of the fat embolism syndrome in trauma patients.[46]

Amniotic fluid embolism occurs in approximately one in 8000 to 80,000 deliveries (spontaneous and cesarean section), with an overall mortality of greater than 80%, accounting for 12% of all maternal deaths.[50]

The diagnosis of amniotic fluid embolism is based on the recognition of the clinical presentation associated with labor or the early puerperium. More convincing evidence may require finding fetal tissue elements in the maternal circulation or sputum during the initial diagnosis and management.[52] However, it is important to remember that fetal squamous cells may also be found in the pulmonary vessels of women without the clinical presentation consistent with amniotic fluid embolism.[53]

Treatment is intense supportive care, including stabilization of the coagulopathy.[50] Heparin, ϵ-aminocaproic acid, cryoprecipitate, fresh frozen plasma, and platelets have all been used in an effort to treat the coagulopathy. Massage of the uterus and the infusion of oxytocin or methylergonovine have been used to control local bleeding, with surgical intervention employed only in refractory situations.

Septic Embolism

Intravenous drug abuse and the expanding use of indwelling catheters are primarily responsible for the rise in the frequency of septic embolization. However, before the unfortunate rise in substance abuse, most cases of septic embolization were related to septic thrombophlebitis, which was generally caused by abortion and postpuerperal uterine sepsis. The rapid growth of critical care units, total parenteral nutrition, and monitoring techniques has increased the incidence of intravenous catheter–related septic embolism.[54] Septic embolization has also developed from the infection of intravenous appliances, such as pacemaker wires and venous filters, as well as from suppurative subcutaneous infections that invade veins.

Regardless of the cause of the venous or endocardial suppurative process, embolization generally results in small vessel pulmonary arterial occlusion with the development of pulmonary parenchymal infection. Scattered lung infiltrates are often found on chest x-ray films, which may cavitate. In severe cases, multiple lung abscesses and empyema can develop. The clinical presentation is very much like that of pneumonia, with some patients complaining of scattered pleuritic chest pain.

In septic embolism, the possibility of endocarditis exists, especially in drug addicts.[55]

The treatment of septic embolism is supportive, with importance placed on the rational use of antibiotic therapy. The concomitant use of heparin should also be considered. When septic embolism is recognized, all intravenous lines should be removed and the catheters should be cultured. If a favorable clinical response does not occur early in the treatment regimen, then antibiotic therapy failure should be considered. Additionally, surgical isolation of the septic vein may be necessary. The removal of intravascular and intracardiac appliances may be necessary to gain control of a persistent septic embolic process.

Other Embolic Processes

Numerous parasitic infections, at some point in their life cycles, can embolize to the lung. Schistosomiasis best exemplifies this problem and can be responsible for severe pulmonary vascular obstruction.[56] Cor pulmonale can develop; this generally occurs with schistosomal liver disease. The success of therapy depends on an early diagnosis, before extensive hepatic and pulmonary involvement occurs.

Cancer cells often find their way into the pulmonary circulation.

Microscopic tumor emboli occlude small pulmonary arteries, arterioles, and capillaries by aggregates of tumor cells that are often entwined in a platelet-fibrin matrix.[57] This process is distinct from large tumor emboli that can cause acute right-sided heart failure and from pulmonary microinvasion that occurs as part of a generalized lymphangitic spread of tumor. Adequate anticoagulation is generally ineffective, constituting one clue that tumor embolization is occurring.

Like cancer cells, sickle cells can often lodge or actually sickle in the pulmonary microvasculature. Acute pulmonary episodes, compatible with either emboli or pneumonia, are common in patients with sickle cell disease, and the difficulty in clinically differentiating one from the other has necessitated the use of the term *acute chest syndrome* to cover the spectrum.[58] In adults, this syndrome is frequently due to pulmonary embolism and thrombosis. In the setting of the acute chest syndrome, anticoagulation is generally not helpful and may be risky. The use of oxygen, hydration, and partial exchange transfusions is now considered to be the treatment of choice. Despite these therapies, progressive obliteration of the pulmonary vasculature bed may occur, resulting in pulmonary hypertension and cor pulmonale.

Finally, in this era of intravenous drug abuse, foreign body emboli and their noninfectious vasculitic-thrombotic complications are being seen with growing frequency. Undissolved particulate emboli lodge in the lung microvasculature, causing vascular inflammation and thrombotic obliteration and at times leading to severe and irreversible pulmonary hypertension and cor pulmonale.

SUMMARY

Deep venous thrombosis and its most serious consequence, pulmonary thromboembolism, are unfortunately common complications of hospitalization. Because the diagnosis is often unsuspected or difficult to make, the best strategy is prevention. Adequate prophylaxis against deep venous thrombosis has now been well defined in high-risk patients and should become a routine component of in-hospital care.

References

1. Dalen JE, Alpert JS. Natural history of pulmonary embolism. *In* Sasahara AA, Sonnenblick EH, Lesch M (eds). Pulmonary Embolism. New York, Grune & Stratton, 1975, pp 77–88.
2. Mueh J, Hebst K, Rapaport S. Thrombosis in patients with the lupus anticoagulant. Ann Intern Med 92:156–159, 1980.
3. Parker BM, Smith JR. Pulmonary embolism and infarction. Am J Med 24:402–427, 1958.
4. Wheeler HB, Anderson FH, Cardullo PA, et al. Suspected deep vein thrombosis: Management by impedance plethysmography. Arch Surg 117:1206–1209, 1986.
5. D'Alonzo GE. Deep venous thrombosis and pulmonary embolism. *In* Dantzker DR (ed). Cardiopulmonary Critical Care, 2nd ed. Philadelphia, WB Saunders, 1991, pp 731–768.
6. Moser KM. Venous thromboembolism. Am Rev Respir Dis 141:235–249, 1990.
7. Philbrick JT, Becker DM. Calf deep venous thrombosis. A wolf in sheep's clothing. Arch Intern Med 148:2131–2138, 1988.
8. Gallus AS, Hirsh J, Hull R, et al. Diagnosis of venous thromboembolism. Semin Thromb Hemost 2:203–231, 1976.
9. Nelson JR, Smith JR. The pathologic physiology of pulmonary embolism: A physiologic discussion of the vascular reactions following pulmonary arterial obstruction by emboli of varying size. Am Heart J 58:916–932, 1959.
10. McIntyre KM, Sasahara AA. Determinants of cardiovascular responses to pulmonary

embolism. *In* Moser KM, Stein M (eds). Pulmonary Thromboembolism. Chicago, Year Book Medical Publishers, 1973, pp 144–159.

11. D'Alonzo GE, Dantzker DR. Gas exchange alterations following pulmonary thromboembolism. Clin Chest Med 5:411–419, 1984.
12. Moser KM. Pulmonary embolism. Am Rev Respir Dis 115:829–852, 1977.
13. Bell WR, Simon TL, DeMets DL. The clinical features of submassive and massive pulmonary emboli. Am J Med 62:355–360, 1977.
14. Overton DT, Bocka JJ. The alveolar-arterial oxygen gradient in patients with documented pulmonary embolism. Arch Intern Med 148:1617–1619, 1988.
15. The Urokinase Pulmonary Embolism Trial: A cooperative study. Circulation 47(Suppl II):1–108, 1973.
16. Hull RD, Hirsh J, Carter CJ, et al. Diagnostic value of ventilation-perfusion lung scanning in patients with suspected pulmonary embolism. Chest 84:819–828, 1985.
17. Hull RD, Hirsh J, Carter CJ, et al. Pulmonary angiography, ventilation lung scanning, and venography for clinically suspected pulmonary embolism with abnormal perfusion lung scan. Ann Intern Med 98:891–899, 1983.
18. PIOPED Investigators. Value of the ventilation/perfusion scan in acute pulmonary embolism: Results of the Prospective Investigation of Pulmonary Embolism Diagnosis (PIOPED). JAMA 263:2753–2759, 1990.
19. Hull RD, Raskob GE, LeClere JR, et al. The diagnosis of clinically suspected venous thrombosis. Clin Chest Med 5:439–456, 1984.
20. Huisman MV, Büller HR, tenCate JW, et al. Serial impedance plethysmography for suspected deep venous thrombosis in outpatients. N Engl J Med 314:823–834, 1986.
21. Huisman MV, Büller HR, tenCate JW, et al. Management of clinically suspected acute venous thrombosis in outpatients with serial impedance plethysmography in a community hospital setting. Arch Intern Med 149:511–513, 1989.
22. Becker DM, Philbrick JT, Abbitt PL. Real-time ultrasonography for the diagnosis of lower extremity deep-venous thrombosis. The wave of the future? Arch Intern Med 149:1731–1734, 1989.
23. NIH Consensus Conference: Prevention of venous thrombosis and pulmonary embolism. JAMA 256:744–749, 1986.
24. Hull RD, Raskob GE, Hirsh J. Prophylaxis of venous thromboembolism. An overview. Chest 89:374S–383S, 1986.
25. Hyer TM, Hull RD, Weg JG. Antithrombotic therapy for venous thromboembolic disease. Chest 95:37S–51S, 1989.
26. Doyle DJ, Turpie AGG, Hirsh J, et al. Adjusted subcutaneous heparin or continuous intravenous heparin in patients with acute deep vein thrombosis. Ann Intern Med 107:441–445, 1987.
27. Hull RD, Delmore TJ, Carter C, et al. Adjusted subcutaneous heparin versus warfarin sodium in the long-term treatment of venous thrombosis. N Engl J Med 306:189–194, 1982.
28. Kakkar VV, Flanc C, Howe CT, et al. Treatment of deep vein thrombosis. A trial of heparin, streptokinase and Arvin. Br Med J 1:806–810, 1969.
29. Arnesen H, Hoiseth A, Ly B. Streptokinase or heparin in the treatment of deep vein thrombosis. Acta Med Scand 211:65–68, 1982.
30. Sidorov J. Streptokinase vs heparin for deep venous thrombosis. Can lytic therapy be justified? Arch Intern Med 149:1841–1845, 1989.
31. Johansson E, Ericson K, Zetterquist S. Streptokinase treatment of deep venous thrombosis of the lower extremities. Acta Med Scand 199:89–94, 1976.
32. Verstraete M, Miller GAH, Bounameaux H, et al. Intravenous and intrapulmonary recombinant tissue-type plasminogen activator in the treatment of acute massive pulmonary embolism. Circulation 77:353–360, 1988.
33. Goldhaber SZ, Heit J, Sharma GVRK, et al. Randomized controlled trial of recombinant tissue plasminogen activator versus urokinase in the treatment of acute pulmonary embolism. Lancet 2:293–298, 1988.
34. Greenfield LJ. Vena caval interruption and pulmonary embolectomy. Clin Chest Med 5:495–505, 1984.
35. Martin B, Martyak TE, Soughton TL, et al. Experience with the Gianturco-Roehm bird's nest vena cava filter. Am J Cardiol 66:1275–1277, 1990.
36. Dailey PO, Johnston GG, Simmons CJ, et al. Surgical management of chronic pulmonary embolism. Surgical treatment and late results. J Thorac Cardiovasc Surg 79:523–531, 1980.
37. DeSoyza NDB, Murphy ML. Persistent postembolic pulmonary hypertension. Chest 62:665–668, 1972.
38. D'Alonzo GE, Bower JS, Dantzker DR. Differentiation of patients with primary pulmonary hypertension and thromboembolic pulmonary hypertension. Chest 84:457–461, 1984.
39. Dantzker DR, Bower JS. Partial reversibility of chronic pulmonary hypertension caused by pulmonary thromboembolic disease. Am Rev Respir Dis 124:129–131, 1981.
40. Lambert MJ. Air embolism in central venous catheterization: Diagnosis, treatment, and prevention. South Med J 75:1189–1191, 1982.
41. O'Quin RJ, Lakshimarayan S. Venous air embolism. Arch Intern Med 142:2173–2176, 1982.

42. Neuman TS, Spragg RG, Wagner PD, Moser KM. Cardiopulmonary consequences of decompression stress. Respir Physiol 41:143–153, 1980.
43. Murphy BP, Harford FJ, Cramer FS. Cerebral air embolism resulting from invasive medical procedures: Treatment with hyperbaric oxygen. Ann Surg 201:242–245, 1985.
44. Coosling H, Pelligrini V. Fat embolism syndrome. Clin Orthop 165:68–92, 1982.
45. Moylan J, Evenson MA. Diagnosis and therapy of fat embolism. Annu Rev Med 28:85–94, 1977.
46. Chastre J, Fagon JY, Soler P, et al. Bronchoalveolar lavage for rapid diagnosis of the fat embolism syndrome in trauma patients. Ann Intern Med 113:583–588, 1990.
47. Eddy AC, Rice CL, Carrico CJ. Fat embolism syndrome: Monitoring and management. J Crit Illness 2:24–37, 1987.
48. Schonfeld SA, Ploysongsang Y, DiLisio R, et al. Fat embolism prophylaxis with corticosteroids: A prospective study in high risk patients. Ann Intern Med 99:436–443, 1983.
49. Morgan M. Amniotic fluid embolism. A review. Anesthesiology 34:20–31, 1979.
50. Hollingsworth HM, Pratter MR, Irwin RS. Acute respiratory failure in pregnancy. J Intensive Care Med 4:11–34, 1989.
51. Clark SL, Montz FJ, Phelan JP. Hemodynamic alterations associated with amniotic fluid embolism: A reappraisal. Am J Obstet Gynecol 151:617–621, 1985.
52. Dolyniuk M, Orfei E, Vania H, et al. Rapid diagnosis of amniotic fluid embolism. Obstet Gynecol 61:20S–30S, 1983.
53. Clark SL, Pavlova Z, Horenstein J, et al. Squamous cells in the maternal pulmonary circulation. Am J Obstet Gynecol 154:104–106, 1986.
54. Hershey CO, Tomford JW, McLaren CE, et al. The natural history of intravenous catheter-associated phlebitis. Arch Intern Med 144:1373–1375, 1984.
55. Julander I. Staphylococcal septicaemia and endocarditis in 80 drug addicts. Scand J Infect Dis 41:49–54, 1983.
56. Jawalurz KI, Karpas CM. Pulmonary schistosomias: A detailed clinicopathological study. Am Rev Respir Dis 88:517–524, 1965.
57. Kane RD, Hawkins HK, Miller JA, Noce PS. Microscopic pulmonary tumor emboli associated with dyspnea. Cancer 36:1473–1482, 1975.
58. Charache S, Scott JC, Charache P. "Acute chest syndrome" in adults with sickle cell anemia: Microbiology, treatment, and prevention. Arch Intern Med 139:67–69, 1979.

43
Sleep and Sleep-Disordered Breathing

Karl L. Yang, M.D.

The alpha-wave has a low amplitude and a high frequency.

Significant progress has been made in the past 15 years in our understanding of the sleep process, including the description of sleep apnea syndrome. Instead of being a passive condition, as externally perceived, sleep is actually a dynamic process during which many physiologic parameters undergo alterations, some of which may even have detrimental effects on an individual's health. Patients with sleep apnea syndrome usually have fairly normal pulmonary mechanics and ventilatory responses to chemical stimuli during wakefulness, but significant degrees of hypoxemia, hypercapnia, breathing pattern irregularities, and hemodynamic instability frequently develop during sleep. This chapter reviews normal alterations in respiratory physiology during sleep and discusses the pathophysiology, clinical features, and treatment of the sleep apnea syndrome.

NORMAL SLEEP PHYSIOLOGY

Wakefulness is a state of cortical activation, which is characterized by alpha-waves on electroencephalographic (EEG) tracings. Sleep replaces the alpha-waves with brain waves of higher amplitude and lower frequency. On the basis of the EEG and electromyographic characteristics, sleep architecture is classified into rapid eye movement (REM) and non-REM (NREM) sleep.[1] NREM sleep is further subdivided into four stages, with stage 1 being light sleep and stage 4 deep sleep. At the onset of sleep, the EEG pattern frequently fluctuates back and forth between wakefulness and stages 1 and 2 of sleep. Eventually, this progresses to a deep and stable sleep and finally to REM sleep. This cycle is repeated several times during the night, with REM sleep occurring approximately every 90 minutes.[2] Each period of REM sleep lasts approximately 15 to 30 minutes, and the duration of REM sleep becomes progressively longer as the night goes on. At the onset of REM sleep, the characteristic delta-waves seen in stages 3 and 4 are suddenly replaced by alpha-waves of wakefulness. In addition, this stage of sleep is associated with bursts of REM and the complete absence of muscular tone. Both the absolute amount and the proportion of sleep time spent in REM sleep progressively decrease throughout a person's life.[3]

During wakefulness, individuals are aware of the surrounding environment and respond to external stimuli by performing complex and meaningful tasks. In sleep, cortical activity is reduced to a minimum; consequently, the responses to external stimuli are also quite simple. The arousal threshold to noxious stimulation is also elevated during sleep.[4] Although skeletal muscle tone is still present during NREM sleep, it is markedly lower than that during wakefulness.[5] With the onset of REM sleep, there is either a complete loss of or a further reduction in muscular activities, which is probably due to the active inhibition at the level of the motoneuron. Dreaming is also a common feature during REM sleep, and sensorimotor responses to external stimuli are actively inhibited. In contrast to NREM sleep, in which body functions tend to remain stable, sudden and wide fluctuations in many physiologic measurements are frequently observed during REM sleep, especially during phasic bursts of REM activity (during the time of REM). It is difficult to make generalizations about physiologic measurements because a true steady state is probably never achieved during REM sleep.[6]

RESPIRATORY PHYSIOLOGY DURING SLEEP

In this section, alterations in minute ventilation; breathing pattern; airway resistance; respiratory muscle function; pulmonary gas exchange; and ventilatory responses to hypoxia, hypercapnia, and resistive loading during sleep are discussed (Table 43–1).

It is well known that minute ventilation is lower during NREM sleep than during wakefulness.[7–9] In one study, the mean minute ventilation was shown to decrease from 6.1 L/min during wakefulness to 5.6 L/min during stage 4 of sleep. This decrease is due in part to the 10 to 30% reduction in the metabolic rate during sleep,[10] but it is also due to suppressed hypercapnic and hypoxic ventilatory responses. Accompanying the reduction in minute ventilation during sleep is an increase in the Pa_{CO_2} of 2 to 7 mm Hg. Hypoventilation during sleep was believed to be primarily due to the resetting of the hypercapnic response threshold to a higher level than that of wakefulness. The higher level of hypercapnic threshold during sleep is also believed to account for the periodic breathing seen occasionally at the onset of sleep. In addition to the suppressed hypercapnic response, increased airway resistance may also be a factor in the development of hypercapnia. Several studies have documented that the airway resistance increases progressively as a person enters deeper stages of sleep and that the tidal volume is significantly lower than that of wakefulness,[11] whereas respiratory frequency remains constant.

During stages 1 and 2 of sleep, oscillations in airflow and tidal volume are frequently observed, but respiratory frequency remains unchanged. This oscillation results from the fluctuations between wakefulness and stage 1 of sleep and the resultant instabilities in chemoregulation during early sleep. As sleep progresses into deeper stages, minute

TABLE **43–1:** Physiologic Changes in Respiration During Sleep

	Non–Rapid Eye Movement Sleep		Rapid Eye Movement Sleep
	Stages I and II	*Stages III and IV*	
Breathing pattern	Periodic	Regular	Irregular
Pa_{CO_2}	Variable	↑ 2–7 mm Hg	Variable
Hypoxic response	↓	↓ ↓	↓ ↓ ↓
Hypercapnic response	↓	↓ ↓	↓ ↓ ↓
Upper airway muscles			
Tonic activity*	Active	Decreased	Inhibited
Phasic activity†	Active	Decreased	Inhibited
Diaphragm			
Tonic activity*	Active	Decreased	Inhibited
Phasic activity†	Active	Decreased	Decreased

↓, Mild reduction; ↓ ↓, moderate reduction; ↓ ↓ ↓, severe reduction; ↑, increase.
*Tonic activity is background electromyographic activity.
†Phasic activity is electromyographic activity during active inspiration.

ventilation, tidal volume, and respiratory frequency usually become very stable and constant. In contrast to that during deep sleep, the breathing pattern during REM sleep shows marked variability. Minute ventilation, respiratory frequency, and tidal volume may increase, remain the same, or decrease, depending on when the measurements are made. A sudden decrease in tidal volume and increase in respiratory frequency are usually associated with periods of REM. However, on the average, the respiratory frequency and tidal volume during REM sleep are about the same as during wakefulness.

Respiratory muscle activity undergoes important changes during sleep as well. The normal activity of skeletal muscle consists of tonic and phasic muscle contractions. Tonic activity represents the background electromyographic activity, and phasic activity represents respiratory muscle contraction during inspiration. The phasic activity of the intercostal muscles increases during NREM sleep, whereas the tonic activity does not change much. On the other hand, diaphragmatic activities show little increase or no change.[12] This relatively greater increase in phasic intercostal muscle activity relative to diaphragmatic activity accounts for the increased rib cage contribution to tidal volume observed during NREM sleep. During REM sleep, in contrast to NREM sleep, both the tonic activity and the phasic activity of the intercostal muscles are totally abolished or markedly reduced.[13] As a result, rib cage expansion becomes a lesser contributor to the overall tidal volume. Much like that of the intercostal muscles, the tonic activity of the diaphragm is also abolished during REM sleep. However, phasic diaphragmatic contraction is generally maintained at its baseline level. This selective reduction in respiratory muscle tone in the intercostal muscles but not in the diaphragm helps to explain the development of paradoxical movement of the rib cage during REM sleep. This lack of both diaphragmatic and intercostal tonic activity, which is necessary to maintain a constant thoracic lung volume, causes a reduction in functional residual capacity, which further predisposes an individual to developing hypoxemia.

Another important group of respiratory muscles, the dilatory muscles that maintain the patency of the upper airway, includes the genioglossus muscle, the pharyngeal veli palatini muscles, and the infrahyoid muscles. The genioglossus is the most frequently studied muscle in this group. During wakefulness, the genioglossus muscle demonstrates both tonic and phasic activities. During the transition from wakefulness to NREM sleep, both tonic and phasic activities decrease, but these activities are not completely abolished.[6] In REM sleep, however, the tonic activity of the upper airway muscles becomes completely silent.[14] Furthermore, phasic contraction of these muscles may be intermittently inhibited for up to 90 seconds.[15] As a result of the decreased upper airway muscle activity, the resistance of the upper airway increases dramatically during sleep. This increase could be as high as 230% over the baseline value and could cause a decrease in mean inspiratory flow and minute ventilation because of the inability of respiratory muscles to handle the increase in inspiratory load. However, a similar degree of external loading in normal subjects during wakefulness did not result in any decrease in minute ventilation or lead to the development of hypercapnia.[16] Most likely, the increase in upper airway resistance is only one of several factors that cause a decrease in ventilation during sleep; its importance varies according to an individual's baseline status. In general, a healthy person should be able to handle the resistive load without difficulties. However, this may be a problem in a patient with chronic obstructive pulmonary disease, who may already be at risk for developing respiratory muscle fatigue.

During wakefulness, the breathing pattern is affected by cortical input, chemical stimuli, and reflexes from pulmonary mechanoreceptors (see Chapter 7). During sleep, the importance of nonchemical inputs gradually diminishes, and the control of breathing is predominantly under the influence of chemical stimuli, specifically the partial pressures of oxygen (Pa_{O_2}) and carbon dioxide (Pa_{CO_2}) in arterial blood.[17] The ventilatory responses to both hypercapnia and hypoxia have been shown to be depressed during NREM sleep when compared with wakefulness,[18, 19] meaning that the increase in minute ventilation in response to hypoxia or hypercapnia is more depressed during sleep than during wakefulness. During REM sleep, the ventilatory response to hypoxia can be as low as one third of the level found during wakefulness. Interestingly, the depressed hypoxic responses appear to occur in male subjects but not in female subjects.[20, 21] Although the idea has not been confirmed, research suggests that hydroxyprogesterone, a respiratory stimulant, may be the reason for this observation. The hypercapnic ventilatory response is also more depressed during REM sleep than during NREM sleep. In addition to the depressed hypercapnic response, the hypercapnic ventilatory response curve during sleep also shifts to the right of that during wakefulness, resulting in a higher apnea threshold during sleep (Fig. 43–1).

Responses to added airway resistance during sleep have not been extensively studied. Preliminary results have suggested that the venti-

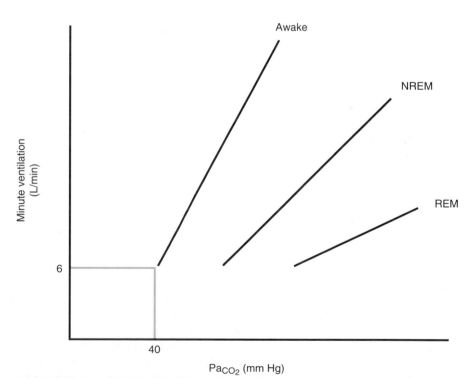

FIGURE 43–1: Hypercapnic ventilatory response curves at various stages of sleep in a normal individual. During sleep, not only is the hypercapnic response depressed, but the response threshold is shifted to the right. The solid lines represent the normal Pa_{CO_2} and minute ventilation during wakefulness. REM, rapid eye movement sleep; NREM, non-REM sleep.

latory response to added resistance is maintained during sleep. Issa and Sullivan reported that in response to airway occlusion, a progressive increase occurs in respiratory effort during NREM sleep and in rapid shallow breathing during REM sleep.[22] In addition to hypercapnia, mild hypoxemia is also observed. Hypoventilation during sleep would account for a 1 to 3% reduction in oxygen saturation. The following factors may also play a part in arterial oxygen desaturation:

- Regional ventilation-perfusion mismatch
- Reduction in thoracic gas volume due to the diminution of diaphragmatic and intercostal muscle activity
- Smaller thoracic gas volume
- The presence of upper airway obstruction during sleep

The arousal response during sleep is an important life-saving mechanism because it terminates an apneic event. A number of studies have shown that hypoxia is a poor arousal stimulus. In the study by Douglas, many subjects remained asleep even though their oxygen saturations fell to as low as 70%.[23] In comparison, hypercapnia is a more potent arousal stimulus. In the same study, the majority of the subjects were aroused when the Pa_{CO_2} increased merely 5 mm Hg over the baseline value. None of the subjects remained asleep when the Pa_{CO_2} was raised 15 mm Hg above the baseline value. Humans also tend to arouse from sleep when the airway resistance suddenly increases. Gleeson and coworkers compared the differences in arousal response under hypoxic, hypercapnic, and resistive loading conditions.[24] They found that the arousal response was highly correlated only with the respiratory effort, regardless of the source of stimulation. Thus, an individual's sleep can be disrupted by increased respiratory effort even in the absence of hypoxemia or hypercapnia (i.e., a heavy snorer). Generally, arousal from REM sleep is far more rapid than arousal from NREM sleep.

SLEEP APNEA

On the basis of our understanding of normal sleep physiology, the pathophysiologic events that lead to the development of sleep apnea syndrome become apparent. Apnea is classified into three types: central, obstructive, and mixed disorders. Central apnea is characterized by the absence of respiratory efforts, whereas obstructive apnea is characterized by the lack of airflow despite continual respiratory efforts. A mixed type is an apnea event that has characteristics of both obstructive and central sleep apnea. Usually, the central event precedes the obstructive event. Obstructive apnea is the most common and the most dangerous of the three types.

Obstructive Sleep Apnea

The classic physical features of patients with sleep apnea syndrome were first described by Charles Dickens in *The Pickwick Papers* as something of an amusement. In more recent years, this syndrome has been increasingly recognized as a potentially lethal illness. If the condition is not properly treated, sleep apnea syndrome can definitely cause many long-term complications. Daytime hypersomnolence frequently interferes with a person's daily functional capacity. Comparing the driving records of sleep apnea patients with those of average drivers, Findley and associates reported that a sleep apnea patient was two and a half times more likely to be involved in a motor vehicle accident than was a person without the disorder.[25]

Although the true prevalence of the sleep apnea syndrome is difficult to ascertain, epidemiologic data are available on the prevalence of snoring. Lugaresi and colleagues found that 40% of men and 28% of women snored, with 24 and 14%, respectively, being habitual snorers.[26, 27] The presence of snoring is both age and weight related. The prevalence of sleep apnea among snorers was estimated to range from 34 to 65%. Fletcher and coworkers reported that as many as 30% of patients with essential hypertension had undiagnosed obstructive sleep apnea syndrome.[28] On the basis of these epidemiologic data, the incidence of sleep apnea in the general population is about 1 to 7%.

Obstructive sleep apnea is characterized by the cessation of airflow despite increased respiratory effort. The site of obstruction is usually in the nasopharynx and oropharynx. The patency of the upper airway depends on the balance of forces between pharyngeal dilatation by the genioglossus and the veli palatini and the negative luminal collapsing pressure generated by the contraction of inspiratory muscles. Obstruction occurs when the negative luminal pressure exceeds the dilatory pressure during inspiration (Fig. 43–2). Once obstruction has occurred, increased respiratory effort would only cause further obstruction. This process continues until the patient awakens and upper airway muscular tone returns. A person is especially vulnerable to obstruction during sleep because hypotonia of the upper airway muscles occurs to a greater degree than that of the inspiratory muscles (mainly diaphragmatic activity).[29] This physiologic hypotonia of the upper airway muscles is particularly prominent during REM sleep. When the obstruction occurs, the

Anatomic conditions leading to obstruction:

- Tonsillar hypertrophy
- Micrognathia
- Macrognathia
- Hypothyroidism
- Thyromegaly
- Acromegaly
- Obesity

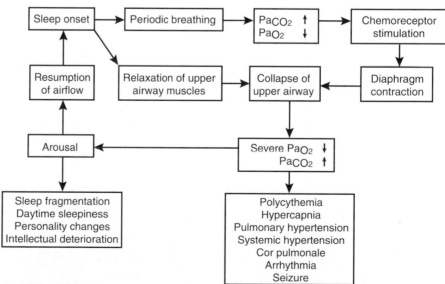

FIGURE 43–2: Pathogenesis of obstructive sleep apnea. A combination of increased diaphragmatic contraction and relaxation of the upper airway muscles during sleep causes the airway to collapse. Recurrent hypoxia and arousal cause most of the symptoms and complications seen in sleep apnea syndrome.

TABLE **43–2:** Anatomic Factors That Predispose to Obstructive Sleep Apnea

Obesity with redundant tissue to reduce pharynx size	Micrognathia
Enlarged adenoid or tonsil	Retrognathia
Elongated uvula	Acromegaly
Deviated nasal septum	Myxedema
	Nasal packing

tongue, soft palate, and posterior oropharyngeal wall form a seal to prevent further airflow. Several anatomic conditions can further increase the risk of obstructive sleep apnea by physically reducing the diameter of the upper airway (Table 43–2). Obesity appears to be an especially important risk factor because of its prevalence in our society, although the precise mechanism by which it causes airway obstruction is not entirely clear. It has been suggested that the obese patient has a narrowed pharyngeal opening because of an excessive amount of soft tissue. Furthermore, deposits of fatty soft tissue increase the airway compliance and the tendency for airway collapse. In addition to anatomic factors, other factors may also influence the upper airway patency. Several medications, such as alcohol, anesthesia, and sedatives, increase the risk of airway obstruction because they have a selective suppressive effect on the upper airway muscles. Sleep deprivation, which is the hallmark of sleep apnea syndrome, also reduces upper airway activity, thus setting up a vicious cycle to perpetuate obstructive sleep apnea.

As already mentioned, arousal is important for terminating an apneic event and is thus a life-saving mechanism in patients with sleep apnea syndrome. Although arousal relieves obstructive sleep apnea by increasing upper airway muscle tone and preventing further arterial oxygen desaturation, it also interferes with the continuity of sleep. Over time, fragmentation of sleep causes the development of excessive daytime somnolence and deterioration in intellectual and psychomotor functions.

Clinical Features

Many clinical manifestations of sleep apnea result directly from sleep fragmentation and nocturnal hypoxemia. Typically, the bed partner describes frequent loud snoring by the patient, which often prevents anyone else from sleeping in the same room or even in adjacent rooms. Often, the snoring is followed by a period of silence lasting anywhere from 10 seconds to 2 minutes. During this time, the patient often appears to be choking and develops severe oxygen desaturation. Excessive tossing and turning are also commonly reported by the patient's bed partner. Because the patient's apneic event is terminated by arousals, sleep fragmentation invariably appears on EEG tracings. Chronic sleep fragmentation causes sleep deprivation and eventually leads to daytime hypersomnolence. In mild cases, hypersomnolence occurs only when external stimulation lessens, leading the patient to sleep while watching television and reading. In more severe cases, sleep can occur even during conversation, driving, and dining. Chronic sleep deprivation is also associated with impairment of intellectual function, memory loss, poor judgment, deterioration of psychomotor skills, and even personality changes. In some patients, sleep apnea may lead to the loss of gainful employment (Table 43–3).

A number of physiologic complications are now recognized in this group of patients (Table 43–4). The most common abnormality is cardiac

Long-term complications of obstructive sleep apnea:

- Chronic hypoxemia
- Pulmonary hypertension
- Cor pulmonale
- Systemic hypertension
- Cardiac arrhythmia
- Respiratory drive depression
- Polycythemia
- Excessive daytime hypersomnolence
- Intellectual deterioration
- Chronic fatigue

TABLE **43–3:**   Clinical Features of Obstructive Sleep Apnea

Loud snoring	Impotence
Excessive daytime sleepiness	Morning headaches
Hypertension	Nocturnal enuresis
Personality changes	Morning nausea

arrhythmias during sleep. Sinus bradytachycardia, sinus arrest, paroxysmal atrial tachycardia, atrial fibrillation, and ventricular tachycardia have all been described in these patients. In one study, more than 80% of the patients had prominent sinus tachycardia-bradycardia arrhythmias.[30] The degree of bradycardia directly relates to the degree of hypoxemia. The most common cardiac arrhythmia was sinus arrest, which can last from 2.5 to 13 seconds. Sinus bradycardia with the heart rate dropping below 30 beats per minute occurred in 7% of the patients. Second-degree atrioventricular block has also been noted during these events. Ventricular ectopy was reported to occur in 57 to 74% of patients with obstructive sleep apnea. It is frequently multifocal, with deterioration into ventricular tachycardia in 1 to 3% of patients. The number of premature ventricular contractions seems to correlate with the severity of oxygen desaturation.[31] These dangerous arrhythmic events have been implicated in some of the unexplained sudden deaths seen in obstructive sleep apnea.

Systemic blood pressure rises transiently during an episode of apnea because of reflex vasoconstriction. The hypertension usually resolves after the apnea stops. On the average, blood pressure increases on the order of 25%. This is proportional to the severity of oxyhemoglobin desaturation. Although hypertension is transient during sleep apnea and quickly returns to baseline, evidence has linked the development of chronic hypertension to the presence of obstructive sleep apnea. The mechanism for this is not clearly understood at this time. In some individuals, adequate treatment has resulted in normalization of blood pressure. Another detrimental consequence of nocturnal hypoxemia is the development of pulmonary hypertension, which once again is usually present only during the sleep apnea event. However, in some patients, persistent pulmonary hypertension develops and leads to cor pulmonale. Other features of obstructive sleep apnea syndrome include polycythemia, cyanosis, and carbon dioxide retention in more severe cases. A lesser known complication of sleep apnea syndrome is anoxic seizure, which

TABLE **43–4:**   Physiologic Complications of Sleep Apnea

	Physiologic Complications
Sleep fragmentation	Excessive daytime sleepiness
	Morning headache
	Personality changes
	Intellectual deterioration
Recurrent apneic events	Hypoxemia
	Hypercapnia
	Depressed hypercapnic response
	Cardiac arrhythmia
	Polycythemia
	Pulmonary hypertension
	Right-sided heart failure
	Systemic hypertension
	Seizure

usually occurs in association with severe oxygen desaturation. Anoxic brain injury is probably the predominant mechanism.

Diagnosis

Sleep apnea syndrome can often be suspected from the clinical history and physical examination findings. In a patient's history, four findings appear to be most discriminatory:

- Periodic absence of breathing identified by the patient's bed partner
- Body mass index
- Hypertension
- Age

Polysomnography—a complete physiologic evaluation of breathing pattern and sleep structure

The diagnosis of sleep apnea is confirmed by polysomnography (Table 43–5). A typical sleep record consists of EEG, electro-oculographic, electromyographic, and electrocardiographic recordings; inductive plethysmographic measurements of rib cage and abdominal motion for respiratory effort; pulse oximetric assessment of the oxygen saturation; and the use of thermistors to detect airflow at the nose and mouth. Airway obstruction can be inferred from the respiratory pattern when paradoxical motion of the rib cage and abdomen occurs (Fig. 43–3). An apneic episode, defined as the absence of nasal or oral airflow for at least 10 seconds, is generally classified by type: central, mixed, or obstructive.

Apnea index—the number of apneic episodes per hour of sleep

The severity of sleep apnea is assessed by calculating the apnea index. An apnea index of 5 or less is considered to be normal. However, an apnea index of 5 episodes/hr is purely an arbitrary criterion of disease. By pooling data from a number of studies, Berry and associates found that the number of apneic occurrences increases with age.[32] In fact, 30% of healthy elderly individuals (older than 65 years of age) who were completely free of symptoms of sleep apnea met the criterion for the diagnosis of sleep apnea syndrome (more than 5 episodes/hr). Without evidence of functional or physiologic impairment, these patients are unlikely to benefit from treatment. Therefore, the polysomnographic findings should be closely correlated with the clinical assessment.

In many patients with classic symptoms of obstructive sleep apnea, the diagnosis can be made readily by directly observing the patient's sleep. Sometimes, overnight oximetry showing periodic desaturation allows identification of the condition. More recently, findings obtained with wrist actigraphy and a static-charged sensitivity bed, which detect movements associated with wakefulness, have been found to correlate very well with sleep-wake events.[33-35] These devices have the potential to be sensitive screening devices. However, none of them should be recommended as diagnostic tools because their accuracies have not been fully

TABLE **43–5:** Routine Polysomnography

Event Monitored	Equipment
Sleep stages	Electroencephalograph
	Electro-oculograph
	Electromyograph (chin, legs)
Cardiac rhythm	Electrocardiograph
Arterial oxygen saturation	Pulse oximeter
Respiration	Inductive plethysmography
	Nasal and oral thermistors
	Pleural pressure monitor
	Electromyograph (surface electromyogram of the intercostal muscle and the diaphragm)

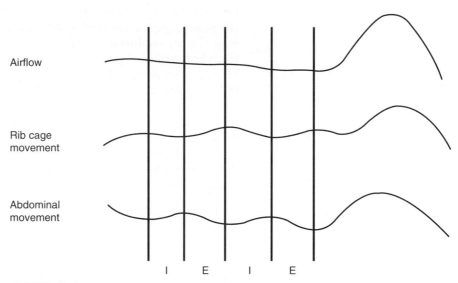

Airflow

Rib cage
movement

Abdominal
movement

I   E   I   E

FIGURE 43–3: An example of polysomnography in a patient with obstructive sleep apnea. Airway obstruction is inferred by the paradoxical motion of the rib cage and abdomen and by the absence of airflow detected by the nasal thermistor. I, inspiration; E, expiration.

validated through clinical trials; polysomnography is still required for an accurate diagnosis of obstructive sleep apnea. A detailed polysomnographic record also allows the physician to identify other causes of excessive daytime sleepiness, such as narcolepsy, nocturnal myoclonus, and restless leg syndrome. In individuals whose polysomnographic findings are negative for sleep apnea, the multiple sleep latency test, which assesses the degree of sleepiness, should be considered. The number of minutes to sleep onset (sleep latency) and the first episode of REM sleep are recorded. In a normal individual, the sleep latency time is about 10 minutes, and REM sleep is rarely observed in early sleep. In sleepy patients, the sleep latency shortens to less than 5 minutes. Narcolepsy is diagnosed when sleep-onset REM appears in two of five naps.

> The multiple sleep latency test consists of five nap studies, each of which is administered at a specific time throughout the day.

Treatment

The indications for and potential benefits of treating sleep-related respiratory disorders remain poorly defined. The demonstration of clinical abnormality should be the key step in initiating treatment. The major morbidity of this disorder is daytime hypersomnolence. Additional useful findings that would justify initiating treatment include the presence of cardiac arrhythmias and hemodynamic instability during sleep and severe oxygen desaturation during sleep. The treatment plan should be tailored to the needs of individual patients.

Since Sullivan and coworkers' first report on nasal continuous positive airway pressure (CPAP) via nasal mask to treat sleep apnea syndrome,[36] it has been widely accepted that nasal CPAP provides the most effective means of therapy. The precise mechanisms by which CPAP relieves airway obstruction remain to be elucidated. The best explanation is that CPAP acts like a pneumonic stent to prevent airway closure at the level of the pharynx by reducing excessive negative intraluminal pressure. Other studies have suggested that CPAP works by causing pressure stimulation of receptors present on the surface of the upper airway, which in turn increases the tone of the upper airway muscles, preventing the collapse of the airway during inspiration. Still other studies have suggested that CPAP prevents sleep apnea by preventing airway closure–induced reflex inhibition. In fact, a study has shown that the application of positive airway pressure during expiration also prevented obstructive sleep apnea. In a study from Australia, more than 90% of patients were effectively treated with nasal CPAP. CPAP is generally well tolerated and has few side effects. Sanders and colleagues found that 85% of their patients were fully compliant with the use of the CPAP mask.[37] However, Guilleminault reported that 29% of 130 patients followed up in the author's clinics stopped using nasal CPAP and requested another form of treatment.[38] Overall, the experience at my institution agrees with the findings of Sanders and colleagues.[37] The rate of compliance seemed to correlate positively with the severity of sleep apnea.

Most pharmacologic agents have not been helpful in relieving obstructive sleep apnea. Progesterone reduces the number of obstructive sleep apnea events in some patients, probably because of its respiratory stimulant properties. However, this agent may also cause an increase in the number of obstructive apnea episodes because it preferentially stimulates the diaphragm over the upper airway muscles.[39] Overall, the effects of progesterone have been disappointing.[40] Protriptyline has been shown to reduce apnea frequency, especially among patients whose apnea is mostly confined to REM sleep, because it reduces the amount of time spent in REM sleep. However, in many patients, it has no effect on the duration of apnea. Strychnine selectively improved the upper airway muscle tone over the diaphragm, thus preventing airway collapse. However, this drug is too toxic for continuous use.[41] Almitrine, a carotid body stimulatory agent available only in Europe, was studied in the setting of obstructive sleep apnea, and again the results were disappointing. Other respiratory stimulants (theophylline and acetazolamide) are equally nonbeneficial. At the current time, there are not sufficient data to recommend any pharmacologic agent.

In some patients, supplemental oxygen is useful in treating sleep apnea, presumably because of its beneficial effect on neural pathways that control the upper airway.[42] In others, nocturnal oxygen actually prolonged apnea duration and caused hypercapnia.[43] Oxygen therapy should be used only if a sleep study demonstrates the continual presence of severe hypoxia despite adequate CPAP treatment.

Tracheostomy, a very effective form of treatment for obstructive sleep apnea syndrome, allows airflow to bypass the site of obstruction in the upper airway. This procedure promptly reverses the symptoms and cures the conditions. However, because tracheostomy is associated with occasional morbidity and frequent psychological disability, this procedure should be reserved for patients with severe conditions that fail to improve with nasal CPAP treatment. Another frequently used surgical procedure is uvulopalatopharyngoplasty (UPPP), in which the soft palate, tonsils, adenoids, and redundant tissue around the oropharynx are removed to enlarge the airway diameter. Approximately 50% of patients who underwent this procedure showed improvement in oxygenation and a reduction in the apnea index.[44] UPPP is an effective treatment if the site of airway obstruction is proximal to the oropharynx. The success rate is about 70% in this subgroup of patients.[44] However, UPPP is not an effective treatment if the site of airway obstruction is distal to the oropharynx. At present, there is no effective way to identify the site of obstruction; thus, the physician finds it difficult to recommend UPPP routinely as a treatment. In a follow-up study of 385 sleep apnea patients that compared the effectiveness of different treatment modalities, patients who underwent UPPP had a mortality rate similar to that of subjects who did not receive any form of treatment.[45] Clearly, UPPP should not be recommended for all patients with sleep apnea; future studies are needed to identify which patients will benefit from this procedure.

The effect of weight reduction on the pharyngeal airway opening has been evaluated, and the results are conflicting. In some studies, the number of apneic episodes and the severity of oxygen desaturation diminished only after massive weight reduction.[46] In other studies, the apnea index decreased after a moderate weight reduction of 20 to 25 kg.[47, 48] In addition, significant improvements in patients' Pa_{O_2} and Pa_{CO_2} values occurred during wakefulness. However, sleep apnea–related events were not completely abolished by weight loss. It is difficult to draw a firm conclusion from this limited number of studies. Weight reduction should be routinely recommended for all sleep apnea patients who are obese, but this form of therapy should not be used as the primary mode of therapy for patients with moderate or severe sleep apnea syndrome. Finally, alcohol, sedatives, and hypnotics can worsen the sleep apnea syndrome; therefore, their use before bedtime should be avoided.

Central Sleep Apnea

Central sleep apnea is characterized by the absence of all respiratory effort due to the reduction in respiratory center output. Central apnea is most frequently observed at the onset of sleep. It can occur intermittently and irregularly or regularly and recurrently. Cheyne-Stokes breathing is perhaps the extreme form of central apnea that occurs at regular intervals and for a well-defined duration. It is hypothesized that central apnea is caused either by the instability of or delay in chemical feedback mechanisms or by the spontaneous intrinsic oscillations in respiratory drive. As mentioned earlier, thresholds and ventilatory responses to hypercapnia and hypoxia differ between wakefulness and stage 1 of sleep. At the onset of sleep, a person's sleep state fluctuates between wakefulness and stages 1 and 2 of sleep; as a result, the breathing pattern fluctuates between hypopnea and hyperpnea. This type of periodic breathing frequently occurs even in young, healthy individuals, especially in a hypoxic environment (e.g., high altitude). Therefore, it is generally not considered pathologic if the central apnea occurs only at sleep onset. However, some patients continue to have long periods of respiratory pause even after the sleep has been established and stabilized. In most cases, a specific cause of central apnea is not found, although it is sometimes associated with neurologic and cardiovascular disorders (Table 43–6). In heart failure patients, prolonged circulation time increases the time lag between the

TABLE **43–6:** Causes of Central Sleep Apnea and Periodic Breathing

Central nervous system	Cardiopulmonary
Brain stem disorders	Congestive heart failure—
Central nervous system	prolonged circulation time
infarction, neoplasm	Hypoxic condition—high
Neuromuscular disorders	altitude
Primary alveolar hypoventilation	Increased chemosensitivity
Sleep onset	

changes in blood gas values and the detection of such changes by central chemoreceptors. This results in overcorrection and undercorrection of Pa_{CO_2} by the respiratory system, thereby causing periodic breathing.

Clinical Features

Clinical features of central sleep apnea similar to those of obstructive sleep apnea include the following:

- Normal sleep is frequently disrupted, resulting in morning headache, chronic fatigue, and daytime hypersomnolence.
- Arterial oxygen desaturation, a common feature of central sleep apnea, can cause persistent pulmonary and systemic hypertension over time if left untreated.

Frequently, the primary underlying illness dominates the clinical manifestations, and apnea is only the incidental finding or the consequence (e.g., Cheyne-Stokes breathing in patients with stroke or congestive heart failure). As in patients with obstructive sleep apnea, cardiac arrhythmias are common during the time of severe arterial oxygen desaturation.

Diagnosis

The diagnosis of central sleep apnea requires full polysomnography to monitor sleep and the breathing pattern throughout the night. The same physiologic parameters are recorded as in the obstructive sleep apnea study. Central apnea is characterized by a lack of airflow and respiratory effort. Frequently, both central and obstructive apnea occur together, with central apnea usually preceding obstructive apnea (Fig. 43–4).

Treatment

Therapy for central sleep apnea has not been as thoroughly evaluated as therapy for obstructive sleep apnea. Obviously, any underlying illness that might precipitate central apnea, such as congestive heart failure or hypoxemia, should be corrected. Supplemental oxygen has been

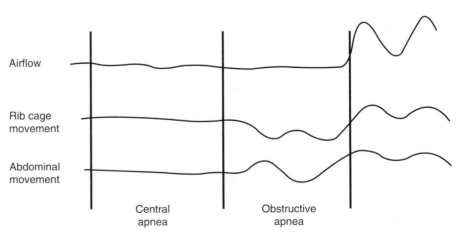

FIGURE 43–4: An example of a mixed event. This episode started as a central event (note the lack of airflow and movement of the rib cage and abdomen) and then developed into obstructive apnea. Note that the onset of diaphragm contraction is more rapid than that of the intercostal muscles, resulting in the paradoxical movement of the rib cage and abdomen during obstructive apnea.

shown to reduce the frequency of periodic breathing in some patients, especially when it is due to hypoxemia. A number of drugs have been studied. Acetazolamide appears to be effective in some patients with central sleep apnea. It stimulates breathing mainly by inducing metabolic acidosis. The results with almitrine, a carotid body stimulant, have been disappointing. Progesterone, a central respiratory stimulant, produces mixed results. At present, none of the medications has been shown to have a consistent effect in relieving central apnea. More recently, nasal CPAP has been shown to be useful in treating patients with central apnea, although extremely high levels of pressure are frequently required. The precise mechanism by which CPAP treatment works, as well as its efficacy, remains to be evaluated. It has been suggested that positive pressure in the airway acts as a respiratory stimulant to prevent reflex inspiratory inhibition due to airway collapse.[49]

> The use of progesterone may precipitate obstructive sleep apnea because progesterone selectively stimulates the diaphragm over the muscles of the upper airway.

SUMMARY

Sleep apnea is a common disorder in the general population. The majority of patients with sleep apnea suffer from the obstructive type. If the disorder is not recognized or properly treated, long-term functional and physiologic impairment may develop. At this time, nasal CPAP is the most effective mode of treatment.

References

1. Rechtschaffen A, Kales A (eds). A Manual of Standardized Terminology: Techniques and Scoring System for Sleep Stages of Human Subjects. Los Angeles, UCLA Brain Information Service/Brain Research Institute, 1968.
2. Douglas NJ. Control of breathing during sleep. Clin Sci 67:465–471, 1984.
3. Williams RL, Karacan I, Hursch CJ. Electroencephalography of Human Sleep. Clinical Applications. New York, John Wiley & Sons, 1974.
4. Whitelaw WA. Disorders of the respiratory pump. *In* Guenter CA, Welch MH (eds). Pulmonary Medicine, 2nd ed. Philadelphia, JB Lippincott, 1982, pp 193–234.
5. Bryan AC, Muller NL. Lung mechanics and gas exchange during sleep. Sleep 3:401–406, 1981.
6. Philipson EA, Bowes G. Control of breathing during sleep. *In* Fishman AP (ed). Handbook of Physiology, sect 3, vol. 2. American Physiological Society, 1986, pp 649–689.
7. Birchfield RI, Sieker HO, Heyman A. Alterations in respiratory function during natural sleep. Lab Clin Med 54:216–222, 1958.
8. Bulow K. Respiration and wakefulness in man. Acta Physiol Scand 59:1–110, 1963.
9. Douglas NJ, White DP, Pickett CK, et al. Respiration during sleep in normal man. Thorax 37:840–844, 1982.
10. Brebbia DR, Altshuler KZ. Oxygen consumption rate and electroencephalographic stage of sleep. Science 150:1621–1623, 1965.
11. Skatrud JB, Dempsey JA, Iber C, Berssenbrugge A. Correction of CO_2 retention during sleep in patients with chronic obstructive pulmonary diseases. Am Rev Respir Dis 124:260–268, 1981.
12. Tabachnik E, Muller NL, Bryan AC, Levison H. Changes in ventilation and chest wall mechanics during sleep in normal adolescents. J Appl Physiol Respir Environ Exercise Physiol 51:557–564, 1981.
13. Muller N, Gulston G, Cade D, et al. Diaphragmatic muscle fatigue in the newborn. J Appl Physiol 46:688–695, 1979.
14. Sauerland EK, Harper RM. The human tongue during sleep: Electromyographic activity of the genioglossus muscle. Exp Neurol 51:160–170, 1976.
15. Harper RM, Sauerland EK. Role of the tongue in sleep apnea. *In* Guilleminault C, Dement WC (eds). Sleep Apnea Syndromes. New York, Liss, 1978, pp 219–223.
16. Daubenspeck JA. Influence of small mechanical loads on variability of breathing pattern. J Appl Physiol 50:299–306, 1981.
17. Sullivan CE, Kozar LF, Murphy E, Philipson EA. Primary role of respiratory afferents in sustaining breathing rhythm. J Appl Physiol 45:11–17, 1978.
18. Douglas NJ, White DP, Weil JV, et al. Hypoxic ventilatory response decreases during sleep in normal men. Am Rev Respir Dis 125:286–289, 1982.

19. Douglas NJ, White DP, Weil JV, et al. Hypercapnic ventilatory response in sleeping adults. Am Rev Respir Dis 126:758–762, 1982.
20. Gothe B, Goldman MD, Cherniack NS, Mantey P. Effect of progressive hypoxia on breathing during sleep. Am Rev Respir Dis 126:97–102, 1982.
21. White DP, Douglas NJ, Pickett CK, et al. Hypoxic ventilatory response during sleep in normal women. Am Rev Respir Dis 126:530–533, 1982.
22. Issa FG, Sullivan CE. Arousal and breathing responses to airway occlusion in healthy sleeping adults. J Appl Physiol 55:1113–1119, 1983.
23. Douglas NJ. Control of ventilation during sleep. Clin Chest Med 6:563–575, 1985.
24. Gleeson K, Zwillich CW, White DP. The influence of increasing ventilatory effort on arousal from sleep. Am Rev Respir Dis 142:289–294, 1990.
25. Findley LJ, Unverzagt ME, Suratt PM. The automobile accidents involving the patients with obstructive sleep apnea. Am Rev Respir Dis 138:337–340, 1988.
26. Lugaresi E, Coccagna G, Cirignotta F. Snoring and its clinical implications. In Guilleminault C, Dement WC (eds). Sleep Apnea Syndromes. New York, Liss, 1978, pp 13–21.
27. Lugaresi E, Cirignotta F, Coccagna G. Some epidemiological data on snoring and cardiocirculatory disturbances. Sleep 3:221–224, 1980.
28. Fletcher EC, DeBehnke RD, Lovoi MS, et al. Undiagnosed sleep apnea among patients with essential hypertension. Ann Intern Med 103:190–194, 1985.
29. Cherniack MS. Respiratory dysrhythmias during sleep. N Engl J Med 305:325–331, 1981.
30. Guilleminault C, Connolly S, Winkie R, et al. Cyclical variation of the heart rate in sleep apnea syndrome. Mechanisms and usefulness of 24h electrocardiography as a screening technique. Lancet 1:126–131, 1984.
31. Shepard JW, Garrison MW, Grither DA, Dolan DF. Relationship of ventricular ectopy to oxyhemoglobin desaturation in patients with obstructive sleep apnea. Chest 88:335–340, 1985.
32. Berry DTR, Webb WR, Block AJ. Sleep apnea syndrome: A critical review of the apnea index as a diagnostic criterion. Chest 86:529–531, 1984.
33. Webster JB, Kripke DF, Messin S, et al. An activity-based sleep monitor system for ambulatory use. Sleep 5:389–399, 1982.
34. Sadeh A, Alster J, Urbach D, Lavie P. Actigraphically based automatic bedtime sleep-wake scoring: Validity and clinical applications. J Ambulatory Monit 2:209–216, 1989.
35. Aubert-Tulkens G, Culee C, Harmant-Van Rijckevorsel, Rodenstein DO. Ambulatory evaluation of sleep disturbance and therapeutic effects in sleep apnea syndrome by wrist activity monitoring. Am Rev Respir Dis 136:851–856, 1987.
36. Sullivan CE, Issa FG, Berthon-Jones M, Eves L. Reversal of obstructive sleep apnea by continuous positive airway pressure applied through the nares. Lancet 1:862–865, 1981.
37. Sanders MH, Cruendl CA, Rogers RM. Patient compliance with nasal CPAP therapy for sleep apnea. Chest 90:330–333, 1986.
38. Guilleminault C. Obstructive sleep apnea syndrome. Psychiatr Clin North Am 10:607–621, 1987.
39. Strohl KP, Hensley MJ, Saunders NA. Progesterone administration and progressive sleep apneas. JAMA 245:1230–1232, 1981.
40. Cook WR, Benich JJ, Wooten SA. Indices of severity of obstructive sleep apnea syndrome do not change during medroxyprogesterone acetate therapy. Chest 96:262–266, 1989.
41. Tobin MJ, Cohn MA, Sackner MA. Breathing abnormalities during sleep. Arch Intern Med 143:1221–1228, 1983.
42. Smith PL, Haponik EF, Bleecker ER. The effects of oxygen in patients with sleep apnea. Am Rev Respir Dis 130:958–963, 1984.
43. Alford AJ, Fletcher EC, Nickson D. Acute oxygen in patients with sleep apnea and COPD. Chest 89:30–38, 1986.
44. Shepard JW, Olsen KD. Uvulopalatopharyngoplasty for treatment of obstructive sleep apnea. Mayo Clin Proc 65:1260–1267, 1990.
45. He J, Kryger MH, Zorick FJ, et al. Mortality and apnea index in obstructive sleep apnea. Chest 94:9–14, 1988.
46. Harman EM, Wynne JW, Block AJ. The effect of weight loss on sleep-disordered breathing and oxygen desaturation in morbidly obese men. Chest 82:291–294, 1982.
47. Rubinstein I, Colapinto N, Rotstein LE, et al. Improvement in upper airway function after weight loss in patients with obstructive sleep apnea. Am Rev Respir Dis 138:1192–1195, 1988.
48. Suratt PM, McTier RE, Findley LJ, et al. Changes in breathing and pharynx after weight loss in obstructive sleep apnea. Chest 92:631–637, 1987.
49. Issa FG, Sullivan CE. Reversal of central sleep apnea using nasal CPAP. Chest 90:165–171, 1986.

44

Respiratory Tract Infections

Victor F. Tapson, M.D., and Peter S. Kussin, M.D.

Despite advances in diagnosis and treatment, respiratory tract infections cause significant morbidity and mortality in the United States. Each year, more than 3 million patients develop pneumonia, with more than 500,000 admitted to the hospital. In addition, a substantial number of patients who are already hospitalized develop pneumonia.

A number of noninfectious entities masquerade as pneumonia. Hospitalized patients, particularly those who are intubated and receiving mechanical ventilation, are at risk for developing pneumonia. The diagnostic and therapeutic approaches to community- and hospital-acquired pneumonia are similar in principle; however, because of the complexity of the conditions of hospitalized patients and the increased incidence of gram-negative pathogens, the diagnosis may require more invasive measures, and empiric coverage must include a broad range of pathogens. This chapter outlines the etiology and pathogenesis of pulmonary infections, the clinical approach to them, and the principles of treatment, with a particular focus on pneumonia. Also discussed are other infectious pulmonary entities, such as bronchitis, bronchiectasis, lung abscess, and empyema.

COMMUNITY-ACQUIRED PNEUMONIA

Etiology and Predisposing Conditions

Pneumonia is defined as pulmonary infection accompanied by a radiographically documented pulmonary infiltrate. Such infections are almost always accompanied by fever and cough. Pneumonia may be associated with classic findings such as fever, chills, a cough productive of purulent sputum, leukocytosis, and a well-defined pulmonary infiltrate. The presentation may, however, be "atypical," with nonproductive cough, headache, myalgias, and bilateral, often diffuse infiltrates. Pneumococcal pneumonia remains the prototype community-acquired pneumonia, and infection with *Streptococcus pneumoniae* appears to be the most commonly documented etiology. Other bacterial pathogens include *Mycoplasma pneumoniae, Chlamydia pneumoniae, Haemophilus influenzae, Staphylococcus aureus, Klebsiella pneumoniae,* and *Legionella pneumophila* (Table 44–1).

Certain epidemiologic trends seem to be appearing:

Unfortunately, Gram's stain and culture yield are relatively low for community-acquired pneumonia. The microbiologic etiology remains elusive in the majority of cases.

TABLE **44–1:** Common Etiologies of Community-Acquired Pneumonia

Streptococcus pneumoniae	*Klebsiella pneumoniae*
Mycoplasma pneumoniae	*Staphylococcus aureus*
Haemophilus influenzae	*Legionella pneumophila*
Chlamydia pneumoniae	

In patients older than 40 years of age who have gram-negative pneumonia, the mortality may be as high as 70%. A gram-negative etiology appears in more than 20% of nursing home patients older than 65 years of age but in fewer than 10% of those younger than 65.

Clues to *Legionella* infection include the predominance of neutrophils on Gram's stain without organisms, hyponatremia, and the failure to respond to beta-lactam and aminoglycoside antibiotics.

The most common viral pneumonia in adults is influenza.

Diabetes may account for as many as one third of patients who develop staphylococcal pneumonia.

Factors that predispose to aspiration include a decreased level of consciousness, neurologic disease, esophageal disorders, and interference with the lower esophageal function caused by nasogastric tubes.

Bronchiectasis is a disease characterized by permanent dilatation of the bronchi. Conditions associated with bronchiectasis include immunoglobulin deficiencies, inherited defects such as cystic fibrosis, and previous infections such as tuberculosis.

- An increasing incidence of gram-negative bacillary pneumonia is being seen, particularly in the elderly. The relationship between increased mortality and advanced age is well established, especially with gram-negative pneumonia.
- The role of *H. influenzae* in bronchitis, as well as in community-acquired pneumonia, is emerging. In patients with chronic obstructive lung disease, oropharyngeal colonization may frequently make it difficult to ascertain the true frequency of community-acquired pneumonia due to this pathogen.
- *Mycoplasma* infections are responsible for 15 to 30% of outpatient pneumonias; they commonly occur in children and young adults.
- *Legionella* pneumonia is caused by a fastidious aerobic gram-negative bacillus. Community-acquired or nosocomial infection can occur, spreading from contaminated air conditioners, cooling towers, or shower heads. Elderly patients have an increased risk of acquiring this disease. A variety of extrapulmonary manifestations present in *Legionella* pneumonia have been described; they vary depending on the series. Relative bradycardia may suggest legionnaires' disease, but this finding is nonspecific. Headache and mental status changes appear to be common, with the latter being the most frequent neurologic abnormality. Diarrhea, abdominal pain, elevated liver function test results, hypophosphatemia, and hematuria are common in legionellosis but may not be more common in this condition than in pneumonia of other causes.
- The emergence of *C. pneumoniae* (TWAR) as a cause of community-acquired atypical pneumonia has more recently been recognized. This organism, particularly in younger patients, together with *Mycoplasma* species, *Legionella* species, and viruses, causes the bulk of atypical pneumonias.
- Viruses as a group rank third behind *S. pneumoniae* and *Mycoplasma* species as causative agents in pneumonia. The type A influenza virus causes local epidemics every few years, particularly in the winter. Superinfection occurs frequently with *S. pneumoniae,* as well as with *Staphylococcus* or *Haemophilus* species. Although most patients with influenzal pneumonia recover, severe infection may lead to adult respiratory distress syndrome.
- Adenovirus frequently causes infections in children and young adults. Respiratory syncytial virus commonly causes infections at the extremes of age. The leading cause of lower respiratory tract disease in infants and young children, it is generally suspected when pneumonia occurs in young infants during a known outbreak. Cytomegalovirus generally causes subclinical infections. In patients with significant immunocompromise, such as those who have had organ transplantation and those who have acquired immunodeficiency syndrome (AIDS), cytomegalovirus may cause pneumonia. Although varicella-zoster virus may cause pneumonia in children with chicken pox, the vast majority of cases of pneumonia occur in adults. Approximately 15% of adults with chicken pox will develop pneumonia. In a minority of patients who develop pneumonia, respiratory failure may result. Measles pneumonia is relatively rare and generally occurs in immunocompromised children.
- Patients with diabetes appear to have an increased rate of colonization with gram-negative bacteria, as well as with *S. aureus.*
- Alcohol alters pulmonary defense mechanisms, and aspiration occurs more commonly in alcoholics. *K. pneumoniae* is a very common and

virulent cause of pneumonia in this population. Although this type of pneumonia may be difficult to differentiate clinically from other bacterial pneumonias, certain features, such as massive consolidation of the upper lobe, bulging fissures, early abscess, and empyema formation, occur frequently with this pathogen.

- Aspiration can be of several types, including gastric acid, particulate matter, and oropharyngeal bacterial aspiration. Bacterial aspiration may result not only in pneumonia but in necrotizing pneumonitis and lung abscess, as well as in empyema. Periodontal disease may increase the bacterial inoculum. The lung segments most commonly involved in aspiration pneumonia are those that are dependent in the supine patient, including the posterior segments of the upper lobes and the superior segments of the lower lobes. Clinical clues to bacterial aspiration include observed aspiration or a predisposition to aspiration, disease in a dependent lung segment, foul-smelling sputum or empyema fluid, and the presence of cavitation or abscess formation. In contrast to patients with community-acquired aspiration pneumonia, hospitalized patients with aspiration pneumonia are often infected primarily with gram-negative bacteria secondary to oropharyngeal colonization, although anaerobic infection may be present in a small minority.

- Patients with anatomic abnormalities in the lung may be predisposed to infection. Patients with bronchiectasis often have chronic sputum production, which may increase in volume and purulence with acute exacerbations. The general approach to patients with bronchiectasis who have either acute flare-ups or pneumonia includes sputum culture, broad-spectrum antibiotic coverage, aggressive pulmonary toilet with nebulized bronchodilators, and chest physical therapy.

Early in the course of HIV infection, bacterial pneumonia occurs frequently.

Patients with known or suspected human immunodeficiency virus (HIV) infection comprise a large group presenting with community-acquired pneumonia. Risk factors for HIV infection, such as homosexuality, intravenous drug abuse, or previous blood transfusions, may not be known at the time of presentation with pneumonia. *Pneumocystis carinii* pneumonia is by far the most common infection diagnosed in these patients, but suspicion must be increased for tuberculosis and fungal pneumonia in HIV-positive patients with community-acquired pneumonia.

Clinical Presentation and Diagnostic Approach

Pneumonia is likely when fever, cough, and pulmonary infiltrates develop acutely; therefore, careful attention should be paid to the history, risk factors, and underlying disease present. Certain clinical features, such as rigors and purulent sputum, suggest a bacterial etiology. The diagnostic approach may be considerably more complicated in patients with significant underlying disease, in those already receiving antibiotics, and in those in whom sputum production is scant. Dry cough, headache, and myalgias suggest atypical pneumonia. Individuals with prior symptoms of pharyngitis, low-grade fever, malaise, headache, and photophobia who subsequently develop a nonproductive cough and pulmonary infiltrates generally have viral pneumonia. Other atypical etiologies include infection with *M. pneumoniae, C. pneumoniae, L. pneumophila,* and *P. carinii.* Patients with bacterial pneumonia are often toxic appearing, and some with atypical pneumonia may be as well. A sputum Gram's stain is performed whenever possible and may be diagnostic. The blood leukocyte count is generally elevated in patients with bacterial pneumonia, but it is often normal in atypical pneumonia. In atypical pneumonia, chest radiography may frequently reveal bilateral diffuse infiltrates, whereas in bacterial pneumonia, a lobar pattern often occurs. However, such patterns are not specific. Clues to the diagnosis of *M. pneumoniae* infection include bullous myringitis, hemolytic anemia, and erythema multiforme. Erythema multiforme may also be caused by certain medications, particularly antibiotics; thus, *M. pneumoniae* is often difficult to implicate with certainty. In rare cases, hepatitis and myocarditis may occur. Certain clinical settings may suggest viral infection. Adenoviruses often cause upper respiratory tract infections in children and young adults. In military recruits, pneumonia caused by adenovirus types 4 and 7 may develop. Respiratory syncytial virus is generally suspected when pneumonia occurs in young infants during a known outbreak. In general, the history, physical examination, and chest radiograph are not sufficient to determine the precise etiology of bacterial or atypical pneumonia.

Adenoviruses have also been associated with pneumonia in immunosuppressed patients, including those with AIDS.

Sputum Analysis

Limitations of sputum processing frequently prevent Gram's stain and culture from being useful. Fewer than 50% of expectorated sputum samples processed by the usual methods yield reliable results, primarily because of upper airway colonization with gram-negative organisms. A poor correlation has been observed between Gram's stain results and sputum culture results. Organisms such as *S. pneumoniae* and *H. influenzae* may be overgrown in culture media by other organisms. Even in pneumococcal pneumonia, false-positive rates of 25 to 44% and false-negative rates of 50% have been reported. Because as many as 50% of healthy persons have oropharyngeal colonization with *S. pneumoniae,* its presence needs to be carefully interpreted. When gram-positive diplococci are present in large numbers and are the predominant organisms and when more than 25 polymorphonuclear leukocytes and fewer than 10 squamous epithelial cells are present per low-power field, true infection is likely. Sputum Gram's stain in the atypical pneumonia syndrome shows few white blood cells and a paucity of organisms. More specific techniques may be applied to the sputum under certain circumstances. When *Legionella* infection is suspected, a direct fluorescent antibody stain can be performed, which has a specificity of 95% and a sensitivity of 70%. Gene probes and antigen detection in urine and sputum are other options that may serve as specific diagnostic tools. Despite drawbacks, sputum Gram's stain and culture remain the time-honored approach to the etiologic diagnosis of community-acquired pneumonia.

Colonization with gram-negative bacteria occurs in fewer than 10% of healthy subjects and in 45 to 100% of patients in medical intensive care units.

Laboratory Examinations

Hematologic and serologic methods are sometimes useful. Elevated cold agglutinin titers support the diagnosis of mycoplasmal infection, with a four-fold or greater increase in complement-fixing antibodies being diagnostic. *Legionella* infection, as well as certain viral infections, may also ultimately be diagnosed by a rise in antibody titers, but such titers are obviously only of retrospective interest.

Blood culture results are positive in only 15 to 25% of patients with community-acquired pneumonia; blood cultures should be drawn, particularly in patients who appear toxic. Whenever pleural effusions are present in community-acquired pneumonia, there are several reasons why thoracentesis should be performed:

- The finding of organisms on Gram's stain or culture of pleural fluid is diagnostic.
- In pneumonia, certain pleural fluid characteristics suggest the need for chest tube placement. These include the presence of pus or organisms on Gram's stain and a pleural fluid pH of less than 7.10. In addition, a very low pleural fluid glucose level may suggest the need for a chest tube.

Transtracheal, bronchoscopic, and transthoracic diagnostic techniques are rarely employed in community-acquired pneumonia unless the patient is an immunocompromised host or unless an unusual infection or another condition such as a neoplasm is suspected.

Treatment

When possible, the treatment of community-acquired pneumonia should be based on Gram's stain and culture results. However, treatment is frequently empiric. In an otherwise normal host, coverage should be included for *S. pneumoniae* and *H. influenzae*. In patients who smoke, these organisms as well as *Moraxella catarrhalis* should be considered. A broad-spectrum second-generation cephalosporin, such as cefuroxime, provides adequate coverage for these organisms. When the sputum is very foul smelling or when the chest radiograph reveals cavitation, particularly in the setting of aspiration, treatment should include high-dose penicillin or clindamycin. The latter appears to be marginally superior in this setting. In young patients, mycoplasmal and chlamydial infections should be considered. Diabetic patients, elderly nursing home patients, and alcoholics need additional gram-negative coverage. Broad-spectrum treatment with an antipseudomonal penicillin provides broad gram-negative coverage with some anaerobic and gram-positive coverage as well. If *S. aureus* infection is suspected, treatment with ticarcillin-clavulanate or ampicillin-sulbactam will be effective and will offer broad-spectrum coverage for gram-positive, gram-negative, and anaerobic organisms. When an atypical pneumonia is suspected or when a patient is particularly ill with a community-acquired pneumonia and no definitive pathogen has been isolated, consideration should be given to adding erythromycin at a dose of 1 g intravenously every 6 hours. This provides coverage for *Legionella* as well as *Mycoplasma* infections. When HIV infection is suspected, bronchoscopy with bronchoalveolar lavage may be necessary to document *Pneumocystis* infection, but there should be a low threshold for early empiric treatment with trimethoprim-sulfamethoxazole. Finally, if tuberculosis is suspected, the patient should be placed in respiratory isolation and begun on empiric antituberculous therapy pending sputum or bronchoscopic diagnosis.

Viral infections may cause atypical pneumonia; the diagnosis may be elusive. Empiric antibacterial therapy may be necessary. Although the treatment of uncomplicated influenzal pneumonia is supportive, amantadine may be used as prophylaxis or therapy for influenza A. It is not active against influenza B. The administration of this drug within 48 hours of the onset of illness reduces the duration of signs and symptoms of influenza, but its use can be associated with mild side effects, including anxiety, insomnia, and tremor. The usual dose is 200 mg daily for adults, but the dose is reduced in elderly patients and in those with renal dysfunction. Neither amantadine nor aerosolized ribavirin has a proven role in established influenzal pneumonia, but these agents are often used in this setting. The treatment of respiratory syncytial virus is also supportive, but ribavirin has been approved for administration via aerosol to infants and young children with severe lower respiratory tract infections. Finally, in the presence of atypical symptoms or in certain high-risk clinical settings, consideration should be given to noninfectious etiologies, such as chemical aspiration pneumonitis, pulmonary or fat embolism, congestive heart failure, bronchiolitis obliterans with organizing pneumonia, collagen vascular disease, vasculitis, and pulmonary hemorrhage. Radiographic improvement in community-acquired pneumonia may take weeks.

Pneumococcal Vaccine

A preventive approach is prudent in certain patients at high risk for the development of pneumonia. The current 23-valent pneumococcal vaccine consists of capsular antigens from the serotypes associated with approximately 90% of pneumococcal infections. Although the vaccine increases antibody levels in some populations at risk for pneumonia, such as those with chronic obstructive lung disease, efficacy has been difficult to prove in clinical trials. Nonetheless, the vaccine is recommended in all persons who are 65 years of age or older and in patients with pulmonary, cardiovascular, and immunosuppressive illnesses, as well as in patients with certain other high-risk conditions, such as diabetes and alcoholism. In certain high-risk patients, a booster inoculation is given 6 years after the initial vaccine.

NOSOCOMIAL PNEUMONIA

Hospitalized patients who are at risk for the development of infections are often critically ill, with multiple potential routes for infection.

Intubation and mechanical ventilation increase the incidence and mortality of nosocomial pneumonia. Despite dramatic advances in medical technology, the incidence of nosocomial infection and the mortality in these patients remain high.

Intubation with mechanical ventilation increases the risk of this complication by more than two-fold, with rates of more than 20% frequently reported. The fatality rate in patients receiving mechanical ventilation is as high as 50 to 75%, compared with a mortality rate of 25 to 29% in mechanically ventilated patients without pneumonia.

The recognition of pneumonia may be difficult in critically ill mechanically ventilated patients with significant underlying disease. The usual features of pneumonia, such as cough, sputum production, fever, and leukocytosis, may be absent or unrelated to pneumonia. The presence of pulmonary infiltrates on the chest x-ray study, the definitive feature of pneumonia, may be absent initially in as many as 36% of granulocytopenic patients with gram-negative pneumonia. Autopsies frequently disclose unsuspected pneumonia in such patients. The recognition of new infiltrates may be difficult in patients with adult respiratory distress syndrome or other underlying pulmonary disease. When new infiltrates are present, noninfectious causes must be considered (Table

---

Unusually slow resolution of the chest radiographic findings, particularly when associated with anorexia, weight loss, hemoptysis, or a heavy smoking history, should prompt further evaluation for malignancy with bronchoscopy.

Nosocomial pneumonia may occur in 0.6% of hospitalized patients and accounts for as many as 10% of nosocomial infections.

The newest definitions of nosocomial pneumonia from the Centers for Disease Control and Prevention do not emphasize a specific period for the onset of infection.

44–2). Drug- and radiation-induced pneumonitis, malignancy, and cardiogenic as well as noncardiogenic pulmonary edema are possibilities. Bleeding in the tracheobronchial tree or alveolar hemorrhage may cause airspace disease, mimicking infection.

Pathogenesis and Risk Factors

Factors that seem to predispose to gram-negative colonization are

- Severity of illness
- Length of hospitalization
- Increased age
- Previous or current use of antibiotics
- Intubation

Medical conditions associated with gram-negative colonization include

- Acidosis
- Alcoholism
- Diabetes
- Hypotension
- Leukopenia
- Underlying lung disease

The supine position, the presence of a nasogastric tube, and the administration of narcotics may contribute to decreased intestinal motility and reflux.

In most instances, oropharyngeal organisms reach the sterile lung by aspiration. A high incidence of aspiration occurs in intubated patients despite the presence of cuffed endotracheal tubes. Other potential mechanisms include bacteremia from other sources and inhalation of aerosols containing microorganisms.

Gram-negative bacilli are infrequently found in pharyngeal culture specimens from normal subjects. Hospitalized patients rapidly become colonized with gram-negative bacteria. Johanson and coworkers (1972) found that 19% of moderately ill and 38% of critically ill patients had positive oropharyngeal culture results within 96 hours of admission. By day 21, at least 41 and 80%, respectively, had positive culture findings. A subsequent prospective study showed that 45% of patients admitted to a medical intensive care unit became colonized with gram-negative bacteria, and 22% of culture results were positive from the first day. Twenty-three percent of colonized patients developed pneumonia, compared with 3.3% of noncolonized patients. Mechanically ventilated patients frequently receive antibiotics that profoundly affect colonization. Inhibition of the growth of streptococci with the use of large doses of penicillin has been shown to permit colonization with gram-negative rods.

The adherence of bacteria to oropharyngeal epithelial cells appears to play a crucial role in colonization. Bacteria appear to attach via pili to oropharyngeal cells. Fibronectin is a high molecular weight glycoprotein that coats normal oropharyngeal epithelial cell surface receptors for gram-negative bacilli. Enzymes, including elastase in the oral secretions of critically ill patients, clear fibronectin from the cell surface, permitting the binding of gram-negative bacilli. Colonization of the gastrointestinal tract may precede oropharyngeal colonization. In addition, critically ill intubated patients are likely to have reflux of gastric secretions. A clinical trial has suggested that the presence of a nasogastric tube may be an independent risk factor for the development of nosocomial pneumonia.

Craven and associates at Boston City Hospital evaluated the specific risks for pneumonia in patients receiving continuous mechanical ventilation. Four independent variables were significantly associated with ventilator-associated pneumonia:

- Presence of an intracranial pressure monitor
- Treatment with cimetidine

TABLE **44–2:** Noninfectious Causes of Pulmonary Infiltrates

Congestive heart failure	Fat embolism
Adult respiratory distress syndrome	Vasculitis
Drug-induced pneumonitis	Collagen vascular disease
Alveolar hemorrhage	Feeding tube misplacement
Gastric (chemical) aspiration	Pulmonary eosinophilic syndromes
Leukemia	Lymphoma
Alveolar cell carcinoma	Pulmonary alveolar proteinosis
Pulmonary embolism	Bronchiolitis obliterans with organizing pneumonia

- Hospitalization during the fall and winter
- Mechanical ventilator circuit changes every 24 hours

In some cases, these risk factors may reflect the severity of the underlying illness in these patients.

The role of exogenous sources of bacteria in the development of nosocomial pneumonia in patients receiving mechanical ventilation has been reviewed in detail by Driks and colleagues. Small particles (less than 4 μm in diameter) can more easily reach the alveoli, and therefore humidifiers or therapeutic nebulizers may impose a risk if their contents become contaminated because they deliver small aerosol particles. Mechanical ventilator tubing and the endotracheal tube itself may become colonized. Significantly increased rates of pneumonia in patients receiving more frequent (every 24 hours) ventilator circuit changes were postulated to result from increased manipulation of the tubing, which may have caused the inadvertent flushing of contaminated condensate into patients' lungs. Severe underlying disease may result not only in an increased susceptibility to colonization by gram-negative bacteria but also in a greater propensity to aspiration. Healthy people frequently aspirate during sleep, but critically ill patients who are in a coma or have depressed gag reflexes are at higher risk for aspiration. Intubation further compromises the barrier between the lower and the upper respiratory tract, allowing colonization of the major airways and introducing difficulty in determining the difference between colonization and a pathogenic state.

Etiology

The National Nosocomial Infections Surveillance System found that *Pseudomonas aeruginosa* was the most commonly isolated agent in nosocomial pneumonia, followed by *S. aureus, Klebsiella* species, and *Enterobacter* species (Table 44–3). An increasing prevalence of especially virulent and resistant organisms has been strongly suggested. The prevalence of *P. aeruginosa* remains high (17%), and increased resistance to broad-spectrum antibiotics has been documented. Other gram-negative organisms, such as *Escherichia coli, Enterobacter* species, and *Klebsiella* species, account for a significant proportion of nosocomial lung infections. Less common isolates include *Proteus, Serratia, Citrobacter,* and *Acinetobacter* species.

Gram-positive organisms, particularly *S. aureus,* cause a significant

TABLE **44–3:** Pathogens in Nosocomial Pneumonia: National Nosocomial Infections Surveillance System

Pathogen	Frequency (%)
Pseudomonas aeruginosa	16.9
Staphylococcus aureus	12.9
Klebsiella species	11.6
Enterobacter species	9.4
Escherichia coli	6.4
Serratia species	5.8
Proteus species	4.2
Candida species	4.0
Enterococci	1.5
Anaerobes	0.3
All others	27.0

minority of nosocomial pneumonias. Predisposing factors include indwelling central venous catheters and recent surgical procedures. Other studies have confirmed that aerobic gram-negative bacilli and *S. aureus* are generally the most common causative agents, being isolated in as many as 80% of cases.

Anaerobic bacterial pneumonias may also be important. Bartlett found that anaerobes were isolated in 35% of nosocomial pneumonias, but they were the exclusive pathogens in only 7%. *Peptostreptococcus, Peptococcus, Fusobacterium,* and *Bacteroides* species were the most common anaerobic isolates. In the majority of patients with anaerobic infections, more than one species was isolated. Viral infections may also occur, but it is not clear how frequently viruses are responsible for nosocomial pneumonia in ventilated patients. *Legionella* species may also cause nosocomial pneumonia in this group of patients.

In immunocompromised patients, gram-negative bacilli remain a frequent cause of nosocomial pneumonia. Invasive fungal infections, such as infection with *Aspergillus* and *Candida* species, and viral infections caused by herpes simplex virus, cytomegalovirus, and varicella-zoster virus may also occur. Infections with *P. carinii* occur in conditions associated with abnormal T lymphocyte function, such as AIDS and immunosuppression after organ transplantation.

Clinical Presentation and Diagnostic Approach

Knowledge of a patient's underlying disease may offer clues to the microbiologic cause of nosocomial pneumonia, but clinical features are usually of minimal benefit in determining the causative agent. Fever patterns are generally not helpful. Elderly patients, patients with hepatic or renal failure, and patients receiving corticosteroids may not develop fever.

An accurate physical examination of the patient receiving mechanical ventilation is important and may prove to be useful. Severely ill patients with pseudomonal bacteremia and tissue invasion may develop ecthyma gangrenosum, a distinctive necrotic skin lesion. A typical lesion is a round, indurated ulcer with a black center that varies from a few millimeters to several centimeters in diameter. The target lesion of erythema multiforme appears in *M. pneumoniae* infection, but it is nonspecific: it may occur in other infections or secondary to drug reactions. Macular skin lesions on an erythematous base may mark the occurrence of hematogenous candidal infection. Herpes zoster and herpes simplex lesions often have a characteristic appearance. Inspection of the nares may reveal the characteristic eschar of mucormycosis in patients with diabetic ketoacidosis or leukemia. Funduscopic examination can reveal single or multiple raised, white fluffy lesions, suggesting candidal endophthalmitis. Funduscopic abnormalities may occur with cytomegalovirus infection and aspergillosis as well. Evidence of extrapulmonary infection, such as meningitis, septic arthritis, or pleural effusion, offers the opportunity to isolate an infectious agent that may be causing pneumonia. As in the setting of community-acquired pneumonia, the history and physical examination findings are usually not suggestive of a specific microbiologic etiology.

The radiographic pattern is sometimes helpful in suggesting an organism. Although lobar consolidation may suggest bacterial or fungal infection, diffuse infiltrates often occur with viral infection or with opportunistic infections such as *P. carinii* infection. However, a great deal of overlap occurs. Although cavitary lesions may occur with *S. aureus* or gram-negative bacillary pneumonia, more unusual infections such as invasive aspergillosis, mycobacterial infection, nocardiosis, and anaerobic infections should also be considered. Cavitation can occur occasionally in patients with *Legionella* pneumonia as well.

Isolation of the microbiologic agent responsible for nosocomial pneumonia is obviously important, but it can be difficult. Blood culture results are diagnostic when they are positive, but this occurs relatively infrequently. Because pleural fluid culture results are specific, pleural fluid culture should be performed if thoracentesis is done.

The utility of endotracheal secretion analysis in the diagnosis of pneumonia in mechanically ventilated patients is controversial. Secretions should be processed for Gram's stain and culture, but the results must be interpreted with care. Because secretions are contaminated by oropharyngeal organisms, it is difficult to differentiate between colonization and true lower respiratory tract infections. Johanson and coworkers (1969) did not find a correlation between the development of true pulmonary infection and sputum bacterial colony counts in a prospective study of 213 intensive care unit patients. However, the sputum was not screened for the presence of epithelial cells, and some of the specimens could therefore have been contaminated by oral secretions.

More invasive approaches have been advocated. The use of transtracheal aspirates may be more reliable than that of expectorated sputum in the diagnosis of pneumonia. A modification of this technique has been suggested for use in intubated patients. Instead of a transtracheal puncture's being used, a 24-inch polyethylene catheter is introduced through the tracheostomy or endotracheal tube. After the catheter has been passed to the full extent, an attempt is made to wedge it in the lung periphery. Specimens are aspirated, and Gram's stain and cultures are performed. Matthay and Moritz studied 20 intubated patients with pulmonary infiltrates who had upper airway cultures. Sterile cultures were obtained from the lower airways in 11 patients. Although this group had some success with this technique, it has not been widely accepted.

Transthoracic needle aspiration has been used to diagnose pulmonary infection. This technique provides samples directly from the lung, avoiding upper airway contamination. The relatively high incidence of pneumothorax, with the additional possibility of tension pneumothorax, deters many physicians from employing this technique in mechanically ventilated patients.

Bronchoscopy has been widely used in an attempt to bypass upper airway colonization. Contamination during passage of the instrument remains a problem. The concept of a protected sterile catheter was refined by Wimberly and coworkers. This device is a retractable brush within a double-sheathed polyethylene catheter with a distal plug of polyethylene glycol in the outer catheter. Once the bronchoscope is in the proper position, the brush remains uncontaminated by the upper airway. The brush is advanced and specimens are obtained under direct vision. Fagon and associates prospectively studied the epidemiologic and bacteriologic aspects of 52 consecutive episodes of pneumonia in patients receiving mechanical ventilation in an intensive care unit. All patients receiving mechanical ventilation for more than 72 hours during the 41-month study period were included. Fiberoptic bronchoscopy with the protected specimen brush (PSB) was performed in all patients, with new and persistent infiltrates being associated with purulent tracheal aspi-

Needle aspiration appears to have its highest yield in localized peripheral lung lesions.

rates. The patients were diagnosed as having pneumonia only if the PSB yielded more than 10^3 colony-forming units (CFU)/mL of at least one organism. Of 111 microorganisms cultured from the PSB during 52 episodes of ventilator-associated pneumonia, 84 were recovered in significant enough concentrations to be considered predominant isolates. Sixty-one percent of the predominant isolates were gram-negative bacilli, and 38% were gram-positive bacteria. Anaerobes accounted for only 1%. In this study, the diagnosis of pneumonia was based on significantly positive culture results by PSB and not solely on clinical criteria. The authors stated that even in the presence of the usual criteria for pneumonia, such as fever, sputum production, and pulmonary infiltrates, quantitative cultures from PSB specimens yielding fewer than 10^3 CFU/mL refute this diagnosis. Verification of false-positive and false-negative results for pneumonia in studies such as these can be difficult because a gold standard would require histologic evidence.

Several disadvantages are inherent in the PSB technique. A small number of false-positive culture findings may result, even when the threshold of 10^3 CFU/mL is used to separate colonization from true lung infection. In addition, culture results require 24 to 48 hours and therefore cannot be used as a guide for initial treatment. Finally, to avoid false-negative results, the catheter must be placed in the area of true lung involvement, which may sometimes be difficult.

BAL has proved to be very effective in diagnosing pneumonia due to *P. carinii*, with sensitivities ranging from 85 to 97% in patients with AIDS.

Bronchoalveolar lavage (BAL) is a safe technique that, in conjunction with quantitative culture of lavage fluid, has been used to distinguish pneumonia from bacterial colonization of the upper airways in intubated, mechanically ventilated patients. The bronchoscope is wedged in a segment corresponding to the radiographic abnormalities. Physiologic solution (approximately 100 mL) is infused through the bronchoscope into the lung. This differs from bronchial washings, which are obtained through a nonwedged bronchoscope and involve small volumes of fluid. BAL is a very simple and safe technique in an intubated, mechanically ventilated patient. Although the culture of organisms such as *Mycobacterium tuberculosis* and *Legionella* species is diagnostic of infection, quantitative cultures of BAL fluid are probably necessary to distinguish infection from colonization in most other bacterial pneumonias. PSB specimens have been compared with those recovered by BAL in mechanically ventilated patients with nosocomial pneumonia; both procedures provided useful and complementary results. The choice should depend on the personal experience of the bronchoscopist, but generally both can be performed quickly during the same bronchoscopy. BAL may be used for diagnosing fungal pneumonia in intubated, mechanically ventilated immunocompromised patients. Isolation of certain fungal organisms, such as *Histoplasma* species in BAL fluid, may be diagnostic of infection. BAL, however, may be less sensitive than transbronchial biopsy for diagnosing histoplasmosis. *Candida* species frequently colonize the respiratory tract of intubated, mechanically ventilated patients. BAL fluid findings are not sufficiently diagnostic of candidal pneumonia. *Aspergillus* species may colonize the air passages of both normal and immunocompromised hosts without causing infection. Thus, a firm diagnosis of invasive aspergillosis pneumonia requires the demonstration of tissue invasion. At present, however, positive BAL fungal stain or culture findings from an immunocompromised host with prolonged neutropenia and focal infiltrates should warrant the initiation of antifungal therapy. When possible, the patient should have direct biopsy evidence of tissue invasion.

The diagnosis of viral pneumonia may be difficult to make by BAL. Although some clinicians may accept the diagnosis if BAL fluid cultures reveal virus, a more conclusive diagnosis requires characteristic cytopathologic findings, such as the intranuclear inclusions of cytomegalovirus infections. It has been found that viral culture findings from the rapid centrifugation of BAL fluid from 33 bone marrow transplant recipients with pneumonia were positive in 96% of specimens. Confirmatory lung tissue culture results were positive in all cases. The sensitivity of BAL was thus 96%, and the specificity was 100%.

Transbronchial biopsy, which has been used to diagnose pulmonary infection, is generally a safe procedure, particularly if guided by fluoroscopy. Critically ill patients may be more susceptible to bleeding, but this procedure can generally be safely performed if the coagulation study results are normal and the platelet count is above 100,000 cells/mm^3. Mechanical ventilation may add significant risk to the procedure, with pneumothorax and the possibility of tension pneumothorax as potential complications. At least one study has suggested that even mechanically ventilated patients can undergo transbronchial biopsy safely if the procedure is performed cautiously. One of 15 patients in this study suffered a tension pneumothorax. The difference between invasive infectious disease, such as with aspergillosis or other fungal infections, and colonization can be determined with biopsy samples but not by simple lavage.

Fiberoptic bronchoscopy was used in 39 renal allograft patients with fever and new pulmonary infiltrates. Transbronchial biopsy was performed in 17 patients, and specific diagnoses were obtained in nine (53%). In three patients (18%), transbronchial biopsy was the only positive bronchoscopic technique. Transbronchial biopsy has no clear advantage over BAL in many cases. Bronchoscopy is a relatively safe technique when it is carefully applied to critically ill patients.

Open-lung biopsy is occasionally required for definitive diagnosis in mechanically ventilated patients with pulmonary infiltrates. This sensitive and specific technique should be considered in selected patients after nondiagnostic bronchoscopy. A frozen section should be obtained, and the tissue should be thoroughly stained and cultured. In a review of 288 open-lung biopsies from different series of immunocompromised patients, 69% of the biopsies were found to yield a specific diagnosis. In another series, 15 patients with acute leukemia who had neutropenia, pulmonary infiltrates, and fever underwent open-lung biopsy. A specific diagnosis was obtained in six (40%) of the patients: four had fungal disease, and two, recurrent leukemia. Although treatment was modified on the basis of the results, only two patients survived the hospitalization. Similarly, in 83 patients, 84% of whom were considered to be immunocompromised hosts, open-lung biopsy led to a change in therapy in approximately one half of the patients; however, even when a specific diagnosis was achieved, no improvement in survival was guaranteed. This should not be surprising in view of the severity of the underlying disease and the pathogenicity of many pulmonary infections in such patients. Thus, management needs to be individualized.

Invasive diagnostic procedures in AIDS patients merit special attention. Increasing numbers of AIDS patients receive mechanical ventilation for respiratory failure. In the appropriate setting of *P. carinii* pneumonia, BAL alone offers a yield of greater than 90%. When the diagnosis is less clear, transbronchial biopsy may enhance the yield somewhat. In 15 patients with AIDS who underwent bronchial washing, transbronchial lung biopsy, BAL, and open-lung biopsy in the same segment of the

Potential complications of bronchoscopy:

- Bronchospasm
- Arrhythmias
- Pneumothorax
- Hemorrhage

In the seriously ill AIDS patient receiving mechanical ventilation, any additional benefit of transbronchial biopsy may be outweighed by the potential complications.

lung under general anesthesia, the sensitivity of BAL was 73%, whereas transbronchial biopsy was 50% sensitive for diagnosing infection. The combination of the two yielded a sensitivity of 85% for opportunistic infection. This yield was comparable to the 88% yield of open-lung biopsy in these patients. Other investigators have also demonstrated the utility of BAL combined with transbronchial biopsy for diagnosing infection in AIDS patients.

Treatment

Appropriate therapy for pneumonia in the mechanically ventilated patient includes specific treatment, such as the use of intravenous antibiotics, as well as supportive measures, including mechanical ventilation, oxygen therapy, and endotracheal suctioning. Other measures, such as bronchodilator inhalation and aminophylline administration, may improve mucociliary clearance and reduce inflammation. The latter measures are certainly indicated in patients with coexisting obstructive airway disease.

When possible, specific antibiotic therapy should be directed at pathogens that have been determined by Gram's stain and culture, but therapy is often empiric. The choice of drugs depends on the underlying disease, the disease severity, and the local sensitivity patterns (Table 44–4). Gram-negative bacilli are frequent pathogens that must always be addressed when empiric treatment is necessary in the patient with nosocomial pneumonia. Antibiotic coverage should initially be aggressive and should include an extended-spectrum penicillin (e.g., piperacillin), a third-generation cephalosporin (e.g., ceftazidime), or a carbapenem (imipenem-cilastatin), often in combination with an aminoglycoside. The combination of an antipseudomonal penicillin with an aminoglycoside offers adequate coverage for most gram-negative rods, including *Pseudomonas* species, and reasonable anaerobic coverage. Although gram-positive coverage is included, the treatment of *S. aureus* infection may be suboptimal. Such combinations have been considered to be the most appropriate therapy in nosocomial pneumonia, but monotherapy has also been considered. Monotherapy may provide suboptimal coverage for *P.*

TABLE **44–4:** Antibiotic Selection in Nosocomial Pneumonia

Drug Class	Examples	Intravenous Dosage
Cephalosporins	Cefotaxime	2 g q 8 hr
	Ceftriaxone	2 g daily
	Ceftazidime	2 g q 8 hr
Extended-spectrum penicillins	Ticarcillin-clavulanate	3.1 g q 4–6 hr
	Piperacillin	4 g q 6 hr
Carbapenems	Imipenem-cilastatin	500 mg q 6 hr
Fluoroquinolones	Ciprofloxacin	200–400 mg q 12 hr IV
		500–750 mg q 12 hr PO
	Ofloxacin	400 mg q 12 hr
Monobactams	Aztreonam	1–2 g q 8 hr
Glycopeptides	Vancomycin	500–1000 mg q 12 hr
Anaerobic coverage	Clindamycin	300–900 mg q 6–8 hr
	Metronidazole	15-mg/kg loading dose, then 7.5 mg/kg q 6 hr
Aminoglycosides	Gentamicin or tobramycin	1.5 mg/kg loading dose, then 1–3 mg/kg q 8 hr
	Amikacin	15 mg/kg/day

IV, intravenously; PO, orally; q, every.

Adequate peak serum aminoglycoside concentrations may be critical in enhancing therapeutic success in gram-negative pneumonia.

Aztreonam appears to be an excellent alternative for pneumonia that is proven to be gram-negative in etiology. Its narrow spectrum, however, renders it inappropriate as empiric monotherapy for nosocomial pneumonia.

aeruginosa, and the mortality associated with infection with this organism may be significantly higher than that associated with other nosocomial pneumonias. In vitro synergism and enhanced in vivo efficacy have been described for the combination of beta-lactam antibiotics and aminoglycosides. Problems with the aminoglycosides include their propensity to cause renal insufficiency. In addition, they penetrate relatively poorly into infected airways, with concentrations less than 40% of those in serum. The acidic pH of infected secretions may contribute to the inactivation of aminoglycosides.

Aztreonam, a monocyclic beta-lactam compound with excellent activity against gram-negative bacteria, including *Pseudomonas* species, has no significant activity against anaerobic or gram-positive organisms. Although its spectrum is similar to that of the aminoglycosides, it is not associated with significant nephrotoxicity. Aztreonam is not hydrolyzed by most beta-lactamases and may be effective against gram-negative bacteria resistant to penicillin or cephalosporins. Synergistic activity between aztreonam and penicillins or cephalosporins appears to be unusual.

The fluoroquinolones are broad-spectrum antibiotics that include ciprofloxacin and ofloxacin, both of which may be used to treat nosocomial pneumonia. These antibiotics have excellent activity against gram-negative bacteria, including *Pseudomonas* species, and against gram-positive cocci, including both methicillin-sensitive and methicillin-resistant strains of *S. aureus.* Coverage for *S. pneumoniae* and anaerobes is less reliable. A multicenter trial evaluating intravenous ofloxacin followed by oral ofloxacin (400 mg every 12 hours) in 100 patients with nosocomial or community-acquired pneumonia requiring hospitalization resulted in cure or improvement in 71 and 24% of patients, respectively. Failure to respond was seen in only 5% of patients. All 12 of the patients with nosocomial pneumonia responded well. However, the results of this trial cannot necessarily be extrapolated to seriously ill patients with nosocomial pneumonia. Advantages of the fluoroquinolones include their activity against beta-lactamase–producing bacteria, high levels in respiratory tract tissue, and relatively few side effects. These antibiotics can be used in patients who are allergic to penicillin or cephalosporins.

When anaerobic or mixed aerobic and anaerobic nosocomial infection is suspected, empiric treatment with clindamycin or metronidazole may be included, although other broad-spectrum antibiotics, such as piperacillin and imipenem, have excellent anaerobic coverage. Such coverage should be considered when overt aspiration is documented, when periodontal or gingival disease is present, or when severe necrotizing pneumonia is present, particularly with empyema formation.

Double–beta-lactam therapy with an antipseudomonal penicillin combined with a third-generation cephalosporin has been used in an attempt to avoid aminoglycoside toxicity. Because these antibiotics are all broad in spectrum, there appears to be little advantage to combining them, and synergy apparently does not occur. In addition, the use of two beta-lactams at once may stimulate the increased production of beta-lactamases, which could result in the increased emergence of resistant organisms. Aminoglycosides are not affected by these enzymes and do not result in their production. A trial consisting of 200 patients with *P. aeruginosa* bacteremia suggested better survival with an antipseudomonal beta-lactam combined with an aminoglycoside than with a beta-lactam alone. Survival was also enhanced when patients had pneumonia. In patients receiving the single agent, mortality was 88% (seven of eight patients), compared with 35% (seven of 20) in those receiving the combination. Our general approach has been to combine a beta-lactam antibiotic with an aminoglycoside pending sputum and other culture results and to monitor aminoglycoside levels carefully.

In addition to the previously mentioned guidelines, erythromycin (1 g intravenously every 6 hours) should be considered in any patient in whom *Legionella* infection appears to be a possibility. It is probably appropriate to add erythromycin to the regimen in any case in which a patient presents with a severe pneumonia, at least until culture results are available. Vancomycin is useful in the presence of a documented staphylococcal infection, particularly in the presence of possible or documented methicillin-resistant infections. Trimethoprim-sulfamethoxazole has excellent activity against gram-negative enteric bacteria, as well as against other gram-negative organisms, such as *Enterobacter* species, *Acinetobacter* species, *Citrobacter* species, *Pseudomonas cepacia,* and *Pseudomonas maltophilia,* which are often resistant to other antibiotics. This antibiotic has excellent activity against many common community-acquired infections, such as streptococcal pneumonia, *H. influenzae* infection, and *Moraxella catarrhalis* infection. It also is effective against opportunistic infections with organisms such as *P. carinii* or *Nocardia* species. Except when the latter infections are suspected, this antibiotic is generally not used for the empiric treatment of nosocomial pneumonia. Clindamycin and metronidazole exhibit potent activity against anaerobic bacteria. Clindamycin also has very good activity against gram-positive organisms. This drug, combined with an antibiotic with gram-negative coverage, serves as appropriate empiric therapy for nosocomial pneumonia. Nebulized aminoglycosides have been used in the treatment of nosocomial pneumonia, but at least one multicenter trial has failed to show any benefit of endotracheal tobramycin when compared with parenteral therapy. In addition to specific antibiotic treatment, immunotherapy for gram-negative pneumonia is currently being investigated.

The prevention of nosocomial pneumonia is logical to attempt; however, improved outcome in the setting of such measures is not always demonstrated. The topical administration of polymyxin has been shown to reduce oropharyngeal colonization and to decrease the incidence of pneumonia in critically ill patients. However, drug-resistant strains of bacteria have been shown to emerge, and the mortality due to pneumonia when it does develop may be increased. Selective decontamination of the digestive tract with oral and nonabsorbable antibiotics and parenteral cefotaxime has been shown to reduce the number of infections, including respiratory tract infections in intensive care unit patients when compared with controls not receiving prophylaxis. Other trials have supported selective gut decontamination, but in general there has been no documented effect on mortality or the length of intensive care unit stay. Although further studies may more clearly delineate the role of this technique, at present it is not recommended as a routine preventive strategy.

SUMMARY

Community-acquired and nosocomial respiratory tract infections result in substantial morbidity and mortality. The diagnostic approach consists of careful clinical assessment, with radiographic studies and use of the microbiology laboratory. Noninfectious entities may occasionally mimic pulmonary infections. The diagnostic and therapeutic approaches to community-acquired and nosocomial pneumonia are similar in principle; however, because of the complexity of the conditions of hospitalized patients and the increased incidence of gram-negative pathogens, the clinical evaluation may require more invasive measures, and empiric coverage must include a broad range of pathogens in the latter setting. Clinical settings such as infection with HIV, organ transplantation, and chemotherapy with prolonged neutropenia may suggest the need for more aggressive diagnostic and therapeutic interventions. The etiology and pathogenesis of pulmonary infections, the clinical approach to them, and the principles of treatment are presented.

Suggested Readings

Bartlett JG. Anaerobic bacterial infections of the lung. Chest 91:901–909, 1987.

Cockerill FR III, Muller SR, Anhalt JP, et al. Prevention of infection in critically ill patients by selective decontamination of the digestive tract. Ann Intern Med 117:545–553, 1992.

Craven DE, Kunches LM, Lichtenberg DA, et al. Nosocomial infection and fatality in medical and surgical intensive care unit patients. Arch Intern Med 148:1161–1168, 1988.

Driks MR, Craven DE, Celli BR, et al. Nosocomial pneumonia in intubated patients given sucralfate as compared with antacids or histamine type 2 blockers. N Engl J Med 317:1376–1382, 1987.

Edelstein PH. The laboratory diagnosis of legionnaires' disease. Semin Respir Infect 3:235–241, 1987.

Fagon JY, Chastre J, Hence A, et al. Detection of nosocomial lung infection in ventilated patients: Use of a protected specimen brush and quantitative culture techniques in 147 patients. Am Rev Respir Dis 138:110–116, 1988.

Faling LJ. New advances in diagnosing nosocomial pneumonia in intubated patients. I. Am Rev Respir Dis 137:253–255, 1988.

Fang GD, Fine M, Orloff J, et al. New and emerging etiologies for community-acquired pneumonia with implications for therapy: A prospective multicenter study of 359 cases. Medicine 69:307–316, 1990.

Feinsilver SH, Fein AM, Niederman MS, et al. Utility of fiberoptic bronchoscopy in nonresolving pneumonia. Chest 98:1322–1326, 1990.

Gastinne H, Wolff M, Delatour F, et al. A controlled trial in intensive care units of selective decontamination of the digestive tract with nonabsorbable antibiotics. N Engl J Med 326:594–599, 1992.

Grayston JT, Diwan VK, Cooney M, et al. Community- and hospital-acquired pneumonia associated with *Chlamydia* TWAR infection demonstrated serologically. Arch Intern Med 149:169–173, 1989.

Hammond JM, Potgieter PD, Saunders GL, et al. A double blind study of selective decontamination in intensive care. Lancet 340:5–9, 1992.

Harkness G, Bentley D, Roughman K. Risk factors for nosocomial pneumonia. Am J Med 89:457–463, 1990.

Huxley EJ, Viroslav J, Gray WR, Pierce AK. Pharyngeal aspiration in normal adults and patients with depressed consciousness. Am J Med 64:564–568, 1978.

Johanson WG, Pierce AK, Sanford JP. Changing pharyngeal bacterial flora of hospitalized patients. N Engl J Med 281:1137–1140, 1969.

Johanson WG, Pierce AK, Sanford JP, et al. Nosocomial respiratory infections with gram negative bacilli: The significance of colonization of the respiratory tract. Ann Intern Med 77:701–706, 1972.

Matthay RA, Moritz ED. Invasive procedures for diagnosing pulmonary infection: A critical review. Clin Chest Med 2:3–18, 1981.

Stover DE, Zaman MB, Hajdu SI, et al. Bronchoalveolar lavage in the diagnosis of diffuse pulmonary infiltrates in the immunosuppressed host. Ann Intern Med 101:1–7, 1984.

Tapson VF, Fulkerson WJ. Infectious complications of mechanical ventilation. Probl Respir Care 4(1):100–117, 1991.

Wimberly N, Faling JC, Bartlett JG. A fiberoptic bronchoscopy technique to obtain uncontaminated lower airway secretions for bacterial culture. Am Rev Respir Dis 199:337–343, 1979.

Woodhead MA, MacFarlane JT. Comparative clinical and laboratory features of legionella with pneumococcal and mycoplasma pneumonias. Br J Dis Chest 81:133–139, 1987.

45 ○

Aspiration Pneumonia

Amal Jubran, M.D.

Key Terms

Adult Respiratory Distress
Syndrome (ARDS)

Aspiration

Aspiration pneumonia refers to the pulmonary consequence resulting from the abnormal entry of endogenous secretions or exogenous substances into the lower airways. Despite the number of reports concerning aspiration pneumonia, much confusion exists about its clinical description and patient management because many practitioners consider it to be a single entity rather than several distinct syndromes. The various forms of aspiration pneumonia are listed in Table 45–1. This chapter deals primarily with pulmonary aspiration of gastric acid contents and oropharyngeal bacteria and briefly with drowning and near-drowning.

PATHOPHYSIOLOGY

The pathophysiologic mechanisms of the various forms of aspiration pneumonia are based on the nature of the inoculum.

pH and Non-pH Effects

The aspiration of gastric contents into the lung can cause severe pulmonary injury. In the past, the acid in the gastric contents was blamed for the pulmonary injury.[1] However, studies have shown that the aspiration of gastric contents causes initial hypoxemia regardless of the pH.[2] If the inoculum is of a relatively high pH (pH of greater than 5.9) and is free of particulate matter, the initial injury is rapidly reversible, whereas an aspirate with a low pH causes parenchymal damage with inflammation, edema, and hemorrhage. The aspiration of foodstuff alone causes an obliterative bronchiolitis with subsequent granuloma formation. In addition to the nature of the gastric aspirate, the volume is also an important determinant of lung injury. Studies have shown that at least 2 to 4 mL/kg is required to produce significant injury in experimental animals.[3]

Pulmonary injury from the aspiration of gastric contents:

- Hypoxemia
- Increased intrapulmonary shunting
- Diffuse pulmonary infiltrates

The physiologic response to gastric acid aspiration occurs in two stages. The early stage is characterized by a rapid development of atelectasis, which is thought to be secondary to the acid denaturation of surfactant, resulting in a dramatic decrease in arterial oxygen tension (Pa_{O_2}). In the later stage, there is an outpouring of fluid into the lung, with the consequent development of adult respiratory distress syndrome (ARDS). Although there is no evidence to suggest that infection plays a

TABLE **45–1:** Classification of Aspiration Pneumonia

Chemical pneumonitis	Bacterial infection
Gastric acid contents	Oropharyngeal bacteria
Oil	Inert substances
Lipoid pneumonia	Solid particles
Hydrocarbons	Liquids
Meconium	
Noxious gases	
Smoke	

role in the initial insult, the aspiration of gastric contents increases susceptibility to subsequent bacterial pneumonia.[4]

Bland Versus Infected

In addition to gastric contents, the aspirated inoculum may also be composed of oropharyngeal bacteria. The bacteriology of the upper airway is quite complex and varies among the locations in the oral cavity. Bacterial counts are higher in the gingival crevice (10^{11} to 10^{12}/mL) than in saliva (10^8 to 10^9/mL). In addition, the ratio of anaerobic to aerobic forms is different: 1000:1 in the gingival crevice, compared with 3:1 to 5:1 in saliva. Consequently, aspiration pneumonitis occurs at an increased incidence in patients with gingivitis and periodontal disease. Bacteriologic studies of aspiration pneumonia show that most infections involve a polymicrobial flora rather than a single organism.

Three major organisms are responsible for infection:

- Anaerobic streptococci (*Peptostreptococcus* species)
- *Fusobacterium nucleatum*
- *Bacteroides melaninogenicus*[5]

Inert Substances

The aspiration of inert substances does not in most cases cause pulmonary injury; however, it occasionally results in airway obstruction or reflex airway closure.[6]

CLINICAL FEATURES

A definitive diagnosis of aspiration pneumonia is extremely difficult to make unless the event is witnessed or gastric contents are suctioned from the airways. Studies have shown that the aspiration of large volumes causes severe pulmonary disease, with a mortality rate of approximately 30%. In contrast, patients who aspirate small volumes do not develop acute progressive pulmonary disease. Most patients fall between these two extremes; thus, significant morbidity probably results.[7]

The initial presentation of an acute episode of aspiration includes

Poor prognostic factors:

- Older patient age
- The presence of apnea
- Shock
- Severe impairment of gas exchange on initial presentation

- Tachypnea
- Fever
- Diffuse crackles
- Severe hypoxemia
- Possibly an asthma-like reaction

These symptoms are generally evident within 1 hour of witnessed aspiration. In the majority of patients, the initial abnormal chest x-ray findings are not associated with any characteristic picture. The subsequent clinical course takes one of three patterns:[8]

- A minority (12%) show progressive worsening of the clinical and radiographic picture and generally die within 24 hours.
- The majority (62%) show rapid clinical and radiographic improvement.
- The remainder (26%) display a rapid initial improvement followed by clinical deterioration, with new or progressive infiltrates and signs of infection suggestive of a superimposed nosocomial pneumonia.

The development of bacterial pneumonia in patients who aspirate gastric contents is an ominous sign because the mortality rate is threefold greater in patients with infection.[8] The mortality rate in aspiration pneumonia has been variably reported to be from 0 to 100%, but studies employing the strictest diagnostic criteria generally report a mortality rate of about 30%.[9] In addition, approximately 30 to 40% of patients with well-documented aspiration pneumonia develop ARDS, a syndrome associated with a high mortality rate.[10]

Although making a definite distinction between lung infection secondary to the aspiration of oropharyngeal bacteria and pneumonia secondary to the aspiration of gastric acid is not always possible, certain clinical features help to distinguish between these two common causes of aspiration pneumonia. Many patients who aspirate oropharyngeal bacteria have an impaired level of consciousness, dysphagia, periodontal disease, or gingivitis. Microbial identification usually reveals anaerobes.[11] About 90% of these pneumonias are localized to the dependent regions of the lung. If a patient was supine at the time of aspiration, the posterior segments of the upper lobes and the superior segments of the lower lobes are most frequently affected. If the patient was in the upright or semirecumbent position, the basilar segments of the lower lobes are most often involved. The right lung is involved twice as frequently as the left because the right mainstem bronchus takes off more directly. More than one segment is commonly involved.

PREDISPOSITION

The aspiration of oropharyngeal contents during sleep takes place in 45% of healthy subjects and in 70% of patients with depressed consciousness.[12] Tracer studies have also demonstrated that the aspiration of small quantities of pharyngeal contents occurs in 55 to 70% of patients with endotracheal[13] and tracheostomy tubes,[14] despite the fact that these tubes are usually placed for the purpose of preventing aspiration. The aspiration of gastric contents occurs less frequently and rarely causes pulmonary disease. After all, the development of pulmonary damage depends on

- The character and volume of the aspirated material
- The frequency with which aspiration occurs
- The adequacy of the pulmonary defenses in addition to a predisposing condition[9]

Conditions associated with an increased risk of aspiration pneumonia can be classified according to neurologic, gastrointestinal, or pulmonary disorders (Table 45–2). Neurologic dysfunction disrupts the normal

Late complications:

- Lung abscess formation
- Necrotizing pneumonia
- Bronchopleural fistula with empyema formation

TABLE **45–2:** Conditions Predisposing to Aspiration Pneumonia

Neurologic disorders
  Decreased level of consciousness: general anesthesia, drug overdose, alcoholism, stroke, head injury, seizures
  Neurologic disease: pseudobulbar palsy, Parkinson's disease, multiple sclerosis, myasthenia gravis
  Local anesthesia to the pharynx
Gastrointestinal disorders
  Gastric disease: protracted vomiting, delayed gastric emptying, gastric distention (e.g., in diabetes mellitus), sphincter incompetency, bowel obstruction
  Esophageal disease: achalasia, stricture, tumor, diverticulum, tracheoesophageal fistula
Pulmonary disorders
  Impaired mechanical barriers: endotracheal tube, tracheostomy tube, nasogastric tube, incompetent larynx
  Impaired mucociliary clearance and cellular defense mechanisms

swallowing mechanism and impairs protective laryngeal closure and cough reflexes.[15] Studies based on retrospective review of hospital files have shown that a disturbance of consciousness was uniformly present in patients with aspiration pneumonia.[8, 16] The risk of aspiration pneumonia in patients undergoing anesthesia is difficult to ascertain, but aspiration pneumonia is estimated to account for 14% of anesthetic deaths[17] and up to 47% of fatalities associated with obstetric anesthesia.[18] Aspiration pneumonia is estimated to occur in about 6% of patients with stroke and in up to 10% of patients with drug overdose.[19] Gastrointestinal disease resulting in increased intragastric pressure (i.e., protracted vomiting) or volume (i.e., delayed gastric emptying or gastric distention) could place the patient at risk for regurgitation, and therefore for aspiration, by overwhelming the normal protective mechanism of the lower esophageal sphincter.[15] In addition, diseases that impede the antegrade propulsion of material in the esophagus are commonly associated with aspiration. Evidence of aspiration pneumonia has been reported in 8 to 16% of patients with esophageal disease;[7] however, one study reported no significant difference in the incidence of aspiration pneumonia between patients with esophageal disease and control subjects.[20] Pulmonary disease necessitating mechanical ventilation requires the use of tracheostomy or endotracheal tubes, which may interfere with normal glottic closure. These factors predispose to aspiration because crevices may form in the cuffs, thus permitting leakage. In addition, the mass effect of the tube may disrupt the swallowing mechanism. Impaired host defenses—mucociliary clearance and immunologic and cellular defense mechanisms—could predispose to infectious complications.[9]

TREATMENT

Local Therapy

Although vigorous suctioning is often recommended after an episode of aspiration, the rapid distribution of the acid material to the lung periphery, together with the instantaneous nature of the injury, limits its potential value.[5, 16] Solid materials should be removed from the pharynx and the major airways with bronchoscopy to provide an adequate airway.[21] Although tracheobronchial lavage with saline or alkaline solutions has been recommended, this procedure will probably not be helpful because endogenous neutralization occurs within minutes. Indeed, this approach is best avoided because lavage can increase the severity of lung injury.

Antibiotics

Pulmonary infection, a significant determinant of clinical outcome, commonly complicates the aspiration of gastric juice. Unfortunately, controlled, prospective studies examining the role of empiric antibiotic therapy in the acute treatment of gastric aspiration do not exist. However, experience gained from retrospective studies has indicated that prophylactic antibiotic therapy does not decrease the incidence of lung infection or improve clinical outcome; in fact, it may instead promote the growth of drug-resistant organisms.[8, 22] Thus, antibiotics should be withheld until clear clinical, microbiologic, or radiographic evidence of bacterial superinfection is apparent. The diagnosis of infection in this setting is extremely difficult because clinical signs such as fever, leukocytosis, purulent secretions, new or progressive radiographic infiltrates, and pathogenic bacteria in tracheobronchial secretions are not specific for infection. In a study of patients with ARDS, Andrews and colleagues found that the use of such criteria resulted in a high incidence of false-positive and false-negative diagnoses.[23] In addition, the high rate of oropharyngeal colonization in critically ill patients makes it difficult to obtain an accurate bacteriologic diagnosis. The microbiologic examination of expectorated sputum is generally misleading. Invasive techniques such as transtracheal or transthoracic aspiration or bronchoscopy using the plugged telescoping-catheter brush technique are required if an accurate etiologic diagnosis is considered necessary.[9]

Most patients with bacterial superinfection are treated empirically on the basis of expected bacteriologic patterns. The likely pathogen depends on whether the aspiration occurred in the community or the hospital setting.[15] Oral anaerobes are the predominant organisms responsible in patients who have community-acquired aspiration pneumonia,[24] whereas hospitalized patients develop mixed aerobic and anaerobic infection.[25] Clindamycin and an aminoglycoside have been recommended to provide broad-spectrum coverage if a mixed aerobic and anaerobic infection is considered to be likely.

Bacterial lung infection secondary to the aspiration of oropharyngeal bacteria requires optimal drug therapy based on a precise etiologic diagnosis. Because most community-acquired aspiration pneumonias are responsive to penicillin, empiric therapy is usually used in this setting. Suggested dosages range from 2 to 20 MU/day. In the presence of allergy to penicillin, chloramphenicol, clindamycin, and metronidazole are alternatives. In a randomized study of patients with lung abscesses, clindamycin proved to be superior to penicillin.[26] In the hospital setting, pneumonia secondary to the aspiration of oropharyngeal contents usually results from a combination of aerobic and anaerobic organisms. Rather than choosing an antibiotic therapy, obtaining a precise bacteriologic diagnosis with the use of invasive procedures may be preferable in deciding on the optimal therapy.

Prolonged therapy over 2 to 4 months is advisable if complications are present. Delayed resolution with the persistence of a cavity on chest radiography after 4 to 6 weeks is no longer considered to be an indication for surgery because most infections resolve with continued antibiotic therapy.[27] Although its value has not been evaluated, chest physiotherapy is sometimes used to enhance drainage. The value of bronchoscopy in assisting drainage is unknown, but it should be performed to exclude the presence of tumor if resolution is delayed. It should also be considered if a lung abscess is found in an edentulous patient because many of these patients have an underlying bronchial carcinoma.[27]

Corticosteroids

Despite the extensive use of corticosteroids, their value in the management of aspiration pneumonia remains controversial. Although the role of steroids in aspiration pneumonia has been evaluated, most studies contain important methodologic flaws, making it difficult to interpret the results.

Much of the clinical experience has been gained in an uncontrolled manner. In the 50 patients reviewed by Bynum and Pierce, 66% received parenteral steroids.[8] No significant effect was observed on clinical outcome. In a randomized, double-blind trial carried out by Sukumaran and coworkers, methylprednisolone sodium succinate (15 mg/kg/day) was compared with a placebo given intravenously in three divided doses for 3 days.[28] Unfortunately, the diagnosis of aspiration pneumonia was based on a history obtained from the family in 12 of the 60 patients included in the trial. The authors divided the patients into two subgroups: a younger group with drug overdose and an older group with neurologic disorders. Steroid administration in the drug overdose group decreased the time taken for improvement in arterial blood gas measurements and chest x-ray study findings, the duration of intubation and mechanical ventilation, and the length of stay in the intensive care unit, but it had no effect on the incidence of complications or mortality. Even though the administration of steroids increased the rate of improvement of the chest x-ray study results and the arterial blood gas measurements in the elderly neurologic patients, the duration of intensive care unit stay was increased in this group. In a subsequent study of pulmonary function 1 year after the episode of aspiration pneumonia, the authors studied 21 survivors.[29] In these patients, all but one of whom developed aspiration pneumonia secondary to drug overdose, pulmonary function was similar whether steroids or placebo had been administered during the acute episode. Thus, improvements in oxygenation and radiologic appearance during the acute period did not translate into a lower complication rate, a reduced mortality rate, or better long-term functional recovery in young patients with drug overdose. In fact, steroids may adversely affect the course in older patients with neurologic disease. In a randomized study, steroids had no effect on the outcome in patients with ARDS of any etiology.[30] Therefore, the use of corticosteroids in patients with ARDS is no longer recommended; their role in the management of aspiration pneumonia will continue to be controversial.

Supportive Care

General supportive measures are the most important factors in the management of aspiration pneumonia. Adequate oxygenation must be maintained by whatever means—supplemental oxygen, mechanical ventilation, or positive end-expiratory pressure. Although some animal models have shown improved survival with prophylactic mechanical ventilation with positive end-expiratory pressure, an evaluation of 92 patients at risk for developing ARDS (10 of whom had aspiration pneumonia) failed to demonstrate any benefit from the early application of positive end-expiratory pressure.[31]

Support of the intravascular volume should be vigorous because these patients are prone to intravascular volume depletion and noncardiogenic pulmonary edema. Early studies suggested a therapeutic role for albumin in limiting the pulmonary edema secondary to increased pulmonary permeability,[32] but more recent studies have found it to be without benefit.[33, 34]

APPROACH TO PREVENTING ASPIRATION

Considerable attention has been focused on the prevention of aspiration pneumonia in high-risk situations. Simple precautions carried out by the allied health personnel are most important.

Supportive care:

- Oxygenation
- Intravascular volume support

The unconscious patient is placed in a head-down position, is turned onto the side, and has pillows inserted behind the legs. The foot of the bed is raised 6 to 9 inches with the use of wooden blocks. This posture promotes the drainage of vomitus or tracheobronchial secretions in a cephalad direction. Similar precautions should be used in the transport of critically ill patients.[9]

Nasogastric tubes are used in patients who are prone to aspiration in an attempt to keep the stomach free of significant volumes of acid. However, nasogastric tubes may increase the risk of aspiration because the presence of such tubes makes both the upper and the lower esophageal sphincters at least partially incompetent. The use of a nasogastric tube should not provide a false sense of security because many patients with a nasogastric tube in place still die of aspiration pneumonia. If a nasogastric tube is used, its patency and function should be frequently checked. Small-bore tubes, which are useless in the removal of solid food particles, are unreliable even in the drainage of fluid contents. Food or mucus may block the suction holes and allow secretions to accumulate, with risk of aspiration. If the tube is also being used for feeding, the rate of administration should be titrated to that of gastric emptying; otherwise, large quantities will accumulate.

Frequent upper airway suctioning is important in patients who have a tracheostomy or endotracheal tubes. Special care should be exercised whenever the cuff is deflated to minimize the risk of aspirating secretions, which are prone to collect above an inflated cuff.[8]

Patients requiring anesthesia for emergency surgery are at increased risk for aspiration because the time interval between food and liquid ingestion and surgery may not be sufficient. The best approach may be awake endotracheal intubation preceding the induction of general anesthesia. Careful preoperative insertion of a nasogastric tube is also advisable. Alternatively, regional anesthesia may be used, or the rapid induction of anesthesia combined with simultaneous pressure on the cricoid cartilage to protect the airway may be attempted.[35]

Numerous investigators have advocated the use of antacids to reduce gastric pH in the hope of decreasing pulmonary injury if aspiration occurs. The prophylactic use of antacids in preventing aspiration pneumonia may be limited by their delayed onset of action (a particular disadvantage in patients requiring emergency surgery); by the layering of antacid, which causes incomplete mixing with gastric contents; and by the possibility of increasing gastric residual volume.[36] In addition, it is clear that gastric juice, independent of its acid concentration, causes lung injury. If an antacid is used, a nonparticulate agent such as sodium citrate should be chosen because severe pulmonary damage has been associated with the aspiration of a particulate antacid.

Cimetidine, 300 mg orally the night before surgery and a further 300 mg intramuscularly 1 to 3 hours before the induction of anesthesia, has been recommended as an alternative prophylactic approach.[18] In general, it produces an increase in gastric pH and a reduction in gastric residual volume.

Although antacids and cimetidine may be helpful before elective surgery, their value is reduced in the acute emergency situation because both trauma and pain reduce gastric emptying. Metoclopramide (Reglan) may be of value in this setting because it accelerates gastric emptying and increases lower esophageal sphincter tone, thus decreasing the risk of regurgitation. In the setting of obstetric anesthesia, evidence that

Preventing aspiration:
- Head-down position
- Nasogastric tube placement
- Drug therapy
- Endotracheal tube placement
- Suctioning

either antacids or cimetidine reduces mortality from gastric aspiration is lacking.[36]

Many surgical procedures have been used in some patients with intractable aspiration. These procedures include an epiglottic-arytenoid flap operation, glottic closure with suture of the vocal cords, cricopharyngeal myotomy, the injection of Teflon into a paralyzed vocal cord, diversion procedures, and even total laryngectomy.[37] Although experience with these surgical procedures has been obtained in a very small number of patients with aspiration pneumonia, the tracheal diversion procedure is preferred because of its reliability in preventing aspiration, its low morbidity, and its potential for reversibility.[38]

DROWNING AND NEAR-DROWNING

In the United States, drowning, the third leading cause of accidental deaths at all ages, causes 6500 deaths a year.[39] Studies have shown that the survival rate for near-drowning victims who are brought to the hospital is 89%. Considerable confusion exists about various terms used in relation to immersion accidents. *Drowning* is defined as submersion in water that results in death from suffocation, whereas the term *near-drowning* refers to survival, even if temporary, after suffocation resulting from submersion in water.[39]

Pathophysiology

When a person is submerged for a time in water, an initial laryngospasm occurs. Death may occur as a result of asphyxia, without aspiration of water into the lungs. However, the vast majority of drowning victims aspirate water into the lungs when involuntary breathing takes place. This can lead to pulmonary edema and increased intrapulmonary shunting and may finally progress to profound hypoxemia accompanied by a clinical picture identical to that of ARDS.

Salt Water Versus Fresh Water

Fresh water, which is hypotonic relative to blood, causes the movement of fluid across the alveolar-capillary membrane into the blood, leading to transient hypervolemia. Salt water, on the other hand, is hypertonic; it draws water from the circulation into the alveoli, leading to hypovolemia. These changes in the blood volume, however, have been shown to depend on the amount rather than the type of the aspirated fluid.[40] Fortunately, the quantity of aspirated fluid is rarely sufficient to produce clinically significant changes in blood volume.

Clinical Features

Pulmonary Insult

Hypoxemia is the single most important consequence of near-drowning in either fresh water or salt water. Although the pathophysiology is similar for both types of near-drowning, the factors contributing to the hypoxemia may differ. After the aspiration of sea water, arterial hypoxemia results from fluid-filled but perfused alveoli. In freshwater near-drowning, hypoxemia is due to alveolar instability and atelectasis. In either case, a large intrapulmonary shunt results.[41]

Nonpulmonary Problems

Prolonged hypoxia secondary to near-drowning causes a profound disturbance of the central nervous system. The degree of this neurologic dysfunction depends on the duration of hypoxia. Neurologic survival after 40 minutes of cold water immersion has been reported.[42] The mechanism for this prolonged survival in cold water is unknown. The lower water temperature may decrease the basal metabolic rate, thereby protecting the brain and the heart from severe hypoxemia. In addition, cold temperatures (lower than 20°C) may activate the diving reflex, producing bradycardia and severe vasoconstriction.[43] The blood redistributes away from the skin and the splanchnic vessels toward the heart and the brain, thus limiting the hypoxic injury. Metabolic acidosis frequently occurs in the near-drowning patient. The cardiovascular system is remarkably stable in near-drowning, with any alterations usually being attributed to hypoxemia or acid-base imbalance. Electrolyte imbalance and hemoglobin alterations are rarely life threatening for either type of near-drowning. Renal function remains intact in most patients, although albuminuria, hemoglobinuria, and oliguria progressing to acute tubular necrosis have been reported.[44]

Treatment

The major determinants of survival in near-drowning depend on

- The pulmonary insult
- The amount of hypoxic brain damage
- The degree of acidosis

As a result, prompt and effective management of hypoxemia and acidosis is essential. The first step, then, is initiating ventilation for the victim as soon as possible. Mouth-to-mouth resuscitation should be started even in the water if it can be accomplished. Attempts to clear the airway of fluid before rescue breathing is started waste valuable time because near-drowning victims rarely aspirate a large volume of water.[7] Closed-chest compression is required if the patient's pulse is absent, but as a general rule it should not be attempted in water. All surviving victims should be evaluated at a medical facility even if they appear to be normal because a significant number of these patients may have life-threatening hypoxemia, which may not be clinically evident. Supplemental oxygen should be continued until the measurement of Pa_{O_2} indicates a satisfactory level of oxygenation. The need for endotracheal intubation and mechanical ventilation should be determined on an individual basis, and these measures should be provided as indicated. Bronchodilators should be administered to treat bronchospasm, and bicarbonate administration may be necessary to correct metabolic acidosis. Electrolyte disturbances, hemolysis, and renal failure should be treated appropriately. Neither prophylactic antibiotic therapy nor steroid therapy is indicated because neither improves survival rates in these patients.[41] The prognosis is excellent for patients who are conscious on arrival at the emergency room, but it is poor for those in coma.

SUMMARY

Three classifications of aspiration pneumonia exist:

- Chemical pneumonitis
- Bacterial infection
- Inert substances

Many neurologic, gastrointestinal, and pulmonary disorders predispose the patient to aspiration pneumonia. Treatment relies on supportive care and preventive therapy, with some treatments being of questionable value.

Acknowledgment

The author gratefully thanks Dr. Martin Tobin for his helpful comments.

References

1. Mendelson CL. The aspiration of stomach contents into the lung during obstetric anesthesia. Am J Obstet Gynecol 52:191–205, 1946.
2. Schwartz DJ, Wynne JW, Gibbs CP, et al. The pulmonary consequences of aspiration of gastric contents at pH values greater than 2.5. Am Rev Respir Dis 121:119–126, 1980.
3. Greenfield LJ, Singleton RP, McCaffree DR, et al. Pulmonary effects of experimental graded aspiration of hydrochloric acid. Ann Surg 170:74–86, 1969.
4. Johanson WG, Jay SJ, Pierce AK. Bacterial growth in vivo. J Clin Invest 53:1320–1325, 1974.
5. Bartlett JG, Gorbach SL. The triple threat of aspiration pneumonia. Chest 68:560–566, 1975.
6. Bartlett JG. Aspiration pneumonia. In Baum GL, Wolinsky E (eds). Textbook of Pulmonary Diseases. Boston, Little, Brown and Company, 1983, pp 583–593.
7. Tobin MJ. Essentials in Critical Care Medicine. New York, Churchill Livingstone, 1989.
8. Bynum LJ, Pierce AK. Pulmonary aspiration of gastric contents. Am Rev Respir Dis 114:1129–1136, 1976.
9. Tobin MJ. Aspiration pneumonia. In Dantzker DR (ed). Cardiopulmonary Critical Care. Orlando, FL, Grune & Stratton, 1986, pp 629–651.
10. Fowler AA, Hamman RF, Good JY, et al. Adult respiratory distress syndrome. Risk with common predispositions. Ann Intern Med 98:593–597, 1983.
11. Bartlett JG. Anaerobic bacterial infections of the lung. Chest 91:901–909, 1987.
12. Huxley EJ, Virslav J, Gray WR, et al. Pharyngeal aspiration in normal adults and patients with depressed consciousness. Am J Med 64:564–568, 1978.
13. Spray SB, Zuidema GD, Cameron JL. Aspiration pneumonia. Am J Surg 131:701–703, 1976.
14. Cameron JL, Zuidema GD. Aspiration in patients with tracheostomies. Surg Obstet Gynecol 136:68–70, 1973.
15. De Paso WJ. Aspiration pneumonia. Clin Chest Med 12:269–284, 1991.
16. Arms RA, Dines DE, Tinstman TC. Aspiration pneumonia. Chest 65:130–139, 1975.
17. Bannister WK, Sattilaro AJ. Vomiting and aspiration during anesthesia. Anesthesiology 23:251–264, 1962.
18. Hodgkinson R, Glassenberg R, Joyce T, et al. Comparison of cimetidine (Tagamet) with antacid for safety and effectiveness in reducing gastric acidity before elective cesarian section. Anesthesiology 59:86–90, 1983.
19. Aldrich T, Morrison J, Cesario T. Aspiration after overdosage of sedation or hypnotic drugs. South Med J 73:456–458, 1980.
20. Vraney GA, Porkorny C. Pulmonary function in patients with gastroesophageal reflux. Chest 76:678–680, 1979.
21. Jubran A, Greenberg SD, Solomon MD, et al. Aspiration injury due to polyacrylamide. Chest 101:576–578, 1992.
22. Cameron JL, Mitchell WH, Zuidema GD. Aspiration pneumonia: Clinical outcome following documented aspiration. Arch Surg 106:49–53, 1973.
23. Andrews CP, Coalson JJ, Smith JD, et al. Diagnosis of nosocomial bacterial pneumonia in acute, diffuse lung injury. Chest 80:254–258, 1981.

24. Bartlett JG, Gorbach SL, Finegold SM. The bacteriology of aspiration pneumonia. Am J Med 56:206–208, 1974.
25. Bartlett JG, O'Keefe J, Tally FP, et al. The bacteriology of hospital acquired pneumonia. Arch Intern Med 146:868–871, 1986.
26. Levison ME, Mangura CT, Lorber B, et al. Clindamycin compared with penicillin for the treatment of anaerobic lung infection. Ann Intern Med 98:466–471, 1983.
27. Bartlett JG, Gorbach SL, Tally FP, et al. Bacteriology and treatment of primary lung abscesses. Am Rev Respir Dis 109:510–514, 1974.
28. Sukumaran M, Granda MJ, Berger HW, et al. Evaluation of corticosteroid treatment in aspiration of gastric contents. A controlled clinical trial. Mt Sinai J Med 47:335–340, 1980.
29. Lee M, Sukumaran M, Berger HW, et al. Influence of corticosteroid treatment on pulmonary function after recovery from aspiration of gastric contents. Mt Sinai J Med 47:341–346, 1980.
30. Bernard GR, Luce JM, Sprung CL, et al. High dose corticosteroids in patients with the adult respiratory distress syndrome. N Engl J Med 317:1565–1570, 1987.
31. Pepe PE, Hudson LD, Carrico CJ. Early applications of positive end-expiratory pressure in patients at risk for the adult respiratory distress syndrome. N Engl J Med 311:281–286, 1984.
32. Tuong TJ, Bordos D, Benson DW, et al. Aspiration pneumonia: Experimental evaluation of albumin and steroid therapy. Ann Surg 183:179–184, 1976.
33. Nanjo S, Bhattacharga J, Staub N. Concentrated albumin does not affect lung edema formation after acid instillation in the dog. Am Rev Respir Dis 128:884–889, 1983.
34. Peitzman PB, Shires GT, Illner H, et al. Pulmonary acid injury: Effects of positive end-expiratory pressure and crystalloid vs colloid fluid resuscitation. Arch Surg 117:662–668, 1982.
35. Wynne JW, Modell JH. Respiratory aspiration of stomach contents. Ann Intern Med 87:466–474, 1977.
36. Moir DD. Cimetidine, antacids, and pulmonary aspiration. Anesthesiology 59:81–83, 1983.
37. Blitzer A, Krespi YP, Oppenheimer RW, et al. Surgical management of aspiration. Otolaryngol Clin North Am 2:743–758, 1988.
38. Eisele DW, Yarrington CT Jr, Lindeman RC. Indications for the tracheoesophageal diversion procedure and the laryngotracheal separation procedure. Ann Otol Rhinol Laryngol 97:471–475, 1988.
39. Shaw KN, Briede CA. Submersion injuries. Drowning and near-drowning. Emerg Clin North Am 7:355–370, 1989.
40. Modell JH, Davis JH. Electrolyte changes in human drowning victims. Anesthesiology 30:414–420, 1969.
41. Modell JH, Graves SA, Ketover A. Clinical course of 91 consecutive near-drowning victims. Chest 30:231–238, 1976.
42. Siebke H, Rod T, Breivik H, et al. Survival after 40 minutes' submersion without cerebral sequelae. Lancet 1:1275–1277, 1975.
43. Gooden BA. Drowning and the diving reflex in man. Med J Aust 2:583–587, 1972.
44. Modell JH. The biology of drowning. Annu Rev Med 29:1–8, 1978.

46

⬛

Key Terms

Barrier Function

Bronchospasm

Cough

Expectorate

Hyperinflation

Microaspiration

Mucus

Stridor

Cough

Leonard J. Rossoff, M.D.

The clinical approach to cough depends on whether it is being evaluated as a protective mechanism, an index of air pollution, or a sign of disease.[1] Healthy people rarely cough, relying instead on lung macrophage and mucociliary transport systems[2] to eliminate the normal mucus production with entrapped debris and microorganisms.[3, 4] The mucus reaches the oropharynx, where it is usually swallowed, not expectorated. This process, unlike cough, rarely reaches the level of consciousness. In the absence of respiratory disease, cough's major role is the elimination of secretions and particulate matter that have somehow bypassed the normal barrier function of the oropharynx. Almost everyone has at some time aspirated fluid or food into the airways; this usually occurs when a person simultaneously attempts to speak, swallows too quickly, or becomes distracted. This results in an effective cough or paroxysm of coughing that eliminates the threat. If the particle, usually food, is large enough and the cough is ineffective, death from asphyxiation may occur in a so-called cafe coronary.[5] The latter is common enough that restaurants are frequently required by law to post signs outlining strategies for the recognition and management of airway emergencies. The normal barrier function may be transiently or permanently impaired (Table 46–1) or overwhelmed. The normal mucociliary transport system also competently deals with the more subtle and frequent "microaspiration" of organism-laden secretions and particulate matter.

PHYSIOLOGY OF COUGH

A cough, whether voluntary or (more commonly) involuntary, usually begins with a rapid inspiration, which is followed by an active forceful contraction of the thoracic and abdominal expiratory muscles, usually against the closed glottis.[6–8] Even as subglottic pressure continues to rise, the glottis suddenly opens with a forceful explosive expulsion of air. The process may even be repeated a number of times during a single expiration until residual volume is approached. In a normal forced expiration, a "maximal" flow rate is achieved at any given lung volume. An effective cough, however, requires an excessive intrathoracic (pleural) pressure, which results in further dynamic compression of the airways[9] and reduction in their diameter. This compression of the airways forces out a small volume of additional gas; more importantly, however, it adds a brief

TABLE **46–1:** Some Common Causes of Altered Barrier Function

Impaired Barrier	Overloaded Barrier
Alcohol	Nausea and vomiting
Drugs	Gastroesophageal reflux
Seizure	Esophageal dysmotility
Coma	Diverticulitis
Topical anesthetics	Tracheoesophageal fistula
Bulbar dysfunction (stroke, Parkinson's disease)	Bowel obstruction
Instrumentation (bronchoscopy, suction)	Instrumentation (nasogastric tube)
Endotracheal tubes	

spike of supramaximal linear flow (peak flow transient) above the normal "maximal" flow in the compressed segment (Fig. 46–1). The posterior membranous portion of the major airways collapses inward, virtually obliterating the lumen, which allows a dramatic increase in the linear rate of flow with no great change in the volume rate of flow.[10] This increased velocity and kinetic energy of the air stream result in the shearing forces required to expel material from the airways.

Closure of the glottis, however, allows higher peak pressures to be achieved at higher lung volumes, resulting in a more effective cough. The major objective of the cough is to move mucus through the tracheobronchial tree toward the mouth. In fact, when compared therapeutically with postural drainage, voluntary cough produced the greater increase in total lung clearance.[11, 12] At these extremely high flow rates, usually achieved only in the larger central airways, mucus is blown off the surface of the mucosa to produce plugs or aerosols. This is the cough that is viewed by patient and clinician to be the "effective" one. However, at somewhat lower flow rates, gas (air) couples with liquid (mucus) to produce a two-phase gas-liquid flow. A "slug" flow of mucus progresses to a wave-like annular flow as flow rates increase. Even at the tidal flow rates of a spontaneously or mechanically ventilated patient, annular flow may be achieved, moving mucus up into the central airways.[13] This mucus and entrapped debris may then be expelled by a cough or removed by a suction catheter. The rheology or stickiness of the mucus, particularly in patients with pulmonary disease such as asthma, bronchitis, or cystic fibrosis, may render the cough less efficient.

Glottic closure is not absolutely necessary for cough;[9] hence an intubated or tracheostomized patient can cough effectively.

COUGH: A REFLEX DEFENSE MECHANISM

An effective cough requires the development of an appropriately timed high expiratory airflow that has an impact on mucus or foreign material. The effectiveness of the cough depends on the integrity of the cough mechanism and the nature of the material to be propelled. In many pulmonary diseases, both may be adversely altered. In chronic airway diseases (e.g., bronchitis, asthma, and cystic fibrosis), mucus may

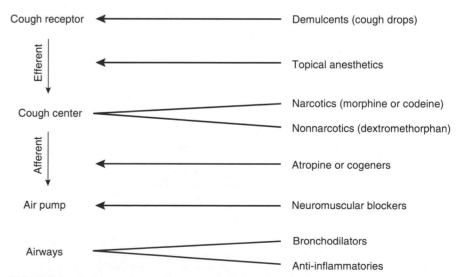

FIGURE 46–1: Antitussives in the interruption of the cough reflex.

be excessive or highly viscid, and patients may have a disadvantaged air pump unable to achieve high flow rates.

The cough mechanism is composed of the air pump and its neural control and integration. The air pump consists mainly of the expiratory musculature and its attachment to the bony-cartilaginous thorax, large and small conducting airways, and glottis. The principal neural components are the cough receptors, afferent nerves, medullary cough center, and efferent nerves. In humans, the cough receptors are located in decreasing concentration from the larynx to the trachea, the carina, and the larger central bronchi.[6–10] These front-line locations are easily comprehensible, but receptors are also located at other thoracic and extrathoracic sites (Table 46–2). The major afferents impinging on the medullary cough center are in the vagus. The vagus also transmits from the pleura, the stomach, and the auditory canal.

INEFFECTIVE COUGH: A COMPROMISED REFLEX DEFENSE MECHANISM

A survey of the linked components of the cough mechanism (Table 46–3) revealed that the ability to mount an effective cough can be compromised at many different levels. Later, this chapter examines pathologic changes in these same components that can result in persistent coughing as a sign of the underlying disease. Possibly the most common disruption of cough receptors' function occurs with the application of topical or regional anesthetics, as in dentistry.[14] This anesthetic may represent a triple threat. It may interfere with the normal reflex physiology of swallowing, simultaneously disrupting normal barrier function (epiglottis and glottis) as well as the "back-up" cough. Patients who receive such anesthetics are thus frequently instructed not to eat or drink for several hours. Even then, normal oropharyngeal secretions (saliva) with microorganisms may be aspirated into the tracheobronchial tree and the lung. An increased risk of aspiration pneumonia has been recognized in these patients.[15]

Alcohol, narcotics, and other drugs can suppress activity in the medullary cough center. The problem, especially with narcotics, may be further compounded by their inducing nausea and vomiting. Patients with strokes, particularly if they are bilateral,[16, 17] are similarly at high risk for both aspiration and ineffective cough.

The inability of the air pump to generate airflows high enough for an effective cough may occur in several ways (see Table 46–3). The efferents to the pump may be disrupted, as with a polyneuropathy (e.g., Guillain-Barré syndrome), spinal cord tumor, or trauma. The interface of nerve to muscle of the air pump (i.e., the myoneural [neuromuscular] junction) may also be affected, as in myasthenia gravis[18] or the use of

The major afferent is the vagus nerve. Other afferents include the trigeminal nerve (nose and sinuses), the glossopharyngeal nerve (pharynx), the phrenic nerve (diaphragm), and the spinal nerve (accessory muscles).

TABLE **46–2:** Locations of Cough Receptors

Thoracic	Extrathoracic
Trachea	Nose
Bronchi	Sinuses
Pleura	Pharynx
Diaphragm	Larynx
Pericardium	Outer ear
	Stomach

TABLE **46–3:** An "Anatomic" Approach to Some Causes of Failure of the Cough Mechanism

Site	Cause
Cough receptor	Topical anesthetic
	Chronic inflammation
Medullary cough center	Anesthesia
	Narcotics or cogeners
	Alcohol
	Stroke
Upper motor neuron	Hemiplegia
	Quadriplegia
	Extrapyramidal disorder
Lower motor neuron	Poliomyelitis
	Amyotrophic lateral sclerosis
	Werdnig-Hoffmann disease
	Postpolio syndrome
Peripheral neurons	Landry-Guillain-Barré syndrome
	Porphyria
	Toxins
	Surgery, trauma, or tumor
	Other polyneuropathies (lupus)
	Critical illness polyneuropathy
Neuromuscular junction	Myasthenia gravis
	Eaton-Lambert syndrome
	Botulism
	Organophosphate poisoning
	Insect bite (tick, black widow spider)
	Drugs
Respiratory muscle	Polymyositis
	Muscular dystrophies
	Acid maltase deficiency
	Carnitine palmitoyl transferase deficiency
	Electrolyte abnormalities
	Corticosteroids
	Malnutrition
Thorax	Obesity
	Kyphoscoliosis or deformity
	Trauma
	Cutaneous disease (burn, scleroderma)
Upper airways	Foreign body
	Epiglottitis
	Trauma
	Vocal cord paralysis
	Edema
	Tumor
	Tracheomalacia or stenosis
	Extrinsic compression (thyroid or tumor)
	Asthma
Small airways/lung	Bronchitis
	Emphysema
	Asthma
	Bronchiectasis
	Pneumonia
	Pulmonary fibrosis
	Edema

curare-like drugs. In addition, unintended neuromuscular blocking properties[19, 20] have been demonstrated in many routinely used drugs (Table 46–4). Congenital and acquired diseases of the muscle[21] can also result in an air pump that is unable to generate an effective cough. Most conditions are unrelentingly progressive, but some are reversible, as is seen with the use of corticosteroids, thyroid disease, and electrolyte abnormalities such as hypophosphatemia.[22] The integrity of the bony-cartilaginous thorax may also be compromised, deformed by acquired conditions (rib fractures) or congenital disease (kyphoscoliosis). With trauma, whole sections of the rib cage may be partially detached, causing a para-

TABLE **46–4:** Some Drugs That May Interfere With Neuromuscular Transmission

Antimicrobials	Psychotropics and Anticonvulsants	Other Agents
Ampicillin	Lithium	Iodinated contrast
Aminoglycosides	Amitriptyline	Amantadine
Tetracycline	Amphetamines	Diphenhydramine
Colistin	Promazine	Emetine
Neomycin	Chlorpromazine	Pindolol
Polymyxin B	Properidol	Sotalol
	Haloperidol	Chloroquine
Cardiac Drugs	Imipramine	D-Penicillamine
Calcium antagonists	Paraldehyde	Oxytocin
Lidocaine	Trichlorethanol	Methoxyflurane
Quinidine	Phenytoin	Tetanus antitoxin
Trimethaphan	Ethosuximide	Adrenocorticotropic hormone
Procainamide		Corticosteroids
Propranolol		Thyroid hormone

Adapted from Argov Z, Mastaeylia FL. Disorders of neuromuscular transmission caused by drugs. N Engl J Med 301:409–413, 1979.

doxical or "flail" movement. Splinting, with the pain of trauma or chest and abdominal surgery, may prevent an effective cough, resulting in atelectasis and pneumonia.[23, 24] The air pump may be restricted by cutaneous disease, such as scleroderma, or scarring from a serious burn. Many different diseases may result in a thickening of the lining of the lung (pleura), the accumulation of pleural fluid, or both.

Adequate airflow in the larger or upper airways may be diminished by paralyzed vocal cords or a glottis and trachea narrowed by edema, inflammation, tumor, or foreign bodies. The removal of an endotracheal tube may result acutely in obstruction, usually because of edema in and around the glottis. The patient may make a characteristic inspiratory noise, or stridor. Delayed complications of endotracheal and tracheostomy tube use include healing with stenosis of the trachea, usually noted weeks to months after decannulation. A loss of elastic recoil of the lung in emphysema and diseases of the more peripheral or smaller airways also reduces airflow and hence effective coughing. The mechanism may be largely or partially reversible, as with spasm of the encircling smooth muscle (bronchospasm), edema, and the inflammation characteristic of asthma. The airways may be permanently narrowed by scarring (bronchitis) or severely deformed (bronchiectasis). Unfortunately, these diseases are also associated with the excessive production of viscid mucus and extensive dysfunction of the normal mucociliary escalator.

Any disease of the lung parenchyma, whether characterized on lung function testing as obstructive or restrictive, can become severe enough to impair an effective cough.

COUGH: AN INDEX OF AIR POLLUTION

The previous discussion largely focused on cough as a defense mechanism. The protection was viewed as being largely directed against the intrusion of ingested food and liquids, as well as normal secretions. Cough can also be viewed as a sentinel of air pollution and may allow retreat from or avoidance of further exposure. Table 46–5 lists some of these pollutants, which may be a consequence of habits that are hard to break (tobacco smoke), of living in an industrial society (sulfur oxides), or of the natural world (pollen). Significant exposure may result in damage to the respiratory system from inflammation (bronchiolitis, bronchoconstriction, or edema), fibrosis, or cancer. The major burden frequently falls on those with pre-existing cardiopulmonary diseases.

TABLE **46–5:**   Some Inhaled Pollutants Resulting in Cough

Tobacco smoke	Oxides of nitrogen
Sulfur oxides	Allergens
Ozone	Airway cooling

COUGH: A SIGN OF DISEASE

The clinician most commonly confronts cough as a symptom or sign of disease. A recollection of the locations of cough receptors and the anatomy of the cough mechanism provides a framework for understanding diseases provoking cough. Table 46–6 lists some of the diseases associated with cough by "anatomic" location. Any such listing is by definition simultaneously incomplete and yet so extensive as to be of limited clinical usefulness. Fortunately, the small number of illnesses likely to be responsible for most cases of cough can be identified by a reasonable clinical approach.[25–27]

History

The history, by far the most important facet of the evaluation of pathologic cough, usually establishes the most probable etiology or at least focuses the physical examination and laboratory investigation.

TABLE **46–6:**   Some Causes of Cough: An "Anatomic" Approach

Site	Cause
Central nervous system	Psychogenic
	Gilles de la Tourette's syndrome
Cough receptors	
Exogenous irritants	Tobacco smoke
	Environmental pollutants
	Occupational exposure
	Allergens
	Foreign body
	Postinfectious hyperreactivity
Endogenous irritants	Postnasal drip
	Gastroesophageal reflux
	Aspiration
	Otitis
	Pleuropericarditis
	Diaphragmatic irritation
Nasopharynx	Rhinitis
	Sinusitis
	Pharyngitis
	Epiglottitis
	Redundant uvula
	Tonsillar enlargement
	Neoplasm
Airways and lung	Asthma
	Hypersensitivity pneumonitis
	Tracheobronchitis
	Chronic obstructive lung disease
	Pneumonia
	Bronchiolitis
	Bronchiectasis
	Drug reaction
	Alveolitis or fibrosis
	Vasculitis
	Neoplasm
	Heart failure
	Others

TABLE **46–7:**   Some Common Causes of Acute and Chronic Cough

Acute	Chronic
Laryngitis	Postnasal drip
Tracheitis	Bronchitis
Bronchitis	Asthma
Bronchiolitis	Bronchiectasis
Pneumonia	Gastroesophageal reflux
Aspiration	Endobronchial tumor
	Restrictive lung disease

Acute or Chronic

Most patients defer medical investigation of their cough unless it becomes chronic or includes another alarming feature. Acute cough (Table 46–7), which is most commonly related to a respiratory tract infection or "cold," is usually self-medicated with a wide variety of over-the-counter medications and folk remedies. Alarming features would include high fever, persistent chills or rigors, purulent sputum, hemoptysis or significant chest pain, and dyspnea. In the absence of these features, clinical help is sought only if the cough worsens or fails to resolve after weeks to months. Cigarette smokers cough frequently but rarely complain unless new symptoms appear. Many times friends and family encourage a smoker to seek help.

In persistent cases in which infection is hard to pinpoint, it must be remembered that many noninfectious inflammatory diseases result in dyspnea, fever, and cough (Table 46–8).

Character and Quality of Cough

An experienced clinician can frequently assess the anatomic location of the cough pathology by virtue of its character or quality and associated features. A bacterial epiglottitis may result in a "barking" cough, and children with *Haemophilus influenzae* infection may have a characteristic "whooping" cough. In adults, there is frequently an associated hoarseness and inability to raise one's voice, with occasional dysphagia, dysp-

TABLE **46–8:**   Some Noninfectious Inflammatory Diseases Causing Dyspnea, Fever, and Cough

Immunologic	**Edema**
Vasculitis or connective tissue disease	Heart failure
Churg-Strauss syndrome	Volume overload
Periarteritis nodosa	Noncardiac disease (adult respiratory distress
Wegener's granulomatosis	syndrome)
Eosinophilic granuloma	**Inhalational**
Goodpasture's syndrome	Berylliosis
Lymphomatoid granulomatosis	Hard metal
Sarcoidal angiitis	Mycotoxicosis
Lupus erythematosus	Drug
Scleroderma	**Traumatic**
Polymyositis	Contusion
Rheumatoid arthritis	Torsion
Bronchopulmonary aspergillosis	Laceration
Hypersensitivity pneumonitis	**Other**
Drug Toxicity	Sarcoidosis
Neoplasia	Aspiration pneumonitis
Bronchioloalveolar carcinoma	Radiation
Lymphoma	Lipoid pneumonia
Lymphangitic carcinomatosis	Eosinophilic pneumonias
Embolic or Thrombotic	Amyloid
Thromboembolic disease	Atelectasis
Fat embolism	Hemorrhage
Amniotic fluid embolism	Lymphocytic interstitial pneumonitis
Sickle cell disease	
Hemagglutination	

nea, and stridor. A "brassy" cough is usually associated with acute tracheobronchitis or chronic smoking and uncommonly with extrinsic compression of the central tracheobronchial tree by a mediastinal mass. A mild "hacking" or throat-clearing cough often suggests a postnasal drip, which is not always detected by the patient, and an associated rhinorrhea or sinusitis. A "stacatto" cough or short, rapid burst of coughing has been described in acute bronchiolitis. An associated intermittent "wheeze" may point to asthma or chronic bronchitis.

Timing and Frequency of Cough

The frequency of cough is usually widely variable and rarely helpful. A young adult with a cold may cough as frequently as once a minute.[28] Cough intensity[29] is quantitatively difficult to assess but probably relates to complications (Table 46–9). An infectious etiology may be suspected if the patient is one of many with similar complaints in a community in which a specific microorganism has been implicated. The time of year may also suggest the pathogen (Table 46–10). This may provide a presumptive diagnosis precluding a detailed investigation. A seasonal variation of a cough may be related to allergic rhinitis and asthma. A relationship to large meals may suggest gastroesophageal reflux, especially if coughing is associated with heartburn and a sour taste in the mouth. An esophageal fistula, a diverticulum, a hiatal hernia, achalasia, or esophageal tumors should also be suspect. Nocturnal coughing may suggest congestive heart failure, especially if coughing is associated with angina, orthopnea, paroxysmal nocturnal dyspnea, or dependent edema. Postnasal dripping is frequently immediately aggravated by the assumption of the supine position. Early morning awakenings (2:00 to 6:00 A.M.) and nocturnal worsening of asthma[30, 31] with cough and allergic rhinitis[32] are well documented. There is even evidence that gastroesophageal reflux, worse at night, may provoke asthma.[33] Rarely, cough may be associated with a specific body position, suggesting a lung abscess or a localized area of bronchiectasis. Recurrent cough (Table 46–11) associated with pneumonia may suggest an underlying disease and the need for investigation.

Sputum Production

The quality of the sputum (if produced) can suggest the underlying cause of cough. Thick, tenacious white sputum may indicate asthma. Purulent, malodorous sputum usually suggests infection. "Rusty" spu-

TABLE **46–9:** Some Complications of Cough

Barotrauma	**Musculoskeletal**
Pneumothorax	Rib fracture
Pneumomediastinum	Vertebral fracture
Pneumopericardium	Ruptured rectus abdominis
Ruptured eardrum	Ventral or inguinal hernia
Cardiovascular	Surgical wound dehiscence
Syncope	Ruptured frenulum
Pulmonary edema	Hoarseness
Ruptured submucosal (nasal and anal) veins	**Other**
Hemorrhoids	Urinary incontinence
Ruptured gastric artery	Psychological distress
Bradycardia and heart block	Headache
	Sleep deprivation
	Mallory-Weiss syndrome
	Emesis

TABLE **46–10:** Seasonal Prevalence of Organisms Commonly Causing Lower
Respiratory Tract Infections in Temperate Climates

Influenza virus	Late fall to winter
Parainfluenza 3	Fall to spring
Parainfluenza 1 and 2	Fall
Respiratory syncytial virus	Winter to early spring
Mycoplasma pneumoniae	Fall to winter
Streptococcus pneumoniae	Winter to early spring

tum has been associated with *Streptococcus pneumoniae* infection; "cur-rant jelly" sputum, with *Klebsiella pneumoniae* infection; "apple green" sputum, with *H. influenzae* infection; and foul-smelling sputum, with anaerobic bacterial infections. A nonproductive cough is much more fre-quent in viral, mycoplasmal, *Pneumocystis carinii,* and *Legionella* infec-tions. A very large volume of sputum may suggest bronchiectasis or lung abscess. Hemoptysis is most frequently associated with a lower respira-tory tract infection (bronchitis), especially if it is associated with puru-lence, but it may signal a malignancy or another serious process (Table 46–12). In the face of a nonmassive bleed[34] and normal chest radio-graphic findings, particularly if fiberoptic bronchoscopy is unrevealing, the cough and hemoptysis will most likely spontaneously resolve without a diagnosis ever being made.[35]

TABLE **46–11:** Diseases Associated With Recurrent Pneumonia

Respiratory	**Neurologic**
Diffuse airway disease	Seizures
Chronic bronchitis	Bulbar dysfunction
Bronchiectasis	**Drug**
Cystic fibrosis	Alcohol
Asthma	Narcotic analgesics
Ciliary dysmotility syndromes	Sedatives
Focal airway disease	Tranquilizers
Bronchogenic carcinoma	**Immune Deficiency**
Carcinoid	Primary
Endobronchial metastasis	B cell
Broncholithiasis	T cell
Foreign body	Complement
Extrabronchial compression (neoplasm,	Phagocytosis
adenopathy)	Secondary
Tracheobronchial fracture	Acquired immunodeficiency syndrome
Endotracheal or tracheostomy tube	Immunosuppressive drugs and sera
Air pump dysfunction	Steroids
Kyphoscoliosis	**Other**
Chest or rib fracture or splinting	Diabetes mellitus
Neuromuscular disorders	Renal failure
Quadriplegia	Sickle cell disease
Other	Multiple antibiotics
Sequestration	Multiple-organ failure
Bronchogenic cyst	Stress
Fibrocystic disease	Burns
Pulmonary Edema	Trauma
Cardiac	Ventilator dependence
Noncardiac (adult respiratory distress	Endotracheal or tracheostomy tubes
syndrome)	
Gastrointestinal	
Bulbar dysfunction	
Motility disorders	
Reflux or emesis	
Tracheoesophageal fistula	
Diverticulum	
Achalasia	

TABLE **46–12:**   Some Causes of Cough and Hemoptysis

Bronchitis	Bleeding diathesis
Bronchiectasis	Congestive heart failure
Lung abscess	Tuberculosis
Necrotizing pneumonia	Mycetoma

Drug History

A history of cough is incomplete unless it includes a detailed drug history,[36] particularly if the previous functional inquiry is unrevealing. As shown earlier, drugs may compromise barrier function (see Table 46–1), resulting in cough, or inhibit an effective cough (see Table 46–3). Drugs may themselves produce pulmonary disease. The mechanism is often poorly understood, and cough is frequently the cardinal sign. It may be idiosyncratic or predictably dose related; it may be an allergic or hypersensitivity reaction but more frequently is not.[37] Regardless of the mechanism of injury, the pattern of clinical presentation is usually a syndrome of chronic pulmonary fibrosis or pneumonitis, acute hypersensitivity pneumonitis, or pulmonary edema. A nonproductive cough is the rule, and its recognition as drug related may prevent unnecessary investigation and treatment. The drug should be discontinued, with the substitution of an alternative medication as indicated. Some of the drugs implicated in lung injury and cough are listed in Table 46–13 on the basis of their therapeutic categories.

Occupational History

> Regardless of the pathogenesis, occupational airway disorders most frequently present with cough as the sole or predominant symptom.

Occupational airway diseases are being reported with an ever-increasing list of agents.[38] The presumed mechanism may be immunologic, as in occupational asthma[39, 40] and allergic alveolitis,[41] or the condition may be a nonatopic reactive airway disease.[42] It may result from nonspecific irritation and inflammation, as in industrial bronchitis,[43] bronchiolitis obliterans,[44] or other disorders such as adult respiratory distress syndrome.[45] There may be associated symptoms, such as wheezing and dyspnea. The diagnosis is usually suspected when the cough is clearly work related, with evidence of exposures to a known pathogen. Unfortunately, the diagnosis may be confounded by concurrent tobacco smoking and atopy.

Physical Examination

> Evidence of air trapping or hyperinflation:
>
> - Barrel chest
> - Limited diaphragmatic excursion
> - Cardiac impulse displaced toward the xiphoid
>
> Evidence of right-sided heart failure:
>
> - Jugular venous distention
> - Hepatojugular reflux
> - Dependent edema

The history and physical examination are the two most important components of the cough investigation and frequently result in a specific etiologic diagnosis. The patient may present with tachypnea, a typical body habitus (leaning forward, elbows on table), and the use of accessory muscles characteristic of chronic bronchitis and emphysema. Nicotine staining of the teeth and fingers and evidence of air trapping or hyperinflation may provide additional confirmation. Bilateral wheezes and hyperinflation associated with prolonged expiration may indicate acute and chronic airflow limitation, whereas a unilateral wheeze and a contralateral tracheal and mediastinal shift suggest a foreign body. A cardiac gallop, bibasilar crackles, and evidence of right-sided heart failure may suggest heart failure. Fine bibasilar, gravity-dependent crackles with a "Velcro" or "cellophane" quality suggest an interstitial lung disease. Evi-

TABLE **46–13:** Drugs Implicated in Lung Injury and Cough

Chemotherapeutic		Immunosuppressants
Cytotoxic	Noncytotoxic	Cyclosporine
Azathioprine	Methotrexate sodium	Interleukin-2
Bleomycin sulfate	Cytosine arabinoside	
Busulfan	Bleomycin	
Chlorambucil	Vinblastine	
Cyclophosphamide		
Etoposide		
Melphalan		
Mitomycin		
Nitrosoureas		
Procarbazine		
hydrochloride		
Vinblastine		

Cardiovascular	Other	Inhalants
Amiodarone hydrochloride	Bromocriptine mesylate	Oxygen
Angiotensin-converting	Dantrolene sodium	Beta-agonists
enzyme inhibitors	Fat emulsions	Cromolyn
Anticoagulants	Methysergide maleate	Pentamidine
Beta-antagonists	Oral contraceptives	Acetylcysteine
Dipyridamole	Tocolytics	Magnesium silicate (talc)
Epinephrine	Tricyclics	Hashish
Fibrinolytics	Calcium	Marijuana
Protamine sulfate	Radiation	Glue
Tocainide hydrochloride	Pituitary snuff	Paint thinner
Hydrochlorothiazide	Hydantoins	Butane
Procainamide	Contrast	Paraquat

Anti-inflammatory	Antimicrobials	Sedative Analgesics and Narcotics
Acetylsalicylic acid	Amphotericin	Ethchlorvynol
Corticosteroids	Nitrofurantoin	Heroin
Gold salts	Sulfasalazine	Methadone hydrochloride
Nonsteroidals	Sulfonamide	Naloxone hydrochloride
Penicillamine	Aminoglycosides or	Propoxyphene hydrochloride
	polymyxin	
	Para-aminosalicylic acid	Cocaine
		Benzodiazepines
		Glutethimide
		Paraldehyde
		Phenobarbital
		Amphetamines

dence of sepsis and consolidation may indicate pneumonia. Clubbing, hypertrophic pulmonary osteoarthropathy, and other paraneoplastic findings may suggest an underlying neoplasm. A basic but comprehensive ear, nose, and throat examination is frequently pivotal. Nasal polyposis, aspirin intolerance associated with wheezing, and dyspnea suggest a nonatopic "adult-onset" asthma. A witnessed paroxysm of coughing after the patient drinks a glass of water may suggest a propensity to aspiration. Several clues point to postnasal dripping as the cough etiology.[46, 47] These include conjunctivitis and bruising from eye rubbing (allergic shiner). There may be boggy nasal mucosa, transverse nasal folds (allergic gape), and a witnessed rubbing of the nose (allergic salute). A cobblestone pattern of the mucosa suggesting lymphoid hyperplasia and sinus tenderness may be additional evidence. Impacted cerumen, foreign bodies, and irritation of the eardrum by hair[48] have been reported as causes of cough.[6]

Diagnostic Clinical Approach

If the history and physical examination findings suggest a specific etiology such as a lung neoplasm, pneumonia, or pulmonary fibrosis, an appropriate diagnostic approach evolves. More commonly, a self-limited lower respiratory tract infection or cold is suggested; for this, the most prudent approach is reassurance, observation, symptomatic therapy, and possibly cough suppression. Antibiotics are reserved for a suspected bacterial superinfection or a more typical pneumonia. The cough of tobacco smoking is usually chronic and unnoticed by the patient unless it is exacerbated by a lower respiratory tract infection. The role of antibiotics in these exacerbations is controversial.[49] Frequently, routine chest radiography and a cell count allay fears of a more serious disorder and avoid the need for more costly and invasive investigations. If the cough persists for more than 1 to 2 months and no clear etiology is evident, then a clinical "anatomic" protocol, as suggested by Irwin and coworkers, appears to be reasonable.[27] Even after this interval, a persistent postinfectious cough may still represent the most likely cause, because abnormal bronchial reactivity has been shown to persist for up to 2 months before resolving spontaneously.[50] This approach usually "rounds up" the most common "suspects." The combination of laboratory investigation and a successful therapeutic trial helps to confirm the diagnosis. In the absence of specific clinical clues, which are usually provided by a detailed personal, occupational, family, and drug history or a physical examination, a laboratory investigation is unlikely to be successful. Fiberoptic bronchoscopy only rarely provides a specific etiology in cough in the absence of a specific clinical suspicion.[51]

COMMON CAUSES OF COUGH

In the case of a persistent cough for which there is no evidence of a recent lower respiratory tract infection, 90% of cases are due to one of four causes:[27] postnasal drip, asthma, chronic bronchitis, and gastroesophageal reflux. A single cause was found in 73% of patients, two causes were found in 23%, and three causes were found in 3%.

Table 46–14 gives a detailed summary of some of the clinical and laboratory clues to their diagnosis.

Postnasal Drip

In two prospective studies, Irwin and colleagues found chronic postnasal drip to be the cause of chronic cough in 40% of patients.[6, 26] A recent prospective study suggested a prevalence of 87%.[27a] This may be due to chronic sinusitis, whether perennial and nonallergic ("vasomotor") or allergic. Postnasal drip is suspected with the history (rarely volunteered) of a drip sensation, frequent voice clearing, hoarseness, and a "hacking" cough. Nasopharyngeal swabs and sinus aspirates for culture are rarely helpful.

Asthma

Mild asthma manifesting with cough,[52] or "cough-equivalent asthma," represents about a third of the cases of persistent cough;[26] in more than a quarter, cough is the sole symptom. Asthma should be considered with an appropriate history and with evidence of reversible airflow limitation, gas trapping, and normal or elevated diffusion for

Bronchial provocation includes

- Aerosols of histamine
- Cholinergic drugs such as methacholine
- Antigen
- Industrial irritants
- Cold air

Histamine, cholinergic, and cold air challenges have been standardized with a predetermined decrease from baseline of flow or conductance as an end-point.

TABLE **46–14:** Clinical Features of Some of the Common Causes of Cough

Cause	History	Physical Examination	Laboratory Tests and Findings
Postnasal drip	Drip sensation	Sinus tenderness	Sinus films (Waters' and Towne's views)
	Nasal speech	Periorbital edema	Nasal smears (polyps, eosinophils)
	Frequent throat clearing	Inflamed pharyngeal mucosa	Ultrasonography
	Hoarseness	Cobblestoned pharyngeal mucosa	Indirect laryngoscopy
	Coryza	Nasal polyps	Fiberoptic endoscopy
	Headache	Enlarged tonsils and adenoids	Computed tomography
	Sinus, jaw, or tooth pain	Epiglottic edema	
	Hypo-osmia		
	Worse in the supine position and in the morning		
Asthma	Family history	Rhonchi	Eosinophils (blood or sputum)
	Seasonal	Prolonged expiration	Reversible airflow obstruction
	Atopy	Hyperinflation	DL_{CO} normal or high
	Dyspnea		Bronchoprovocation response
	Wheeze		Normal radiographic findings
	Sticky sputum		
	Nocturnal awakening		
Gastro-esophageal reflux	Heartburn		Barium swallow
	Sour taste		pH probe
	Burping		Fiberoptic endoscopy
	Dysphagia		
	Nocturnal awakening		
Chronic bronchitis	Smoking	Typical body habitus	Lung function
	Perennial	Accessory muscle use	Minimally reversible airflow obstruction
	Dyspnea	Barrel chest	DL_{CO} normal or low
	Excessive sputum	Rhonchi	"Dirty lung" on radiography

DL_{CO}, diffusing capacity of the lung for carbon monoxide.

carbon monoxide on lung function testing. If the results of standard spirometry are normal, exercise testing or bronchial provocation[53] with a variety of inhaled agents may be used.

Gastroesophageal Reflux

Irwin and colleagues found reflux to account for up to 21% of cases of chronic cough, and cough was the sole symptom in 43%.[26] The pathophysiology is uncertain and may include the stimulation by refluxed material of cough receptors in the hypopharynx, larynx, or tracheobronchial tree. It might also provoke bronchoconstriction and nocturnal asthma associated with cough. Alternatively, inflammation of the esophageal mucosa may trigger a vagally mediated cough reflex. Reflux may also be simply a complication of cough or an incidental finding.

Chronic Bronchitis

Even with the improved pathologic descriptions available,[55, 56] the diagnosis of chronic bronchitis is almost purely a clinical one of cough

Suspect reflux with

- Complaints of heartburn
- Atypical chest pain and dysphagia
- Radiographic evidence of reflux of barium
- Symptoms supported by esophagoscopy, scintiscanning, or esophageal pH electrode monitoring

Chronic bronchitis has been defined as "a condition associated with prolonged exposure to nonspecific bronchial irritants accompanied by mucus hypersecretion and certain structural alterations in the bronchi."[26]

and excessive mucus production. In smokers, cough becomes both a sign of disease and possibly the most important mode of mucus clearance.[57] Classically, chronic bronchitis is the expectoration of sputum most days for at least 3 months a year for 2 successive years.[58, 59] Additionally, other causes of cough and sputum, such as asthma and bronchitis, must be excluded. Spirometry may reveal mild to severe minimally reversible or nonreversible airflow obstruction, with a normal to low diffusion to carbon monoxide.

OTHER CAUSES OF COUGH

Neuropsychological Causes

Cough may occasionally be seen in individuals

- As an expression of an anxiety state, particularly if a family member or friend has suffered a serious disorder, such as lung cancer.
- Representing a form of speech pathology or a speech habit. The latter is commonly noted in the normal voids of speech or when conversation is socially suppressed, such as in the theater.
- Associated with a more serious resistant depression, frequently resulting in multiple unsuccessful medical consultations and therapies. The coughing, especially if vigorous, may become self-sustaining by damaging the airway cords or the glottis. Endoscopy may reveal edema and inflammation of these structures, which may be mistaken for the primary process. Suspicion is aroused by a failure of the cough to improve with time or treatment. The cough may be unusually loud, honking, and easily interrupted by speech, and it does not awaken the patient from sleep. The patient frequently seems unconcerned or ambivalent about its investigation.

Cough has been associated rarely with neurologic disorders such as Gilles de la Tourette's syndrome.[6] Increasingly recognized causes of cough resulting in an increased load to and depression of the protective barrier (see Table 46–1) are the neurologic sequelae of conditions such as Parkinson's disease and stroke. As many as one third of stroke patients aspirate on barium swallow,[17, 60] which is usually associated with cough, an abnormal gag reflex, and a delayed swallowing reflex. This risk doubles if the stroke is bilateral.[17] The consequent increased risk of aspiration pneumonia becomes a major factor in morbidity and mortality.

Pneumonia

Pneumonia in the immunocompetent host frequently presents with cough. If the cough is nonproductive and associated with minimal radiographic findings, the pneumonia is referred to as "atypical." Atypical pneumonias are common and suggest a viral, mycoplasmal, chlamydial, or *Legionella* pneumonia. If segmental or lobar radiographic infiltrates and a mucopurulent cough are present, a "typical," usually bilateral pneumonia such as *S. pneumoniae* infection is diagnosed. Recurrent cough and pneumonia should prompt a thorough investigation for an underlying predisposition (see Table 46–11), such as a lung carcinoma.

Lung abscess,[61] which is usually a consequence of the aspiration of secretions, food, or foreign material, is usually associated with impaired or overwhelmed barrier function. It may be associated with a known event such as an alcoholic binge, a drug overdose, the use of an anesthetic, dental work, or a seizure disorder.

Bronchiectasis

The diagnosis of bronchiectasis is suggested by persistent cough, excessive mucopurulent sputum, and occasional, usually transient hemoptysis. The most reliable confirmatory imaging technique appears to be thin-section computed tomography.[67]

Bronchiectasis,[62] or severe irreversible deforming damage to the bronchial wall, may result from several causes. Frequently, the patient has a history compatible with a prior necrotizing pneumonia. Cystic fibrosis, also a form of bronchiectasis, has milder variants of the disease that are increasingly being reported in later life and are confirmed by genetic analysis.[63] Bronchiectasis is also rarely associated with ciliary dysfunction,[64] barrier malfunction, and immune deficiency.[65] A variant of bronchiectasis associated with asthma involves only the proximal airways.[66] This has been described in bronchopulmonary aspergillosis.

Neoplasm

Primary carcinomas of the lung commonly present with cough. Lung carcinoma, the most frequently diagnosed cancer in both sexes,[68] is almost invariably associated with tobacco smoke. Suspicion increases with abnormalities on chest radiography and computed tomography. The etiologic diagnosis may be made at the time of or before surgery with sputum cytology, bronchoscopy, or percutaneous needle biopsy guided by fluoroscopy, computed tomography, or sonography. If a pleural effusion exists, thoracentesis or pleural biopsy is indicated. Thoracoscopy[69] allows direct inspection of most of the pleural surface and significantly improves the diagnostic yield.

TREATMENT OF COUGH

Specific Therapy

Cough is best treated when a specific etiology is identified. A viral respiratory tract infection may require just time and reassurance, whereas a frank pneumonia may require specific antimicrobials. A foreign body in the external ear or the tracheobronchial tree should be removed. A neoplasm or mass should be treated with surgical resection, chemotherapy, or irradiation. The better and more specific the treatment, the more likely the elimination of cough. The latest studies have suggested that an etiologic diagnosis can be made and successful treatment effected in almost all cases.[27]

Rhinitis medicamentosa—shortening durations of benefit with a medication and rebound on discontinuation of the medication.

Postnasal Drip

In postnasal drip, an antibiotic is indicated only if a purulent sinus infection is suspected. A patient with allergic rhinitis might benefit from the avoidance of allergens and the inclusion of an air filtration system.[70] Antihistamines (H_1 antagonists), frequently in conjunction with a decongestant,[71, 72] may be helpful; occasionally, even systemic steroids are useful. Currently, most medications are applied topically by an intranasal route. Topical decongestants, widely sold over the counter, should be restricted to occasional use for several days because they lead to rhinitis medicamentosa.[73] More promising are topically applied glucocorticoids, cromolyn sodium, nedocromil sodium, and ipratropium bromide.[74, 75] Specific immunotherapy[76] is available, although with some risk, including death.[77] Surgery may also play an adjuvant role.[78] Many of these strategies, with the exception of immunotherapy, are useful in nonallergic and vasomotor rhinitis as well. A good response to treatment is an essential part of the diagnosis of postnasal drip because no "gold standard" diagnostic test exists. Postnasal drip may also coincide with other causes of cough (e.g., asthma, gastroesophageal reflux), but initial treatment of it alone may be sufficient.[27a]

Asthma

In the case of cough-equivalent asthma, a good response may be expected with conventional therapy. Emphasis has been placed on the treatment of the inflammatory component, which also appears to play a role in airway hyper-reactivity and damage. The current commonly used bronchodilators and anti-inflammatory agents are listed in Table 46–15, but exciting new agents are now being tested. If possible, factors provoking cough (Table 46–16) should be identified.

Gastroesophageal Reflux

The treatment for gastroesophageal reflux as a cause of cough may simply entail weight reduction, smoking cessation, raising the head of the bed, and instituting an antireflux diet that is high in protein and low in fat and in which snacking is avoided, particularly 2 to 3 hours before retiring.[27] The use of antacids, H_2 receptor antagonists, proton pump inhibitors, sucralfate, anticholinergics, a variety of prostaglandins, and metoclopramide has also been advocated. The success of therapy, however, may not be apparent until the patient has had more than 5 months of continuous treatment.[79] Several surgical antireflux strategies may also be helpful.[80]

Chronic Bronchitis

The definitive treatment of cough in chronic bronchitis is smoking cessation. Many strategies for quitting smoking have been proposed; most have a high failure rate.[81] Strategies for preventing chronic bronchitis, although unproven, may also include influenza and pneumococcal vaccination. The use of bronchodilators and steroids closely resembles their use in asthma, with an emphasis on quaternary anticholineric agents.[82] The use of antibiotics and expectorants is also of unclear value.

Nonspecific Therapy (Cough Suppression)

The role and efficacy of nonspecific antitussive therapy have been reviewed in detail elsewhere.[83, 84] Long-term success is unlikely unless

TABLE **46–15:** Some Drugs Used in the Treatment of Asthma

Bronchodilators	Anti-inflammatories
Beta-adrenergic agonists	Steroids (systemic, inhaled)
Theophylline	Cromolyn sodium
Anticholinergics	Nedocromil sodium
	Others

TABLE **46–16:**   Some Factors That May Provoke Cough-Equivalent Asthma

Viral respiratory infection (respiratory syncytial virus, rhinovirus, influenza virus)
Allergens (dander, mold, dust mites)
Occupational factors (toluene, wood dust, anhydrides)
Exercise (running)
Physical factors (cold, humidity)
Medications (beta-blockers, aspirin, nonsteroidal anti-inflammatory drugs)
Irritants (ozone)
Stress
Nocturnal reflux

the underlying pathophysiology is uncovered or is self-limited. Reasonable indications for cough suppression (Table 46–17) occasionally include the need to avoid or contain cough complications (see Table 46–9), such as lessening the pain of a rib fracture or decreasing hemoptysis in the setting of bronchitis, bronchiectasis, pneumonia, and neoplasm. Cough suppression might also reduce the risk of barotrauma, most commonly pneumothorax, particularly in the mechanically ventilated patient. Paroxysmal cough may also prevent adequate ventilation. Antitussives might diminish the embarrassment of stress incontinence and allow for gainful employment, especially while a patient awaits the benefits of more specific therapy. The interruption of the "cough cycle" (see Fig. 46–1) might also prove to be therapeutically useful by reducing edema and inflammation. In addition, it may play a role in a small subgroup of patients who prove to have a sensitized cough receptor or reflex.[85] Cough suppression is also important during certain diagnostic procedures, such as fiberoptic bronchoscopy; during endotracheal intubation, corneal transplantation, and neurosurgery; and in the case of impending wound dehiscence. Excessive and continuous suppression of the cough reflex, however, may impair barrier functions, diminish the ability to eliminate excessive sputum production, or both.

A review of the previously described cough reflex and mechanism (see Table 46–3) suggests the classification of antitussives and where and how they might work to diminish the frequency and severity of cough. This might include a modification of the stimulus environment of the cough receptor or of the receptors themselves.[83] Antitussives may affect the threshhold, latency,[84] or both of the afferents, the efferents, and the cough center itself. They might also diminish the strength of contraction of the air pump, as well as the diameter and tone of the airways. Proprietary over-the-counter cough preparations or demulcents largely contain sugar, but they have been shown to decrease the frequency and severity of cough,[86] possibly at the level of the cough receptor.[83] Local anesthetics[87] such as lidocaine are also effective, most likely at the level of the afferent limb. Anesthetics are topically applied as a jelly, a spray, an aerosol, or a liquid, usually in preparation for instru-

TABLE **46–17:**   Some Indications for Cough Suppression

Presence of or increased risk of cough complication
Severe hemoptysis
Interruption of the cough cycle
Interference with gainful employment
Awaiting benefit of specific therapy
Decrease the risk of instrumentation or surgery
Postoperative (neurosurgery, cataract surgery, risk of dehiscence)
Cerebral edema
"Bucking" or "fighting" ventilator

TABLE **46–18:** Cough Induction for Sputum Collection

Spontaneous cough (instruction)
Induced cough
    Nebulized sodium chloride
    Nebulized amiloride
    Nebulized acetylcysteine
    Bronchodilators
    Hydration
    Chest physiotherapy
    Postural drainage
    Nasotracheal suction

mentation (bronchoscopy or intubation). Their use in the management of ongoing cough is limited by their transient action and side effects. Opiates, whether narcotics such as morphine or codeine[88] or analogues such as dextromethorphan, are also effective, possibly on the opiate receptors in the medullary cough center. Their side effects are similar at equally effective antitussive doses. Interestingly, they are not in high enough concentration in proprietary cough mixtures to suppress cough reliably.[89] Modified anticholinergic compounds such as ipratropium bromide and glycopyrrolate may exert their antitussive effect at the efferent limb.[90] The use of neuromuscular blocking agents has no role in the spontaneously breathing patient. These agents may be used in mechanically ventilated patients with paroxysms of cough resulting in inadequate ventilation (i.e., "bucking" or "fighting" the ventilator), hemodynamic compromise, or barotrauma.

Cough Induction and Enhancement (Protussive Therapy)

In the clinical setting, therapy may be useful to the patient with an ineffective cough mechanism. This form of cough enhancement or induction (protussive therapy) may include simple instructions on how to cough effectively while minimizing pain and discomfort. Bronchodilators, although used extensively, have not been evaluated specifically in this role. Although the receptors for cough and bronchoconstriction can be separated,[91, 92] their role in patients with and without hyper-reactive airways is unknown. Drugs that enhance the ciliary transport system, mucus rheology, and possibly sputum volume might also be expected to be helpful.

Only aerosolized hypertonic saline in bronchitis[93] and amiloride in cystic fibrosis[94] have systematically demonstrated improvement in mucociliary clearance. Several inhaled agents may be useful in the induction of cough in the collection of a sputum specimen (Table 46–18), but their use in increasing cough frequency has not been explored as a therapeutic strategy.

SUMMARY

In health, cough can be viewed as a sensitive reflex defensive barrier and a sentinel of atmospheric irritants. In illness, it may be both the sign of disease and the only effective mechanism of clearing bronchial secretions. This chapter outlined the physiology of cough and the clinical approach to the identification of a specific etiology and reviewed specific management strategies and methods of cough suppression and induction.

References

1. Loudon RG. Cough: A symptom and a sign. Basics Respir Dis 9:1–6, 1981.
2. Sleigh MA. The nature and action of respiratory tract cilia. *In* Brain JD, Proctor DF, Reid LM (eds). Respiratory Defense Mechanisms—Part I. Lung Biology in Health and Disease, vol 5. New York, Marcel Dekker, 1977, pp 247–288.
3. King M. Mucus and mucociliary clearance. Basics Respir Dis 11:1, 1982.
4. Smaldone GC, Itoh H, Swift DL, et al. Effect of flow-limiting segments and cough on particle deposition and mucociliary clearance in the lung. Am Rev Respir Dis 120:747–758, 1979.
5. Brooks JW. Foreign bodies in the air and food passages. Ann Surg 175:720–732, 1972.
6. Irwin RS, Rosen MJ, Braman SS. Cough: A comprehensive review. Arch Intern Med 137:1186–1191, 1977.
7. Loudon RG, Shaw GB. Mechanisms of cough in normal subjects and in patients with obstructive respiratory disease. Am Rev Respir Dis 96:666–677, 1969.
8. Leith DE. *In* Lenfant C, Brain JD, Proctor DF, et al (eds). Respiratory Defense Mechanisms—Part II. Lung Biology in Health and Disease, vol 5. New York, Marcel Dekker, 1977, p 545.
9. Knudson RJ, Mead J, Knudson DE. Contribution of airway collapse to supramaximal expiratory flows. J Appl Physiol 36:653–667, 1974.
10. Murray JF. The Normal Lung. The Basis for Diagnosis and Treatment of Pulmonary Disease, 2nd ed. Philadelphia, WB Saunders, 1986, p 103.
11. Oldenburg FA Jr, Dolovich MB, Montgomery JM, Newhouse MT. Effects of postural drainage, exercise and cough on mucus clearance in chronic bronchitis. Am Rev Respir Dis 120:739–745, 1979.
12. DeBoeck C, Zinman R. Cough versus chest physiotherapy: A comparison of the acute effects on pulmonary function in patients with cystic fibrosis. Am Rev Respir Dis 129:182–184, 1984.
13. Sackner MA. Cough. *In* Murray JF, Nadel JA (eds). Textbook of Respiratory Medicine, vol 2. Philadelphia, WB Saunders, 1988, p 397.
14. Fuller RW, Jackson DM. Physiology and treatment of cough [Editorial]. Thorax 45:425–430, 1990.
15. Bartlett JG, Gorbach SL. The triple threat of aspiration pneumonia. Chest 68(4):560–566, 1975.
16. Groher ME, Bukatman R. The prevalence of swallowing disorder in two teaching hospitals. Dysphagia 1:3–6, 1986.
17. Horner J, Massey W, Brazer SR. Aspiration in bilateral stroke patients. Neurology 40:1686–1688, 1990.
18. Ringqvist I, Ringqvist T. Respiratory mechanics in untreated myasthenia gravis with special reference to the respiratory forces. Acta Med Scand 190:499–508, 1971.
19. Argov Z, Mastaeylia FL. Disorders of neuromuscular transmission caused by drugs. N Engl J Med 301:409–413, 1979.
20. Hunter JM. Adverse effects of neuromuscular blocking drugs. Br J Anaesth 59:46–60, 1987.
21. Aldrich TK, Aldrich MS. Primary muscle diseases: Respiratory mechanisms and complications. *In* Kanholz SL (ed). Pulmonary Aspects of Neurologic Disease. New York, SP Scientific and Medical Books, 1986.
22. Gravelyn TR, Brophy N, Siegert C, Peters-Golden M. Hypophosphatemia—Associated respiratory muscle weakness in a general inpatient population. Am J Med 84:870–876, 1988.
23. Tisi GM. Preoperative evaluation of pulmonary function: Validity, indications and benefits. Am Rev Respir Dis 119:293–309, 1979.
24. Garibaldi RA, Britt MR, Coleman ML, et al. Risk factors for postoperative pneumonia. Am J Med 70:677–680, 1981.
25. Irwin RS, Rosen MJ, Braman SS. Cough: A comprehensive review. Arch Intern Med 137:1186–1191, 1977.
26. Irwin RS, Corrao WM, Pratter MR. Chronic persistent cough in the adult: The spectrum and frequency of causes and successful outcome of specific therapy. Am Rev Respir Dis 123:413–417, 1981.
27. Irwin RS, Curley FJ, French CL. Chronic cough: The spectrum and frequency of causes, key components of the diagnostic evaluation, and outcome of specific therapy. Am Rev Respir Dis 141:640–647, 1990.
27a. Pratter MR, Bartter T, Akers S, DuBois J. An algorithmic approach to chronic cough. Ann Intern Med 119:977–983, 1993.
28. Woolf CR, Rosenberg A. Objective assessment of cough suppressants under clinical conditions using a tape recorder system. Thorax 19:125–130, 1964.
29. Rashkin MC, Loudon RG, Jackson JL. Cough intensity [Abstract]. Am Rev Respir Dis 131:A96, 1985.
30. Hetzel MR, Clark TJH. Comparison of normal and asthmatic circadian rhythms in peak expiratory flow rate. Thorax 35:732–738, 1980.
31. Smolensky MH, Barnes PJ, Rheinberg A, McGovern JP. Chronobiology and asthma. Day-night differences in bronchial patency and dyspnea and circadian rhythm dependencies. J Asthma 23:321–343, 1986.
32. Rheinberg A, Gervais P, Levi F, et al. Circadian and circannual rhythms of allergic

rhinitis: An epidemiological study involving chronobiological methods. J Allergy Clin Immunol 81:54–62, 1988.

33. Larrain A, Carrasco E, Galleguillos F, et al. Medical and surgical treatment of non-allergic asthma associated with gastroesophageal reflux. Chest 99:1330–1335, 1991.
34. Conlan AA, Hurwitz SS, Kriege L, et al. Massive hemoptysis. Review of 123 cases. J Thorac Cardiovasc Surg 85:120–124, 1983.
35. Gong H Jr, Salvatierra C. Clinical efficacy of early and delayed fiberoptic bronchoscopy in patients with hemoptysis. Am Rev Respir Dis 124:221–225, 1981.
36. Rosenow EC III. The spectrum of drug-induced pulmonary disease. Ann Intern Med 77:977–991, 1972.
37. Cooper AD Jr, White DA, Matthay RA. Drug induced pulmonary disease. Am Rev Respir Dis 133:321–340, 1986.
38. Cullen MR, Cherniak MG, Rosenstock L. Occupational medicine. N Engl J Med 322:594–601, 1990.
39. Brooks SM. Occupational asthma. *In* Weiss EB, Segal MS, Stern M (eds). Bronchial Asthma: Mechanisms and Therapeutics. Boston, Little, Brown and Company, 1985, pp 461–493.
40. Chan-Yeun M, Lam S. State of the art: Occupational asthma. Am Rev Respir Dis 133:686–703, 1986.
41. Hunninghake GW, Garrett KC, Richardson HB, et al. State of the art: Pathogenesis of granulomatous lung disease. Am Rev Respir Dis 130:476–496, 1984.
42. Brooks SM, Weiss MA, Bernstein IL. Reactive airways dysfunction syndrome: Case reports of persistent airways hyperreactivity following high-level irritant exposures. J Occup Med 27:473–476, 1985.
43. Morgan WKC. Industrial bronchitis and other nonspecific conditions affecting the airways. *In* Occupational Lung Diseases, 2nd ed. Philadelphia, WB Saunders, 1984, pp 521–540.
44. Horvath EP, DoPico DGA, Barkie RA, Dickie HA. Nitrogen dioxide induced pulmonary disease. J Occup Med 20:103–110, 1978.
45. Simpson DL, Goodman M, Spector SL, Petty TL. Long-term follow-up and bronchial reactivity testing in survivors of the adult respiratory distress syndrome. Am Rev Respir Dis 117:449–454, 1978.
46. Irwin RS, Pratter MR. Postnasal drip and cough. Clin Notes Respir Dis 14:11–12, 1980.
47. Irwin RS, Pratter MR, Holland PS, et al. Postnasal drip causes cough and is associated with reversible upper airway obstruction. Chest 85:346–352, 1984.
48. Wolff AP, May M, Nuelle D. The tympanic membrane: A source of cough reflex. JAMA 223:1269, 1973.
49. Anthonisen NR, Manfreda J, Warren CPW, et al. Antibiotic therapy in exacerbations of chronic obstructive pulmonary disease. Ann Intern Med 106:196–204, 1987.
50. Empey DW, Laitinen LA, Jacobs L, et al. Mechanisms of bronchial hyperactivity in normal subjects after upper respiratory tract infection. Am Rev Respir Dis 113:131–139, 1976.
51. Poe RH, Israel RH, Utell MJ, Hall WJ. Chronic cough: Bronchoscopy or pulmonary function testing. Am Rev Respir Dis 126:160–162, 1982.
52. Corrao WM, Braman SS, Irwin RS. Chronic cough as the sole presenting manifestation of bronchial asthma. N Engl J Med 300:633–637, 1979.
53. Cockroft DW, Killian DN, Mellon JJA, et al. Bronchial reactivity to inhaled histamine. A method and clinical survey. Clin Allergy 7:235–243, 1977.
54. Pulmonary terms and symbols: A report of the ACCP-STS Joint Committee on pulmonary Nomenclature. Chest 67(5):583–593, 1975.
55. Reid LM. Measurement of bronchial mucous gland layer. A diagnostic yardstick in chronic bronchitis. Thorax 15:132–141, 1960.
56. Thurlbeck WM, Angus GE. A distribution curve for chronic bronchitis. Thorax 19:436–442, 1964.
57. Lauque D, Aug F, Puchelle E, et al. Efficiency of mucociliary clearance and cough in bronchitis. Bull Eur Physiopathol Respir 20:145–149, 1984.
58. American Thoracic Society. Chronic bronchitis, asthma and pulmonary emphysema. Am Rev Respir Dis 85(4):762–768, 1962.
59. Medical Research Council Committee on the Etiology of Chronic Bronchitis. Definition and classification of chronic bronchitis for clinical and epidemiological purposes. Lancet 1:775–779, 1965.
60. Linden P, Siebens AA. Dysphagia: Predicting laryngeal penetration. Arch Phys Med Rehabil 64:281–284, 1983.
61. Bartlett JG, Gorbach SL, Finegold SM. The bacteriology of aspiration pneumonia. Am J Med 56:202–207, 1974.
62. Barker AF, Bardana EJ. Bronchiectasis: Update of an orphan disease. Am Rev Respir Dis 137:969–978, 1988.
63. Iannuzzi MC, Collins FS. Reverse genetics and cystic fibrosis. Am J Respir Cell Mol Biol 2:309–316, 1990.
64. Sturgess JM, Turner JAP. Recurrent illness due to immotile cilia syndrome. J Respir Dis 3:48, 1982.
65. Reynolds HY. Host defense impairments that lead to respiratory infections. Clin Chest Med 8:339–358, 1987.

66. Schuyler MR. Allergic bronchopulmonary aspergillosis. Clin Chest Med 4:15–22, 1983.
67. Grenier P, Maurice F, Musset D, et al. Bronchiectasis: Assessment by thin-section CT. Radiology 161:95, 1986.
68. Stollev PD. Lung cancer in women: Five years later situation worse. N Engl J Med 309:428, 1983.
69. Menzies R, Charbonneau M. Thoracoscopy for the diagnosis of pleural disease. Ann Intern Med 114:271–276, 1991.
70. Platts-Mills TAE, Chapman MD. Dust mites: Immunology, allergic disease, and environmental control. J Allergy Clin Immunol 82:841, 1988.
71. Simons FER. H1-receptor antagonists: Clinical pharmacology and therapeutics. J Allergy Clin Immunol 84:845–861, 1989.
72. Fraser CM, Potter P, Venter JC. Adrenergic agents. I. Adrenergic receptors. *In* Middleton E Jr, Reed CE, Ellis E, et al (eds). Allergy: Principles and Practice, vol 1. St. Louis, CV Mosby, 1988, pp 636–647.
73. Weiner N. Norepinephrine, epinephrine and the sympathomimetic amines. *In* Gilman AG, Goodman LS, Rall TW, Murad F (eds). Goodman and Gilman's the Pharmacological Basis of Therapeutics, 7th ed. New York, Macmillan, 1985, pp 145–180.
74. Welsh PW, Stricker WE, Chu CP, et al. Efficacy of beclomethasone nasal solution, flunisolide, and cromolyn in relieving symptoms of ragweed allergy. Mayo Clin Proc 62:125–134, 1984.
75. Mygind N, Borum P. Anticholinergic treatment of watery rhinorrhea. Am J Rhinol 4:1–5, 1990.
76. Ilipoulos O, Proud D, Adkinson NF Jr, et al. Effects of immunotherapy on the early, late, and rechallenge nasal reaction to provocation with allergen: Changes in inflammatory mediators and cells. J Allergy Clin Immunol 87:855–866, 1991.
77. Normal PS. Safety of allergen immunotherapy. J Allergy Clin Immunol 84:438–439, 1989.
78. Binder E, Holopainen E, Malmberg H, Salo OP. Clinical findings in patients with allergic rhinitis. Rhinology 22:255–260, 1984.
79. Irwin RS, Zawacki JK, Curley FJ, et al. Chronic cough as the sole presenting manifestation of gastroesophageal reflux. Am Rev Respir Dis 140:1294–1300, 1990.
80. Pairolero PC, Trastek VF, Spencer Payne W. Esophagus and diaphragmatic hernias. *In* Schwartz SI, Shires GT, Spencer FL (eds). Principles of Surgery, vol 1, 5th ed. New York, McGraw-Hill Book Company, 1989, pp 1103–1156.
81. Chapman KR. Therapeutic algorithm for chronic obstructive pulmonary disease. Am J Med 91(Suppl 4A):4A–16S, 1991.
82. Gross NJ, Skorodin MS. Anticholinergic, antimuscarinic bronchodilators. Am Rev Respir Dis 129:856–870, 1984.
83. Fuller RW, Jackson DM. Physiology and treatment of cough. Thorax 45:425–430, 1990.
84. Irwin RS, Curley FJ. The treatment of cough. Chest 99:1477–1484, 1991.
85. Fuller RW, Choudry NB. Patients with a non-productive cough have increased cough reflex [Abstract]. Thorax 43:225, 1988.
86. Packman EW, London SJ. The utility of artificially induced cough as a clinical model for evaluating the antitussive effects of aromatics delivered by inhalation. Eur J Respir Dis 110:101–109, 1980.
87. Karlsson J-A. Airway anesthesia and the cough reflex. Bull Eur Physiopathol Respir 23(Suppl 10):29–36S, 1983.
88. Sevelius H, Lester PD, Colmore JP. Objective evaluation of antitussives 71:1209–1212, 1969.
89. Eddy NB, Friebel H, Hahn K-J, Halbach H. Codeine and its alternatives for pain and cough relief. 3. The antitussive action of codeine—Mechanism, methodology and evaluation. Bull World Health Organ 40:425–454, 1969.
90. Chafouri MA, Datil KD, Kass I. Sputum changes associated with the use of ipratropium bromide. Chest 86:387–392, 1984.
91. Sheppard D, Rizk NW, Boushey HA, et al. Mechanism of cough and bronchoconstriction induced by distilled water aerosol. Am Rev Respir Dis 127:691–694, 1983.
92. Eschenbacher WL, Boushey HA, Sheppard D. Alteration in osmolarity of inhaled aerosols causes bronchoconstriction and cough, but absence of a permeant anion causes cough alone. Am Rev Respir Dis 129:211–215, 1984.
93. Clarke SW, Lopez-Vidriero MT, Pavia D, Thomson ML. The effect of sodium 2-mercaptoethane sulphonate and hypertonic saline aerosols on bronchial clearance in chronic bronchitis. Br J Clin Pharmacol 7:39–44, 1979.
94. App EM, King M, Helfesrieder R, et al. Acute and long-term amiloride inhalation in cystic fibrosis lung disease: A rational approach to cystic fibrosis therapy. Am Rev Respir Dis 141:605–612, 1990.

47
◉

Key Terms

Cor Pulmonale and Pulmonary Hypertension

David R. Dantzker, M.D.

Cor Pulmonale

Diuretics

Primary Pulmonary
Hypertension (PPH)

Pulmonary Artery Pressure
(PAP)

Pulmonary Vascular
Resistance (PVR)

Vasodilators

Vascular resistance = inflow
pressure − outflow pressure ÷
blood flow
The pulmonary vascular resistance
(PVR) is thus

$$PVR = \frac{PAP - LAP}{Q}$$

where PAP is the mean pulmonary
artery pressure, LAP is the left atrial
pressure, and Q is cardiac output.

Cor pulmonale is defined as right ventricular hypertrophy and pulmonary hypertension occurring secondary to pulmonary parenchymal or pulmonary vascular disease. Right ventricular failure, as demonstrated by peripheral edema, jugular venous distention, and hepatomegaly, need not be present, although if the underlying lung disease is allowed to progress, it is inevitable. Pulmonary hypertension may result from numerous causes, its onset is often insidious, and it is difficult to recognize until heart failure develops.

PHYSIOLOGIC CONSIDERATIONS

The normal pulmonary vascular bed is a high-compliance, low-resistance network through which the entire cardiac output flows, driven by pressures that are only 10 to 20% of those found in the systemic vasculature (Fig. 47–1). The relationship between pressure and flow in any vascular bed is quantitated by calculating the vascular resistance.

When cardiac output increases in normal individuals, as might be seen during exercise, pulmonary artery pressure (PAP) rises, but only by a small amount, despite three- or four-fold increases in flow. This is accomplished by the distention of already-open vessels and a recruitment of new vessels in the lung. Both of these mechanisms serve to decrease PVR as flow increases.[1] The maintenance of a low PAP in the face of an increase in blood flow is an important mechanism for preventing the development of pulmonary edema because the movement of fluid from the pulmonary vasculature into the lung depends, to a great degree, on pulmonary vascular pressure (see Chapter 37).

The physiologic behavior of the pulmonary vascular bed is reflected in its anatomy. The normal pulmonary arteries are thin walled and contain only a small amount of smooth muscle. Unlike the systemic vessels, they have little or no resting smooth muscle tone. The right ventricle, a relatively nonmuscular compliant chamber with a large surface-volume ratio, serves mainly as a capacitance chamber for blood returning from the systemic veins.[2] As long as the pulmonary vascular bed is normal, blood moves from the systemic veins through the lungs to the left side of the heart, mainly because of the action of the left side of the heart and phasic changes in intrathoracic pressure. Contraction of the left ventricle and interventricular septum pulls the free wall of the right ventricle against the septum, producing a roller pump–like action, as opposed to the piston pump action of the left ventricle. In experimental studies, the free wall of the right ventricle has been replaced with a nonelastic material without interfering with cardiac output as long as

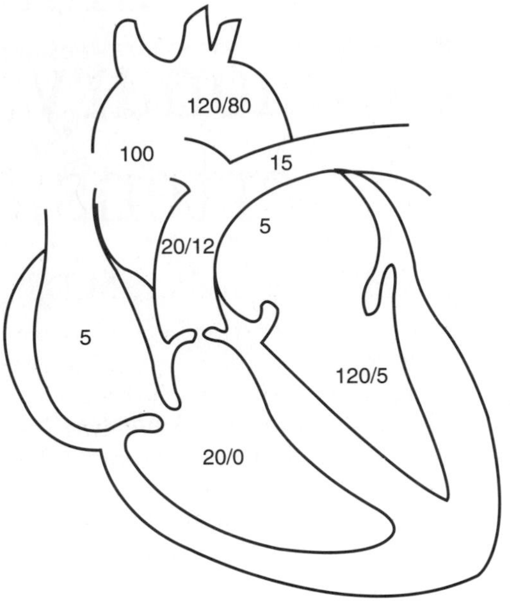

$$\text{Vascular resistance} = \frac{\text{Inflow pressure} - \text{outflow pressure}}{\text{cardiac output}}$$

$$\text{Pulmonary vascular resistance} = \frac{15 - 5}{5} = 2.0$$

$$\text{Systemic vascular resistance} = \frac{100 - 5}{5} = 19$$

FIGURE 47–1: Typical cardiac pressures in a normal adult.

PVR remains normal.[3] The forward movement of blood is further assisted by the fall in intrathoracic pressure, which tends to suck blood into the pulmonary circulation from the systemic veins, and is ensured by the one-way direction of the tricuspid and pulmonary valves.

A number of factors can influence the magnitude and distribution of blood flow in the pulmonary vascular bed. Some of these are direct mechanical effects caused by the anatomic positioning of the pulmonary vessels within the lung, which exposes them to both alveolar and intrathoracic pressure. Because of its influence on these two pressures, lung volume is an important determinant of PVR since it alters the diameter of the pulmonary vessels. Two types of pulmonary vessels can be defined:

- Intra-alveolar vessels lie within the alveolar walls and consist mainly of the pulmonary capillaries. As lung volume increases above functional residual capacity, the distending alveoli compress the vessels, increasing their contribution to vascular resistance.
- Extra-alveolar vessels comprise the remainder of the pulmonary vessels. Because of their location in the lung interstitium, increasing lung volume increases their diameter since they are tethered to the lung in all axes.

Because of these opposing effects, the influence of lung volume on PVR is complex. However, as a general rule, PVR tends to fall as lung volume increases during normal breathing because of the fall in resistance in the extra-alveolar vessels. At high lung volumes, or when lung volume increases by positive pressure ventilation, PVR may actually increase owing to compression of the intra-alveolar vessels.[4]

The distribution of blood flow in the lung also depends on the influence of alveolar and intrathoracic pressure (Fig. 47–2). In the normal upright adult, because of gravity, a difference in vascular pressure exists between the top and the bottom of the lung that is equal to about 20 mm Hg. This is a large difference in the very low pressure pulmonary vascular bed. At the very top of the lung, where PAP may fall below alveolar pressure, no blood flow occurs because of the collapse of the intra-alveolar vessels. This so-called zone 1 condition, unusual in normal individuals, may be seen when vascular pressures are very low, as in shock, or when alveolar pressure is increased during positive pressure mechanical ventilation. As one moves down the lung, pulmonary vascular pressure increases; it eventually exceeds alveolar pressure, and the vessels open (zone 2). However, because pulmonary venous pressure is still less than alveolar pressure, blood flow through zone 2 depends on the difference between arterial and alveolar pressure rather than the arterial-venous pressure difference. As arterial pressure increases down the lung in zone 2, the increasing gradient between arterial and alveolar pressure increases blood flow. As one continues toward the lung base, a point is reached at which pulmonary venous pressure also exceeds alveolar pressure and blood flow depends on the arterial-venous pressure difference, as it does elsewhere in the body (zone 3). Even though the arterial-venous difference stays constant as one continues down zone 3, blood flow continues to increase because of vascular distention. When measuring left atrial pressure with a pulmonary artery catheter, the practitioner must be sure that the catheter is in zone 3. If the catheter is in zone 2, alveolar rather than left atrial pressure may be sampled. Under some

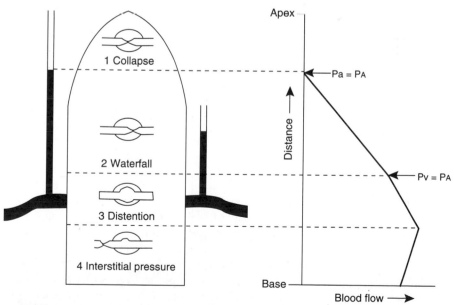

FIGURE 47–2: The four-zone model of pulmonary blood flow distribution. Blood flow is controlled by the relative values of arterial (Pa), alveolar (PA), and venous (Pv) pressures (see the text for a complete description). (From Hughes JMB, Glazier JB, Maloney JE, West JB. Effect of lung volume on the distribution of pulmonary blood flow in man. Respir Physiol 25:701–712, 1968.)

circumstances, a fall in blood flow can be seen at the very bottom of the lung (zone 4). This is due to an increase in interstitial pressure, perhaps as a result of fluid transudating into the interstitium, which compresses the extra-alveolar vessels.[5]

Changes in the alveolar P_{O_2} can influence the pulmonary vessels. A decrease in the alveolar P_{O_2} from about 150 to 25 mm Hg leads to a concomitant decrease in blood flow to those lung units (Fig. 47–3).[6] At an alveolar P_{O_2} of less than 25 mm Hg, vasodilatation may occur, although this degree of alveolar hypoxia would be very unlikely. Pulmonary hypoxic vasoconstriction is a way to preserve normal pulmonary gas exchange in the face of ventilation-perfusion inequality (see Chapter 6). A reduction in the ventilation-perfusion ratio results in alveolar hypoxia, which in turn causes a decrease in perfusion, bringing the ratio back toward normal. The effectiveness of hypoxic vasoconstriction in preserving pulmonary gas exchange, however, is incomplete. For example, a significant degree of hypoxemia is seen in patients with pneumonia, indicating that the poorly ventilated areas of lung are still being perfused.

In the setting of generalized alveolar hypoxia, whether due to diffuse lung disease or exposure to high altitude, the pulmonary hypertension caused by hypoxic vasoconstriction is often detrimental to the individual because it leads to cor pulmonale. Hypoxic vasoconstriction is probably most useful during intrauterine life, when constriction of the pulmonary vasculature in the unventilated fetal lungs is necessary to ensure that most of the blood flow returning well oxygenated from the placenta bypasses the lungs through the ductus arteriosus.

Pulmonary vasoconstriction is also seen in response to acidosis and hypercapnia. The hypercapnic response is probably secondary to the development of acidosis. The vasculature of the lung also responds to a

Factors that appear to interfere with pulmonary hypoxic vasoconstriction:

- Inflammation
- Increased pulmonary vascular pressures
- Vasodilating drugs

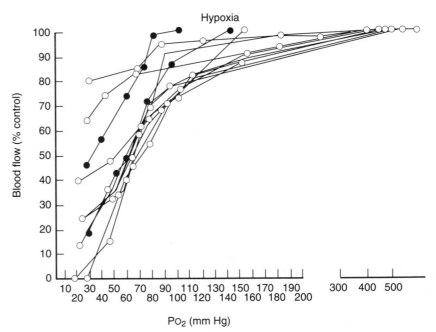

FIGURE 47–3: Stimulus-response curves of hypoxic pulmonary vasoconstriction in a cat lung. The abscissa shows alveolar P_{O_2}. Note the decrease in blood flow as alveolar P_{O_2} falls. (From Barer GR, Howard P, Shaw JW. Stimulus-response curves for the pulmonary vascular bed to hypoxia and hypercapnia. J Physiol [Lond] 211:139–155, 1970.)

large number of circulating substances, whether produced endogenously or used as therapeutic agents (Table 47–1). What role these substances play in the regulation of vascular tone in health and disease is unclear.

The pulmonary vessels are innervated by alpha- and beta-adrenergic efferent nerves, which in experimental animals can be shown to constrict and dilate the vessels, respectively. However, it is unclear to what degree this neural innervation participates in the control of pulmonary vascular tone and how it influences the development of pulmonary hypertension.

A final influence on the pulmonary vascular bed must be understood in order to appreciate the changes that are seen during disease. Anatomic remodeling of the small pulmonary arteries inevitably accompanies a prolonged increase in PAP from any etiology.[7] The changes consist of proliferation of the intimal lining cells; hypertrophy of the medial smooth muscle, with extension of this muscle into smaller and smaller arteries; and finally, the development of angiodestructive lesions that may culminate in marked reductions in the cross-sectional area. These anatomic alterations lead to a further worsening of the pulmonary hypertension. It has been suggested that anatomic remodeling may be caused by the abnormal elaboration of growth factors, implying that it may in part be a primary event in the development of pulmonary hypertension and not just a response to the elevated pressure.

The phenomenon of anatomic remodeling has been best studied in the setting of chronic hypoxia, in which the anatomic changes begin soon after the onset of hypoxic vasoconstriction and progressively amplify the increase in PAP. When the hypoxic stimulus is removed, the PAP remains elevated until the anatomic lesions gradually resolve. In normal humans born at high altitude, this resolution can take as long as 2 years after moving to sea level.

PULMONARY HYPERTENSION

The causes of pulmonary hypertension are easily grouped on the basis of the predominant mechanisms (Table 47–2). These mechanisms can be most easily defined if the PVR equation is rearranged to emphasize the determinants of PAP:

$$PAP = (PVR \times Q) + LAP$$

Thus, PAP increases with an increase in PVR, cardiac output (Q), or left atrial pressure (LAP). An increased left atrial pressure is most commonly due to the presence of heart failure or mitral valve disease. Increased pulmonary blood flow usually accompanies congenital heart disease associated with left-to-right shunting. Because these problems are not caused by an abnormality of the lung or pulmonary vasculature, they would not qualify as a cause of cor pulmonale.

Pulmonary hypertension is said to exist when the mean PAP is greater than 25 mm Hg at rest or 30 mm Hg during exercise.

An increase in PVR may result from

- Vascular destruction as a result of diffuse lung disease
- Embolic occlusion of the vessels
- Narrowing secondary to some primary pulmonary vascular disease

Alternatively, it may arise secondary to vasoconstriction as seen with alveolar hypoxia.

TABLE **47–1:** Effect of Vasoactive Agents on the Pulmonary Vascular Bed

Vasoconstriction	Vasodilation
Angiotensin II	Bradykinin
Endothelin	Prostacyclin
Thromboxane	Isoproterenol
Leukotrienes	Acetylcholine
Serotonin	
Tumor necrosis factor	

TABLE **47–2:**   Mechanisms of Pulmonary Hypertension

Passive: due to increased left atrial pressure
    Left ventricular failure
    Mitral stenosis
    Constrictive pericarditis
Hyperkinetic: due to increased pulmonary blood flow
    Intracardiac left-to-right shunt
    Patent ductus arteriosus
Obliterative: due to structural abnormalities involving the vessels or lung parenchyma
    Interstitial lung disease
    Pulmonary vasculitis
    Embolization and thrombosis
    Primary pulmonary hypertension
Vasoconstrictive: due to increased smooth muscle tone
    Hypoxia
    Acidosis and hypercapnia

SPECIFIC CAUSES OF PULMONARY HYPERTENSION

Chronic Obstructive Pulmonary Disease

Perhaps the most common setting for pulmonary hypertension is chronic obstructive pulmonary disease (COPD). Although factors such as the loss of pulmonary capillaries due to emphysema may contribute to the development of pulmonary hypertension, the most important inciting cause in patients with COPD is chronic alveolar hypoxia and the resultant hypoxic pulmonary vasoconstriction.[8] With time, the development of anatomic remodeling of the pulmonary vessels further augments the pulmonary hypertension. The development of cor pulmonale, common in this setting, contributes to the typical characteristics of the "blue and bloated" patient. Cor pulmonale often develops in these patients at PAPs much lower than those seen with other causes of pulmonary hypertension, suggesting that other factors might contribute to the appearance of right-sided heart failure (e.g., excessive retention of salt and water by the kidney).

Hypoventilation Syndromes

A number of disorders are characterized by a decreased Pa_{O_2} and an elevated Pa_{CO_2} secondary to an inappropriate minute ventilation (Table 47–3). The hypoventilation may be due to abnormal ventilatory control, neuromuscular disease, or abnormal chest wall configuration. Like patients suffering from COPD, these patients develop pulmonary hypertension and eventual cor pulmonale secondary to pulmonary hypoxic vasoconstriction. Disorders associated with the development of hypoventilation should be considered in any patient with pulmonary hypertension and no other obvious cause.

Restrictive Lung Diseases

Restrictive lung diseases (Table 47–4), which are characterized by gross disruption of lung architecture and vascular destruction, are complicated by pulmonary hypertension in about one quarter of patients as a late consequence of the loss of pulmonary cross-sectional area. Hypoxic pulmonary vasoconstriction may play a contributing but not a necessary role in the development of pulmonary hypertension in this setting.

TABLE 47–3: Causes of Hypoventilation

Central nervous system depression
  Drugs
  Anesthesia
  Myxedema
Disorders affecting the medullary respiratory center
  Trauma
  Vascular disease
  Encephalitis
  Idiopathic
Neuromuscular disease
  Spinal cord trauma
  Poliomyelitis
  Multiple sclerosis
  Amyotrophic lateral sclerosis
  Guillain-Barré syndrome
  Muscular dystrophy
  Myasthenia gravis
Thoracic cage abnormalities
  Trauma
  Kyphoscoliosis
  Thoracoplasty
  Ankylosing spondylitis
Upper airway disease
  Sleep apnea
  Laryngeal or tracheal stenosis

Pulmonary Vasculitis

The development of pulmonary vasculitis accompanies a number of systemic disorders (Table 47–5).[9] In most cases, the pulmonary manifestations of the disease are a relatively minor component of the systemic problem. In some cases, however, particularly with scleroderma, pulmonary vascular disease with resultant pulmonary hypertension may play a prominent role and may even be the major source of disability.

Primary Pulmonary Hypertension

Primary pulmonary hypertension (PPH), an unusual cause of pulmonary hypertension, may be seen in patients of all ages, although female patients predominate and a peak incidence exists in the third and fourth decades of life.[10] Although the etiology of PPH is unknown, the end-result is marked anatomic alteration of the pulmonary vessels, leading to narrowing and occlusion as well as an increase in pulmonary vascular tone. This causes marked elevations in PAP, which may reach levels found in the systemic circulation. The clinical manifestations of PPH are almost entirely limited to the pulmonary vasculature. Symptoms of shortness of breath and exercise intolerance are often present for a considerable time before PPH is successfully diagnosed. The development of obvious signs of cor pulmonale is often a late development and is always a signal of a very poor prognosis.[11]

TABLE 47–4: Diffuse Lung Diseases Associated With Pulmonary Hypertension

Adult respiratory distress syndrome	Sarcoidosis
Drug-induced pulmonary fibrosis	Rheumatoid arthritis
Pneumoconiosis: silicosis, asbestosis	Scleroderma
Hypersensitivity pneumonitis	Idiopathic pulmonary fibrosis

TABLE **47–5:** Disorders Associated With Pulmonary Vasculitis

Rheumatoid arthritis	Leukocytoclastic vasculitis
Systemic lupus erythematosus	Wegener's granulomatosis
Scleroderma	Behçet's disease
Polymyositis and dermatomyositis	

Pulmonary Thromboembolism

Persistent pulmonary hypertension is an unusual manifestation of pulmonary thromboembolism.[12] Although pulmonary hypertension may be seen immediately after the acute event, PAPs uniformly fall toward normal within hours to days owing to recanalization of the clot by the intrinsic thrombolytic activity of the body; this occurs as long as the diagnosis is made and further episodes are prevented. In a small subgroup of patients with thromboembolic disease, long-standing elevations in PAP are an important pathophysiologic finding.[13] However, these are almost always patients in whom the acute event was never recognized. Whether this represents silent, recurrent embolism or a disorder that is entirely different from the typical acute thromboembolic event is uncertain.

SIGNS AND SYMPTOMS OF PULMONARY HYPERTENSION

The symptoms and signs of the underlying disorder often obscure the manifestations of pulmonary vascular disease. However, in patients in whom the pulmonary vascular disease is the predominant manifestation, a characteristic constellation of abnormalities is found.[10] The chief symptom is dyspnea, which is markedly worsened during exercise. This is usually accompanied by complaints of fatigue and occasionally by a nonspecific chest pain. When the pulmonary hypertension is far advanced, syncope may occur. In view of these nonspecific symptoms, it is not surprising that the diagnosis is often missed until the disease is far advanced.

The physical examination is often unrevealing. Examination of the heart may demonstrate a sternal lift suggestive of right ventricular hypertrophy, a loud pulmonic component of the second heart sound, or the systolic murmur of tricuspid regurgitation. Even in severe pulmonary hypertension, however, these may be seen in only 20 to 30% of cases. As the disease worsens, evidence of right-sided heart failure, including elevated jugular venous pressure and peripheral edema, may become increasingly apparent.

Although a definitive diagnosis depends on right-sided heart catheterization, noninvasive tests can often indicate pulmonary hypertension. Cardiopulmonary exercise testing is a useful screening test for the patient presenting with nonspecific complaints of exercise intolerance or dyspnea on exertion. It can document the presence of exercise limitation and can often separate a cardiac from a pulmonary etiology.[14]

Electrocardiography and chest roentgenography may demonstrate the presence of right ventricular hypertrophy. Echocardiography can confirm right ventricular hypertrophy, and Doppler studies of the heart can be used to estimate PAP.[15]

TREATMENT OF PULMONARY HYPERTENSION

Whenever pulmonary hypertension results from a clearly definable underlying disorder, the emphasis should be on treating that problem.

This is clearly the case when pulmonary hypertension is secondary to heart failure or to valvular or congenital heart disease. However, because most causes of cor pulmonale are not directly approachable, treatment is often directed at the pulmonary hypertension itself.

Oxygen Therapy

Because hypoxic vasoconstriction is a potent cause of pulmonary hypertension, its correction should be an important part of the management of hypoxemic patients with pulmonary hypertension.

However, in patients with chronic hypoxemia, O_2 therapy often fails to lower PAP rapidly because of the anatomic remodeling of the vessels. Just as people growing up at high altitude in the mountains need prolonged sea level exposure before the PAP returns to normal, prolonged treatment with O_2 is necessary before a fall in PAP can be expected. Even with long-term O_2 therapy, the fall in PAP is often less than dramatic, either because of irreversible anatomic changes or because patients fail to use the O_2 for a sufficient amount of time during the day. Animal studies have shown that as little as 6 hours a day of alveolar hypoxia is sufficient to prevent resolution of the anatomic changes induced by hypoxia in the first place.[16]

This feature of O_2 therapy was clearly demonstrated in two large clinical trials of patients with COPD and cor pulmonale.[17, 18] After prolonged O_2 therapy that increased the arterial P_{O_2} to above 60 mm Hg for various amounts of time during the day, ranging from about 10 to 20 hours, only minimal regression of the pulmonary hypertension was seen. Fortunately for the patients, however, the use of supplemental O_2 on a long-term basis did have an effect on mortality, with a significant improvement seen in the O_2-treated patients. This beneficial survival advantage appeared to be directly related to the daily duration of therapy. This benefit is thought to be due to the improvement in tissue oxygenation resulting from the increased peripheral O_2 delivery. Although this beneficial effect of prolonged O_2 therapy on survival has only been proved thus far in COPD patients with stable hypoxemia, similar effects may eventually be shown in other patients with chronic hypoxemia and even in patients with intermittent hypoxemia, such as that which often occurs during sleep in patients with marginal daytime arterial blood gas measurements.

Vasodilators

A large number of drugs have been shown to dilate pulmonary vessels (Table 47–6). However, because of considerations of both potency and side effect profile, most clinical interest now centers around the use of calcium channel blocking agents and prostacyclin. Most of the clinical

TABLE **47–6:**   Pulmonary Vasodilators

Calcium channel blockers	Angiotensin-converting enzyme inhibitors
Prostacyclin	Hydralazine
Beta-sympathomimetic agents	Phentolamine
Nitroglycerin	Prazosin
Nitroprusside	Tolazoline

trials of these drugs have been carried out in patients with COPD and PPH.

About one third of patients with PPH decrease their PVR in response to vasodilators, at least on initial testing.[19] This usually results in an improvement in exercise tolerance and a reduction in the other symptoms and signs of pulmonary hypertension. The best clinical responses have been reported with very high doses of the calcium channel blockers. In some patients, this has resulted in long-term reductions in pulmonary pressures and even a regression in the right ventricular enlargement.[20] In most cases, however, the response to vasodilators gradually wanes or patients require continuously increasing doses to maintain a reduction in PVR. This has led to the generally held belief that at best, vasodilators should be considered to be a bridge to lung transplantation (see later discussion).

In selected patients with COPD, vasodilators have also been shown to reduce PVR. However, in these patients, in contrast to patients with PPH, it is difficult to demonstrate that this translates into an improvement in functional ability because patients with COPD are limited predominantly by their impaired ventilatory function.[21] Therefore, any improvement in cardiovascular function that might occur secondary to vasodilatation is not likely to be as apparent. In addition, no evidence exists, as of yet, that the reduction in pulmonary pressures by vasodilators in patients with COPD alters the natural history of the disorder.

There have been sporadic reports of vasodilator use in other clinical settings of pulmonary hypertension, such as restrictive lung disease and pulmonary vasculitis. However, because the data conflict, at this time no clear consensus has emerged as to the effectiveness of these agents.

Vasodilators must be used with great care and only after a carefully monitored trial during which pulmonary pressures and cardiac output are continuously measured because these drugs may have serious side effects. The major side effect is systemic hypotension because each of these drugs has an equal or greater effect on the systemic vasculature. A fall in systemic vascular resistance may result in a drop in systemic blood pressure and worsening oxygen delivery leading to organ failure. In addition, vasodilators interfere with the matching of ventilation and blood flow in the lung. Increased ventilation-perfusion inequality is an inevitable consequence of their use; significant hypoxemia may result, especially in patients with COPD.

To summarize, vasodilators should probably be reserved for patients with PPH and used only after a carefully monitored trial. The use of these drugs in all other forms of pulmonary hypertension, at this point in time, should be considered experimental and relegated only to clinical trial protocols.

Other Drugs

Digitalis

Cardiac glycosides have been shown to improve the contractility of the failing left ventricle. However, it is unclear if there is a similar beneficial effect with isolated right ventricular failure associated with cor pulmonale. In addition, these patients have an increased risk of digitalis-induced arrhythmias.

Diuretics

Peripheral edema is a common finding in patients with cor pulmonale. A careful use of diuretics is appropriate to improve patient comfort. However, it takes a higher right ventricular filling pressure to maintain flow through the abnormal pulmonary vessels. Thus, excessive diuresis may result in a drop in the already insufficient cardiac output; this must be avoided.

Anticoagulants

Some patients with PPH have evidence of low-grade coagulation activity. Because the pathology in certain patients suggests that thrombosis may play either a primary or an amplifying role in the vascular obstructive process, it has been hypothesized that this coagulation activity is the marker of that process. In addition, a retrospective study has suggested that patients with PPH who are placed on long-term warfarin therapy have a longer survival.[22] Because of these two pieces of somewhat circumstantial evidence, it is generally recommended that unless a contraindication exists, patients with PPH receive long-term anticoagulation.

Lung Transplantation

In 1981, heart-lung transplantation was introduced as the first really viable option for the treatment of PPH. Single-lung transplantation was then developed and successfully used in patients with end-stage interstitial lung disease. This is a technically easier operation with a lower perioperative mortality and morbidity, but it was believed to be inappropriate for patients with pulmonary hypertension because the recovery of right-sided heart function was thought to be unlikely. Subsequent studies have shown these fears to be unfounded, and single-lung transplantation virtually replaced heart-lung transplantation for the definitive treatment of PPH; this procedure is even being used in selected patients with far-advanced COPD.[23] Recently, new questions have been raised with regard to the long-term outcome of single lung transplantation in the setting of PPH, and a re-evaluation is under way.

Although lung transplantation holds out hope for the successful treatment of many patients with pulmonary hypertension, the large number of potential candidates and the limited number of donors force the imposition of strict selection criteria. Among these are younger age (usually less than 60 years) and the absence of significant comorbidity (e.g., coronary artery disease).

SUMMARY

Because of its anatomic location and complex physiology, the pulmonary vascular bed is difficult to access and monitor. As a consequence, a diagnosis of pulmonary hypertension is usually made only after signs of right-sided heart failure are already present. If we are to make progress against this condition, it is mandatory that the diagnosis be considered in all cases of unexplained dyspnea or decreased exercise tolerance and when the degree of physiologic impairment in patients with underlying lung disease appears to be out of proportion to the degree of pulmonary dysfunction.

References

1. Fishman A. Pulmonary circulation. *In* Fishman AP, Fisher AB (eds). The Respiratory System, vol 1. Bethesda, MD, American Physiological Society, 1985, pp 93–166.
2. McFadden ER, Braundwald E. Cor pulmonale and pulmonary thromboembolism. *In* Braundwald E (ed). Heart Disease. Philadelphia, WB Saunders, 1980, pp 1643–1682.
3. Kagan A. Dynamic responses of the right ventricle following extensive damage by cauterization. Circulation 5:816–822, 1952.
4. Permutt S, Brower RG. Mechanical support. *In* Crystal RG, West JB (eds). The Lung: Scientific Foundations. New York, Raven Press, 1991, pp 1077–1086.
5. Hughes JMB, Glazier JB, Maloney JE, West JB. Effect of lung volume on the distribution of pulmonary blood flow in man. Respir Physiol 25:701–712, 1968.
6. Barer GR, Howard P, Shaw JW. Stimulus-response curves for the pulmonary vascular bed to hypoxia and hypercapnia. J Physiol (Lond) 211:139–155, 1970.
7. Reid L. The pulmonary circulation remodelling in growth and disease. Am Rev Respir Dis 119:531–546, 1979.
8. Harris P, Heath D. The Human Pulmonary Circulation. New York, Churchill Livingstone, 1986.
9. Leavitt RY, Fauci AS. Pulmonary vasculitis. Am Rev Respir Dis 134:149–166, 1986.
10. Rich S, Dantzker DR, Ayres SM, et al. Primary pulmonary hypertension: A national prospective study. Ann Intern Med 107:216–223, 1987.
11. D'Alonzo GE, Barst RJ, Ayres SM, et al. Survival in patients with primary pulmonary hypertension. Ann Intern Med 115:343–349, 1991.
12. Riedel M, Stanck V, Widimsky J, Prevosky I. Long-term followup of patients with pulmonary thromboembolism: Late prognosis and evaluation of hemodynamic and respiratory data. Chest 81:151–158, 1982.
13. Moser KM, Auger WR, Fedullo PF. Chronic major-vessel thromboembolic pulmonary hypertension. Circulation 81:1735–1743, 1990.
14. D'Alonzo GE, Gianotti L, Dantzker DR. Noninvasive assessment of hemodynamic improvement during chronic vasodilation therapy in obliterative pulmonary hypertension. Am Rev Respir Dis 133:380–384, 1986.
15. Yock PG, Popp RL. Noninvasive estimation of right ventricular systolic pressure by Doppler ultrasound in patients with tricuspid regurgitation. Circulation 70:657–662, 1984.
16. Kay JM. Effect of intermittent normoxia on chronic hypoxic pulmonary hypertension, right ventricular hypertrophy and polycythemia in rats. Am Rev Respir Dis 121:993–1001, 1980.
17. Report of the Medical Research Council Working Party: Long term domiciliary oxygen therapy in chronic hypoxic cor pulmonale complicating chronic bronchitis and emphysema. Lancet 1:681–685, 1981.
18. Nocturnal Oxygen Therapy Trial Group. Continuous or nocturnal oxygen therapy in hypoxemic chronic obstructive lung disease. Ann Intern Med 93:391–398, 1980.
19. Reeves JT, Groves BM, Turkevich D. The case for treatment of selected patients with primary pulmonary hypertension. Ann Rev Respir Dis 134:342–346, 1986.
20. Rich S, Brundage BH. High-dose calcium channel blocking therapy for primary pulmonary hypertension: Evidence for long-term reduction in pulmonary arterial pressure and regression of right ventricular hypertrophy. Circulation 76:135–141, 1987.
21. Dal Nogare AR, Rubin LJ. The effects of hydralazine on exercise capacity in pulmonary hypertension secondary to chronic obstructive pulmonary disease. Ann Rev Respir Dis 133:385–389, 1986.
22. Fuster V, Steele PM, Edwards WD, et al. Primary pulmonary hypertension: Natural history and the importance of thrombosis. Circulation 70:580–587, 1984.
23. Carere R, Patterson GA, Liu P, et al. Right and left ventricular performance after single and double lung transplantation. J Thorac Cardiovasc Surg 401:115–122, 1991.

48 Neuromuscular Disorders

Michael A. DeVita, M.D., and Sunil Hegde, M.D.

Weakness is defined as a decrease in the capacity of a rested muscle to perform work.[1] This should be distinguished from fatigue, which is a decrease in the ability of a muscle to contract that is caused by muscular activity and correctable by rest. It is not difficult to understand that a weak muscle is more susceptible to fatigue.

Patients with neuromuscular diseases frequently manifest some respiratory dysfunction, the severity of which tends to correlate with the severity of the disease. Although each disorder has a somewhat different spectrum of ventilatory impairment, all cause muscular weakness to some degree.

The material covered in this chapter includes

- A description of most of the neuromuscular diseases
- A discussion of the impact of these diseases on the respiratory system
- A discussion of the spectrum of therapeutic modalities available to the practitioner, from early therapy through full mechanical ventilatory support to issues surrounding the discontinuation of support

EFFECTS OF NEUROMUSCULAR DISORDERS ON MUSCLES

Most neuromuscular diseases exert the same overall effect on ventilation: respiratory muscle weakness.

The causes of muscle weakness vary. Table 48–1 lists causes of either acute exacerbations of respiratory muscle weakness or chronic decline in respiratory muscle function that are not neuromuscular diseases per se. Some of these disorders can be solely responsible for respiratory failure in an otherwise stable patient. For example, severe hypophosphatemia can cause respiratory failure. On the other hand, a mild electrolyte abnormality in a patient with myasthenia gravis can have catastrophic results. Correcting any of these factors can result in a dramatic improvement in pulmonary function.

Nutritional deficiencies may cause neural dysfunction or muscular weakness, impair energy storage and utilization, and diminish function of the central nervous system. The provision of adequate nutrition, including the correction of calorie and protein depletion and the treatment of vitamin and mineral deficiencies, is necessary for patients to perform optimally. A discussion of these entities is beyond the scope of this chapter, but pertinent information is available in most nutrition and critical care texts.

Respiratory muscles become weak in patients with neuromuscular disorders. However, all muscles do not weaken to the same extent or at the same rate. Inspiratory and expiratory muscle strengths may decline independently of each other.[2] Initially, the ventilatory problems are

TABLE **48–1:** Causes of Acute Exacerbation of Respiratory Muscle Weakness

Hypercapnia	Hypomagnesemia
Acidosis	Hypophosphatemia
Hyponatremia	Alcohol ingestion
Hypokalemia	Acute myopathy (e.g., steroid induced)
Hypocalcemia	Use of certain drugs (e.g., aminoglycosides)

caused by weakness and hypoventilation. These are compounded by weakness of the intercostal muscles, which allows inward bulging of these muscles. The intrathoracic volume decreases and opposes the generation of negative thoracic pressure, thus decreasing the inspiratory force and volume.[1] After prolonged weakness, secondary changes occur, including scoliosis, fibrosis, and shortening of the muscles. These alterations all decrease compliance and increase the work of breathing, which impairs ventilation, causing atelectasis, ventilation-perfusion imbalance, and hypoxemia.

Muscle strength decreases as the disease progresses. Weakness of the inspiratory and expiratory muscles, which have different functions, causes different ventilatory problems. Inspiratory weakness causes a decrease in the vital capacity and the functional residual capacity, promoting atelectasis and intrapulmonary shunting. The tidal volume decreases as inspiratory weakness worsens, leading to hypoventilation, hypoxemia, and hypercapnia. Expiration is usually passive, so patients may not notice weakness of these muscles. In fact, because effort-independent expiratory flow is related to lung elasticity and airway compliance, the flow may be increased because of markedly diminished compliance. Because the expiratory muscles are not used as often, they may weaken at a faster rate. However, forced exhalation is effort dependent and is markedly decreased in these patients. It is first noticeable as a weakened force of cough, which may be attributed to a diminished vital capacity. However, even when the vital capacity is kept constant, the peak flow remains diminished.[2]

PRIMARY DISORDERS OF NEUROMUSCULAR FUNCTION

Muscular weakness may be a manifestation of pathology that occurs anywhere along the neuromuscular axis. This includes disorders of the central or peripheral nervous system, the neuromuscular junction, and the muscles themselves. Table 48–2 lists common causes of ventilatory failure. Classification according to the site of the defect is used only to facilitate the study of the causes of ventilatory pump failure and does not necessarily mean that in each disease state the pathophysiologic process is restricted to a single target area. More than one site along the neuromuscular axis may be involved in the same disease process. For example, in inflammatory myopathies, the primary target is the muscle. However, the terminal nerves may also be involved.

TABLE **48–2:** Neuromuscular Causes of Ventilatory Failure

Disorders of the Central Nervous System	**Disorders of the Neuromuscular Junction**
Parkinsonism	Myasthenia gravis
Spinal cord injuries	Eaton-Lambert syndrome
Motor neuron disease	Drug-induced disorders (e.g., D-tubocurarine, penicillamine)
Amyotrophic lateral sclerosis	Botulism
Poliomyelitis and postpolio syndrome	**Disorders of the Muscles**
Spinal muscular atrophy	Myopathies, both inflammatory and noninflammatory
Tetanus	Muscular dystrophy
Disorders of the Peripheral Nervous System	Myotonia congenita
Critical illness polyneuropathy	Myotonic dystrophy
Guillain-Barré syndrome	
Phrenic nerve injury	
Diphtheria	

Disorders of the Central Nervous System

Parkinson's Disease

Parkinson's disease, which is a disorder of the extrapyramidal system, leads to the loss of motor control. Generally occurring between the fourth and the seventh decades of life, it affects about 1% of the population in the United States.

In the early 1900s, most cases of Parkinson's disease occurred after a viral encephalitis. Parkinson's disease is idiopathic, but a parkinsonian syndrome can be caused by drugs such as phenothiazines or reserpine. Patients suffer a loss of dopaminergic pigmented cells in the substantia nigra, locus coeruleus, and dorsal motor nucleus of the vagus.

The symptoms fall mainly into three broad groups:

- Loss of movement
- Resting tremor
- Rigidity

Loss of movement (bradykinesia or hypokinesia) is characterized by an expressionless face, the loss of arm swing, and a short, shuffling gait. The tremor is most obvious in the hands, diminishing with purposeful movements. The movement has been classically described as a "pill-rolling" tremor. Rigidity, the third major symptom, has been classically described as having a "cog-wheeling" character.

Pulmonary complications have been described.[3, 4] Obstructive ventilatory defect, which is frequently seen in patients with Parkinson's disease, persists even after treatment and control of the neurologic symptoms. The pathophysiology of this process has not yet been defined,[3, 4] although parasympathetic overactivity has been postulated.

There is no known established treatment to reverse the disease process of parkinsonism, so therapy is directed toward controlling the symptoms. Levodopa, currently the preferred drug, is usually given with a decarboxylase inhibitor to prevent its rapid destruction peripherally. Other drugs that have beneficial effects are amantadine and bromocriptine.

Spinal Cord Injury

Pulmonary complications are a leading cause of death in patients with spinal cord injuries.

Spinal cord injury, a devastating event, occurs in 28 to 50 persons per 1 million every year. Motor vehicle accidents, diving injuries, falls, and gunshot wounds are responsible for the bulk of spinal cord injuries. A significant proportion of these injuries involve the cervical cord, which may result in ventilatory insufficiency. Cervical cord injury above the level of C3 results in immediate and complete cessation of respiration because of the loss of motor control of the diaphragm, which is innervated by roots C3 through C5 via the phrenic nerve. Cervical cord injuries between C3 and C5 lead to partial loss of motor function of the diaphragm and most of the expiratory muscles that are supplied by thoracic nerve roots. Cervical injuries below C5 spare most of the important inspiratory muscles but paralyze most of the expiratory muscles. The pectoralis major is the only expiratory muscle preserved in a cervical cord injury.[5]

Abnormalities in pulmonary function resulting from cervical cord injury include a loss in vital capacity caused by (1) a loss of inspiratory force, (2) an increase in residual volume, and (3) an increase in the workload caused by decreased thoracic compliance.[6] Both the maximal inspiratory and expiratory pressures are reduced, particularly the latter.[7] Vital capacity may approach tidal volume. When inspiration is maintained with increased effort, patients are easily fatigued. Ventilatory failure may occur. It is important to measure the vital capacity and the maximal inspiratory pressure repeatedly during the acute phase. Expiration becomes exclusively a passive process, with subsequent loss of an effective cough. These abnormalities result in the accumulation of pulmonary secretions, atelectasis, and infectious complications.

Pulmonary function improves with time as muscle flaccidity changes to spasticity, thereby reducing the opposing motion ("flail") of the intercostal muscles. The vital capacity may improve, as do the maximal inspiratory and expiratory pressures.

Atelectasis and pneumonia occur more often in the lower left lobe because of inadequate drainage of this segment of the lungs.[8] Deep breathing, positive pressure insufflation, chest percussion, and assisted "quad" cough may help to mobilize secretions. Early therapeutic bronchoscopy for the clearing of secretions may be indicated in persistent atelectasis.

Resistive inspiratory exercises can help to strengthen the diaphragm.[10] The use of an abdominal binder improves diaphragm function by stabilizing the insertion of that muscle on the abdominal muscles, which in turn increases the vital capacity. Full-time ventilatory support by phrenic nerve pacing, which has been effective, is discussed later in this chapter.

Amyotrophic Lateral Sclerosis

Occurring in adults, amyotrophic lateral sclerosis (ALS) is a progressive disease characterized by degeneration of the anterior horn cells with associated degeneration of the descending motor pathways.[11] Although primarily the motor system is involved, nonmotor pathways are increasingly being recognized as having a role in the pathology of this disease.[12]

ALS is characterized by motor neuron degeneration and loss with gliosis, an extensive loss of Betz's cells and other pyramidal cells from the postcentral cortex, as well as loss of the spinal motor neurons. The corticospinal tracts show a preferential loss of myelinated fibers, especially in the anterior and lateral columns and to a lesser extent in the ventral spinal roots. The disease is progressive, resulting in ventilatory failure and death. Death would usually occur in 2 to 3 years, but the life span may be prolonged.

Weakness, the chief complaint in ALS, may involve any skeletal muscle. Early weakness occurs in the limb musculature, especially that of the upper extremity. The pattern of weakness and atrophy, which is focal and asymmetrical, varies from patient to patient. Unilateral diaphragmatic paralysis may occur at presentation. Extraocular muscle involvement is almost never symptomatic. Control of bowel and bladder functions is preserved even late in the disease course. Although ventilatory pump failure is predominant, in the late stages severe bulbar involvement is a common feature. The resultant muscular weakness may lead to secondary symptoms such as dysphagia or aspiration of saliva, which may exacerbate or cause ventilatory insufficiency. In addition, patients may complain of cramps, pain, and paresthesia, although clinical findings of sensory symptoms are rare.

The diagnosis, which is based on clinical features and electrophysiologic study findings, is mainly a diagnosis of exclusion. Electrophysiologic studies show a loss of motor units with fibrillations and positive sharp waves. Subsequent reinnervation of the denervated muscle fibers results in large polyphasic motor unit potentials. Clinically, these are observed as fasciculations. These typical findings indicate a scattered distribution

"Quad" cough is assisted expectoration in which a rapid force is applied to the epigastric area during expiration to force the secretions from the alveoli and bronchioli into the trachea, from which they can then be suctioned.

ALS can occur randomly or be hereditary. The annual incidence in the United States is 0.4 to 1.8 cases per 100,000, with a predominance in men. There is some geographic correlation, with higher rates in the Western Pacific.

Pulmonary function testing reveals a restrictive defect caused by muscle weakness and a reduction in chest wall compliance.

involving many nerves. Nerve conduction studies may show a small motor amplitude with a conduction velocity that is more than 70% of normal. The sensory conductions are normal.[13, 14]

Treatment is primarily supportive because no known cure exists. Cramps and paresthesias may respond to quinine, phenytoin, baclofen, or combinations of all three.[11] Pyridostigmine may alleviate the fatigue. The pseudobulbar symptoms may be helped by levodopa, lithium, or amitriptyline.

Aerobic and submaximal strengthening exercises help to maintain optimal endurance and strength in the uninvolved and partially involved muscle groups. However, care should be taken not to overexercise the muscles. Early ventilatory support has been advocated because it not only prevents nocturnal hypoventilation but also may improve the quality of life.[15] Ventilatory support may be intermittent, nocturnal, or full-time support with positive or negative pressure ventilation.[14]

With the use of mechanical ventilatory support, life may be greatly prolonged.[16]

Poliomyelitis and Postpolio Syndrome

Poliomyelitis is a rare entity in the United States today. However, recently more cases are being reported because of lower immunization rates. The disease is caused by the enterovirus poliovirus, a small, single-stranded RNA virus. The human intestinal tract is the only known habitat for this virus. In most cases, the primary manifestations are non-neurologic, usually consisting of a mild flu-like syndrome or gastroenteritis. In the early phase of neurologic involvement, meningeal signs may be seen. Most patients demonstrate rapidly developing muscular weakness, which usually peaks in 48 hours or less. Any of the limb, bulbar, or cranial nerves may be involved. The clinical progression may halt at any stage or the disease may progress to complete paralysis of all involved muscles.

The loci of primary involvement are the motor nuclei of the brain stem and the spinal gray matter, where affected nerve cells are completely destroyed. The thalamus, hypothalamus, and brain stem reticular formation are involved to a lesser extent. Lesions of the cortex are not clinically significant.

Treatment in the acute phase is supportive. In patients with respiratory failure, assisted ventilation is required. Most patients recover from the ventilatory paralysis; however, a few patients may need continued ventilatory support.

Postpolio syndrome is a more recently recognized entity. Postpolio syndrome typically presents with progressive fatigue and muscular weakness. Occasionally, patients also have sensory complaints, including pain.

The pathophysiologic process causing the syndrome has not yet been identified. The commonly accepted hypothesis is that the weakness results from a gradual, progressive loss of motor units in patients with prior exposure to poliovirus.[17] A loss of motor units occurs normally with aging; however, this process seems to be accelerated in patients with postpolio syndrome. Patients who have had poliovirus infection have a smaller reserve of motor units because of previous loss. The further loss of motor units manifests as muscle weakness, which in turn leads to functional loss. Overwork of the remaining motor units may also lead to the acceleration of motor unit aging and loss. Other investigators have hypothesized that the pathophysiologic process of the postpolio syndrome may be due to defects in neuromuscular transmission or in the contractile mechanism.[17] However, no hypothesis has been conclusively proved. Electrodiagnostic studies typically show an unstable motor unit with evidence of ongoing denervation and reinnervation.[17, 18]

Pulmonary function testing reveals a restrictive pattern. Maximal inspiratory force, vital capacity, and expiratory reserve volume may be compromised. The compliance of the chest wall is reduced. Respiratory decompensation may be due to progressive weakness of the ventilatory muscles or to a loss of ventilatory capacity, which is a normal process of aging in patients with marginal respiratory reserve.

Patients typically present with nocturnal hypoventilation, sleep apnea during the rapid eye movement phase, or progressive ventilatory insufficiency with the need for increasing levels of mechanical assistance. Pneumonia or the use of general anesthesia may result in respiratory decompensation.

The management of poliomyelitis and postpolio syndrome is supportive. Titrated mechanical ventilatory assistance may be needed.[19, 20] Rest therapy may help the ventilatory muscles to recover from fatigue. In patients whose muscle strength is at least capable of moving against gravity, an aerobic training program may help to improve work capacity as well as minute ventilation.[21] Care should be taken, however, not to overexercise these weak muscles.

Spinal Muscular Atrophy Types I, II, and III

Spinal muscular atrophy type I (acute Werdnig-Hoffmann disease), a degenerative disease of the anterior horn cells and the cranial nerve motor nuclei, is an autosomal recessive disorder. The disease presents during infancy and may be clinically evident in the first 2 or 3 months of life. It has a progressive course and usually results in death in 2 to 3 years.[22]

Spinal muscular atrophy type II (chronic Werdnig-Hoffmann disease) becomes clinically evident at about 6 months of age, delaying the child's motor development. The weakness is predominantly in the trunk and limbs. Proximal muscles are more affected than distal muscles. Cranial nerves are relatively spared. Asymmetrical weakness of the trunk muscles predisposes the child to skeletal deformities. Kyphoscoliosis is a predominant feature.

The clinical course of the disease may be prolonged, and patients may survive to early adulthood. Death is usually due to respiratory complications.[23] The supportive management follows the same principles outlined later in this chapter for Duchenne's muscular dystrophy.

Spinal muscular atrophy type III (Kugelberg-Welander disease) is clinically evident between 5 and 15 years of age. The disease usually presents with muscular weakness of the hip and shoulder girdles and difficulty with walking. The distal muscles are involved late in the disease. The cranial muscles are usually spared, although they may be involved in the later stages. In chronic cases, kyphoscoliosis and joint contractures develop, especially after the patient is confined to a wheelchair. Laboratory studies may show an increase in the level of creatine phosphokinase of two to (rarely) 10 times the normal level. Muscle biopsy shows the grouping of similar muscle fibers (e.g., clusters of only fast or only slow fibers) and loss of the heterogeneity that is normally present. Electromyography (EMG) shows muscle fibrillation and positive sharp waves with large polyphasic motor unit potentials and reduced recruitment.

The management of spinal muscular atrophy type III follows the pattern outlined for Duchenne's muscular dystrophy, with bracing and limiting of the range of motion of the spine to prevent contractures and to limit the progression of scoliosis.[24] Spinal fusion may be indicated. Aggressive pulmonary management with ventilatory support may be needed.

Tetanus

The etiologic agent is tetanospasmin, which is produced by *Clostridium tetani.*

Tetanus is a disease characterized by muscular stiffness and rigidity. Tetanospasmin prevents the release of the inhibitor neurotransmitters glycine and gamma-aminobutyric acid in the brain stem and spinal cord. This loss of central inhibition leads to rigidity.[25] The toxin also affects sympathetic neurons and the hypothalamus, which may explain the autonomic instability that frequently occurs. Tetanus can be localized, cephalic, or generalized.

Early in the disease, facial rigidity (colloquially called lockjaw) is the predominant symptom. In the generalized phase, trismus, dysphagia, rigidity of the entire body, and opisthotonos may be seen. Reflex spasms may be stimulated by any external stimulus. Involvement of the autonomic nervous system causes hypertension, tachycardia, fever, sweating, labile blood pressure, and even cardiac arrest. During the spasms, respiratory arrest may ensue. Sustained muscular contraction causes chest wall rigidity and effectively halts ventilation.

The diagnosis is usually based on the history and on clinical manifestations because the culture of *Clostridium tetani* occurs in only 30% of cases. There are no clinical syndromes that closely mimic tetanus.

Treatment is with human tetanus antitoxin, antibiotics for *Clostridium tetani* infection (e.g., penicillin), and local wound débridement. The antitoxin does not block tetanospasmin already bound to neurons, so it does not reverse symptoms already present, but it does prevent progression. The patient should be kept in a quiet room and sedated. In generalized tetanus, a tracheostomy may be indicated to facilitate the clearance of secretions. If the spasms continue, the patient should receive a neuromuscular blocking agent and be placed on mechanical ventilatory support.[25]

Disorders of the Peripheral Nervous System

Critical Illness Polyneuropathy

Critical illness polyneuropathy is one of the major causes of weaning difficulty,[26] with an incidence as high as 50% in patients who have been septic for longer than 2 weeks.[27]

Critical illness polyneuropathy is a sensorimotor axonopathy seen in patients who are critically ill with multiorgan failure. The clinical features include loss of muscle mass, symmetrical weakness or flaccid paralysis that is worse distally, and diminished or absent deep tendon reflexes. The sensory examination may reveal a compromised sensation of pinprick, temperature, and vibration.

Laboratory investigations show normal biochemical values as well as normal levels of calcium, phosphorus, and magnesium.[28] Cerebrospinal fluid findings are normal. Electrodiagnostic studies show preservation of the distal latency, conduction velocity, and "F" latency. There have been some reports of a demyelinating component with reduced conduction velocity in the motor and sensory nerves. However, the predominant components are axonopathy and a reduction in the amplitude of the compound motor and sensory evoked responses.[27, 28] In severe cases, studies of phrenic nerve conduction may show a small or an absent evoked response or a prolongation of the latency. EMG shows fibrillation and positive sharp waves with a decreased number of motor units that are polyphasic. The distribution of the abnormalities on EMG is multifocal.

Recovery usually does occur, but it requires time. A mean of 67 days before patients are weaned from mechanical ventilation has been observed.[29] Treatment is supportive, with prevention of secondary problems and aggressive rehabilitation.

Guillain-Barré Syndrome

Guillain-Barré syndrome is a symmetrical ascending areflexic paralysis characterized by demyelination of motor and sensory axons. In severe cases, there is paralysis of all peripheral and cranial nerves.

Although motor deficit predominates, a significant sensory involvement occurs as well. Patients experience dysesthesias, pain, and some autonomic instability. Treatment of the most severe cases is supportive: that is, it consists of the provision of ventilatory, nutritional, and cardiovascular therapy. Respiratory support in the form of meticulous endobronchial hygiene, incentive spirometry, and airway protection is necessary. Patients with Guillain-Barré syndrome develop alveolar hypoventilation, and a restrictive pattern (a low vital capacity and a normal ratio of forced expiratory volume to forced vital capacity) is indicated by pulmonary function testing. Paradoxical motion of the abdomen and thorax indicates diaphragm paralysis. Patients with Guillain-Barré syndrome may have involvement of cranial nerves IX and X, which causes dysphagia and an inability to control secretions, predisposing the patient to aspiration and pneumonitis. In patients with borderline respiratory function, the aspiration of even small volumes of saliva can be catastrophic. Although decreases in oxygenation and ventilation are gradual, these patients should be considered for intubation before blood gas abnormalities or overt respiratory insufficiencies occur. These patients are at great risk for aspiration caused by the dysphagia.[30, 31] Most patients, once intubated, require at least 2 weeks, and usually more, of mechanical ventilation.[30] The duration of ventilation appears to be shorter than in the past, with 23 days required from 1970 to 1978 as opposed to 14 days from 1979 to 1983.[32]

The survival of patients with Guillain-Barré syndrome has changed over the past 20 years. From 1970 to 1983, 56 of 210 (26.7%) patients with Guillain-Barré syndrome required mechanical ventilation.[32] In 1970, five of five (100%) ventilated patients with Guillain-Barré syndrome died. From 1971 to 1977, 15 of 25 (60%) died, whereas from 1978 to 1983, three (12%) died. This improvement was thought to be a consequence of better critical care. The complications and causes of death in these patients seem to support this interpretation. Complications were due to thromboembolism, cardiovascular events (including arrhythmia and cardiac failure), bronchopneumonia, gastrointestinal bleeding, and renal failure, with pulmonary and cardiac complications being the most frequent. Deaths were most commonly caused by cardiac complications, followed by pulmonary embolism and pneumonia. Stress ulcer prophylaxis, cardiac monitoring, treatment of infection, and nutritional support have greatly enhanced survival. It is interesting to note that the mortality rate for these patients decreased from 100% in 1970 to 0% in 1983. Currently, with optimal critical care, death occurs in less than 5% of this population.[32, 33]

Most cases of Guillain-Barré syndrome follow a viral or mycoplasmal infection, surgery, or immunization, but an inciting event is not present in all cases.

Early tracheostomy has been recommended for enhanced safety, comfort, and ease of maintaining endobronchial and oral hygiene.

In the early stages of the disease, plasmapheresis decreases both the severity of the attack and its duration.[33] This improvement is most obvious in patients in the most severe stages of the disease.

Hypothermic Phrenic Nerve Injury

Local hypothermia has become a mainstay of myocardial preservation during open heart surgery because it reduces cardiac morbidity with little increase in risk. However, as early as 1963, local hypothermia was related to an increased risk of pulmonary pathology.[34] The term *frostbitten phrenic* was coined to characterize the injury to the phrenic nerve that was postulated to result from prolonged exposure to hypothermic cardioplegic solution. Four patients were documented to have "diaphragm paralysis," as indicated by inspiratory and expiratory radiographs. Two of them died as a result of the pulmonary dysfunction. A pathologic diagnosis of hypothermic injury to the phrenic nerve was made in one patient.

Since then, other studies[35–37] in humans have demonstrated that hypothermic phrenic nerve injury is common, occurring in 9[38] to 85%[39] of patients exposed to hypothermic solutions; injury occurred mostly on the left side (probably as a result of the phrenic nerve's location on the pericardium). There have been cases of bilateral diaphragmatic paralysis, which is far less common (10 to 20% of the cases) but carries a higher morbidity rate and a graver prognosis.[34, 39, 40]

Patients suffering from hemidiaphragmatic dysfunction have increased pulmonary complications, with more than 80% having pneumonia, pulmonary effusion, atelectasis, pulmonary edema, or the need for prolonged mechanical ventilation. The incidence of and prognosis for hypothermic phrenic nerve injury were studied at the University of Pittsburgh Medical Center.[41] After open heart surgery, patients were evaluated with chest roentgenography, diaphragmatic ultrasonography, and electrophysiologic testing of the phrenic nerve. Immediately after surgery, 46% had abnormal motion of the diaphragm, and 26% had abnormal function of the phrenic nerve as well. Patients with hypothermic phrenic nerve injury tended to have longer mechanical ventilation times and longer hospital stays than did patients without injury. Respiratory symptoms were present in a significantly greater number of patients with phrenic nerve injury than in those without it. During the 12 months after surgery, normal phrenic nerve function returned in all patients. Treatment is supportive, and a good outcome is achieved in most patients once nerve function returns.

Diphtheria

Diphtheria is an infectious disease caused by *Corynebacterium diphtheriae*. The symptomatology is related both to the direct bacterial invasion and to the effects of its exotoxin. The exotoxin is directly toxic to the peripheral nerves, affecting myelin production and leading to multifocal paranodal demyelination. EMG shows a significant decrease in conduction velocity about 2 weeks after infection.

The clinical features of diphtheria include fever, listlessness, and a membranous pharyngitis. This membrane may involve the glottis and larynx, causing upper respiratory obstruction. Neurologic features first manifest around the first week as paralysis of the soft palate, which may progress to involve other cranial nerves (V, VII, X, and XI). Myocarditis has been described in two thirds of diphtheria cases, although clinical

In about 6 to 8 weeks, some patients may develop a sensorimotor polyneuropathy that includes the nerves supplying the respiratory muscles; ventilatory failure may result.

evidence is much less frequent. Arrhythmias and conduction defects are the most common manifestations of cardiac involvement.

Treatment is supportive, although antitoxin may help in decreasing the severity of the clinical course.[25]

Disorders of the Neuromuscular Junction

Myasthenia Gravis

Myasthenia gravis is caused by a defect in transmission at the neuromuscular junction. The incidence has a bimodal distribution, with the first peak occurring at 20 years of age and the second peak occurring at around 40 years of age.

The pathophysiologic process in myasthenia gravis is a reduction in the quantity of the acetylcholine receptors at the neuromuscular junction. These problems with transmission at the neuromuscular junction lead to either a delay in the generation of the action potential or a block in conduction.

The diagnosis is based on clinical findings of ocular and bulbar muscle weakness, positive edrophonium test results, characteristic electrophysiologic findings, and acetylcholine receptor antibody identification. Anti–acetylcholine receptor antibody may be seen in up to 93% of patients.

Cranial nerve involvement is seen very early in the disease and may present as diplopia, ptosis, or dysphagia. The extremities are involved next. Weakness, which is exercise induced, becomes less severe with rest. Myasthenic crisis, manifested by respiratory failure, is a serious complication with a 10% mortality rate. The crisis typically presents in the setting of increasing bulbar muscle paresis, leading to aspiration of secretions. Respiratory muscle weakness and respiratory failure may ensue. Respiratory failure is also commonly seen after a transsternal thymectomy.

Repetitive stimulation of a nerve at 2 to 3 Hz results in a characteristic decrease in the amplitude of the motor evoked response in myasthenia gravis. This decrease is exacerbated by fatiguing exercise and by warming the limb. An improvement in neuromuscular transmission and a return of the response to normal amplitude may also be seen with brief, nonfatiguing exercise.[42] A diagnostic technique that has gained popularity is the study of "jitter" using single-fiber electrodes. This technique assesses the neuromuscular junction with greater sensitivity.[42]

Treatment with cholinesterase inhibitors such as pyridostigmine or neostigmine results in the rapid recovery of muscle strength. Steroids may produce a marked improvement. Plasma exchange also produces rapid improvement, but this effect is short lived. Thymectomy has produced a longer-term improvement in most patients. It is difficult, however, to predict which patients will have improvement. In addition, it may take months before the improvement is seen.[43]

Several predictors of respiratory failure have been suggested. These include severe bulbar involvement[44] and the degree of compromise of maximal static expiratory pressure.[45]

The mainstay of treatment is assisted ventilation. High-dose steroids and plasmapheresis have been found to be effective.[46] Frequently, several exchanges of plasma are required for improvement. Cholinesterase inhibitors are started at low doses during the recovery phase, and then the dosage is optimized. Prethymectomy plasma exchange has been advocated by some authors.[47]

Myasthenic Syndrome (Eaton-Lambert Myasthenic Syndrome)

Eaton-Lambert myasthenic syndrome (ELMS) is a disorder of the neuromuscular junction that results in muscular weakness. ELMS presents with weakness of the limbs and limb girdles. The deep tendon reflexes are hypoactive. The extraocular muscles and other muscles innervated by the cranial nerves may be mildly involved. One characteristic of this disease is an improvement in the deep tendon reflexes and muscle strength immediately after brief exertion.[48] ELMS is frequently associated with malignancy (70% of cases in men and 25% of cases in women), with small cell carcinoma of the lung being the most common neoplasm.

Histopathologic studies have shown a paucity of active zones in the motor nerve terminals and a disorganization of their arrangement. The microanatomy of the neuron and myocyte portions of the neuromuscular junction is altered.[48] Study of the neuromuscular junction using microelectrodes has shown postjunctional acetylcholine receptors to be intact. The lesion is due to the inadequate release of acetylcholine quanta from the prejunctional neuron. Repetitive stimulation at rates of 20 to 40 Hz potentiates the release of acetylcholine, and there is progressive improvement in the amplitude of the recorded response. A potentiation of greater than 200% of the original response is pathognomonic for ELMS.[49]

If a malignancy is present, treatment with chemotherapy, radiation therapy, or resection can produce a transient improvement in transmission at the neuromuscular junction.[50] Guanidine hydrochloride (10 to 35 mg/kg/day), which increases the release of acetylcholine, has been found to be effective. Other treatment options include 3,4-diaminopyridine, azathioprine, corticosteroids, and plasmapheresis. Respiratory support is the same as with other types of flaccid paralysis.

Botulism

Botulism, a disease caused by *Clostridium botulinum* and its exotoxin, mimics ELMS. The toxin affects primarily the prejunctional nerve endings at the neuromuscular junction, where it interferes with the release of acetylcholine quanta. The sensory neurons are not affected.

Clinical symptoms are seen very early, usually within 12 to 24 hours after infection. Nausea and vomiting are the initial symptoms, with progression to weakness of the extraocular muscles. Patients may have diplopia, ptosis, or other symptoms caused by these weakened muscles. Weakness spreads to the muscles supplied by the other bulbar nerves and then to the muscles supplied by the peripheral nerves. Patients ultimately develop a flaccid paralysis and may develop ventilatory failure.

Electrodiagnostic studies show a small motor evoked response. Repetitive stimulation at a frequency of 20 to 50 Hz may show a characteristic improvement in the amplitude of the motor evoked response.[42] The cerebrospinal fluid is normal.

Treatment is with trivalent antitoxin. Guanidine hydrochloride can alleviate the symptoms. Supportive ventilation is an important component of definitive care that results in a positive outcome. Antibiotics are used only when there is invasive infection. Magnesium should be avoided because it may potentiate the neuromuscular blockade.

ELMS occurs predominantly in men, with a 5:1 male to female ratio.

Disorders of the Muscles

Polymyositis and Dermatomyositis

Polymyositis usually occurs in the fifth or sixth decade of life. The prominent feature of this disease is a symmetrical weakness of the limb girdle and neck flexor muscles that progresses over weeks to months. Dysphagia and respiratory muscle weakness may occur.[51] Discoloration of the eyelids; periorbital edema; and an erythematous, scaly dermatitis of the face, neck, upper trunk, dorsum of the hands, and extensor surfaces of the knees and elbows may be seen.[52]

The disease may run a variable course, involving

- Complete recovery
- A relapsing illness with imperfect recovery between bouts
- A chronic, indolent form[53]

In the later stages of this disease, fibrosing alveolitis may be seen.[54] Pulmonary function is compromised, with death usually resulting from pulmonary complications.

Laboratory studies show an increase in the level of serum creatine kinase. Biopsy reveals evidence of segmental myonecrosis, muscle fiber regeneration, and the infiltration of inflammatory cells (predominantly mononuclear cells) into the connective tissue within the muscular fascicles or blood vessels. Early in the disease process, EMG shows short-duration, small-amplitude, polyphasic motor unit potentials; positive sharp waves; and fibrillations. These findings predominate in the paraspinal muscles.[55] In the chronic phase, large polyphasic motor units may be evident.[52]

Treatment consists of steroid administration or immunosuppression with azathioprine or methotrexate. A combination of these drugs has also been tried.[51] Respiratory management is similar to that for the other disorders that are characterized by muscular weakness.

Muscular Dystrophy

Duchenne's muscular dystrophy is a rapidly progressing disease characterized by weakness and "pseudohypertrophy" of the muscles, predominantly those in the calf. The disease has an X-linked recessive inheritance; however, about one third of cases are due to spontaneous mutation.

The disease usually presents in the second year of life. Early developmental milestones are achieved; however, when ambulation is attempted, the first abnormalities are noted. The infant walks on tiptoe and is unable to rise from a kneeling position without the support of his or her hands, using them virtually to "walk" up the body in order to stand erect (Gowers' sign). Up to about 10 years of age, the muscle strength is sufficiently maintained to enable ambulation, but as the child ages, the weakness becomes severe enough to require a wheelchair. Once the child is confined to a wheelchair, complications, including joint contractures, kyphoscoliosis, and respiratory compromise, can rapidly appear and progress.

Pulmonary function testing shows a restrictive pattern. The maximal inspiratory force, the vital capacity, and the total lung volume show a progressive decrease. The decrease in vital capacity is due to a decrease in both the inspiratory force and the compliance of the chest wall and lungs. Residual volume may increase.

The ratio of forced expiratory volume in 1 second to forced vital capacity is maintained at or above normal because the forced expiratory volume in 1 second depends mainly on the recoil of the lung and not on muscular force, whereas the maximal expiratory flow rate at peak volumes is effort dependent and therefore reduced.

Biochemical tests show an increased level of serum creatine phosphokinase and myoglobin. EMG demonstrates myopathy with fibrillation, positive sharp waves, and small polyphasic motor unit potentials with increased recruitment of motor units for a given effort. Biopsy of the muscle shows variation in fiber size, and areas of muscle atrophy and necrosis may be adjacent to hypertrophic fibers. There is a proliferation of connective tissue and an inflammatory reaction as well.

Although the disease is primarily muscular, a low IQ is common. In addition, electrocardiographic abnormalities may exist.[56] Duchenne's muscular dystrophy usually results in death by the third decade of life.

There is no specific treatment to abort the course of the disease. Treatment is therefore directed at preventing complications, prolonging muscular function, and improving the quality of life. Every effort is made to prolong the ambulatory phase by bracing or appropriate surgery.[57] Ambulation maintains the spine in lordosis, thereby locking the spinal facets and preventing scoliosis. Adequate wheelchair seating and spinal bracing help to slow the progression of scoliosis.

Aggressive pulmonary management, including the early and prolonged use of ventilators and an aggressive rehabilitation program, has been advocated.[59] Chronic ventilatory insufficiency typically presents first at night, with retention of carbon dioxide, fitful sleep, morning headache, narcolepsy, and a general decrease in vigor during the day. Nighttime ventilation and rest therapy may help to improve daytime oxygenation and decrease hypercarbia. In later stages, supplemental ventilation may be required in the daytime as well.[60]

Becker's dystrophy is a slowly progressive X-linked recessive muscular dystrophy. The disease onset occurs much later than that of Duchenne's dystrophy; patients are usually ambulatory until approximately 16 years of age. They normally survive until middle adulthood. Cognitive disability is less common. All the other clinical features and the management of this disease follow the same course as with Duchenne's muscular dystrophy.

Myotonia

Myotonias (myotonia congenita and myotonia dystrophica) are rare muscular disorders that can result in respiratory deficiencies similar to those of the muscular dystrophies. Respiratory care of these patients is supportive and is comparable to that used for muscular dystrophy.

RESPIRATORY MANAGEMENT FOR PATIENTS WITH NEUROMUSCULAR WEAKNESS

Although a variety of diseases result in respiratory muscle weakness, the management remains relatively similar. Table 48–3 outlines the principles of pulmonary therapy. Most patients manifest muscular weakness, fibrosis, diminished compliance, impaired central drive, high infectious risk, atelectasis, and respiratory failure. Because increased rates of morbidity and mortality are caused by respiratory complications,

Spinal fusion may partially correct scoliosis or prevent its progression; however, it has no effect on the decline of respiratory function.[58]

TABLE **48–3:**   Principles of Pulmonary Rehabilitation

Treatment and prevention of parenchymal and airway disease	Exercise conditioning
Delivery of oxygen	Rest therapy
Chest physiotherapy	Patient education
Pulmonary muscle training	Psychological support

Because of its appearance, glossopharyngeal breathing has been called "frog breathing." By using this technique, a patient may obtain 80 mL of air per stroke, and by performing an average of 20 strokes per breath, the patient can maintain a tidal volume of about 1.33 L.[61, 62]

therapy must be directed at maximizing respiratory function. This includes decreasing the work of the respiratory muscles by increasing compliance and lessening demand. Exercising the respiratory muscles may increase their strength and improve their functional status. Providing adequate pulmonary toilet should decrease the number of infectious complications. The importance of resting fatigued muscles is being realized by clinicians, so this practice is increasing. The pharmacologic management of individual diseases was discussed previously. However, some agents may enhance performance for various disorders. The facilitation of pulmonary toilet by humidification of the air, chest percussion, postural drainage, suctioning, and assisted "quad" cough can be vital in preventing atelectasis and pneumonia.[7]

Glossopharyngeal breathing coordinates movement of the tongue, cheeks, and pharynx to force air from the mouth into the lungs. Inspiration is active and voluntary, whereas exhalation is passive. Glossopharyngeal breathing may provide adequate ventilation for short periods in patients with ventilatory failure. This technique may give an additional tidal volume and may produce a deep breath in patients who are able to ventilate on their own.

Assessment

The various ways of measuring respiratory function that are available to the practitioner are covered in more detail elsewhere in this text. However, certain variables are particularly useful as indicators of respiratory function in this group of patients (Table 48–4).

Because it is affected by changes in thoracic compliance, vital capacity is an easily obtained and reproducible measurement of respiratory muscle strength. Vital capacity measures both strength and (indirectly) compliance; however, it does not discriminate between alterations in one or the other. Many argue that vital capacity is the best clinical indicator of respiratory impairment.[63] Vital capacity may be a better predictor of the ability to generate an effective cough. This ability to cough is important for pulmonary toilet with respect to both the clearance of secretions and the prevention of atelectasis. Despite all this predicted benefit, vital capacity has been shown to correlate poorly with weaning from mechanical ventilation in patients with Guillain-Barré syndrome and myasthenia gravis.[64]

Inspiratory force is thought to approximate inspiratory muscle strength[65] and transdiaphragmatic pressure (Pdi) during inspiration.[64]

TABLE **48–4:**   Useful Measures of Respiratory Function

Tidal volume	Maximal voluntary ventilation
Vital capacity	Inspiratory time/respiratory cycle
Minute volume	time (t_i/t_{tot})
Inspiratory force	

In the study by Borel and coworkers, the Pdi correlated best with weaning; however, these investigators recognized that the ability to generate a single large force (inspiratory force or Pdi) may lack correlation with the ability to sustain ventilation for a prolonged period. These two measurements evaluate only inspiratory muscle function. However, it is recognized that the generation of expiratory flow is important as well. For this reason, peak expiratory flow may be measured. This variable can help to predict the ability to cough, the amount of expiratory resistance, and the response to bronchodilator therapy.

The ability to sustain ventilation for prolonged intervals is the single most important characteristic in weaning weak patients from mechanical ventilation. However, accurate measurement of this ability is difficult. Single-breath measurements of force, volume, and flow are unreliable predictors of long-term success in weaning. Measurements of diaphragmatic work and reserve have been studied in patients recovering from respiratory failure due to neuromuscular disease.[64] In addition to the measurements of inspiratory force and vital capacity described earlier, the ratio of Pdi to maximal Pdi (Pdi/Pdi_{max}), inspiratory time (t_i), and the percentage of the ventilatory cycle spent in inspiration (t_i/t_{tot}) were measured. The intention was to determine whether the diaphragmatic tension-time integral (TTIdi), a measure of the diaphragmatic fatigue threshold, would predict weaning in this population.

Other measurements of reserve and fatigue thresholds have been studied. Measurement of the ability of patients to breathe in excess of the minute work has been advocated. Maximal minute volume by forced ventilation (MVV) is easily measured by spirometry. If the MVV is divided by the minute volume at rest ($MVV/\dot{V}E$), the quotient reflects the amount of respiratory reserve a patient has. A $MVV/\dot{V}E$ of greater than 2 is considered to be indicative of a favorable outcome.[65] However, the sensitivity and specificity of this ratio are low.[67]

Because none of these variables reliably predicts success in weaning a patient from mechanical ventilation, probably the most useful benefit of measuring respiratory muscle function is the ability to monitor performance trends over time. For the prediction to be accurate, the measurement must be reproducible. For instance, a vital capacity that has a tendency to decrease continually becomes a good predictor of poor performance, poor response to treatment, or worsening disease. The best measurements for this purpose are those that are simple and reliable. Typically, inspiratory force and vital capacity have been used in this way. To date, no other measurements have been shown to be as simple, reproducible, or predictive of ventilatory strength.

Electrodiagnostic Studies

The neural axis, which mediates its function through the muscle pump, controls the ventilatory system. Ventilatory pump failure can be due to either a focal lesion involving the neural axis or a primary muscle disease. Electrodiagnostic studies may help to assess the neurophysiologic status of the ventilatory pump and to verify the presence of a lesion.

The phrenic nerves are accessible for percutaneous or transcutaneous stimulation in the neck; it is possible to conduct to the ipsilateral hemidiaphragm with this method.[68, 69] Lesions in the phrenic nerve that cause slowed conduction also prolong the distal latency, as is seen in Guillain-Barré syndrome. The loss of axons in the phrenic nerve results

$$TTIdi = t_i/t_{tot} \times Pdi/Pdi_{max}$$

All muscles become fatigued when work (demand) exceeds a particular threshold. For the diaphragm, fatigue occurs when the TTIdi goes above 0.15.[66] However, the TTIdi was not a good predictor of weaning because patients did not exceed the threshold during spontaneous breathing but were not capable of being weaned from mechanical ventilation.

There are two parts to electrodiagnostic study: the nerve conduction study and EMG.

Electrodiagnostic studies are useful in evaluating the generalized neuromuscular causes of ventilatory pump failure and in helping to diagnose and classify the peripheral neuropathies, radiculopathies, and myopathies.

in a small amplitude of evoked response, as is the case with critically ill polyneuropathy.

EMG of the hemidiaphragm involves inserting a monopolar or concentric needle electrode into the hemidiaphragm at the eighth intercostal space in the anterior axillary line. The electrode can also be inserted under the xiphoid process into the anterior crural attachment. The risk of pneumothorax is small. If there is axonal loss in the phrenic nerve, fibrillation and positive sharp waves may be seen in the diaphragm. During inspiration, the motor units are recruited, and the morphology of this potential is analyzed. The motor unit potentials are normally triphasic. Polyphasic motor unit potentials are seen after a neuropathic lesion of the phrenic nerve or a myopathic lesion of the diaphragm.

Computer-aided analysis has introduced a new dimension to electrodiagnostic studies. Even though this method is still investigational, early reports have suggested that it may enable the assessment of fatigue in the muscles involved. Analysis of the power frequency spectrum shows a loss of high-frequency components with a shift toward the lower-frequency components of the EMG signal during fatigue. Study of the phrenic nerve and the diaphragm is important not only for diagnostic purposes but also for therapeutic reasons; for example, an intact nerve is essential to permit implantation of a phrenic nerve pacer.

Mechanical Ventilatory Assistance

Mechanical ventilatory assistance is frequently necessary in the treatment of patients with neuromuscular disease. A variety of modalities are available to the practitioner (Table 48–5). All are effective to some degree; however, respiratory support will not reverse the primary process. Rather, mechanical ventilatory assistance either provides temporary respiratory support until the process resolves, as in the Guillain-Barré syndrome, or is permanently supportive, as in a ventilator-dependent patient with ALS. Decisions to use mechanical support must take into account the potential goals of the therapy.

The most commonly used form of mechanical ventilation is positive pressure ventilation. Various authors have supported the use of continuous mandatory ventilation, intermittent mandatory ventilation, pressure support ventilation, mandatory minute ventilation, and extended minute ventilation; however, none of these modes has been demonstrated to be consistently superior to any other for purposes of ventilatory weaning or support. These modes of ventilation are discussed at length elsewhere in this text.

Intermittent Positive Pressure Ventilation

Atelectasis is a common complication of neuromuscular disorders.[70] Patients with weakness of the respiratory muscles develop decreased

TABLE **48–5:**   Methods of Mechanical Ventilatory Assistance

Intermittent positive pressure ventilation	Negative pressure ventilation
Continuous positive airway pressure	Body ventilation
Face mask ventilation	Electrophrenic respiration
Nasal ventilation	BiPAP

respiratory compliance because of a variety of factors. Diminished excursions of the chest wall cause hypoventilation, which predisposes to atelectasis. In addition, after a time, the muscles involved in the neuromuscular disorder become stiff and shortened, and the joints may become less flexible as well. Therefore, energy expenditure increases for a given amount of chest wall movement. This increased work of breathing exacerbates the tendency to fatigue and hypoventilate, which increases atelectasis and the work of breathing.

Poor strength also diminishes the effectiveness of the patient's cough. Although the maximal rate of flow at midexpiration is only slightly effort dependent, peak flow at the height of inspiration is very effort dependent. In patients with weakened respiratory muscles, peak flow is greatly diminished, which may result in an ineffectual cough. This allows secretions to be retained, causing obstruction, loss of pulmonary compliance, an increased tendency to infection, and ventilation-perfusion mismatch. A decrease in oxygenation creates the need for greater ventilation, thereby increasing the work of breathing and the tendency to respiratory failure.

Patients with respiratory muscle weakness require therapy directed at decreasing the work of breathing (increasing efficiency) or increasing muscle strength. Intermittent positive pressure ventilation (IPPV) has been thought to reverse atelectasis and increase chest wall compliance by repeatedly stretching the chest muscles and bony articulations. Few data exist to support this, however. In fact, studies have demonstrated the lack of effect of IPPV on lung compliance.[71, 72] A mean IPPV pressure of 29 cm H_2O for 30 minutes has resulted in no effect on pulmonary compliance or work of breathing.[72] The effect of a single IPPV treatment in patients with quadriplegia and muscular dystrophy has been studied.[71] An IPPV pressure of 22 cm H_2O resulted in inspiratory volumes that were at least three times patients' resting tidal volumes, but no difference was found in lung, chest wall, or respiratory system compliance after the maneuver.

The poor response to IPPV is believed to be multifactorial. Some explanations are

- Failure of the patient to create an adequate seal around the mouthpiece
- Failure of the volume of air to enter the trachea (esophageal insufflation)
- Muscular resistance to the positive pressure, causing increased airway pressure and termination of the breath at a low delivered tidal volume
- Rapid derecruitment after termination of the treatment
- An inequitable distribution of the positive pressure breath to better-ventilated rather than atelectatic areas of the lungs
- An altered pressure-volume relationship (decreased compliance) in the lung parenchyma that is not improved by IPPV[71, 72]

At this time, there appear to be no significant data that support the use of IPPV in this patient population, although the practice remains prevalent. Further studies using larger volumes may demonstrate benefit, although patient compliance may become a factor.

Continuous Positive Airway Pressure

Continuous positive airway pressure has been advocated as a method of increasing functional residual capacity and thus preventing atelectasis in patients with weak respiratory muscles. However, few data exist to support its use in this population. Nasal continuous positive airway pressure is now gaining in popularity for use in diseases such as obstructive sleep apnea and in those that cause upper airway obstruction due to muscular laxity. Continuous positive airway pressure, which does not protect against aspiration, may be contraindicated in patients who are unable to maintain the airway well.

A newer form of continuous positive airway pressure (CPAP), termed BiPAP, is now available (Respironics, Murraysville, PA). BiPAP is delivered via a face mask or, more commonly, a nasal mask. It has all the advantages of CPAP and the additional improvement of allowing the physician to manipulate inspiratory and expiratory pressures independently. Adjusting inspiratory airway pressure to be higher than expiratory pressure decreases the inspiratory work of breathing, thereby augmenting "spontaneous" tidal volume. Although the effectiveness of BiPAP has not been demonstrated specifically in patients with neuromuscular disease, benefit has been observed in other classes of patients with respiratory insufficiency. Thus, it is reasonable to expect that this therapy may be useful in selected patients with neuromuscular disorders.

Respiratory Muscle Training

Muscles that are weak are prone to fatigue. As weak muscles have chronic work imposed on them, they progressively lose reserve capacity and ultimately fail. Two methods of therapy have been advocated to help prevent this cycle: respiratory muscle training and rest therapy.

Respiratory muscle training has been advocated for patients with chronic obstructive pulmonary disease,[73] quadriplegia,[10] or postpolio syndrome[21] and for those who are in or approaching respiratory failure. Respiratory muscle training can increase both strength and endurance beyond that accomplished with routine breathing or exercise with the use of a protocol that incrementally adds inspiratory resistance to a breathing circuit. Intermittent use of an inspiratory resistor increases the vital capacity and the maximal inspiratory pressure generated by a patient with muscular dystrophy.[74] With the use of either strength or endurance (resistive work) training, both strength and endurance could be improved independently of each other.[75] Selecting an appropriate amount of resistance is important. Appropriate levels of exercise may result in improved function or weaning from the ventilator, whereas excessive exercise can damage respiratory muscle fibers.[73]

Both strength and endurance training have been effective in some patients under experimental conditions; however, some researchers have questioned the utility of respiratory muscle training.[77] Currently, some patients can be expected to exhibit a functional improvement with a combined approach of rest and resistive training.

Rest and Nocturnal Ventilation

As neuromuscular disease progresses, muscles become weaker, with an increased tendency to fatigue. Muscles that are continuously stressed can develop chronic fatigue, decreasing function and respiratory reserve, which in turn can increase the likelihood of respiratory decompensation.

Respiratory muscle training is effective for patients who have not yet developed respiratory failure[76] and for those who are ventilator dependent.[74]

TABLE **48–6:** Effect of Respiratory Rest on Respiratory Function in Patients With Chronic Airflow Limitation

	Before	After	P
FEV_1	27%	31%	NS
Vital capacity	36%	53%	.001
PI_{max}	36%	58%	.001
Maximal voluntary ventilation	21%	28%	.02
Pa_{CO_2}	54 mm Hg	45 mm Hg	.001
Class	5	3	.001
Admissions	2.8	0.4	.001

Data from Braun N, Marino W. Effect of daily intermittent rest of respiratory muscles in patients with severe chronic airflow limitation (CAL). Chest 85:59S, 1984.
FEV_1, forced expiratory volume in 1 second; NS, not significant.

To prevent the onset of fatigue and forestall adverse respiratory events, some authors have advocated intermittently resting the muscles of respiration with mechanical support.[78, 79]

Rest therapy for respiratory muscles may be defined as the removal of all work from the muscles of respiration for a period of time. Mechanical ventilators (either positive or negative pressure ventilators) perform the work of breathing and relieve the respiratory muscles of the obligation to work. To prove that muscles are resting, EMG of the diaphragm may be performed to demonstrate an absence of electrical activity. More commonly, this is determined by observing a lack of inspiratory effort by the patient.

Rest therapy increases the performance of the respiratory muscles after rest. This therapy has been examined in patients with chronic airflow limitation.[78] Although airway resistance did not change, vital capacity, maximal inspiratory pressure, and maximal voluntary ventilation did improve (Table 48–6). The arterial partial pressure of carbon dioxide (Pa_{CO_2}) decreased to near-normal values, and the functional class improved from dyspnea at rest to dyspnea with exertion. Most importantly, patients were hospitalized less frequently. Patients with Duchenne-type muscular dystrophy who had daily rest therapy had improvement as well.[80, 81] After 1 to 3 months of therapy, these patients had a significant improvement in forced vital capacity and Pa_{CO_2} (Table 48–7). Although the patients' ventilation ultimately worsened, there was a demonstrated clinical improvement, with chronic mechanical support being delayed. The mode of ventilatory support does not appear to be as important as the provision of rest. Body ventilation,[81] negative pressure ventilation,[80, 88] and positive pressure ventilation via tracheostomy[78, 80] or via mask[86, 89] have all been demonstrated to be beneficial.

Although intermittent rest therapy benefits patients with slowly progressive neuromuscular disease, weakness, and fatigue, it is probably not the modality of choice for patients with severe and rapidly progressive disorders, such as Guillain-Barré syndrome. However, this therapy

Rest therapy has been beneficial in patients with postpolio syndrome,[82] myopathy,[83] polymyositis,[84] motor neuron disease,[85] surgical phrenic nerve injury,[82] and ALS.[86, 87]

TABLE **48–7:** Effect of Intermittent Mechanical Respiratory Support in Ventilation for Patients With Duchenne-Type Muscular Dystrophy

	Initiation	After 1 to 3 Months	Change (%)
Forced vital capacity	603 mL	693 mL	+15
Pa_{CO_2}	63 mm Hg	45 mm Hg	−29
Ventilator use	0 hr/day	8 hr/day	—

Data from Mohr C, Hill N. Long-term follow-up of nocturnal ventilatory assistance in patients with respiratory failure due to Duchenne-type muscular dystrophy. Chest 97:91, 1990.

may be useful during the recovery phase or if this disease progresses slowly.

Mask Ventilation

As neuromuscular disease progresses, a patient's ability to breathe spontaneously waxes and wanes. For this reason, as patients approach permanent respiratory failure, there tend to be episodes of respiratory failure separated by long periods of unassisted ventilation. To improve patient comfort and decrease the invasiveness of care, ventilation without intubation has been used. There are two methods of assisting ventilation without intubation: negative pressure ventilation and positive pressure ventilation with an occlusive mask.[90] Negative pressure ventilation is effective, but problems can occur, including airway obstruction and inadequate ventilation in patients who have kyphoscoliosis or are not supine.

Positive pressure ventilation via a face or nasal mask is convenient and effective. It has been used frequently and without complication for long-term ventilation of patients at home.[15, 89] Nasal positive pressure ventilation can entirely relieve the respiratory muscles of all effort involved in the work of breathing.[91] Thus, patients need not be intubated to utilize rest therapy effectively. Patients starting positive pressure ventilation via a mask may begin with intermittent rest therapy; they then progress to increased frequency as needed for acute decompensations and finally to continual use for long-term ventilatory therapy. It is generally well tolerated, especially because patients remain able to talk and eat; the need for tracheostomy is obviated. Complications include aspiration, aerophagia, transient hypoxemia (if the mask is removed), sores from facial pressure, and patient anxiety.[92]

Negative Pressure and Body Ventilation

Mechanical ventilation, which is possible without using positive intrathoracic pressure, has been effective in the treatment of patients with respiratory failure. From its first use in 1929[93] until the 1960s, when positive pressure ventilators gained greater acceptance, the iron lung was a mainstay in ventilatory assistance.

Negative pressure ventilators work by applying a subatmospheric pressure about the thorax, causing an outward expansion of the chest and subsequent airflow into the lungs. Release of the pressure and the elastic recoil of the lungs and thorax cause passive exhalation. From the prototype iron lung, a cuirass or shell evolved. The apparatus consists of a rigid plastic shell that is placed over the thorax or the thorax and abdomen and is connected by a hose to a negative pressure generator. The ventilator, which is set to create a subatmospheric pressure of about -10 to -40 cm H_2O at a rate of 10 to 25 cycles per minute, can generate tidal volumes of roughly 300 to 1000 mL.

Body or belt ventilators work by displacing the abdominal contents inward and upward against the diaphragm, forcing it to move up, which causes exhalation. Release of the abdominal pressure allows the diaphragm to fall, generating an inspiration. In order to facilitate the downward motion of the diaphragm, the patient must be sufficiently upright

Severe kyphoscoliosis or obesity may preclude the use of body or shell ventilators.

to take advantage of gravity. The patient should be sitting at an angle of no less than 30 degrees and optimally of 75 degrees.

Both body and shell ventilators require fitting. With an inappropriate fit, the shell ventilator will leak and be unable to generate an effective pressure, whereas the belt ventilator will ineffectively move the diaphragm, thereby generating an inadequate tidal volume. These ventilators may have other problems as well. They must be synchronized to the patient's respiratory rate, completely assuming control of ventilation. The apparatus may cause pain or irritation at sites of contact, or abdominal pain may be caused by excessive motion of the abdomen. These effects can be lessened by gradually accustoming the patient to the ventilator. Finally, because the ventilators create a subatmospheric endotracheal pressure, any upper airway obstruction may be exacerbated, thereby precluding their use. Patients may prefer one type of ventilation to another, so it is appropriate to try several methods, allowing the patient to select the most advantageous one.[94]

The use of shell and body ventilators is common in patients with neuromuscular disorders, including

- Poliomyelitis[93, 95]
- Muscular dystrophy[95, 96]
- ALS[86]
- Guillain-Barré syndrome[97]
- Nonspecific myopathy[95]
- Multiple sclerosis[96]
- Friedreich's ataxia[96]

Furthermore, these ventilators have been used in a variety of clinical settings, including

- Nocturnal ventilation[95, 98]
- Home mechanical ventilation[95, 96]
- Acute ventilatory assistance[97]

Home Mechanical Ventilation

Because many patients with neuromuscular impairment have an intact sensorium and irreversible ventilatory insufficiency, long-term mechanical ventilation is often needed. In these patients, it is as important to choose the best setting as it is to choose the best ventilatory mode for providing the mechanical support. There is now considerable experience with ventilating patients at home for prolonged periods.[16, 19, 20, 80, 99–101] Home mechanical ventilation has been successfully provided for patients with polio,[16, 99, 100] myasthenia gravis,[99] ALS,[99, 101] myopathy,[20, 100] spinal cord injury,[19] and muscular dystrophy.[80] Table 48–8 lists these and other disorders for which home mechanical ventilation is appropriate. In many cases, providing the care at home is preferable because of the improved quality of life, improved pulmonary status, and greatly decreased cost of medical care. Patients prefer to be at home despite the effort involved because they have increased autonomy and ability to participate in the community.[19]

Patients may enter into the home program when the need for mechanical ventilation becomes stable. Oxygen is unnecessary because the parenchymal function of the lungs is often preserved, despite the loss of muscular function. The home ventilation program is of necessity multi-

TABLE **48–8:** Neuromuscular Disorders for Which Long-Term Home Mechanical Ventilation Has Been Advocated

Spinal cord disorders
  Tumor
  Trauma
Neural disease
  Amyotrophic lateral sclerosis
  Poliomyelitis
  Phrenic nerve injury (traumatic or
    hypothermic)
  Multiple sclerosis
Muscular and neuromuscular junction disorders
  Myasthenia gravis
  Myopathy
  Muscular dystrophies

disciplinary.[99] Table 48–9 lists the professionals involved in home mechanical ventilation, along with the types of assistance they provide. The decision to provide home mechanical ventilation involves all the caregivers and the family or the family support group. Once the decision has been made to provide care at home, an emphasis is placed on education. The patient and family need to be aware of the responsibilities of each member of the care team. The caregivers need to ensure that safe care can be provided at home by the patient, the family, the appropriate home health services, and the primary physician. The time leading up to the patient's discharge may be difficult and stressful. There is much to learn, and confidence in the ability to care for the patient at home wanes. Psychological support should be as much of a priority as teaching skills. A nurse and a respiratory care practitioner should visit the home to assess the likelihood of success and ensure continuity of care. Understanding the home environment allays fears and improves planning. After patient discharge, frequent follow-up is necessary. Telephone contact and visits to the home can provide solutions to care problems and alleviate any fears.

Various ventilators have been used in home care, including positive pressure, body, and mask ventilators. The type used depends on the physical structure of the home, the support provided by the medical caregivers and the family, and the physiologic needs of the patient. Long-term home ventilatory support may be equivalent to or more successful than care provided in a hospital or a long-term care facility.

Diaphragm Pacing

Neural control of ventilatory function may be impaired in the central nervous system, the peripheral nerves, or the neuromuscular junction. When neural control is blocked, an electrical stimulus may be used to

TABLE **48–9:** Home Mechanical Ventilation: Health Professionals and Their Roles

Respiratory care practitioner	Teaching, ventilator care, pulmonary therapy
Nurse (hospital, home care)	Teaching, tracheostomy care, general nursing care, physiotherapy, pulmonary therapy
Social worker	Psychological support, mobilization of resources
Physician	Medical therapy, coordination of care
Family	Psychological support, provision of some basic care

induce diaphragmatic contraction and assist ventilation. This technique is termed electrophrenic respiration.

It has long been recognized that electrical stimulation of the phrenic nerve results in contraction of the diaphragm. However, it was not until 1966 that long-term electrophrenic respiration was used in humans.[102] The initial problems encountered included diaphragmatic fatigue, damage to the phrenic nerve, inability to ventilate adequately, and electromechanical (equipment) failure. Since that time, much work has been done to refine the equipment and the type of stimulation and to prevent diaphragmatic fatigue.

Currently, the most common form of electrophrenic respiration is phrenic nerve pacing. It is possible to pace the diaphragm directly; however, this technique has not been as popular. Consequently, the amount of experience with this technique is limited.

The system consists of a unipolar or multipolar electrode that is surgically implanted adjacent to the phrenic nerve in the thorax. One or both phrenic nerves may have electrodes placed at the same time. The electrode is connected to a subcutaneously implanted receiver. In addition to the electrodes and the receiver, a radio transmitter and a power supply are required. The transmitter emits radiofrequency waves that are picked up by the subcutaneous receiver. The receiver then converts this energy to electrical impulses, which are sent to the phrenic electrodes. The frequency and the duration of the impulses determine the strength of muscular contraction. In addition, the inspiratory time, the respiratory rate, and to some extent the tidal volume can be controlled. The transmitter is external because the large energy requirement for diaphragm pacing necessitates frequent changing of the energy source, usually a battery.

Training of the diaphragm should not begin until about 2 weeks after surgical implantation, in order to allow the perineural edema to resolve and the incisions to heal.[102–104] The training then commences with a gradual increase in the duration of the pacing. Pacing starts at a low respiratory rate for a duration of about 15 min/hr several times a day. When there is no evidence of fatigue during a trial, as measured by tidal volume, inspiratory force, and level of carbon dioxide, the duration may be gradually lengthened as needed up to 24 hours.

Diaphragm pacing has been successfully used in patients with tetraplegia,[102–108] primary alveolar hypoventilation,[109] and central sleep apnea.[110] When it has been used as a method of ventilation, some patients have become ventilator independent within several months, enabling them to be moved on to a rehabilitation facility. It has been reported that 53% of patients tolerated 24-hour diaphragm pacing. An additional 22% tolerated 12-hour pacing, greatly increasing the patients' independence.[105] Pacing helped to condition the diaphragm successfully in quadriplegic patients[102] and in a patient with primary alveolar hypoventilation.[109] Diaphragm muscle fibers convert from fast-contracting (fatigue-sensitive) to slow-contracting (fatigue-resistant) ones.[102] Through the use of a multipolar electrode and stimulation of quadrants of the nerve in succession, this conversion can be augmented with a low pulse-cycle frequency (11 Hz or less). This ability is important because the most frequent complication of pacing is fatigue, which precludes continuous pacing. Nocturnal pacing conditions the diaphragm, causing a marked improvement in daily function.[109] Other unexpected benefits have been reported with electrophrenic respiration, including improved arterial oxygenation despite a decreased alveolar ventilation[107] and longer survival in patients with spinal cord injury.[106]

Complications of electrophrenic respiration, which are relatively uncommon with the exception of battery failure, include

- Pacing failure due to mechanical system failure or electrode placement
- Phrenic nerve damage resulting from overstimulation or surgery
- Fatigue of the diaphragm due to an overly aggressive pacing schedule
- Wound infection
- Upper airway obstruction caused by negative pressure ventilation

In the last instance, patients who may have obstruction should be considered for tracheostomy before phrenic pacing is started. Other possible contraindications include phrenic nerve injury, severe parenchymal dysfunction requiring high minute volumes or end-expiratory pressure, and chest wall damage, which greatly reduces compliance.

The benefits of electrophrenic respiration in patients with neuromuscular disease, particularly those with high cervical spinal cord trauma, are freedom from positive pressure ventilators, shorter time before moving to a rehabilitation facility, increased independence, and improved performance of the remaining muscular units.

Diaphragmatic Inotropic Support

It has long been recognized that the contractility of the heart can be augmented pharmacologically and that this improves myocardial performance. However, not until 1981 was it demonstrated that diaphragmatic contractility can be augmented as well.[111] Theophylline, for example, increases the fatigue resistance in the diaphragm. For years, it was thought that theophylline improved ventilation as a result of decreased airway resistance. However, improved ventilation persisted even when there was no decrease in airway resistance, and theophylline's effect was discovered to result instead from an augmentation of diaphragmatic contractility and fatigue resistance.[112] Digoxin[113, 114] and dopamine[115] also improve diaphragmatic strength, even when cardiac output remains constant.

There is no current controversy about whether pharmacologic agents can enhance diaphragmatic strength and endurance. However, it remains to be shown whether these agents have a positive clinical effect. It is not known whether a diaphragmatic inotrope should be used in any patient with a weak or fatigue-sensitive diaphragm. If no contraindication to therapy exists, then using digoxin or theophylline seems to be reasonable at this time.

ETHICAL ISSUES IN NEUROMUSCULAR DISEASE

Providing mechanical ventilatory support to patients with neuromuscular disease is not technically difficult. Most frequently, gas exchange in the lung is preserved. Thus, the support is directed primarily at ventilation. The patient's cognition is usually preserved as well. It would thus seem simple to provide ventilation to these patients and allow them to continue living as normally as possible. However, the situation is rarely this clear. Patients tend to have a gradual decline in function interspersed with periods of increasing severity, often making it

TABLE **48–10:** Stresses Encountered by Patients Receiving Long-Term Mechanical Ventilatory Assistance

Feeling tied to the machine, dependency
Infections: treatment, isolation, activity restriction
Inadequacy: cannot reach potential
Social stigma: personal and by others
Isolation, inability to participate
Decreased involvement in recreational activities

difficult to determine which decompensation will result in long-term ventilation. Further, defining the goals of both the patient and the physician is very important in determining what level of support to provide to the patient. For example, a patient with early ALS who is rendered unable to breathe after a motor vehicle accident but who has a good prognosis for recovery and independent function is viewed differently than a patient with ALS who has ventilatory insufficiency because of disease progression.

Patients and their families have been studied to determine the impact of providing mechanical ventilation to patients with neuromuscular disease.[116] The age of the patients ranged from 16 to 31 years, making this a very young reference group. Tables 48–10 and 48–11 list sources of stress for the patient and the family, respectively. Of interest, most were generally pleased with the decision to use mechanical support, despite the stress involved. Issues raised in deciding to use mechanical ventilation centered on factors related to decision making. Adequate education of the family and the patient must be provided. Everyone involved must be aware of the medical prognosis, the amount of work involved, the financial considerations, and the prediction of what daily life will be like for both patients and their families. It is important to initiate discussion before mechanical support is needed so that all concerned can comprehend and discuss the issues and formulate a decision. The physician, respiratory care practitioner, nurse, and social worker may all be involved in the educational plan for the family.

The issues related to starting mechanical support are the same as those for discontinuing it (Table 48–12), although for each situation these issues will differ. The issues must be identified and discussed and the relative priorities clarified. The patient and family must be educated about the disease and its prognosis, what life will be like with or without the machine, how death will occur, and whether there will be discomfort (with either mechanical ventilation or death). All need to be aware of the distinction between active euthanasia (causing death by some direct action) and allowing a patient to die of the underlying disease process without intervention (e.g., forgoing ventilator support in a patient with irreversible respiratory failure). The legal environment must be taken

TABLE **48–11:** Stresses Encountered by Families of Patients Receiving Mechanical Ventilatory Assistance

Feeling tied to the machine
Providing continuous care (no rest)
Having less time for other family members
Alterations in the family's schedule (e.g., altering or eliminating vacations)
Diminished social activities
Equipment breakdown
Ambiguous future
Presence of "strangers" in the home (nurses, therapists)
Loss of privacy

TABLE **48–12:** Major Issues Involving the Provision of Mechanical Ventilatory Support

Identification of the primary decision maker
Formulation of goals for providing ventilatory support
Education of the patient and family
Identification of the ethical issues
Advance directives (living will, health care proxy)
Quality of life after mechanical ventilation
Course of neuromuscular disease after mechanical ventilation
Legal factors (state, federal, statute)
Religious considerations

into account as well. Most states have either legislation or case law that permits withholding life-supporting medical treatment. There is now federal case law for this as well. Currently in the United States, the burden of decision making resides with the patient, family, and physician. A US Supreme Court ruling[117] has supported the concept of persons having the right to refuse medical treatment, even if the refusal results in the patient's death (see Chapter 58). However, the court reaffirmed that the state has an interest in preventing suicide and homicide and in upholding the integrity of the medical profession. The state may place some restrictions on the practice of withholding treatment: it may require clear and convincing evidence of a patient's wishes. This is most important when families and physicians are making decisions for a person who cannot and has not expressed his or her own preferences. This issue is discussed in more detail elsewhere.[118, 119]

The patient, family, and physician must identify a primary decision maker, although in most situations decisions are made by consensus. Specific ethical issues may include reconciling diverse opinions about what an appropriate quality of life is, whether the potential outcome is worth the burden of continued support, religious beliefs, and medical care. Sensitive discussion of these issues must take place; when everyone comprehends and agrees, a decision may be made.

SUMMARY

Treatment of the underlying process is, of course, the primary goal of medical therapy. When preventing or postponing the need for ventilatory support is no longer possible, most patients can benefit from a variety of respiratory modalities. Decisions about whether to provide support, when to provide it, and which type of support to use for optimal ventilation must be carefully considered by the patient, family, and physician. Once the decision to provide ventilatory support has been made, the care of the respiratory system includes the efforts of a trained medical team.

References

1. Macklem P, Chairman. NHLBI workshop summary: Respiratory muscle fatigue. Am Rev Respir Dis 142:474, 1990.
2. Smith P, Calverley P, Edwards R, et al. Practical problems in the respiratory care of patients with muscular dystrophy. N Engl J Med 316:1197, 1987.
3. Neu H, Connolly J, Schwertley F, et al. Obstructive respiratory dysfunction in parkinsonian patients. Am Rev Respir Dis 95:33, 1967.

4. Obenour W, Stevens P, Cohen A, McMutchen J. The causes of abnormal pulmonary function in Parkinson's disease. Am Rev Respir Dis 105:382, 1972.
5. Troyer A, Estenne M, Heilporn A. Mechanism of active expiration in tetraplegic subjects. N Engl J Med 314:740, 1986.
6. Carter E. Medical management of pulmonary complications of spinal cord injury. Adv Neurol 22:261, 1979.
7. Mansel J, Norman J. Respiratory complications and management of spinal cord injuries. Chest 97:1446, 1990.
8. Fishburn M, Marino R, Ditunno J. Atelectasis and pneumonia in acute spinal cord injury. Arch Phys Med Rehabil 71:197, 1990.
9. Kirby N, Barnerias M, Siebens A. An evaluation of assisted cough in quadriparetic patients. Arch Phys Med Rehabil 47:705, 1966.
10. Gross D, Ladd H, Riley E, et al. The effect of training on strength and endurance of the diaphragm in quadriplegia. Am J Med 68:27, 1980.
11. Williams D, Windebank A. Motor neuron disease (amyotrophic lateral sclerosis). Mayo Clin Proc 66:54, 1991.
12. Tandan R, Bradley W. Amyotrophic lateral sclerosis: Part 1. Clinical features, pathology, and ethical issues in management. Ann Neurol 18:271, 1985.
13. Daube J. EMG in Motor Neuron Diseases. American Association of Electromyography and Electrodiagnosis. AAEE minimonograph 18, Rochester, MN, June 1982.
14. Howard R, Wiles C, Loh L. Respiratory complications and their management in motor neuron disease. Brain 112:1155, 1989.
15. Bach J, Alba A, Mosher R, Delaubier A. Intermittent positive pressure ventilation via nasal access in the management of respiratory insufficiency. Chest 92:168, 1987.
16. Sawicka E, Loh L, Branthwaite M. Domiciliary ventilatory support: An analysis of outcome. Thorax 43:31, 1988.
17. Einarsson G, Grimby G, Stalberg E. Electromyographic and morphological functional compensation in late poliomyelitis. Muscle Nerve 13:165, 1990.
18. Ravits J, Hallett M, Baker M, et al. Clinical and electromyographic studies of postpoliomyelitis muscular atrophy. Muscle Nerve 13:667, 1990.
19. Fischer D. Long-term management of the ventilator patient in the home. Cleve Clin J Med 52:303, 1985.
20. Peters S, Viggiano R. Home mechanical ventilation. Mayo Clin Proc 63:1208, 1988.
21. Jones D, Speier J, Canine K, et al. Cardiorespiratory responses to aerobic training by patients with postpoliomyelitis sequelae. JAMA 22:3255, 1989.
22. Russman B, Melchreit R, Drennan J. Spinal muscular atrophy: The natural course of disease. Muscle Nerve 6:179, 1983.
23. Dubowitz V. Benign infantile spinal muscular atrophy. Dev Med Child Neurol 16:672, 1974.
24. Piasecki J, Mahinpour S, Levine D. Long-term follow-up of spinal fusion in spinal muscular dystrophy. Clin Orthop 207:44, 1986.
25. Bennett D, Bleck T. Diagnosis and treatment of neuromuscular causes of acute respiratory failure. Clin Neuropharmacol 11:303, 1988.
26. Witt N, Zochodne D, Bolton C, et al. Peripheral nerve function in sepsis and multiple organ failure. Chest 99:176, 1991.
27. Zochodne D, Bolton C, Wells G, et al. Critical illness polyneuropathy: A complication of sepsis and multiple organ failure. Brain 110:819, 1987.
28. Coronel B, Mercatello A, Couturier J, et al. Polyneuropathy: Potential cause of difficult weaning. Crit Care Med 18:486, 1990.
29. Bolton C. Weaning failure due to acute neuromuscular disease [Letter to the editor]. Crit Care Med 15:180, 1987.
30. Loh L. Neurological and neuromuscular disease. Br J Anaesth 58:190, 1986.
31. Prakash U. Neurologic diseases. *In* Baum G, Wolinsky E (eds). Textbook of Pulmonary Diseases, 4th ed. Boston/Toronto, Little, Brown and Company, 1989, p 1409.
32. Krull F, Schuchardt V, Haupt W. Prognosis of acute polyneuritis requiring artificial ventilation. Intensive Care Med 14:388, 1988.
33. McKhann G, Griffin J, Cornblath D, et al. Plasmapheresis and Guillain-Barré syndrome: Analysis of prognostic factors and the effect of plasmapheresis. Ann Neurol 23:347, 1988.
34. Scannell J. Results of open heart operation for acquired aortic valve disease. J Thorac Cardiovasc Surg 45:64, 1963.
35. Benjamin J, Cascade P, Rubenfire M, et al. Left lower lobe atelectasis and consolidations following cardiac surgery: The effect of topical cooling on the phrenic nerve. Radiology 142:11, 1982.
36. Rousou J, Parker T, Engelman R, Breyer R. Phrenic nerve paresis associated with the use of iced slush and the cooling jacket for topical hypothermia. J Thorac Cardiovasc Surg 89:921, 1985.
37. Wheeler W, Rubis L, Jones C, Harrah J. Etiology and prevention of topical cardiac hypothermia-induced phrenic nerve injury and left lower lobe atelectasis during cardiac surgery. Chest 88:680, 1985.
38. Dajee A, Pellegrini J, Cooper G, Karlson K. Phrenic nerve palsy after topical cardiac hypothermia. Int Surg 68:345, 1983.
39. Kohorst W, Schonfeld S, Altman M. Bilateral diaphragmatic paralysis following topical cardiac hypothermia. Chest 85:65, 1984.

40. Chandler K, Rozas C, Kory R, Goldman A. Bilateral diaphragmatic paralysis complicating local cardiac hypothermia during open heart surgery. Am J Med 77:243, 1984.
41. DeVita M, Robinson L, Rehder J, Hattler B, Cohen C. Incidence and natural history of phrenic neuropathy occurring during open heart surgery. Chest 103:850, 1993.
42. Litchy W, Albers J. Repetitive stimulation. Symposium Proceedings, American Association of Electromyography and Electrodiagnosis, Rochester, Minnesota, May 1984.
43. Perlo V, Arnason B, Pokanzer D, et al. The role of thymectomy in the treatment of myasthenia gravis. Ann N Y Acad Sci 183:308, 1971.
44. Gracey D, Divertie M, Howard F, Payne W. Postoperative respiratory care after transsternal thymectomy in myasthenia gravis. Chest 86:67, 1984.
45. Younger D, Braun N, Jaretzki A, et al. Myasthenia gravis: Determinants for independent ventilation after transsternal thymectomy. Neurology 34:336, 1984.
46. Sellman M, Mayer R. Treatment of myasthenia crisis in late life. South Med J 78:1208, 1985.
47. d'Empaire G, Hoaglin D, Verlo V, Pontoppidan H. Effect of prethymectomy plasma exchange on postoperative respiratory function in myasthenia gravis. J Thorac Cardiovasc Surg 89:592, 1985.
48. Jablecki C. Lambert-Eaton Myasthenic Syndrome. Muscle Nerve 7:250, 1984.
49. Keesey J. Electrodiagnostic Approach to Defects of Neuromuscular Transmission. American Association of Electrodiagnostic Medicine. AAEM minimonograph 33, Rochester, MN, August 1989.
50. Chalk C, Murray N, Newsome-Davis J, et al. Response of the Lambert-Eaton myasthenic syndrome to treatment of associated small cell lung carcinoma. Neurology 40:1552, 1990.
51. Metzger A, Bohan A, Goldberg L, et al. Polymyositis and dermatomyositis: Combined methotrexate and corticosteroid therapy. Ann Intern Med 81:182, 1974.
52. Whitaker J. Inflammatory myopathy: A review of etiologic and pathogenetic factors. Muscle Nerve 5:573, 1982.
53. Brook M. Inflammatory myopathies. In McSherry-Collins N (ed). A Clinician's View of Neuromuscular Disorders. Baltimore, Williams & Wilkins, 1986, p 216.
54. Ansell B. Management of polymyositis and dermatomyositis. Clin Rheuma Dis 10:205, 1984.
55. Mitz M, Chang G, Albers J, Sulaiman A. Electromyographic and histologic paraspinal abnormalities in polymyositis/dermatomyositis. Arch Phys Med Rehabil 62:118, 1981.
56. Slucka C. The electrocardiogram in Duchenne progressive muscular dystrophy. Circulation 38:933, 1968.
57. Kingston W, Moxley R. Treatment of muscular dystrophies and inflammatory myopathies. Clin Neuropharmacol 9:361, 1986.
58. Miller R, Chalmers A, Dao H, et al. The effect of spine fusion on respiratory function in Duchenne muscular dystrophy. Neurology 41:38, 1991.
59. Bach J, Alba A, Pilkington L, Lee M. Long-term rehabilitation in advanced stage of childhood onset, rapidly progressive muscular dystrophy. Arch Phys Med Rehabil 62:328, 1981.
60. Curran F, Colbert A. Ventilator management in Duchenne muscular dystrophy and postpoliomyelitis syndrome: 12 years' experience. Arch Phys Med Rehabil 70:180, 1989.
61. Dail C. Glossopharyngeal breathing by paralyzed patients. Calif Med 75:217, 1951.
62. Affeldt J, Dail C, Collier C, Farr A. Glossopharyngeal breathing: Ventilation studies. Calif Med 8:111, 1955.
63. Rideau Y, Jankowski L, Grellet J. Respiratory function in the muscular dystrophies. Muscle Nerve 4:155, 1981.
64. Borel C, Tilford C, Nichols D, et al. Diaphragmatic performance during recovery from acute ventilatory failure in Guillain-Barré syndrome and myasthenia gravis. Chest 99:444, 1991.
65. Sahn A, Lakshminarayan S. Bedside criteria for discontinuation of mechanical ventilation. Chest 63:1002, 1973.
66. Bellemare F, Grassino A. Force reserve of the diaphragm in patients with chronic obstructive pulmonary disease. J Appl Physiol 55:8, 1983.
67. Tahvanainen J, Salmenpera M, Nikki P. Extubation criteria after weaning from intermittent mandatory ventilation and continuous positive airway pressure. Crit Care Med 11:702, 1983.
68. Markand O, Kincaid J, Pourmand R, et al. Electrophysiologic evaluation of diaphragm by transcutaneous phrenic nerve stimulation. Neurology 34:604, 1984.
69. MacLean I, Mattioni T. Phrenic nerve conduction studies: A new technique and its application in quadriplegic patients. Arch Phys Med Rehabil 62:70, 1981.
70. Schmidt-Nowara W, Altman A. Atelectasis and neuromuscular respiratory failure. Chest 85:792, 1984.
71. McCool F, Mayewski R, Shayne D, et al. Intermittent positive pressure breathing in patients with respiratory muscle weakness. Chest 90:546, 1986.
72. DeTroyer A, Deisser P. The effects of intermittent positive pressure breathing on patients with respiratory muscle weakness. Am Rev Respir Dis 124:132, 1981.
73. Braun N, Faulkner J, Hughes R, et al. When should respiratory muscles be exercised? Chest 84:76, 1983.

74. Aldrich T, Uhrlass R. Weaning from mechanical ventilation: Successful use of modified inspiratory resistive training in muscular dystrophy. Crit Care Med 15:247, 1987.

75. Estrup C, Lyager S, Noerra N, Olsen C. Effect of respiratory muscle training in patients with neuromuscular diseases and in normals. Respiration 50:36, 1986.

76. Stern L, Martin A, Jones N, et al. Training inspiratory resistance in Duchenne dystrophy using adapted computer games. Dev Med Child Neurol 31:494, 1989.

77. Rodillo E, Noble-Jamieson C, Aber V, et al. Respiratory muscle training in Duchenne muscular dystrophy. Arch Dis Child 64:736, 1989.

78. Braun N, Marino W. Effect of daily intermittent rest of respiratory muscles in patients with severe chronic airflow limitation (CAL). Chest 85:59S, 1984.

79. Levine S, Henson D, Levy S. Respiratory muscle rest therapy. Clin Chest Med 9:297, 1988.

80. Mohr C, Hill N. Long-term follow-up of nocturnal ventilatory assistance in patients with respiratory failure due to Duchenne-type muscular dystrophy. Chest 97:91, 1990.

81. Curran F. Night ventilation by body respirator for patients in chronic respiratory failure due to late stage Duchenne muscular dystrophy. Arch Phys Med Rehabil 62:270, 1981.

82. Garay S, Turino G, Goldring R. Sustained reversal of chronic hypercapnia in patients with alveolar hypoventilation syndrome. Am J Med 70:269, 1981.

83. Braun N, Rochester D. Muscular weakness and respiratory failure. Am Rev Respir Dis 119:123, 1979.

84. Rochester D, Braun N, Laine S. Diaphragmatic energy expenditure in chronic respiratory failure. Am J Med 63:223, 1977.

85. Sivak E, Streib E. Management of hypoventilation in motor neuron disease presenting with respiratory insufficiency. Ann Neurol 7:188, 1980.

86. Braun S, Sufit R, Giovannoni R, et al. Intermittent negative pressure ventilation in the treatment of respiratory failure in progressive neuromuscular diseases [Abstract]. Neurology 37:1874, 1987.

87. Kerby G, Mayer L, Pingleton S. Nocturnal positive pressure ventilation via nasal mask. Am Rev Respir Dis 135:739, 1987.

88. Cropp A, DiMarco A. Effects of intermittent negative pressure ventilation on respiratory muscle function in patients with severe chronic obstructive pulmonary disease. Am Rev Respir Dis 135:1056, 1987.

89. Ellis E, Bye P, Bruderer J, Sullivan C. Treatment of respiratory failure during sleep in patients with neuromuscular disease. Am Rev Respir Dis 135:148, 1987.

90. Meduri G, Conoscenti C, Menashe P, Nair S. Noninvasive face mask ventilation in patients with acute respiratory failure. Chest 95:865, 1989.

91. Carrey Z, Gottfried S, Levy R. Ventilatory muscle support in respiratory failure with nasal positive pressure ventilation. Chest 97:1150, 1990.

92. Meduri G, Abou-Shala N, Fox R, et al. Noninvasive face mask mechanical ventilation in patients with acute hypercapnic respiratory failure. Chest 100:445, 1991.

93. Drinker P, McKhann C. The use of a new apparatus for the prolonged administration of artificial respiration. JAMA 92:1658, 1929.

94. Hill N. Clinical applications of body ventilators. Chest 90:897, 1986.

95. Kinnear W, Hockley S, Harvey J, Shneerson J. The effects of one year of nocturnal cuirass-assisted ventilation in chest wall disease. Eur Respir J 1:204, 1988.

96. Splaingard M, Frates R, Jefferson L, et al. Home negative pressure ventilation: Report of 20 years of experience in patients with neuromuscular disease. Arch Phys Med Rehabil 66:239, 1985.

97. Lands L, Zinman R. Maximal static pressures and lung volumes in a child with Guillain-Barré syndrome ventilated by a cuirass respirator. Chest 89:757, 1986.

98. Bach J, Alba A. Intermittent abdominal pressure ventilator in a regimen of noninvasive ventilatory support. Chest 99:630, 1991.

99. Kopacz M, Moriarty-Wright R. Multidisciplinary approach for the patient on a home ventilator. Heart Lung 13:255, 1984.

100. Dunkin L. Home ventilatory assistance. Anaesthesia 38:644, 1983.

101. Leger P, Jennequin J, Gerard M, et al. Home positive pressure ventilation via nasal mask for patients with neuromusculoskeletal disorders. Eur Respir J 2:640S, 1989.

102. Glenn W, Hogan J, Loke J, et al. Ventilatory support by pacing of the conditioned diaphragm in quadriplegia. N Engl J Med 310:1150, 1984.

103. DeBoeck H, Vincken W, Cham B, Opdecam P. Diaphragmatic pacing in the treatment of chronic respiratory insufficiency of quadriplegic patients. Acta Chir Belg 89:276, 1989.

104. Sharkey P, Halter J, Nakajima K. Electrophrenic respiration in patients with high quadriplegia. Neurosurgery 24:529, 1989.

105. Baer G, Talonen P, Hakkinen V, et al. Phrenic nerve stimulation in tetraplegia. Scand J Rehabil Med 22:107, 1990.

106. Carter R, Donovan W, Halstead L, Wilkerson M. Comparative study of electrophrenic nerve stimulation and mechanical ventilatory support in traumatic spinal cord injury. Paraplegia 25:86, 1987.

107. Vincken W, Corne L. Improved arterial oxygenation by diaphragmatic pacing in quadriplegia. Crit Care Med 15:872, 1987.

108. Vanderlinden R, Epstein S, Hyland R, et al. Management of chronic ventilatory insufficiency with electrical diaphragm pacing. Can J Neurol Sci 15:63, 1988.

109. Wilcox P, Paré P, Fleetham J. Conditioning of the diaphragm by phrenic nerve pacing in primary alveolar hypoventilation. Thorax 43:1017, 1988.
110. Yernault JC. Mechanical assistance in chronic respiratory insufficiency due to neuromuscular disease. Bull Eur Physiopathol Respir 20:467, 1984.
111. Aubier M, Troyer A, Sampson M, et al. Aminophylline proves diaphragmatic contractility. N Engl J Med 305:249, 1981.
112. Aubier M. Effect of theophylline on diaphragmatic muscle function. Chest 92:27S, 1987.
113. Aubier M, Viires N, Murciano D, et al. Effects of digoxin on diaphragmatic strength generation. J Appl Physiol 61:1767, 1986.
114. Aubier M, Murciano D, Viires N, et al. Effects of digoxin on diaphragmatic strength generation in patients with chronic pulmonary disease during acute respiratory failure. Am Rev Respir Dis 135:544, 1987.
115. Aubier M, Murciano D, Meno Y, et al. Dopamine effects on diaphragmatic strength during acute respiratory failure in chronic obstructive pulmonary disease. Ann Intern Med 110:17, 1989.
116. Miller J, Colbert A, Schock N. Ventilator use in progressive neuromuscular disease: Impact on patients and their families. Dev Med Child Neurol 30:200, 1988.
117. Cruzan v Director, Missouri Department of Health, 110 SCt 2841 (1990).
118. Annas G. Sounding board: Nancy Cruzan and the right to die. N Engl J Med 323:670, 1990.
119. Annas G, Arnold R, Aroskar M, et al. Occasional notes: Bioethicists' statement on the U.S. Supreme Court's Cruzan decision. N Engl J Med 323:686, 1990.

49

◼

Key Terms

Chemical Pleurodesis

Empyema

Exudate

Pleural Effusion

Starling's Law

Thoracentesis

Thoracoscopy

Transudate

Starling's law depends on the balance of the capillary hydrostatic pressure (Pc), capillary and pleural colloid osmotic pressure (πc and πpl), and intrapleural tissue pressure (Ppl) as follows:

$$F = K ((Pc - Ppl) - (\pi c - \pi pl))$$

On physical examination one may find:

- Decreased movement of the affected hemithorax
- Dullness to percussion of the chest
- Decreased tactile fremitus
- Absent or reduced breath sounds in the affected area.

In large pleural effusions (greater than 1500 ml of fluid), shifting of the mediastinum and trachea can be present.

Pleural Effusion

Rodolfo C. Morice, M.D.

Pleural effusion, the abnormal accumulation of fluid in the pleural space, is not a specific disease but the manifestation of an underlying systemic or intrathoracic pathologic condition. Pleural effusion is among the most frequently encountered problems in pulmonary medicine. The incidence of this condition varies with the clinical setting, but congestive heart failure, pneumonia, malignancy, and pulmonary embolism account for at least 90% of all pleural effusions.[1]

PHYSIOLOGY OF THE PLEURAL SPACE

The pleural space is a virtual cavity between the visceral pleura, which covers the surface of the lungs, and the parietal pleura, which covers the internal surface of the thoracic cage, mediastinum, and diaphragm. Within the visceral and parietal pleura, a thin layer of fluid (to 27 μm thick) lubricates the pleural surfaces, thereby decreasing the work of breathing.

The formation and absorption of fluid within the pleural cavity follows Starling's law (Fig. 49–1). This law explains the fluid formation in the parietal pleura. F represents the pressure that forces fluid out of the parietal pleura into the pleural space.[2] This pressure results from the balance of the hydrostatic pressure of the systemic capillaries that supply that membrane (Pc = 30 cm H_2O), the pleural pressure (Ppl = -5 cm H_2O at functional residual capacity), the capillary oncotic pressure (πc = 34 cm H_2O), and the pleural oncotic pressure (πpl = 5 cm H_2O). This results in a net gradient of 6 cm H_2O, favoring the movement of fluid from the parietal pleura into the pleural space.

The Starling equation is also used to explain the movement of fluid across the visceral pleura. Most capillaries in the visceral pleura are supplied by the pulmonary circulation with a hydrostatic pressure (Pc) of 11 cm H_2O. With all other factors in the Starling equation being the same as listed for the parietal pleura, there would be a 13-cm H_2O net force (F) for fluid to move from the pleural space into the visceral pleural capillaries. The net balance between fluid formation at the parietal pleura and its absorption at the visceral pleura would indicate an essential fluid free state. In addition to the movement of fluid regulated by the Starling law, other mechanisms of fluid transfer play an important role in maintaining the homeostasis of the pleural space.[3] Passage of fluid, electrolytes, and small particles occurs through intercellular junctions between the mesothelial cells. The lymphatics remove cells, larger particles, and protein through stoma located on the parietal pleura of the lower chest wall, mediastinum, and diaphragm. Respiratory movements and regional variations in pleural pressure facilitate the clearance of fluid and particles by the lymphatics.

CLINICAL CONSIDERATIONS

The clinical manifestations of pleural effusion relate primarily to the underlying disease responsible for the abnormal pleural process. In large

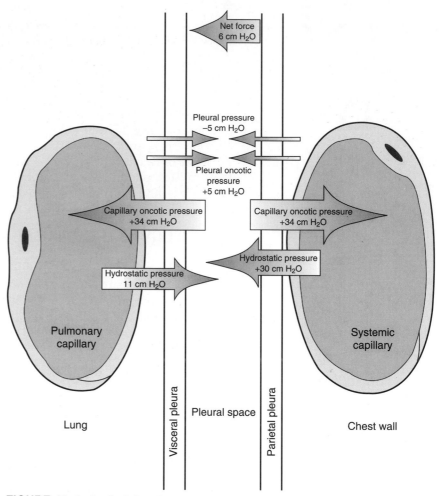

FIGURE 49–1: Starling's law: formation and absorption of fluid within the pleural cavity.

pleural effusions, manifestations may be related to compression of lung parenchyma but most importantly to the effects of fluid accumulation on the work of breathing. Large amounts of fluid can displace the diaphragm downward, impairing its ventilatory function.[4]

DIAGNOSTIC PROCEDURES

The chest x-ray film may show no abnormalities if the amount of fluid is less than 250 ml.[5] However, as little as 10 ml of pleural fluid can show if a lateral decubitus chest x-ray film or an ultrasound of the chest is obtained (Figs. 49–2 and 49–3). Thoracentesis consists of introducing a needle or thin catheter percutaneously into the pleural space to sample (diagnostic) or evacuate (therapeutic) a pleural effusion.

Clinical correlation is crucial when ordering biochemical and other special tests on the pleural fluid. Based on the biochemical characteristics, the fluid can be classified as an exudate or a transudate (Table 49–1).[6] This categorization is important because the presence of a transudate indicates a lack of abnormality of the pleural space, suggesting that only an alteration in the normal equilibrium of the forces stated in the Starling equation is present. When the clinical presentation suggests

A diagnostic thoracentesis is indicated in virtually all patients with free pleural effusions. Exceptions include a clinical course consistent with uncomplicated congestive heart failure or the presence of only a small amount of fluid on lateral decubitus chest x-ray films (less than 10 ml). In this instance the patient requires close observation.

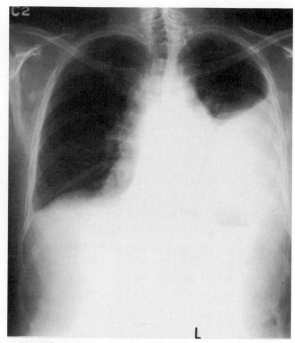

FIGURE 49–2: Posteroanterior chest roentgenogram. A large pleural effusion occupies the lower half of the left hemithorax.

that a transudative pleural effusion is highly likely, the most cost-effective method of diagnosis is to analyze the fluid for protein and lactate dehydrogenase (LDH) first. Other tests should be ordered if the results indicate that the fluid is an exudate. Table 49–2 lists the differential diagnoses of transudative effusions. Further investigation or treatment should be directed to the specific underlying condition.

Exudative pleural effusions, in contrast, have multiple causes (Table 49–3). Further analysis of pleural fluid, if indicated, is based on the clinical context of each case. The majority of exudative effusions appear in association with pneumonia, malignancy, and pulmonary emboli.

In general, an undiagnosed exudative effusion should be analyzed by performing a differential cell count, cytologic examination, and microbiologic studies, as well as glucose, LDH, and amylase determinations. More specific tests, such as pH determination, lipid analysis, and determination of lupus erythematosus cells, complement levels, antinuclear antibody, and rheumatoid factor levels, may be ordered depending on the clinical suspicion (Table 49–4).

Based on the analysis of the fluid alone, a definitive cause can be established in only a minority of cases. These situations include:

TABLE **49–1:** Differential Characteristics of Transudative and Exudative Effusions

	Protein (Fluid-Serum)	LDH (Fluid-Serum)	LDH (Fluid)
Transudate	<0.5	<0.6	<200
Exudate	>0.5	>0.6	>200

LDH, lactate dehydrogenase.

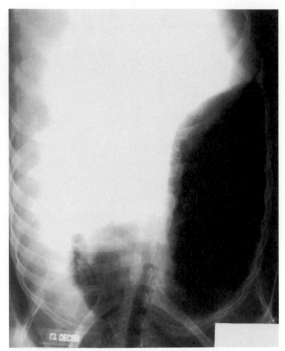

FIGURE 49–3: Left lateral decubitus chest roentgenogram. A free-flowing pleural effusion layers along the side of the left costal wall.

- Presence of malignant cells
- Positive stain or culture result for a specific infection
- Presence of lupus erythematosus cells in lupus pleuritis
- Low pH and high amylase levels in cases of esophageal rupture
- High triglyceride concentration in chylothorax
- Low pH transudate with a pleural fluid–to–serum creatinine ratio greater than 1 in urinothorax

Needle pleural biopsy is most useful in the diagnosis of tuberculous pleuritis (95% with biopsy specimen culture).[7] In malignant pleural effusions, needle pleural biopsy gives positive results in only 40% of cases.[8]

A pleural biopsy should be performed in patients with exudative pleural effusions of undetermined cause. Most frequently, pleural biopsies are performed blindly with a biopsy needle (Cope or Abrams needle). The diagnostic yield of needle pleural biopsy varies with the underlying condition.

Thoracoscopy allows the direct inspection and biopsy of the pleural surface. Any endoscope that can be sterilized and passed through an intercostal space can be used. However, specifically designed rigid metal

TABLE **49–2:** Causes of Transudative Pleural Effusions

1. Congestive heart failure
2. Pericardial disease
3. Liver disease
4. Obstructive uropathy
5. Following childbirth
6. Myxedema
7. Peritoneal dialysis
8. Superior vena cava syndrome
9. Misplacement of central venous catheter
10. Hypoalbuminemia
11. Nephrotic syndrome
12. Atelectasis

TABLE **49–3:** Causes of Exudative Pleural Effusions

1. Parapneumonic
2. Malignancy
3. Pulmonary embolism
4. Tuberculous pleurisy
5. Other infections (fungal, actinomycetes, viral, parasitic, Q fever)
6. Empyema
7. Collagen vascular disease (rheumatoid arthritis, systemic lupus erythematosus, Wegener's granulomatosis)
8. Postcardiac injury syndrome
9. Gastrointestinal disease (pancreatic disease, esophageal rupture, following laparotomy)
10. Asbestos-related
11. Lipid pleural effusion (chylothorax, pseudochylothorax)
12. Drug-related (nitrofurantoin, methysergide, procarbazine)
13. Radiation therapy
14. Hemothorax
15. Uremia
16. Meigs' syndrome
17. Yellow nail syndrome

The diagnostic accuracy of thoracoscopy for malignant and tuberculous effusions is more than 90%.[9, 10] The value of thoracoscopy for the diagnosis of other conditions has not been systematically analyzed.

Some other therapeutic uses for thoracoscopy in the management of pleural diseases include:[11, 12]

- Removal of foreign objects (sheared catheters)
- Evaluation of patients with penetrating chest injuries
- Breakage of loculation in empyema following pneumonia
- Electrocauterization of bleeding pleural adhesions

thoracoscopes are usually employed in the adult population. This procedure is commonly performed with local anesthesia, although general anesthesia is preferred with extensive examinations or therapeutic interventions.

Thoracoscopy is also useful in therapeutic procedures such as chemical pleurodesis, which consists of the intrapleural instillation of a sclerosing substance for the purpose of ablating the pleural space by fusing together the visceral and parietal pleurae. This procedure is indicated in the palliative treatment of symptomatic, recurrent malignant pleural effusions. Inspection of the pleural space, breakage of pleural loculations, and direct instillation of the sclerosing substance by thoracoscopy results in improved pleurosymphysis.

SPECIFIC ENTITIES

Transudative Pleural Effusions

Congestive heart failure, the most common cause of transudative pleural effusion, occurs with increased venous capillary hydrostatic pres-

TABLE **49–4:** Differential Characteristics of Various Pleural Effusions

Diagnosis	Usual Gross Appearance	Protein (g/dL)	LDH (IU/L)	pH	Glucose (mg/dL)	Amylase Fluid-Serum	Leukocytes Count (cells/mm³)	Predominance
Congestive heart failure	Serous	<3	<200	>7.4	= Serum	≤1	<1000	Mono
Malignancy	Bloody	>3	>500	> or <7.3	<60	> or <1	3000	Mono
Tuberculosis	Serous	>5	>200	> or <7.3	<60	≤1	100–50,000	PMN (early) Mono (late)
Pulmonary embolism	Clear, bloody	> or <3	>200	>7.3	= Serum	≤1	100–50,000	PMN or Mono
Parapneumonic, complicated	Cloudy, purulent	>3	>1000	<7	<50	≤1	5000–100,000	PMN
Parapneumonic, uncomplicated	Clear, cloudy	>3	<1000	>7.2	>50	≤1	5000–10,000	PMN
Pancreatitis	Serous, bloody	>3	>200	>7.3	= Serum	>2	1000–50,000	PMN
Rheumatoid arthritis	Serous, cloudy	>3	>700	<7.3	<30	≤1	1000–20,000	PMN (early) Mono (late)
Systemic lupus erythematosus	Serous, cloudy	>3	<500	>7		≤1	5000	PMN (early) Mono (late)

LDH, lactate dehydrogenase; PMN, polymorphonuclear; mono, mononuclear.

sure, the main mechanism by which such effusions develop.[1] Other factors, however, such as impaired lymphatic drainage and altered capillary permeability due to tissue hypoxia also play a role in the genesis of these effusions.

Congestive heart failure tends to produce bilateral effusions with greater accumulation of fluid in the right hemithorax. Unilateral effusions related to cardiac failure, which are uncommon (less than 10%), tend to be right-sided. Pericardial disease, in contrast, shows predominantly unilateral left-sided effusions or bilateral effusions with larger amounts of fluid in the left hemithorax.[13] Although the mechanisms for the variable distribution of fluid are not known, this finding may be useful in the differential diagnosis.

Occasionally these transudative effusions can transform into exudates after a long-standing process that results in associated inflammatory changes of the pleura. This also can occur following intensive diuretic therapy resulting in greater free water elimination.

In liver disease, the main mechanism of abnormal pleural fluid formation is the transfer of ascitic fluid through the diaphragm via lymphatics or diaphragmatic defects. Other factors responsible for pleural effusion in liver disease include hypoalbuminemia and azygos venous hypertension.[14]

Pleural effusion secondary to obstructive uropathy is called urinothorax. Urinary tract obstruction results in hydronephrosis followed by extravasation of fluid into the perirenal space. The extravasated urine then passes the peritoneal and retroperitoneal spaces into the thoracic cavity. The effusion is usually ipsilateral to the affected kidney and resolves rapidly (days) on removal of the urinary obstruction. The diagnosis of urinothorax is confirmed by the presence of a pleural fluid–to–creatinine ratio greater than 1 and a low pH transudate.

Small amounts of pleural fluid have been roentgenographically documented in up to 50% of patients in the immediate postpartum period.[16] They resolve rapidly; therefore, therapeutic or diagnostic intervention is not indicated except in the symptomatic patient.

Pleural effusions can occur in patients with myxedema even without cardiovascular or renal complications. These effusions, frequently associated with pericardial effusion, are more commonly transudates.[17] Exudative effusions have also been reported in this condition.

Rapidly developing large pleural effusions can occasionally be associated with peritoneal dialysis. Their presence has been attributed to the passage of fluid through diaphragmatic defects in a manner similar to that seen in hydrothorax related to ascites.[18]

Superior vena cava obstruction as a cause of transudative pleural effusion is presumably due to elevated venous pressure.[19] However, malignant pleural involvement commonly occurs when a neoplasm causes superior vena cava obstruction.

Rapidly developing pleural effusions can occur as a complication of a misplaced central venous catheter. Although these effusions are frequently associated with a pneumothorax, they can present without one. The pleural fluid may have the same characteristics of the fluid being infused or it may be bloody when vascular rupture occurs.

Exudative Pleural Effusions

Parapneumonic Effusions

A parapneumonic pleural effusion develops as a result of a bronchopulmonary infection. Parapneumonic effusions, which occur in approxi-

Other processes leading to pleural transudation include the nephrotic syndrome, hypoalbuminemia (decreased colloid osmotic pressure), and reduced intrapleural pressure occurring in the early period after atelectasis.

The characteristics of complicated parapneumonic effusions include:

- Pleural fluid glucose level less than 50 mg/dL
- Pleural fluid pH less than 7 and 0.15 U lower than arterial pH

In borderline cases or when pleural fluid pH is between 7 and 7.2 and pleural fluid LDH levels are greater than 1000 IU/L, close observation and serial thoracentesis are recommended. If the LDH level increases and the pH and glucose level decrease, a tube thoracostomy is indicated.

An undrained empyema will not resolve; in fact, it may cause lung necrosis, leading to pulmonary infection or patient death from pus filling the airways.

mately 40% of pyogenic pneumonias, are associated with higher morbidity and mortality.[20] Parapneumonic effusions occur when capillary permeability increases in response to the inflammatory reaction. Other factors contributing to the development of these effusions include impaired clearing of fluid and protein by fibrin deposition and thickening of the pleural membranes. The term *complicated parapneumonic effusion* is used for those effusions that require chest tube drainage for their resolution.

Empyema

By definition, empyema is the presence of pus in the pleural space; in a broader and more practical clinical context, empyema denotes the presence of microorganisms in an exudative pleural fluid. In addition to the selection of appropriate antibiotic therapy, the decision about whether or not to initiate chest tube drainage must be based on the analysis of the fluid. A tube thoracostomy is indicated when an empyema or a complicated parapneumonic effusion is present.[20]

If not appropriately drained, a complicated parapneumonic effusion can rapidly form adhesions and loculations. When this occurs, insertion of additional chest tubes, guided by an ultrasonogram, or instillation of intrapleural streptokinase may be attempted. Open drainage or full thoracotomy with lung decortication may be required in cases in which the organizing pleuritis becomes multiloculated or the lung becomes encased in a fibropurulent pleural peel.

Malignant Pleural Effusions

Malignant pleural effusions are the second most common cause of exudative pleural effusions.[1] Pleural effusions associated with malignant neoplasms can be seen as a result of direct malignant invasion of the pleural space or indirect alteration of the mechanisms responsible for the formation and clearance of pleural fluid.[21] Effusions associated with malignancy but not due to direct pleural tumor extension are termed *paramalignant*. Impaired lymphatic drainage due to mediastinal lymph node invasion and bronchial obstruction resulting in atelectasis or pneumonia are examples of modes by which paramalignant effusions occur. This distinction is important in the staging and treatment of lung cancer because the presence of malignant cells in the fluid defines a malignant effusion and indicates inoperability and a much worse prognosis.

Primary lung cancer and breast carcinoma are the most common causes of malignant pleural effusion. These lesions are followed in order of frequency by metastatic adenocarcinomas from the ovary and gastrointestinal tract.[21] Malignant mesothelioma, the primary neoplasm of the pleura, is a much less common cause of pleural effusion. The incidence of malignant mesothelioma in North America has been reported to be approximately 2.2 per million population per year.[22] Its development is closely linked to occupational or environmental asbestos exposure.

Pleural effusions in patients with hematologic malignancies are common.[23] Direct malignant pleural involvement is rare. The effusions are usually related to infection, chemotherapy or radiation therapy, lymphatic obstruction (lymphoma), or pulmonary parenchymal infiltration resulting in increased capillary permeability (leukemias).

Multiple myeloma can produce pleural involvement by direct extension of a chest wall tumor (plasmacytoma), rib destruction and ensuing chest wall invasion, pulmonary parenchymal myelomatous infiltration, and altered oncotic hydrostatic pressure balance because of paraproteinemia.

The fluid in pleural malignancies is usually a serosanguineous exudate. Frankly hemorrhagic fluid indicates direct pleural tumor invasion. In addition to red cells, there are moderate numbers of leukocytes (2000 to 3000 cells/mm³) with a predominance of lymphocytes (50%). The diagnostic yield of cytologic examination in diagnosing malignant pleural effusions is approximately 60%.[8] Malignant cells suspended in the pleural fluid degenerate and alter their morphology. Therefore, since new cells are continuously shed into the pleural fluid, the accuracy of the diagnosis increases with repeated thoracentesis. Unguided needle pleural biopsies have a lower diagnostic yield than pleural fluid cytologic examination, but occasionally the pleural biopsy results are positive in a patient with nondiagnostic pleural fluid cytologic features.[8] Pleuroscopy or thoracotomy with pleural biopsy should be considered in the symptomatic patient in whom less invasive attempts to establish a diagnosis have failed.

Transudative pleural effusions have been reported in up to 19% of pleural effusions of patients with malignancies. These transudates are thought to be related to congestive heart failure or early lymphatic obstruction. A low glucose level (<60 mg/dL) and pH (<7.3) is found in approximately 30% of patients with malignant effusions. This correlates with high tumor burden, poor prognosis, and poor response to chemical pleurodesis.[24] Determination of hyaluronic acid levels in pleural fluid has been proposed as useful in patients with suspected mesothelioma. A fluid hyaluronic acid level of greater than 0.8 mg/dL is suggestive of mesothelioma. A definitive diagnosis of mesothelioma requires histologic confirmation. Electron-microscopic or histochemistry analysis is usually required in differentiating mesotheliomas from other pleural malignancies, especially adenocarcinomas.

The treatment of malignant pleural effusions usually depends on the patient's symptoms. Chemotherapy is unrewarding except in selected cases of breast cancer, lymphoma, or small cell carcinoma of the lung. Radiation therapy is useful only in the treatment of paramalignant effusions secondary to mediastinal lymphomas.

Obliteration of the pleural space by chemical pleurodesis is indicated for palliation of symptomatic recurrent pleural effusions. The majority of pleurodesis procedures are performed in malignant effusions in which specific tumor therapy is unavailable or ineffective. Complete evacuation of the pleural fluid, breakage of any loculations, and full approximation of the pleural membranes are essential for a successful pleural symphysis. This is best accomplished by chest tube drainage or pleuroscopy. Once the fluid has been evacuated, the sclerosing agent is instilled in the pleural space and the chest tube is clamped. The patient's position is then sequentially rotated to ensure a homogenous distribution of the sclerosing substance. Appropriate analgesia and intrapleural local anesthetic instillation are necessary to reduce the pain associated with the local inflammatory reaction.

The effectiveness of the sclerosing agent depends on its ability to induce an inflammatory fibrotic reaction. Doxycycline and talc are the two substances most frequently used.[25] Antineoplastic agents, such as bleomycin, 5-fluorouracil, and thiotepa, are also effective, but their utility is limited by bone marrow toxicity related to systemic absorption.

Pulmonary Embolism

Pleural effusions can be present in 30 to 50% of patients with pulmonary thromboembolic disease.[26] The incidence of pulmonary embolism in the United States has been estimated to be 500,000 cases per year;[27] therefore, pulmonary emboli as a cause of pleural effusion should be much higher than the 5% figure commonly reported. The formation of pleural effusion in pulmonary embolism results from an increased capillary permeability secondary to ischemic injury or pulmonary infarction. The pleural fluid is usually a bloody exudate with widely variable leukocyte counts (100 to 50,000 cells/mm^3). The biochemical profile of the fluid demonstrates no distinctive characteristics. This diagnosis should be considered in any patient with a pleural effusion of undetermined cause. Transudative effusions can occur in pulmonary emboli and are thought to form because of increased negative pleural pressure resulting from atelectasis, which is frequently associated with the embolic process. The presence of an effusion in cases of pulmonary emboli is not a contraindication to anticoagulation or thrombolytic therapy, and specific therapy for the effusion is not required.[28]

Mycobacterial Infections

Pleural effusions associated with mycobacterial infections account for approximately 9% of all effusions.[29] The most common form of effusion seen with *Mycobacterium tuberculosis* infections is a hypersensitivity reaction. This occurs following the primary phase of the initial infection (first 6 months) concomitantly with the development of cell-mediated immunity. Associated parenchymal infiltration is usually lacking in this entity. More rarely, effusions develop in reactivation tuberculosis. Tuberculous empyemas can also occur when parenchymal infection breaks through the visceral pleura.

Exudative effusions seen in the primary phase of pulmonary tuberculosis usually resolve spontaneously. However, approximately 40 to 65% of patients acquire active pulmonary tuberculosis within 5 years if not treated with antituberculous therapy.[30] The number of bacilli responsible for the inflammatory pleural reaction is low; thus, pleural fluid smears and cultures will produce positive results in only 20 to 25% of cases.

The presence of a positive tuberculin skin test in a patient with an undiagnosed exudative pleural effusion is highly suggestive of tuberculous pleurisy. Since this entity occurs early in the development of the immune response to the tuberculous infection, a single negative skin test result does not exclude this diagnosis. In this case, the test should be repeated in 1 month with appropriate test controls for anergy. Another characteristic of tuberculous pleural effusion is lymphocyte predominance, amounting to more than 50% of the total white cell count. Eosinophils are rarely present unless the patient has had a previous thoracentesis or pneumothorax. A low pleural fluid glucose level (<30 mg/dL) is suggestive of tuberculous pleurisy if bacterial pneumonia, rheumatoid disease, and malignancy can be excluded.

A definitive diagnosis can be made in 60 to 90% of cases if a needle pleural biopsy is performed and the specimen is examined histologically and cultured for tuberculosis.[7]

As with *M. tuberculosis,* pleural effusions are present in approximately 5% of chronic nontuberculous mycobacterial infections. *M. kansasii* and the *M. avium-intracellulare* complex are the most common organisms in the United States.[31]

Fungal Infections

Pleural effusions due to fungal infections account for about 1% of all effusions.[29] They can be caused by true fungal pathogens in an otherwise

The most common inherently pathogenic fungi causing pleural disease are *Histoplasma capsulatum, Blastomyces dermatitidis,* and *Cryptococcus neoformans.*

normal subject or by opportunistic fungi in an immunocompromised patient.

In primary histoplasmosis, pleural effusion is present in only 2% of cases.[32] When it occurs, it is usually unilateral, small, and on the same side as the parenchymal infiltration. In the chronic forms of histoplasmosis, pleural involvement is usually in the form of localized fibrous thickening. The pleural fluid characteristics in primary histoplasmosis are indistinguishable from those found in tuberculous effusions. Thus, this diagnosis should be considered in patients who live in areas of endemic histoplasmosis with a clinical presentation suggestive of tuberculous pleurisy in whom *M. tuberculosis* cannot be isolated.

Although clinically significant pleural effusions related to pulmonary blastomycosis are rare, small pleural effusions can be detected by chest roentgenograms in almost 90% of cases.[33] The diagnosis can usually be made by identifying the organism in the pleural fluid or lung tissue biopsy specimen. The fluid is an exudate with lymphocytic predominance similar to that found in other granulomatous effusions.

Approximately 7% of patients with coccidiodomycosis experience pleural effusions.[34] The usually small effusions that accompany primary coccidioidal infections resolve without specific therapy. In the chronic forms, however, rupture of a parenchymal cavity may result in the formation of a bronchopleural fistula with ensuing hydropneumothorax or coccidioidal empyema. In these cases, the prognosis is guarded; treatment requires chest tube placement and systemic amphotericin B administration. Surgical resection of the bronchopleural fistula is indicated if it fails to resolve with conservative management.

Effusions caused by *C. neoformans* are uncommon.[35] Classically, they are associated with a well-circumscribed, homogenous parenchymal density, usually in the lower lobes. Culture results are positive in about 50% of cases. Identification of cryptococcal antigen in the fluid or peripheral blood is helpful, but the diagnosis is most commonly made by histologic examination or culture of the infected lung tissue.

Pulmonary infections caused by *Aspergillus* are frequent in immunocompromised patients, especially in those with hematologic malignancies. The pneumonic process usually presents as a peripheral rounded or wedge-shaped infiltrate or in the form of a necrotizing process. Effusions associated with this presentation are usually parapneumonic. Invasion of the pleural space by *Aspergillus* can occur when a parenchymal abscess ruptures. It can also develop as a secondary infection of empyema cavities after lung resection and in patients with a history of tuberculosis who had been treated with artificial pneumothorax.[36]

Actinomycetes Infections

Pleuropulmonary infections caused by *Actinomyces* and *Nocardia* species resemble those produced by fungal and mycobacterial infections. However, these organisms are branching, filamentous, gram-positive bacteria that respond to therapy with common antibiotics (i.e., penicillin, sulfonamides) and not antifungal agents (amphotericin B).

Actinomycosis, a chronic suppurative process, initially involves the lung in the form of pneumonia followed by abscess formation. The infection can extend into the pleural space, producing an empyema. From there it can penetrate the parietal pleura, resulting in rib osteomyelitis and subcutaneous chest wall abscess formation. Multiple draining sinus tracts and abscesses in distant sites can occur. More than 50% of patients with pulmonary actinomycosis present with pleural involvement.[37]

The clinical presentation of actinomycosis can be confused with other granulomatous infections or lung neoplasms. The diagnosis is confirmed by fluid analysis showing the presence of gram-positive, filamentous, branching organisms or characteristic hard, yellow concretions within the purulent exudate called *sulfur granules*. Superimposed pyogenic infection can be present; thus, the fluid should be cultured aerobically and anaerobically. Prolonged (6 to 12 months) high-dose penicillin administration is the treatment of choice.

Pleuropulmonary infections caused by *Nocardia* species usually occur in immunocompromised individuals. Pleural involvement occurs in approximately 20% of patients with pneumonia resulting from *Nocardia* infection.[38] The appearance of the pleural fluid can vary from a serous parapneumonic effusion to a frank empyema. Although the organisms can be identified by Gram stain or aerobic culture of the pleural fluid, the diagnosis is more commonly made by analysis of airway secretions or lung tissue obtained by bronchoscopy. Sulfonamides or trimethoprim-sulfamethoxazole is the antibiotic therapy of choice.

Collagen Vascular Diseases

Approximately 5% of patients with rheumatoid arthritis experience pleural effusions.[39] They classically present in elderly men with a long-standing history of active rheumatoid arthritis. They occur more often in patients with subcutaneous rheumatoid nodules. The effusions are usually unilateral, but bilateral effusions can present in approximately 25% of cases. The pleural fluid is frequently clear and pale yellow. However, a turbid appearance can occur in long-standing effusions because of the accumulation of cholesterol crystals. The pleural fluid in rheumatoid arthritis is an exudate with the distinctive triad of:

- A glucose level less than 30 mg/dL
- A pH less than 7.3
- An LDH level higher than 700 IU/L[40]

Other characteristics of the fluid include a high rheumatoid factor titer (≥1:320) and decreased complement levels.

Most rheumatoid effusions are small and resolve spontaneously within 3 months, but they can occasionally have a chronic course leading to progressive pleural fibrosis. Steroidal therapy is recommended for persistent effusions, especially if LDH levels increase on sequential fluid analyses. Surgical decortication may be required in symptomatic patients with dyspnea secondary to pleural thickening.

Pleural effusions develop in up to 75% of patients during the course of systemic lupus erythematosus.[41] This condition commonly affects women; pleuritis usually occurs during episodes of exacerbation of the disease. Although the effusions seen in lupus pleuritis are usually small, the patients are symptomatic because of the systemic manifestations of the disease (fever, arthralgias) and pleuritic chest pain due to the local pleural inflammatory reaction. Lupus pleurisy that presents in patients with drug-induced lupus is indistinguishable from the native form. Hydralazine, procainamide, isoniazid, and diphenylhydantoin are the drugs most commonly associated with this condition.[1]

The fluid is a straw-colored or a serosanguineous exudate with leukocyte counts usually less than 20,000 cells/mm³. These cells are mostly polymorphonuclear leukocytes during the acute phase, but lymphocytes predominate in more protracted presentations. A pleural fluid glucose level greater than 50 mg/dL and a pH greater than 7.3 occur in 80% of patients with lupus pleurisy. This can be useful in differentiating this condition from a similar one in a patient with arthritis and pleural effusion due to rheumatoid arthritis. The finding of lupus erythematosus cells in the pleural fluid is diagnostic of lupus pleuritis. High levels of antinuclear antibody titers ($\geq$1:160), a pleural fluid–to–serum antinuclear antibody ratio of greater than or equal to 1, and decreased levels of complement are presumptive diagnostic features. Lupus pleurisy responds well to corticosteroid therapy.

Wegener's granulomatosis is a disease characterized by necrotizing granulomatous vasculitis of the upper and lower respiratory tracts and the kidneys. Pleural effusions have been described in up to 55% of cases.[42] The usually small effusions are associated with the classic nodular or cavitating pulmonary lesions described in Wegener's granulomatosis. The effusions resolve spontaneously or in response to therapy with cyclophosphamide for the underlying condition.

Postcardiac Injury Syndrome

Postcardiac injury syndrome refers to the development of pleuropericardial and pulmonary parenchymal inflammatory symptoms that can occur following a variety of myocardial and pericardial injuries. It usually develops 3 weeks after the initial injury, but occurrences ranging from 2 to 86 days following the injury have been described.[43]

Originally described by Dressler[44] in patients with a history of myocardial infarction, injury following cardiac surgery is a more frequent cause of this condition. Other causes of postcardiac injury syndrome include blunt chest trauma, percutaneous puncture of the left ventricle, and implantation of a pacemaker. Patients present with fever, dyspnea, and pleuritic and pericardial chest pain. The chest roentgenogram characteristically shows a unilateral, usually left-sided pleural effusion and an adjacent basilar pulmonary infiltrate. Enlargement of the cardiac silhouette because of pericardial effusion is also commonly found.

The fluid is usually a serosanguineous exudate with leukocyte counts of approximately 10,000 cells/mm^3. Polymorphonuclear cells predominate if the sample is obtained within 10 days of the onset of symptoms. After 20 days, the differential cell count shows mononuclear cell predominance. Pleural fluid pH and glucose levels are normal.

Patients with postcardiac injury syndrome respond well to aspirin or nonsteroidal, anti-inflammatory therapy. In more severe cases, corticosteroid therapy is indicated.

Gastrointestinal Disease

Esophageal rupture is a relatively rare entity but an important one to consider in the differential diagnosis of pleural effusions because of its high mortality if not promptly treated.[45] Esophageal perforation is most commonly seen as an iatrogenic complication of esophagoscopic examination. It can also be seen during the removal of esophageal foreign bodies, dilatation of esophageal strictures, or insertion of a Sengstaken-Blakemore tube for treatment of esophageal varices.

Spontaneous rupture of the lower esophagus can occur from vomiting (Boerhaave's syndrome). These patients characteristically present with a history of prolonged vomiting followed by tearing pain of the chest and upper abdomen. The chest roentgenogram classically shows a unilateral, small, left-sided pleural effusion; widened mediastinum; and subcutaneous, pleural, and mediastinal air. Spontaneous rupture can be initially silent, with symptoms not developing until infectious complications occur.

The findings on the analysis of the pleural fluid depend on the timing of the thoracentesis and the extent of the esophageal perforation. It classically shows a low pH (<6) and high amylase level (salivary origin). Squamous epithelial cells and food particles can also be found. Immediate confirmation of the diagnosis needs to be accomplished with an esophagogram using a water-soluble contrast medium. Computed tomographic scanning of the chest is also useful in the diagnosis of esophageal rupture.[46] Mediastinitis and empyema usually develop within 12 hours of the perforation. In addition to antibiotic therapy, urgent surgical exploration should be performed. The surgical procedure includes drainage of the mediastinum and pleura, as well as repair of the esophageal tear.

Pleural effusions in pancreatic diseases are seen as a complication of acute pancreatitis, chronic pancreatic pseudocyst, and pancreatic ascites. The inflammatory reaction in acute pancreatitis results in the formation of an enzyme-rich exudate. This fluid reaches the pleural space through lymphatic vessels that cross the diaphragm.[47] In a chronic pancreatic pseudocyst, the effusion is caused by a direct sinus tract communicating with the pleural space.[48] As in other forms of ascites, peritoneal fluid secondary to pancreatic disease can reach the pleural space through diaphragmatic defects. The pleural fluid in pancreatic effusions is an exudate with high LDH levels. High amylase levels in the pleural fluid are found in 90% of these patients and are usually higher than those in serum. The leukocyte count ranges from 1000 to 50,000 cells/mm^3, with a polymorphonuclear predominance. Pleural fluid glucose levels are similar to those in serum.

Pleural effusions related to acute pancreatitis resolve as the pancreatic inflammatory response subsides. Treatment of the chronic pleural effusion associated with pancreatic pseudocyst usually requires laparotomy with ligation and excision of the fistulous tract and drainage of the pancreatic pseudocyst.

Other causes of exudative pleural effusion associated with intraabdominal processes include splenic, liver, and subdiaphragmatic abscesses and postlaparotomy and strangulated diaphragmatic hernias.

Asbestos Pleural Effusions

The term *asbestosis* refers to pulmonary parenchymal fibrosis secondary to the inhalation of asbestos fibers.

Benign pleural effusions are the most common and earliest manifestation of asbestos-related pleuropulmonary diseases. These pleural effusions usually appear during the first 20 years after exposure to asbestos.[49] Most effusions are small and patients are usually asymptomatic. Characteristically, effusions resolve spontaneously within several months, leaving a residual, small, localized pleural thickening. Occasionally, large or recurrent effusions are seen in asbestos pleurisy. Other pleural conditions associated with asbestos are pleural plaques, rounded atelectasis, progressive pleural fibrosis, and malignant mesothelioma.

The analysis of the pleural fluid does not provide any specific differentiating characteristics. The diagnosis of benign asbestos pleurisy is one of exclusion. Bronchogenic carcinoma and malignant mesothelioma need to be considered in an asbestos worker with recurrent or progressive pleural disease.

Lipid Pleural Effusions

The presence of lipids in the pleural fluid can occur in two situations:

- A disruption of the thoracic duct with extravasation of dietary fats and lymphatic cellular elements in the pleural cavity (chylothorax)
- An accumulation of cholesterol and lecithin-globulin complexes in chronic pleural effusions (pseudochylothorax)

This distinction is important because the treatment, prognosis, and underlying disease are entirely different in these two situations. In cases of chylothorax, the lipids present in the pleural fluid are mostly long-chain triglycerides. They are absorbed by intestinal lymphatics and transported to the cisterna chyli in the abdomen and then to the thoracic duct in the posterior mediastinum. The thoracic duct finally drains its contents into the venous system at the junction of the left jugular and subclavian veins.

More than half of the cases of chylothorax result from malignancies, mostly lymphomas.[50] The second most common cause of chylothorax is iatrogenic disruption of the thoracic duct following cardiovascular surgery. Other less frequent causes of chylothorax are congenital lymphangiectasia and pulmonary lymphangioleiomyomatosis.

Pseudochylothorax is a much less common cause of lipid pleural effusions, presenting in patients with long-standing pleural effusions, probably because of the impaired passage of lipids through a thickened pleura. Pseudochylous effusions are seen mostly in cases of tuberculous or rheumatoid pleuritis. The presence of lipids in the pleural space gives the characteristic milky, cloudy appearance to the fluid. However, the presence of serous or serosanguineous effusion does not exclude this diagnosis. The presence of an elevated triglyceride level (>110 mg/dL) is the main criterion for the diagnosis of chylothorax. Lipoprotein analyses that demonstrate the presence of chylomicrons may be required for the diagnosis of borderline cases. Pseudochylous effusions demonstrate elevated levels of cholesterol (>250 mg/dL) but low levels of triglycerides (<110 mg/dL).[51]

Treatment of chylothorax is aimed at the management of the underlying condition. However, other measures need to be taken to relieve respiratory symptoms and avoid intravascular volume depletion and malnutrition. These measures include drainage of the pleural space, parenteral nutrition, and resting the gastrointestinal tract. In patients with pseudochylous effusions, an attempt should be made to exclude an active infectious process (tuberculosis).

SUMMARY

The evaluation of patients with pleural effusions presents a frequent and interesting challenge. The clinical manifestations are usually related to the underlying disease responsible for the effusion. Although dyspnea or hemodynamic compromise can occur in large effusions, thoracentesis and analysis of the fluid is indicated in most patients with pleural effusions. The analysis of the fluid yields a specific diagnosis in only a minority of cases.

Clinical correlation is crucial when ordering specific tests and interpreting the results of the fluid analysis. Based on the protein and LDH values, the pleural fluid can be characterized as a transudate or an

More than 90% of all effusions are caused by congestive heart failure, pneumonia, malignancy, and pulmonary embolism.

exudate. This categorization constitutes the basis for further work-up and differential diagnosis. A pleural biopsy, indicated in patients with exudative effusions of undetermined cause, can be performed blindly with a needle or by direct inspection with a thoracoscope.

The treatment of the pleural effusion is most commonly directed at the underlying condition responsible for the effusion. Evacuation of the pleural fluid is indicated when the effusion causes ventilatory compromise or the fluid characteristics indicate frank infection or the likelihood that adhesions or loculations will form.

Sclerosis of the pleural space by chemical pleurodesis is indicated in the management of symptomatic effusions when successful treatment for the underlying disease (i.e., malignancy) is not available.

References

1. Light RW. Pleural Diseases. Philadelphia. Lea & Febiger, 1983.
2. Starling EH. On the absorption of fluids from the connective tissue spaces. J Physiol (Lond) 19:312–326, 1896.
3. Fedorko ME, Hirsch JG, Fried B. Studies on transport of macromolecules and small particles across mesothelial cells of the mouse omentum. II. Kinetic features and metabolic requirement. Exp Cell Res 69:313–323, 1971.
4. Light RW, Stansbury DW, Brown SE. The relationship between pleural pressures and changes in pulmonary function after therapeutic thoracentesis. Am Rev Respir Dis 133:658–661, 1986.
5. Felson B. Chest Roentgenology. Philadelphia, WB Saunders, 1973.
6. Light RW, Macgregor MI, Luchsinger PC, et al. Pleural effusions: The diagnostic separation of transudates and exudates. Ann Intern Med 77:507–513, 1972.
7. Levine H, Metzger W, Laccera D, Kay L. Diagnosis of tuberculous pleurisy by culture of pleural biopsy specimen. Arch Intern Med 126:269–271, 1970.
8. Prakash UBS, Reiman IIM. Comparison of needle biopsy with cytologic analysis for the evaluation of pleural effusion: Analysis of 414 cases. Mayo Clin Proc 60:158–164, 1985.
9. Boutin C, Viallat JR, Cargnino P, Farisse P. Thoracoscopy in malignant pleural effusions. Am Rev Respir Dis 124:588–592, 1981.
10. Loddenkemper R, Mai J, Scheffler N, Brandt H-J. Prospective intraindividual comparison of blind needle biopsy and of thoracoscopy in the diagnosis and differential diagnosis of tuberculous pleurisy. Scand J Respir Dis 102(Suppl):196–198, 1978.
11. Hausheer FH, Yarbro JW. Diagnosis and treatment of malignant pleural effusion. Semin Oncol 12:54–75, 1985.
12. Hutter JA, Harari D, Braimbridge MV. The management of empyema thoracis by thoracoscopy and irrigation. Ann Thorac Surg 39:517–519, 1985.
13. Weiss JM, Spodick DH. Association of left pleural effusion with pericardial disease. N Engl J Med 308:696–699, 1983.
14. Liberman FL, Hindemura R, Peters RL, Reynolds TB. Pathogenesis and treatment of hydrothorax complicating cirrhosis with ascites. Ann Intern Med 64:341–351, 1966.
15. Stark BD, Schanes JG, Baron RL, Koch DD. Biochemical features of urinothorax. Arch Intern Med 142:1509–1511, 1982.
16. Hughson WG, Friedman PJ, Feigin DS, et al. Postpartum pleural effusion: A common radiologic finding. Ann Intern Med 97:856–858, 1982.
17. Aelony Y. Myxedematous effusions. Arch Intern Med 144:857–861, 1984.
18. Spadaro JJ, Thakur V, Nolph KD. Technetium-99m labelled macroaggregated albumin in demonstration of transdiaphragmatic leakage of dialysate in peritoneal dialysis. Am J Nephrol 2:36–38, 1982.
19. Good JT, Moore JB, Fowler AA, et al. Superior vena cava syndrome as a cause of pleural effusion. Am Rev Respir Dis 225:246–247, 1982.
20. Light RW, Girard WM, Jenkinson SG, George RB. Parapneumonic effusions. Am J Med 69:507–511, 1980.
21. Chernow B, Sahn SA. Carcinomatous involvement of the pleura: An analysis of 96 patients. Am J Med 63:695, 1977.
22. Legha SS, Muggia FM. Pleural mesothelioma: Clinical features and therapeutic implications. Ann Intern Med 87:613–616, 1977.
23. Weick JK, Kiely JM, Harrison EG Jr, et al. Pleural effusion in lymphoma. Cancer 371:848–851, 1973.
24. Good JT, Taryle DA, Sahn SA. Pleural fluid pH in malignant effusions: Pathophysiologic and prognostic implications. Chest 74:338–343, 1978.
25. Rubinson R, Bolooki H. Intrapleural tetracycline for control of malignant effusions. South Med J 65:847–850, 1972.

26. Bynum LJ, Wilson JE III: Radiographic features of pleural effusions in pulmonary embolism. Am Rev Respir Dis 117:829–834, 1978.
27. Moser KM. Pulmonary embolism—State of the art. Am Rev Respir Dis 115:829–852, 1977.
28. Bynum LJ, Wilson JE. Characteristics of pleural effusions associated with pulmonary embolism. Arch Intern Med 136:159–162, 1976.
29. Storey DD, Dines DE, Coles DT. Pleural effusion: A diagnostic dilemma. JAMA 236:2183–2186, 1976.
30. Roper WH, Waring JJ. Primary serofibrinous pleural effusion in military personnel. Am Rev Respir Dis 71:616–632, 1955.
31. Rosenzweig DY. "Atypical" mycobacterioses. Clin Chest Med 1:273–284, 1980.
32. Goodwin RA Jr, Loyd JE, Des Prez RM. Histoplasmosis in normal hosts. Medicine 60:221–266, 1981.
33. Busey J (Chairman). Blastomycosis cooperative study of the Veterans Administration: Blastomycosis—I. A review of 198 collected cases in Veterans Administration hospitals. Am Rev Respir Dis 89:659–672, 1965.
34. Salkin D, Birsner TW, Tarr AD, et al. Roentgen analysis of coccidioidomycosis. *In* Ajello L (ed). Coccidioidomycosis. Tucson, University of Arizona Press, 1967.
35. Young EJ, Hirsch DD, Fainstein V, et al. Pleural effusions due to *Cryptococcus neoformans*: A review of the literature and report of two cases with cryptococcal antigen determinations. Am Rev Respir Dis 212:743–747, 1980.
36. Hillerdal G. Pulmonary *Aspergillus* infection invading the pleura. Thorax 36:745–751, 1981.
37. Bates M, Cruickshank G. Thoracic actinomycosis. Thorax 12:99–124, 1957.
38. Palmer DL, Harvey RL, Wheeler JK. Diagnostic and therapeutic considerations in *Nocardia asteroides* infection. Medicine 53:391–401, 1974.
39. Horler AR, Thompson M. The pleural and pulmonary complications of rheumatoid arthritis. Ann Intern Med 51:1179–1203, 1959.
40. Halla JT, Schrohenloher RE, Volanakis JE. Immune complexes and other laboratory features of pleural effusions. Ann Intern Med 92:748–752, 1980.
41. Israel HC. The pulmonary manifestations of disseminated lupus erythematosus. Am J Med Sci 226:387–392, 1953.
42. Goodman GC, Churg J. Wegener's granulomatosis: Pathology and review of the literature. Arch Pathol 58:533–553, 1954.
43. Stelzner TJ, King TE Jr, Anthony VB, Sahn SA. The pleuropulmonary manifestations of the postcardiac injury syndrome. Chest 84:383–387, 1983.
44. Dressler W. The post-myocardial-infarction syndrome: A report of 44 cases. Arch Intern Med 103:28–42, 1959.
45. Bladergroen MR, Lowe JE, Postlethwait RW. Diagnosis and recommended management of esophageal perforation and rupture. Ann Thorac Surg 42:235–239, 1986.
46. Parkin GJ. The radiology of perforated oesophagus. Clin Radiol 24:324–331, 1973.
47. Kaye MD. Pleuropulmonary complications of pancreatitis. Thorax 23:297–306, 1968.
48. Anderson WJ, Skinner DB, Zuidema GD, et al. Chronic pancreatic pleural effusion. Surg Gynecol Obstet 137:827–830, 1973.
49. Cohen BA, Effemidis A, Chahinian AP, et al. Computed tomography of the chest in diffuse malignant pleural mesothelioma. Am Rev Respir Dis 123:131–134, 1981.
50. Williams KR, Burford TH. The management of chylothorax. Ann Surg 160:131–140, 1964.
51. Hillerdal G. Chyliform (cholesterol) pleural effusion—Eleven new cases. Chest 86:426–428, 1985.

50

Pulmonary Rehabilitation

Nelson E. Leatherman, Ph.D.

Key Terms

Aerobic Metabolism

Anaerobic Threshold

Exercise Stress Testing

Pulmonary Rehabilitation

Respiratory Muscle
Endurance Training

Resting Energy Expenditure
(REE)

Vo_{2max}

In the early 1950s, the standard therapy for patients with chronic obstructive lung disease was rest and avoidance of physical activity. As a result, Barach's published comment in 1952 suggesting that patients with disorders of oxygen transport could actually benefit from an exercise training program was met with skepticism that was appropriate for the time.[1]

Rest and inactivity remained central in the management of chronic obstructive pulmonary disease (COPD) for a full decade. In the early 1960s, studies challenged this standard therapy by demonstrating that exercise training in COPD patients not only resulted in training effects similar to those observed in normal subjects but also promoted a state of well-being. Numerous investigations followed that supported these initial findings. Almost universally, the early investigations supported three conclusions:

1. Exercise training in patients with COPD increases exercise capacity.
2. Exercise training improves the patient's psychological state.
3. Exercise training *does not* improve pulmonary function.

Evaluation of the effectiveness of exercise training as a therapeutic modality, however, focused predominantly on the changes in the results of pulmonary function tests. Failing to demonstrate statistical improvements in the pulmonary function tests, the investigators, and the clinical community, had no way to explain the improvements in exercise capacity. As a result, some studies concluded that exercise training was of little benefit to the patient. As reports of improved functional capacity and increased sense of well-being continued to grow, however, an evolution in clinical thought redirected the focus from the results of laboratory tests to what the patients were feeling and experiencing. This new focus on the patient's quality of life made it possible to justify the costs of exercise training as a therapeutic modality.

DEFINITION OF PULMONARY REHABILITATION

The decade of the 1970s witnessed an explosion in the number of pulmonary rehabilitation programs offering exercise training. These programs became multidisciplinary and increasingly comprehensive, incorporating psychological, nutritional, and vocational support; oxygen therapy; bronchial hygiene; education; and, of course, the new component, exercise. The concept of a comprehensive rehabilitation program that draws support from multiple disciplines was recognized in 1974, when an ad hoc committee of the American College of Chest Physicians developed the following definition of pulmonary rehabilitation.

Pulmonary rehabilitation may be defined as an art of medical practice wherein an individually tailored multi-disciplinary program is formulated which, through accurate diagnosis, therapy, emotional support, and education, stabilizes or reverses both the physio- and psychopathology of pulmonary diseases and attempts to return the patient to the highest possible functional capacity allowed by his pulmonary handicap and overall life situation.

In response to the proliferation of pulmonary rehabilitation programs in the United States and the recognized need for guidelines for improved management of the growing numbers of patients with chronic lung disease, the American Thoracic Society (ATS) formally published its official position statement on pulmonary rehabilitation in 1981.[2] This statement, which incorporated the definition of the American College of Chest Physicians, signaled the acceptance of pulmonary rehabilitation by the medical community as a recognized component in the management of patients afflicted with chronic lung disease.

This definition was the formal conceptualization of today's pulmonary rehabilitation program and, as such, has proved vital to its success. It recognized the extreme complexity of the pulmonary patient's medical situation and then succeeded in molding the bits and pieces of medical management into a concept of total care. The definition not only states the goal of pulmonary rehabilitation but also prescribes a path to attaining that goal.

After 40 years of evolution, pulmonary rehabilitation is now accepted in both the United States and Europe as an important component in the medical management of patients with chronic respiratory disease. Pulmonary rehabilitation is still evolving today—not toward an identity or toward recognition by the medical community but toward ways to refine and improve on the individualization of each program and to increase the magnitude of the known benefits.

This chapter presents guidelines for the establishment of pulmonary rehabilitation programs based on current knowledge in the field while attempting to present the essential elements of a comprehensive program.

MECHANISMS OF FUNCTIONAL DETERIORATION IN CHRONIC LUNG DISEASE

Without a sudden event to stimulate a change in lifestyle, pulmonary patients, unlike cardiac patients, generally have a long, slow, downhill course. Chronic lung disease progressively damages lung tissue and airways and, over a period of years, ultimately results in a depletion of ventilatory reserves. Complicating this physiologically are abnormalities in gas exchange and elevations in pulmonary vascular pressures that lead to right ventricular dysfunction. All these factors contribute to the sensation of dyspnea and the resultant limitation on physical activity.

As dyspnea and exercise capacity worsen, the need for medical care increases and the patient's ability for self-care decreases; a confusing combination of functional limitations and dependence on others is thrust on the patient. The net effect is a profound sense of "loss of control," with consequent depression and anxiety.

Although the limitation to exercise imposed by the lung disease is generally considered irreversible, the additional functional deterioration caused by physiologic and psychological changes associated with the cycle of inactivity are considered reversible.

These factors are further worsened by the vicious cycle of inactivity (Fig. 50–1). The cycle begins when the patient starts to associate exertional dyspnea with the disease and no longer recognizes dyspnea as a normal response to exertion. In this setting, exertional dyspnea promotes increased levels of anxiety, depression, and fear of exertion, all of which generally lead to an exertion phobia and physical inactivity. The lack of exercise, in turn, leads to both central and peripheral deconditioning and, ultimately, to decreased endurance and weakness, and often to muscular atrophy. As a result of deconditioning, the patient experiences greater dyspnea, an even greater intolerance to exertion, and further loss of functional capacity. As the cycle continues, the patient's exercise capacity spirals progressively downward while the levels of fear, anxiety, and depression increase unabated. As the patient becomes progressively

Vicious Cycle of Inactivity

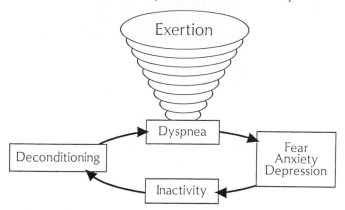

FIGURE 50–1: Vicious cycle of inactivity.

more physically and psychologically incapacitated, the consumption of medical resources increases dramatically. The progressive loss of exercise capacity resulting from the vicious cycle of inactivity is superimposed on the underlying functional reduction caused by the lung disease.

Pulmonary rehabilitation activities attempt to break the cycle at the point of fear and lack of exertion by providing capable, caring supervision of rehabilitation activities. Once the level of fear of exertion has been reduced, the patient is able to tolerate more exercise and thereby reverse the cycle of inactivity.

GOAL OF PULMONARY REHABILITATION

The goal of pulmonary rehabilitation is to improve the quality of life of patients with chronic lung disease by increasing their functional capacity and sense of well-being.

PROGRAM STRUCTURE

The basic elements of today's pulmonary rehabilitation program have not changed significantly from those outlined by the 1981 ATS Statement on Pulmonary Rehabilitation. The recommended sequence of steps for a pulmonary rehabilitation program, the components, and the list of required services provide guidelines for developing a pulmonary rehabilitation program. Even within these established guidelines of the ATS recommendations, however, the potential exists for diversity in the structure of pulmonary rehabilitation programs. This potential diversity results from consideration of several factors at the time the pulmonary rehabilitation program is under development, including the patient population, the available physical facilities, and the available pool of allied health professionals.

The extent to which these factors have influenced program structure is apparent from a recent national survey of pulmonary rehabilitation programs by Bickford. This survey showed that enrollment at any given time in pulmonary rehabilitation programs ranged from one to 48 patients (average of six), that contact time ranged from 1 to 8 hours per day (average, 2.2 hours) with a frequency of 1 to 7 days per week (average, 2.6 days), and that program duration ranged from 1 to 52 weeks (average, 8.3 weeks). In addition, the survey assessed the professional background of the health care team. No less than 18 different health specialties were represented in the programs surveyed. The specialists ranged from a physician, who was the most frequently represented (88% of programs), to a home care individual, a massage therapist, and a speech therapist, each of whom were represented in less than 1% of the programs.

The health care team is frequently described as a multidisciplinary team that consists of a pulmonary physician and a number of allied health professionals, including a respiratory therapist, a physical therapist, a psychologist, a nutritionist, an occupational therapist, a social worker, a chaplain, and a respiratory nurse, among others. Although this implies the necessity for a large, diverse team, the recommended services for pulmonary rehabilitation may be provided by far fewer personnel if the individuals are appropriately trained in the evaluation and management of pulmonary patients. The ultimate provider of the essential services depends on the allied health professionals available to the program and the size of the facility and likely varies from program to program.

The pulmonary rehabilitation programs at Duke University Medical Center typify the diversities in structure. The Duke program consists of two programs: (1) a short-term, intensive program designed to accommodate participants from outside the local area and provide an intense focus on pulmonary rehabilitation, and (2) a long-term maintenance program that is less time-intensive. These programs are referred to, respectively, as the intensive program and the graduate program.

Intensive Program

The intensive program operates ten 4.5-week sessions over the course of a year. Each intensive session has a maximum enrollment of 12 patients, approximately half of whom are from outside the local area. These participants meet 4 to 5 hours per day, 5 days per week, for the 4.5-week program. The primary health care team consists of the patient, a pulmonary physician, two respiratory therapists, two physical therapists, and a psychologist. The emphasis of the intensive program is on exercise training, education, medication optimization, bronchial hygiene, and psychological support. Other health care specialists who contribute regularly to the program through the educational component include an exercise physiologist, a clinical pharmacist, a nutritionist, a pulmonary nurse clinician, and an occupational therapist. Individual consultations with specialists in nutrition, psychology, and smoking cessation are common. The intense focus of this program produces recognized benefits sooner than less intensive programs—a factor that enhances patient motivation.

Graduate Program

The graduate program serves primarily as a medically supervised home program for pulmonary patients who reside locally. Enrollment in the graduate program is limited to patients who have successfully completed the intensive program. These participants usually meet for 2 hours per day 3 days per week and are enrolled on a yearly basis, although quarterly enrollment is possible. Medical supervision of the graduate program is provided by a physical therapist and a respiratory therapist. Although program emphasis is on exercise conditioning, all intensive program services are available to these participants as needed. The long-term social interaction with peers and the formation of support groups is a major advantage of the graduate program.

Each of the Duke programs was designed to provide the necessary rehabilitation services to a particular patient population and, as a result, major differences exist between the two programs in enrollment numbers, staff to patient ratio, contact hours per week, and program cost. The functional relationship between the two programs is noteworthy and may serve as a national model. The concept is one in which the patient may be intensely engaged in the rehabilitation process at a regional medical center initially, benefiting from its extensive resources, and then return to a local setting to continue the rehabilitation process with a local maintenance program. The importance of this relationship lies in the continuation of supervised training, which has been shown to be essential in sustaining the patients' motivation to continue the rehabilitation process over the long term.

At Duke, as elsewhere, program diversity is also apparent in component emphasis, which may differ, depending on the training, experience, and interest of the members of the health care team. As a result, certain programs emphasize nutrition and others emphasize activities of daily living, exercise, or psychological support. This diversity gives each program a character and appeal of its own while providing a comprehensive, individualized pulmonary rehabilitation program.

To individuals engaged in the process of developing a pulmonary rehabilitation program, these structural differences between programs that share the same basic elements can be bewildering. These differences, however, are the end result of tailoring programs with given resources to a particular population of pulmonary patients.

Belman has stated: "The encouraging finding is that despite the wide range of practice prevalent in the community, it is difficult if not impossible to find a rehabilitation program that fails."[3]

THE SEQUENCE OF PULMONARY REHABILITATION

The recommended sequence for a pulmonary rehabilitation program and the list of services used in implementing a program are virtually unchanged from a decade ago. Following the recommended sequence described in the ATS statement provides the greatest likelihood for successfully achieving the goals of pulmonary rehabilitation.

Patient Selection

Any patient with stable chronic respiratory disease who is symptomatic and experiences dyspnea on exertion should be considered a candidate for pulmonary rehabilitation. In addition, candidates must be free of acute illness and motivated to lead a more active life.

The clinical description of patients who potentially may benefit from pulmonary rehabilitation has broadened over the years. In the position statement published by the ATS in 1981, the section on patient selection

Patients with complicating conditions in which exercise is contraindicated, such as coronary artery disease and life-threatening arrhythmias, may be addressed more appropriately by other therapies or programs.

mentions only patients with COPD, excluding any mention of patients without COPD. As recently as 1988, 23% of the programs in the United States still limited patient selection to those with COPD. Recent evidence has demonstrated that multidisciplinary pulmonary rehabilitation programs are also of value in the management of patients with restrictive pulmonary diseases. These findings should encourage acceptance of patients with non-COPD pulmonary diseases as well as those with COPD into pulmonary rehabilitation programs.

The observation that patients with limited ventilatory capacity may be unable to exercise with sufficient intensity to receive a training effect has raised concern over whether benefits could be derived from a comprehensive pulmonary rehabilitation program. Although evidence of a true training effect in this group of patients remains controversial, at a minimum they can benefit from a program designed to improve coordination, muscle strength, suppleness, and state of well-being. Even exercise capacity may be improved in patients with limited ventilatory capacity, since the standard training effect is only one of several ways in which exercise capacity is known to increase.

Concern that exercise might precipitate respiratory failure by overloading weakened respiratory muscles leads to speculation that exercise training might be contraindicated in hypercapnic COPD patients. It has been shown, however, that hypercapnic COPD patients with severe ventilatory impairment and respiratory muscle weakness tolerate exercise and benefit significantly from intensive pulmonary rehabilitation. Similarly, exercise hypoxemia has been considered by some to be a contraindication to an exercise program. Our experience, however, has been that appropriate supplemental oxygen and proper monitoring (e.g., oximetry) allow such patients to participate fully in all aspects of the exercise program.

> Patient motivation plays a key role in optimizing the benefits received by the participant.

The pulmonary rehabilitation patient is subjected to many demands on time, energy, and finances, not to mention the commitment to an altered lifestyle. Motivational aspects of the selection process may be self-limiting in that individuals unwilling to face these demands will not, in general, pursue the pulmonary rehabilitation experience. Regardless, the patient selection process should carefully evaluate the patient's motivation or lack thereof.

Patient Assessment

A comprehensive patient evaluation essential to attaining the goals of pulmonary rehabilitation is the foundation on which the individually tailored program is constructed. Any condition or attitude that potentially limits the patient's ability to perform desired activities or grasp essential information must be identified by the health care team, assessed, and ultimately addressed. All members of the primary health care team are vital participants in the process of gathering and evaluating information from patient questionnaires, interviews, and a variety of clinical evaluations.

Ultimately the assessment process provides answers to a seemingly endless list of questions concerning the patient's condition.

Will this patient benefit from aerosol therapy or chest physical therapy, or both?

Will supplemental oxygen be necessary during exercise?

Must the exercises be modified to accommodate a limited range of motion or a weak extremity?
Should a particular mode of exercise be avoided or emphasized?
Is the patient motivated?
Is the patient compliant?
Does the patient need counseling on smoking cessation?

The interviewer must also determine the patient's level of knowledge about the disease and its management and assess the patient's level of independence.

What activities of daily living are difficult to perform?
What activities cannot be performed?
What is the patient's current state of mind?
What support systems and coping mechanisms currently exist for the patient's benefit?

Throughout the assessment process, the functional and physiologic severity of the patient's condition should be documented as an aid to selection of appropriate components of rehabilitation and to serve as a baseline in determining the effectiveness of the rehabilitation process in reaching both short- and long-term goals. Several important aspects of the assessment process are now discussed.

Accurate Diagnosis

The first step in this assessment is for the physician to make an accurate diagnosis of the patient's pulmonary problem and any complicating medical problems. The diagnosis should be substantiated by history, physical examination, chest roentgenography, pulmonary function testing, and any indicated laboratory tests. The importance of this initial step is evidenced by the inability of many patients to report a correct diagnosis. In one study, 64% of the patients entering a pulmonary rehabilitation program reported an incorrect diagnosis of their pulmonary problem.

Other diseases or medical problems that have a potential impact on the rehabilitation process must also be identified. As many as 91% of the patients entering a pulmonary rehabilitation program were identified as having other medical problems such as rhinitis-sinusitis (52%), hypertension (34%), gastrointestinal conditions (30%), and arrhythmias or coronary artery disease (27%). Other potentially complicating diseases include diabetes, obesity, osteoporosis, and stroke.

Evaluation of Exercise Capacity

Timed Walking Test. A timed 6- or 12-minute walking test is a simple and convenient way to evaluate the patient's ability to perform walking activities. The test may be performed in a measured corridor, on a track, or on a treadmill. The patient is instructed to walk as far as possible in the allotted time, stopping only if symptoms require, and is encouraged to continue as soon as possible. Encouragement must be provided throughout the duration of each test. For severely impaired patients, the 6-minute walking test may be more appropriate. Indeed, since the primary purpose of the 6- or 12-minute walking test is to establish a baseline for assessing progress, an initial 6-minute test is recommended to familiarize the patient with the test and to assess the patient's walking potential.

Exercise Stress Testing. Exercise stress testing commonly has been

Extremely anxious or fearful patients may be less likely to perform to their potential, and patients who recently have had traumatic experiences, such as a death of someone close or a divorce, may be limited in their performance and at poor risk for completion of a program of rehabilitation.

Without identification of the secondary problems, individualization of the patient program is incomplete and the likelihood of ever reaching full rehabilitation potential is greatly reduced.

As a guideline in avoiding truncation of a patient's walking performance, it is recommended that when the initial 6-minute distance exceeds 1500 feet (457 m), the patient should be re-evaluated with the 12-minute walking test.

used to assess an individual's functional capacity and establish the safety of exercise by providing a risk assessment of cardiac status. With exercise training being increasingly advocated in the management of chronic pulmonary disease, information provided by exercise stress testing is becoming essential in the comprehensive patient assessment. Exercise testing can provide valuable information concerning the mechanisms limiting the patient's exercise capacity, the presence of resting or exercise-induced hypoxemia (Pa_{O_2} <55, O_2 saturation <88%), exercise-induced hypertension (systolic pressure >250 mm Hg), and exercise-induced bronchospasm (comparison of pre- and postexercise FEV_1 maneuvers). It identifies problems, such as arthritis or limited range of motion, that might be associated with certain modes of exercise. Information gained from the stress test is also useful in prescribing the initial exercise intensity for bicycle and arm ergometry and in determining the resting energy expenditure (REE) necessary for an appropriate nutritional intervention.

The physiologic response to exercise is obtained by performing progressive exercise on a treadmill or stationary bicycle. The bicycle offers the advantage of being less frightening to some patients, less costly, and more accurate in quantifying the workload. In addition, electrically braked bicycles maintain work rates despite fluctuations in pedaling speed, and they can be programmed to provide true ramping protocols. Regardless of the mode of exercise used, the test should be performed to exhaustion or to a symptom limitation while measuring oxygen uptake (V_{O_2}), heart rate (HR), exercise ventilation (VE), and oxygen saturation. Arterial blood gases determined at rest and immediately following exercise remain the standard for evaluating resting hypoxemia, exercise-induced hypoxemia, and hypercapnia. Arterial blood samples also allow evaluation of the development of a significant lactic acidosis that would be indicative of reaching an anaerobic threshold (AT).

After an initial rest period, the workload is increased progressively at a rate that provides a test of sufficient duration, that is, 6 to 12 minutes. To facilitate selecting the rate at which the load is increased, it has been proposed that the workload should be increased each minute by 10% of the maximum predicted workload (Wmp). This is particularly convenient with the programmable bicycle ergometers in use today. It should be noted that the same load profile should be used in all subsequent tests on that patient.

Several mechanisms exist by which patients with chronic lung disease are limited in their ability to engage in physical activity, including:

- Cardiovascular limitation
- Ventilatory limitation
- Gas exchange limitation
- Psychological limitation

Knowledge of the specific limitation is important in tailoring the rehabilitation program to the individual patient. For instance, a different approach and different expectations would be contemplated for a patient limited by fear of exertion than for a patient with a cardiovascular limitation. Before discussing the specific exercise limitations that can be revealed by the abnormal exercise responses of patients with chronic lung disease, it is useful to review the exercise response typical of healthy individuals.

Healthy Subjects. When an individual performs progressive exercise, the

---

In some pulmonary patients, a good correlation does not exist between pulse oximeter measurements of oxygen saturation and those determined by arterial blood analysis. By having both measures during the stress test, a comparison may be made prior to extensive use of the oximeter during the rehabilitation process.

Wmp = 1.7 × Wt (kg) + 40 × FEV_1 (L) − 25.

The increase in V_{O_2} with exercise is due to increases in HR, stroke volume (SV), and the arterial-venous oxygen difference $[(a - V)\, O_2]$.

$$V_{O_2} = HR \times SV \times (a - V)O_2$$

$V_{O_{2max}}$ within the normal predicted range implies a normal exercise capacity, whereas reduction in $V_{O_{2max}}$ suggests an exercise-limiting impairment.

V_{O_2} increases until the individual can no longer perform the workload. The healthy, motivated subject stops exercise because of an inability to maintain aerobic metabolism; V_{O_2} is maximal in this situation (Fig. 50–2A) and is referred to as the aerobic capacity ($V_{O_{2max}}$). The V_{O_2} response thus provides information as to whether or not the exercise capacity is impaired. If impaired, the factors limiting the exercise (e.g., reduced cardiac or ventilatory reserves) must then be determined from the HR and VE responses.

The HR response (Fig. 50–2B) provides a means of assessing the cardiac reserve during progressive exercise. Since the stroke volume is maximized at relatively low work rates, the increase in cardiac output necessary to meet the demands of progressive exercise depends primarily on increases in HR. When HR increases to a physiologic maximum (i.e., predicted maximal HR), cardiac output is also maximal. At HR_{max}, there is no cardiac reserve to support the increasing workload (cardiovascular limitation). Depletion of cardiac reserves, therefore, is signaled by the

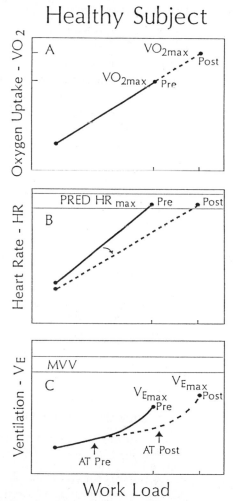

Physiologic Response to Exercise
Healthy Subject

FIGURE 50–2: Physiologic response to progressive exercise in healthy subjects. *A* to *C,* Oxygen uptake (V_{O_2}), heart rate (HR), and minute ventilation (VE), respectively, versus workload. The solid line represents the response prior to physical training. The dotted line represents the response after physical training.

The magnitude of the ventilatory reserve is determined by comparing the peak exercise ventilation to the maximum voluntary ventilation (MVV) obtained during pulmonary function testing.

HR increasing during exercise to the predicted maximal HR, as shown in Figure 50–2B.

The ventilatory response (Fig. 50–2C) provides a means of assessing ventilatory reserve. VE increases with work rate—slowly at first but more rapidly toward the end of the exercise. The acceleration in ventilation in the later phases of exhausting exercise is caused by the additional CO_2 load resulting from buffering of excess lactic acid produced by anaerobic metabolism (AT, Fig. 50–2C). As shown in Figure 50–2C, VE_{max} is usually only 50 to 80% of the MVV in the healthy, motivated individual at the end of exhausting exercise, implying that the ventilatory reserves are not depleted and that there is no ventilatory limitation to exercise.

In summary, healthy subjects have a normal VO_{2max} and a cardiovascular limitation to exercise. Although they may experience exertional dyspnea, at exhaustion they still have significant ventilatory reserve. These responses are in marked distinction to those observed in patients with chronic pulmonary disease.

Pulmonary Patients. When the pulmonary patient performs progressive exercise, the maximum level achieved, which is usually less than predicted, results in a lower maximal measured VO_2. The mechanisms for this limitation are multifactorial:

The actual measured VO_2 at peak exercise is thus sometimes referred to as the "symptom-limited" VO_2 (VO_{2sl}).

1. Ventilatory factors are manifested by an inability to increase the minute ventilation (VE) commensurate with metabolic demands. These patients usually have either mechanical limitations to ventilation (e.g., flow obstruction or reduced compliance) or muscle weakness. Thus, the MVV is reduced. The patient with limited ventilatory capacity terminates exercise when the VE approaches the MVV. In these patients, the maximal VO_2 is often not reflective of the true VO_{2max}, since the cardiovascular system does not reach its maximum capacity (i.e., HR is not maximal).

2. Gas exchange factors are manifested by hemoglobin desaturation during exercise. Patients with pulmonary disease may or may not have significant pulmonary mechanical abnormalities but all will have abnormalities in ventilation-perfusion matching that worsens when ventilation and perfusion increase with exercise.

As with the patient with limited ventilatory capacity, the actual measured VO_2 at peak exercise in patients with limited gas exchange is sometimes referred to as the "symptom-limited" VO_2 if the maximal HR is not achieved.

3. Cardiovascular factors are manifested by attaining a cardiovascular maximum (i.e., maximal predicted HR) at a lower than predicted maximal VO_2. This is sometimes expressed as a low oxygen pulse (VO_2/HR). Cardiovascular limitations in pulmonary patients may reflect deconditioning from inactivity or underlying ventricular dysfunction, especially right ventricular dysfunction.

4. Other factors include a severe sense of subjective dyspnea, fear of exertion, or lack of motivation. These factors are suspected whenever there is no indication of a cardiovascular limitation (HR less than 80% of predicted maximum), a ventilatory limitation (VE less than 80% of MVV), or a gas exchange limitation (O_2 saturation less than 88%).

In summary, the abnormal physiologic response for the pulmonary patient may show

- An impaired oxygen uptake because of a ventilatory limitation
- A cardiovascular limitation
- A gas exchange limitation
- A nonspecific limitation such as a lack of motivation, fear of exertion, or hypersensitivity to dyspnea

Each of these limitations may occur singly or in combination. After the exercise evaluation has determined that a particular limitation exists, the patient's program may be tailored according to the particular limitation. For instance, a gas exchange limitation requires consideration of the use of supplemental oxygen during the rehabilitation process. A ventilatory limitation de-emphasizes the endurance training effect and places more emphasis on improvements in strength, coordination, suppleness, and sense of well-being. Improvements in the functional capacity of patients with limited ventilatory capacity may be possible by

- Reducing hyperventilation that may result from anxiety, fear, or diet (high respiratory quotient, high V_{CO_2})
- Raising the ventilatory limit (MVV) through bronchial hygiene and medication optimization
- Improving respiratory muscle function specifically in patients with limited ventilatory capacity who show signs of ventilatory muscle fatigue, that is, hypercapnia

A cardiovascular limitation stresses the importance of an exercise training effect with an increased AT and, in some cases, improvements in efficiency of performance. A psychological limitation requires further assessment to determine the probable cause for the patient's inability to reach a physiologic limitation.

Inspiratory Muscle Function Assessment

There are two compelling reasons to evaluate respiratory muscle function in patients participating in pulmonary rehabilitation programs. First, inspiratory muscle function evaluation provides a baseline on which to evaluate improvements in respiratory muscle function that occur as a result of the rehabilitation process. Respiratory muscle weakness often occurs in patients with chronic lung disease and is particularly common in malnourished patients and those with hypercapnia. Since hypercapnic respiratory failure has been associated with values of respiratory muscle strength less than 30% of that predicted, patients with respiratory muscle weakness must be considered at increased risk of respiratory failure. Any demonstrated improvement in strength and endurance of the respiratory muscles of these patients during rehabilitation is an asset in potentially delaying respiratory muscle fatigue and the subsequent onset of respiratory failure during an acute pulmonary exacerbation. The additional functional reserve would theoretically provide more time for standard therapeutic modalities to be effective.

Second, evaluation of respiratory muscle function allows assessment of respiratory muscle weakness or fatigue as a potential factor limiting exercise. Reduction of respiratory muscle strength after the exercise stress test is indicative of respiratory muscle fatigue, which implicates respiratory muscle dysfunction as a possible factor limiting the patient's exercise capacity. The validity of this observation is enhanced in the presence of exercise-induced hypercapnia.

Inspiratory Muscle Strength Evaluation. Inspiratory muscle strength may be estimated by measuring maximal inspiratory mouth pressure, PI_{max}. The measurements are made by having the seated patient exhale to residual volume and then inspire maximally against a closed airway. A small resistive leak prevents facial muscles from producing significant pressure. After a few practice maneuvers, the best of a minimum of three values, reproducible to within 10%, is taken as PI_{max}. Each maneuver must be sustained for a minimum of 1 second. Predicted normal values

Male patients with measured PI_{max} values less than 70% of those predicted (females, 60% PI_{max}) should receive inspiratory muscle training (see Inspiratory Muscle Training).

for PI_{max} can be calculated from the regression equations shown in Table 50–1.

Inspiratory Muscle Endurance Evaluation. Changes in respiratory muscle endurance are frequently measured as a change in the maximum sustainable ventilatory capacity (MSVC). This is the highest level of ventilation that can be sustained for a given duration, usually 10 to 15 minutes. Determination of this level requires several hyperventilation trials and, consequently, is both time-consuming and uncomfortable to the patient.

A reported simple approach to inspiratory muscle endurance evaluation uses inspiratory flow resistive loads (IFRL) or inspiratory pressure threshold loads (IPTL) with a controlled pattern of breathing. The endurance of the patient is tested with an inspiratory load set at 60 to 70% of the maximum inspiratory mouth pressure, PI_{max}, while controlling the breathing pattern with visual feedback. A pressure time index ($PI/PI_{max} \times ti/t_{tot}$) of 0.3 has been shown to produce fatigue in 10 to 15 minutes. A breathing pattern that successfully accomplishes this has an inspiratory time of 3 seconds, an expiratory time of 4 seconds, and an inspiratory mouth pressure 70% of PI_{max}. It should be noted, however, that it is not clear if endurance measured under these resistive-loaded conditions is reflective of actual endurance capabilities under less loaded exercise hyperventilation.

Nutritional Assessment

Although the evidence for improvements in exercise capacity resulting from nutritional intervention during pulmonary rehabilitation remains controversial, it is increasingly clear that an adequate nutritional status is necessary in maintaining adequate ventilatory muscle function. At a time when the exercise component of the rehabilitation program is attempting to improve skeletal muscle strength and endurance, including that of the respiratory muscles, it is imperative that the nutritional requirements of the muscles be met. If not, there is reason to believe the therapeutic intervention will be less than optimal.

The need for nutritional intervention may be assessed by simply obtaining the patient's body weight as percent ideal body weight based on the Metropolitan Life Insurance height and weight tables, and a history of weight loss or gain. Patients with a percent ideal body weight less than 90 should be further evaluated for nutritional repletion and those with a percent ideal body weight greater than 110 should receive dietary support if the additional weight has a potential impact on exercise performance. Additional information as to the extent of malnutrition is obtained from serum albumin levels and total lymphocyte count.

Nutritional repletion requires determination of the patient's resting energy expenditure. This may be estimated by the equations presented

---

The research data suggest a reasonably good correlation between peak inspiratory flow rate (PIFR) and MSVC, which may allow approximating MSVC from measurements of PIFR using the following equation:

MSVC (L/min) = 14.8 × PIFR (L/sec)

Since expiration is predominantly effort-independent in COPD patients, improvement in MSVC has been hypothesized to result from increasing the PIFR, which is highly effort-dependent. If the correlation between MSVC and PIFR withstands further verification, it offers the possibility that changes in respiratory muscle endurance might be estimated by simply measuring PIFR.

Albumin levels less than 3.5 g/dL suggest a significant protein depletion, whereas a lymphocyte count less than 1500 cells/mm^3 suggests deficiency in the immune system.

If a patient has a history of recent weight gain or loss, a 3-day dietary diary is useful in evaluating average caloric intake. Comparison with REE provides an estimate of the net caloric gain or loss.

TABLE **50–1:** Predicted Normal Values for PI_{max} (cm H_2O)

	Age (yr)				
	20–54	*55–59*	*60–64*	*65–69*	*70–74*
Male	124 ± 44	103 ± 32	103 ± 32	103 ± 32	103 ± 32
Female	87 ± 32	77 ± 26	73 ± 26	70 ± 26	65 ± 26

From Black LF, Hyatt RE. Am Rev Respir Dis 99:696–702, 1969.

in Table 50–2 or calculated directly from the resting V_{O_2} determined during an exercise test. In the latter case,

$$REE = 6.91 \times V_{O_2}$$

where REE is in kcal/24 hour and V_{O_2} is in milliliters per minute.

REE (kcal/24 hr) = 4.8 (kcal/L O_2) $\times$ 0.001 (L/ml) $\times$ V_{O_2} (mL O_2/min) $\times$ 1440 (min/24 hr)

Psychological Assessment

Psychological disturbances are common in patients with chronic lung disease. The most common emotional consequences of COPD are depression and anxiety, which can further reinforce social isolation and inactivity. Cognitive function has also been shown to be impaired in these patients, perhaps as a consequence of chronic hypoxemia.

These problems need to be addressed in a comprehensive rehabilitation program. A number of simple tests can be given to provide insight into a patient's psychological status. Techniques to address these problems range from formal psychological-psychiatric consultations to group sessions. The Duke program has a formal psychologist team member to provide the initial assessment, arrange individual treatment programs for those who need it, and coordinate periodic group sessions.

Implementing the Program

Education

A primary purpose of the educational component of pulmonary rehabilitation is to provide the framework for self-care. Through an educational process of instruction, supervision, and practice patients can acquire an awareness of their disease and its management that allows them to begin to take responsibility for their own care. Through increased use of several treatment modalities, pulmonary patients have demonstrated the ability to recognize and treat symptoms of chronic bronchitis and emphysema. Greater independence requires that patients acquire confidence in their knowledge and abilities to perform techniques of self-care. That confidence is developed and reinforced by providing repeated opportunities to demonstrate (practice) their capabilities in a supervised setting.

The educational process usually consists of a combination of lectures, discussions, demonstrations, and practice sessions. During all program activities, the patient's knowledge and ability to perform self-management techniques are continually reinforced. Topics typically covered in formal lectures and discussion sessions include the anatomy and physiology of the lung, the pathophysiology of chronic lung disease, pulmonary medications, nutrition, physiologic responses to exercise, sexual con-

A spouse, family member, or close friend also participates in the educational activities to provide familial understanding of the disease process and to reinforce the recommended self-care techniques in the home setting.

TABLE **50–2:** Resting Energy Expenditure Equations for Chronic Obstructive Pulmonary Disease Patients (REE, kcal/24 hr)

| Male | REE = 11.5 $\times$ BW (kg) + 952 |
| Female | REE = 14.5 $\times$ BW (kg) + 515 |

From Moore JA, Angellillo VA. Chest 94:1260–1263, 1988.
REE, resting energy expenditure; BW, body weight.

The use of a pulse oximeter to provide visual feedback of improvements in blood oxygenation during pursed-lip breathing has been shown to be useful in teaching that particular technique. Auscultation has also been used successfully to enhance breathing retraining by allowing patients to listen to their own chest while breathing with and without pursed-lip breathing. The significant difference in airflow is readily recognized by the patient and serves to reinforce the value of the technique.

Pulse oximetry should be used to monitor all patients during exercise sessions, but particularly those receiving supplemental oxygen or those with a history of arterial desaturation.

The exercise training prescription is individualized for each patient by specifying four characteristics of exercise: mode, intensity, duration, and frequency.

cerns, travel concerns, coping with chronic lung disease, early recognition of infections and exacerbations, and psychosocial issues. Respiratory therapy and physical therapy techniques are more appropriately presented in either individual or group demonstrations and in practice sessions. These topics include cleaning and care of equipment, proper use of metered-dose inhalers and spacers, relaxation techniques, clearing of secretions using techniques of controlled coughing, postural drainage, percussion and vibration, and supplemental oxygen therapy. Educational material in the form of pamphlets, booklets, and books is available from a multitude of sources, including the American Lung Association. This additional information should be used to support and reinforce the information the patient receives in the lectures, discussions, and demonstrations.

Breathing retraining traditionally has been a key aspect of the educational component of a pulmonary rehabilitation program. Pursed-lip breathing and diaphragmatic breathing are commonly used concomitantly to reduce shortness of breath and improve gas exchange. By using pursed-lip breathing, patients may be able to maintain adequate oxygenation without supplemental oxygen.

The success of the program's educational process may be assessed by providing testing of didactic information before and after instruction and by requiring each patient to satisfactorily demonstrate the recommended management techniques.

Supplemental Oxygen Considerations

All exercise training should be performed under conditions of adequate arterial oxygenation (PaO_2 >55 mm Hg, O_2 saturation >88%). If the initial patient assessment has determined that the resting oxygenation is low, or that significant desaturation occurs with exertion, supplemental oxygen must be provided to the patient to maintain adequate oxygen saturation. Usually, oxygen delivered at 2 L per minute via nasal cannula is sufficient. In some cases, however, it may be difficult to provide adequate oxygenation during exertion with even a partial rebreathing system. When adequate oxygenation cannot be maintained, either the intensity of the exercise must be reduced or the patient must be instructed to stop exercising until oxygenation is again adequate. Besides reducing the medical risk associated with low oxygenation, supplemental oxygen often allows the patient who needs oxygen to exercise for a longer duration at a higher intensity, thereby enhancing the beneficial effects of the exercise.

Exercise Training Prescription

In general, the exercise training experience provided by the pulmonary rehabilitation program should expose the patient to a balance of three types of exercise: stretching and flexibility exercises, strengthening exercises, and endurance exercises. Stretching and flexibility exercises are usually part of a floor exercise routine that develops suppleness, improves range of motion, and helps provide a general warm-up. Strength training may be obtained as part of the floor exercise routine by performing exercises with dumbbells, cuff weights, or a stretch band. Pulmonary patients also do well with free weights and weight machines, such as Nautilus equipment, for strength training. Strength exercises require a stimulus of high intensity and low frequency. General endurance training involves exercises that produce a cardiopulmonary stress that results in elevated HR and ventilation. Such exercises include walking, rowing, swimming, water aerobics, cycling (arm or leg), stair climbing, and so on, provided that the exercise intensity produces sufficient cardiopulmonary stress. Compared with strength training, endurance training is of lower intensity and higher frequency.

Mode (Specificity of Training). The benefits of exercise training are, for the most part, specific to the muscles and tasks involved in training. For instance, a walking program will produce significant improvement in walking performance but not in swimming or biking performance. It is important, therefore, to consider the particular mode of exercise in conjunction with the needs and goals of the patient. If a patient has a stated goal that requires improvement in stair climbing, this should be one of the modes of exercise in the prescription. Walking is generally considered an essential exercise because of its prevalence in daily activities and, probably for that reason, most exercise training prescriptions use predominantly lower extremity exercises.

Many patients with chronic airway obstruction experience marked shortness of breath when they use their arms for even simple tasks. Arm exercise is thought to contribute to the dyspnea by contributing to ventilatory muscle fatigue, by placing a load on an already stressed system, and by placing a nonventilatory demand on shoulder girdle muscles that have been recruited to act as accessory muscles of respiration. Improvement in upper extremity function as a result of specific upper extremity exercises has been demonstrated in patients with COPD. Improvement in upper extremity function has been observed to carry over to self-care, leisure, and other arm activities. By combining arm and leg exercises in a training program for patients with chronic airway obstruction, others have shown not only increased exercise performance in both upper and lower extremities but also a significantly improved state of well-being that was greater in the combined training than in either arm or leg training alone. The conclusion is that leg and arm exercise should be combined in exercise programs for patients with chronic airway obstruction.

Upper extremity exercise training may be accomplished through simple games or activities that use the arms above shoulder height (e.g., passing an object overhead) or gravity-resistive exercises (e.g., performing arm circles at shoulder height or walking with exaggerated arm movement—possibly with hand weights). Upper extremity strength training may be achieved by performing exercises with free weights, pulley systems, or weight machines. Arm endurance training may be accomplished with an arm ergometer, rowing machine, combined arm/leg bicycle, or cross-country ski machine.

Intensity. Well-established guidelines exist for prescribing the intensity of endurance exercise for normal subjects as well as for cardiac patients. These guidelines are based on target exercise heart rates expressed as a percent of the predicted maximum HR. Application of these guidelines, however, is generally not appropriate to pulmonary patients because the ventilatory impairment may prevent the patient from reaching the predicted maximum HR.

The initial load prescription should be of sufficiently low intensity that it can be accomplished by the patient without discomfort. Nothing destroys the patient's motivation faster than failure to complete the initial exercise or experiencing significant discomfort during or after the first exercise session. The initial loads used by the Duke intensive pro-

Specificity of training provides the incentive for including upper as well as lower extremity exercises in the training program.

Few guidelines currently exist for prescribing exercise intensity in patients with lung disease.

gram for the stationary bicycle and arm ergometer are based on the maximum workload reached during the exercise stress test (W_{max}). The initial bicycle workload (W_{bike}) is set at 50% of the maximum workload ($0.5 \times W_{max}$). This value is based on data suggesting that an individual can be expected to work for 8 hours at 50% of maximum work capacity without undue fatigue. The initial load prescription for arm exercise is 30% of W_{max} (or 60% of W_{bike}) and is based on studies showing that the aerobic power of the arms ranges from 50 to 70% of the maximum power output of the legs.

Whenever the patient experiences significant symptoms of fatigue or dyspnea, instead of stopping exercise, the load is reduced while the patient is encouraged to complete the exercise if possible. When the initial load is already the lowest possible, the patient stops until the symptoms subside and then continues the exercise to completion. The duration of the rest period is considered part of the exercise period. The short-term goal then becomes reducing the number of rests during the exercise period.

Workloads must be reassessed each exercise session and adjusted according to the patient's progress. The appropriate intensity for the target workload (the desired training load) has been an area of controversy. Evidence now shows, however, that patients with severe lung disease, particularly those with a ventilatory limitation to exercise, may tolerate training at a much higher percentage of their maximum exercise tolerance than was previously thought. Target intensities reaching the highest level attained on the initial exercise stress test have been used successfully in exercise training regimens.

High-intensity exercise training is based on the observation that patients with ventilatory limitation can tolerate exercise at levels near their maximum exercise HR (personal observation) and sustain a ventilation near their maximum voluntary ventilation. The principle of high-intensity endurance training is ultimately to exercise the patient at, or as close as possible to, the AT. If a significant lactic acidosis does not develop during the initial exercise stress test, the target intensity is set at the maximum workload reached. If a significant lactic acidosis does develop, the target intensity is set at the workload associated with the AT.

The process of increasing the exercise intensity from the initial intensity to the target intensity is as much art as science. So as not to overstress the patient and create a negative impact on motivation, it becomes necessary to prescribe loads based at least in part on the patient's assessment of the severity of symptoms.

To accomplish the transition from the relatively low initial loads to the higher target loads, the Duke University intensive program relies on the Borg Scale of Perceived Exertion as a measure of perceived stress, and the exercise heart rate as a measure of cardiopulmonary stress. If the patient was unable to reach the AT during the exercise stress test, the desired target HR is the maximum HR achieved on the exercise stress test. If the AT was reached, the target HR is the HR at the AT. If the Borg rating of the previous exercise session exceeds 17 and the HR during exercise approximates the target HR, consideration is given to reducing the intensity. If the rating is less than 15 and the HR during exercise is less than the desired target HR, consideration is given to increasing the intensity. Whenever the patient is capable of performing a given load for the duration of the exercise session, the load is increased by 0.25 kilopond for the bicycle ergometer (about 12.5 watts) and 50

The desired Borg rating is 15 to 17 on a scale of 6 to 20.

kilopond/min for the arm ergometer (about 9 watts). After approximately six exercise sessions, most patients will have attained an exercise level representing a high percentage of the target workload.

Duration and Frequency. The recommended minimum duration and frequency of endurance exercise is no less than 20 minutes, three times per week. Increasing the duration and frequency beyond this minimum must take into consideration the motivation and goals of the patient, and balance the time spent in training against the benefits derived from a more intense training regimen. The primary benefits of spending additional time on training are faster and greater improvement in physical capacity.

Inspiratory Muscle Training

Supporting Evidence. Since it has been reported that both the endurance and strength of respiratory muscles could be improved in normal subjects by specific training of these muscles, application of respiratory muscle training techniques to patients with chronic lung disease has been of considerable interest. Many studies have now demonstrated that the respiratory muscles of pulmonary patients also respond to physical training with significant increases in strength and endurance. Although nonspecific training programs that demand increased ventilation and provide general body conditioning (e.g., running and swimming) have demonstrated improved respiratory muscle endurance, this form of training is not as effective in producing improvements in ventilatory muscle function as specific respiratory muscle training. The effects of inspiratory muscle training on exercise capacity and performance of activities of daily living have been reviewed and remain controversial.

Despite the questionable effects of respiratory muscle training on the patient's functional capacity, the convincing evidence that ventilatory muscle strength and endurance can be increased is sufficient reason to provide specific respiratory muscle training as a component of pulmonary rehabilitation. Since adequate strength and endurance are necessary for muscle performance without fatigue, it is reasonable to believe that improving the strength and endurance of respiratory muscles will provide additional functional reserve during periods of increased ventilatory load. At this time, there are no studies to support the hypothesis that respiratory muscle training will delay the onset of respiratory failure or reduce its severity.

Respiratory Muscle Strength Training. Respiratory muscle strength training requires a strength-training regimen—a forceful contraction maintained for a brief period (stimulus of high intensity and low frequency). Typically the subject makes repeated maximal static efforts against a closed airway. Inspiratory efforts (Mueller maneuvers) train inspiratory muscles, whereas expiratory efforts (Valsalva maneuvers) train expiratory muscles. Inspiratory muscle strength also may be increased by the techniques to be described to improve ventilatory muscle endurance.

Respiratory Muscle Endurance Training. Two forms of specific endurance training of ventilatory muscles have been used to improve respiratory muscle endurance.

- Voluntary isocapnic hyperpnea
- Inspiratory loading

Inspiratory loading involves either of two methodologies. The first uses an inspiratory flow-resistive load (IFRL) and the second an inspiratory pressure threshold load (IPTL).

Voluntary Isocapnic Hyperpnea. This type of endurance training requires the patient to maintain levels of ventilation on the order of 60 to 70% of the MVV for 15 minutes twice a day. Decreases in Pa_{CO_2} subsequent to the hyperventilation are prevented by having the patient rebreathe through an appropriate dead space or by using more complex equipment to maintain a constant Pa_{CO_2} and supply adequate O_2 to prevent hypoxemia.

Inspiratory Flow-resistive Loading. Currently, IFRL is probably the most common form of specific respiratory muscle training. This form of endurance training is achieved by inspiring against an external resistive load (usually an orifice of adjustable size). A number of flow-resistive devices have been used to provide this type of training.

Inspiratory Pressure Threshold Loading. IPTL devices have also been used successfully to provide endurance training in respiratory muscles. This training regimen requires that the patient exert sufficient inspiratory pressure to overcome a predetermined threshold in order to initiate an inspiratory breath. Inspiration is made progressively more difficult by adjusting a weight or spring. As with IFRL, the training is performed for 15 minutes twice a day.

Of the two forms of training, inspiratory loading, using either IFRL or IPTL, is more applicable to the rehabilitation setting because of patient comfort, time constraints, and technical requirements. As mentioned previously, respiratory muscle training with either type of inspiratory load, IFRL or IPTL, should be performed for 15 minutes twice a day. To achieve a reliable training effect, it is vital that the patient use a controlled (targeted) breathing pattern that defines inspiratory pressure as well as the duration of inspiration and expiration. Without such a ventilatory target, the patient may circumvent fatiguing inspiratory loads by inspiring more slowly. The target pressure is generally expressed as a percentage of PI_{max}. Target pressures ranging from 30 to 70% of PI_{max} have been reported in the literature. A target pressure of 70% PI_{max} with an inspiratory time of 3 seconds and an expiratory time of 4 seconds has been used in training and has been reported to be fairly well tolerated. Justification of the higher target was based on a tension time index of 0.3 (ti/t_{tot} 0.43, PI/PI_{max} 0.7), a value that has been shown to result in diaphragmatic fatigue in 10 to 15 minutes.

Nutritional Intervention

Supporting Evidence. There has been renewed interest in the nutritional aspects of chronic lung disease since 1980. The prevalence of chronic malnutrition and weight loss in patients with COPD, particularly emphysema, has been reported to range from 24% to as high as 60%, confirming that a significant number of patients seeking pulmonary rehabilitation may experience the effects of malnutrition.

The most obvious effect of chronic undernourishment is respiratory muscle atrophy with loss of muscle mass. It should be noted, however, that younger patients with asthma or cystic fibrosis often have respiratory muscle hypertrophy and normal strength in spite of significant weight loss. Loss of strength due to weight loss, coupled with the loss of strength due to alterations in the size and length of the diaphragm often seen in COPD, may predispose the patient to respiratory failure. In pulmonary patients, physical activity with weakened limb muscles causes increased ventilatory demands on a system with impaired ventilatory capacity. This increased ventilatory load is placed on respiratory muscles that may well be equally weakened by the effects of malnutrition. The resulting increase in symptoms decreases physical activity and the patient gets pulled further into the cycle of inactivity.

The effect of malnutrition on the exercise capacity of pulmonary patients, in contrast, is less clear than its effect on ventilatory muscle function. Although reductions in functional capacity have been reported in underweight COPD patients, other evidence suggests that moderate weight loss in COPD does not affect 6-minute walking distance, dyspnea index, and quality of life scores.

Likewise, effects of nutritional intervention on the functional capacity of stable, ambulatory COPD patients have been substantiated by several studies, but not by others, and thus remain controversial. A compilation of the results of six of these investigations suggests that the degree of nutritional repletion is critical in achieving benefits. Patients repleted to more than 1.5 times the REE ($1.5 \times REE$) showed significant improvement in hand grip strength or inspiratory muscle strength and also improved significantly on 6- and 12-minute walking tests. Other studies concur with the assessment that adequate nutritional intervention requires a 50% increment in caloric intake above the REE.

Nutritional repletion is not without potential problems. Although overfeeding can cause increased production of CO_2 with concomitant increases in ventilation that are undesirable, it is more likely that difficulty will be encountered in attaining the recommended caloric intake. Donahoe and Rogers have reviewed various factors commonly attributed to limiting caloric intake and the potential therapeutic strategies.[4] The success of the various strategies is reportedly dependent on both patient and staff motivation.

Nutritional Repletion. All patients with a body weight less than 90% of ideal body weight should be considered for nutritional repletion, particularly those with respiratory muscle dysfunction (indicated by a low PI_{max}). Under normal circumstances, the recommended caloric intake for repletion is 1.5 times the REE, but with the additional energy demands of a pulmonary rehabilitation program, caloric intake in the range of 1.5 to 1.7 times the REE is recommended. Repletion is accomplished in the following proportions: 15% protein, 50% carbohydrate, and 35% fat. However, if a patient is retaining CO_2, the carbohydrate and fat proportions may be reversed to 35% carbohydrate and 50% fat to minimize the effect of respiratory quotient on the production of CO_2.

EVIDENCE THAT PULMONARY REHABILITATION PROGRAMS REVERSE FUNCTIONAL DETERIORATION

Some of the most recent data supporting the concept that pulmonary rehabilitation reverses functional deterioration come from our own program at Duke University Medical Center. The psychological and physiologic data to be presented here were obtained from 79 pulmonary patients participating in the intensive outpatient pulmonary rehabilitation program.

Psychological Changes

Psychological changes resulting from the Duke pulmonary rehabilitation program are assessed by the Psychological General Well-Being Index (PGWB) designed by Dupuy.[5] The PGWB is a 22-item, self-report questionnaire tapping six dimensions of psychological functioning, including anxiety, depressed mood, positive well-being, self-control, general health, and vitality. Individual items are scored from 0 to 5, with higher scores indicating greater well-being. In addition, a summary score having a maximum of 110 is derived by summing the individual item scores.

Figure 50–3 shows the changes in the mean PGWB index and the means of the six subscales of the 79 patients expressed as a percent of the normal score as the result of completion of the rehabilitation program. The average raw PGWB index was 60 (73%) on entry into the Duke program and 78 (95%) on discharge, compared with 82 (100%) in the normal population, a 30% improvement in the psychological index. Scores on all six subscales increased after rehabilitation, with many approaching the norm by the end of the program. Major contributions to the total index came from the subscales of vitality, positive well-being, anxiety, and general health. The general health subscale, although showing significant improvement, remained notably below normal, suggesting that as a whole the patients retain a view of their state of health that is consistent with their condition. They have a chronic lung disease, they recognize that fact, and yet they are able to deal better with their chronic disease after the rehabilitation process.

The documented changes in the PGWB index and its subscales suggest that the patients' improved sense of well-being and self-esteem may be related to positive changes in their psychological state. It is plausible that these same changes in the psychological state may also account for the improved exercise capacity by improving motivation, reducing fear of exertion, and desensitizing the patient to shortness of breath.

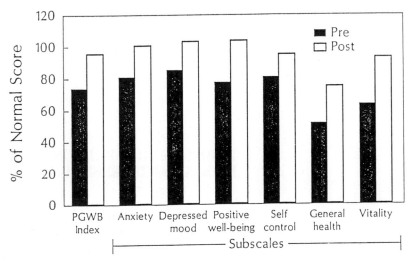

FIGURE 50–3: Results of administering the Psychological General Well-Being (PGWB) schedule before *(solid bars)* and after *(open bars)* intensive pulmonary rehabilitation.

Physiologic Changes

Figure 50–4 shows a preliminary compilation of data illustrating the effects of pulmonary rehabilitation on a variety of physiologic measurements. There was a 44% increase in the distance covered during the 12-minute walking test and a 20% improvement in the workload obtained during a progressive cardiopulmonary stress test; this reflected a statistically significant increase in exercise capacity. The improvement in workload represents a 41% increase in the total work performed.

Data derived from the pulmonary function tests (i.e., the forced expired volume in 1 second [FEV_1], forced vital capacity, and MVV) showed that there was no significant change in either the forced vital capacity or the FEV_1 as a result of pulmonary rehabilitation. Although the MVV increased about 9%, this increase also was not statistically significant. It should be noted that some individuals did experience improvement in pulmonary function; this improvement was considered the direct result of optimizing the individual's pulmonary medications during the course of the program.

As a result of the rehabilitation program VO_{2sl} increased 15% and VE_{sl} increased 13%; however, there was no significant change in symptom-limited HR (HR_{sl}) after completion of the program. Our findings of a significant increase in O_2 uptake without a significant change in maximum HR strongly suggest that the patients, on average, are indeed experiencing a physical training effect. Such a training effect may be one of the mechanisms by which pulmonary rehabilitation helps to reverse functional deterioration in pulmonary patients.

MECHANISMS WHEREBY PULMONARY REHABILITATION ACCOMPLISHES THE REVERSAL IN FUNCTIONAL DETERIORATION

How might the documented psychological and physiologic changes just described for patients in our program be explained? The remainder

Effects of Pulmonary Rehabilitation

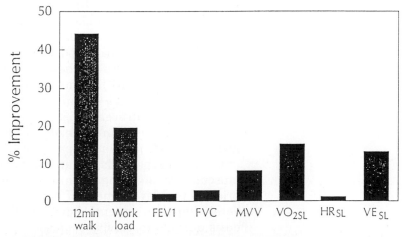

FIGURE 50–4: Percent change in various measures of exercise capacity and pulmonary function after intensive pulmonary rehabilitation.

of this chapter considers some of the real and hypothetic mechanisms that may be at work here.

Five mechanisms have been proposed to account for the observed improvement in exercise tolerance:

- Improved aerobic capacity
- Increased motivation
- Desensitization to the sensation of dyspnea
- Improved ventilatory muscle function
- Improved techniques of performance

Although numerous studies have provided evidence supporting one or more of these factors, none has yet emerged as the predominant mechanism. Indeed, these mechanisms probably operate in combination, depending on both the patient's limiting factors and the specific strengths of the rehabilitation program. In this discussion, we consider specifically the hypothetical role of exercise training, increased motivation, decreased hyperventilation, and increased efficiency in the production of the psychological and physiologic changes seen in our patients undergoing pulmonary rehabilitation.

Exercise Training

Prior to discussing exercise training in pulmonary patients, it is informative to consider the physiologic changes resulting from physical training in healthy subjects. After physical training, the healthy subject has a greater maximal oxygen uptake (VO_{2max}) as shown by the dotted line in Figure 50–2A, and thus can exercise to a higher workload. The increase in VO_{2max} is the result of an increased maximum cardiac output (O_2 transport) and a greater arterial-venous oxygen difference (O_2 extraction). The maximum cardiac output increases solely as a result of an increase in the stroke volume, since the maximum HR does not change significantly with physical training, as shown by the dotted line in Figure 50–2B. The slope of the HR response, however, decreases so that at any submaximal workload, a lower HR is required after training. The combination of an increase in VO_{2max} without a change in HR_{max} causes the O_2 pulse to increase (O_2 pulse = VO_{2max}/HR_{max}). The ventilatory response (Fig. 50–2C, *dotted line*) shows that after physical training the AT occurs at a higher workload, both in absolute terms and as a percentage of the maximum work that can be attained. Although VE_{max} may increase after training, there is still ventilatory reserve. These physiologic changes are typical of the training response in healthy individuals. They probably also reflect the types of changes seen in pulmonary patients having primarily cardiovascular limitations.

The existence of a training effect in patients with limited ventilatory capacity is a controversial issue. Since it is generally considered necessary to exercise at an intensity approximating the AT to experience a training effect, pulmonary patients with moderate to severe ventilatory impairment reportedly are unable to experience either cardiovascular or muscular conditioning because they may become limited by symptoms prior to the development of a significant lactic acidosis. Many less severely impaired patients, however, do experience a significant lactic acidosis during progressive exercise, and still others may experience localized metabolic acidosis that is sufficient to promote a training effect. If sufficient exercise can be performed so that the AT occurs at a higher

VO_2, the reduced CO_2 production can allow for more efficient use of ventilation VE and thus lower the VE/VO_2 requirement.

Increased Motivation

Lack of motivation is a factor that similarly may reduce exercise tolerance and limit exercise. Characteristically, this factor is important whenever the physiologic response demonstrates neither a cardiovascular, ventilatory, nor gas exchange limitation to exercise. Under these conditions, neither cardiac nor ventilatory reserves would be depleted. Increased motivation after the rehabilitation intervention would allow the patient to use these reserves. HR_{sl} would increase toward the predicted HR_{max}, and VE_{sl} would increase toward the MVV without a change in the AT. The O_2 pulse would not change significantly with this mechanism because VO_{2sl} would increase in proportion to HR_{sl}.

Decreased Hyperventilation

Anxiety in the pulmonary patient is often expressed as pronounced fear of exertion or shortness of breath and may be evidenced by hyperventilation during any form of exertion. During progressive exercise, the MVV would be reached earlier because of this hyperventilation, thereby limiting the maximum workload attained. This situation can be identified by the development of a respiratory alkalosis during exercise. After rehabilitation, reduction in anxiety would allow ventilation to increase more slowly and in accord with metabolic demand. Ventilation would be reduced at any given work rate, thereby reducing the respiratory alkalosis, and VE_{sl} would increase toward the limiting MVV. The HR_{sl} would increase, thereby providing the increment in maximum cardiac output necessary for the increase in VO_{2sl} and, consequently, there would be no change in the O_2 pulse.

Increased Efficiency

Another mechanism that might be associated with pulmonary rehabilitation is increased efficiency. This mechanism would allow the individual's exercise capacity to improve without a corresponding increase in VO_{2sl}. At any given workload, the patient would be able to exercise with a lower O_2 consumption than prior to rehabilitation. Since the energy requirements (VO_{2sl}) and, consequently, maximum cardiac output would remain unchanged, no significant change would be expected in HR_{sl} or the O_2 pulse. Although the ventilatory response would also be more efficient (lower ventilation required for a given submaximum work rate) after rehabilitation, the AT would not increase with improved efficiency, and VE_{sl} would be unable to change because of the fixed ventilatory limit.

In addition to the increase in exercise tolerance resulting from the four mechanisms described, several other factors probably contribute to the patient's increased feeling of well-being. Among them are a better understanding of the disease process, a firmer grasp on the role of medications and how to adjust them, and a realistic outlook for the future. All these factors tend to return control to the patient, lessen dependence, and improve the patient's ability to cope.

SUMMARY

Both rationale and evidence exist for considering physiologic and psychological mechanisms for the functional benefits derived from pulmonary rehabilitation. The rationale lies in the sequence of physiologic and psychological changes that constitute the vicious cycle of inactivity and consideration of how best to reverse that cycle. Evidence abounds in the form of both psychological and physiologic data obtained before and after a rehabilitation intervention. Having now identified numerous plausible mechanisms, we must develop our skills in analyzing and interpreting the data to better define the patient's limitations and then decide how to individualize the pulmonary rehabilitation program to facilitate the appropriate mechanisms.

References

1. Barach AL, Bickerman HA, Beck G. Advances in the treatment of non-tuberculous pulmonary disease. Bull NY Acad Med 28:353–384, 1952.
2. American Thoracic Society official statement. Pulmonary Rehabilitation. Am Rev Respir Dis 124:663–666, 1981.
3. Belman MJ. Exercise in patients with COPD. Thorax 48:936–946, 1993.
4. Donahoe M, Rogers RM. Nutritional assessment and support in chronic obstructive pulmonary disease. Clin Chest Med 11:487–504, 1990.
5. Dupuy HJ. The psychological general well-being (PGWB) index. *In* Wenger N, Mattson ME, Furboug KD, Elinson J (eds). Assessment of Quality of Life in Clinical Trials of Cardiovascular Therapies. New York, LeJacq Publishing, 1984, pp 170–183.

Suggested Reading

Bickford LS, Hodgkin JE. National Pulmonary Rehabilitation Survey. J Cardiopulmonary Rehabil 11:473–491, 1988.
Hodgkin JE, Connors GL, Bell CW (eds). Pulmonary Rehabilitation: Guidelines to Success. 2nd ed. Philadelphia, Lippincott, 1993.
Jones NL. Clinical Exercise Testing. Philadelphia, WB Saunders, 1988.
Ries AL. Position paper of the American Association of Cardiovascular and Pulmonary Rehabilitation: Scientific basis of pulmonary rehabilitation. J Cardiopulmonary Rehabil 10:418–441, 1990.
Ries AL, Archibald CJ. Endurance exercise training at maximal targets in patients with chronic obstructive pulmonary disease. J Cardiopulmonary Rehabil 7:594–601, 1987.
Rochester DF. Nutritional repletion. Semin Respir Med 13:44–52, 1992.
Shephard RJ. Test of maximum oxygen intake: A critical review. Sports Med 1:99–124, 1984.

51

Home Care

Susan L. McInturff, R.C.P., R.R.T.

Key Terms

Oxygen Concentrator
Transtracheal Catheter

Home care is an aspect of comprehensive respiratory care that is sometimes overlooked because it occurs after the acute stage of an illness. It can involve the patient who has spent time in the intensive care unit with highly trained clinicians and the latest technology. As the patient improves and leaves the intensive care unit, he or she will still need highly trained clinicians and more of the same technology. This patient may be discharged still requiring the same services. What can home care offer this patient? A comprehensive program of education, assessment, medical devices, and a team to provide needed expertise is available in a home care situation.

Because of financial incentives such as the prospective payment system, patients are being discharged sooner from the hospital.[1-3] Simply put, the sooner a hospital can discharge a patient the better it is for that hospital financially. The patients who are being discharged may still have medical needs that require outside assistance for the duration of their convalescence, for example, the patient who, because of myriad medical conditions, may require medical assistance in the home for the remainder of his or her life (e.g., continuous ventilator care). A patient who, during the outpatient visit to the physician, may exhibit signs and symptoms of a condition that could be treated at home if the proper medical devices were available, for example, intravenous antibiotic therapy for pneumonia. Through a well-developed home care program, these patients can continue to receive the required medical care. Technology and the financial incentive to create medical devices that can be used in the home have allowed the home care industry to evolve to the point that almost any patient—from infant to adult, from acute and requiring "intensive care" to chronic and stable—can receive home care services. Respiratory care practitioners (RCPs) play an essential role in the treatment of pulmonary patients who use home care, whether short-term or long-term.

This chapter provides an overview of the types of services and equipment available to treat a patient at home and discusses several key areas of home care: patient selection, equipment selection, assessment, and the role the RCP plays in the discharge process and management of the patient once he or she is home.

BENEFITS AND GOALS

One of the primary benefits of home care is also one of the primary goals: assistance in the reduction of total medical dollars spent by third-party payors such as Medicare and private insurance carriers. This can be achieved by decreasing total days spent in acute and long-term care facilities. Individuals requiring ventilator assistance and technology-dependent pediatric patients can be treated at home instead of having to spend a lifetime being institutionalized.

Studies show that treating these types of patients at home presents a significant cost savings. In one study, patients requiring ventilator assistance who were treated in a long-term facility had expenses reimbursed at $718 per day, as opposed to treating the patient at home for $235 per day.[4] High-technology cases, such as pediatric patients requiring complex equipment, offered potential savings of $4 million every year when the cost of home versus institutional care was compared in a 50-patient study.[5] Other sources cite cost comparisons of $2000 to $3000 per day for inpatient hospital care versus $500 to $1000 per day for care provided in the home.[6]

Patients with chronic pulmonary diseases offer a real challenge in attaining cost savings because of repeated hospitalizations, longer hospital stays, and frequent emergency room visits. Careful management of these patients at home can reduce these acute admissions; however, cost savings are not as significant because of the use of professional services, such as nursing and RCPs.[7]

Home care also allows patients to stay in an environment familiar to them and, in most cases, one that is preferable to an unpleasant hospital environment. Allowing patients the "comforts of home" is conducive to better healing, allowing them some dignity and control over their environment.

The goals of home care are

- To encourage optimal quality of life, comfort, and independence within the confines of the patient's disease state
- To keep the patient from having to be admitted to the acute care facility

This is accomplished through the use of various professional services, such as nursing, respiratory care, and other allied health specialties, as well as the provision of any number of medical devices to treat the patient.

PATIENT SELECTION

Numerous areas should be considered when discharging a patient to a home care program in order to meet those goals and achieve the benefits of home care. Not every patient is a candidate for home care and not every patient who needs home care receives it. What is appropriate for one may not be indicated for another, so a "prepackaged" program will not meet the needs of many patients. Home care must be individualized for each patient, but there are guidelines to help with this customization.[8]

As stated earlier, many factors must be considered when determining the feasibility of home care for a particular patient. These factors are most usually assessed by a hospital discharge planner or an RCP knowledgeable in discharge planning. This process begins when the physician determines that the patient may be able to go home. The discharge planner starts by evaluating the patient to determine if he or she is a candidate for home care. The patient who has been hospitalized frequently for a recurring problem, such as chronic obstructive pulmonary disease, is an ideal candidate for a home care program. The ongoing assessment and re-education that is provided can identify and prevent problems before they become unmanageable and require hospitalization. A home care program can be beneficial for

- Patients requiring wound care, intravenous therapy, enterostomal therapy, or assessment to prevent postoperative complications such as infection or pneumonia

- Patients needing physical and pulmonary rehabilitation
- Patients who require home medical equipment

Table 51–1 lists additional examples of the types of patients who can benefit from a home care program.

The Discharge Process

Contrary to what many believe, a patient is not discharged instantaneously once the physician writes an order to "discharge to home." Depending on the patient's needs, it may take hours, days, or even weeks to make all the necessary arrangements and complete all the training required to care for the patient in the home. This is particularly true when a patient is discharged with a mechanical ventilator.

Several other factors need to be considered once it has been established that home care is required in order for a patient to be discharged. Is the patient willing to accept the professionals required in the home? There are patients with a sense of privacy that is so strong they may decline home care rather than have that privacy invaded. Other patients may not feel they require the additional assistance despite efforts to educate them to the contrary. Some patients who are unwilling to be compliant with the prescribed therapy may not benefit from home care. Home visits made by health professionals have to be justified according to a plan of care with specific goals of therapy in order to be reimbursed by third-party payors. The noncompliant patient cannot meet those goals, so home visits might not be justified. Some patients even refuse to have medical equipment in their home.

The Home Environment

Is the home environment conducive to home care? Sometimes the patient's home is unsuitable for the medical equipment required for treatment because of space restrictions (such as the patient who lives in a single-wide mobile home), electrical requirements, or safety reasons, such as a fire hazard or lack of cleanliness. An assessment of the home prior to ordering many types of home medical equipment or other professional services is extremely helpful to determine if modifications are necessary to ensure proper use, safety, and maximum benefit.[9] A home may need ramps installed or doors widened for improved access. Many times furniture must be removed to allow room for medical equipment. For electrical problems, additional wiring or grounding of existing circuitry may be required, particularly if the medical devices are being used

TABLE **51–1:** Patients Who Can Benefit From Home Care

Patients who are not completely recovered from an acute illness
Patients requiring repeated hospitalizations for the same illness
Patients who are technology-dependent (i.e., ventilator, oxygen therapy, intravenous or enteral therapy)
Patients who require wound care (i.e., stoma or decubitus)
Patients who are unable to manage medication schedules or other treatments
Patients with an acute illness that can be treated without hospitalization (e.g., pneumonia, mild congestive heart failure)
Patients who require diagnostic testing, such as oximetry, blood tests, blood pressure checks, on a repeated basis

in the same electrical circuit as home appliances. Patients with major physical impediments in their homes that cannot be altered, such as inadequate wiring that they cannot afford to repair, may not be candidates for home care and may require alternative placement. An inspection of the home prior to discharge to identify any such potential problems is standard procedure with most home medical equipment providers when the patient requires high-technology equipment, such as mechanical ventilators.

Does the patient live in an area in which home care is available? Patients living in extremely remote areas may not have professional services such as home nursing or other allied health professions available to them, or there may not be a home medical equipment supplier servicing the area. Most medical equipment suppliers have policies regarding their response time in the event of an emergency, so they may decline a patient in a remote area. This problem does not occur often, but if it does, alternative living arrangements are required if continuing care is essential.

Are there other people living in the home who may make provision of home care difficult? Are they supportive about the patient coming home? Some family members have difficulty dealing with their loved one's high degree of medical needs accompanied by a number of strangers in white coats and lots of frightening medical equipment. In many cases, informing families of common difficulties and continually monitoring for dysfunction will be necessary.

A patient's spouse or other caregivers may have difficulty providing care for both the patient and other persons in the home, such as small children. Trying to meet the needs of a patient requiring "intensive care," along with caring for the needs of other family members, quickly becomes exhausting. It may be necessary to isolate equipment from small children. Finding alternate care for children may also be necessary. In rare instances, the abusive family member or the noncompliant caregiver may necessitate evaluation by social services so that a safe home environment may be provided for the patient.

> All caregivers must be able to demonstrate competency in all nursing and respiratory therapy modalities to be used in the treatment of the patient. If that competency does not exist, it would be unwise and unsafe to discharge the patient to that type of home care program.

Consideration must be given to whether the patient and the caregivers are trainable in the techniques required. Some patients and caregivers are unwilling or unable to learn how to suction a tracheostomy tube, how to properly administer medications or, particularly, how to care for a home mechanical ventilator or oxygen delivery equipment. Assessment of patient readiness to learn is important, since patients and caregivers may say almost anything in order to go home as soon as possible. The RCP in the hospital can help in the assessment of competency for many of these procedures.

Reimbursement Issues

Insurance coverage is one of the most important areas to consider when selecting a patient and a home care program. Most of the professional services and equipment delivered in home care are costly; they may not always be covered by the patient's insurance. Most of the professionals who provide these services are not willing or able to provide them free of charge. Many patients are unable to pay for these services themselves, so establishing insurance coverage is essential.

Third-party payors have coverage guidelines and criteria that must be met before they authorize payment for services rendered, particularly

Medicare and Medicaid. For example, a patient must have a P_{O_2} of 55 mm Hg or less for both Medicare and Medicaid to reimburse for use of oxygen equipment in the home without requiring additional documentation of need.[10, 11] Simply having a physician's order for home oxygen therapy will not assure that patient payment from the insurance company. Patients who require something as basic as a hospital bed must have a specific medical need such as occurs with certain diagnoses, for example, arthritis of the hips and knees or congestive heart failure, in order for entities such as Medicare and Medicaid to provide reimbursement. It is essential to contact individual carriers for their current guidelines for reimbursement, since each carrier may have different criteria. Many of the modalities used on a patient (e.g., bathroom safety equipment) while in the hospital may not be covered, although they may be assumed to be. The home care program that is developed for a patient may have to be altered to fit the guidelines of the carrier, particularly when it comes to home nursing care and medical equipment.

Customizing the Program

Once the patient has been identified as a candidate for home care, is willing to cooperate with the providers, and has insurance to pay for home care, the program can be fully customized. The medical needs of the patient determine the types of professional services required. A multidisciplinary team of home care experts is often involved in providing the nursing, therapy, and equipment services that may be ordered by the physician. Table 51–2 lists the members of the professional home care team.

The home care program developed for the patient with end-stage chronic obstructive pulmonary disease may require home oxygen therapy for the treatment of hypoxemia, bronchodilator therapy via a compressor nebulizer, and visits by the RCP or home health nurse, or both, for assessment, evaluation of compliance, and re-education as necessary. This patient may also require physical and occupational therapy for training in activities of daily living and physical conditioning, a home health aide for assistance with bathing and personal care, and visits by a social worker for assessment of psychosocial issues such as chronic depression. The home care program developed for the patient requiring mechanical ventilation may be much more complicated but will use the same health professionals, whereas the home care program developed for the patient recovering from pneumonia may not require all the team members or services available. The length of service is established by medical necessity, which is determined by the physician but may also be guided by insurance coverage.

TABLE **51–2:** The Home Care Team

┌──────────── Patient ────────────┐	
Caregiver	Physician
Nurse	Social worker
Physical therapist	Home health aide
Respiratory care practitioner	HME provider
Occupational therapist	

HME, home medical equipment.

EQUIPMENT SELECTION

In conjunction with the professional services available in the home, many types of home medical equipment can be used to treat the patient. Durable medical equipment, such as walking aids, bathroom safety aids, hospital beds, and wheelchairs, is used to promote the health and comfort of the patient with pulmonary disease and to assist the patient in performing normal daily activities (Table 51–3). This equipment is generally provided by a home medical equipment supplier. Patients may be assessed concerning their need for any of these items, prior to discharge, after they are home, or if their condition changes. The RCP who visits the patient at home may determine that he or she is unable to tolerate standing in the shower because of dyspnea, so bathing is no longer possible. This may indicate that a shower chair and hand-held shower attachment are necessary to allow the patient to bathe and conserve energy. The RCP may find that a patient is sleeping in a chair because he or she is too dyspneic to lie flat in bed; therefore, a hospital bed capable of raising the head in a Fowler's position would help this patient. These needs may even be identified by the hospital RCP before the patient goes home, so knowledge of this equipment is useful.

Statistics have shown that chronic obstructive pulmonary disease ranks second only to coronary disease as a cause of disability in persons older than 40 years of age.[12] It is no wonder that between these two diseases, a very large population of patients require medical assistance at home. Many medical devices are available to treat pulmonary and coronary diseases.

Oxygen therapy, aerosol therapy, and ventilatory assistance devices are the major categories of home respiratory equipment used for coronary and pulmonary patients.

Oxygen Therapy

Many studies[13–17] indicate that when compared with chronically hypoxic patients who did not receive oxygen therapy, patients with chronic hypoxia secondary to lung disease who receive oxygen therapy at least nocturnally have

- A greater survival rate
- Improved cognitive function
- Better tolerance to exercise

These patients benefit from long-term oxygen therapy, sometimes lasting for the duration of their lives. This oxygen can be provided at home. Three methods of delivering oxygen to a patient in the home exist: liquid oxygen, concentrator, and gaseous systems.

Home oxygen systems are safe to use; however, all patients need to be instructed about common oxygen safety techniques. Cigarette smoking while using oxygen should be expressly forbidden, as should handling

TABLE **51–3:**   Types of Home Medical Equipment

Walking Aids	Bathroom Safety Equipment	Durable Medical Equipment	Respiratory Care Equipment	Other Equipment
Walker	Commode	Hospital bed	Oxygen therapy devices	Enteral therapy
Wheeled walker	Shower chair	Trapeze bar	Home ventilators	IV therapy
Hemiwalker	Bath bench	Patient lift	Cardiorespiratory monitors	Pain-management devices
Forearm crutches	Bathtub transfer bench	Wheelchair	Aerosol therapy devices	
Cane	Grab bars	Seat-lift chair	Suction equipment	
	Hand-held shower attachment			

any flame or electrical device, such as an electric shaver, while wearing oxygen. High-pressure cylinders need to be secured in tank stands or placed horizontally on the floor to prevent their falling. Patients must also be instructed not to increase the liter flow unless ordered by their physician; they must understand the hazards of doing this against medical advice.

Liquid Oxygen

The LOX vessel, which is 3 to 4 feet tall and approximately 18 inches in diameter, holds approximately 70 to 90 pounds of oxygen in its liquid state at −273°F. Depending on the manufacturer and the internal pressure (normally 22 to 50 psi), the stationary LOX vessel can generate flow rates of 0.25 to 15 L/min.

The home liquid oxygen system (LOX) is a smaller version of the bulk liquid system used by hospitals.[18] The LOX can also be used to power other delivery systems such as a large-volume nebulizer. The LOX stationary vessel can be accompanied by a "portable" unit, and herein lies liquid oxygen's major advantage over other systems. This portable unit, which is very light (weighing 8 to 10 pounds when full), will last approximately 8 hours when used at 2 L/min continuously. The patient can easily fill the portable unit by attaching it to the stationary unit. The fact that the patient can fill his or her own portable unit whenever needed and can spend an entire day away from home greatly enhances the ability to participate in activities outside the home. Portable gaseous cylinders cannot hold as much oxygen nor allow the same amount of use time as the LOX at the same flow rate. For example, a LOX portable unit running at 2 L/min lasts about 8 hours compared with a gaseous E cylinder, which lasts only 4 to 5 hours. Figure 51–1 shows an example of stationary and portable LOX systems.

LOX systems are not without disadvantages. Because of the nature of the system, continual evaporative loss occurs whether the system is being used or not. In fact, a full LOX reservoir would run "dry" in

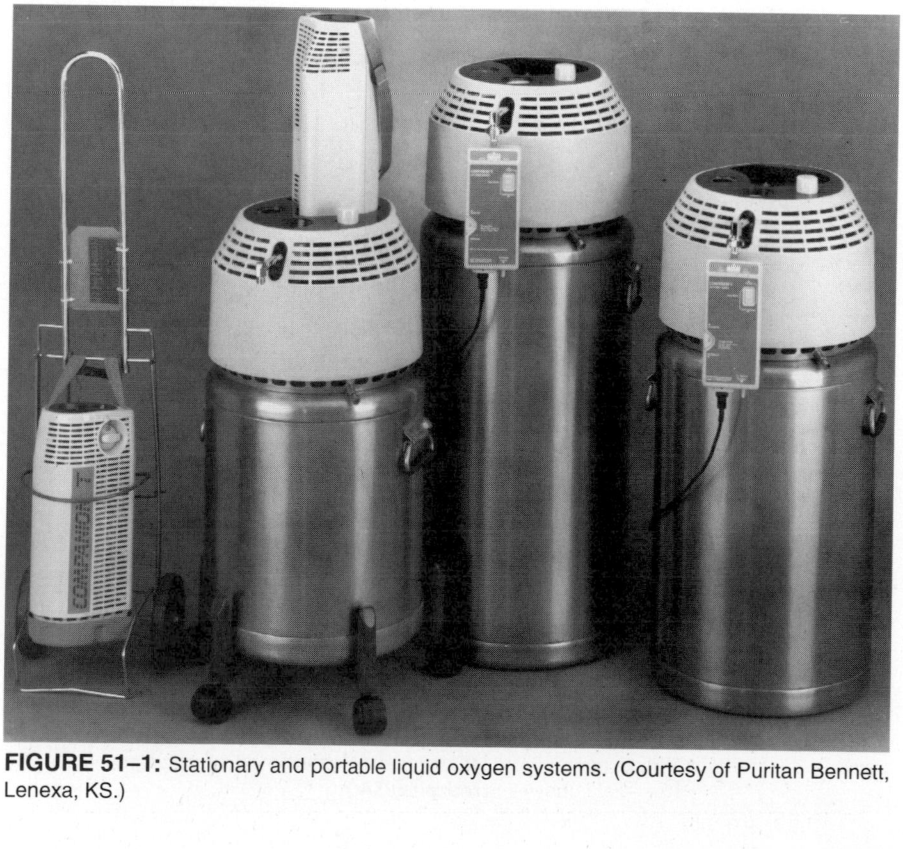

FIGURE 51–1: Stationary and portable liquid oxygen systems. (Courtesy of Puritan Bennett, Lenexa, KS.)

approximately 30 days if it were not used. For this reason liquid oxygen can be considered somewhat wasteful. The LOX system also requires periodic refilling by the medical equipment supplier (average weekly fills); these refill deliveries are at a substantial cost to the supplier. Liquid oxygen, which is considered the most expensive oxygen delivery system, is typically used when the patient exhibits a need for portability or is unable to manage a tank system (i.e., an E cylinder).

Oxygen Concentrator

The oxygen concentrator is an electrical device that draws in room air and passes it through a molecular "sieve." This "sieve" filters out the nitrogen molecules, water vapor, and other trace gases that are in the room air and allows the oxygen molecules to pass through, delivering a concentrated oxygen gas via a flowmeter.[18]

The concentrator is an ideal home oxygen delivery system because of its ability to continually produce oxygen without replenishing the supply; however, because it is using electricity to continually produce this oxygen, a power failure renders the system inoperable. A back-up source of oxygen, usually an H size gaseous cylinder, is necessary whenever a concentrator is placed in the home. Concentrators, which are fairly small "console" devices about the size of an end table, are sometimes made to look like a piece of furniture, depending on the manufacturer (Fig. 51–2).

Patients who require portability obviously cannot use the concentrator. In this case, portable gaseous tanks (usually E and D sizes) are used, often with a wheeled cart or carrying pouch (Fig. 51–3). The concentrator and portable tank system is cost-effective, easy to use, and ideal for patients who leave home infrequently.

A molecular sieve-canister within the machine containing sodium-aluminum silicate pellets. Concentrators are capable of delivering up to 5 L/min at 4 to 10 psi at concentrations of usually 90 to 96%, depending on the flow rate (the higher the flow rate the lower the concentration).

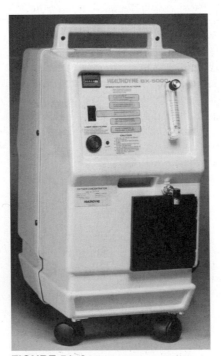

FIGURE 51–2: Oxygen concentrator. (Courtesy of Healthdyne Technologies, Marietta, GA.)

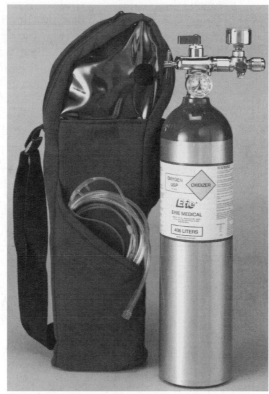

FIGURE 51–3: Portable gas cylinder with carrying pouch. (Courtesy of Erie Manufacturing, Milwaukee, WI.)

One disadvantage of the concentrator is that it increases the patient's electric utility bill approximately $50 per month depending on the utility rates in the area. The patient can submit a special application to the utility company for reduced rates when using life support devices such as a concentrator. Another disadvantage is that concentrators produce a level of noise and heat that patients may find somewhat bothersome. This can be alleviated by placing the concentrator in another room. The concentrator, which weighs approximately 50 pounds, usually has casters, making its movement to multiple locations in the home feasible. A final disadvantage is that the concentrator system cannot be used to power other devices such as large-volume nebulizers because of its low operating pressure. It can be used to "bleed-in" oxygen into aerosol delivery systems, however.

Gaseous Systems

An H cylinder lasts only about 3 days at 2 L/min of continuous use.

Hospital-based RCPs are familiar with gaseous systems, such as the H and E cylinders. These cylinders contain a volume of oxygen pressurized to 2200 psi, which is reduced to 50 psi via a pressure regulator. A flowmeter adjusts the amount of oxygen that reaches the patient. Because of the limited volumes these cylinders contain when compared with concentrators or LOX systems, they are not regularly used as the primary source of oxygen for the patient at home.

Cylinders require frequent changing, which is difficult for the patient to accomplish. Many cylinders would have to be in the home to reduce the frequency of supplier deliveries. Gaseous systems are an ideal back-up system to a concentrator or LOX system, since they do not evaporate, maintaining their volume for an indefinite time (assuming the regulator and flowmeter are functioning properly). They are not usually used to power aerosol therapy devices because of the high liter flow required to do so; they empty quickly and require frequent replacement.

Regardless of the system, the delivery devices used at home are essentially the same as those used in the hospital. Cannulas, simple masks, and nonrebreathing and Venturi masks are all used, although masks are used less frequently in the home.

Humidifiers may or may not be used with oxygen systems, depending on the liter flow. The criteria for placement of a humidifier at home are similar to those used in hospitals.[19] For liter flows less than 4 L/min, a humidifier should be used if the patient complains of a dry nose or mouth, nasal irritation, or bleeding. Otherwise, humidifiers are avoided because they need to be cleaned and disinfected routinely. They also may leak, particularly if the humidifier has a plastic fitting connected to a metal fitting at the oxygen source. The plastic fitting threads are easily stripped, creating leaks in the system and thereby reducing the oxygen flow to the patient. Some equipment vendors supply prefilled, disposable humidifiers. These humidifiers are relatively expensive compared with plastic humidifiers that are filled with distilled water and reused; most insurance companies will not pay for the disposable units.

Oxygen-Conserving Devices

Oxygen-conserving devices were developed to reduce the total volume of oxygen used or to decrease the liter flow required by the patient. Three major types are available today, and they are being used both in the hospital and in the home: (1) the cannula-reservoir device, (2) the electromechanical-pulsing device, and (3) the transtracheal catheter. The first two are most frequently used with liquid oxygen and gaseous cylinder systems, whereas the transtracheal catheter can be used with all systems.

Cannula-Reservoir Device

The nasal cannula-reservoir device is a cannula with either a pendant reservoir that hangs at the chest (Fig. 51–4) or a "mustache" reservoir that sits directly under the nose (Fig. 51–5). Oxygen fills the reservoir during the patient's exhalation, becoming available to the patient on inspiration (similar to the function of the nonrebreathing mask).

One major disadvantage of the reservoir-type cannula is that it may be viewed as cosmetically unappealing. The tubing is larger than that on a conventional cannula, and the "mustache" reservoir is somewhat unsightly. Patients who already have concerns about their appearance with a conventional cannula may not want to wear this device. Some patients may prefer to use the reservoir-type cannula in the privacy of the home and use a conventional cannula at a higher liter flow when out in public.

Electromechanical-Pulsing Devices

Electromechanical-pulsing oxygen-conserving devices are small box-shaped units that are attached to the outlet of the liquid or gaseous oxygen tank (Fig. 51–6). They generally provide oxygen on demand by sensing the decrease in pressure when the patient inhales, which opens a valve and produces a "pulsed" volume of 15 to 35 ml of oxygen. Some

If a patient requires a mask, he or she is probably too unstable to be a good candidate for home care.

A patient using oxygen at a rate of 2 L/min with a conventional cannula will require approximately 0.5 L/min with the reservoir-type cannula to achieve the same level of oxygenation.[20] This presents a significant savings in total oxygen usage, increasing the length of time the oxygen source lasts.

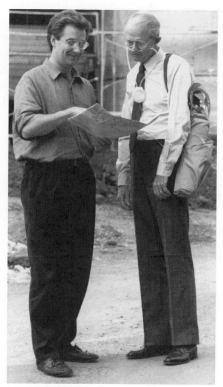

FIGURE 51–4: Nasal cannula-reservoir device. (Courtesy of Chad Therapeutics, Chatsworth, CA.)

make oxygen available for the patient who has brief periods of apnea. Since these devices do not provide a continuous flow, as do the conventional or reservoir-cannula systems, their major advantage is that oxygen is being used only when it is actually needed. This reduces the amount of oxygen usage by 35 to 70%, producing a 7:1 savings compared with continuous-flow systems.[21] They are also useful on portable cylinders to increase the length of time a cylinder will last. Several manufacturers make units for use with the piped-in oxygen systems in hospitals to help conserve the use of bulk liquid.

Pulsing devices do have some disadvantages. The demand valve can produce a noisy "clicking" sound, which the patient may find irritating.

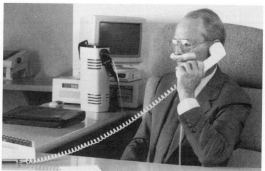

FIGURE 51–5: Mustache-type cannula. (Courtesy of Chad Therapeutics, Chatsworth, CA.)

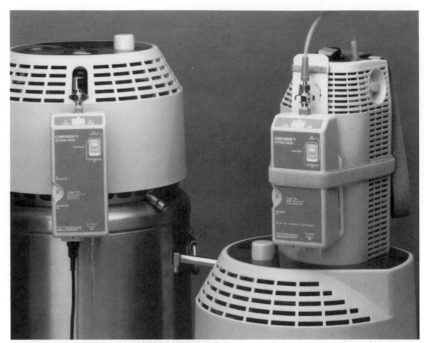

FIGURE 51–6: Electromechanical oxygen-conserving device attached to a liquid system. (Courtesy of Puritan Bennett, Lenexa, KS.)

They are also quite costly (usually several hundred dollars); the patient's insurance may not cover the cost. The oxygen supplier may not provide one free of charge because of the significant cost. For patients receiving liquid oxygen at greater than 4 L/min, however, there can be a financial incentive for the oxygen supplier to place a unit on the LOX system to reduce the number of oxygen deliveries. This could also apply to patients living in remote areas where frequent deliveries would be time-consuming.

Transtracheal Catheters

Studies show that transtracheal oxygen administration reduces the oxygen flow required by 50% when compared with the nasal cannula.[22, 23]

Another type of oxygen-conserving device is the transtracheal catheter. This narrow-lumen catheter (resembling an angiocatheter) is inserted directly into the trachea. The oxygen delivery tubing is attached to a small fitting at the neck (Fig. 51–7). The oxygen bypasses the naso-

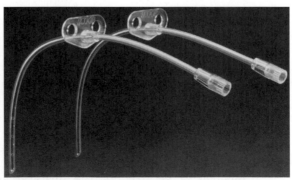

FIGURE 51–7: Transtracheal catheter. (Courtesy of Transtracheal Systems, Englewood, CO.)

pharynx and goes directly into the trachea, decreasing the liter flow required to oxygenate the patient. The transtracheal catheter can be useful for patients receiving very high liter flows; however, patients requiring such high liter flows may not be good candidates to undergo the invasive procedure necessary to place the catheter because of the severity of their illness.

Transtracheal catheters have the primary advantage of reducing the liter flow a patient needs. They are also more cosmetically appealing because there is nothing on the face and the catheter can be easily hidden beneath a shirt collar. This device is helpful for increasing patient compliance because of this benefit. The catheter may also enhance continuous use during sleep because it does not become dislodged as readily as a cannula when the patient moves in bed.

Before using a transtracheal catheter, consideration must be given to its disadvantages. Because it is invasive, there is the increased risk of infection and subcutaneous emphysema when the patient undergoes the procedure. Since the device also can become plugged with mucus, it must be cleaned religiously by the patient on a daily basis. The entire catheter must be replaced periodically (generally every 3 months). This can represent a substantial ongoing expense to the patient, since the cost of these catheters is not covered by many insurance companies. Patients who receive the transtracheal catheter must have a conventional cannula on hand at all times to use in the event that the catheter becomes kinked or plugged. They must also be instructed about the specific higher liter flow that must be used with the cannula.

Aerosol Therapy

Patients who have chronic lung disease frequently require topical treatment with aerosol therapy. The major types of equipment used to deliver aerosol therapy in the home include compressor nebulizers and compressors used to power large-volume nebulizers.

Compressor Nebulizers

A compressor nebulizer capable of delivering an oxygen flow at 12 to 15 L/min at about 15 to 20 psi is used to power a hand-held nebulizer for medication delivery to the lungs.

Compressor nebulizers are one of the most commonly used aerosol delivery devices in the home. Patients receiving nebulizer treatments in the hospital frequently go home with a compressor nebulizer in order to continue therapy. The oil-free compressor is housed in a small box-like casing that is lightweight and electrically powered (Fig. 51–8). Patients who are unable to use metered-dose inhalers when they are away from home can use battery-powered compressor nebulizers, which allow about 60 minutes of treatment time on a fully charged battery (Fig. 51–9). Some units can also be plugged into the cigarette lighter in a car. The types of medication nebulizers used with either device are the same as those used in the hospital.

For patients using medications such as pentamidine, the basic compressor nebulizer will not be adequate. These medications require a greater pressure (20 to 26 psi) to nebulize properly. There are "table-top" compressors available for this purpose. Medication nebulizers with filters such as those used in the hospital are also used at home for these treatments.

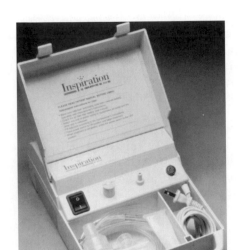

FIGURE 51–8: Compressor nebulizer. (Courtesy of Healthdyne Technologies, Marietta, GA.)

High-Output Compressors

Patients with tracheostomies frequently require aerosol therapy at home to help keep their secretions thin. This is accomplished by using a large-volume nebulizer driven by a high-output compressor. This compressor, which is larger than a compressor nebulizer or table-top compressor, is capable of delivering up to 50 psi with a variable adjustment (Fig. 51–10). A large-volume nebulizer, like the type used in hospitals, is attached to the outlet of the compressor. Oxygen, if needed, is usually "bled in" at the outlet of the nebulizer. Corrugated tubing, an aerosol drainage bag, and tracheostomy mask complete the circuit.

Suction Equipment

Suction equipment must be available for the patient who receives aerosol therapy and cannot remove secretions by coughing. Small table-

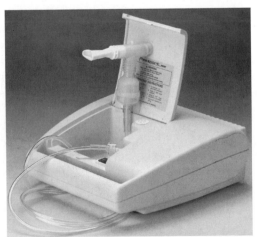

FIGURE 51–9: Battery-operated compressor nebulizer. (Courtesy of Invacare, Elyria, OH.)

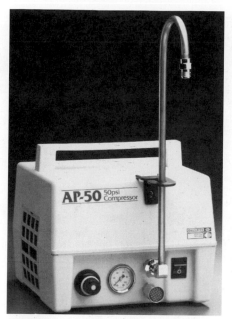

FIGURE 51–10: High-output compressor.
(Courtesy of DeVilbiss Health Care,
Somerset, PA.)

top suction machines can accomplish this (Fig. 51–11). Home suction units are electrically powered and capable of generating suction pressures up to −300 mm Hg. For patients who require portability, battery-operated suction units are available (Fig. 51–12). A battery-operated suction machine is essential as a back-up unit for patients who depend on suction to clear the airway.

Suction catheters run the gamut of types found in a hospital. Some patients sterilize rubber suction catheters and reuse them, particularly if their insurance will not pay for them. Suction catheters attached inline to the ventilator circuit typically are not used in the home because of their high cost compared with conventional catheters. Suction catheters with sleeves attached are ideal because

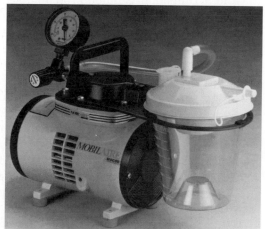

FIGURE 51–11: Tabletop suction machine.
(Courtesy of Invacare, Elyria, OH.)

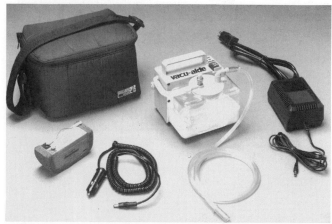

FIGURE 51–12: Battery-operated suction machine. (Courtesy of DeVilbiss Health Care, Somerset, PA.)

- They can be reused for several suctioning periods
- They do not require gloves, which saves on the cost of supplies
- They are much easier to teach caregivers to use when sterile technique is desired

Ventilatory Assistance Devices

Many types of equipment are available to treat patients with ventilatory insufficiency—from intermittent positive pressure breathing to home ventilators to continuous flow devices that treat obstructive apnea. Patients who once might have been kept in an acute facility for the remainder of their lives can go home with one of these devices.

Home Ventilators

One of the most rewarding aspects of home care is the successful use of a ventilator in this setting. Planning the discharge of a patient who will use a home ventilator is extremely complicated and requires more discussion than this overview allows. Many details must be considered and arrangements made prior to discharge to ensure a safe and positive experience for the patient and his or her caregivers. Continuous monitoring and assessment must occur once the patient arrives home.[24] Much consideration must be given to whether a patient would be a good candidate for home ventilation because of the "intensive care" involved.

Many disorders can now be treated at home with mechanical ventilation, for example, end-stage chronic obstructive pulmonary disease, neuromuscular diseases, and spinal cord lesions.[25] Some patients are assisted by family only, whereas others have the benefit of paid skilled help such as nurses.[26] Even with paid nursing care, studies indicate that there is substantial cost savings in keeping a patient at home on a ventilator as opposed to keeping such a patient institutionalized.[4]

Home ventilators are small enough to sit on a bedside table. They can also be mounted under a wheelchair, allowing the user great portability (Figs. 51–13 and 51–14). These devices are capable of conventional ventilation modes such as assist-control and synchronized intermittent mandatory ventilation. Oxygen can be used when necessary. These ven-

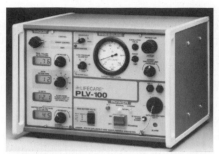

FIGURE 51–13: Portable volume ventilator used in the home. (Courtesy of Lifecare, Lafayette, CO.)

tilators run on 110-V wall current and use a 12-V deep-cycle battery for external power, such as that needed when the patient leaves home or in the event of a power failure. Depending on the battery size, the patient may have several hours or several days of battery time on a full charge.

Humidification is accomplished with heated cascade-type humidifiers, wick-type humidifiers, heated wire circuits, or artificial noses. Heated wire circuits are seen most often in neonatal and pediatric home ventilator care; most adults do not require this form of humidification.

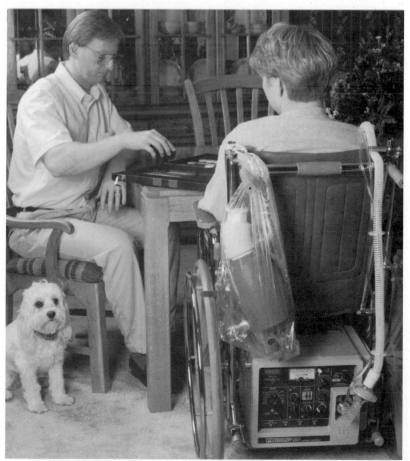

FIGURE 51–14: Portable volume ventilator mounted to a wheelchair. (Courtesy of Puritan Bennett, Lenexa, KS.)

Ventilator circuits are either permanent or disposable, depending on the needs of the patient or the payment guidelines of the insurance company. Permanent circuits are ideal because they constitute a one-time charge to a patient and can be washed and disinfected repeatedly. Also, the exhalation valve is easy to troubleshoot because the valve is clear and all the parts are easily seen. Disposable circuits are a costly, recurring charge to the patient and are not to be reused. In addition, the exhalation valve is difficult to troubleshoot because it is not made of clear plastic and is hard to take apart. Disposable circuits should be chosen only when cleaning and disinfecting permanent circuits is not feasible.

Another type of home mechanical ventilation is noninvasive ventilation. Ventilation by nasal mask is commonly used to treat respiratory insufficiency.[27] This procedure may cause enough improvement in the patient so that a tracheostomy is avoided. Patients using nasal mask ventilation most commonly require it only at night.

Negative pressure ventilators are also being used in the home for long-term nocturnal ventilation. A chest shell or coat-like suit is employed (Fig. 51–15). The cycle rate and depth of negative pressure are set to create the desired respiratory rate and tidal volume. Although somewhat cumbersome, negative pressure ventilation can be a satisfactory method of ventilation for selected patients.[18]

Although not used often, intermittent positive pressure breathing has a place in home ventilation. It is used most frequently to treat patients in chronic respiratory failure from neuromuscular disorders, such as muscular dystrophy and kyphoscoliosis. The fairly small compressor-driven unit is used to give intermittent positive pressure breathing treatments several times a day (Fig. 51–16). It is hoped that the use of this device will delay the need for more continuous ventilation.

With proper planning, home mechanical ventilation is a viable option for patients requiring ventilator care. There is a great deal of written material available to help in the process of discharging a patient home on a mechanical ventilator and determining equipment needs.[24–26, 28–31]

Obstructive Apnea

Another area that is receiving a great deal of attention is the treatment of obstructive breathing problems during sleep. It is estimated that 70 million individuals in the United States have sleep disorders.[32] There are many devices available to treat them. A common method of treatment is with nasal continuous positive airway pressure (CPAP).

Nasal CPAP uses an electrically powered blower that delivers a high flow of air at a preset pressure to a nasal mask (Figs. 51–17 and 51–18). This pressurized airflow acts as a "pneumatic splint" that helps keep the

Pressures usually range from 3 to 20 cm H$_2$O pressure; the pressure setting is frequently determined during a sleep study to ensure that it is therapeutic.

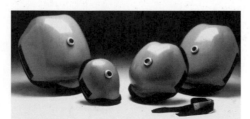

FIGURE 51–15: Chest shells used for negative pressure ventilation. (Courtesy of Lifecare, Lafayette, CO.)

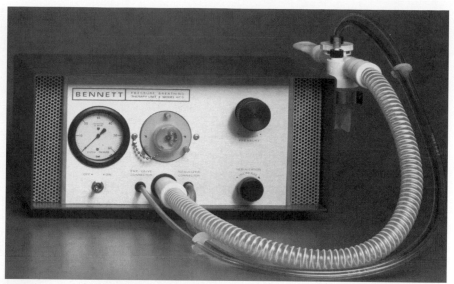

FIGURE 51–16: Electrically powered intermittent positive pressure breathing machine. (Courtesy of Puritan Bennett, Lenexa, KS.)

tissues in the hypopharynx stable and open when the patient inhales. There are numerous units manufactured with many different features, but they are all small, quiet, and effective in relieving the snoring and repeated awakenings typical in the patient with obstructive apnea. There are devices available that can deliver different pressures for inspiration and expiration, called Bi-Level, which are indicated for patients who are unable to tolerate CPAP. Some patients cannot tolerate exhaling against the continuous pressure with CPAP. For these patients, a reduced pressure during the expiratory phase may make it easier for them to exhale. Bi-Level pressure therapy is also being used to treat some types of ventilatory insufficiency.

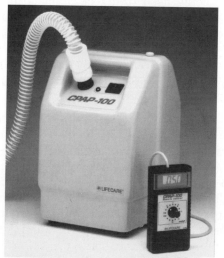

FIGURE 51–17: Home continuous positive airway pressure unit. (Courtesy of Lifecare, Lafayette, CO.)

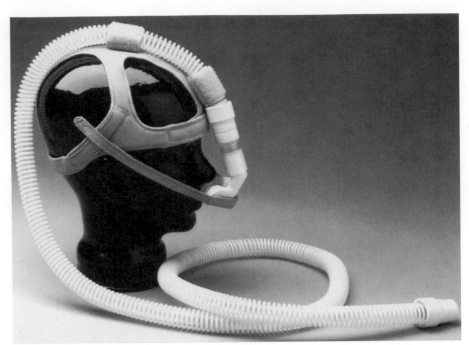

FIGURE 51–18: "Nasal Pillows" nasal mask for use with continuous positive airway pressure. (Courtesy of Puritan Bennett, Lenexa, KS.)

Other Ventilation Assistance Devices

To be complete, it is important to mention other devices that can be useful in the treatment of ventilatory problems at home. Cardiorespiratory monitors (Fig. 51–19) are helpful in detecting apnea with concomitant bradycardias, particularly in infants who are at risk of sudden infant death syndrome. They are also used with children and adults who need monitoring to detect life-threatening apneic events. Oximeters are used to monitor oxygen saturation levels either for "spot-checks" or on a continuous basis. Continuous monitoring is most often performed in infants whose needs are more critical. Nocturnal screening equipment is now being used to detect changes in oxygen and carbon dioxide levels during sleep. Any positive results are evaluated by a complete study in a sleep laboratory.

PATIENT ASSESSMENT AND LONG-TERM CARE

Once the process of patient and equipment selection is complete and the patient is at home, ongoing evaluation must occur. The RCP plays an important role in the patient's long-term care.[8]

Most home medical equipment suppliers employ RCPs to assist in the management of the pulmonary patient; many hospitals use their RCPs to evaluate patients in the home. Home care therapists perform important functions, including patient-caregiver education, ongoing assessment and decision-making, and equipment maintenance.

Commonly, the home care therapist trains the patient and caregivers on procedures such as tracheostomy tube maintenance and changing, suctioning, infection control, and evaluating signs and symptoms. These caregivers will frequently include home care nurses who may not

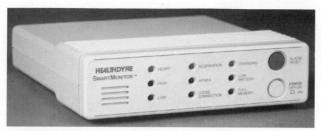

FIGURE 51–19: Home cardiorespiratory monitor. (Courtesy of Healthdyne Technologies, Marietta, GA.)

have experience with such procedures. Patients and caregivers must also be instructed in the use of the many types of equipment described in this chapter.

Plan of Care

Once the patient has been instructed, the RCP must develop a plan of care, which may involve nothing more than visits when problems arise or for scheduled equipment maintenance. More frequently, however, the plan of care involves evaluation of many criteria, which may include physical examination, self-management, psychosocial issues, and oximetry and forced vital capacity measurements.[33] The plan of care must be approved by the patient's physician prior to implementation. Results of the plan of care are communicated to the physician for interpretation and change of treatment as indicated. The RCP can play a valuable role in identifying problems in their early stages and implementing new orders to treat the patient at home, hopefully preventing a hospitalization. This is one of the most valuable and rewarding aspects of home care.

The home care therapist also plays an essential role in equipment maintenance. All the equipment described in this chapter requires periodic maintenance to keep it performing according to the manufacturer's specifications. A large portion of the maintenance is carried out in the patient's home, such as changing filters and checking settings on ventilators, analyzing oxygen concentration and flow rates on concentrators, and checking output pressures on CPAP devices. Assessment is also carried out to see if the patient and caregiver are performing the minor maintenance they are responsible for; if not, reinstruction is indicated.

The RCP will also assess whether the equipment is meeting the patient's needs and will recommend changes if it is not. For example, a patient may be using a concentrator and portable E system. During a home visit, the RCP may determine that the patient is not performing prescribed walking because the E system is too difficult to use. The RCP, who can communicate this to the physician, would recommend a liquid system with its portable unit to allow the patient to continue with the prescribed walking regimen.

Patients who are not compliant with their prescribed therapy or who will not use the equipment properly pose another challenge for the RCP. These patients may require frequent reinstruction to ensure that they understand the implications of their noncompliance and improper use of the equipment. The RCP may call on the other professionals on the home care team to assist in the evaluation and education of the difficult pa-

All home care equipment must be exchanged periodically (usually annually) for preventive maintenance and electrical safety checks. The therapist may assist in the testing, repair, and replacement of equipment.

tient. Good communication with the physician will also aid in the treatment of this type of patient.

SUMMARY

Home care is a challenging field of expertise that requires exactly that—experts. Although many of the modalities are the same, the rules are different. Items that the hospital therapist may take for granted, for example, saline vials, disposable circuits, and sterile water, may not be available for home use because of the lack of insurance coverage for these items. Quantities of these supplies may be limited when they are covered. Even oxygen therapy is not possible for every patient; it may be difficult for hospital-based therapists to understand why their patients cannot have oxygen at home. Other adjuncts, such as oxygen analyzers, respirometers, or oximeters, may not be necessary or indicated in the home setting, which would be considered unthinkable in a hospital setting. The RCP must be able to understand the sometimes nonsensical rules and keep up with the continual changes in these rules.[11, 34] The home care therapist can assist the hospital therapist in determining the most appropriate method of delivering therapy within the confines of those rules.

It takes expert therapists to be able to use their well-honed skills to consider many details that may have been completely out of the scope of their formal respiratory therapy training, such as feeding tubes, urologic devices such as bladder catheters, and enteral therapy. The therapist must also be able to work alone, assess the patient, and make a decision without being able to ask the opinion of the therapist down the hall. The therapist must be willing to accept the fact that he or she is on the patient's "turf" and that the patient is in control. In addition, the therapist must also be willing to accept the fact that for all the education and assessment made available to the patient, he or she is going to live according to his or her desires. It is our responsibility to give these patients all the information and assistance they need and then allow them the right to make their choices.

References

1. Kane NM. The home care crisis of the nineties. Gerontology 29(1):24–31, 1989.
2. American Geriatrics Society Public Policy Committee. Home care and home care reimbursement. JAGS 37(11):1065–1066, 1989.
3. Shamansky SL. Providing home care services in a for-profit environment. Nurs Clin North Am 29(2):387–398, 1988.
4. Bach JR, Intinola P, Alba AS, Holland IE. The ventilator-assisted individual. Cost analysis of institutionalization vs rehabilitation and in-home management. Chest 101(1):26–30, 1992.
5. Fields AI, Rosenblatt A, Pollack M, Kaufman J. Home care cost-effectiveness for respiratory technology-dependent children. Am J Dis Child 145:729–733, 1991.
6. Tompkins C. The ventilator dependent child. Continuing Care May 28–31, 1992.
7. Haggerty MC, Stockdale-Woodley R, Nair S. Respi-Care: An innovative home care program for the patient with chronic obstructive pulmonary disease. Chest 100(3):607–612, 1991.
8. Dunne PJ, McInturff SM, Darr C. The role of home care. *In* Hodgkin JE, Connors GL, Bell CW (eds). Pulmonary Rehabilitation: Guidelines to Success, 2nd ed. Philadelphia, JB Lippincott, 1992.
9. US Consumer Product Safety Commission: Safety for older consumers: Home safety checklist. Washington, DC, June 1986.
10. Medicare Benificiary Services: Oxygen used in a beneficiary's home—Revised coverage guidelines and documentation requirements. Medicare Bull 91(3):11–15, 1991.

11. Shigeoka JW, Shults BM. Home oxygen therapy under Medicare—A primer. West J Med 156(1):39–44, 1992.
12. Bergner M, Hudson LD, Conrad DA, et al. The cost and efficacy of home care for patients with chronic lung disease. Med Care 26(6):566–579, 1988.
13. Petty TL. Home oxygen therapy. Mayo Clin Proc 62:841–847, 1987.
14. Tiep BL. Long-term home oxygen therapy. Clin Chest Med 11(3):505–521, 1990.
15. Herrick TW, Yeager H. Home oxygen therapy. Am Fam Phys 39(2):157–162, 1989.
16. Howard P. Cost effectiveness of oxygen therapy. Eur Respir J 2 (Suppl 7):637s–639s, 1989.
17. Nocturnal Oxygen Therapy Trial Group. Continuous or nocturnal oxygen therapy in hypoxemic chronic obstructive lung disease. An Intern Med 93(3):391–398, 1980.
18. McPherson SP. Gas delivery devices. *In* McPherson SP. Respiratory Home Care Equipment. Iowa, Kendall Hunt, pp 1–36.
19. Estey W. Subjective effects of dry versus humidified low flow oxygen. Respir Care 25(11):1143–1144, 1980.
20. Tiep BL. Oxygen conserving devices: Efficiency and cost advantages. Choice Respir Management 21:114–118, 1991.
21. Tiep BL, Christopher KL, Spofford BT, et al. Pulsed nasal and transtracheal oxygen delivery. Chest 97(2):364–368, 1990.
22. Tiep BL, Brooke Nicotra M, Carter R, et al. Low-concentration oxygen therapy via a demand oxygen delivery system. Chest 87(5):636–638, 1985.
23. Reinke LF, Hoffman LA. Transtracheal oxygen: Patient management strategies. RT 5(3):66–71, 1992.
24. American College of Chest Physicians. Discharge planning resources and equipment for home care of ventilator-assisted individuals. Park Ridge, IL, 1985.
25. Gilmartin ME, Make BJ (eds). Mechanical ventilation in the home—Issues for health care providers. Probl Resp Care 1(2):155–295, 1988.
26. Peters SG, Viggiano RW. Home mechanical ventilation. Mayo Clin Proc 63:1208–1213, 1988.
27. Leger P, Jennequin J, Gerard M, Robert D. Home positive pressure ventilation via nasal mask for patients with neuromuscular weakness or restrictive lung or chest-wall disease. Resp Care 34(2):73–78, 1989.
28. Patient Care and Home Care Committee. Respiratory Home Care Procedure Manual. Pittsburgh, Pennsylvania Society for Respiratory Care, 1983.
29. Plummer AL, O'Donohue WJ, Petty TL. Consensus conference on problems in home mechanical ventilation. Am Rev Respir Dis 140:555–560, 1989.
30. Make BJ, Gilmartin ME. Care of ventilator-assisted individuals in the home and alternative community sites. *In* Burton G, Hodgkin JE (eds). Respiratory Care: A Guide to Clinical Practice, 3rd ed. Philadelphia, JB Lippincott, 1991.
31. Jackson NC. Pulmonary rehabilitation for the mechanically ventilated patient. Crit Care Nurs Clin No Am 3(4):591–600, 1991.
32. Smith R. Building a sleep program. RT 5(3):53–58, 1992.
33. American Thoracic Society. Standards of nursing care for adult patients with pulmonary dysfunction. Am Rev Respir Dis 144(1):231–236, 1991.
34. O'Donohue WJ. New problems in home oxygen therapy. Am Rev Respir Dis 140:1813, 1989.

52

Respiratory Care Pharmacology

E. Neil Schachter, M.D., and
Theodore J. Witek, Jr., Dr. P.H., R.R.T.

Pharmacology plays a critical role in respiratory care. Inhaled anti-inflammatory drugs and bronchodilators have emerged as first-line treatment in bronchospastic disorders; therefore, their delivery is frequently a primary responsibility of the respiratory care practitioner. In addition, practitioners work in a progressively more complex and interrelated environment. In intensive care, home care, and rehabilitative care, as well as in diagnostic pulmonary disease, the practitioner is frequently asked to evaluate and treat patients as a primary caregiver. Such responsibility requires a broad and full understanding of the agents that affect the respiratory system.

Several classes of drugs are used in respiratory therapeutics and diagnostics (Table 52–1). This chapter provides the practitioner with an overview of the mechanisms of their action and their role in therapeutics.

BETA-ADRENERGIC AGONISTS

Mechanism of Action

The autonomic nervous system is made up of the sympathetic and parasympathetic branches. Each of these two pathways is composed of preganglionic and postganglionic neurons. All functions in these systems are mediated through neurotransmitter substances. In the sympathetic nervous system, transmission of postganglionic impulses is mediated by norepinephrine, which is structurally similar to epinephrine released from the adrenal medulla. Thus, adrenergic function involves sympathetic nerves, which secrete norepinephrine, and the adrenal medulla, which secretes epinephrine. These naturally occurring transmitters, along with synthetic drugs that reproduce their action, are now widely used in respiratory care.

The actions of drugs that mimic the sympathetic nervous system (i.e., sympathomimetics) are mediated by two major classes of receptors, termed *alpha-adrenergic* and *beta-adrenergic*. In addition, two subtypes of each receptor are clinically recognized—$alpha_1$ and $alpha_2$ and $beta_1$ and $beta_2$.

Adrenergic receptors are widely distributed in numerous tissues. In the lung, relaxation of airway smooth muscle following stimulation of

TABLE **52–1:** Classes of Respiratory Care Drugs

Beta-adrenergic agonists	Mediator antagonists
Methylxanthines	Mucokinetic agents
Anticholinergic drugs	Antitussives
Corticosteroids	Ventilatory stimulants
Antiallergic drugs	

beta$_2$-adrenergic receptors is the basis for adrenergic bronchodilator therapy. The ability of alpha-agonists to contract vascular smooth muscle is the basis for their use as nasal vasoconstricting decongestants.

Adrenergic receptors on cells of the respiratory tract are recognized by hormones, neurotransmitters, or synthetic drugs. By a process referred to as signal transduction, these receptors convert an external stimulus to intracellular events that result in a response by the target tissue.

Receptors

Recent studies at the molecular level have provided significant insight into the structure and function of adrenergic receptors. Several adrenergic receptors have been cloned and shown to consist of stretches of amino acids that span the cell membrane seven times; the amino terminus ($-NH_2$) is located extracellularly and the carboxyl ($-COOH$) terminus is located intracellularly.[1] A simplified diagram of an adrenergic receptor is seen in Figure 52–1.

In addition to the *receptor* that binds the drug, the active functional unit is composed of a coupling protein, known as a *G protein* and one or more *second messenger systems*, which are involved in the biochemical events that produce a response.

Agonist interaction with a receptor results in an alteration of the receptor and its coupled G protein, leading to an exchange of guanosine triphosphate for guanosine diphosphate. In the case of the beta-receptor, the guanosine triphosphate–activated G protein then activates a membrane-bound adenylate cyclase, leading to the formation of intracellular cyclic adenosine monophosphate (cAMP) (Fig. 52–2). In this model, cAMP serves as a second messenger. Since an increased intracellular concentration of cAMP results in relaxation of airway smooth muscle, these events provide an explanation for why inhaled beta-agonists cause bronchodilation.

Effects of Adrenergic Agonists

Beta-adrenergic agonists have numerous therapeutic effects, the most important being relaxation of airway smooth muscle. Additionally,

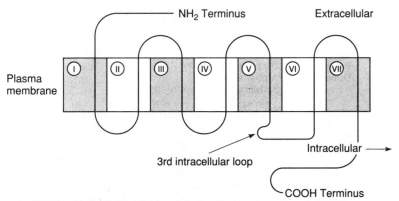

FIGURE 52–1: A simplified schematic representation of the membrane organization of plasma membrane receptors, such as the adrenergic receptor. Structural features include an extracellular amino terminus, an intracellular carboxyl terminus, and seven membrane spanning regions. (Adapted from Insel PA. Structure and function of the alpha adrenergic receptor. Am J Med 87(Suppl 2A):155, 1989.)

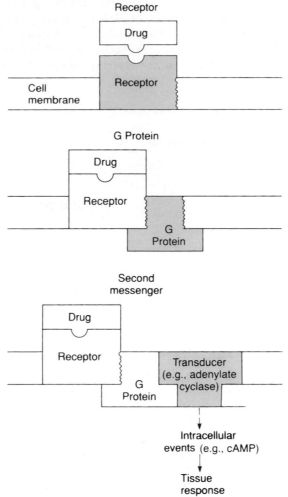

FIGURE 52–2: The active functional unit involved in producing a receptor-mediator biologic response. (From Witek TJ Jr, Schachter EN. Pharmacology and Therapeutics in Respiratory Care. Philadelphia, WB Saunders, 1994, p 142.)

beta-agonists have been shown to prevent mediator release, increase mucus secretion, increase mucociliary transport, inhibit bronchial edema, inhibit cholinergic transmission, and decrease airway hyperresponsiveness.[2]

Undesired effects of therapy with beta-adrenergic agonists are influenced by the dose and the route of administration of these agents as well as by clinical factors in the individual patient. Such adverse effects include

- Skeletal muscle tremor
- Tachycardia
- Various metabolic effects that are mediated by beta-adrenergic receptor stimulation[3] (e.g., hypokalemia)

Other side effects that are potentially serious problems in some susceptible patients include cardiac arrhythmias and hypoxemia. Nevertheless, the therapeutic benefit of adrenergic bronchodilators generally outweighs these relatively uncommon side effects.

Clinical Utility of Adrenergic Agonists

Subcutaneous or intravenous administration of beta-agonists may be indicated in acute, severe cases of asthma.

Beta-adrenergic agonists are the most widely used pharmacologic agents in respiratory care (Table 52–2). Long-acting, selective beta$_2$-adrenergic agonists have a rapid onset of action when given by inhalation and are the treatment of choice for acute exacerbations of asthma. Although oral therapy is associated with increased adrenergic side effects, sustained-release preparations may be useful in treating specific symptoms, such as nocturnal asthma. Beta-agonists are effective in the treatment of airway obstruction in chronic bronchitis and emphysema; however, evidence suggests that anticholinergic agents should be tried prior to (or in conjunction with) beta-agonist therapy in these conditions (see Antimuscarinic Agents).

The once common clinical practice of prescribing beta-agonist therapy three to four times a day for asthma has come under scrutiny, with current recommendations suggesting the use of these agents on an intermittent basis.[4] Long-acting, potent agents such as salmeterol may also change current standard therapy. Clinical trials will provide further insight into the role of beta-agonists in airway obstruction.

METHYLXANTHINES

Theophylline and related agents are in a stage of transition in terms of their role in the treatment of airway disease. As an effective bronchodilating agent, however, theophylline remains important and useful in airway obstruction.

Theophylline is closely related to the other well-known methylxanthines caffeine and theobromine (Fig. 52–3). These naturally occurring alkaloids are found in a variety of plants distributed throughout the world and routinely consumed in a variety of drinks and foods. All of the natural methylxanthines (caffeine, theobromine, and theophylline) are capable of eliciting airway responses, such as airway smooth muscle relaxation.[5] Although theophylline is probably the most potent bronchodilator among these agents, both theobromine and caffeine have significant airway-dilating effects.

TABLE **52–2:** Approximate Onset and Duration of Action of Sympathomimetics with Beta-adrenergic Properties

Drug	Route of Administration	Onset (M)	Duration (H)
Albuterol	Oral,	Within 30	4–8
	inhalation	Within 15	3–4
Bitolterol	Inhalation	3–4	5–8
Ephedrine	Oral	15–60	3–5
Epinephrine	Subcutaneous,	6–15	<1–4
	inhalation	3–5	1–3
Isoetharine	Inhalation	1–6	1–3
Isoproterenol	Inhalation,	2–5	0.5–2
	intravenous	Immediate	<1
Metaproterenol	Oral,	15–30	4
	inhalation	1–5	3–4
Pirbuterol	Inhalation	Within 5	5
Terbutaline	Oral,	30	4–8
	subcutaneous,	6–15	1.5–4
	inhalation	5–30	3–6

From Cada DJ, Covington TR, Hussar DA, et al (eds). Drug Facts and Comparisons, 45th ed. Philadelphia, JB Lippincott, 1991.

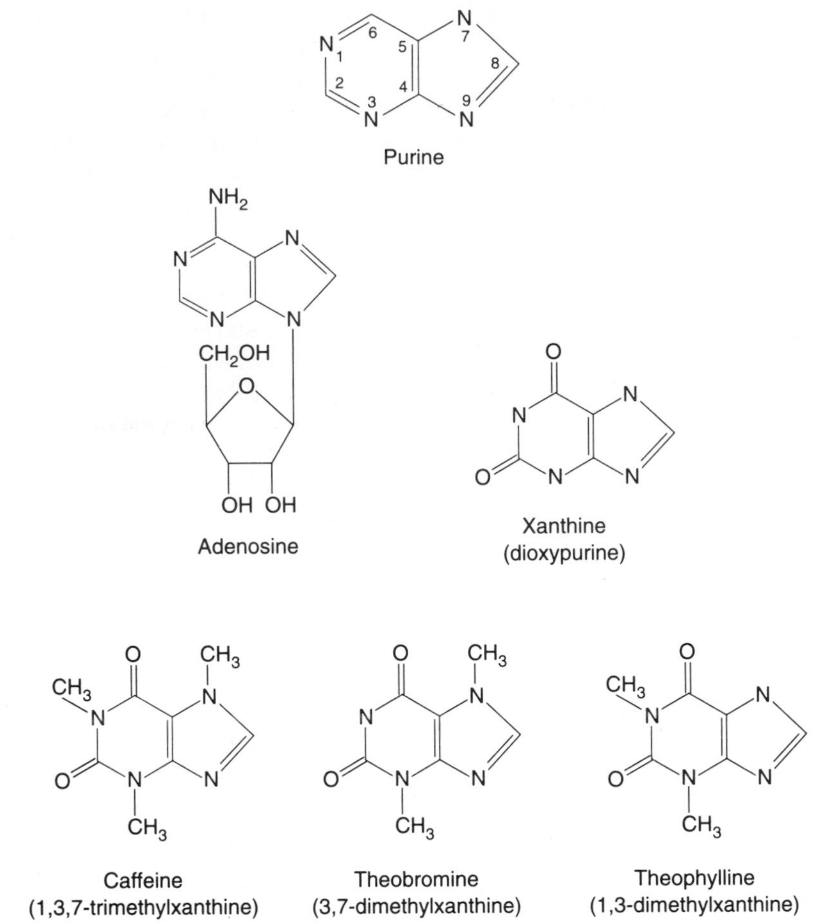

Purine

Adenosine

Xanthine
(dioxypurine)

Caffeine
(1,3,7-trimethylxanthine)

Theobromine
(3,7-dimethylxanthine)

Theophylline
(1,3-dimethylxanthine)

FIGURE 52–3: Principal, pharmacologically active methylxanthines: caffeine, theobromine, and theophylline compared and contrasted to related biochemical structures: purine nucleus, adenosine, and xanthine. (From Witek TJ Jr, Schachter EN. Pharmacology and Therapeutics in Respiratory Care. Philadelphia, WB Saunders, 1994, p 184.)

Mechanisms of Action

The original unifying concept of smooth muscle relaxation used to explain the bronchodilating effect of theophylline was introduced by Sutherland and Roll.[5a] In their scheme, intracellular cAMP is synthesized by membrane-bound adenyl cyclase and subsequently hydrolyzed by the enzyme phosphodiesterase (Fig. 52–4).

Relief or amelioration of bronchospasm by theophylline and related compounds has been hypothesized to result from their ability to inhibit intracellular cyclic 3'5' nucleotide phosphodiesterase in smooth muscle and mast cells. Inhibition of phosphodiesterase enzymes (by a methylxanthine) would reduce the breakdown of cyclic 3'5' AMP and result in increased levels of intracellular cyclic 3'5' AMP, thus favoring smooth muscle relaxation and mast cell stability.

In spite of this attractive theory, a number of in vivo and in vitro observations suggest that the serum levels of theophylline necessary for significant phosphodiesterase inhibition would be toxic and that at standard therapeutic levels, theophylline barely increases intracellular cAMP.[6]

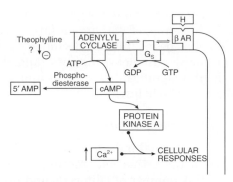

FIGURE 52–4: Cyclic AMP (cAMP) as the second messenger for smooth muscle relaxation. Possible role of theophylline as a phosphodiesterase inhibitor. ATP, adenosine triphosphate; GDP, guanosine diphosphate; GTP, guanosine triphosphate. (Adapted from Goodman AG, Roll TW, Nies AS, Taylor P. Goodman and Gillman's: The Pharmacologic Basis of Therapeutics, 8th ed. Elmsford, NY, Pergamon Press, 1990, p 109.)

Because of the present uncertainty about phosphodiesterase inhibition as the sole, or even the main, mechanism explaining theophylline's ability to relax airway smooth muscle, other theophylline-related mechanisms have been invoked, including

- Inhibition of the airway smooth muscle constrictor agent adenosine
- The enhanced release of catecholamines by methylxanthines
- Prostaglandin inhibition by theophylline[7, 8]

As yet none of these theories is considered established.

Clinical Utility of Methylxanthines

A number of clinical syndromes associated with airway obstruction respond to methylxanthines.

Nocturnal Asthma Symptoms

Nocturnal symptoms, which are particularly prominent in the early morning hours, have long been recognized as a major component of asthma, affecting most asthmatics with clinically significant disease. Continuous treatment with theophylline can provide significant relief of these symptoms as well as a reduction in diurnal fluctuations of lung function.[9]

Mucociliary Function

Mucociliary dysfunction is a relatively constant feature of many airway illnesses (e.g., asthma, chronic bronchitis, cystic fibrosis). In vivo studies show that radiolabeled aerosol is more rapidly cleared under the influence of theophylline and that this response is dose-dependent.

Enhancement of Diaphragm Function

Administration of theophylline for 1 week in patients with chronic obstructive pulmonary disease (COPD) who experienced respiratory insufficiency resulted in a significant (20%) increase in diaphragm strength and a lessening of diaphragm fatigability.[10] The effect of theophylline in COPD has been clinically documented. Improvements in minute ventilation, blood gas measurements, and dyspnea have been demonstrated without a significant change in lung function, suggesting enhanced respiratory muscle function.

Treatment of Asthma

The original indication for theophylline, its role in the treatment of status asthmaticus, has recently been challenged in controlled clinical trials.[11] A number of editorials and reviews argue that theophylline has been superseded as an effective, rapid-acting bronchodilator by inhaled beta-agonists.[12] The use of the latter in this context is not enhanced by the administration of theophylline, even in patients with severely compromised lung function. At present, it would appear that under these acute conditions, theophylline adds little if anything to clinical improvement and may contribute to unwanted side effects.

Patients with chronic, stable asthma are known to benefit from therapy with theophylline both alone and in combination with beta-agonists. In asthmatics dependent on systemic steroids, judicious use of theophylline may offer a steroid-sparing strategy.

Treatment of Chronic Obstructive Pulmonary Disease

The use of theophylline in patients with COPD has equivocal objective support. Theophylline improves mucociliary clearance and stimulates the respiratory center—actions that would be expected to improve pathophysiologic abnormalities in COPD.

Intravenous aminophylline reduces pulmonary vascular pressure and pulmonary vascular resistance and improves cardiac output while lowering right and left ventricular end-diastolic pressures independent of changes in oxygen saturation. These findings, along with data on right ventricular ejection fraction, suggest that theophylline can improve cardiovascular function in COPD.

Finally, in a recent review of seven randomized double-blind studies on the overall effectiveness of theophylline in stable COPD, a trend in symptomatic improvement in the treated groups was noted but was unaccompanied by objective changes in lung function.[13]

The methylxanthines are rapidly absorbed by the oral and parenteral routes. In recent years, efforts to improve formulation have been directed at reducing the frequency of dosing by providing slow-release oral formulations. Many preparations are now available (Table 52–3). Dosing schedules vary from every 8 hours to twice daily to once every 24 hours.

Elimination of theophylline depends on a number of patient and pharmacologic variables, some of which are listed in Table 52–4. Because the liver is central to theophylline metabolism, factors that affect its function such as disease (e.g., cirrhosis, congestive heart failure, prematurity) can reduce a patient's ability to metabolize and hence lower the clearance of theophylline. Conversely, drugs that enhance hepatic enzyme systems (e.g., phenobarbital) can accelerate clearance.

The methylxanthines in general and theophylline in particular are recognized to have a narrow therapeutic index. The availability of a wide variety of laboratory methods capable of rapidly determining serum concentrations of theophylline has led to a greater appreciation of the close

In the generally accepted therapeutic range of 10 to 20 mg/L, many patients experience side effects that may disrupt compliance or, in rare instances, jeopardize the patient. By contrast, toxic side effects are almost always experienced when theophylline is administered in doses greater than the therapeutic range, particularly at levels of 30 mg/L or more. Most side effects that clinicians recognize tend to be self-limited and involve the gastrointestinal tract (nausea, diarrhea, pain), the nervous system (nervousness) and the cardiovascular system (tachycardia), but severe life-threatening events do occur.

TABLE **52–3:** Commonly Used Oral Methylxanthine Preparations

Generic Compound	Brand Name	Formulation	Recommended Dosing Schedule
Theophylline			
	Aerolate	Aerolate	q 8–12 hr
		Aerolate Sr (260 mg)	q 8–12 hr
		Aerolate Jr (130 mg)	q 8–12 hr
		Aerolate III (65 mg)	q 8–12 hr
	Bronkodyl	100, 200 mg	
	Constant-T	200, 300 mg	q 12 hr
	Elixophyllin	Capsules (100, 200 mg)	q 6–8 hr
		SR (125, 250 mg)	q 6–8 hr
	Quibron-T	300 mg (divisible)	Children, adults q 8 hr
	Quibron T/SR	300 mg (divisible)	Children, adults q 8 hr
	Respbid	250, 500 mg	q 8–12 hr
	Slo-bid	50, 75, 100, 125, 200, 300 mg	q 8–12 hr
	Slo-phyllin	100, 200 mg	Children, adults q 8 hr
	Theo-24	100, 200, 300 mg	q 12 or 24 hr
	Theobid	130 (JR), 260 mg	q 8–12 hr
	Theo-Dur	100, 200, 300, 450 mg	q 12 hr
	Theo-Dur Sprinkle	50, 75, 125, 200 mg	q 12 hr
	Theolair	125, 250 mg	
	Theolair-SR	200, 250, 300 mg	
	Theospan-SR	130, 260 mg	
	Uniphyl	400 mg	q 24 hr*
Dyphylline			
	Lufyllin	200 mg	q 6 hr
	Lufyllin-400	400 mg	q 6 hr
Oxtriphylline			
	Choledyl	100, 200 mg	q 6–8 hr
	Choledyl SA	400, 600 mg	q 12 hr
Theophylline, ephedrine, guaifenesin, barbiturates†	Bronkolixir		2–4 times daily
	Bronkotabs		2–4 times daily
	Quibron Plus		2–4 times daily
Theophylline, ephedrine, hydroxyzine†	Marax		2–4 times daily
Theophylline, ephedrine, phenobarbital†	Tedral		q 4 hr
	Tedral SA		q 12 hr
Theophylline, guaifenesin†	Asbron-G		q 6–8 hr
	Elixophyllin-GG		q 6–8 hr
	Quibron		q 6–8 hr

Adapted from Drug Information for the Health Care Professional, vols IA and B. Rockville, MD, United States Pharmacopeia—Dispensing Information, 1990; Physician's Desk Reference, 44th ed. Oradell, NJ, Medical Economics, 1990.

*Recommended for patients whose daily dose is less than 800 mg/day.

†Combination products, particularly those containing ephedrine, a barbiturate, and antihistamines are not recommended for the therapy of obstructive airway diseases. They are currently under review by the Food and Drug Administration.

relationship between concentration and toxicity and to frequent monitoring in clinical practice.

Among the most serious toxic effects, theophylline therapy may be associated with prolonged focal motor seizures that are difficult to control.[14] Theophylline-induced seizures may result in death or permanent neurologic damage. In the face of actual seizures, intravenous diazepam (Valium) is used as a treatment of choice while supporting all other vital functions.

ANTIMUSCARINIC AGENTS

In the parasympathetic nervous system, postganglionic fibers release acetylcholine. The effect of this mediator has been classified as

TABLE **52–4:** Effect of Patient and Pharmacologic Variables on Total Body Clearance and Half-Life (t½) of Theophylline

	Characteristic	Effect on Clearance	Effect on Half-Life
Age	Premature (3–15 days)	0.5*	3.7
	Children (4–12 yr)	2.5	—
	Elderly (nonsmoker)	0.6	1.2
Illness	Febrile illness	—	0.9
	CHF	0.5	2.3
	COPD	0.8	—
	Cystic Fibrosis	1.9	0.7
	Cirrhosis	0.5	3.9
Smoking		—	0.5
Drugs	Allopurinol, cimetidine, erythromycin, influenza vaccine, Tao, oral contraceptives, beta-blocking agents, quinolones, calcium channel blockers	↓	↑
	Phenobarbital, phenytoin, rifampin, carbamazepine (Tegretol), lithium	↑	↓

Adapted from Hendeles L, Massanari M, Weinberger M: Theophylline. *In* Middleton E Jr, Reed CE, Elliott E, et al (eds). Allergy: Principles and Practice, vol I, 3rd ed. St. Louis, CV Mosby, 1989. (In this review, the average clearance for healthy nonsmoking adults was 0.63 ± 0.19 ml/kg/min and the average half-life was 8.2 hours [range of 6.1 to 12.8]).

*Fraction compared with healthy nonsmoking adult.

muscarinic because transmission can be mimicked by the drug of muscarine. Muscarinic effects are blocked by atropine.

Mechanism of Action

Muscarinic receptors are located on airway smooth muscle, secretory cells, and the cholinergic nerve cells themselves. Mapping studies have shown that muscarinic receptors are widely distributed in the human lung, including the airway smooth muscle of large and small airways as well as the alveolar walls.[15, 16] Muscarinic receptors are also present on nasal glands and vasculature.

Like the alpha$_2$-, beta$_1$-, and beta$_2$-receptors, the muscarinic receptor is a transmembrane receptor that binds the ligand (e.g., drug) outside the cell. At least five muscarinic receptor subtypes exist, with three of these subtypes (M1, M2, M3) capable of being distinguished pharmacologically. The clinical implications of each of these subtypes is the focus of current research. Highly selective drugs for these receptor subtypes are not currently available.

Postreceptor Events

The mode of action of antimuscarinic bronchodilators has until recently been described as simply preventing the increase in intracellular concentration of cyclic guanosine monophosphate following receptor stimulation. The postreceptor events are now believed to be more complex (Fig. 52–5).

Activation of the muscarinic receptor may decrease adenylate cyclase activity, leading to a fall in the intracellular cAMP content. Such a decrease would favor contraction of airway smooth muscle. Another signal transduction mechanism, associated with a different G protein, involves the activation of phospholipase C, which breaks down the membrane lipid phosphatidylinositol 4,5-biphosphate (PIP2) to inositol

M1 receptors are present in parasympathetic ganglia. M2 receptors are found on the cholinergic nerve terminals themselves, and M3 receptors are found on airway smooth muscle and mucous glands.

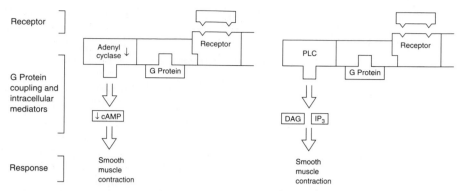

FIGURE 52–5: Schematic representation of the effector systems associated with the muscarinic receptor. PLC, phospholipase; DAG, diacylglycerol. (From Witek TJ Jr, Schachter EN. Pharmacology and Therapeutics in Respiratory Care. Philadelphia, WB Saunders, 1994, p 172.)

Airway provocation studies with cholinergic agonists such as methacholine have shown that atropine and atropine-like drugs provide uniform protection against bronchoconstriction.

1,4,5-triphosphate (IP3). This releases calcium from intracellular stores, resulting in contraction of airway smooth muscle. Receptor activation also leads to the formation of diacylglycerol; this second messenger causes protein kinase C to become associated with the cell membrane, where it becomes activated. There is evidence that protein kinase C may contribute to a slow (sustained) contractile response in airway smooth muscle, whereas IP3 may have a primary role in initiating contraction.

Atropine and atropine-like drugs are competitive antagonists of the bronchoconstrictor acetylcholine. These drugs promote bronchodilation in situations in which parasympathetic activity is present.[17, 18] In the normal airway, resting bronchomotor tone is due to endogenous acetylcholine release, which regulates airway caliber in health and disease. As a result, antimuscarinic drugs usually cause bronchodilation in normal subjects as well as in asthmatics and patients with COPD.

Antimuscarinic drugs can also inhibit reflex cholinergic bronchoconstriction, which can be elicited by a variety of chemical (e.g., gases) and physical (e.g., cold, dry air) stimuli and can arise from irritation of sensory fibers in a variety of locations, including the nasopharynx, larynx, and subglottic airways.

Unlike their protective effect on irritant and sulfur dioxide challenges, antimuscarinic agents do not consistently protect against provocation with histamine, prostaglandins, leukotrienes, or serotonin in humans. In addition, antimuscarinic agents are not particularly effective against antigen-induced bronchoconstriction, nor do they inhibit mediator release from mast cells. These observations highlight the fact that antimuscarinic agents work primarily by inhibiting the cholinergic component of airway constriction as opposed to any direct effect on bronchoconstriction caused by other mediators.

Atropine and related belladonna alkaloids can inhibit airway secretions, causing a drying of the mucous membranes of the respiratory tract. Atropine is used in general anesthesia specifically for this purpose.

Ipratropium bromide lacks the negative effects on mucociliary function that are reported for atropine. Therefore, it can be used as a bronchodilator without significant risk to airway clearance mechanisms.

Clinical Utility of Antimuscarinic Agents

Many clinical studies of inhaled antimuscarinic drugs (primarily ipratropium bromide) that have been reported over the past 10 to 20 years, provide a rationale for their selective use in present-day respiratory care.

Asthma

The bronchodilation produced by ipratropium bromide in asthmatics is usually less effective than that produced by beta-agonists, as evidenced by a slower onset to peak effect (30 to 90 minutes following inhalation) as well as a smaller peak effect. Nevertheless, the duration of action persists beyond 6 hours for both types of drugs. Although the slower onset and lower peak effects of ipratropium bromide often make it less desirable as first-line asthma therapy, it has been used in combination with beta-agonists, which provides an additive benefit.

Antimuscarinic drugs have been shown to block psychogenic asthma and asthma caused by therapy with beta-adrenergic–blocking agents; therefore, these agents should be considered in such clinical situations, particularly those associated with stress.

Chronic Bronchitis and Emphysema

In most patients with COPD, antimuscarinic agents provide greater bronchodilation and fewer side effects than do beta-agonists or theophylline. Additionally, the effectiveness of these agents remains evident with continued use. Current practice dictates antimuscarinic agents as the primary bronchodilator in COPD.[19, 20]

It has been suggested that the difference in response between asthmatics and COPD patients is a reflection of the lack of response to adrenergic agents in chronic bronchitis-emphysema. In these diseases, destructive changes and impaired airway mechanics probably play more of a role than inflammatory mediators in the airway obstruction, thus limiting the value of adrenergic agonists. The reversal of normal physiologic cholinergic tone, which accounts for the antimuscarinic-induced bronchodilation in both health and disease, provides (at least in part) a rationale for the use of ipratropium bromide in treating airway obstruction. When no additional factors cause obstruction (e.g., as in emphysema), inhaled antimuscarinic agents will provide maximal bronchodilation.

Ipratropium Bromide

Ipratropium bromide, currently the only antimuscarinic agent approved for inhalational respiratory care in the United States, is available in a metered dose inhaler that delivers 18 μg per actuation with a recommended dose of two actuations (36 μg) four times a day. Although patients may take additional inhalations as required, the package insert states that the total number of inhalations should not exceed 12 in 24 hours. Ipratropium bromide is also available in a solution for nebulizer administration (500 μg/dose).

Because of its lack of systemic absorption, side effects following ipratropium bromide administration occur less often than with atropine. Unlike adrenergic agents, antimuscarinic agents do not reduce arterial oxygen tension or cause tremor. Prolonged dilation of the pupils can occur if ipratropium bromide is sprayed into the eye, an effect that both the practitioner and the patient should know about. Patients may also complain of bad taste from inhaler use, a factor that could affect compliance.

GLUCOCORTICOIDS

Adrenal cortical hormones that demonstrate biologic activity have been classified according to their predominant effects in the body. The mineralocorticoids, which display principally salt-retaining activities, are responsible for maintaining electrolyte balance and extracellular fluid volume. A second major group of corticosteroids is composed of the glucocorticoids. Glucocorticoids, which generally exert a variety of effects on intermediary metabolism (e.g., the metabolism of carbohydrates, proteins, and fats), are pharmacologically useful because of their anti-inflammatory qualities and their ability to suppress immunologic activity in the body.

The normal regulation of adrenocortical hormones is under complex control. The pituitary gland stimulates glucocorticoids via a peptide hormone, adrenocorticotropic hormone, which is, in turn, released under the influence of corticotropin-releasing factor, a peptide produced in the hypothalamus. Adrenocorticotropic hormone is suppressed by high levels of circulating glucocorticoids (both endogenous and pharmacologic). This latter phenomenon is responsible for the adrenal atrophy and dysfunction seen in patients maintained for extended periods on pharmacologic doses of glucocorticoids.

Mechanisms of Action

The major effects of glucocorticoid hormones are felt to be at the genetic level in the cell nucleus, influencing protein synthesis. The common pathway of biologic action of these hormones can be summarized as shown in Figure 52–6. The steroid hormone is transported through the circulation bound to either corticosteroid-binding globulin or albumin. It reaches a target organ and the following occurs:

1. The steroid hormone is taken up by the target cell and binds to a specific cytoplasmic receptor protein.

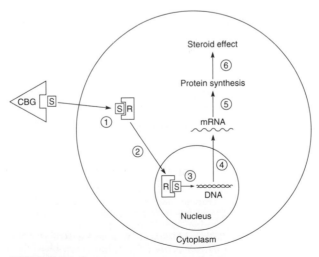

FIGURE 52–6: Cellular mechanism of steroid action. S, steroid hormone; R, cytoplasmic receptor; CBG, corticosteroid binding globulin. (From Witek TJ Jr, Schachter EN. Pharmacology and Therapeutics in Respiratory Care. Philadelphia, WB Saunders, 1994, p 213.)

2. The steroid-receptor complex is transported (translocation) to the nucleus of the cell.

3. The steroid-receptor complex binds to specific receptor sites on the genome (DNA and chromatin).

4. Following binding there is activation of the process of transcription, resulting in specific messenger RNA molecules being formed.

5. The newly synthesized messenger RNA is transported to the cytoplasm where, binding to ribosomes, it results in new protein synthesis.

6. The newly synthesized proteins bring about the cellular responses associated with the steroid.[21]

Table 52–5 outlines the physiologic and pharmacologic effects of glucocorticoids.

Clinical Utility of Glucocorticoids

Glucocorticoids are extremely useful in a broad variety of lung diseases (Table 52–6).

Asthma

Much of the current research in asthma suggests that it represents a persistent bronchitis in which the inflammation involves the mucosal layers. Because of their diversified effects on inflammatory reactions, glucocorticoids would be expected to modify the course of both acute attacks and sustained disease. Until the advent of aerosolized steroid preparations, treatment of asthma with glucocorticoids tended to be conservative, particularly when chronic administration was involved. The established safety and versatility of aerosol preparations have greatly extended the usefulness of steroids in this disease.[22]

Chronic Obstructive Pulmonary Disease

The spectrum of COPD is wide, stretching from emphysema to chronic bronchitis. The approach to therapy in this disorder must in many cases be empiric, based on clinical evaluation and observed response to therapy. It is not surprising that many of the published studies give widely different pictures of the effectiveness of corticosteroids in COPD.[23]

Upper Respiratory Disease

Disease of the upper airways, particularly rhinitis, may require therapy with glucocorticoids. The indications are similar and parallel those

> Steroids are commonly used in patients with acute exacerbations of their disease, particularly with impending or established respiratory failure.

TABLE **52–5:** Physiologic and Pharmacologic Actions of Glucocorticoids

Intermediate Metabolism: Controls the rate of synthesis and the storage and the transformation of proteins, sugars, fats

Electrolyte Balance: Influences the kidney's handling of salts (Na^+, K^+) through its mineralocorticoid properties

Calcium Balance: Influences gastrointestinal absorption and renal secretion of calcium

Gastrointestinal Tract: Influences blood flow to gastrointestinal mucosa

Cardiovascular System: Influences (indirectly) blood pressure by its action on salt and water

Central Nervous System: Excess glucocorticoids associated with euphoria; apathy and depression associated with decreased levels

Anti-inflammatory and Anti-immunologic Actions

TABLE **52–6:** Pulmonary Diseases Treated With Corticosteroids

Obstructive Lung Disease	Interstitial Lung Disease	Vasculitis
Asthma	Usual interstitial lung disease	Bronchocentric granulomatosis
Status asthmaticus	Connective tissue diseases	Hypersensitivity vasculitis
Chronic asthma	Systemic lupus erythematosus	Lymphomatoid granulomatosis
COPD	Rheumatoid arthritis	Wegener's granulomatosis
Acute exacerbations	Sjögren's syndrome	**Infections**
Stable COPD	Dermatomyositis-polymyositis	Miliary tuberculosis
Inhalational airway injury	Mixed connective tissue disease	Severe PCP
Toxic gases (e.g., sulfur dioxide;	Drug-induced pneumonitis (e.g., from	**Miscellaneous**
nitrogen dioxide)	bleomycin, methotrexate, busulfan,	Goodpasture's syndrome
Toxic fumes	amiodarone)	Pulmonary eosinophilic syndromes
Bronchiolitis obliterans	Radiation pneumonitis	(e.g., Loeffler's syndrome)
Bronchopulmonary aspergillosis	Sarcoidosis	
Upper airway diseases	Eosinophilic granuloma	
Allergic rhinitis	Hypersensitivity pneumonitis	
Laryngitis		
Tracheitis		

PCP, *Pneumocystis carinii* pneumonia.

of obstructive airway disease at other levels of the airways. Corticosteroids may be indicated for the relief of symptoms. Topical therapy in particular is preferred, but as with severe airway disease, topical therapy alone may not control symptoms sufficiently, so systemic steroids may be necessary.

Pulmonary Fibrosis

Pulmonary fibrosis is not a distinct clinical entity; rather, it is the final common pathway of many diseases. A patient with rapidly deteriorating disease is a candidate for therapy. The guidelines for therapy remain highly empiric, since some of these diseases remit spontaneously (e.g., sarcoidosis) or progress slowly. The efficacy of steroid therapy in pulmonary fibrosis is often difficult to assess.

Pulmonary Vasculitis

Vasculitis such as that associated with Wegener's granulomatosis or lymphomatoid granulomatosis has been successfully treated with combinations of glucocorticoids and immunosuppressive agents. Therapy may be required for long periods, since vasculitis diseases are only suppressed by these agents and tend to recur when treatment is discontinued prematurely.

Pulmonary Infections

The use of glucocorticoids has been advocated in the treatment of miliary tuberculosis to slow down or reverse the consequences of rapidly progressive exudative disease. Impending respiratory failure or involvement of other critical systems (e.g., tuberculous meningitis, tuberculous pericarditis) are indications for glucocorticoid therapy. Treatment with glucocorticoids should not be initiated unless the diagnosis is firmly established and until adequate antituberculous therapy is initiated.

Pneumocystis carinii pneumonia (PCP) is currently the single most important cause of reversible morbidity and mortality in acquired immunodeficiency syndrome (AIDS). Recent studies document that in patients with AIDS, PCP, and impending respiratory failure, the early adjunctive use of glucocorticoids reduces the risk of respiratory failure and death.[24]

After prolonged therapy, glucocorticoid drugs must be withdrawn gradually to prevent the onset of symptoms related to adrenal insufficiency. Alternate-day oral therapy is a strategy that minimizes disturbances in normal adrenal function. During alternate-day therapy, twice the daily dosage of a glucocorticoid (previously taken every day) is administered every other day, preferably in the morning.

There is little doubt that the glucocorticoids are among the most powerful pharmacologic agents available for treating asthma and many of the other major obstructive and interstitial lung diseases. Because of their unpleasant and often dangerous side effects, however, they are reserved for use in patients who fail to respond to theophylline compounds or adrenergic amines with beta$_2$ activity, or both. For sustained use, glucocorticoid drugs are administered in the lowest effective dose possible. Complete relief of symptoms may ultimately have untoward consequences; therapeutic dose levels are empiric in that requirements vary. Therapy must be individualized. Once symptoms are under control, glucocorticoid doses are gradually tapered by small decrements until the lowest dose producing adequate clinical results is reached.

Early attempts to treat asthma with aerosols of hydrocortisone or prednisolone proved ineffective. The development of lipid-soluble corticosteroids suitable for inhalational therapy has transformed the management of moderately severe steroid-dependent asthma. With the success of aerosolized steroid preparations in severe asthma, there has been a growing consensus on the use of corticosteroid aerosols as the primary management for mild asthma (in conjunction with beta-agonists).

Side effects of aerosolized steroid preparations are primarily local, including oropharyngeal candidiasis and dysphonia. Higher doses appear to be more likely to cause these complications. Topical antifungal agents (e.g., nystatin) and simple techniques such as mouth rinsing are usually effective in protecting against and eliminating these local problems.

Table 52–7 lists glucocorticoids commonly employed for the control of symptoms in asthma and other respiratory diseases. The selection of a specific agent depends on the relative anti-inflammatory effect, mineralocorticoid activity, and preferred route of administration.

H$_1$-RECEPTOR ANTAGONISTS AND OTHER MEDIATOR-MODIFYING AGENTS

At present, the major agents available for modifying inflammatory responses include specific mediator antagonists (e.g., antihistamines) and agents felt to modify the inflammatory response by preventing the release of mediators from active cells. Antagonists to many of the recently characterized inflammatory mediators (e.g., leukotrienes, prostaglandins) are under investigation, but as yet few are available for clinical

TABLE **52–7:**   Properties of Commonly Administered Glucocorticoids in Asthma

Steroid	Relative Anti-inflammatory Strength	Relative Mineralocorticoid Strength	Routes of Administration	Duration of Action (Systemic)
Hydrocortisone	1	1	IV, IM, oral	Short
Cortisone	0.8	0.8	IV, IM, oral	Short
Prednisone	2.5–3.5	0.8	Oral	Intermediate
Prednisolone	3–4	0.8	IV, IM, oral	Intermediate
Methylprednisolone	4–5	0–0.8	IV, IM, oral	Intermediate
Triamcinolone	4–5	0	IV, IM, oral	Intermediate
Dexamethasone	20–40	0	IV, IM, oral, aerosol	Long
Betamethasone	20–30	0	IV, IM, oral, aerosol	Long
Beclomethasone	500 (topical)	0	Aerosol	

IV, intravenous; IM, intramuscular.

use. In general, those tested have not shown a clear-cut advantage over conventional therapy.

H₁-RECEPTOR ANTAGONISTS

Mechanism of Action

H₁-receptor antagonists, often referred to as antihistamines, are competitive antagonists of histamine at the H₁-receptor site. In particular, they block the constrictor effects of histamine on respiratory smooth muscle and the inflammatory action of histamine that results in increased capillary permeability, edema, and wheal formation. They are commonly used in respiratory care

- As therapy for allergic disorders such as rhinoconjunctivitis
- For symptomatic treatment of upper respiratory tract infections
- For the treatment of asthma

Some newer agents may offer mild benefits.

H₁-receptor antagonists have been available for some 50 years. A second generation of agents has been introduced over the past decade.[25] This family of newer agents distinguishes itself by the absence of sedation as a side effect.[26]

Many of the second-generation compounds reflect slight modifications of the structure of the first-generation parent.

Clinical Utility of Antihistamines

The major role for antihistamines in airway disease has been in the treatment of allergic rhinitis, acute upper respiratory infection, and asthma.

Allergic Rhinitis

The complex of symptoms associated with allergic rhinitis includes sneezing, nasal and palatal itching, nasal congestion, and watery rhinorrhea. Eye, ear, or sinus involvement is not uncommon, especially in severe cases.

Histamine is associated with many of these pathologic features of allergic rhinitis. For example, itching is caused by stimulation of H₁-receptors at sensory nerve endings. Mucosal edema and its associated nasal obstruction can be caused by H₁ stimulation; sneezing is due to an H₁-mediated neural reflex; and nasal mucus secretion can be triggered by histamine both directly and indirectly through muscarinic discharge.[27]

Acute Upper Respiratory Tract Infection

H₁-receptor antagonists are widely used for the symptomatic treatment of upper respiratory tract infections ("the common cold"). Their use in reducing rhinorrhea is probably due to their anticholinergic activity; however, the role of histamine in the common cold is not entirely clear and remains controversial.

Asthma

Airway mast cells contain most of the histamine found in the lung. A variety of physical (e.g., exercise, cold air) as well as chemical (e.g., allergens) insults can stimulate its release. Increased plasma levels of histamine have been associated with both allergen-induced and spontaneous bronchoconstriction. Antihistamines may be of benefit in certain types of asthma.[28]

MEDIATOR-MODIFYING COMPOUNDS

Sodium cromoglycate (SCG) (Fig. 52–7) is the first of a series of antiallergy medications introduced for the therapy of asthma and related allergic diseases.

Mechanism of Action

The mechanism by which SCG produces its therapeutic effect is poorly defined but continues to intrigue pharmacologists (Table 52–8). This mechanism appears to be unique and distinct from that of other classes of compounds used in airway disease. Initial characterization of SCG by Cox[29] suggested that inhibition of IgE-dependent mediator release from mast cells was the most likely mechanism for SCG's therapeutic effect in asthma (Fig. 52–8). Subsequently developed agents, however, with mast cell stabilizing effects similar to or greater than those of SCG have not been shown to have the therapeutic efficacy of SCG.

Clinical Utility of SCG

SCG is available in three formulations for clinical use in airway disease: "spin caps," solution for nebulizer administration, and pressurized metered dose inhaler.

In clinical studies in humans, SCG blocks both the immediate and the delayed response to antigen challenge of atopic asthma. Additionally, in asthmatics it blocks the response to exercise, to inhaled adenosine, hypotonic saline aerosol, cold air and hyperventilation, sulfur dioxide and industrial agents such as toluene diisocyanate (TDI). It also protects against challenge with aspirin and other agents that inhibit prostaglandin synthesis. Although all of these clinical effects suggest a wide range of useful applications for this agent, particularly in the case of targeted irritants (Table 52–9), the main rationale for its use remains the treatment of airway hyperreactivity. Regular administration has been shown to reduce airway responses to histamine in asthma. Enthusiasm for this agent appears greatest among pediatricians in the treatment of young atopic asthmatics.[30] This agent is infrequently prescribed for the management of adults, however, perhaps because of the more complex pathophysiology and associated contributing factors (e.g., bronchitis due to smoking) in this population.

Cromolyn sodium is available for the treatment of other allergic disorders, namely allergic rhinitis and allergic conjunctivitis (currently this preparation is not available in the United States).

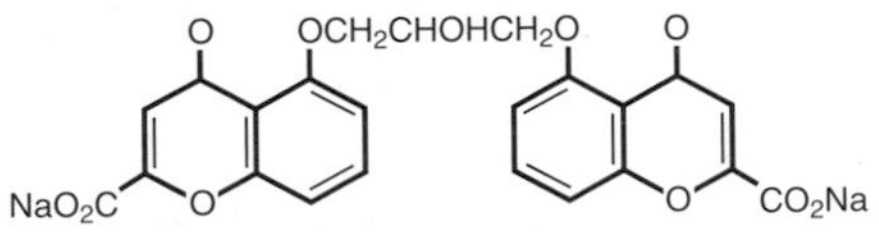

FIGURE 52–7: Chemical structure of sodium cromoglycate.

TABLE **52–8:** Postulated Mechanisms of Disodium Cromoglycate Action

Inhibition of IgE-mediated, mast cell degranulation	Alteration of intracellular calcium mobilization
Phosphodiesterase inhibition	Inhibition of neural irritant receptors

In humans, inhalation of the solution is not infrequently associated with a transient cough. Anaphylaxis has also been reported. Other allergic reactions include generalized dermatitis, facial dermatitis, myositis, and gastroenteritis. Pulmonary infiltrates with eosinophilia have also been described. Overall, however, this agent is well tolerated.

Two cromolyn-like agents have been widely tested and used in the treatment of asthma—nedocromil (Tilade) and ketotifen. (Nedocromil is currently approved for use in asthma. Ketotifen is not currently approved for use in the United States.)

MUCOKINETIC AGENTS AND ANTITUSSIVES

Abnormal quantities of mucus can be troublesome to patients with respiratory conditions, and numerous agents are available to improve its mobilization and clearance.[31, 32] Although widely used in clinical practice, well-controlled clinical trials demonstrating effectiveness are lacking for many of these agents. Nevertheless, Table 52–10 lists several terms to describe pharmacologic agents used to alter mucokinetic activity. The most commonly used agents are discussed here.

Hydrating Agents and Diluents

Bland aerosols include water and saline. Both can serve to hydrate or dilute mucus. Hydration refers to the situation in which water mole-

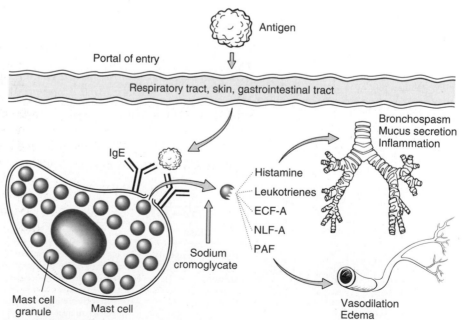

FIGURE 52–8: Postulated action of sodium cromoglycate on IgE-mediated mast cell degranulation. (Adapted from Stites DB, Stobo JD, Fudenberg HH, Wells JV. Basic Clinical Immunology, 5th ed. Los Altos, CA, Lange Medical Publications, 1984.)

TABLE **52–9:** Indications for Sodium Cromoglycate

Bronchial asthma (prophylactic management)
Prevention of exercise-induced asthma
Prevention of bronchospasm induced by environmental allergens and pollutants as well as
    toluene diisocyanate
Allergic rhinitis
Mastocytosis

cules are incorporated into the mucoprotein matrix of mucus, whereas diluents act to produce a dispersion of the solid mucoid constituents of mucus within the watery medium.

Sputum from patients with lung disease may have a lower water content than sputum from healthy individuals (i.e., 90 to 95% water). However, the benefit of increased fluid intake on the mechanical properties of sputum in such patients lacks objective evidence.

Inhaled aerosols of water offer limited mucokinetic effects. Coughing can occur following inhalation of these water aerosols, which may indirectly increase mucus production. However, bronchoconstriction can also result, which will hamper mucus flow.

Hypertonic saline aerosols have been shown to enhance mucociliary clearance in patients with chronic bronchitis. For diagnostic studies in patients who cannot spontaneously expectorate, hypertonic saline can be effective in inducing sputum.

Expectorants

Expectorants are drugs taken orally to promote or facilitate the removal of secretions from the respiratory airways. The pharmacologic basis for therapy with expectorants involves activation of the gastropulmonary mucokinetic vagal reflex. In this reflex, stimulation of the gastric mucosa initiates the secretion of mucus from bronchial glands, and the mucus is ultimately expectorated.

Guaifenesin

Now known as guaifenesin, this agent was initially referred to as glycerol guaiacolate or glyceryl guaiacolate. It has a short plasma half-life of about 1 hour.

In patients with chronic bronchitis and asthma, clinical improvement and decreases in sputum adhesiveness have been reported with this agent, and subjective improvements in sputum characteristics have been observed during acute upper respiratory tract infection. Subjective improvements have also been documented in stable bronchopulmonary

TABLE **52–10:** Primary Mucokinetic Drugs Used in Respiratory Care

Class	Action	Examples
Hydrating agent	Causes water to be incorporated into the structure of respiratory secretions	Water Salt water solutions
Diluent	Dilutes respiratory secretion by the addition of water	Water Salt solutions
Expectorant	Acts reflectively on bronchial glands to increase output of secretion	Guaifenesin Potassium salts
Mucolytic	Breaks up glycoproteins, other proteins, DNA, and macromolecules into smaller components	Acetylcysteine

disease, but such findings have not been universal. Likewise, improvements have been observed in mucociliary clearance rates.

Although the effectiveness of guaifenesin has been debated, subjective improvements in conditions characterized by abnormal sputum have been observed following treatment. There appears to be some evidence suggesting that such improvements are associated with changes in sputum characteristics.

Guaifenesin is available in many products, including a host of non-prescription cold products. The recommended dose for adults and children 12 years of age and older is 200 to 400 mg every 4 hours not to exceed 2400 mg in 24 hours. For children aged 6 to 12 years, the oral dosage is 100 to 200 mg every 4 hours, not to exceed 600 mg in 24 hours. Extended-release preparations of guaifenesin are also available.

Iodine-Containing Agents

Iodine is a nonmetallic halide element whose ion (iodide) may have several effects on the respiratory system, including increased mucus secretion, improved ciliary beating, mucolytic effects, and expectoration. Both inorganic and organic preparations of iodine have mucokinetic properties.[33] *Inorganic iodide* is used as an expectorant primarily in the form of potassium iodide (KI) and is given in a saturated solution (SSKI). It is a clear, odorless liquid with a salty, metallic taste. In addition to its emetic-like actions as an expectorant, mucolytic action has been demonstrated; it may improve mucociliary clearance. Clinical benefit, including looser phlegm, has been reported. A saturated solution of potassium iodide is available on a prescription basis (SSKI) and contains 1 g of potassium iodide per milliliter.

The organic iodine used for respiratory therapeutics is iodinated glycerol (Organidin). The product is a viscous stable liquid that does not contain inorganic iodide or free iodine. Renewed interest in the drug followed a relatively recent multicenter study of patients with stable bronchitis in which improvement in expectoration with therapy was reported.[34]

Iodinated glycerol (or propylene glycol) is available in solution, tablets, and elixir. The recommended adult dose of the 5% solution, which is added to fruit juice or other liquid, is 20 drops four times a day (one drop of solution equals approximately 3 mg iodinated glycerol). The recommended adult dose of the 30-mg tablets is two tablets four times a day with liquid; the adult dose for the 1.2% elixir is one teaspoonful four times a day. Recommended children's doses are up to one half the adult doses based on the child's weight.

Mucolytics

Agents capable of modifying the chemical composition of mucus to improve its physical properties are called mucolytics.

Acetylcysteine. Acetylcysteine (*N*-acetyl-L-cysteine or NAC) is the *N*-acetyl derivative of the natural amino acid, L-cysteine. The basis for the therapeutic action of NAC as a mucolytic is the ability of its free sulfhydril group to interact with disulfide bonds in mucoprotein.[31] This interaction causes rupture of disulfide bonds that bind mucoprotein molecules to each other and to DNA. This lysis results in less viscous mucus. Reduced viscosity of sputum has been demonstrated in patients with cystic fibrosis, asthma, emphysema, bronchitis, and silicotuberculosis.

NAC has been delivered by direct instillation into endotracheal tubes to break up inspissated tracheobronchial secretions. Its beneficial use with fiberoptic bronchoscopy to relieve mucus plugging in asthma and atelectasis has been reported.

Nebulization of NAC has been shown to be effective in increasing sputum volume and decreasing sputum viscosity as well as in relieving postoperative atelectasis.

Inhalation of NAC aerosol (mainly the 20% solution) results in reported side effects in a few patients, usually mild nausea and stomatitis. Airway obstruction can follow NAC inhalation in susceptible patients, particularly those with airway hyperresponsiveness. Airway obstruction induced by NAC can be relieved by a bronchodilator.

rhDNase. High concentrations of DNA, derived from disintegrating inflammatory cells, contribute to the thick, viscous secretions in conditions such as cystic fibrosis. Recently, recombinant human DNA I (rhDNase, Genentech, San Francisco, CA), a 37-kd glycosylated enzyme produced in Chinese hamster ovary cells,[35] has been approved in the management of cystic fibrosis patients. The purpose of this therapy is to assist in reducing the frequency of respiratory infections requiring parenteral antibiotics and to improve pulmonary function. A preliminary study in cystic fibrosis patients has shown that although treatment with aerosolized rhDNase did not increase the volume of sputum more than a placebo, it was effective in improving lung function.[36] Biologic activity of the aerosolized rhDNase on respiratory tract secretions was demonstrated by the detection of cleaved DNA in sputum after treatment. The clinical utility of this agent in other airway diseases, such as bronchitis and bronchiectasis is currently under investigation.

Antitussive Agents

Agents that reduce coughing act either peripherally or centrally. Numerous agents are available.

Codeine. Like morphine, codeine is derived from opium, and is therefore termed an opiate, or more generally, an opioid. Because it can produce sedation and cause dependence, codeine is also classified in the legal context as a narcotic.

Morphine and related opioids affect primarily the central nervous system and gastrointestinal system. Such effects provide the basis for the use of morphine and related opioids such as codeine for the symptomatic treatment of pain, cough, and diarrhea. Morphine suppresses respiratory drive; death from morphine poisoning is nearly always due to hypoventilation and respiratory arrest.

Clearly the benefit of cough suppression needs to be weighed against the risk of potential side effects. Codeine, the most common opioid antitussive, has several advantages over morphine, including less addiction potential and less tendency to cause respiratory depression, bronchospasm, or constipation. Furthermore, such opioid side effects can be reduced or avoided by the use of nonopioid nonaddictive antitussives.

Dextromethorphan. A methylated dextroisomer of levorphenol, dextromethorphan

- Does not possess significant analgesic effect
- Does not suppress respiration
- Is not associated with addiction

• Is one of the most widely used antitussive agents in the United States

In adults, the recommended dose is 10 to 30 mg every 4 to 8 hours, not to exceed 120 mg in 24 hours. In children 6 to 12 years, the recommended dose is 5 to 10 mg every 4 hours or 15 mg every 6 to 8 hours, not to exceed 30 mg in 24 hours. Individual product instructions should be consulted for exact dosage and frequency.

Miscellaneous Antitussives. Diphenhydramine, a first-generation H_1-receptor antagonist (antihistamine), is regarded as an effective antitussive. Its action is due to a central mechanism involving the medullary cough centers with possible peripheral action as well.

ANTIMICROBIAL AGENTS

Antibiotics act directly on microorganisms and do not increase the normal defense mechanisms of patients receiving them. These drugs inhibit (bacteriostatic) or kill (bactericidal) microorganisms by selectively interfering with the function of certain of their vital constituents, such as enzymes, ribosomes, and nucleic acids.

Mechanism of Action

An understanding of the mechanisms of action of common antimicrobials requires a knowledge of the structure and metabolic activity of microorganisms.

The bacterial cell is surrounded by a series of complex biochemical layers beginning with a *cytoplasmic membrane*. This membrane, like the membrane of higher organisms, consists primarily of phospholipids in which proteins are embedded.

Many bacteria, both gram-positive and gram-negative, have an additional layer surrounding them, *the capsule*, which is composed of complex polysaccharides. This capsule may enhance the virulence of certain bacteria (e.g., type III *Pneumococcus*) by making them more difficult to ingest by white blood cells.

In addition to the preceding structures in the outer coating of bacteria, there are two additional structures commonly present in bacteria:

• *Flagella*, which serve the purpose of locomotion
• *Pili*, which allow bacteria to join and transfer genetic material, in particular information allowing them to resist various classes of antibiotics

Bacterial metabolism is controlled by genetic material DNA, which is synthesized from nucleic acids and stores information for the "coding" of bacterial peptides and proteins. This information is transferred to RNA by copying of nucleic acid "messages" (transcription). Peptides are synthesized along bacterial polyribosomes where messenger RNA establishes a cellular "production line" (translation). Antibiotics exert their antibacterial effects by one of six mechanisms (Table 52–11 and Fig. 52–9).

The toxic selectivity of antimicrobial agents for infectious microorganisms (and not human cells) depends on certain key structural and functional differences between microorganisms and human cells. In spite

TABLE **52–11:**   Modes of Action of Antibiotics

Inhibition of cell wall synthesis	Inhibition of DNA replication
Interference with cell membrane function	Inhibition of DNA transcription
Interference with nucleic acid synthesis	Inhibition of protein synthesis (translation)

of great differences between humans and microbes, not all anti-infectious substances are harmless to human cells.

Many bacteria are either naturally resistant to certain classes of antibiotics (e.g., erythromycin for gram-negative bacilli) or can develop resistance as a result of biochemical or genetic changes during treatment.[37] The latter development is particularly common with staphylococci, gram-negative bacilli, and *Mycobacterium tuberculosis*. Bacterial resistance represents a major therapeutic problem because it significantly restricts the usefulness of many antibiotics, often necessitating the substitution of toxic and less potent drugs when the more acceptable antimicrobials are found to be ineffective. Table 52–12 lists examples of some of the most common bacterial mechanisms for drug resistance.

Whenever possible, antibiotics are administered orally, but the effectiveness of this route is limited in general to milder infections or infections that have initially been treated by a course of parenteral antibiotics.

When high serum concentrations are required, as in sepsis, the parenteral route, and intravenous dosing in particular, is indicated. Measurements of serum levels of antibiotics, particularly the aminoglycosides, have been used to monitor the minimal effective dosage and the potential for toxicity, particularly in patients with kidney or liver disease.

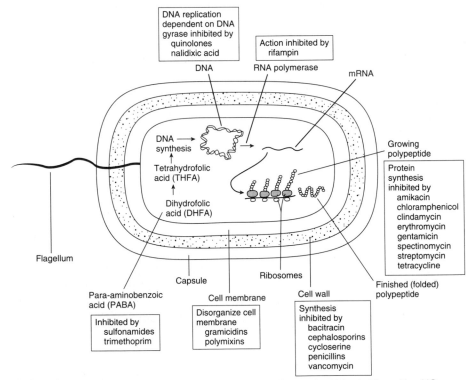

FIGURE 52–9: Mechanisms of action of major antibiotic agents. (Adapted from Neu HC. Antimicrobial chemotherapy. *In* Baron S (ed). Medical Microbiology, 3rd ed. New York, Churchill Livingstone, 1991, p 180.)

TABLE 52–12: Mechanisms of Microbial Resistance to Antibiotics

Mechanism	Example
Lack of specific bacterial receptors necessary to bind antibiotics	*Streptococcus pneumoniae (Pneumococcus)* resistance to penicillin
Lack of metabolic pathway inhibited by drug or adaptation of other pathways	Change in bacterial dihydrofolate reductase, rendering it less susceptible to trimethoprim
Inadequate permeability of antibiotics through the cell wall	Tetracycline penetration into otherwise susceptible organisms (gram-negative) is impaired
Synthesis of an enzyme that destroys the antibiotic	Beta-lactamase enzymes cleave the central ring
Alteration of cell structures to which the antibiotic binds	Change in 30s and 50s ribosomes, preventing binding with macrolides (erythromycin) and aminoglycosides
Inactivation of drug by bacterial metabolism	Acetylation of chloramphenicol by enzyme (chloramphenicol transacetylase)

Treatment of respiratory infections with aerosolized antibiotics was advocated as early as the 1940s. The presence of thick airway and parenchymal exudates, especially in localized sites of infection, is considered to be a formidable diffusion barrier for these agents to overcome. The rationale for antibiotic aerosol therapy originated with the idea that these diffusion barriers could at least be partially bypassed by direct topical application of antimicrobial drugs onto the tracheobronchial tree. Currently, antibiotic therapy administered by aerosol is used primarily in three specific situations.

1. The prophylactic therapy of PCP in patients with AIDS[38]
2. The treatment of respiratory syncytial virus disease in young children with severe lower respiratory tract infections[39]
3. The treatment of *Pseudomonas* respiratory infections in patients with cystic fibrosis

Despite these relatively recent indications for aerosolized antibiotics, many problems arise from their use (Table 52–13).[40]

Clinical Utility of Antimicrobials

Nine major classes of antibiotics provide a wide selection of agents, which allows the clinician to balance potential organisms and severity of infection against the hazards of side effects and the risk of bacterial resistance.[41]

Penicillins

The penicillins are among the most important of the bactericidal antibiotics. For pulmonary infections, penicillins occupy a central role in antimicrobial therapy for pneumococcal pneumonia, nonhospital-acquired aspiration pneumonia, and pulmonary suppuration (lung abscess). Currently, five groups of penicillin exist: (1) penicillin G and V, (2) penicillinase-resistant penicillins (methicillin), (3) aminopenicillins (ampicillin), (4) carboxypenicillins (carbenicillin), and (5) ureidopenicillins (piperacillin).

Cephalosporins

Cephalosporins resemble the penicillins in several major respects, including:

TABLE 52–13: Disadvantages of Antibiotics Delivered by Aerosol to the Respiratory Tract

Bronchospasm is a frequent complication.
Deposited antimicrobial agents may be inactivated by mucous constituents.
Effective dose ranges are not established.
Aerosolized drugs may not penetrate or be retained at the site of infection.
Airborne antimicrobials may contribute to the development of hospital microorganisms that demonstrate selective resistance.
Untoward systemic effects are not necessarily eliminated.
The most appropriate method of aerosolization of antimicrobials has not been established.
Techniques that have been employed in the nebulization of antimicrobials often involve expensive equipment and considerable time for the respiratory therapist.
Individuals other than the intended recipient are exposed to airborne antimicrobial agents (e.g., nurses administering ribavirin).

- *Structurally*: by the presence of a beta-lactam ring
- *Mechanism of action*: inhibition of cell wall synthesis

Like the penicillins, the cephalosporins are bactericidal. By contrast, these antibiotics, which resist the action of penicillinase, are active against both gram-positive and gram-negative bacteria. Since their discovery, a large number of semisynthetic derivatives have been added to this class of antimicrobials. For historical as well as therapeutic reasons, the new additions to this family have been classified into three "generations." Table 52–14 lists representative compounds.

Carbapenems

The only currently available representative of this class of antibiotics is imipenem. It is the broadest spectrum agent available with only a

TABLE 52–14: Selected Cephalosporins, Route of Administration, Dose, Frequency Indication

Antibiotic	Route of Administration	Single Dose	Frequency (Hr)	General Indications
First Generation				
Cephalothin	IM, IV	1–2 g	4	Gram-positive *(Staphylococcus)* susceptible infections
Cefazolin	IM, IV	1–1.5 g	6	Gram-positive *(Staphylococcus)* susceptible infections
Cephalexin	PO	1 g	6	Surgical prophylaxis Gram-positive susceptible infections
Second Generation				
Cefamandole	IM, IV	2 g	4	Gram-positive *Haemophilus influenzae*
Cefuroxime	IM, IV, PO	0.75–1.5 g	8	Community-acquired pneumonia (penetrates the cerebrospinal fluid)
Cefaclor	PO	1 g	8	
Third Generation				
Cefotaxime	IM, IV	2 g	4	Gram-negative infections (not *Pseudomonas*)
Ceftriaxone	IM, IV	2 g	12–24	Gram-negative infections (not *Pseudomonas*)
Cefoperazone	IM, IV	1.5–4 g	6–12	Most active against *Pseudomonas* (does not penetrate cerebrospinal fluid)
Ceftazidime	IM, IV	2 g	8	Most active against *Pseudomonas*

IM, intramuscular; IV, intravenous; PO, by mouth.

few select organisms currently showing resistance, including *P. cepacia* and *maltophilia*, and most methicillin-resistant staphylococci. This drug is not absorbed through the gastrointestinal tract, so it must be given parenterally. Severe infections respond to this antibiotic, but it should be used conservatively to prevent the emergence of resistant strains.

Monobactams

Currently, only one agent in the monobactam group is commercially available, aztreonam. Its activity, which is directed against gram-negative organisms only, is particularly useful against organisms resistant to other antibiotics. Because it does not cover gram-positive organisms, it is not used alone for the treatment of sepsis of unknown cause. Despite its chemical structure, it does not appear to have significant cross-reactivity with the penicillins.

Aminoglycosides

The aminoglycosides continue to represent a major group of parenteral antimicrobial drugs used in the treatment of serious respiratory tract infections. Serious toxicity, particularly ototoxicity and nephrotoxicity, occurs with all the members of this group. Antibiotics from this group demonstrate a broad antibacterial spectrum, including many gram-negative organisms. Important drugs in the aminoglycoside family that are used in respiratory tract infections include gentamicin, amikacin, kanamycin, tobramycin, and streptomycin.

Quinolones

The quinolones are a newer group of agents with a broad spectrum of activity. The number of approved quinolones for use in the United States is rapidly increasing (e.g., ciprofloxacin, ofloxacin). These agents currently enjoy a broad spectrum of action against hard to treat organisms including *P. aeruginosa*, resistant gram-negative organisms, and methicillin-resistant *Staphylococcus aureus*. They can be administered orally, and their pattern of side effects is relatively mild. Parenterally administered quinolones may have an important role to play in the treatment of nosocomial pneumonia, particularly gram-negative pneumonias in immunocompromised hosts. In patients with cystic fibrosis, oral ciprofloxacin has been used successfully for the control of pulmonary exacerbations with *P. aeruginosa*.

Macrolide Antibiotics

Erythromycin, the best known macrolide antibiotic, has been available for more than 30 years. This agent continues to enjoy extensive use in respiratory infection. Macrolide antibiotics, which work by interfering with bacterial synthesis of proteins, in general are bacteriostatic. Erythromycin is most effective against gram-positive bacteria, including beta-hemolytic streptococci and *Streptococcus pneumoniae*. It is the drug of choice for *Mycoplasma pneumoniae* and *Legionella*. This spectrum makes it a drug of choice for community-acquired pneumonia in the noncompromised host who can be treated on an outpatient basis. It is also used as an alternative drug in the penicillin-sensitive patient. A number of newer macrolide antibiotics are now in use, including clarithromycin and azithromycin. The advantages of these agents include better activity against erythromycin-resistant strains, fewer gastrointestinal side effects, and less frequent dosing.

Sulfonamides

Sulfonamides are chemotherapeutic agents that are bacteriostatic against many gram-positive and gram-negative bacteria (excluding *Pseudomonas* organisms). Their effectiveness against respiratory pathogens, in particular *Haemophilus influenzae*, *Diplococcus pneumoniae*, and *Klebsiella*, is generally less than that of other antibiotics, with their use generally being limited to urinary tract infections.

Since 1968, the combination drug trimethoprim-sulfamethoxazole (TMP-SMX) has found wide therapeutic application. The TMP-SMX combination has high activity against *H. influenzae* and *S. pneumoniae*. This antibiotic is commonly used for respiratory infections in patients with chronic bronchitis and cystic fibrosis.

TMP-SMX is currently the agent of choice for patients with PCP. Patients with AIDS require a 3-week course of treatment. These patients are particularly susceptible to adverse reactions with this agent (> 50% in some studies), thereby requiring alternative therapy with pentamidine, trimetrexate, or dapsone. Prophylaxis of AIDS patients has been recommended by a National Institutes of Health task force on *P. carinii* prophylaxis for AIDS patients with a history of at least one *P. carinii* infection or a CD4 (lymphocyte) cell count of less than 200/mm^3. These patients may receive oral TMP-SMX twice daily on a continuous basis, although some authors recommend intermittent treatment (3 days a week).

Pentamidine

Pentamidine is a chemotherapeutic agent of the diamidine group. The major use of this drug currently is as an alternative to TMP-SMX in the treatment of PCP as well as a prophylactic agent in immunocompromised patients at risk for this disease (e.g., those with AIDS). The drug can be administered either intramuscularly or intravenously.

Serious pancreatitis and hypoglycemia may occur as side effects, as may renal dysfunction, thrombocytopenia, and hypocalcemia. (Because of these side effects and the availability of other agents, pentamidine is no longer the drug of choice for PCP.)

Pentamidine is also administered by aerosol as a prophylactic agent in patients at risk for PCP, particularly AIDS patients. Prophylaxis consists of a single aerosol treatment of 300 mg once a month. Care must be taken to administer the appropriate particle size, as great differences in success have been attributed to different nebulizer systems. Unlike parenterally administered pentamidine, aerosolized pentamidine has virtually no serious toxic effects. It is, however, less effective than TMP-SMX and is usually reserved for patients who cannot tolerate TMP-SMX.

Antituberculous Agents

The treatment of pulmonary tuberculosis (caused by *M. tuberculosis* as well as the atypical mycobacteria, particularly *M. avium* and *M. kansasii*) involves a complex approach of evaluation and care because of the nature of the organisms, characteristics of the disease process, and the possible immunocompromise of patients with these infections (particularly AIDS patients). Antituberculosis drugs inhibit the multiplication of these bacilli, but their intracellular invasion complicates eradication. Drugs have traditionally been considered "first"- and "second"-line based on efficacy and side effects. Table 52–15 lists these agents. Additionally, new investigational agents are currently being evaluated, including clofazimine, rifabutin (Ansamycin), quinolones, and newer macrolides.

To reduce the development of mycobacterial resistance and to produce a synergistic antituberculous effect, two to three of the first-line drugs are administered concurrently. In patients with nonresistant *M. tuberculosis* who are compliant, regimens of isoniazid and rifampin given for 6 or 9 months (possibly with the addition of pyrazinamide or ethambutol) results in effective cure.

Drug-resistant tuberculosis is an issue of increasing concern to the health community. A recent review by Snider and colleagues[42] demonstrated that from 1982 to 1986, 5.3% of never treated and 19.4% of previously treated tuberculosis patients were resistant to isoniazid. Primary drug resistance had risen from 6.9% in a previous survey to 9% in the current survey.[42] Of perhaps even greater concern is the concurrence of human immunodeficiency virus (HIV) infection and tuberculosis. HIV-infected patients have an excess of tuberculous infection. In the United States, this has been notable among drug abusers and Haitian immigrants. Fortunately, treatment of drug-sensitive organisms with standard regimens has been effective. The American Thoracic Society suggests that therapy should be continued for at least 6 months beyond sputum conversion.[43] Additionally, isoniazid prophylaxis is recommended for HIV-infected individuals with positive tuberculin skin tests as well as HIV-infected patients who were formerly tuberculin-positive. The increasing prevalence of drug resistance both in the general population and in HIV-infected persons may require the initiation of multiple-drug regimens (four drugs or more) for patients with smear-positive disease in whom the sensitivity of the organism is not known. If the organism is later found to be not resistant, a standard regimen could be continued.

Antiviral Therapy

Therapy for viruses presents a fundamentally different problem for chemotherapy in that viruses, unlike most other microorganisms, do not have an independent metabolic system, as do bacteria or fungi, but rely on the host (human) cells to provide the machinery for their fundamental processes. These processes include replication of viral genetic material and production of viral protein necessary for the viral shell. Most of the available agents are related structurally to purines and pyrimidines that viruses must incorporate into their genetic structure. These analogues ultimately interrupt the viral genetic message or interfere with enzymes that synthesize viral genetic material. Specific agents of particular interest to respiratory practitioners include amantadine, ribavirin, and zidovudine (AZT).

TABLE **52–15:** First- and Second-Line Antituberculous Agents

First Line	Second Line
Isoniazid	Ethionamide
Rifampin	Para-aminosalicylic acid
Ethambutol	Cycloserine
Pyrazinamide	Kanamycin
Streptomycin	Amikacin
	Capreomycin

TABLE **52–16:** Compendium of Respiratory Care Drugs Administered by Inhalation

Drug Class	Drug Name	Brand Name*	Dose Form	Usual Adult Dosage†
Sympathomimetic	Albuterol	Proventil or Ventolin	Inhalation aerosol (90 μg/puff) Solution (0.5%)	2 Inhalations q4hr to q6hr Nebulize 2.5 mg (0.5 mL) t.i.d. to q.i.d.
		Ventolin Rotacaps	(200 μg/cap)	1 Capsule q4hr to q6hr
	Bitolterol	Tornalate	Inhalation aerosol (0.37 mg/puff)	2 Inhalations q8hr
	Epinephrine	Primatene	Inhalation aerosol (0.16 mg/puff)	1 Inhalation; 2 if needed (wait 3 hrs before reuse)
	Isoetharine	Bronkosol	Inhalation aerosol (0.34 mg/puff) Solution (1%)	1–2 Puffs not >q4hr Nebulize (0.25–0.5 mL) not >q4hr
	Isoproterenol	Isuprel	Inhalation aerosol (131 μg/puff) Solution (1% & 0.5%)	Individualize Individualize
	Metaproterenol	Alupent	Inhalation aerosol (0.65 mg/puff) Solution (5%)	2–3 Inhalations q3hr to q4hr Nebulize (0.3 mL) not >q4hr
	Pirbuterol	Maxair	Inhalation aerosol (0.2 mg/puff)	2 Inhalations q4hr to q6hr
	Racemic epinephrine	Vaponefrin	Solution (2.25%)	0.25–0.5 mL, 4–6 times daily
	Terbutaline	Brethaire	Inhalation aerosol (0.2 mg/puff)	2 Inhalations q4hr to q6hr
	Salmeterol	Serevent	Inhalation aerosol (25 μg/puff)	2 Inhalations b.i.d.
Antimuscarinic	Ipratropium bromide	Atrovent	Inhalation aerosol (18 μg/puff) Solution (0.02%)	2 Inhalations q.i.d. Nebulize 2.5 mL t.i.d. to q.i.d.
Corticosteroids	Beclomethasone	Beclovent, Vanceril	Inhalation aerosol (42 μg/puff)	2 Inhalations t.i.d. or q.i.d.
	Dexamethasone	Decadron Respihaler	Inhalation aerosol (0.084 mg/puff)	3 Inhalations t.i.d. or q.i.d.
	Flunisolide	AeroBid	Inhalation aerosol (250 μg/puff)	2 Inhalations b.i.d.
	Triamcinolone	Azmacort	Inhalation aerosol (100 μg/puff)	2 Inhalations t.i.d. to q.i.d.
Miscellaneous antiasthma	Cromolyn sodium	Intal	Capsule (20 mg) Solution (20 mg/2 mL) Inhalation aerosol (800 μg/puff)	1 Capsule q.i.d. Nebulize 1 ampule q.i.d. 2 Inhalations q.i.d.
	Nedocromil sodium	Tilade	Inhalation aerosol (1.75 mg/puff)	2 Inhalations q.i.d.
Mucoregulators	N-acetylcysteine	Mucomyst	Solution (10% & 20%)	Nebulize 3–5 mL t.i.d. or q.i.d.
	rhDNase	Pulmozyme	Inhalation solution (2.5 mg)	1 Ampule (0.1%) q.i.d.

*Brand name or representative brand name.
†Consult package insert of products for current dosage information, including recommendations for individualized dosages.

Amantadine. This agent inhibits replication of influenza A virus. Clinically it is effective in preventing disease in patients exposed to persons with active disease. Patients who are at high risk for the development of complications of the disease (e.g., elderly individuals) are treated for the duration of the epidemic. Patients can be vaccinated at this time.

The dose for adults is 200 mg daily, which is well absorbed orally. Side effects tend to include mild disturbances of the central nervous system.

Because of the potential teratogenic effects of ribavirin, respiratory personnel administering or preparing this agent should wear respiratory protection capable of filtering the aerosol.

Ribavirin. Structurally related to the pyrimidines, ribavirin has a broad spectrum of antiviral activity, with its primary usefulness being against respiratory syncytial virus. Administered by aerosol to hospitalized infants with documented lower respiratory tract infection, the drug is mixed in sterile water at a concentration of 20 mg/mL. It is delivered as an aerosol over 12 to 18 hours, with treatments continuing for 3 to 7 days. Deterioration of respiratory function has been observed in treated infants.

Zidovudine. Treatment of infection by HIV has become a priority of antiviral therapy in the 1990s.

The exact mechanism by which zidovudine influences the life cycle of HIV is not completely understood, but it is generally accepted that the drug can selectively incorporate into the viral genome under the influence of retroviral reverse transcriptase, causing the viral DNA chain to prematurely terminate. Zidovudine is felt to lower the immediate mortality of AIDS and prolongs life expectancy. In patients infected with HIV but without overt disease, the onset of AIDS can be delayed. Side effects are common, the most serious being hematologic, including anemia and neutropenia.

SUMMARY

The respiratory care practitioner is a key member in the management of some of the most critically ill patients treated inside and outside the hospital setting. In addition to administering a constantly expanding list of aerosolized medications, the therapist needs to know and understand

- The wide variety of pharmacologic agents used in the management of patients with respiratory diseases
- Their mechanism of action
- Their side effects

The classes of agents reviewed in this chapter are among those most frequently encountered by the respiratory care practitioner (Table 52–16). It is anticipated that this list will continue to grow with the advances made in the management of these patients. Keeping up with these developments requires a sound foundation in the principles of basic pharmacologic science and medical therapeutics.

References

1. Strader CD, Sigal IS, Dixon RAF. Mapping the functional domain of the beta adrenergic receptor. Am J Respir Cell Mol Biol 1:81–86, 1989.
2. Barnes PJ. Airway pharmacology. *In* Murray JF, Nadel JA (eds). Textbook of Respiratory Medicine. Philadelphia, WB Saunders, 1988, pp 249–268.
3. Lulich KM, Goldie RG, Ryan G, Paterson JW. Adverse reactions to B-2 agonist bronchodilators. Med Toxicol 1:286–299, 1986.
4. Lofdahl CG. Basic pharmacology of new long-acting sympathomimetics. Lung 168(Suppl):18–21, 1990.
5. Becker AB, Simons KJ, Gillespie CA, Simons FER. The bronchodilator effects and pharmacokinetics of caffeine in asthma. N Engl J Med 310:743–746, 1984.
5a. Sutherland EW, Roll TW. The relation of adenosine 3'5'-phosphate and phosphorylase to the actions of catecholamines and other hormones. Pharmacol Rev 12:263–299, 1960.
6. Kolbeck RC, Speir WA Jr, Carrier GO, Bransome ED Jr. Apparent irrelevance of cyclic nucleotides to the relaxation of tracheal smooth muscle induced by theophylline. Lung 156:173–183, 1979.

7. Cushley MJ, Tattersfield AE, Holgate ST. Adenosine induced bronchoconstriction in asthma: Antagonism by inhaled theophylline. Am Rev Respir Dis 129:380–384, 1984.
8. Mackay AD, Baldwin CJ, Tattersfield AE. Action of intravenously administered aminophylline on normal airways. Am Rev Respir Dis 127:609–613, 1983.
9. Barnes PJ, Greening AP, Neville L, et al. Single dose slow release aminophylline at night prevents nocturnal asthma. Lancet 1:299–301, 1982.
10. Murciano D, Aubier M, Le Cocguic Y, Pariente R. Effects of theophylline on diaphragmatic strength and fatigue in patients with chronic obstructive pulmonary disease. N Engl J Med 311:349–353, 1984.
11. Appel D, Shim C. Comparative effect of epinephrine and aminophylline in the treatment of asthma. Lung 159:243–254, 1981.
12. Littenberg B. Aminophylline treatment in severe acute asthma. JAMA 259:1678–1684, 1988.
13. Hill NS. The use of theophylline in "irreversible" chronic obstructive pulmonary disease. Arch Intern Med 148:2579–2584, 1988.
14. Tsiu SJ, Self TH, Burns R. Theophylline toxicity update. Ann Allergy 64:241–257, 1990.
15. Barnes PJ, Basbaum CB, Nadel JA. Autoradiographic localization of autonomic receptors in airway smooth muscle: Marked differences between large and small airways. Am Rev Respir Dis 127:758–762, 1983.
16. Murlas C, Nadel JA, Roberts JM. The muscarinic receptors of airway smooth muscle: Their characterization in vitro. J Appl Physiol 52:1084–1091, 1982.
17. Gross NJ, Skorodin MS. Anticholinergic, antimuscarinic bronchodilators. Am Rev Respir Dis 129:856–870, 1984.
18. Mann JS, George CF. Anticholinergic drugs in the treatment of airway disease. Br J Dis Chest 79:209–228, 1985.
19. Braun SR, McKenzie WN, Copeland C, et al. A comparison of the effect of ipratropium and albuterol in the treatment of chronic obstructive airway disease. Arch Intern Med 149:544–547, 1989.
20. Tashkin DP, Ashutosh K, Bleecker ER, et al. Comparison of the anticholinergic bronchodilator ipratropium bromide with metaproterenol in chronic obstructive airway disease: A 90 day multicenter study. Am J Med 81(Suppl 5A):81–90, 1986.
21. Munck A, Mendel DB, Smith LI, Orti E. Glucocorticoid receptors and actions. Am Rev Respir Dis 141:S2–S11, 1990.
22. Reed CE. Aerosol glucocorticoid treatment of asthma. Am Rev Respir Dis 141:S82–S88, 1990.
23. Callahan CM, Dittus RS, Katz BP. Oral corticosteroid therapy for patients with stable chronic obstructive pulmonary disease. Ann Intern Med 114:216–223, 1991.
24. Borzette SA, Sattler FR, Chia J, et al. A controlled trial of early adjunctive treatment with corticosteroids for *Pneumocystis carinii* pneumonia in the acquired immunodeficiency syndrome. N Engl J Med 323:1451–1457, 1990.
25. Simons FER, Simons KJ. Second generation H1-receptor antagonists. Ann Allergy 66:5–19, 1991.
26. Metzler EO. Performance effects of antihistamines. J Allergy Clin Immunol 86:613–619, 1990.
27. White MV. The role of histamine in allergic disease. J Allergy Clin Immunol 86:599–605, 1990.
28. Holgate ST, Finnerty JP. Antihistamines in asthma. J Allergy Clin Immunol 83:537–547, 1989.
29. Cox JSG. Disodium cromoglycate (FPL 670, 'Intal'), a specific inhibitor of reaginic antigen-antibody mechanisms. Nature 81:1328–1329, 1967.
30. Toogood JH, Lefcoe NM, Wonnacott TM, et al. Cromolyn sodium therapy: Predictors of response. Adv Asthma Allergy Pulmonary Dis 5:2–15, 1978.
31. Ziment I. Agents that affect respiratory mucus. *In* Witek TJ Jr, Schachter EN (eds). Problems in Respiratory Care, vol 1. Philadelphia, JB Lippincott, 1988, pp 15–41.
32. Ziment I. Help for an overtaxed mucociliary system: Managing abnormal mucus. J Respir Dis 12:21–33, 1991.
33. Ziment I. Inorganic and organic iodides. *In* Bragga PC, Allegra L (eds). Drugs in Bronchial Mucology. New York, Raven Press, 1989, pp 251–260.
34. Petty TL. The national mucolytic study. Results of a randomized, double blind, placebo-controlled study of iodinated glycerol in chronic obstructive bronchitis. Chest 97:75–83, 1990.
35. Shak S, Capon DJ, Helimiss R, et al. Recombinant human DNase I reduces the viscosity of cystic fibrosis sputum. Proc Natl Acad Sci USA 87:9188–9192, 1990.
36. Hubband RC, McElvaney NG, Birrer P, et al. A preliminary study of aerosolized recombinant human deoxyribonuclease I in the treatment of cystic fibrosis. N Engl J Med 326:812–815, 1992.
37. Farrar WE. Bacterial resistance. *In* Lambert HP, O'Grady FW (eds). Antibiotic and Chemotherapy. Edinburgh, Churchill Livingstone, 1992, pp 303–312.
38. Leoung GS, Feigal DW, Montgomery AB, et al. Aerosolized pentamidine for prophylaxis against *Pneumocystis carinii* pneumonia. N Engl J Med 323:769–775, 1990.
39. Keating MR. Antiviral agents. Mayo Clin Proc 67:160–178, 1992.
40. Hodson ME. Antibiotic treatment. Aerosol therapy. Chest 94(Suppl):156S–160S, 1988.

41. Wilkowske CJ. General principles of antimicrobial therapy. Mayo Clin Proc 66:931–941, 1991.
42. Snider DE, Canthen GM, Farer LS, et al. Drug resistant tuberculosis. Am Rev Respir Dis 144:732, 1991.
43. Lambert HP, O'Grady FW. Tuberculosis and leprosy. *In* Lambert HP, O'Grady FW (eds). Antibiotic and Chemotherapy. Edinburgh, Churchill Livingstone, 1992, pp 471–480.

53

Pediatric Respiratory Care

Shekhar T. Venkataraman, M.D., Al Saville, R.R.T., Drew Wiltsie, R.R.T., John Frank, R.R.T., and Charles W. Boig, Jr., R.R.T.

Key Terms

Asynchrony

Extracorporeal Membrane Oxygenation (ECMO)

High-Frequency Ventilation

Respiratory care is an integral part of the treatment of infants and children with cardiorespiratory disease. Respiratory disease is one of the major causes of morbidity and mortality in infants and children.[1, 2] Respiratory failure is the leading cause of admissions to the pediatric intensive care unit.[3] Children are neither miniature adults nor big infants, and infants are not miniature children. Respiratory care in infants and children requires special skills and an understanding of the developmental differences in the anatomy, physiology, and pharmacology of the airways and lung parenchyma. This chapter discusses some of the essential aspects of these developmental issues and provides a state-of-the-art approach to selected topics in pediatric respiratory care. The topics reviewed in this chapter are

- Conventional and unconventional methods of support of gas exchange
- Aerosol administration
- The role of the respiratory care practitioner in interhospital transport
- Home care

DEVELOPMENTAL ISSUES

Alveoli increase in number in the first few years of life and then increase in size until adulthood. An infant's diffusing capacity for oxygen is lower than that of the adult because of the lower surface area for gas exchange; this results in a lower arterial oxygen tension (Pa_{O_2}) in the infant compared with the adult with the same fraction of inspired oxygen (FI_{O_2}).[4, 5] The diffusing capacity for oxygen increases with age, height, and body surface area.[5] With age, the airways increase in both diameter and length, with a concomitant decrease in airway resistance.[6] Distal airway development lags behind the proximal airways during the first 5 years of life[7] and therefore contributes to the higher distal airway resistance in the infant and the young child. During infancy, the airway resistance is almost equally distributed between the upper and the lower airways, whereas in the adult, the majority of the airway resistance resides in the upper airway. The amount of cartilage in the tracheobronchial tree also increases with age[6] and thus increases the stiffness of the airways. The airways of the infant are, therefore, more collapsible than those of the older child, resulting in dynamic compression of the intrathoracic airways during forced expiration in the younger age group. Airway reactivity to bronchoconstrictor stimuli also increases with age.[8]

Functional residual capacity is maintained by the balance between elastic recoil of the lung, which tends to promote alveolar collapse, and elastic recoil of the chest and surfactant, which tend to oppose it. An infant's chest wall is compliant, with a decreased elastic recoil. Closing capacity, the lung volume at which distal airways close, is higher than the functional residual capacity in infants and children less than 5 years of age.[9] In an infant, the mechanisms by which the functional residual capacity is maintained during normal expiration include active glottic narrowing, increased respiratory muscle tone, and incomplete expiration with earlier onset of inspiration. A compliant chest wall, a higher closing capacity, and the potential for dynamic collapse of distal airways during forced expiration contribute to the tendency of the infant and the young child to experience atelectasis and a higher risk of respiratory failure compared with older children and adults.

PHYSIOLOGY OF INFLATION AND DEFLATION

The lungs resist inflation. The factors that contribute to this impediment to lung inflation are

- Elasticity of the lung and thoracic structures
- Resistance to airflow in the airways
- Inertia of the gas molecules in the airway
- Frictional resistance to deformation of the lung and thoracic structures[10]

Elastance, a measure of elasticity, is defined as the change in transmural pressure of an inflatable structure with a unit change in volume. Compliance is the reciprocal of elastance and is defined as the change in volume of any inflatable structure per unit change in transmural pressure of that structure. Lung compliance is defined as the change in lung volume for a unit change in transalveolar pressure (alveolar pressure − pleural pressure). Chest compliance is the change in thoracic cage volume produced by a unit change in transthoracic pressure (ambient pressure − pleural pressure). Specific lung compliance refers to lung compliance that is normalized to the lung volume or body weight and is similar in children and adults.[4] Airway resistance is defined as the change in transpulmonary pressure (proximal airway pressure − alveolar pressure) required to produce a unit flow of gas through the airways of the lung. During normal tidal breathing, the pressure required to overcome inertia of the inspired gas and frictional resistance is negligible. Pulmonary edema, interstitial lung disease, and pulmonary fibrosis may increase frictional resistance. The rate of inflation and deflation of the lung is monoexponential and is dependent on the compliance and resistance. Time constant is the product of compliance and resistance and defines the time taken to cause a given change in lung volume with a constant distending pressure. One time constant is the time taken to cause a 63% change in volume, and three time constants is the time taken to cause a 95% change in volume.[10] Normal expiration is passive and is entirely due to the elastic recoil of the lung. During normal breathing, almost all of the work is performed during inspiration. Most of the work of breathing during inspiration is dissipated as heat.[10] Increased airway resistance and decreased chest and lung compliances increase the workload on the respiratory muscles and increase the work of breathing. Breathing is predominantly diaphragmatic in infants and children. Therefore, any impedance to downward diaphragmatic movement during inspiration will increase the work of breathing. Conditions that impede diaphragmatic movement during inspiration include moderate to severe hepatomegaly, ascites, and gastrointestinal obstruction. In infants and young children, an increase in diaphragmatic contraction coupled with a compliant chest wall can result in paradoxical breathing and ineffective ventilation. An infant's metabolic rate adjusted for weight is about twice that of an adult.[1] A higher ventilatory demand, a decreased respiratory reserve caused by the tendency for paradoxical breathing, and a propensity for premature airway closure and atelectasis make respiratory illnesses more life threatening in the very young. When the oxygen supply to the respiratory muscles is insufficient to meet the workload demand, respiratory muscles fatigue, resulting in ventilatory failure.

MECHANICAL VENTILATION OF INFANTS AND CHILDREN

Indications for Mechanical Ventilation

The primary indication for assisted ventilation is apnea, respiratory arrest, or respiratory failure. Respiratory failure is defined as the presence of inadequate oxygenation or inadequate ventilation, or both. Inadequate oxygenation is defined as an arterial oxygen tension (Pa_{O_2}) less than 60 mm Hg with an inspired oxygen fraction ($F_{I_{O_2}}$) of 0.6, an alveolar to arterial oxygen tension gradient (PA_{O_2}–Pa_{O_2}) greater than 300 mm Hg with an $F_{I_{O_2}}$ of 1, or an intrapulmonary shunt fraction greater than 15%. Measurement of intrapulmonary shunting requires pulmonary artery catheterization and is not available in all pediatric patients. Ventilation-perfusion mismatching is the most likely mechanism of inadequate oxygenation in patients with respiratory disease. Inadequate ventilation is defined as an arterial carbon dioxide tension (Pa_{CO_2}) greater than 50 mm Hg in the absence of chronic hypercapnia and results from a minute alveolar ventilation that is insufficient to meet the metabolic production of CO_2. Impending respiratory failure, which is characterized by a rapidly rising Pa_{CO_2}, or a Pa_{CO_2} out of proportion to the respiratory effort, is usually associated with progressive respiratory distress or fatigue of respiratory muscles. It is preferable to intubate and institute mechanical ventilation before respiratory failure develops. Acute neurologic disorders associated with decreased ventilatory drive, decreased ventilatory effort, and loss of airway protective reflexes, such as gag and cough reflexes, are also indications for intubation and mechanical ventilation. Moderate to severe cardiovascular dysfunction is another indication for assisted ventilation. Cardiovascular dysfunction can result in increased work of breathing and a decreased ability to meet the metabolic demands of the respiratory muscles. Under these circumstances, institution of mechanical ventilation can decrease the workload on the heart by decreasing the work of breathing. Mechanical ventilation may also be instituted in patients with intracranial hypertension or pulmonary hypertension to produce hypocapnia and respiratory alkalosis by deliberately hyperventilating the patient.

Principles of Pediatric Mechanical Ventilation

Selection of Parameters

The first parameter to select is the tidal volume. A practical approach to determining an adequate tidal volume is to evaluate the degree of chest expansion while manually ventilating the patient with a resus-

Children with chronic lung disease may not grow well because of an increased work of breathing. By decreasing the work of breathing, mechanical ventilation may allow these children to grow.

The effective tidal volume, which is the tidal volume actually delivered to the patient, is the difference between the volume delivered by the ventilator and the volume of gas that fills the ventilator circuit.

The compressible volume lost in the circuit can be calculated by multiplying the compliance of the ventilator circuit by the difference between peak inspiratory pressure and positive end-expiratory pressure (PEEP). The compliance of the ventilator circuit is determined by delivering a preset tidal volume to the circuit with the patient connection occluded while observing the pressure change in the circuit. The volume used to inflate the occluded tubing circuit divided by the pressure change produced in the circuit is the compliance of the ventilator circuit (mL/cm H_2O).

In infants with bronchiolitis and children with asthma, the expiratory time may have to be lengthened to avoid air trapping.

citation bag and to reproduce that when the patient is connected to the ventilator. An adequate chest rise must be produced! Although this may seem to be a simplistic statement, patients may be underventilated because of the fear of inducing barotrauma. Such underventilation may result in atelectasis, hypercapnia, and hypoxemia and increase the work of breathing. The normal tidal volume, for spontaneously breathing patients, regardless of age, is 6 to 8 mL/kg. During mechanical ventilation, it may often be necessary to deliver an effective tidal volume of 8 to 10 mL/kg. Volume monitors such as the Bear NVM (Bear Medical Systems, Inc, Riverside, CA) (neonates and infants), the Ohmeda volume monitor (Ohmeda Inc, Madison, WI) (children and adults), and the Bird Partner (Bird Products Corp, Palm Springs, CA) volume monitor are capable of measuring the patient's effective tidal volume directly via a pneumotachometer placed at the hub of the endotracheal tube. Ventilator circuit compliance does not effect this form of measurement. Direct measurement of effective tidal volume, which can be used with all types of conventional ventilators, is the only form of effective tidal volume measurement available for continuous flow ventilators such as the Infant Star (Infrasonics Inc, San Diego, CA), Sechrist IV-100 (Sechrist Industries, Inc, Anaheim, CA), Bear Cub (Bourns BP200), Bird VIP (Bird Products Corp), and Babybird 1 and 2 (Bird Products Corp). Measurements may be obtained intermittently or continuously with the ability to set high and low alarms. In volume-regulated ventilators, effective tidal volume can be estimated by subtracting the compressible volume lost in the ventilator circuit from the tidal volume delivered by the ventilator. When the lung compliance decreases, proportionately more volume may be lost in the ventilator circuit because of an increase in peak inspiratory pressure. Infants and children less than 10 years of age are usually intubated with uncuffed endotracheal tubes. Therefore, it is not uncommon for some of the delivered tidal volume to leak around the endotracheal tube, especially at higher peak airway pressures. In the presence of a leak around the endotracheal tube, exhaled tidal volume should be substituted for the delivered tidal volume in the calculation of effective tidal volume. Patients with normal lung compliance may require a preset tidal volume of 12 to 13 mL/kg to produce an effective exhaled tidal volume of 8 to 10 mL/kg. Patients with lung disease may require a preset tidal volume of 14 to 15 mL/kg to produce an effective tidal volume of 8 to 10 mL/kg, since more volume will be lost in the ventilator circuit because of higher inflating pressures.

The ventilator rate is the next parameter to be selected. When mechanical ventilation is initiated, it is often preferable to provide controlled mechanical ventilation. The rate selected depends on the age and ventilatory requirements of the patient, with subsequent adjustments made according to the Pa_{CO_2}. The initial ventilator rate for a newborn infant usually ranges from 25 to 30 breaths/min; for a 1-year-old child, it is between 20 and 25 breaths/min; and for an adolescent, it is from 15 to 20 breaths/min. The inspiratory time is selected to provide an inspiratory to expiratory time ratio of 1:2. Inspiratory time can be set either as a percentage of the total respiratory cycle or as a fixed time in seconds, depending on the ventilator. Inspiratory time must be selected to allow sufficient time for all lung segments to be inflated. In heterogeneous lung disease with varying regional time constants, a short inspiratory time may not be sufficient to inflate all lung segments, thereby contributing to underventilation and underinflation. Similarly, sufficient expiratory time must be provided for all lung segments to empty. When inspiration starts before the lung has completely emptied, air trapping and inadvertent positive end-expiratory pressure result.

PEEP is the next parameter to be selected. The level of PEEP depends on the clinical circumstance. The goals of PEEP include

- Increasing the functional residual capacity above closing volume to prevent alveolar collapse
- Maintaining stability of alveolar segments
- Improving oxygenation
- Reducing work of breathing

The optimum PEEP is the level at which there is an acceptable balance between the desired goals and undesired adverse effects. The desired goals are

- Reduction in inspired oxygen concentration to "nontoxic" levels (usually less than 50%)
- Maintenance of Pa_{O_2} or Sa_{O_2} of greater than 60 mm Hg or greater than 90% respectively
- Improvement of lung compliance
- Maximal oxygen delivery[11-13]

Arbitrary limits cannot be placed on the level of PEEP or mean airway pressure needed to maintain adequate gas exchange. When the level of PEEP is high, peak inspiratory pressure may be limited to prevent it from reaching dangerous levels that contribute to air leaks and barotrauma. The level of PEEP selected for patients with lower airway obstruction is usually low (3 to 5 cm H_2O). High levels of PEEP are not recommended in respiratory failure due to lower airway diseases because of concern for pulmonary barotrauma from air trapping and alveolar hyperinflation. In adults with severe asthma, however, high levels of PEEP have been shown to decrease the magnitude of air trapping and work of breathing without significant complications.[14-16] In children with tracheomalacia or bronchomalacia, PEEP decreases the airway resistance by distending the airways and preventing dynamic compression during expiration.

Modes of Ventilation

In pediatric patients, the most common mode of ventilation is time-cycled ventilation. The two forms of time-cycled ventilation used in infants and children are volume-regulated and pressure-limited ventilation. In volume-regulated time-cycled ventilation, the tidal volume delivered is regulated by controlling the inspiratory flow and time with no limit on the peak inspiratory pressure. In pressure-limited time-cycled ventilation, the inspiratory flow rate is high (4 to 10 L/kg/min) to allow the peak inspiratory pressure to reach the predetermined limit before the end of inspiration; the peak inflation pressure is held at that level until the onset of expiration. Time-cycled, volume-regulated ventilation may be accomplished with a variety of "adult" ventilators provided that the delivered tidal volume is adjustable down to 100 mL, with fine manipulation including flow rate adjustment to permit inspiratory times of 0.5 to 1 second. The tidal volume setting should range between 12 and 15 mL/kg. In infants and children, it is possible to use a continuous flow ventilator as a volume-regulated time-cycled ventilator. The tidal volume delivered depends on the inspiratory flow rate and the inspiratory time. The inspiratory flow rate required to produce an effective tidal volume of

8 to 10 mL/kg is usually about 1 to 3 L/kg/min. The peak inspiratory pressure is not limited; rather the peak pressure is usually set to cause an alarm at 10 to 15 cm H_2O higher than that which generates an adequate tidal volume. If the patient's compliance worsens, secretions accumulate, or the endotracheal tube kinks, the peak pressure automatically increases. This mode of ventilation provides relatively consistent tidal volumes despite minor changes in the patient's compliance or resistance. The mean airway pressure with this mode of ventilation is lower than pressure-limited time-cycled ventilation with similar tidal volumes and ventilator rate. In volume-regulated ventilators with both inspiratory and expiratory valves, the patient must open the inspiratory valve during spontaneous breathing to obtain a tidal volume. In infants and children, this may impose additional work of breathing, resulting in asynchrony and fatigue. By providing a constant flow of gas during the expiratory phase, continuous flow ventilators can facilitate spontaneous breathing in infants and children and decrease the work of breathing. This style of ventilation is most applicable to patients weighing approximately 6 to 20 kg.

Time-cycled pressure-limited ventilation may be accomplished via a variety of previously listed, continuous flow ventilators and with the Siemens-Elema Servo 900C (Siemans-Elema Medical Systems, Danvers, MA) ventilator in the pressure control mode. Most continuous flow ventilators using time-cycled, pressure-limited ventilation are designed for patients weighing less than 20 kg. Notable exceptions are the Newport Wave (Newport Medical Instruments, Newport Beach, CA), which can ventilate infants, children, and adults using continuous flow, and the Siemens-Elema Servo 900C/300, which can also ventilate larger patients in the pressure control mode without continuous flow. During time-cycled, pressure-limited ventilation, the inspiratory flow is usually 4 to 10 L/kg/min. The desired peak inspiratory pressure limit is reached early in inspiration because of the higher inspiratory flow. The excess flow is vented through a pressure limit valve in continuous flow ventilators. In the Siemens-Elema Servo 900C ventilator, the inspiratory valve closes when the preset peak inspiratory pressure is reached. The preset peak pressure is then held for the remainder of the inspiratory time. Tidal volume measurements may be accomplished by direct inline measurement as previously described. As with volume ventilation, an effective exhaled tidal volume of 8 to 10 mL/kg is desirable, although changes in compliance of the patient or secretions in the airway result in variation in the effective tidal volume, whereas the airway pressure remains constant.

Weaning and Extubation

When the underlying disease process is improving and the patient is able to breathe effectively, weaning should be started. Improvement of the underlying disease process is signaled by improvement in gas exchange, pulmonary mechanics, and ventilation-perfusion relationships. Patients cannot be arbitrarily forced to wean. Inspired oxygen tensions should be decreased to less than 0.5, minute ventilation provided by the ventilator reduced to a minimum by decreasing the ventilatory rate and tidal volume, and PEEP–continuous positive airway pressure (CPAP) reduced to 3 to 5 cm H_2O. When the ventilator rate, PEEP, and FI_{O_2} have been decreased to the desired levels, mechanical ventilation is discontinued and the patient is extubated.

Note: Unless continuous flow ventilation has provisions to allow higher flow rates during the expiratory phase for spontaneous breathing, the preset flow rate may not be sufficient.

Factors that determine a patient's ability to wean include respiratory muscle strength, work of breathing, nutritional status, and stability of the cardiovascular system.

Inflation with a large tidal volume prior to extubation may prevent laryngospasm, which occasionally occurs during extubation.

Intermittent mandatory ventilation was first introduced as a technique to aid weaning from mechanical ventilation in adults.[17-19] Despite theoretical advantages, intermittent mandatory ventilation has not been conclusively shown to be beneficial or superior to other techniques of weaning. In infants, continuous flow through the ventilator circuit decreases the work of breathing; this may aid in weaning.[20] Weaning may be delayed because of slow resolution of the underlying disease process, decreased ventilatory drive, and ventilatory pump failure. Decreased ventilatory drive may result from respiratory center dysfunction from sedation, neurologic disease affecting the brain stem, sleep deprivation, and metabolic alkalosis. Phrenic nerve injury as a complication of birth trauma or operative procedures involving the heart and other thoracic structures[21-24] may result in either paresis or paralysis of one or both hemidiaphragms. When muscle weakness is present, weaning should generally be slow, allowing sufficient time for muscle strength and endurance to return. Techniques for muscle training used in adults have not been studied in children. Ventilatory requirements can be reduced by decreasing carbon dioxide production by lowering excess caloric intake. Muscle loading may occur during intermittent mandatory ventilation because of patient asynchrony. Asynchrony between the patient's breathing and the mechanical breaths, which may occur during both phases of the respiratory cycle, increases the work of breathing. Prolonged asynchrony may result in muscle fatigue, and contribute to prolonged weaning. Tracheostomy may aid in weaning by

Immediate complications of tracheostomy include bleeding and pulmonary air leaks. Long-term complications include infections, subglottic stenosis from scarring, and bleeding from erosion into a major thoracic vessel.

- Decreasing airway resistance, thus decreasing the work of breathing
- Increasing patient and nursing comfort
- Allowing better interaction between the patient and the caretakers

UNCONVENTIONAL MODES OF MECHANICAL VENTILATION

Pressure Support Ventilation

Pressure support ventilation allows better synchrony between the patient and the ventilator than does intermittent mandatory ventilation, volume-assisted ventilation, or pressure control ventilation in adults.[25]

Pressure support ventilation is a form of assisted ventilation in which the ventilator assists the patient's own spontaneous effort with a mechanical breath with a preset pressure limit. Pressure support mainly has been used to wean patients from mechanical ventilation. Recently, it has been used as the primary mode of ventilation during the acute phase of respiratory failure in adults.[26, 27] Although this method of weaning is theoretically attractive, its benefit in the weaning process has yet to be established in infants and children. A relative contraindication to the use of pressure support ventilation is a high baseline spontaneous respiratory rate. There is a finite lag time involved from the initiation of a breath to the sensing of this effort and from the sensing to the delivery of a mechanical breath. In infants breathing at a relatively fast rate (40 to 50 breaths/min), this lag time may be too long, resulting in asynchrony between the patient and the ventilator.

Independent Lung Ventilation

Unilateral or asymmetrical lung disease in infants and children poses special problems during mechanical ventilation. Because of regional differences in compliance and resistance, the time constants for inflation and deflation may vary widely between lung segments. During conventional ventilation, tidal volume delivered tends to preferentially inflate the more compliant lung and underventilate the stiffer, more affected lung. This may result in overinflation of the relatively "normal" lung, causing redistribution of pulmonary blood flow away from the hyperinflated lung and thus exaggerating the ventilation-perfusion mismatching. Such overinflation may contribute to further barotrauma. In such circumstances, with unilateral or asymmetrical lung disease, simultaneous independent lung ventilation (SILV) may allow each lung to be ventilated according to its needs without affecting the opposite lung. SILV requires a biluminal tube, with one side being the longer "bronchial" tube and the other side the shorter "tracheal" tube. Usually, the bronchial tube is advanced into the right main stem bronchus so that both lungs can be ventilated separately. In adults, SILV has been shown to be useful in the treatment of unilateral lung disease.[28-31] In infants and children, SILV has been limited because of the lack of a suitable biluminal tube. Marraro[32] recently reviewed his experience with SILV in infants and children younger than 1 year of age with a biluminal tube developed at his institution but currently available through Portex Ltd., Mythe, Kent, England. The indications for this technique included bronchopneumonia with a monolateral prevalence, unilateral pneumonia, lobar atelectasis, and diaphragmatic hernia. Nine of 41 patients treated with SILV had rapid improvement in the lung pathologic condition with SILV, whereas the other 32 patients recovered more slowly. No major complications were attributed to SILV.

High-Frequency Ventilation

High-frequency ventilation refers to diverse modes of ventilation characterized in general by supraphysiologic ventilatory frequencies and low tidal volumes (less than or equal to physiologic dead space during conventional ventilation). High-frequency positive pressure ventilation refers to ventilation with a tidal volume of 3 to 4 mL/kg at a frequency of 60 to 100 cycles/min using a ventilator with a small internal dead space, low internal compliance, and minimal compression of gases.[33] High-frequency jet ventilation refers to delivery of inspiratory gases at a high velocity through a jet injector introduced into the endotracheal tube, usually at rates of 100 to 400 cycles/min, with inspiratory times of 20 to 30% of the duty cycle.[34] High-frequency oscillatory ventilation refers to ventilation at frequencies of 900 to 3600 cycles/min, using an alternating positive and negative pressure produced by a piston pump or a diaphragm.[35] With this form of ventilation, there is no net change in lung volume. High-frequency chest wall oscillation refers to a method of ventilation in which a rigid harness surrounds the chest. High-frequency body surface oscillation refers to a method of ventilation whereby the whole body is encased in an airtight tank that oscillates at a frequency of 180 to 600 cycles/min. The minute ventilation is controlled by adjusting the inflation pressure and frequency.[36] Only the first three forms of high-frequency ventilation have been used extensively in patients. Mechanisms involved in gas transport during high-frequency ventilation include

- Accelerated axial dispersion

- Increased collateral flow through the pores of Kohn
- Intersegmental gas mixing or pendulluft phenomenon
- Taylor dispersion
- Asymmetrical gas flow profiles
- Gas mixing within the airway due to the nonlinear pressure-diameter relationship of the bronchi

The theoretical advantage of high-frequency ventilation is its ability to ventilate effectively at low airway pressures. High-frequency ventilation has been found useful in the operating room for airway surgery in which airway movement has to be reduced to a minimum.[37] Studies using high-frequency ventilation in premature infants with idiopathic respiratory distress syndrome have shown improvement in gas exchange with lower airway pressures and amelioration of interstitial emphysema.[38–43] A large multicenter trial of high-frequency oscillation did not show any advantage over conventional mechanical ventilation in premature newborns with idiopathic respiratory distress syndrome.[44] A more recent study demonstrated that newborn infants with respiratory distress syndrome treated with high-frequency oscillation had a decreased incidence of chronic lung disease.[45] Although the role of high-frequency ventilation in pediatric respiratory failure is unclear, it may be useful in the management of bronchopleural fistula.[46]

Extracorporeal Cardiorespiratory Support

Extracorporeal oxygenation by direct bubbling of oxygen into blood was achieved by Hill and Gibbon.[47] Development of a semipermeable membrane oxygenator in which gas exchange occurs by diffusion across the membrane greatly facilitated prolonged extracorporeal support.[48] When maximal conventional respiratory support fails to maintain adequate oxygenation and ventilation, adequate gas exchange can be achieved by extracorporeal techniques such as extracorporeal membrane oxygenation (ECMO) and extracorporeal carbon dioxide removal ($ECCO_2R$). ECMO is used to fully support both oxygenation and ventilation, whereas $ECCO_2R$ is used primarily to support ventilation. All extracorporeal techniques of gas exchange require venous blood to be withdrawn from the patient through a cannula placed in the right internal jugular vein. The blood is circulated through a semipermeable membrane by a flow pump and then returned to the patient. Gas exchange occurs across the membrane primarily by diffusion. In venoarterial ECMO, the blood is returned to the patient through a cannula placed in a major artery, usually the right common carotid artery. In venovenous ECMO, blood may be returned to the patient through a double-lumen cannula placed in the right internal jugular vein or through a separate cannula placed in the femoral vein. In $ECCO_2R$, the blood is returned to the patient through a separate cannula placed in the femoral vein.

Extracorporeal Circuit

Venous drainage is usually accomplished by cannulating the internal jugular vein. In patients who have intractable myocardial dysfunction after cardiac surgery, the venous cannula may be placed through a sternotomy in the right atrium. Systemic venous blood drains into the extracorporeal circuit aided by gravity. Using a roller pump or a centrifugal pump, the venous blood is driven across the semipermeable membrane oxygenator. The oxygenator consists of a membrane envelope that is usually made of silicone and wound around a polycarbonate spool. Blood flows between the turns and the gas flows countercurrent through the interior of the membrane envelope. Gas exchange across the membrane is affected by

- Diffusion coefficients for oxygen and carbon dioxide
- Membrane surface area
- Blood flow across the membrane
- Gas flow through the membrane
- Composition of the gas
- Time of contact between the blood and gas in the membrane interface

The pump controls the blood flow whereas the gas flow can be controlled using flow regulators. Blood or gas flow in excess of the manufacturer's specifications may cause the membrane to rupture, resulting in air embolism. The maximum pump flow rate that can be achieved depends entirely on the venous drainage. If there is insufficient venous drainage, increasing the pump flow rate results in collapse of the venous system and entrainment of air in the circuit. A reservoir or "bladder box" is usually placed in the venous side of the circuit to monitor the venous drainage. When the pump flow exceeds the available venous return, the bladder collapses and the pump momentarily stops. A photoelectric oxygen sensor monitors the venous oxygen saturation. The blood leaving the membrane flows through a heat exchanger in which it is warmed to body temperature before returning to the patient. In venoarterial ECMO, blood returning from the oxygenator is returned to the arterial system through a cannula placed in the common carotid artery. In venovenous ECMO, blood returning from the oxygenator is returned to the venous system in one of two ways: (1) in neonates and young children, it is returned to the internal jugular vein via a double-lumen catheter and (2) in older children and adolescents, blood may be returned via the femoral vein. In $ECCO_2R$, venous drainage may be accomplished by cannulating either the internal jugular or the femoral vein. The blood from the circuit is returned to the patient via the femoral vein.

Physiology of Gas Exchange in the Membrane

As the desaturated venous blood flows across the membrane, oxygen diffuses into the blood resulting from the gradient in partial pressures between the two sides of the membrane. The amount of oxygen that diffuses into the blood depends on the initial oxygen saturation of hemoglobin in the venous blood, the hematocrit, the oxygen-dissociation curve of hemoglobin, the gradient in partial pressures of oxygen across the membrane, the solubility of oxygen, and the pump flow. The oxygen concentration of the gas that flows through the membrane oxygenator is adjusted to maintain the oxygen saturation of the blood, leaving the oxygenator between 95 and 98%. The Pa_{O_2} depends on the admixture of blood returning to the systemic circulation from the extracorporeal circuit and the patient's own cardiac output. If the lungs are atelectatic, the blood traversing through the pulmonary circulation remains desaturated with the Pa_{O_2}, reflecting this venous admixture. The amount of carbon dioxide exchanged across the membrane depends primarily on

- Gas flow
- Gradient in partial pressures across the membrane
- Solubility of carbon dioxide

- Diffusion coefficient for carbon dioxide
- Acid-base status of the blood

The Pa_{CO_2} can be maintained in the desired range by adjusting the gas flow through the membrane.

Indications for Extracorporeal Cardiorespiratory Support

The major indication for extracorporeal support is intractable respiratory failure or myocardial dysfunction, or both. The primary aim of extracorporeal support is to supplant the patient's cardiopulmonary support until the underlying disease can improve. As the primary disease improves, extracorporeal support is withdrawn and the patient is switched to conventional cardiopulmonary support. Viral pneumonias, adult respiratory distress syndrome, and hydrocarbon ingestion with acute lung injury are the major respiratory indications for non-neonatal extracorporeal support. Intractable myocardial dysfunction immediately after surgical repair of congenital heart disease is a major cardiac indication for extracorporeal support. This type of support is also used in intractable myocardial dysfunction as a bridge to heart or lung transplantation. Here, the aim of extracorporeal support is to supplant the patient's cardiopulmonary support until the transplantation is performed.

Respiratory Care During Extracorporeal Circulation

To rest the lungs or not to rest the lungs—that is the question! Respiratory care during extracorporeal circulation depends on the underlying disease process and the mode of extracorporeal support. With severe lung disease, the goal of extracorporeal respiratory support is to provide adequate gas exchange and to prevent or reverse barotrauma. Most centers decrease the ventilator support by decreasing the inflating pressures, PEEP, and rate. This results in a reduction in mean airway pressures. The consequence of reducing airway pressures with severe lung disease is atelectasis. It is not uncommon to find bilateral opacification of the lungs on a chest X-ray film[49, 50] with a reduction in lung volumes and compliance.[51] High levels of CPAP/PEEP prevent atelectasis while reportedly reducing the duration of extracorporeal support in neonates requiring ECMO.[52] Atelectatic lungs require high inflating pressures for reinflation and prolong the duration of extracorporeal support. In children placed on extracorporeal support for severe myocardial dysfunction, atelectasis may increase pulmonary vascular resistance and right ventricular afterload. Therefore, we prefer to maintain the lung volume and avoid collapse of the lung by judicious application of PEEP, a relatively higher ventilator rate, and a tidal volume of at least 6 to 8 mL/kg. It is often impossible to achieve this goal without using excessive airway pressures. In such circumstances, the lungs may be allowed to collapse for a few days. Attempts are then made to recruit the lung. Surfactant administration during extracorporeal support has been shown to improve lung mechanics and aid in earlier discontinuation of ECMO in neonates.[53] Whether surfactant administration would benefit older infants and children is unknown. It is interesting to speculate that surfactant or liquid ventilation may aid in respiratory support during extracorporeal support in the future.

Complications

The most common complication during extracorporeal support is bleeding. This may result from excessive heparinization or consumption of coagulation factors. Intracranial bleeding is the most serious complication during extracorporeal support and may be an indication to discontinue it. In infants with an open anterior fontanelle, alternate-day ultrasound of the head is performed to monitor intracranial bleeding. Bacterial and fungal nosocomial infections are the second most common complication during extracorporeal support. Routine prophylactic antibiotics are of no use and in fact may encourage infections with resistant organisms. Another major concern during extracorporeal support is significant neurologic injury. This may occur from air embolism during cannulation or from the circuit, intracranial bleeding, or alteration in regional cerebral blood flows resulting from carotid artery ligation. Neurologic outcome in neonates after ECMO shows that the majority ($>75\%$) are neurologically normal.[54, 55]

Weaning From Extracorporeal Support

The first step in weaning from extracorporeal support is establishment of adequate lung volume. If lung volume is not adequate, gas exchange suffers. When the lung mechanics improve, the extracorporeal support is reduced in decrements. If the patient's lung is able to maintain adequate gas exchange at relatively low airway pressures, the cannulas are removed and the patient is switched to conventional management. The ventilator settings are set to deliver an effective tidal volume of 6 to 10 mL/kg, a rate appropriate for age, with a peak inspiratory pressure less than 35 cm H_2O, and a PEEP of 5 to 8 cm H_2O. Weaning from venoarterial ECMO requires reducing oxygen concentration, the flow of the sweep gas, and the ECMO flow. Weaning from venovenous ECMO and $ECCO_2R$ requires only reduction of sweep gas flow and oxygen concentration.

SPECIAL TECHNIQUES OF RESPIRATORY SUPPORT

Altering Inspired Oxygen and Carbon Dioxide Concentration

Alveolar oxygen tension affects pulmonary vascular resistance; administration of supplemental oxygen decreases pulmonary vascular resistance. In newborns with certain types of congenital heart disease, such as hypoplastic left heart syndrome, it is critical to control pulmonary blood flow. One approach is to decrease the FI_{O_2} to less than 0.21. As the FI_{O_2} is decreased, pulmonary vascular resistance increases and limits pulmonary blood flow. This can be achieved by bleeding in nitrogen. The exact FI_{O_2} delivered must be monitored frequently to avoid administering excessively low inspired oxygen. The other approach, both preoperatively and postoperatively, and especially in mechanically ventilated patients, is to increase the inspired carbon dioxide concentration (FI_{CO_2}). Increased FI_{CO_2} also increases pulmonary vascular resistance. During mechanical ventilation, increasing the FI_{CO_2} allows the patient to be hyperventilated and prevents atelectasis without producing hypocarbia. We found that these two approaches facilitate management of these infants. One of the difficulties with increased FI_{CO_2} is increased ventilatory drive because of an increased Pa_{CO_2}. This increases the work of breathing and with marginal cardiac reserve imposes undue strain on the heart. Therefore, increased FI_{CO_2} should be used judiciously, avoiding an increased workload on the heart.

Helium-Oxygen Mixture

A helium-oxygen mixture, which has much lower density when compared with an oxygen-nitrogen mixture, offers reduced resistance to breathing. This property has been used in the successful treatment of upper airway obstruction after extubation in children.[56] We have used helium-oxygen mixture in upper airway obstruction from laryngotracheobronchitis and postextubation subglottic edema in infants and children. Use of an oxyhood is not indicated, since helium tends to separate and layer at the top of the oxyhood, with the patient breathing very little helium. Recently, helium-oxygen mixtures have been shown to improve gas exchange in neonates with respiratory distress syndrome.[57] Oxygenation should be monitored during administration of a helium-oxygen mixture to avoid hypoxia, especially in neonates.[58] In adults, helium-oxygen mixtures have also been used in the management of severe lower airway obstruction in asthma.

Inhaled Nitric Oxide

The endothelium modulates the tone of the vascular smooth muscle by its ability to release endothelial-derived relaxant factor and endothelin. Nitric oxide or a nitroso compound is thought to be the endothelial-derived relaxant factor. Nitric oxide is endogenously produced in endothelial cells and causes relaxation of vascular smooth muscle. Inhaled nitric oxide produces selective pulmonary vasodilatation in lambs.[59] In newborn infants with pulmonary hypertension of the newborn, inhaled nitric oxide at a concentration of 6 to 80 ppm in 90% oxygen improved oxygenation and overall gas exchange without any untoward systemic effects.[60, 61] Nitric oxide binds to hemoglobin to produce methemoglobin; therefore, methemoglobin levels should be monitored during administration of nitric oxide. At present, inhaled nitric oxide is investigational in infants and children. Future indications for this therapy might include use in diaphragmatic hernia, pulmonary hypertension after repair of congenital heart disease, primary pulmonary hypertension, and isolated right-sided heart failure.

AEROSOL THERAPY

A beta$_2$-agonist is the most common therapeutic aerosol prescribed for infants and children. Other less common drugs used as aerosol agents include atropine, ipratropium bromide, cromolyn sodium, antiviral agents, corticosteroids, antibiotics, surfactant, pentamidine, and mucolytics.

Aerosolized drug administration is perhaps the most widely used therapy in the treatment of respiratory diseases in infants and children. Until recently, drug aerosols have been primarily directed toward reversible lower airway obstruction. Drug aerosols are now being used for the treatment of parenchymal lung diseases such as *Pneumocystis carinii* pneumonia, respiratory syncytial virus, and hyaline membrane disease. The following sections discuss the salient physiologic and technical factors affecting aerosol delivery and examine current trends and practices in infants and children.

A Dosing Paradigm

The unique challenge in drug aerosol therapy in patients with respiratory illness is to identify the most effective and practical method of delivery to ensure optimal therapeutic effect without compromising the safety of the patient. By delivering drugs as aerosols, the therapeutic index may be enhanced by their delivery directly to the site of action, with minimal side effects. Compared with adults, deposition of aerosolized particles in infants and children is poor. Anatomic and physiologic factors that contribute to the poor deposition of aerosols in the airways of infants and children are[62–64]

- Small-caliber airway size with greater airway resistance
- High respiratory rate with a short inspiratory time
- Increased chest wall compliance
- Ineffective coordination effort
- Inconsistent breath-holding maneuvers

Despite poor aerosol deposition, a clinical response to inhaled medications can often be seen. Optimal dosing varies among patients, depending on the type of delivery devices used, the procedure used to deliver the medication, and the type of drug used. Knowing that a physiologic response to inhaled medications is determined by the amount of drug that reaches the site of action in the respiratory tract, the goal would be to control as many variables as possible responsible for ensuring this response. To ensure a good response, the dose and the delivery method should be individualized to each patient. This may necessitate aerosol doses greater or lesser than those recommended by the manufacturer or the Food and Drug Administration. Effective aerosol administration requires a complete understanding of these variables to determine optimal dosing regimens. Often, the dosages and treatment recommendations for these medications are the product of clinical experience at an institution and rarely conform to the drug manufacturer's recommended guidelines or have the consent for pediatric use by the Food and Drug Administration.[65–67]

Beta$_2$-agonists, which are the mainstay in the treatment of bronchospasm, dilate the distal airways by relaxing the airway smooth muscle. Because of concern about the systemic side effects seen with intravenous bronchodilators, the inhaled route is currently the preferred route of administration of bronchodilators in mild to moderate bronchospasm. In patients with moderate to severe acute bronchospasm, the use of aerosols in doses larger than those recommended for age and nebulized more frequently has been shown to be safe and more effective. Schuh and coworkers[68] have shown that 0.3 mg/kg up to a maximum of 10 mg/hr (recommended dose being 0.1 mg/kg) given every 20 minutes was very effective and safe when given to children with acute asthma. Compared with smaller and less frequent doses, large doses of beta$_2$-agonists delivered by metered inhaler (as high as 20 inhaler activations per treatment period) every 20 to 30 minutes produces a favorable response in patients with exacerbation of asthma. Use of larger doses nebulized at more frequent intervals has become an accepted practice in many institutions today.

This trend in frequent administration of beta$_2$-agonists with larger doses has stimulated the use of continuously nebulized beta-agonists in the treatment of status asthmaticus. Our experience, as well as that of several published studies,[69–71] shows that continuous administration of nebulized beta$_2$-agonists is effective and safe in the treatment of severe bronchospasm. A controlled, randomized trial at our institution has found that patients improved more rapidly with continuous nebulization and were discharged from the intensive care unit sooner than patients receiving the standard intermittent therapy, even though the cumulative hourly doses were similar in both groups.[72] Additionally, continuous nebulization has demonstrated a considerable savings in cost and labor in comparison with intermittent therapy. This form of therapy is more effective than intermittent nebulization because it provides sustained stimulation of beta$_2$ receptors, thereby preventing the rebound bronchospasm that can occur when aerosols are delivered intermittently. When considering the many variables that impede effective delivery of aerosols in children, continuous delivery of aerosol offers a greater chance that the medication will be inhaled, thereby increasing the likelihood of better deposition. Although the majority of experience with continuous nebulization has been limited to severe asthma conditions, it is speculated that continuous nebulization will expand beyond the treatment of severe asthma, becoming a routine therapy for patients hospitalized for the treatment of bronchospasm. This may limit intermittent nebulization to less labor-intensive, short-lived episodes of bronchospasm, preventive treatment, or home therapy.

Delivery Devices

Controversy exists regarding the optimal method of delivery of drug to the airways. Particle size has to be at least 1 to 5 μm for deposition in the distal airways. Currently, four types of delivery systems are clinically available to generate medication aerosols: jet nebulizers (small-volume and large-volume nebulizers), ultrasonic nebulizers, metered dose inhalers, and dry powder inhalers.[73] Small-volume jet nebulizers are the most common aerosol generators used in infants and children. Many technical and patient-related factors must be considered when using small-volume nebulizers for intermittent therapy.[11] The type of nebulizer, flow rate, nebulizer volume fill, patient breathing pattern, airway geometry, and mouth or nose breathing during treatment periods are critical to nebulizer performance. Variations can significantly alter the efficacy of the nebulizer therapy. The aerosol deposition in the lungs when these nebulizers are used with a mouthpiece or face mask is about 8 to 12%, with almost 30% remaining in the nebulizer. Large-volume nebulizers use a jet nebulization principle like that found in the small-volume nebulizer but with a larger medication basin (240 mL). The larger nebulizers can be used for longer periods. Duration of therapy depends on the output performance and the amount of medication available in the basin. This type of nebulizer has been developed primarily for continuous aerosol use. Until the large-volume nebulizer became available, continuous nebulization was accomplished with a modified small-volume nebulizer. This nebulizer had been modified with a small hole taped into the nebulizer basin and received a continuous drip of medication from an infusion pump. The pump delivered a medication solution through a pressure line that attached to the nebulizer. This modified method has been effective in the treatment of severe asthma in children. To date, no data have been reported verifying the effectiveness of the large-volume nebulizers in pediatric patients. The ultrasonic nebulizer, which uses a piezoelectric crystal that produces a highly concentrated output of aerosol particles, has historically been used for cough and sputum production or bronchoprovocational challenges. Rarely have ultrasonic nebulizers been used for medication delivery in infants or children (mainly because of the concentrated mist produced). However, by replacing the saline solution with medication, the highly concentrated output from the ultrasonic nebulizer may perform better than a small-volume nebulizer in accomplishing greater deposition of medications in children. Little information exists comparing the ultrasonic nebulizer's capabilities to small-volume nebulizers.

Metered dose inhalers use a pressurized canister that dispenses a single bolus of aerosolized medication. They are convenient, cost-effective, and versatile and generally have an effective deposition rate of 10 to 15%. To optimize the delivery of the drug, the patient must be able to coordinate a series of inspiratory maneuvers while activating the canister. Low inspiratory flow rates, inspiratory pause, or sustained maximal inflation maneuvers facilitate better deposition. Lower flow rates reduce aerosol impaction on the oropharynx and inner walls of the airway, whereas breath holding improves deposition by gravity. In our experience, many young children are unable to master the technique required for proper aerosol delivery, especially during episodes of respiratory distress. A spacer device can be a valuable attachment if the metered dose inhaler is used by children. By adding a spacer device to the inhaler, the synchronized effort is less of a concern, whereas drug delivery is maximized. The canister is activated into the spacer, with the medication remaining suspended in the chamber until the patient inhales. In addition to overcoming the synchronized challenge, the chamber improves airway deposition and reduces oropharynx impaction by reducing particle size and travel velocity of the aerosol. When used properly, the spacer is an added benefit to the delivery of medication from a metered dose inhaler; however, when poor conditions exist, such as improper technique, rapid shallow breathing, or delay in inhaling the collection of aerosol in the chamber, it is doubtful that any value is gained from the spacer. For younger children or infants, a mask is added to the spacer for delivery. In our experience, we have found this technique to be cumbersome in the younger patient, and it increases the level of anxiety for the patients and their families. Therefore, we replaced the metered dose inhaler with a small-volume nebulizer in these children.

Many children older than 5 years of age do well with the spacer and metered dose inhaler when used for preventive treatment.

A dry powder inhaler delivers a large bolus of medication during a single inspiration maneuver and produces therapeutic effects similar to a metered dose inhaler and an aerosol nebulizer. The dry powder medication, released from a capsule and deposited into a small canister, is delivered to the lungs during inspiration. The inspired flow rate causes a turbulent state within the canister directing the powder toward the respiratory tract. Children having difficulty mastering the synchronized technique and breath-holding maneuver find this form of therapy useful. As long as these patients can generate the inspiratory flow rate necessary to move the medication from the capsule to the lower respiratory tract, this device becomes a reasonable alternative.

Aerosols Delivered Through Ventilators

Aerosolized medications are often delivered through mechanical ventilators for the treatment of bronchospasm. Aerosol delivery is not very efficient when delivered through a ventilator.[74] The endotracheal tube is the most significant barrier to effective delivery. Endotracheal tube sizes range from 3 mm to 6 mm in infant and pediatric care. The smaller the inner diameter of the tube, the less efficient is the aerosol delivery. Drug delivery beyond endotracheal tubes with an internal diameter of 3 and

3.5 mm has been reported to be as low as 0.02% of the total dose.[12] These reported values have been obtained under controlled experimental conditions; therefore, actual delivery rates at the bedside may be even lower. In addition to the endotracheal tube, several other factors have an impact on the delivery of aerosols by mechanical ventilators. The nebulizer is most effective when placed near the manifold of most ventilators. The premise is that allowing the inspiratory limb of the circuit to fill with aerosolized particles during the exhalation phase of ventilation improves the delivery of medication during the subsequent inspiration. The inspiratory portion of the circuit serves as a space chamber, similar to the spacer used for metered dose inhalers. The aerosolized particles remain suspended in the inspiratory limb waiting to be delivered with the ensuing ventilator breath. With this practice, the nebulizer mode becomes a critical part of maximizing aerosol delivery. Aerosols must be generated during the expiratory phase of the ventilator cycle to fill the inspiratory limb; therefore, a synchronized nebulizer mode is essential. Some modern day ventilators offer a synchronized nebulization capability in which a portion of the preset inspiratory gas is diverted to power the nebulizer. Most institutions find it necessary to modify their ventilators, since the ideal method would have the nebulizer functioning intermittently during the expiratory phase of the ventilator cycle. Even if the nebulizer was activated during the expiratory phase, however, the amount of nebulizer gas priming the ventilator circuit between mechanical breaths may contribute to the tidal volumes delivered to the patient. This becomes a real concern when ventilating patients with small tidal volumes.

To minimize the effects of added volume and to prime the inspiratory limb during the expiratory phase, a one-way valve must be inserted between the ventilator circuit and nebulizer setup (Fig. 53–1). The nebulizer setup consists of a nebulizer driven from a separate gas source and a pressure relief valve set to release at a pressure 2 to 3 cm H_2O, slightly higher than the baseline pressure of the ventilator circuit. The gas flow to the nebulizer is turned on to allow the nebulizer to run

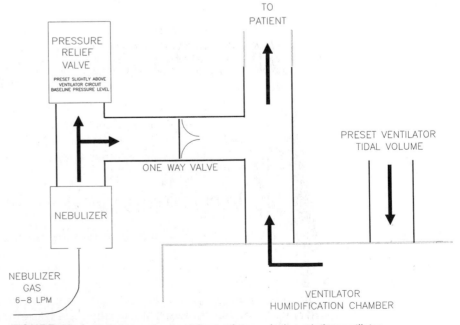

FIGURE 53–1: Nebulizer setup for delivery of aerosols through the ventilator.

continuously. During the ventilator inspiratory phase, the circuit pressure rises above the pressure relief valve setting, and the aerosol particles from the nebulizer are diverted out through the pressure relief valve. With the expiratory phase of ventilation, the circuit pressure drops back to baseline and the aerosol particles travel through the one-way valve into the inspiratory limb of the circuit. Because the circuit pressure is lower than the relief valve's preset pressure, aerosols are no longer exiting the pressure relief valve. This method offers significant advantages to aerosol delivery in smaller patients. The one-way valve is a baffle to the nebulizer particles and reduces the number of particles delivered to the inspiratory limb of the circuit. Although this technique has been demonstrated to be effective with demand-style ventilators, continuous flow (pressure-limited) ventilators, commonly used with infants, appear to be less compliant with this process. Usually, the continuous flow of gas washes the nebulized aerosol through the ventilator circuit into the expiratory limb before the mechanical breath begins. A nebulizer gas flow of 6 to 8 L/min may often contribute significantly to the patient's small tidal volumes or to the pressure-limited phase. To minimize flow-related problems, nebulizers driven by lower flow rates (2 L/min) are commercially available; however, no data exist regarding their effectiveness.

Many practitioners are concerned about modifying ventilators. Adding a bias gas flow to modern day ventilators can damage expiratory transducers, create added resistance to expiration, make it more difficult for patients to generate a breath during pressure support and synchronized intermittent mandatory ventilation modes, and exhibit misleading volume or pressure readings on the ventilator display panel. Furthermore, aerosolized particles collected in expiratory filters increase the expiratory resistance or cause complete blockage of the expiratory port. Filters must be monitored and changed frequently to avoid obstruction or added resistance. In such a circumstance, airway pressures and tidal volumes delivered to the patient should be measured at the hub of the endotracheal tube.

Caution should be taken when using metered dose inhalers with small infants who have tidal volumes less than 100 mL.

Metered dose inhalers are equally effective as nebulizers in adults requiring mechanical ventilation. Several activators and chambers are commercially available for inhaler use with ventilators. Like nebulizers, these activators, which vary widely in performance, can alter the amount of medication delivered from the inhaler. Some activators connect to the endotracheal tube and deliver the medication directly down the tube. Because of the high velocity established on activation, the major portion of medication contacts the upper walls of the endotracheal tube. Spacer devices inserted into the inspiratory limb help reduce this problem of tube impaction and improve the chances for lower deposition. Connecting a metered dose activator and chamber to a custom-made pediatric or infant heated wire circuit requires a great deal of modification to the circuit. Furthermore, the spacer becomes ineffective when ventilating infants, since the bias flow from the continuous flow ventilator washes out the chamber. The chlorofluorocarbon mixture dispensed from the inhaler can potentially lead to hypoxic events during metered dose activations.

The most promising method of delivery was described by Taylor and Lerman.[75] A 19-gauge catheter is inserted into the endotracheal tube and the inhaler contents are delivered through the catheter, achieving delivery rates of up to 96.7%. This clearly shows the need for a delivery system capable of bypassing the endotracheal tube completely. With further study and modification, this practice of bypassing the ventilator circuit and endotracheal tube may have an unprecedented advantage in administering medications to smaller patients. Whether a small-volume nebulizer or metered dose inhaler is used for delivering medications through ventilators, it becomes evident that the efficiency of the process is poor. Drug dosages may need to be doubled and delivered continuously in order to generate a physiologic response in these patients. Whatever delivery device is chosen, the method of delivery and dosage should be tailored to the patient's response. Because of the hazards associated with these types of ventilator modifications, great caution and additional monitoring devices should be used.

INTERHOSPITAL TRANSPORTS

Indications

Interhospital transport involves the transfer of patients who have received initial stabilization at the referring hospital. The priorities for interhospital transport differ from ambulance runs. The primary goals of interhospital transport are

- Maintaining stability
- Preventing morbidity and mortality
- Safe transfer of critically ill patients to the appropriate tertiary care center

Ongoing monitoring appropriate to the severity of illness is crucial in achieving these goals. Table 53–1 shows the diagnostic categories that result in interhospital transport for infants and children. Geographic location, capabilities of the referring and receiving hospitals, and availability of transport vehicles all influence the type of patient transported

TABLE **53–1:** Indications for Interhospital Transport of Children[76-79]

Respiratory
Airway obstruction (croup, epiglottitis, asthma, bronchiolitis)
Parenchymal lung disease (pneumonia, aspiration, ARDS)
Apnea or respiratory arrest
Neurologic
Infections (meningitis, encephalitis)
Acute encephalopathies (Reye's syndrome, poisoning)
Hypoxic-ischemic encephalopathy (drowning, SIDS, shaken baby syndrome)
Mass lesions (tumors, bleeding)
Seizures
Guillain-Barré syndrome
Miscellaneous
Cardiovascular
Congenital heart disease
Dysrhythmias
Cardiac failure and cardiogenic shock
Acute myocardia
Cardiomyopathy
Myocardial infarction (rarely)
Trauma
Other
Hematologic diseases (acute anemia, ITP, leukemia)
Renal (renal failure, hemolytic-uremic syndrome)
Gastrointestinal (obstruction, peritonitis, pancreatitis)
Hepatobiliary (hepatic failure, biliary obstruction)

ARDS, adult respiratory distress syndrome; SIDS, sudden infant death syndrome; ITP, idiopathic thrombocytopenic purpura.

by a particular institution.[76–79] Unlike neonatal transport teams, pediatric teams must care for a wider range of illnesses.

Composition of the Transport Team

The American Academy of Pediatrics guidelines state that "transport team members should be chosen for both their medical skill and their ability to behave responsibly when interacting with personnel at the referring and receiving hospital, parents, and with each other" and "transport team members should be dually trained and competent, not only in pediatric critical care but also in transport medicine, managing the supplies and equipment required by the transport vehicle, the physiologic effects of transport on the patient, and the limitations imposed by the transport equipment."[80] Many critically ill patients transported to a tertiary care center require intensive care during transport or soon after arrival at the receiving hospital.[81–85] Therefore, at the time of the initial contact between the referring hospital and the receiving institution, the child's severity of illness must be assessed. This will determine the level of support required during transport and will facilitate the selection of team members with the appropriate skills. The National Leadership Conference on Pediatric Interhospital Transport[86] stated that an interhospital transport triage system must satisfy the following requirements:

- Classify patients based on severity of illness with the available phone information
- Classify patients based on the need for skilled care during transport, including specialized monitoring and additional major interventions
- Classify patients based on the potential for morbidity

Each receiving institution must form its team in a manner that will bring the highest quality of care to the patient and assure his or her safe return to the center. In order to achieve this goal, there must be a firm commitment by the institution to the transport system. Adequate resources must be available from the institution and the local community. Qualified team members must be recruited and trained appropriately. Once an institution has made the commitment to a designated transport team, the medical director, transport team manager, and administrator must develop guidelines for selecting the team members. Because of the high level of support required on transport and the technical aspects of the equipment, the team must be able to provide the highest level of care possible.

Utility of a Therapist During Transport

Respiratory care during transport of the critically ill neonate and pediatric patient has brought the field into a highly specialized focus. Respiratory illnesses are the most common indication for interhospital pediatric transport.[79] A respiratory therapist is a valuable member of a dedicated transport system.[77, 79, 85] The role of the respiratory therapist in pediatric interhospital transport has been reviewed in detail elsewhere.[87] This section briefly reviews the salient aspects of the role of the respiratory therapist in interhospital transport. Respiratory care during interhospital transport may range from administration of bronchodilator aerosols to providing mechanical ventilation. Patients who might benefit from the presence of a respiratory therapist during transport include all mechanically ventilated children and patients who require drug aerosol administration during transport. The presence of an additional team member must be weighed against the benefit of having a skilled individual who can perform a specialized function.

Responsibility of the Respiratory Therapist During Transport

The respiratory therapist is responsible for providing respiratory care during transport. First, a thorough assessment of the patient is essential to determine the severity of illness. Care must be coordinated among team members at the referring hospital, en route during transport, and on arrival at the receiving hospital. The therapist must secure the artificial airways, check proper functioning of the respiratory care equipment and aid in monitoring the patient's respiratory status. Dislodgement of artificial airways or malfunction of mechanical ventilators poses a tremendous risk to the patient. The primary goal of the team must be quick and safe transfer of the patient, not an exhaustive diagnostic evaluation; therefore, only immediate management plans should be addressed.

Training

Table 53–2 lists the requirements necessary for a respiratory therapist to be considered for interhospital transport at Children's Hospital of Pittsburgh. Following the selection of the transport therapist, an extended period of training must occur prior to his or her participation as the primary caregiver. This program should consist of didactic lectures, clinical hands-on training, evaluation of clinical performance, and monitoring of that performance. Every respiratory therapist involved in pediatric transport should undergo a training orientation (Table 53–3). Following completion of the transport training module, the transport therapist orientee should be able to

- Assemble and apply all respiratory care–related equipment
- Verify the performance of gas cylinders and regulators
- Secure the patient and equipment
- Assess the patient's respiratory status and overall clinical condition
- Participate in the stabilization of the patient prior to transport
- Monitor the patient throughout transport

TABLE **53–2:** Requirements for a Transport Respiratory Therapist at Children's Hospital of Pittsburgh

1. RRT by the NBRC (RRT-eligible considered)
2. 1 year minimum critical care experience (NICU-PICU)
3. High performance evaluations
4. AHA Basic Provider (Course C—Health Care Provider)
5. Pediatric Advanced Life Support (PALS)
6. Neonatal Resuscitation Program—AHA-AAP
7. Demonstrated ability to provide intrahospital transports
8. No medical conditions that exclude traveling in team vehicles

RRT, Resistered Respiratory Therapist; NBRC, National Board of Respiratory Care; NICU, Neonatal Intensive Care Unit; PICU, Pediatric Intensive Care Unit; AHA, American Heart Association; AAP, American Academy of Pediatrics.

TABLE **53–3:** Training Components for a Transport Therapist

Advanced training in the maintenance of a patent airway
Advanced skills in airway stabilization
Assessment and evaluation of patient's clinical condition
In-depth knowledge of anatomy and physiology of the respiratory tract
Understanding of congenital cardiac anomalies
Understanding of abdominal and chest wall defects
Understanding of neonatal transport ventilators
Ability to manipulate the mechanical ventilator parameters to obtain maximal (optimize) oxygenation and physiologic ventilation
Specialized training and understanding of noninvasive monitoring to assess patients
Certification in the Neonatal Resuscitation program
Certification in the Pediatric Advanced Life Support program
Unique understanding of aviation physiology
Demonstration of proper scoring of all patients and patient care equipment
Maintenance of safety inservices every 6 months on rotocraft and fixed wing aircraft
Provision of precise documentation of each transport on transport logs

- Assist in the safe transfer of the patient from referral hospital to vehicle and from vehicle to home hospital
- Document and provide an accurate and pertinent patient status report on arrival
- Restock all used equipment

It has been our experience that the candidate should not be assigned as the primary caregiver until he or she has been observed on a transport by a preceptor. Continuous ongoing monitoring and review of each transport should be conducted by the transport team coordinator and medical director. Data and statistics must be gathered to determine that team members are participating in enough out-of-house transports to maintain their skill levels. Multidisciplinary team meetings should be scheduled to discuss patient management and strategies. This will also promote a "team" approach and develop further rapport among team members. It is crucial that a team functions at maximal efficiency and that each member complements the others.

HOME CARE

The survival of children with chronic respiratory failure is increasing. In 1984, the Ad Hoc Task Force on Home Care of Critically Ill Infants stated that "the goal of a home care program for infants, children, or adolescents with chronic conditions is the provision of comprehensive, cost-effective health care within a nurturing home environment that maximizes the capabilities of the individual and minimizes the effects of disabilities."[88] Respiratory care requirements in these children may range from supplemental oxygen to long-term mechanical ventilation. Long-term care in a tertiary care center is expensive. Such long-term respiratory care can alternatively be provided in a specialized chronic care rehabilitation center or at home. Chronic care centers, which traditionally have cared for children with musculoskeletal disorders, are increasingly managing children with chronic respiratory failure. However, not all rehabilitation centers are capable of caring for children on mechanical ventilation. Home care is therefore becoming an increasingly feasible option for these patients. Home care is psychosocially more acceptable to families and less expensive; it also may provide a better quality of life. In 1986, the American College of Chest Physicians published guidelines for the management of ventilator-dependent patients in the home and at alternate community sites.[89] In 1976, Pinney and Cotton[90] reported on the feasibility of home care for infants with bronchopulmonary dysplasia requiring supplemental oxygen. In the late 1970s and early 1980s, home care was reported to be as safe as hospital care for infants with tracheostomies and infants and children requiring mechanical ventilation.[91-96] The diagnoses included neuromuscular disease, spinal cord trauma, and respiratory failure from chronic cardiorespiratory disease.[91-96] Several investigators have reported that home care for respiratory technology–dependent children is cost-effective for children who required only supplemental oxygen and for those who were ventilator-dependent.[97, 98]

Indications for Home Respiratory Care

The goals of long-term home respiratory care include

- Provision of comprehensive, cost-effective respiratory care
- Enhancement of the quality of life
- Reduction of morbidity whenever possible
- Extension of life

The major indication for home respiratory care is chronic respiratory failure, which may occur in children with parenchymal or airway disease or in children with normal lungs. In the latter case, respiratory failure is usually due to central or peripheral nervous system dysfunction, neuromuscular disorders, or chest wall abnormalities. Patients who require home respiratory care generally fall into the following categories:

- Patients whose underlying disease will most likely resolve and therefore these patients would need respiratory care during the recovery phase, such as infants with bronchopulmonary dysplasia and children recovering from adult respiratory distress syndrome
- Patients whose underlying disease is irreversible but not progressive, such as patients with spinal cord injury
- Patients whose underlying disease is irreversible and progressive, such as patients with muscular dystrophy

The approach to home care planning depends on the natural course of the underlying disease.

Home care requires a team approach with interaction among several health care personnel, that is, a primary physician, home care nurses, respiratory therapists, social workers and sometimes the state health agency, and the family and the patient (Table 53–4). First, the patient must be ready for home care.[96, 99, 100] A stable tracheostomy with a mature stoma is essential for patients who require an artificial airway. The inspired oxygen requirement should not be greater than 35%. The Pa_{O_2} should be greater than 60 to 70 mm Hg with a Pa_{CO_2} less than 60 mm Hg with a normal arterial pH at relatively low ventilator settings. The family must demonstrate not only a desire to provide home care but also a minimal ability to provide various aspects of home care. Health care personnel must be available in the local community to assist the family in providing care. The home must have adequate facilities to maintain and run all necessary equipment and store supplies. Contingency plans must be made for emergencies.

TABLE **53—4:**   Factors to be Considered in Home Care for Children

---

A. Patient selection
- Medical assessment
- Cardiopulmonary stability
- Positive trend in weight gain and growth curve
- Freedom from frequent respiratory infection and fever

B. Characteristics of the family and child
- Awareness
- Motivation
- Commitment

C. Home requirements
- Safe electrical, plumbing, and heating systems
- Telephone
- Space

D. Health care support personnel
- Nurses
- Aides
- Family and friends

E. Funding
- Third party
- State
- Other

F. Multidisciplinary home care team from the discharging institution
- Physician specializing in respiratory disease
- Nurse specializing in respiratory disease
- Social worker
- Respiratory therapist

G. Other services
- Occupational therapy
- Physical therapy
- Speech therapy
- Dietary services
- Psychologist

H. Responsibilities of the health care team
- Coordinator
- Physician available on a 24 hour basis
- Referral to a local durable medical equipment (DME) company
- Instruction of parents and caretakers
- Assistance to family in securing funding

I. Family preparation
- Training in CPR
- Instruction in all aspects of home care plan
- Instruction in use and maintenance of equipment
- Psychological impact
- Techniques of instruction

J. Responsibility of the respiratory therapist

CPR, cardiopulmonary resuscitation.

Home Location and Atmosphere

The location of the home has major implications for home care. It must be easily accessible by standard transportation. Durable medical equipment companies must be able to respond to emergencies in a timely fashion. Emergency calls from the family to the durable medical equipment company most often are equipment-related. For medical emergencies, families generally tend to contact the discharging hospital or physician or nurse coordinator. Ideally, a coordinator from the medical equipment company should be available on a 24-hour basis to respond to emergencies, a requirement for accreditation by the Joint Commission on the Accreditation of Healthcare Organizations (JCAHO). There are many durable medical equipment companies that provide medical equipment for home care that are not certified by JCAHO. Some families live in areas that are not readily covered by durable medical equipment companies or nursing agencies. There are many areas of the United States that do not have home nursing agencies that can be caretakers for children for long periods. The services provided by durable medical equipment companies depend not only on the location of the home but also on their level of sophistication. When the home is not easily accessible, the response time tends to be longer. This may affect the margin of safety in relation to the time of response. The home must have adequate space to accommodate all the caretakers and the required equipment. If it does not, alternative arrangements must be found. The home must have a telephone and adequate utilities, such as electricity and gas. The structure of the family and the commitment of its members are major factors in the success of home care. Single parents or parents who do not want to be involved cause caretaking problems at home. Single parents who work may not be able to absent themselves from their place of employment without the risk of losing their jobs. Some children have many medical concerns, and parents need time for themselves and may pose problems if the number of caretakers is insufficient. The frequency of visiting by other caretakers must be arranged and planned before discharge so that the family members can structure their lives optimally.

Medical Support and Caretaker Training

Discharge planning must be thorough and take into account all the factors listed in Table 53–4. The more complicated the medical needs of the home-based child, the more difficult the training and the more difficult it is to find caretakers. There must be educators available who can teach all aspects of home care. It would be ideal if all parents and caretakers were able to understand all the equipment and care that the child needs. Discharge planning requires that the parents and the caretakers have at least a reasonable understanding of all the procedures that are to be performed at home. The home's psychosocial atmosphere must be taken into account during discharge planning, as it will have a significant impact on caring for a medically dependent household member.

Equipment and Supplies

Since a detailed description of the various kinds of respiratory care equipment used for pediatric home care is beyond the scope of this chapter, the reader is referred elsewhere.[101] A thorough knowledge of the limitations of various devices is essential for the respiratory care personnel coordinating home care. Even though many types of oxygen delivery are available, such as portable cylinders, liquid systems, and concentrators, the choice of a particular oxygen source depends on the clinical circumstance. For example, portable small oxygen cylinders may be insufficient and not cost-effective for patients who need oxygen 24 hours a day on a ventilator. Most home ventilators are electrically driven. This provides the safety of the ventilator continuing to function even if the oxygen source fails. Compressed oxygen would be required only to provide supplemental inspired oxygen and not to power the ventilator. Oxygen flow is adjusted to provide the desired concentration. PEEP-CPAP can usually be provided by external PEEP valves attached to the ventilator circuit. Parents who are motivated to provide home care for their children are willing to take on the cumbersome responsibility of carrying all the necessary equipment from place to place just to have the benefit of having the child at home.

SUMMARY

Respiratory care of infants and children poses unique challenges for the practitioner. Developmental differences need to be considered when respiratory care is provided to infants and children. What is applicable in adults may not necessarily be applicable to children, and what is applicable to children may not be applicable to infants. Newer modes of ventilation such as pressure support ventilation have not been studied in children. The small size makes independent lung ventilation difficult. ECMO has been much more valuable in infants and children than in adults with cardiorespiratory failure. The respiratory therapist is critical in developing a dosing paradigm for aerosol administration, providing support in interhospital transport of mechanically ventilated children, and home care of children with chronic cardiorespiratory disease.

References

1. Wohl MEB, Mead J. Age as a factor in respiratory disease. *In* Chernick V (ed). Kendig's Disorders of the Respiratory Tract in Children. Philadelphia, WB Saunders, 1990, p 175.
2. Loda FA, Glezen WP, Clyde WA Jr. Respiratory disease in group day care. Pediatrics 49:428, 1972.
3. Gregory GA. Respiratory failure in the child. Clin Crit Care Med 3:vii, 1981.
4. Nelson NM. Respiration and circulation after birth. *In* Smith CA, Nelson NM. The Physiology of the Newborn Infant. Springfield IL, Charles C Thomas, 1976, p 117.
5. Bucci G, Cook C, Barrie H. Studies of respiratory physiology in children. J Pediatr 58:820, 1961.
6. Thurlbeck WM. Postnatal growth and development of the lung. Am Rev Respir Dis 111:803, 1975.
7. Hogg JC, Williams J, Richardson JB, et al. Age as a factor in the distribution of lower airway conductance and in the pathologic anatomy of obstructive lung disease. N Engl J Med 282:1283, 1970.
8. Sander RA, McNicol KJ, Stecenko AA. Effect of age on lung mechanics and airway reactivity in lambs. J Appl Physiol 61:2074, 1986.
9. Mansell A, Bryan AC, Levison H. Airway closure in children. J Appl Physiol 33:711, 1972.
10. Nunn JF. Resistance to gas flow and airway closure. *In* Nunn JF. Applied Respiratory Physiology, 3rd ed. London, Butterworths, 1987, p 460.
11. Suter PM, Fairley HB, Isenberg MD. Optimal end-expiratory airway pressure in patients with acute pulmonary failure. N Engl J Med 292:284, 1975.
12. Civetta JM, Barnes TA, Smith LO. "Optimal PEEP" and intermittent mandatory ventilation in the treatment of respiratory failure. Respir Care 20:551, 1975.
13. White MK, Galli SA, Chatburn RL, Blumer JL. Optimal positive end-expiratory pressure therapy in infants and children with acute respiratory failure. Pediatr Res 24, 217, 1988.
14. Beasley JM, Jones SEF. Continuous positive airway pressure in bronchiolitis. Br Med J 283:1506, 1981.
15. Pontoppidan H, Geffin B, Lowenstein E. Acute respiratory failure in the adult. N Engl J Med 287:690, 743, 799, 1972.
16. Martin JG, Shore S, Engel LA. Effect of continuous positive airway pressure on respiratory mechanics and pattern of breathing in induced asthma. Am Rev Respir Dis 126:812, 1982.
17. Downs JB, Perkins MH, Modell JH. Intermittent mandatory ventilation. Arch Surg 109:519, 1974.
18. Downs JB, Klein EF, Jr, Desautels D, et al. Intermittent mandatory ventilation: A new approach to weaning patients from mechanical ventilators. Chest 64:331, 1973.
19. Klein EF Jr. Weaning from mechanical breathing with intermittent mandatory ventilation. Arch Surg 110:345, 1975.
20. Kirby RR, Robinson E, Schultz J, DeLemos RA, et al. Continuous flow ventilation as an alternative to assisted or controlled ventilation in infants. Anesth Analg 51:871, 1972.

21. Greene W, L'Heureux P, Hunt CE. Paralysis of the diaphragm. Am J Dis Child 129:1402, 1975.
22. Zhao HX, D'Agostino RS, Pitlick PT, et al. Phrenic nerve injury complicating closed cardiovascular procedures for congenital heart disease. Ann Thorac Surg 39:445, 1985.
23. Lynn AM, Jenkins JG, Edmonds JF, Burns JE. Diaphragmatic paralysis after pediatric cardiac surgery. A retrospective analysis of 34 cases. Crit Care Med 11:280, 1983.
24. Mickell JJ, Oh KS, Siewers RD, et al. Clinical implications of postoperative unilateral phrenic nerve paralysis. J Thorac Cardiovasc Surg 76:297, 1978.
25. MacIntyre NR. Pressure-support ventilation. In Grenvik A, Downs JB, Rasanen J, Smith R (eds). Contemporary Management in Critical Care. New York, Churchill Livingstone, 1991, p 51.
26. MacIntyre NR, Leatherman NE. Ventilatory muscle loads and the frequency-tidal volume pattern during respiratory pressure assisted (pressure supported) ventilation. Am Rev Respir Dis 141:327, 1990.
27. MacIntyre NR. Respiratory function during pressure support ventilation. Chest 89:677, 1986.
28. Powner DJ, Eross B, Grenvik A. Differential lung ventilation with PEEP in the treatment of unilateral pneumonia. Crit Care Med 5:170, 1977.
29. Carlon GC, Ray C, Klein R, et al. Criteria for selective positive end-expiratory pressure and independent synchronized ventilation of each lung. Chest 74:501, 1978.
30. Rivara D, Burgain JL, Rieuf P, et al. Differential ventilation in unilateral lung disease: Effects on respiratory mechanics and gas exchange. Intensive Care Med 5:189, 1979.
31. Baehrendtz S, Santesson J, Bindselv L, et al. Differential ventilation in acute bilateral lung disease. Influence on gas exchange and central haemodynamics. Acta Anaesthesiol Scand 27:270, 1983.
32. Marraro G. Simultaneous independent lung ventilation in pediatric patients. Crit Care Clin 8:131, 1992.
33. Oberg PA, Sjostrand U. Studies of blood pressure regulation. Common carotid artery clamping in studies of the carotid-sinus baroreceptor control of the systemic blood pressure. Acta Physiol Scand 75:276, 1969.
34. Sanders RD. Two ventilating attachments for bronchoscopes. Dev Med 39:170, 1967.
35. Lunkenheimer P, Rafflenbeul W, Keller H, et al. Application of transtracheal pressure oscillations as modification of "diffusion respiration." Br J Anaesth 44:627, 1972.
36. Zidulka A, Gross D, Minami H, et al. Ventilation by high frequency chest wall compression in dogs with normal lungs. Am Rev Respir Dis 127:709, 1983.
37. Klain M. Clinical applications of high frequency jet ventilation in high frequency ventilation in intensive care and during surgery. In Carlon GC, Howland WS (eds). Lung Biology in Health and Disease. New York, Marcel Dekker, 1985, pp 137–150.
38. Bohn D. High frequency oscillation. Br J Anaesth 63(7 Suppl 1):16S–23S, 1989.
39. Bryan AC. Use of high frequency ventilation in HMD. Acta Anaesth Scand 90:124, 1989.
40. Frantz ID, Werthammer J, Stark AR. High frequency ventilation in premature infants with lung disease: Adequate gas exchange at low tracheal pressure. Pediatrics 71:483, 1983.
41. Marchak BE, Thompson WK, Duffty P, et al. Treatment of RDS by high frequency oscillatory ventilation: A preliminary report. J Pediatr 99:287, 1981.
42. Harris TR. High frequency jet ventilation treatment of neonates with life-threatening restrictive lung disease. Pediatr Res 17:316A, 1983.
43. Ng NPK, Easa D. Management of interstitial emphysema by high frequency low positive pressure hand ventilation in the neonate. J Pediatr 95:117, 1979.
44. HiFi Study Group. High frequency oscillatory ventilation compared with conventional mechanical ventilation in the treatment of respiratory failure in preterm infants: Assessment of pulmonary function at 9 months of corrected age. J Pediatr 116:933, 1990.
45. Clark RH, Gerstmann DR, Null DM Jr, et al. Prospective randomized comparison of high frequency oscillatory and conventional ventilation in respiratory distress syndrome. Pediatrics 89:5, 1992.
46. Turnbull AD, Carlon G, Howland WS, Beattie EJ. High frequency ventilation in major airway or pulmonary disruption. Ann Thorac Surg 32:468, 1980.
47. Hill JD, Gibbon JH Jr. Development of the first successful heart lung machine. Ann Thorac Surg 34:337, 1982.
48. Kolobow T, Bowman RL. Construction and evaluation of an alveolar membrane artificial lung. Trans Am Soc Artif Intern Organ 9:243, 1963.
49. Hall JA Jr, Hartenberg MA, Kodroff MB. Chest radiographic findings in neonates on extracorporeal membrane oxygenation. Radiology 157:75, 1985.
50. Taylor GA, Lotze A, Kapur S, Short BL. Diffuse pulmonary opacification in infants undergoing extracorporeal membrane oxygenation: Clinical and pathologic correlation. Radiology 161:347, 1986.
51. Koumbourlis AC, Motoyama EK, Mutich RL, et al. Lung mechanics during and after extracorporeal membrane oxygenation for meconium aspiration syndrome. Crit Care Med 20:751, 1992.

52. Keszler M, Ryckman FC, McDonald JV Jr, et al. A prospective, multicenter, randomized study of high versus low positive end-expiratory pressure during extracorporeal membrane oxygenation. J Pediatr 120:107, 1992.

53. Lotze A, Knight GR, Martin GR, et al. Improved pulmonary outcome after exogenous surfactant therapy for respiratory failure in term infants requiring extracorporeal membrane oxygenation. J Pediatr 122:261, 1993.

54. Adolph V, Ekelund C, Smith C, et al. Developmental outcome of neonates treated with extracorporeal membrane oxygenation. J Pediatr Surg 25:43, 1990.

55. Griffin MP, Minifee PK, Landry SH, et al. Neurodevelopmental outcome in neonates after extracorporeal membrane oxygenation: Cranial magnetic resonance imaging and ultrasonography correlation. J Pediatr Surg 27:33, 1992.

56. Kemper KJ, Ritz RH, Benson MS, Bishop MS. Helium-oxygen mixture in the treatment of postextubation stridor in pediatric trauma patients. Crit Care Med 19:356, 1991.

57. Elleau C, Galperine RI, Guenard H, Demarquez JL. Helium-oxygen mixture in respiratory distress syndrome: A double-blind study. J Pediatr 122:132, 1993.

58. Butt WW, Koren G, England S, et al. Hypoxia associated with helium-oxygen therapy in neonates. J Pediatr 106:474, 1985.

59. Roberts JD Jr, Chen TY, Kawai N, et al. Inhaled nitric oxide reverses pulmonary vasoconstriction in the hypoxic and acidotic newborn lamb. Circ Res 72:246, 1993.

60. Kinsella JP, Neish SR, Shaffer E, Abman SH. Low-dose inhalation nitric oxide in persistent pulmonary hypertension of the newborn. Lancet 340:819, 1992.

61. Roberts JD, Polaner DM, Lang P, Zapol WM. Inhaled nitric oxide in persistent pulmonary hypertension of the newborn. Lancet 340:818, 1992.

62. Tabachnik E, Levison H. Infantile bronchial asthma. J Allergy Clin Immunol 67:339, 1981.

63. Gergen PJ, Mullally DI, Evans R. National survey of prevalence of asthma among children in the United States, 1976 to 1980. Pediatrics 81:1, 1988.

64. Siegel SC, Rachelefsky GS. Asthma in infants and children. J Allergy Clin Immunol 76:1, 1985.

65. Canny GJ, Levison H. Aerosols—Therapeutic use and delivery in childhood asthma. Ann Allergy 60:11, 1988.

66. Kelly HW. When and how to use bronchodilators in infants. Respir Ther 14:47, 1984.

67. Sly RM. Unlabeled use of approved drugs. J Allergy Clin Immunol 71:515, 1983.

68. Schuh S, Reider MJ, Canny G, et al. Nebulized albuterol in acute childhood asthma: Comparison of two doses. Pediatrics 86:509, 1990.

69. Portnoy J, Aggarwal J. Continuous terbutaline nebulization for the treatment of severe exacerbations of asthma in children. Ann Allergy 60:368, 1988.

70. Moler FW, Hurwitz ME, Custer JR. Improvement in clinical asthma score and Pa_{CO_2} in children with severe asthma treated with continuously nebulized terbutaline. J Allergy Clin Immunol 81:1101, 1988.

71. Calcone A, Wolkove N, Stern E, et al. Continuous nebulization of albuterol in acute asthma. Chest 97:693, 1990.

72. Papo MC, Frank JA, Thompson AE. A prospective randomized study of continuous vs. intermittent nebulized albuterol for severe status asthmaticus in children. Crit Care Med 21:1479, 1993.

73. Newman S. Aerosol generators and delivery systems. Respir Care 36:939, 1991.

74. Arnon S, Grigg J, Nikander K, Silverman M. Delivery of micronized budesonide suspension by metered dose inhaler and jet nebulizer into a neonatal ventilator circuit. Pediatr Pulmonol 13:172, 1992.

75. Taylor R, Lerman J. High-efficiency delivery of salbutamol with a metered-dose inhaler in narrow tracheal tubes and catheters. Anesthesiology 74:360, 1991.

76. Black RE, Mayer T, Walker ML, et al. Air transport of pediatric emergency cases. N Engl J Med 307:1465, 1978.

77. Dobrin RS, Block B, Gilman JI, Massaro TA. The development of a pediatric emergency transport system. Pediatr Clin North Am 27:633, 1980.

78. Frankel LR. The evaluation, stabilization and transport of the critically ill child. Int Anesthesiol Clin 25:77, 1987.

79. Smith DF, Hackel A. Selection criteria for pediatric critical care transport teams. Crit Care Med 11:10, 1983.

80. American Academy of Pediatrics Committee on Hospital Care: Guidelines for air and ground transportation of pediatric patients. Pediatrics 78:943, 1986.

81. Mayer TA, Walker ML. Severity of illness and injury in pediatric air transport. Ann Emerg Med 13:108, 1984.

82. Kanter RK, Tompkins JM. Adverse events during interhospital transport: Physiologic deterioration associated with pretransport severity of illness. Pediatrics 84:43–48, 1989.

83. Orr RA, Venkataraman ST, Singleton CA. Pediatric risk of mortality score (PRISM): A poor predictor in triage of patients for pediatric interhospital transport. Crit Care Med 22:101, 1994.

84. Owen H, Duncan AW. Towards safer transport of sick and injured children. Anaesth Intensive Care 11:113, 1983.

85. McCloskey K, Faries G, King W, et al. Variables predicting the need for major interventions during pediatric critical care transport. Pediatr Emerg Med 8:1, 1992.

86. Day S, McCloskey K, Orr R, et al. Pediatric interhospital critical care transport: Consensus of a national leadership conference. Pediatrics 88:696, 1991.
87. Salyer JW. Respiratory care in the transport of critically ill and injured infants and children. Respir Care 36:720, 1991.
88. Ad Hoc Task Force on Home Care of Chronically Ill Infants: Guidelines for home care of infants, children and adolescents with chronic disease. Pediatrics 74:434, 1984.
89. O'Donohue WJ Jr, Giovanni RM, Keens TG, Plummer AL. Long-term mechanical ventilation. Guidelines for management in the home and at alternate community sites. Report of the Ad Hoc Committee, Respiratory Care Section, American College of Chest Physicians. Chest 90:1S, 1986.
90. Pinney MA, Cotton EK. Home management of bronchopulmonary dysplasia. Pediatrics 58:856, 1976.
91. Okamoto E, Fee WE Jr, Boles R, et al. Safety of hospital vs home care of infant tracheostomies. Trans Am Acad Ophthalmol Otolaryngol 84:92, 1977.
92. Foster S, Hoskins D. Home care of the child with a tracheostomy tube. Pediatr Clin North Am 28:855, 1981.
93. Alexander MA, Johnson EW, Petty J, Stauch D. Mechanical ventilation of patients with late stage Duchenne muscular dystrophy: Management in the home. Arch Phys Med Rehabil 60:289, 1979.
94. O'Leary J, King R, Leblanc M, et al. Cuirass ventilation in childhood neuromuscular disease. J Pediatr 94:419, 1979.
95. Schraeder BD. A creative approach to caring for the ventilator-dependent child. MCN 4:165, 1979.
96. Splaingard ML, Frates RC Jr, Harrison GM, et al. Home positive pressure ventilation. Twenty years experience. Chest 84:376, 1983.
97. Burr BH, Guyer B, Todres ID, et al. Home care for children on respirators. N Engl J Med 309:1319, 1983.
98. Fields AI, Rosenblatt A, Pollack MM, Kaufman J. Home-care effectiveness for respiratory technology–dependent children. Am J Dis Child 145:729, 1991.
99. Gioia FR, Wetzel RC, Rogers MC. Home mechanical ventilation in pediatric patients. Crit Care Med 11:216, 1983.
100. Goldberg AI, Faure EAM, Vaughn CJ, et al. Home care for life-supported persons: An approach to program development. J Pediatr 104:785, 1984.
101. McPherson SM. Respiratory home care equipment. Daedalus Enterprises, Kendall/Hunt Publishing, Dubuque, IA, 1988.

54

Pathophysiology-Based Approach to Neonatal Respiratory Care

Jon N. Meliones, M.D., Barbara G. Wilson, R.R.T., M.Ed., R. Alan Leonard, R.R.T., and Alan R. Spitzer, M.D.

Key Terms

Respiratory System Development

Neonatal Respiratory Care

Neonatal Ventilatory Support

High-Frequency Ventilation

Extracorporeal Membrane Oxygenation

Surfactant

Since 1970, advances in newborn respiratory care have been instrumental in improving neonatal survival. This chapter discusses the principles of respiratory physiology and pathophysiology because these principles provide the basis for determining respiratory support for infants with respiratory disease. The initial sections focus on the respiratory physiology that is critical to pulmonary gas exchange in newborns and include neonatal respiratory development and developmental considerations. The next section discusses respiratory care for neonates, emphasizing the differences between approaches used for neonates and those used for children and adults. The final sections focus on respiratory support for common pathophysiologic disturbances that occur in neonates and the complications that result from respiratory interventions.

NEONATAL RESPIRATORY DEVELOPMENT

During gestation, the placenta is the primary organ of gas exchange. After the birth of the infant, a complex series of changes within the lungs and the circulation promote oxygen uptake and carbon dioxide elimination within the lung. In fact, the ultimate respiratory viability of the infant is directly proportional to the degree of lung maturation and the capability for gas exchange present at birth. In an infant with inadequate lung development, respiratory distress syndrome (RDS) is commonly the end-result. RDS may result from surfactant deficiency in the lung, and the less mature the infant, the more likely that RDS will be present.

Pulmonary development in the fetus is, however, a complex process. In contrast to the premature infant, the infant born post-term (at greater than 42 weeks of gestation) may be exposed to involution and infarction of the placenta. These events can result in chronic hypoxemia and hypertrophy of the muscular layer of pulmonary blood vessels. This process, referred to as primary pulmonary hypertension, causes severe hypoxemia in the large postmature baby. An understanding of fetal lung development is therefore essential in the diagnosis and treatment of neonatal lung disease.

The development of the lung begins at approximately 24 to 25 days of gestation, as an outpouching of the primitive gut (Fig. 54–1). Within 2 days, primary branches appear, which subsequently become the right and the left mainstem bronchi. During the remainder of the first trimester, lung growth consists of further branching of the endodermal tube into the surrounding mesenchyme. This period of pulmonary maturation is referred to as the glandular stage.

At approximately 16 weeks of gestation, the canalicular stage of lung development begins. During this stage, the primitive airways display the first signs of subsequent tubular development. Throughout this stage of lung maturation, the airspaces are lined by simple cuboidal epithelium. Before approximately 24 weeks of gestation, airway and capillary proliferation within the lung is insufficient for gas exchange. The abundance of connective tissue also interferes with oxygen uptake and carbon dioxide elimination. As a result, the lower limit of viability for the human neonate is at 24 weeks after conception.

After 24 weeks of gestation, the final period of prenatal lung development, the alveolar stage, begins. During this stage, preparation for air breathing occurs. The cuboidal epithelium begins to attenuate, the amount of connective tissue decreases, and capillaries increase in number, moving closer to the terminal airspaces. At approximately 28 weeks, alveoli begin to proliferate from alveolar ducts, and the potential for the viability of the fetus increases rapidly.

During the midtrimester, in the canalicular stage of lung development, two distinct pulmonary cells can be seen in the terminal airspaces: a nonvacuolated cell, similar to that found in other connective tissue (type I cell), and a larger, vacuolated cell containing lipoidal material (type II cell). The type II cell contains cytoplasmic inclusion bodies, which appear concurrently with the synthesis and secretion of pulmonary surfactant. Because surfactant inadequacy plays such a central role in the understanding of neonatal lung disease, it is critical to understand the concept of surface tension.

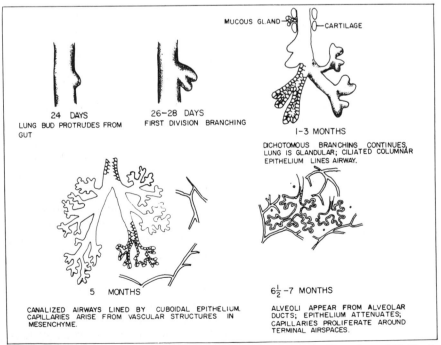

FIGURE 54–1: The stages of lung development during gestation. (From Avery ME. The Lung and Its Disorders in the Newborn Infant. Philadelphia, WB Saunders, 1985, p 5.)

Surface tension refers to the sum of the cohesive forces that hold a liquid together. Within this liquid, the forces exerted on a single molecule are equal in all directions because each molecule attracts and is in turn attracted by other molecules of the liquid with an identical strength. At the interface of the liquid with air, however, the liquid molecules exert a net force that is directed inward, reducing the surface to its minimal area. This force is expressed per unit length (dynes per centimeter) and is called surface tension.

Within the lung, a similar situation exists, with an air-liquid interface at the lining of the terminal airspace, or alveolus. The net tendency of the lung is to reduce the alveolar surface to a minimal area (atelectasis). The design of the lung, therefore, must decrease the net force that tends to collapse the alveolus (surface tension). This reduction of surface tension is achieved by surface-active materials within the lung.

Surface-active materials lower surface tension by forming an insoluble surface film that expands spontaneously on the liquid surface. The molecules of the surface-active material have a lower surface tension than do the bulk of the molecules of the liquid to which they are added, and they usually consist of a polar and a nonpolar group. The polar group, possibly through hydrogen bonding, is drawn toward the liquid, whereas the nonpolar group turns toward the gas phase. The dispersion of surface-active molecules thereby reduces the surface tension at the air-liquid interface, and the liquid no longer tends to shrink to its minimal area. In the lung, the presence of surfactant counteracts a tendency to collapse at the end of a breath, allowing a volume of gas to remain in the lung at the end of expiration (functional residual capacity). Subsequent breaths therefore require far less effort to inflate the lung. In the child with surfactant deficiency and RDS, an inadequate amount of surface-active material is present, and progressive atelectasis occurs as the alveolar surfaces become increasingly adhesive.

The primary components of surfactant are dipalmitoylphosphatidylcholine, to a lesser extent phosphatidylglycerol, and protein. An important feature of these phospholipids is their high degree of fatty acid saturation, which enables them to be densely packed at a surface interface and exclude water. Although dipalmitoylphosphatidylcholine is the main functional component of surfactant, phosphatidylglycerol is believed to stabilize the surfactant, a feature of critical biomedical significance. Several surfactant replacements are commercially available and are used extensively in patients with surfactant deficiency.

Macklin first described the role of the type II cell, or granular pneumonocyte, in 1954. Subsequent studies have confirmed its role in the production of surface-active phospholipids. Since this first description of the type II cell, much research in fetal lung maturation has focused on the role of this cell. In 1955, Pattle described the existence of a surface-active material in the lung that reduced surface tension. Clements, in 1957, isolated an extract of surfactant from lung tissue and showed that this preparation had surface-active properties. Subsequently, Avery and Mead found that infants who died of RDS had a decreased amount of surfactant in the lung. In 1967, Clements and Tooley attempted to administer surfactant to infants dying of RDS, but this effort was unsuccessful. In 1980, Fujiwara and coworkers, working with a new preparation of surfactant derived from cows' lungs, found a marked improvement in oxygenation after surfactant administration in babies with RDS. Since the mid-1980s, work toward developing effective surfactant replacement has proceeded rapidly (see later sections).

Fetal Lung Fluid

The first recognition of the importance of fetal lung fluid occurred in 1948, when Jost and Policard performed a series of studies on fetal rabbits that demonstrated an increase in lung volume after tracheal ligation. They concluded that fetal fluid contributed to the volume of amniotic fluid. Before these experiments, lung fluid was thought to be the product of in utero aspiration of amniotic fluid. Subsequent studies have confirmed these observations and have substantiated the fact that fetal lung fluid is actually an important contributor to the composite volume of amniotic fluid. The volume of fetal lung fluid in amniotic fluid is relatively small, however, compared with the contribution of the fetal genitourinary system.

The net outward flow of fetal lung fluid into the uterine cavity is aided by the process of fetal breathing. The fetus demonstrates respiratory activity of a rapid, irregular nature beginning at the end of the first trimester. Through the studies of Dawes, these activities have been shown to be crucial to the development of respiratory muscle tone, preparing the chest wall and diaphragm for air breathing after birth. Infants who have no fetal breathing, as in the case of congenital absence of the diaphragm, have severe lung hypoplasia.

At term, the amount of fetal lung fluid present within the lung is about 20 to 30 mL/kg body weight, which is approximately equal to the postnatal functional residual capacity of the lung. Fetal lung fluid appears to be removed from the birth canal through circumferential chest compression at the time of birth, an important but not critical event. Hormonal and other factors also play a role in this process. At birth, approximately two thirds of fetal lung fluid is expressed upward through the trachea, and one third is absorbed by pulmonary capillaries and lymphatics. A child born by cesarean section, therefore, may have some delay in the reabsorption of fetal lung fluid and may have respiratory symptoms for some time after birth. This disease process, commonly referred to as transient tachypnea of the newborn, is a self-limited disease that usually lasts about 2 to 3 days.

These investigations of fetal lung fluid have provided obstetricians with a window for assessing lung maturation. Because there is a net flow of fetal lung fluid outward into the amniotic cavity, biochemical determination of surfactant concentration can be used to assess the risk of RDS in a preterm infant. In 1971, Gluck and coworkers demonstrated that a lecithin-sphingomyelin ratio of greater than 2:1 was associated with pulmonary maturity and a low risk of RDS. Subsequently, they developed a lung profile that evaluates several additional factors and provides a better estimate of lung maturation.

Several alternative tests have been developed for more rapid assessment of fetal lung maturation. The lung profile, which requires high-pressure liquid chromatography, has in many institutions been replaced by simple bedside determinations, such as the shake test, or the fluid foam stability test devised by Clements. In this test, a rapid bedside evaluation is performed by diluting amniotic fluid with 95% alcohol. The tester shakes a series of diluted tubes and observes the ring of bubbles at the surface of the liquid to assess lung maturation. At present, a number of commercially available kits provide similar information on lung maturation.

Lung maturation can be enhanced by several techniques. Prominent among these is the prenatal administration of glucocorticoids, particularly betamethasone or dexamethasone, to the mother. This technique, first attempted by Liggins and Howie in 1972, was effective in babies from 26 to 34 weeks of gestation. In addition to surfactant effects, anatomic effects, such as thinning of the alveolar septa and a decrease in the amount of connective tissue of the lung, also occur. Subsequent trials have indicated that glucocorticoids are more effective in female infants than in male infants. It is thought that this difference may be due to the presence of androgens in the male fetus. There may also be some nonspecific positive benefits of the administration of glucocorticoids, such as the reduction of intraventricular hemorrhage in the preterm infant. Bronchopulmonary dysplasia, a primary consequence of mechanical ventilation in the newborn infant, may be reduced by the prenatal administration of glucocorticoids. The administration of glucocorticoids often requires the administration of tocolytic agents to inhibit preterm labor because glucocorticoids appear to take at least 24 hours to exert their effectiveness. Glucocorticoids are avoided if any potential exists for infection of the mother or the infant.

Thyroid hormone may also mature the fetal lung. Because it does not cross the placenta, it must be given intra-amniotically. Work in this area is still very preliminary.

DEVELOPMENTAL CONSIDERATIONS

Effective respiratory support in infants requires a fundamental understanding of the developmental changes in the static and dynamic components of respiratory mechanics. Respiratory rate, inspiratory time, inspiratory flow, tidal volume, and mechanical properties of the respiratory system for a given age are the principal determinants of respiratory support in neonates. These developmental features of respiratory physiologic parameters limit the applicability of ventilatory equipment and approaches designed primarily for adults.

Respiratory Rate

The respiratory rate in newborns ranges from 30 to 60 breaths per minute. The respiratory rate does not decrease to the adult value of 12 to 16 breaths per minute until adolescence. Higher respiratory rates in neonates and young children are reflected in shorter inspiratory times. The normal inspiratory time in infants is between 0.3 and 0.5 second. The shorter inspiratory time is a result of the decreased time constant that occurs in neonates versus adults.

Tidal Volume

Tidal volume relative to body weight changes little during development (i.e., it is 6 to 8 mL/kg). On an absolute basis, however, the range of tidal volume encountered in neonates changes by orders of magnitude with advancing age (e.g., it is 18 mL per breath in the newborn versus 500 mL per breath in the adult).

Inspiratory Flow

Although the average inspiratory flow encountered in neonates is approximately 1.9 L/min, peak inspiratory flows during periods of respiratory distress can approach 20 L/min. This is in contrast to older children and adults, who can generate instantaneous peak flows of 300 to 600 L/min, despite a normal average inspiratory flow of 24 L/min.

Total Respiratory Compliance

Total respiratory compliance is the change in respiratory system volume per unit change in distending pressure. The absolute value of total respiratory compliance increases by a factor of 20 from the neonatal period through adolescence. When total respiratory compliance is expressed on a relative basis as a function of lung volume or body weight (i.e., specific respiratory compliance), infant and adult values are remarkably similar (approximately 0.06 mL/cm H_2O/mL lung volume).

Total Respiratory Conductance

Total respiratory conductance, which is the reciprocal of total resistance, is flow per unit pressure change across the respiratory system. Total respiratory conductance increases from infancy to adulthood by a factor of 15. As is the case with total compliance, airway conductance normalized for unit lung volume or body weight is similar for infants and adults.

Respiratory compliance and conductance define the mechanical forces required to inflate the lungs during positive pressure ventilation. Although the absolute values of compliance and conductance are much lower in the infant, when they are indexed to relative size, inspiratory flow, and tidal volume, they are similar to values found in adults. Therefore, comparable inspiratory pressures are required in infants and adults to ensure adequate volume during positive pressure ventilation. The low absolute compliance and high absolute resistance of the developing respiratory system require special attention in designing systems to deliver physiologic tidal volumes to children. Pediatric ventilators must deliver low inspiratory volumes under pressures comparable to those used in adults; consequently, estimates of tidal volume delivered during positive pressure ventilation in children are subject to gross error because of the relatively large volume of the ventilator systems. The distribution of volume delivered by a positive pressure ventilator between the ventilator circuit (i.e., compressible volume) and the patient is determined by the relative compliance of the circuit and the patient. If the compliances of the ventilator circuit and the patient are equal, the volume distributed to the patient and the circuit is the same. This could result in gross errors in estimating the actual delivered tidal volume. These large circuit compliance characteristics also give rise to decreased sensitivity of ventilator valve systems to spontaneous inspiratory efforts and delays in the delivery of assisted or synchronized positive pressure breaths.

RESPIRATORY INTERVENTIONS

Inhaled Medical Gases

Medical gases are inspired into the airways and distributed to the alveoli to allow gas exchange. The inhaled medical gases described here include oxygen, carbon dioxide, and nitric oxide.

OXYGEN

Increased concentrations of inspired oxygen are administered to patients who have inadequate oxygen delivery as a result of decreased systemic arterial saturation. Oxygen administration is less helpful if decreased oxygen delivery is due to decreased cardiac output, decreased hemoglobin concentration, or excessive tissue oxygen needs. The presence of an alveolar-arterial oxygen tension gradient [$P(A - a)O_2$] is the primary indication for oxygen administration. The goal of oxygen administration is to improve the oxygen saturation of hemoglobin while minimizing oxygen toxicity.

In general, care should be taken to administer the lowest fraction of inspired oxygen (FI_{O_2}) to maintain an Sa_{O_2} of greater than 90 to 92%. Oxygen for neonates is usually administered via oxy-hood oxygenators or nasal cannulas. Oxy-hood oxygenators are Plexiglas chambers that deliver a set FI_{O_2} to the head and face. FI_{O_2} and temperature should be continuously monitored to prevent hypoxia or hyperoxia and cooling or overheating of the infant. Nasal cannulas can be used with low-flow flowmeters for more precise titration of oxygen in stable infants because small changes in the oxygen flow rate or spontaneous breathing may result in dramatic changes in oxygenation.

CARBON DIOXIDE

Carbon dioxide is rarely used as an inhaled gas in the neonatal intensive care unit. It has, however, been used in patients with single-ventricle physiology to reduce pulmonary blood flow. Increasing the inspired carbon dioxide concentration results in an increase in PA_{CO_2} and Pa_{CO_2}. Increasing the PA_{CO_2} results in an increase in pulmonary vascular resistance, which leads to a reduction in pulmonary blood flow and stabilization of shunt flow in patients with single-ventricle physiology.

Carbon dioxide is administered into the inspiratory limb of the ventilator after it is blended with oxygen and air. To evaluate the concentration of the administered carbon dioxide, an inline capnograph is placed in the inspiratory limb. The inspired carbon dioxide is then titrated to achieve the desired hemodynamic effect, which usually yields a Pa_{CO_2} of approximately 40 mm Hg. Monitoring during carbon dioxide administration primarily consists of evaluating inspired end-tidal carbon dioxide concentrations, arterial blood gas values, and indicators of systemic perfusion (including peripheral pulses and perfusion) and of oxygen delivery.

NITRIC OXIDE

Nitric oxide, or endothelial-derived relaxing factor, can be administered as an inhaled gas. It is a nonselective vasodilator that is rapidly inactivated by hemoglobin. When inhaled, nitric oxide results in rapid vasodilation of the pulmonary arteries and a reduction in pulmonary vascular resistance. Inhaled nitric oxide has virtually no effect on the systemic circulation because it is rapidly inactivated by hemoglobin. A prompt reduction in pulmonary vascular resistance has been demonstrated after the inhalation of nitric oxide in newborns with pulmonary artery hypertension and in patients with pulmonary artery hypertension after surgery for congenital heart disease. In the perioperative period, patients with congenital heart disease and pulmonary artery hypertension may benefit from the addition of nitric oxide because of the favorable decrease in pulmonary vascular resistance. A reduction in pulmonary vascular resistance may reduce right ventricular work and improve cardiac output and oxygen delivery in this clinical setting.

Nitric oxide administration is generally initiated at concentrations of 10 ppm. This gas is administered through an oxygen–nitric oxide blender. A reduction in the inspired oxygen to 90% or less is required. If the desired cardiorespiratory effects are not achieved, the nitric oxide concentration is gradually increased to a maximum of 80 ppm. Higher levels of inspired nitric oxide should be considered in selected patients only. Once the desired cardiorespiratory effects have been achieved, the most toxic therapy is weaned first. In many instances, this is the inspired oxygen concentration, airway pressures, or inotropes. When the patient has demonstrated improved cardiorespiratory performance, the nitric oxide dosage should be reduced to the lowest therapeutic level. Nitric oxide administration should be terminated when the patient's condition has improved and a reduction in nitric oxide can be accomplished without significant increases in pulmonary artery pressures. Nitric oxide therapy should be terminated in patients who are nonresponders and in those who develop hypotension after nitric oxide initiation. Methemoglobinemia is the most frequently demonstrated side effect, and methemoglobin levels should be measured after 6 hours of nitric oxide administration and every 12 hours thereafter.

Classification of Positive Pressure Ventilators

A mechanical ventilator is a life-support system designed to replace or support lung function. Nomenclature to classify the essential features of positive pressure ventilators has been described by many authors. A sound classification system provides a common knowledge-base of terms and concepts to facilitate the understanding, interpretation, and assessment of ventilator operating systems and performance characteristics. The classification system must be clinically relevant and must accurately reflect the pattern of respiratory support a patient receives. This section presents ventilator classification as it supports the clinical practice of neonatal ventilatory care.

A ventilator is designed to alter, transmit, and apply energy directly in a predetermined way to perform the work of the thorax and lungs. A ventilator classification system presented in Table 54–1 addresses five basic categories: power input, power transmission, control schemes, output parameters, and alarm systems.

POWER INPUT AND TRANSMISSION

Ventilator power input is either electrical or pneumatic (compressed gas). The transmission of input power is a function of the drive and control mechanisms of the ventilator. Ventilator classification focuses on the control variables, output parameters, and alarm systems as applied to their clinical utility. More specifically, clinicians focus on breath types and breath limits to describe the type of respiratory support a patient may be receiving.

CONTROL SCHEMES AND CONTROL VARIABLES

Ventilator control variables address the physical qualities adjusted, measured, or used to manipulate various phases of the ventilatory cycle.

TABLE **54–1:** Ventilator Classification System

Power input	Control scheme
Pneumatic	Control circuit
Electrical	Control variables
Power transmission or conversion	Phase variables
(drive mechanism)	Conditional variables
External compressor	Output waveforms
Internal compressor	Pressure
Output/control valves	Volume
	Flow
	Alarm systems

The four common types of control variables are flow, pressure, volume, and time. Typically, the functioning of the control variables remains constant despite changes in ventilatory load. Therefore, the ventilator sacrifices all other preset variables to keep the control variables constant, despite changes in the patient's compliance and resistance. Each manufacturer develops and refines its control scheme for the manipulation of these variables. However, commonalities arise among ventilators that allow clinicians to describe the resultant respiratory patterns with common terminology.

Flow

The inspiratory flow pattern determines the characteristics of the gas flow delivery during a positive pressure breath and the distribution of that breath within the patient's respiratory system. Airway pressures depend on the mechanical properties of the lungs and the movement of gas into the lungs. The airway pressures (peak inspiratory and mean airway) generated during inspiration increase as flow enters the respiratory system and encounters the resistance of the airways. The gas volume must also overcome the elastic recoil of the lung. Therefore, peak pressure = flow × RAW + tidal volume × elastance. The shape of the inspiratory flow pattern as it delivers the positive pressure breath determines the shape of the pressure curve and the peak pressure generated. This can be predicted, given knowledge of the characteristics of the various flow patterns and the pneumatic characteristics of the patient's lungs, as is described later.

Figure 54–2 illustrates tracings typical of the inspiratory flow patterns available with positive pressure ventilators. A sine wave pattern has a variable flow with an increase during the early phase of inspiration, a peak at midinspiration, and then a decrease in flow until end-inspiration. A square wave pattern is produced by a constant flow of gas throughout inspiration. Ascending flow patterns produce a ramp pattern with low flow at the beginning of inspiration, linear increases in flow throughout inspiration, and peak flow delivered at end-inspiration. Descending flow is a waveform characterized by peak flow at the beginning of inspiration and linear decreases until end-inspiration. The functional performance of the various types of inspiratory flow patterns remains constant across manufacturers but may be produced by dramatically different control schemes.

Pressure

The flow pattern characteristics of a specific mechanical ventilator significantly influence the airway pressure. Gas flow always takes the path of least resistance. Flow pattern alterations affect this distribution based on the underlying pathophysiology and anatomic considerations of the patient. Ascending flow patterns deliver the highest flow at end-

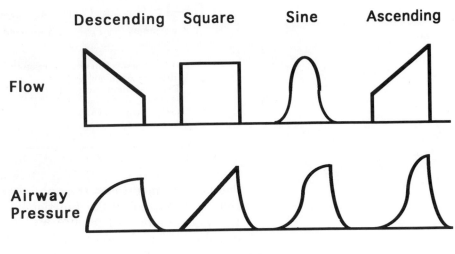

FIGURE 54–2: Tracings typical of the various inspiratory waveforms available with mechanical ventilators. Pressure control ventilation uses a descending wave that results in lower peak and higher mean airway pressures. Volume control ventilation uses a square waveform. (Adapted from Rau JL. Inspiratory flow patterns: The shape of ventilation. Respir Care 38[1]:132–140, 1993.)

inspiration, when the effects of resistance and elastance are increased. Ascending flow patterns produce higher peak pressures than do other flow patterns. A descending or decelerating flow pattern has several advantages over an ascending pattern. Descending flow patterns deliver the highest flow at the beginning of inspiration, when volume and elastance are low. Flow then decreases during inspiration as delivered volume increases. Therefore, peak pressures are lower but the mean pressure is higher with this flow pattern. The various flow patterns may generate different airway pressures. In general, as the maximal flow moves from the beginning to the end of the inspiratory cycle, peak pressure increases and mean airway pressure decreases. Flow patterns should therefore be matched to the clinical condition of the patient.

In neonatal clinical situations in which the patient has low lung compliance as a result of decreased surfactant, the square wave flow pattern provides consistent flow levels throughout inspiration to recruit collapsed alveoli.

BREATH TYPES AND BREATH LIMITS

Phase Variables

Factors that affect the phases of the ventilatory cycle are called phase variables. These factors address the initiation, duration, and termination of inspiration and expiration. Trigger variables are parameters that initiate inspiratory flow, whereas cycle variables are parameters that terminate inspiration. All ventilators measure variables associated with the delivery of the positive pressure breaths (time, pressure, and volume). Inspiration begins when one of these variables, historically time or pressure, reaches a preset value called the trigger variable. Several newer neonatal and pediatric ventilators offer flow triggering, which increases the sensitivity of the ventilator to the patient's spontaneous demands and decreases the response time of breath delivery. Therefore, mechanical breaths may be pressure, time, or flow triggered. Some neonatal ventilators trigger inspiration via an external sensor taped to the abdomen of the infant to sense respiratory movement, initiate inspiration, and synchronize the delivery of the mechanical breath with the patient's spontaneous efforts. Under these conditions, the mechanical breath could be considered an "impedance" trigger.

The cycle variable determines when inspiration ends. This variable is used as a feedback signal to terminate gas flow and allow the patient to exhale passively. Time is currently the neonatal standard cycle variable; therefore, most ventilators are considered time cycled.

Limit Variables

Limit variables, which are safety checks in the ventilator system, prevent selected ventilatory parameters from exceeding predetermined values. During inspiration, pressure, volume, and flow increase above the end-expiratory values. Limit variables allow the clinician to control the upper limits of pressure and volume of the mechanical breath a patient receives: hence, the descriptions "pressure limited" and "volume limited." A baseline variable describes the parameter controlled during the expiratory phase of the ventilatory cycle. The most commonly manipulated expiratory variable is pressure. This pressure is most often positive and consists of positive end-expiratory pressure (PEEP) or continuous positive airway pressure (CPAP).

VENTILATORY MODES

With this terminology, a system can be developed that describes the ventilatory modes and specific breathing patterns used during positive pressure ventilation. Ventilatory modes may include spontaneous breaths, mechanical breaths, or combinations of both.

Spontaneous breaths may be supported with CPAP, a mode that maintains a constant positive airway pressure above baseline throughout inspiration and expiration. The CPAP mode differs from normal CPAP because the patient is intubated. A preset expiratory pressure limit prevents the patient from exhaling down to atmospheric pressure at end-expiration. Continuous or demand flow during inspiration maintains airway pressure above atmospheric pressure. Raising the expiratory pressure above the atmospheric pressure traps a volume of gas in the lungs that is proportionate to the pressure applied and lung compliance. This gas volume augments the expiratory reserve volume of the lung and increases the functional residual capacity. The CPAP mode can be used alone or in conjunction with mechanical breaths.

Pressure support ventilation is also a spontaneous breathing mode that can be used alone or in combination with other modes (synchronized intermittent mandatory ventilation [SIMV] or CPAP). A preset level of inspiratory pressure is delivered above the baseline pressure with each spontaneous effort. Pressure support ventilation is initiated when pressure or flow is dropped during inspiration to the preset threshold level. When this trigger is sensed by the ventilator, flow accelerates into the breathing circuit, which increases proximal airway pressure to the preset pressure level. The pressure support breath is terminated when approximately 25% of peak flow is reached. The tidal volume delivered in this mode varies with changes in lung compliance, airway resistance, and pressure support settings. Inspiratory time can be fixed or variable during pressure support ventilation, depending on the design configuration.

Volume support ventilation combines the benefits of pressure support ventilation with the safety of a volume guarantee during spontaneous breathing. The ventilator monitors airway resistance and compliance of the lung and adjusts the pressure support level using a predetermined algorithm to deliver a preset volume.

Positive pressure breaths may be delivered in a controlled or an assisted-controlled manner. During controlled breaths, a preset ventilator rate is delivered to the patient. Inspiratory and expiratory times are fixed in this mode and are dependent on the ventilator rate and the inspiratory-expiratory ratio. The clinical usefulness of controlled mode is limited because the patient cannot trigger additional positive pressure breaths. Controlled ventilation is best achieved by sedating or paralyzing the patient to prevent spontaneous breathing or by adjusting the ventilator rate above the patient's native rate to "capture" and control the ventilation and limit patient-ventilator dyssynchrony. Assisted breaths deliver a patient-triggered ventilator rate with each spontaneous effort. In assisted mode, the ventilatory rate is determined by the patient and may be in excess of the controlled rate. Still, the positive pressure ventilator is providing the entire work of breathing. The ventilator "sensitivity" determines the degree of effort a patient must exert to trigger the ventilator into inspiration. Ideally, this should be adjusted to -0.5 to -1.5 cm H_2O of pressure or 0.2 to 5.0 L/min of flow to minimize the patient's work of triggering.

Controlled and assisted breaths may be limited by either volume or pressure. Combining this terminology provides a better classification of the ventilatory mode. A patient may receive volume control ventilation, in which a predetermined breath rate is delivered and breaths are volume limited, or volume assist ventilation, in which mechanical breaths are also volume limited but the patient triggers breaths in excess of the preset rate. A patient may also receive pressure control ventilation, in which a preset breath rate is delivered along with a preset pressure value. Pressure assist ventilation describes a breathing pattern in which the patient may trigger the breath rate in excess of a preset rate and breaths are pressure limited.

Intermittent mandatory ventilation (IMV) modes combine mechanical breaths with spontaneous breathing. In these modes, the spontaneous volume and rate are a function of the patient's inspiratory effort and stimulus to breathe. Flow for spontaneous breathing may be provided by a continuous flow of oxygen through the breathing circuit, a demand valve, or a combination of both. If PEEP is applied with continuous and demand flow, the spontaneous breaths become CPAP breaths. Pressure support may also be administered in conjunction with SIMV, as previously described. SIMV differs from IMV in that the initiation of the mechanical breaths is synchronized with the patient's spontaneous efforts to prevent stacking of positive pressure and spontaneous breaths.

NEONATAL VENTILATION

Neonatal ventilators have traditionally been classified as continuous-flow, time-cycled, pressure-limited IMV systems. Examples of this type of ventilator are the Sechrist and Bear Cub ventilators. Under the new classification system, the mechanical breaths produced by a neonatal ventilator would be considered to be flow-controlled, time-triggered, time-cycled pressure control breaths. The spontaneous breaths provided by these ventilators would be flow-controlled positive expiratory pressure breaths (CPAP). Recent advances in neonatal ventilator design now provide the option of volume control SIMV breaths. Improvements in calibration and the measurement of smaller volumes facilitate volume as-

TABLE **54–2:** Classification of Modes of Positive Pressure Ventilation

Mode	Mechanical Breath Variables			Spontaneous Breath Variables		
	Trigger	*Cycle*	*Limit*	*Trigger*	*Cycle*	*Limit*
Continuous mechanical ventilation	Time	Time	Volume*	—	—	—
Assisted-controlled ventilation	Time	Time	Volume*	—	—	—
	Pressure	Time	Volume*	—	—	—
Intermittent mandatory ventilation	Time	Time	Volume*	Patient	Patient	Flow
Synchronized intermittent mandatory ventilation	Time	Time	Volume*	Patient	Patient	Flow
	Pressure	Time	Volume*	Pressure	Flow	Pressure
				Flow		
Pressure control ventilation	Time	Time	Pressure	—	—	—
	Pressure	Time	Pressure	—	—	—

*Flow may also be a limit variable.

sisted mechanical SIMV breaths with CPAP or pressure support of the spontaneous breaths. Mechanical breaths can be pressure- or flow-triggered, time-cycled volume assist breaths. Spontaneous breaths are flow-controlled CPAP or flow-variable pressure support breaths. Table 54–2 contains the common classifications of mechanical ventilator breaths by mode of ventilation.

OUTPUT WAVEFORM ANALYSIS

Before waveform graphics became integral components of ventilator systems, ventilator monitoring was restricted to reading the ventilator's controls, digital monitors, and mechanical gauges and to physical assessment. Detailed analysis of the patient-ventilator interface was therefore impossible. Technologic advances now permit continuous respiratory mechanics monitoring, including graphic displays of gas flow, volume, and airway pressure. Output waveforms are a useful tool for studying the characteristics of ventilator operation and providing a graphic display of the various modes of ventilation. Waveform analysis can be used to optimize mechanical ventilatory support and analyze ventilator incidents and alarm conditions. With the use of this technology, it is now possible to shape the form of ventilatory support to improve patient-ventilator synchrony, reduce the work of breathing, and calculate various physiologic parameters related to respiratory mechanics.

The most commonly reported waveforms are flow, pressure, and volume. Convention dictates that positive values correspond to inspiration and negative values correspond to expiration; horizontal axes represent time in seconds and vertical axes represent the measured variable in its common units of measurement. Optimal measurements are obtained when the pressure- and flow-monitoring device is positioned between the patient and the ventilator circuit. The integration of intrapleural pressure from an esophageal balloon further enhances graphic data and enables assessment of the patient's work of breathing. During spontaneous breathing, patient effort, the work of breathing, and the level of intrinsic PEEP are best evaluated via esophageal pressure measurements.

Flow Graphics

Flow may be measured in the ventilator circuit at the patient WYE connector or in the inspiratory or expiratory limb. Flow sensors should be capable of measuring a wide range of flows (-300 to $+150$ L/min)

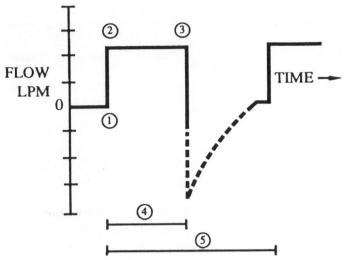

FIGURE 54–3: Inspiratory flow graphic of a square wave mechanical breath. Positive deflections indicate flow from the ventilator to the patient. 1, the initiation of flow from the ventilator; 2, peak inspiratory flow; 3, end-inspiration; 4, inspiratory time; 5, total cycle time. LPM, liters per minute. (Adapted from MacIntyre NR. Graphical Analysis of Flow, Pressure, and Volume During Mechanical Ventilation, 3rd ed. Riverside, CA, Bear Medical Systems, 1991, p 2–1.)

and should be reasonably resistant to motion artifact, moisture, and respiratory secretions. The flow graphic has two distinct parts (inspiratory flow and expiratory flow), which should be analyzed separately. The inspiratory flow graphic displays the magnitude, duration, and flow pattern of the positive pressure breath or spontaneous breath. Figure 54–3 is a theoretical inspiratory flow pattern of a continuous-flow mechanical breath. In actual application, flow delivery mechanisms have response times that alter the shape of the flow graphic. These response times result in a positive slope at the start of inspiration and a negative slope at end-inspiration (Fig. 54–4). Graphic flow analysis can also be affected

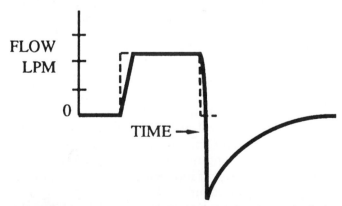

FIGURE 54–4: Constant inspiratory flow graphic of a mechanical breath, modified by ventilator response time. Note the phase shift and the alteration in the shape of the flow curve during inspiration. LPM, liters per minute. (Adapted from MacIntyre NR. Graphical Analysis of Flow, Pressure, and Volume During Mechanical Ventilation, 3rd ed. Riverside, CA, Bear Medical Systems, 1991, p 2–2.)

by back pressure in the patient-ventilator circuit. Third-generation ventilators with low internal compliance and increased driving pressures are less responsive to changes in back pressure, but significant alterations in lung compliance and airway resistance may affect the shape of the flow graphic.

The flow graphic of a spontaneous breath is demonstrated in Figure 54–5. The characteristic of the flow graphic is determined by the characteristics of the patient's inspiratory demand and the ventilatory support provided to the spontaneous breath (i.e., continuous-flow CPAP, demand-flow CPAP, or pressure support).

The expiratory flow graphic is a passive movement for both mechanical and spontaneous breaths. The magnitude, duration, and pattern of the expiratory graphic are determined by the compliance and resistance of both the patient's respiratory mechanics and the ventilator circuit. Important features of the ventilator circuit that affect the flow graphic include the size and length of the endotracheal tube, the internal diameter and length of the ventilator circuit, the resistance of the expiratory valve, and the distensibility of the circuit itself. Figure 54–6 shows a typical expiratory flow graphic for a positive pressure breath. The expiratory flow by convention is shown below the zero baseline. Because the characteristics of the patient circuit that affect the expiratory flow pattern are generally fixed, dramatic changes in the expiratory flow curve may be attributable to changes in the patient's compliance, resistance, or activity. For example, an increase in airway resistance due to obstructive disease or secretions may result in decreased peak expiratory flow, increased duration of flow, or failure of flow to return to baseline (Fig. 54–7).

Pressure Graphics

During graphic analysis, pressure is measured in the ventilator circuit at the patient Y connector or at the inspiratory or expiratory limb. Although resistance of the endotracheal tube is a component of the pressure graphic, pressures reported are generally considered to reflect airway pressure (P_{AW}). Pressure graphics for positive pressure and spontaneous breaths are very different and are considered separately here. The type of breath a patient receives (positive pressure versus spontaneous) can easily be identified by examination of the pressure graphic. In a typical spontaneous breath from a demand-flow valve (Fig. 54–8), there is a slight pressure drop at the beginning of inspiration, the mag-

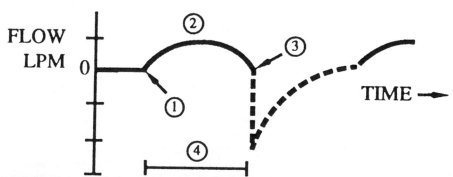

FIGURE 54–5: Inspiratory flow graphic of a spontaneous breath. Inspiratory flow from the ventilator to the patient is by convention shown as a positive deflection. 1, the start of inspiration; 2, peak inspiratory flow; 3, end-inspiration; 4, inspiratory time. LPM, liters per minute. (Adapted from MacIntyre NR. Graphical Analysis of Flow, Pressure, and Volume During Mechanical Ventilation, 3rd ed. Riverside, CA, Bear Medical Systems, 1991, p 2–4.)

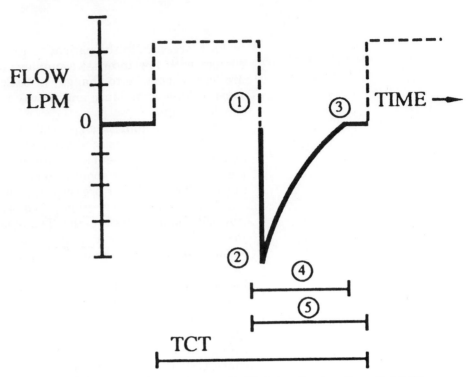

FIGURE 54–6: Normal expiratory flow graphic. Expiratory flow from the patient to the ventilator is by convention shown as a negative deflection. 1, the start of expiration; 2, peak expiratory flow; 3, end-expiratory flow; 4, duration of expiratory flow; 5, expiratory time. LPM, liters per minute; TCT, total cycle time. (Adapted from MacIntyre NR. Graphical Analysis of Flow, Pressure, and Volume During Mechanical Ventilation, 3rd ed. Riverside, CA, Bear Medical Systems, 1991, p 2–5.)

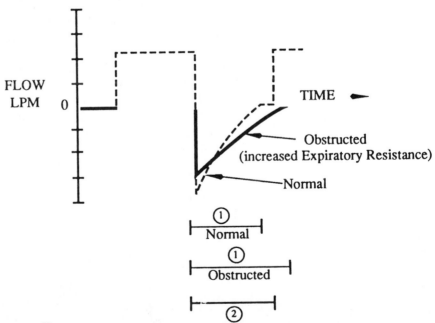

FIGURE 54–7: Abnormal expiratory flow graphic in a patient with airway obstruction. The expiratory flow exceeds the available expiratory time because exhalation is not complete. 1, duration of normal expiratory flow; 1, duration of obstructed expiratory flow; 2, duration of mechanical expiratory time. If expiratory time is short (as occurs in the expiratory waveform marked "obstructed"), premature termination of exhalation occurs with resultant gas trapping and an increased dead space–tidal volume ratio. LPM, liters per minute. (Adapted from MacIntyre NR. Graphical Analysis of Flow, Pressure, and Volume During Mechanical Ventilation, 3rd ed. Riverside, CA, Bear Medical Systems, 1991, p 2–6.)

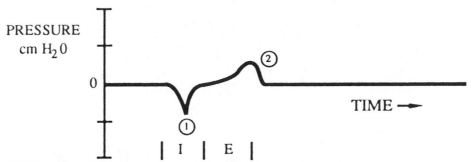

FIGURE 54–8: Spontaneous breath pressure graphic. 1, the pressure drop during inspiration (I); 2, the pressure rise during expiration (E). (Adapted from MacIntyre NR. Graphical Analysis of Flow, Pressure, and Volume During Mechanical Ventilation, 3rd ed. Riverside, CA, Bear Medical Systems, 1991, p 2–7.)

nitude of which is proportionate to the patient's peak inspiratory flow rate, the sensitivity of the demand valve, and the response of the flow delivery system. This drop is followed by a pressure rise toward baseline as flow enters the circuit and the patient. The graphic curve then increases above baseline as the patient exhales. The increase in pressure is due to flow resistance in the expiratory limb, the expiratory valve, or both. The magnitude of the pressure rise varies, depending on the peak expiratory flow. In contrast, during a typical positive pressure breath, the peak inspiratory pressure is determined by the patient and circuit compliance, resistance, delivered tidal volume, and inspiratory flow (Fig. 54–9). Baseline pressure reflects the expiratory pressure in the circuit (i.e., PEEP or CPAP settings).

Volume Graphics

Volume is generally measured by integrating the flow signal with inspiratory time (Fig. 54–10). The upsweep of the graphic represents the volume delivered to the patient or the circuit. The downsweep of the graphic represents the total expiratory volume. Typically, the inspiratory and expiratory volumes should be equal. However, in infants and chil-

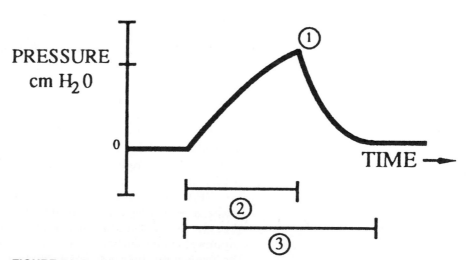

FIGURE 54–9: Pressure graphic of a valved-control mechanical breath. 1, peak inspiratory pressure; 2, inspiratory time; 3, duration of positive pressure. (Adapted from MacIntyre NR. Graphical Analysis of Flow, Pressure, and Volume During Mechanical Ventilation, 3rd ed. Riverside, CA, Bear Medical Systems, 1991, p 2–8.)

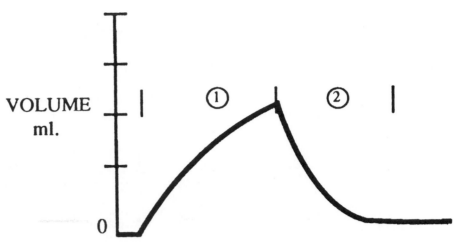

FIGURE 54–10: Volume graphic of a volume control mechanical breath. The volume that is delivered to the patient during inspiration is the delivered inspiratory volume. The volume that returns during expiration is the expiratory volume. 1, time for inspiration; 2, expiratory time. (Adapted from MacIntyre NR. Graphical Analysis of Flow, Pressure, and Volume During Mechanical Ventilation, 3rd ed. Riverside, CA, Bear Medical Systems, 1991, p 2–14.)

dren with uncuffed endotracheal tubes, it is not uncommon for the expiratory volume to be less than the inspiratory volume. An actual percentage leak can be calculated and reported under these conditions and may aid in the decision to change endotracheal tube size. If flow is measured at the patient Y connector in the absence of an endotracheal leak, measurement of the difference between inspiratory and expiratory volumes reflects the loss of volume due to the compliance of the circuit.

The timing sequence of various respiratory events can be determined by displaying volume, flow, and pressure simultaneously over time (Figs. 54–11 and 54–12). Comparison of all three graphics simultaneously facilitates analysis of ventilator-patient interaction. Ventilator dyssynchrony becomes evident when the timing and magnitude of flow, pressure, and volume are disproportionate or delayed.

CPAP

CPAP has become a standard part of neonatal ventilatory care. CPAP is also referred to as PEEP when it is applied with a mechanical ventilator. CPAP can be applied to spontaneously breathing infants via nasal prongs, or nasopharyngeal CPAP may be administered via an endotracheal tube. The neonatal response to CPAP may be variable, depending on the clinical status of the infant at the time that it is applied. CPAP does appear to increase the functional residual capacity of the lung and result in an increase in dynamic lung compliance. Excessive CPAP can result in decreased compliance and decreased tidal volume with resultant acidosis. Excessive levels of CPAP can also decrease cardiac output, reduce pulmonary perfusion, and enhance ventilation-perfusion mismatch, leading to a lower Pa_{O_2}.

CPAP has some additional effects on neonatal ventilation. It produces a more regular breathing pattern in preterm neonates and is thought to stabilize the chest wall, reduce thoracic distortion, and reopen collapsed upper airway structures. The highly compliant chest wall of the premature infant is easily distorted during spontaneous breathing, especially with increased respiratory effort. This breathing pattern may become disorganized and lead to a variety of apnea patterns. Nasal CPAP effectively reverses this process.

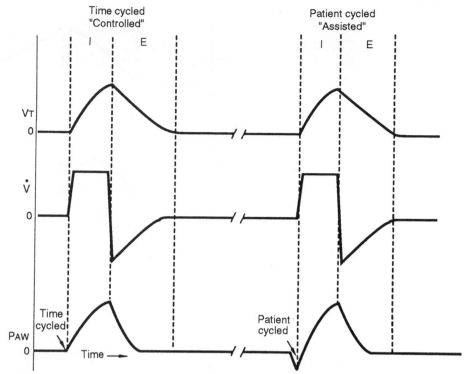

FIGURE 54–11: Volume, flow, and pressure of mechanical volume control and volume assist breaths. E, expiration; I, inspiration; PAW, airway pressure; V̇, flow; VT, tidal volume. (Adapted from MacIntyre NR. Graphical Analysis of Flow, Pressure, and Volume During Mechanical Ventilation, 3rd ed. Riverside, CA, Bear Medical Systems, 1991, p 2–16.)

Airway obstruction due to airway collapse may be eliminated by the application of CPAP, and surfactant release may also be improved with CPAP. CPAP, however, should be used judiciously in treating the neonate with lung disease. A CPAP level of less than 2 to 3 cm H_2O is usually of little value because normal partial closure of the glottis generates these levels of "physiologic PEEP." In general, a CPAP of 4 to 7 cm H_2O appears to be optimal for most infants. Higher levels result in decreased tidal volumes and overdistention of the lung. Early nasal CPAP has shown promise in limiting the need for mechanical ventilation in selected patient populations.

VENTILATOR PARAMETERS

The primary control for tidal volume on most infant ventilators is the peak inflating pressure (PIP). Since the introduction of mechanical ventilation for neonatal respiratory care, the optimal PIP has been a controversial topic. Different management strategies for mechanical ventilation use various approaches to PIP.

When mechanical ventilation is initiated, several physiologic changes occur in the infant. Tidal volume and minute ventilation increase, and mean airway pressure may vary. Mean airway pressure has been shown to correlate directly with oxygenation. However, because mean airway pressure can be changed by altering the ventilatory pattern, these differences produce a variety of effects on oxygenation and carbon dioxide elimination.

The role of PIP in barotrauma is unclear. At present, no studies have

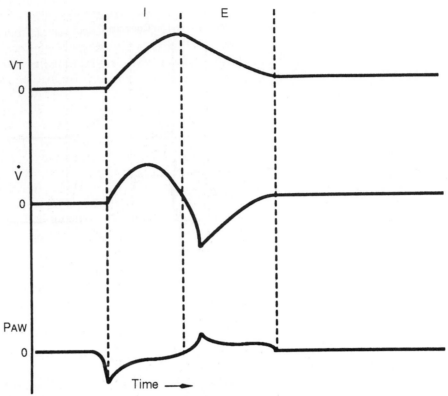

FIGURE 54–12: Volume, flow, and pressure of a spontaneous breath. E, expiration; I, inspiration; PAW, airway pressure; V̇, flow; VT, tidal volume. (Adapted from MacIntyre NR. Graphical Analysis of Flow, Pressure, and Volume During Mechanical Ventilation, 3rd ed. Riverside, CA, Bear Medical Systems, 1991, p 2–17.)

substantiated the theory that PIP is the critical pressure variable that causes pulmonary barotrauma. The size and gestational age of the infant, the underlying lung disease, and the inherited predisposition of the infant may all determine the injury potential from PIP. In general, most clinicians attempt to reduce PIP to the lowest level at which adequate gas exchange occurs. It should be noted again, however, that PIP should not be arbitrarily reduced just to avoid barotrauma. If gas exchange worsens, this erroneous approach may lead to respiratory acidosis, pulmonary vasoconstriction, and further hypoxemia.

Although a high peak inspiratory pressure is ordinarily contraindicated because of the risks of pulmonary barotrauma, many clinical situations warrant the use of high pressures to achieve adequate gas exchange. For example, in the infant with decreased compliance or decreased lung volume associated with atelectasis, a high inspiratory pressure may be required to re-expand atelectatic areas and achieve acceptable arterial carbon dioxide levels. In addition, hyperventilation, in which arterial carbon dioxide levels are intentionally decreased below 35 mm Hg, may be valuable in treating some infants with persistent pulmonary hypertension of the newborn.

Ventilatory rate is one of the factors that determines minute ventilation:

$$\text{Minute ventilation} = \text{frequency} \times \text{tidal volume}$$

As noted previously, tidal volume is primarily determined on pressure ventilators by the pressure differential between the PIP and the positive end-expiratory pressure (PEEP). The optimal ventilatory rate for the newborn period has not been determined. Many studies have shown value in both slow-rate and high-rate mechanical ventilation. With slower-rate ventilation, however, the clinician usually needs to increase the inspiratory time to achieve adequate oxygenation. This approach may reduce venous return from the central nervous system and cause an increase in intraventricular hemorrhage. High-rate positive pressure ventilation has also been useful in the hands of some investigators. This technique has its drawbacks: it may cause air trapping and pulmonary interstitial emphysema. It may also decrease venous return and cardiac output. In the majority of cases, therefore, ventilator rates of between 20 and 40 breaths per minute for the newborn seem to be optimal. Rates above 40 to 60 breaths per minute may exceed the time constant of the lung, resulting in decreased emptying and hyperinflation. The time constant of the lung is a measure of how rapidly equilibration between proximal airway and alveolar pressure occurs. In other words, the time constant expresses how quickly an infant can move air in or out of the lung. The time constant is expressed by the equation:

$$\text{Time constant} = \text{compliance} \times \text{resistance}$$

Studies by Bancalari and colleagues have demonstrated that with a compliance of 0.005 L/cm H_2O and a resistance of 30 cm/L/sec, one time constant is approximately 0.15 seconds. A single time constant is defined as the time required to discharge 63% of the tidal volume delivered to the terminal airspace. Three time constants, the time required for the alveolus to discharge 95% of the gas delivered, would therefore be approximately 0.45 seconds in the spontaneously breathing infant. In the diseased lung, therefore, effects of compliance and resistance must be considered in applying mechanical ventilation. For neonates with significantly reduced compliance, the time constant of the lung may be very short. During that disease stage, higher rates can be used to ventilate an infant because gas exit from the lung is so rapid. Similarly, if a slower rate with a prolonged inspiratory phase is used, the short time constant allows the stiff lung to eliminate gas rapidly. As the lung heals, however, this situation changes, and gas elimination may not occur as rapidly. It is imperative, therefore, that a different ventilatory rate be used at this point, so that gas trapping is minimized.

Mean Airway Pressure. Mean airway pressure is defined as the mean of instantaneous readings of pressure within the airway during a single ventilatory cycle. In waveform terminology, the mean airway pressure equals the integral of the area under the pressure curve during a single respiratory cycle. Mean airway pressure is higher in square wave ventilation if inspiratory time and PIP are equal. Increasing mean airway pressure, in general, increases oxygenation. As noted previously, this relationship may not hold for all methods of increasing mean airway pressure. The primary factors that influence mean airway pressure are (1) PIP, (2) waveform, (3) inspiratory-expiratory ratio, and (4) PEEP.

Work by Boros and coworkers has confirmed the value of increasing mean airway pressure to improve oxygenation. As mean airway pressure increases, right-to-left shunting and the alveolar-arterial oxygen gradient decrease. A high mean airway pressure may improve oxygenation during acute phases of neonatal lung disease, although the continued use of high mean airway pressures during recovery may lead to pulmonary barotrauma, as noted previously.

In general, mean airway pressure is not directly dialed into mechanical ventilators but is the result of the previously noted variables. With some types of high-frequency oscillatory ventilators, however, mean airway pressure can be directly controlled. Of the factors that contribute to mean airway pressure, end-expiratory pressure has the most direct effect because a 1-cm H_2O increase in end-expiratory pressure results in a similar increase in mean airway pressure.

Inspiratory-Expiratory Ratio. The manipulation of the inspiratory-expiratory ratio has also been controversial in neonatal ventilation. At present, few data support the use of one inspiratory-expiratory ratio versus another. On some neonatal ventilators, the inspiratory-expiratory ratio can be selected directly. On others, the clinician chooses the inspiratory time and the rate to achieve the desired inspiratory-expiratory ratio. In general, inspiratory-expiratory ratios of 1:1 to 1:2 seem to be most natural and appropriate for achieving the desired oxygenation and carbon dioxide elimination in neonatal mechanical ventilation.

Reversal of the inspiratory-expiratory ratio, indicating an inspiratory time that is longer than the expiratory time, has been advocated for improving oxygenation (through an increase in mean airway pressure). Although this technique may be of some value, it also impedes venous return from the central nervous system and leads to an increased incidence of intraventricular hemorrhage. It is no longer part of the standard care of the neonate.

Inspiratory time is selected by the bedside clinician to facilitate patient comfort and synchronous breathing during positive pressure ventilation. The patient's age and breathing pattern are major considerations in the selection of inspiratory time. The recommended inspiratory time for newborns is between 0.3 and 0.5 second.

Peak Flow. Peak flow should be titrated to the spontaneous demands of the patient and the desired tidal volumes.

Positive End-Expiratory Pressure. PEEP is produced by early closure of the ventilator expiratory valve, which traps exhaled gas in the lung and increases the expiratory pressure above baseline. The volume of gas trapped in the lung is proportionate to the end-expiratory pressure setting and the patient's compliance. Increasing the volume of trapped gas increases expiratory reserve volume and functional residual capacity, as previously described for CPAP.

FI_{O_2}. The FI_{O_2} should be analyzed continuously, with high and low alarm limits set to prevent inadvertent hypoxemia or hyperoxia. The FI_{O_2} should be aggressively weaned to reduce the risk of oxygen toxicity or the retinopathy of prematurity.

Nonconventional Modes of Ventilation

HIGH-FREQUENCY POSITIVE PRESSURE VENTILATION

High-frequency positive pressure ventilation was first developed in 1978 by Peckham and Fox for treating persistent pulmonary hypertension of the newborn. They demonstrated that oxygenation in some infants can be improved by intentionally reducing the Pa_{CO_2} to 15 to 30 mm Hg. Hyperventilation was first introduced with rates of 60 to 80 breaths per minute but was subsequently increased to rates as high as

150 breaths per minute. It should be noted, however, that although some ventilators are capable of delivering rates of 150 breaths per minute, ventilator efficiency often falls off significantly at higher rates. Therefore, hyperventilation can usually be provided by using PIPs at rates of 60 to 100 breaths per minute. In addition, high-frequency positive pressure ventilation requires very short inspiratory times, so that dead space ventilation increases, especially when rates of 120 to 150 breaths per minute are approached. Furthermore, gas trapping is a commonly associated phenomenon with this form of therapy, leading to a high incidence of pulmonary air leaks. When applied in infants with RDS, high-frequency positive pressure ventilation can often be disastrous, leading to acute tension pneumothorax and severe intraventricular hemorrhage. In view of the availability of true high-frequency devices, this therapy appears to have reduced importance in current intensive care nursery management.

HIGH-FREQUENCY VENTILATION

High-frequency ventilation is a form of mechanical ventilation that uses extremely small tidal volumes and high frequencies to provide gas exchange. The apparent advantage of this form of therapy is that it can potentially reduce pulmonary barotrauma while maintaining oxygenation and ventilation. The mechanism by which high-frequency ventilation produces gas exchange is not understood at present. One of the primary difficulties in describing the physiologic effects of high-frequency ventilation derives from the fact that with most forms of high-frequency ventilation, tidal volume is near or less than dead space volume. Because alveolar ventilation equals the product of ventilatory frequency and tidal volume minus the dead space volume, alveolar ventilation would seem to approach zero! Alternative mechanisms must therefore operate during high-frequency ventilation to enable adequate gas exchange.

Several theories have been proposed to explain the mechanism of high-frequency ventilation. One is spike formation, in which a high-energy wave impulse of gas penetrates the center of the airway, both enhancing the bulk flow of gas in the upper airway and providing a more expansive area for gas mixing in the more distal lung. This mechanism appears to rely, to some extent, on the rigidity of the airway. In a more compliant airway, as in the premature infant, the spike appears to be less effective. Data have indicated that the position of the high-frequency device (especially with jet ventilation) within the endotracheal tube may also be important in spike formation and gas mixing. The presence of secretions and debris in the airway also reduces spike effectiveness. A second theory is augmented diffusion, in which the frequencies used in this form of therapy enhance molecular activity of the gas, thereby increasing gas exchange of the alveolar-capillary membrane. A third theory is helical diffusion, a variant of the spike theory in which fresh gas enters the lung through a spike generated in the center of the airway while gas exits from the lung along the periphery of the airway. One corollary of this theory is that carbon dioxide removal occurs in a spiral fashion, producing a whirlpool effect in which fresh gas is drawn deeper down the center of the airway while gas exits the lung. To date, there has been essentially no substantiation of any of these theories.

Two basic types of high-frequency ventilation exist at present. In high-frequency jet ventilation (HFJV) (Fig. 54–13), a positive pressure gas flow to the patient is intermittently interrupted, followed by a pas-

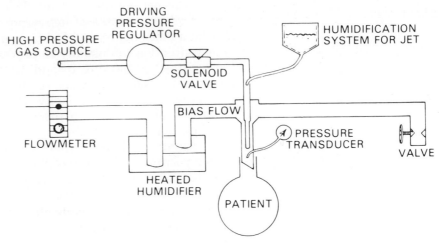

FIGURE 54–13: High-frequency jet ventilation. (From Bancalari E, Goldberg RN. High frequency ventilation in the neonate. Clin Perinatol 14:583, 1987.)

sive expiratory relaxation of the lung; in high-frequency oscillatory ventilation (HFOV) (Fig. 54–14), a piston or a vibrating diaphragm creates a bidirectional sine wave movement of gas within the airway (Tables 54–3 and 54–4). Entrainment appears to assist in gas exchange in both forms of high-frequency ventilation. Entrainment refers to the process by which additional gas molecules are drawn or "dragged" into the airway in the vicinity of the orifice of the high-frequency device. Thus, an additional gas volume is delivered beyond what is directly injected by the high-frequency ventilator. As a result, gas exchange at a given level of airway pressure seems to be greater with high-frequency ventilation than with more conventional modes of ventilatory support.

High-Frequency Jet Ventilation

Physiologic Effect on Gas Exchange

During positive pressure ventilation, manipulations in minute ventilation, through changes in ventilatory rate and tidal volume, allow

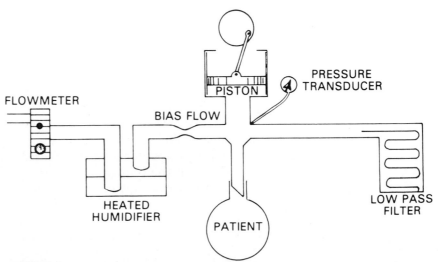

FIGURE 54–14: High-frequency oscillatory ventilation. (From Bancalari E, Goldberg RN. High frequency ventilation in the neonate. Clin Perinatol 14:585, 1987.)

TABLE **54–3:** Characteristics of High-Frequency Ventilators

	Delivery System	Frequency (Breaths per Minute)	Tidal Volume	Expiratory	Inspiratory-Expiratory Ratio	Special Endotracheal Tube	Second Ventilator	PIP Versus PPV	Paw Versus PPV
High-frequency jet ventilation	Solenoid	150–900	≤Vᴅ	Passive	Variable	Yes	Yes	↓	↓
High-frequency oscillatory ventilation	Piston or diaphragm	180–900	<Vᴅ	Active	Variable	No	No	↓	↑

Paw, mean airway pressure; PIP, peak airway pressure; PPV, positive pressure ventilation; Vᴅ, dead space volume.

alterations in carbon dioxide elimination. During HFJV, carbon dioxide elimination is governed by the relationship $V_T^a \times f^b$, where V_T is tidal volume and f is frequency. In this relationship, a has a value from 1.5 to 2.5, and b has a value from 0.5 to 1.0. Because a is greater than b, alveolar ventilation during HFJV has a greater dependency on alterations in tidal volume than on those in frequency. During HFJV, the tidal volume is dependent on the respiratory frequency, which also confounds carbon dioxide elimination. When the respiratory frequency is increased, a reduction in tidal volume can occur, which results in a decrease in alveolar ventilation. Therefore, under certain conditions, increasing the respiratory frequency actually results in a reduction in alveolar ventilation. For these reasons, manipulations of tidal volume remain the most important determinant of alveolar ventilation during HFJV.

In premature patients, HFJV is initiated at frequencies of 350 to 450 insufflations per minute. This can be accomplished because the premature lung has a short time constant and b approximates 1.0. In premature infants, increasing the respiratory frequency results in improved alveolar ventilation. In older patients and those with compliant lungs, the lung has a longer time constant and b approaches 0.5. Unlike in premature patients, increasing the respiratory frequency in older patients and in patients with normal compliance results in a reduction in the delivered tidal volume and an overall reduction in alveolar ventilation. For these reasons, HFJV is usually begun at a frequency of 250 insufflations per minute in pediatric patients with respiratory or cardiovascular dysfunction.

TABLE **54–4:** Advantages and Disadvantages of High-Frequency Ventilation

	Advantages	Disadvantages
High-frequency jet ventilation	↓ Airway pressures (PIP/Paw) versus PPV Improved hemodynamics versus PPV (if Paw ↓) ↓ Barotrauma	Requires separate endotracheal tube and additional ventilator
High-frequency oscillatory ventilation	↓ ΔP, ↓ FIO₂ (↓ barotrauma) versus PPV	↑ Paw
	Single ventilator	Air trapping with high airway resistance
	FDA approved for neonates and children	Patient positioning

Paw, mean airway pressure; PIP, peak airway pressure; PPV, positive pressure ventilation; ΔP, peak pressure minus end-expiratory pressure; FDA, US Food and Drug Administration.

Carbon Dioxide Elimination

The primary method of eliminating carbon dioxide during HFJV is by increasing the delivered tidal volume. Increasing the delivered tidal volume can be accomplished by raising the inspiratory pressures during HFJV. This results in an increase in alveolar ventilation and in improved ventilation-perfusion matching. If atelectasis develops, the PEEP can be increased to recruit lung volume and maintain functional residual capacity. PEEP is initiated during HFJV by adjusting the PEEP level on the tandem ventilator. The tandem ventilator is usually adjusted to allow "sigh" breaths to be delivered at a rate of between 5 and 10 breaths per minute. Some centers recommend using the sigh breath at a peak pressure that is less than that set on the high-frequency jet ventilator (HFJV breaths are not interrupted), whereas others utilize sigh breaths that are at higher peak pressures than those on the high-frequency jet ventilator (HFJV breaths are interrupted). In patients with congenital heart disease, sigh breaths are designed to prevent atelectasis and are adjusted to interrupt the HFJV breath and allow for appropriate recruitment of lung volume. When the Pa_{CO_2} becomes elevated, increasing the tidal volume and the rate of the sigh breaths may be necessary to increase alveolar ventilation.

Lung Volumes

During HFJV, lung volumes do not change dramatically because peak pressures are low and inspiratory time is short. Therefore, lung volumes remain static around the mean lung volume. Mean lung volume is determined by mean airway pressure. Therefore, during HFJV, oxygenation is primarily dependent on mean airway pressures, and increasing mean airway pressures increases lung volume, improving ventilation-perfusion matching and oxygenation. Mean airway pressure can be increased by raising peak inspiratory pressure, PEEP, and the tidal volume and rate of the sigh breaths.

Physiologic Effect on Respiratory Parameters

The primary physiologic effect of HFJV is a reduction in mean airway pressure due to the reduced peak airway pressures generated. In general, this results in improved ventilation compared with similar mean airway pressures developed during positive pressure ventilation. During HFJV, the mean airway pressures measured in the trachea accurately reflect mean alveolar pressure when ventilatory frequencies of 600 breaths per minute or lower are used.

Cardiovascular Effects

HFJV strategies in patients with congenital heart disease differ from those in infants with RDS, primarily because of differences in the compliance of the two patient populations. Attempts to optimize cardiorespiratory interactions in infants and children who have had surgery for congenital heart disease have focused on the use of high-frequency ventilation to improve cardiac function.

Evaluations of HFJV after surgery for congenital heart disease have been encouraging. One study by Meliones of 13 patients who had the Fontan procedure compared HFJV with conventional positive pressure ventilation. When HFJV was compared with standard positive pressure ventilation, there was a 50% reduction in mean airway pressure, a 59% reduction in pulmonary vascular resistance, and a 25% increase in cardiac index. These results indicate that HFJV may be a preferable means of ventilation in patients who have had the Fontan procedure and that HFJV may be useful in certain patients with cardiac dysfunction.

Clinical Trials

Results have indicated that improved gas exchange occurs at lower peak inflating pressures and lower mean airway pressures with HFJV than with conventional ventilation. In particular, carbon dioxide elimination is more effective at lower peak pressures, so that theoretically, high-frequency jet ventilators may provide a safer modality of therapy in the infant with severe neonatal lung disease. To date, HFJV has not produced a significant reduction in the incidence of chronic lung injury, although the resolution of pulmonary air leakage does appear to be enhanced with HFJV. In addition, infants with respiratory failure that is refractory to treatment with conventional mechanical ventilation often appear to have improvement on HFJV. Hyperventilation for persistent pulmonary hypertension of the neonate can also be achieved through the use of HFJV.

Clinical Indications

HFJV should be considered in patients in whom high airway pressures are present and in patients who are unusually sensitive to airway pressures (Table 54–5). HFJV is indicated for neonates who fail to respond to conventional therapy despite high peak airway pressures. These patient populations frequently include patients with infantile RDS, those with barotrauma (especially patients with pulmonary interstitial emphysema), and those with refractory pulmonary artery hypertension. In neonatal patients, HFJV should be considered when the patient requires a mean airway pressure of 15 to 20 mm Hg or higher or when a significant air leak is present.

Technique

The Life Pulse ventilator is designed to be used in parallel with a conventional mechanical ventilator. To accomplish this synchronization, a specially designed endotracheal tube needs to be inserted into the infant's airway. This endotracheal tube, referred to as the Hi-Lo tube (Mallinckrodt), must be placed before HFJV is started. This tube is a triple-lumen tube. The main port is connected to the conventional ventilator. The remaining two ports are the pressure-sensing port, which is located near the tip of the endotracheal tube, and the jet delivery port, which is located in the midportion of the tube. Distal tracheal airway pressure is constantly sensed through the pressure port, resulting in real-time adjustment of PIP during treatment. Jet pulsations are delivered by the opening and closing of a solenoid valve on a piece of plastic tubing, which lies in the patient box, near the infant's head. This interruption of flow produces spike-like jets of gas in the airway, resulting in "jet ventilation."

TABLE **54–5:** Clinical Indications for High-Frequency Ventilation

	Demonstrated Efficacy	Undetermined Efficacy
High-frequency jet ventilation	Respiratory distress syndrome Barotrauma Bronchopleural fistula	Pulmonary hypertension During thoracic surgery
High-frequency oscillatory ventilation	Infant respiratory distress syndrome Barotrauma Bronchopleural fistula	Congenital diaphragmatic hernia Pulmonary hypertension

If the patient to be treated with HFJV does have a pulmonary air leak, HFJV alone is started. PEEP is provided through the main port, which connects to the conventional ventilator. For infants with RDS, the starting PIP on HFJV is approximately 80% of the PIP that was used on conventional mechanical ventilation. For infants with diseases other than RDS, or if pulmonary hypertension is a significant component of the child's illness, the same initial PIP is used on HFJV. Ventilation with the Life Pulse ventilator is initiated at a rate of 420 breaths per minute. Empiric observations and animal studies have indicated that rates of 400 to 500 breaths per minute are optimal for neonatal patients with short time constants. In the presence of an air leak, 6 to 24 hours of HFJV alone is performed before background ventilation with the conventional ventilator is added.

In the neonate, one of the common complications of HFJV is atelectasis. Because of the restrictive lung disease that is typically treated, along with the very compliant chest wall, the reduced tidal volumes of HFJV often lead to progressive atelectasis. As a result, failure to provide some associated positive pressure conventional breaths usually results in a deterioration in the infant's status. Because the Life Pulse ventilator has a sensing mechanism that cuts off pressure delivery if a pressure greater than the designated airway pressure is sensed, background ventilation with the conventional mechanical ventilator is usually delivered at a pressure that is 5 cm H_2O below the pressure of the jet ventilator. This design is currently being revised, however, to allow a pressure equal to that on the jet ventilator, which may further improve oxygenation. The rate for such ventilation is 5 to 10 breaths per minute. This technique improves oxygenation and reduces the atelectasis of the lung during HFJV. Pressures dissipate rapidly with this approach, so that the airway is not exposed to unusually high pressures.

The jet valve is set at 0.02 second for an "on time." This is the shortest time possible and equates to inspiratory time. It appears that the shorter the "jet," the more effective the use of HFJV. Prolonging inspiration during HFJV does not improve oxygenation. The primary ways to improve oxygenation during HFJV are (1) increasing the FI_{O_2}, (2) increasing the mean airway pressure by increasing PEEP, and (3) increasing the rate of background sighing to 15 to 20 breaths per minute or higher.

Carbon dioxide elimination is extremely effective during HFJV. It is not uncommon to see Pa_{CO_2} levels in the range of 20 to 35 mm Hg during HFJV. As a result, once adequate oxygenation has been obtained, further removal of carbon dioxide is usually not necessary. In practice, it is more common to have to raise Pa_{CO_2} because of concerns about the autoregulation of cerebral blood flow and ischemic neurologic injury. The Pa_{CO_2} can be increased by (1) increasing PEEP, (2) decreasing the background sigh rate, and (3) decreasing the background sigh pressure. In some cases, prolonging the background sigh time may be valuable if the Pa_{CO_2} is too low. A reduction in PIP in this situation often leads to an unacceptable drop in oxygen saturation, again indicating the enhanced effectiveness of carbon dioxide removal during HFJV. It is therefore not uncommon to treat an infant with pressure settings that are impossible to use during conventional mechanical ventilation, with relatively high PEEP for a given PIP, in order to achieve the desired arterial blood gas values. Decreasing the jet ventilator rate may increase the Pa_{CO_2}. It also typically decreases oxygenation, however, as ventilator effectiveness is reduced, and it is therefore not recommended as an initial approach.

Weaning from HFJV again concentrates on reducing the factors primarily responsible for bronchopulmonary dysplasia. FI_{O_2} and PIP are the two variables that are reduced initially once improvement is noted. As oxygenation improves, the FI_{O_2} is decreased; for a low Pa_{CO_2}, PIP is decreased. With HFJV, the clinician must be extremely cautious during the weaning process. The most common mistake during HFJV treatment is to wean too rapidly, leading to "flip-flop" and a need to increase settings above a prior level in order to achieve previous arterial blood gas results. This weaning error is often difficult to pick up because it occurs several hours after the change in ventilatory support has been made. It appears that decreasing pressure with HFJV may lead to a gradual, progressive atelectasis that is not reflected in arterial blood gas values for several hours. To reinflate the lung, increased pressure is needed. Weaning should therefore be approached cautiously, and changes should not be made more frequently than every 1 to 2 hours.

Side Effects

The primary side effect of HFJV therapy is necrotizing tracheobronchitis from the high velocity of gas that is pulsed into the trachea [16]. Necrotizing tracheobronchitis has contributed to significant morbidity and mortality, especially in premature infants who are at an increased risk because of their small tracheas. It has been demonstrated that necrotizing tracheobronchitis occurs with all forms of ventilation and is far less common with present high-frequency jet ventilator models. Earlier prototypes of the Life Pulse ventilator had a less effective method of humidifying gas, so that airway injury may have occurred not only from the shear forces on the airway but also from the dryness of the gases. Improvements in humidification in newer HFJV systems have significantly reduced this problem. A second side effect is the development of large areas of atelectasis during HFJV. The low airway pressures generated during HFJV result in a reduction in alveolar pressures and a tendency for alveolar collapse. This can lead to a worsening of oxygenation and increased ventilatory requirements. Atelectasis can be prevented by maintaining adequate levels of PEEP and sigh breaths that are large enough to allow alveolar recruitment (a delivered tidal volume of 10 to 15 mL/kg). One final side effect is the risk of extubation or destabilization during reintubation with the triple-lumen endotracheal tube.

High-Frequency Oscillatory Ventilation

HFOV differs from HFJV in various technical and physiologic components (see Tables 54–3 and 54–4). HFOV uses an electrically powered piston or diaphragm to alternate positive and negative pressures in the airway. With the use of this technique, tidal volumes of between 1 and 3 mL/kg and cycles ranging from 180 to 3000 breaths per minute are generated. The main difference between HFOV and other modes of ventilation is that inspiration and expiration are both active during HFOV and occur above and below the mean airway pressure (Fig. 54–15). One advantage of HFOV over HFJV is that a single ventilator is used and a special endotracheal tube (or adapter) is not required (see Tables 54–3 and 54–4). The adjustments during HFOV consist of changes in bias flow, which regulates mean airway pressure, oscillatory amplitude (via alterations in power), inspiratory time, and frequency.

The SensorMedics 3100A system (SensorMedics, Yorba Linda, CA) is a high-frequency oscillatory ventilator that has been approved by the US Food and Drug Administration for use in patients weighing 540 g to

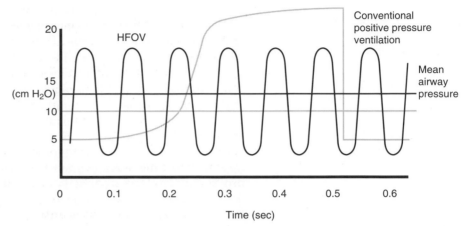

FIGURE 54–15: Conventional positive pressure ventilation (*cross-hatched lines*) and high-frequency oscillatory ventilation (HFOV; *solid lines*). The airway pressures from a typical conventional positive pressure breath for a neonate are shown. During HFOV, both inspiration and expiration are active and occur above and below the mean airway pressure. As a result of the active inspiration and expiration, the mean airway pressure that occurs during HFOV (*solid horizontal line*) is higher than the mean airway pressure that occurs during conventional positive pressure ventilation (*cross-hatched horizontal line*). The amplitude during HFOV is the difference between the peak inspiratory pressure and the peak end-expiratory pressure.

4.6 kg. Approval is pending in other weight categories. During HFOV, the ventilator does not supply any fresh gas, and a humidified blended gas is supplied through the bias flow, which ranges up to 40 L/min. The mean airway pressure is controlled by adjusting the resistance of the mean airway pressure control valve or more frequently, by altering the bias flow. Mean airway pressure values range from 10 to 45 cm H_2O. The oscillatory amplitude or ΔP (peak inspiratory airway pressure minus peak end-expiratory pressure) is altered by changing the power. The power, the amount of energy utilized to drive the piston to and fro, ranges from 0 to 100%. The inspiratory time determines the percentage of the time the piston is in the inspiratory position, and it can be altered from 33 to 50%. The final adjustment is frequency, which can be altered on the SensorMedics 3100A from 3 to 15 Hz (150 to 900 breaths per minute).

Physiologic Effect on Gas Exchange, Lung Volumes, and Respiratory Parameters

The mechanism of gas exchange during HFOV differs from that during other modes of ventilation because both inspiration and expiration are active. These technologic differences result in HFOV's creating unique properties of gas exchange, lung volumes, and respiratory parameters. During HFOV, the active inspiration and expiration result in alveoli being continually open. Inspiration and expiration therefore occur around a set mean lung volume. The mean lung volume is determined by the set mean airway pressure and does not vary as widely as occurs during conventional positive pressure ventilation. The peak inspiratory pressures and peak end-expiratory pressures occur around the set mean airway pressure and above and below the baseline mean airway pressure and mean lung volume (see Fig. 54–15). In comparison to conventional positive pressure ventilation, HFOV results in increased mean airway pressure and peak end-expiratory pressure. There is, however, a reduction in peak inspiratory pressure. Additionally, there is a reduction in ΔP and a resultant decrease in shear forces.

Airway pressures are measured at the airway during HFOV. Alveolar pressures differ from those measured at the airway for a variety of reasons. The amplitude or ΔP at the alveolar level is lower than that measured at the airway. This may result from attenuation of the pressure differential through the loss of energy of the gas as it traverses the endotracheal tube and trachea. In addition, the decreased inspiratory time may limit the time available for the pressure swings to occur and may also contribute to attenuation of the phasic changes. When the inspiratory time is short, the mean airway pressure measured at the airway is similar to that measured at the alveolus. However, when the inspiratory time is increased to 50%, the alveolar mean airway pressure is higher than the airway pressure measured at the airway, and inhomogeneity of alveolar pressures develops. Alterations in the frequency during HFOV do not significantly alter the relationship between alveolar and airway pressure measurements.

The unique properties of HFOV allow clinicians to manipulate oxygenation and carbon dioxide elimination independently. Oxygenation during HFOV is determined by both the inspired oxygen concentration and the mean airway pressure. During HFOV, oxygenation is critically dependent on the mean airway pressure because inspiration and expiration occur around the set mean airway pressure. The mean airway pressure is primarily determined by the bias flow, and alterations in bias flow allow changes in mean airway pressure from 10 to 45 cm H_2O. When HFOV is initiated, the mean airway pressure is set 1 to 6 cm H_2O higher than that used during conventional positive pressure ventilation. The mean airway pressure is then adjusted to achieve the desired oxygenation. The mean airway pressure is reduced once there has been recruitment of appropriate lung volume, as indicated by an ability to wean the FI_{O_2} to less than 0.65.

Carbon dioxide elimination during HFOV is governed by the same relationship as occurs during HFJV: $VT^a \times f^b$, where VT is tidal volume and f is frequency. During HFOV, the tidal volume can be altered directly by altering the amplitude. In addition, because the tidal volume decreases as the frequency increases, an increase in the frequency also reduces the tidal volume. An increase in the frequency during HFOV therefore results in a reduction in alveolar ventilation and carbon dioxide elimination. Improved carbon dioxide elimination can be achieved by increasing the amplitude or decreasing the frequency, whereas a reduction in carbon dioxide elimination can occur with a decrease in amplitude or an increase in frequency.

Cardiovascular Effects

The cardiovascular effects of HFOV are not well defined. HFOV by design results in a higher mean airway pressure, which could theoretically decrease cardiovascular performance. In several animal studies, HFOV was associated with a reduction in cardiac output. However, in pathophysiologic conditions with abnormal compliance, the increased mean airway pressure is not as readily transmitted to the cardiovascular structures. In an animal study with lung injury, HFOV did not result in a reduction in cardiovascular performance, despite an increase in mean airway pressure. In addition, in a small clinical study, oxygen delivery was not altered, despite an increase in mean airway pressures. It should be noted, however, that as compliance improves, mean airway pressure is more easily transmitted to the cardiovascular structures and results in a reduction in cardiac output. Once compliance begins to improve, mean airway pressure should be reduced in order to minimize the cardiovascular effects. As a result of the inconclusive data, the role of HFOV in patients with cardiovascular dysfunction remains unclear.

Side Effects

HFOV employs an active expiratory phase; therefore, its use in conditions in which there is a prolongation of expiration or an obstruction to expiration may result in overexpansion of lung segments. When this occurs, barotrauma can develop. HFOV is therefore not recommended in conditions in which airway obstruction occurs because of the increased risk of barotrauma. Another disadvantage of HFOV is that patient positioning is relatively fixed because of the rigid nature of the HFOV circuit configuration. This can result in the development of pressure sores when HFOV is used for extended periods. Suctioning is also difficult during HFOV because there is a loss of airway pressure. During HFOV, the mean lung volume and airway pressure are kept relatively constant. When suctioning is performed, the patient is disconnected from the ventilator, and massive atelectasis can result from the precipitous loss of airway pressures. To reduce the risk of atelectasis, suctioning is kept to a minimum: it is usually performed once in a 24-hour period.

Clinical Trials

Clinical trials have been performed with HFOV. HFOV has been shown to be beneficial in neonatal patients with various conditions, including infantile RDS, pulmonary artery hypertension, and congenital diaphragmatic hernia. No benefit was found for HFOV over conventional positive pressure ventilation in a clinical trial using HFOV for preterm infants with infantile RDS. In addition, the patients begun on HFOV were noted to have an increased incidence of intracranial hemorrhage. The study has been criticized because lung volumes were maintained in a low range in order to minimize airway pressures. This approach may have compromised alveolar recruitment during HFOV and led to lower oxygenation. In an infant trial, an increased lung volume and alveolar recruitment strategy was employed. With this approach, a decreased incidence of chronic lung disease was found when HFOV was compared with conventional therapy. These data suggest that HFOV may be useful in selected neonatal conditions, provided that high lung volumes are maintained.

Clinical Indications

HFOV should be considered in patients in whom oxygenation is impaired and in those in whom barotrauma has occurred (see Table 54–5). HFOV is indicated for neonates with infantile RDS, barotrauma, refractory pulmonary artery hypertension, air leakage, and diaphragmatic hernia. In pediatric patients, the primary indication for HFOV is in patients with RDS who have decreased oxygenation despite high levels of support (oxygenation index of greater than 30; oxygenation index $= [FI_{O_2} \times$ mean airway pressure$]/Pa_{O_2} \times 100$) or who develop significant barotrauma. Clinical indications for HFOV in adult patients await elucidation, which will be forthcoming after the completion of adult trials. Conditions in which HFOV may be beneficial include adult RDS. Adult RDS has a pathophysiology similar to that of pediatric RDS, in which HFOV has been shown to be beneficial. Adults who have injury to the airway and those who have had surgical intervention in the airway may also benefit from HFOV. In conditions in which air leakage, bronchopleural fistula, or both are present, HFOV has been shown to enhance resolution of the air leakage in selected patient populations. These patients benefit from the maintenance of a more constant lung volume, the reduction in peak inspiratory pressure, and the attenuation of airway pressure swings that can be achieved with HFOV. Postsurgical patients who are at high risk for pneumonitis or aspiration may also benefit from HFOV because mucus clearing from the distal airways is enhanced and airway pressure and volume swings are reduced. These beneficial effects may decrease the risk of aspiration by minimizing fluctuations in intrathoracic processes.

Set-Up

The patient is begun on HFOV at an $F_{I_{O_2}}$ of 1.0, a mean airway pressure that is 1 to 6 cm H_2O greater than that on conventional positive pressure ventilation, and a rate of 10 to 15 Hz. In larger patients, the frequency is reduced to 5 to 7 Hz. The amplitude is adjusted to allow for adequate chest wall excursions. Chest radiography is invaluable and allows determination of the adequacy of lung volumes. The mean airway pressure is increased until alveolar recruitment allows appropriate lung volumes. This can be demonstrated by radiography, pulmonary function testing, or improvements in oxygenation. Manipulations in the various parameters are as previously described.

Surfactant Replacement Therapy

One of the most significant advances in neonatal respiratory care has been the ability to administer exogenous surfactant to newborns with surfactant deficiency. Multiple studies have conclusively demonstrated that surfactant administration reduces the length of ventilation, the development of air leakage, and the length of hospital stay while increasing survival in the preterm infant. Surfactant is composed of phospholipids, neutral lipids, proteins, and carbohydrates. As previously described, some preterm and term infants suffer from inadequate surfactant production. With the development of exogenous surfactant preparations, it has become possible to instill surfactant directly into the infant's trachea. Surfactant can be synthetically produced, or it can be extracted from human or animal sources. These preparations have individual advantages and disadvantages. Preliminary data suggest that animal surfactant provides greater benefit than synthetically produced surfactant, although conclusive data are pending.

Clinical conditions that benefit from surfactant replacement therapy can be divided into two categories: those that benefit from prophylactic therapy and those that benefit from rescue therapy. Prophylactic therapy is administered immediately after birth and is indicated in patients who are at high risk for respiratory distress. These infants include those less than 32 weeks of gestation, those less than 1.3 kg, those with a lecithin-sphingomyelin ratio of less than 2:1, those with bubble stability test results indicating lung immaturity, and those with an absence of phosphatidylglycerol. Rescue or therapeutic treatment is indicated in patients with increased work of breathing, increasing oxygen requirements, an $F_{I_{O_2}}$ of greater than 0.40, chest radiographic results consistent with RDS, and a mean airway pressure of greater than 7 cm H_2O. Contraindications for the use of surfactant consist of life-threatening chromosomal abnormalities, a mature lecithin-sphingomyelin ratio, the presence of phosphatidylglycerol, and bubble stability.

Delivery of surfactant requires a coordinated effort between caregivers. Surfactant should be administered as soon as the patient is identified as being at risk for the development of surfactant deficiency or as having surfactant deficiency. The patient must be intubated and initially stabilized. Frequently, surfactant is administered in the delivery room. In this case, confirmation of the proper placement of the endotracheal tube is not possible. Therefore, care must be taken to ensure that the endotracheal tube is in the proper location before surfactant is administered. Once the patient has been identified and stabilized, surfactant is administered. Surfactant dosing depends on the individual preparation. Synthetic surfactant (Exosurf, Burroughs Welcome, Research Triangle Park, NC) is initially administered at a dose of 5 mL/kg, with repeated doses 12 and 24 hours later. Bovine surfactant (Survanta, Ross Laboratories, Columbus, Ohio) is administered at a dose of 3 mL/kg for infants who are from 24 to 26 weeks of gestation and at 4 mL/kg for older infants. Retreatment consists of 4 mL/kg to a total dose not to exceed four doses over a 24-hour period. The administration of surfactant requires patient repositioning during the instillation to ensure homogeneous distribution. Several groups recommend partitioning the surfactant into four quarter doses, which are administered in four separate instillations. The first two are performed with the patient's head and body down, with the head first in the right and then in the left position. The final two doses are given with the head and body inclined up slightly, with the head first to the right and then to the left. After surfactant administration, suctioning is not performed for 1 to 2 hours.

The delivery of surfactant is not without risk. Potential complications include the development of plugging of the endotracheal tube; pulmonary hemorrhage; an increased incidence of patent ductus arteriosus; desaturation episodes during and shortly after administration, resulting in the need for an increase in oxygen; arrhythmias; apnea; an increased incidence of retinopathy of prematurity; barotrauma resulting from an increase in lung compliance after surfactant administration with a failure to decrease ventilatory support; and unilung delivery of surfactant.

A successful outcome is primarily determined by outcome measures, which include a reduced incidence of air leakage, a reduced length of ventilation, and improved survival. Individual benefit is determined by an improvement in lung compliance, as demonstrated by a reduction in the work of breathing; improved chest radiographic findings; a reduction in airway pressures; and improved gas exchange, as demonstrated by an improvement in the alveolar-arterial oxygen tension ratio.

Extracorporeal Membrane Oxygenation in the Neonate

Extracorporeal membrane oxygenation (ECMO) has proved to be a valuable therapy for larger (greater than 2 kg) neonates with severe intractable lung disease. Although it was attempted periodically in the past, not until the mid-1980s, with the introduction of new technologies, did ECMO became practical.

ECMO has been successfully used as a form of cardiorespiratory support in more than 6000 neonates since the mid-1980s. This procedure is applied when conventional and nonconventional modes of ventilatory support have failed and when patients have an expected mortality exceeding 80%. Diseases in which ECMO is often used include meconium

TABLE **54–6:** Differences Between Venovenous and Venoarterial Extracorporeal Membrane Oxygenation

	Technical			Cardiac		Pulmonary			
	Ligation of the Carotid	Rapid Stabilization	Recirculation	Cardiac Support	Cardiac Do_2	Ventilatory Support	Sao_2	Pulmonary Do_2	Pulsatile Flow
Venoarterial	Yes	Yes	No	Yes	↑	↓	↑	↓	No
Venovenous	No	No	Yes	No	No	↓ but < venoarterial	↑ but < venoarterial	↑	Yes

Do_2, oxygen delivery; Sa_{O_2}, oxygen saturation.

aspiration syndrome, persistent pulmonary hypertension of the newborn, congenital diaphragmatic hernia, and neonatal sepsis.

ECMO can be applied with either a venoarterial approach or a venovenous approach (Table 54–6). Access for neonatal venoarterial ECMO requires dissection and cannulation of the right internal jugular vein and the right common carotid artery. Access for venovenous ECMO involves cannulation of the right internal jugular vein with a double-lumen cannula. Perfusion and gas exchange are maintained by means of an external membrane oxygenator and a roller or centrifugal pump. After the placement of catheters in the appropriate vessels, extracorporeal support is initiated. A heat exchanger rewarms the blood before its reinfusion.

SELECTION CRITERIA

The selection criteria for ECMO are constantly being re-evaluated in the intensive care unit. ECMO criteria are listed in Table 54–7. The oxygenation index is calculated as follows:

$$\text{Oxygenation index} = \frac{(\text{MAP} \times \text{Fi}_{O_2})}{\text{Pa}_{O_2}} \times 100$$

A value of 40 or greater has been historically associated with a mortality rate of approximately 80%. ECMO has not been routinely used in infants who are less than 2000 g or 34 weeks of gestation at the time of birth because of the increased risk of intracranial hemorrhage since ECMO requires anticoagulation. The evaluation of heparin-bonded circuits, which would avoid anticoagulation, is under way.

Before the initiation of ECMO, extensive evaluation is required. Echocardiography is needed to eliminate the possibility of congenital heart disease. Head ultrasonographic and electroencephalographic studies evaluate the neurologic status of the infant. Extensive hematologic, electrolyte, renal, and liver function studies are also used throughout the

TABLE **54–7:** Indications and Contraindications for Neonatal Extracorporeal Membrane Oxygenation

Indications	Contraindications

Persistent hypoxia
  Oxygenation index > 40 for
    > 4 hr
  P(A −a)O_2 > 610 mm Hg
    for > 4 hr
  Pa$_{O_2}$ < 50 mm Hg for > 2–4 hr
Persistent barotrauma
Persistent acidosis
  pH < 7.25 for 2 hr
	Gestational age < 34 wk, birthweight < 2 kg
	> Grade I intraventricular hemorrhage
	> 7–10 days of mechanical ventilation
	Major chromosomal abnormalities
	Grossly abnormal neurologic examination findings

course of ECMO. Daily blood cultures and circuit cultures are used to anticipate infection.

MANAGEMENT

After the initiation of ECMO, patient improvement is often rapid and dramatic. Ventilator support is reduced to minimal settings. Some degree of ventilatory support must be maintained to prevent atelectasis. It has been shown that the use of high PEEP, in the range of 8 to 15 cm H_2O, can reduce the lung consolidation that is associated with the initiation of ECMO and can hasten recovery. This massive alveolar atelectasis appears on radiographic evaluation. A massive outpouring of fluid into the alveoli occurs, similar to a shock lung situation.

Activated clotting times are monitored hourly to titrate the heparin dose. Blood products are given as needed to replace red blood cells and platelets. The hematocrit is usually maintained in the range of 40%, and the platelet count at greater than 100,000. Laboratory determinations of hemoglobin, hematocrit, electrolytes, clotting factors, and renal and liver function continue during the course of ECMO.

Weaning from ECMO occurs when reversal of the disease process can be demonstrated. This consists of the elimination of pulmonary artery hypertension and improved respiratory compliance. A "trial off" is then performed, which consists of the infant's being isolated from the ECMO circuit while the cannulas remain in place. The infant's ventilator support is increased to determine if mechanical ventilation alone can support the infant's clinical condition, and such support is considered to be successful if the infant can be maintained at an FI_{O_2} of less than 0.50, a PIP of less than 30 to 35 cm H_2O, and a mean airway pressure of less than 12 to 15 cm H_2O. If the infant's condition can be successfully maintained for 4 to 8 hours, the cannulas are removed. The average ECMO run is approximately 140 hours.

Currently, the Extracorporeal Life Support Registry data demonstrate a survival rate of 81% for all infants. Infants with meconium aspiration syndrome (93%) and primary pulmonary hypertension (83%) have the highest survival rates. The survival rate for infants with sepsis syndrome is lower (76%), and those with congenital diaphragmatic hernia have the lowest survival rate (58%).

Until recently, the initiation of ECMO required the permanent sacrifice of the infant's right common carotid artery. Several centers now repair the carotid artery after ECMO has been discontinued. Further follow-up, however, is required to assess the utility of this technique.

Long-term follow-up of ECMO patients is essential. It appears that 60% of infants will recover from ECMO with no significant complications, 20% of infants will have mild to moderate neurologic problems, and 20% will show severe neurologic deficits after ECMO. It is unclear at present if this subsequent development is due to complications related to ECMO or to the perinatal and early neonatal therapy used before ECMO.

Liquid Ventilation

Liquid ventilation is a new technique that offers promise as a method for life support during the neonatal period. Liquid ventilation uses inert nonbiotransformable liquids (perfluorochemicals), which have a high solubility for respiratory gases under atmospheric conditions.

These are substituted for nitrogen as a vehicle for delivering oxygen and removing carbon dioxide. In a manner similar to that in ECMO, roller pumps circulate liquid to and from the lung, and through a membrane oxygenator, to continuously add oxygen and remove carbon dioxide. Air-liquid interfaces are eliminated, which increases lung compliance and eliminates pulmonary barotrauma. Because the perfluorochemicals can be distributed through the lung at low pressure, liquid ventilation may permit the distribution of surfactant and other active biologically acting agents while assisting in the removal of pulmonary debris. At present, this technique is highly experimental, although one report has indicated some utility of the treatment in neonates with severe RDS.

Follow-up studies have shown that perfluorochemical liquids are minimally absorbed, are removed by vaporization through the lungs, and do not cause adverse histologic or biochemical effects. Ventilation with liquids effectively supports cardiopulmonary stability and minimizes the trauma of positive pressure ventilation. In the previously mentioned trial with liquid ventilation, an improvement in lung compliance, with no change in cardiovascular status, occurred in all infants. Although the infants died of underlying respiratory disease, this trial does demonstrate that liquid breathing can support gas exchange and improvement in pulmonary function. Further studies are indicated for this form of therapy.

RESPIRATORY EVALUATION OF THE NEONATAL PATIENT

In neonates with cardiorespiratory dysfunction, evaluation of the respiratory system requires both invasive and noninvasive assessment.

Noninvasive Evaluation

CLINICAL EXAMINATION

The primary clinical signs of respiratory failure include an increased respiratory rate; an altered respiratory pattern, including deep, shallow, or irregular breaths; the use of accessory muscles with flaring of the nares; and expiratory grunting. Crackles can be demonstrated during auscultation of the respiratory system in many pathologic conditions. Airway obstruction can also occur in neonates and is suggested by wheezing and prolonged expiration. Physical examination is also helpful during the initiation of positive pressure ventilation and can help to determine the adequacy of the delivered tidal volume, the appropriate inspiratory and expiratory times, and patient-ventilator synchrony.

CHEST RADIOGRAPHY

Chest radiographic evaluation is helpful in determining the presence of respiratory pathophysiology. A systematic evaluation of chest radiographs is recommended in infants because the differential diagnosis includes congenital heart disease. The lung fields should be evaluated for the adequacy of lung volumes and the presence of areas of under- or overexpansion. The lung parenchyma should be examined to determine if edema, atelectasis, or pneumonia is present. A careful examination of the pleura-diaphragm interface is essential to determine the presence of a pleural effusion, pneumothorax, or phrenic nerve paralysis. The cardiac silhouette is then evaluated. Finally, the locations of the various catheters, wires, and endotracheal tubes are determined.

PULSE OXIMETRY

One of the most important advances in the noninvasive evaluation of gas exchange is pulse oximetry technology. Pulse oximetry allows the determination of the percentage of hemoglobin saturated with oxygen (Sp_{O_2}). By infrared light absorption, pulse oximetry compares saturated and unsaturated hemoglobin, and Sp_{O_2} is derived from changes in curves. Pulse oximetry–derived oxygen saturations (Sp_{O_2}) correlate closely with co-oximeter (Sa_{O_2}) values for saturations between 70 and 100% when normal cardiac output is present. At low saturations, the curves approximate, reducing the accuracy. A discrepancy between the Sp_{O_2} and the Sa_{O_2} can occur in various conditions, including when low cardiac output is present. This is frequently a result of inadequate distal perfusion to the extremity where the pulse oximetry probe is located. Moving the probe to a different site or warming the extremity may improve the correlation. In conditions in which an abnormal hemoglobin level is present, Sp_{O_2} may not reflect Sa_{O_2}, and direct measurement of Sa_{O_2} may be required. Sp_{O_2} monitoring should be provided for all patients who require positive pressure ventilation, supplemental oxygen, or cardiac pacing.

CAPNOGRAPHY

Capnography is the graphic display of airway carbon dioxide during the respiratory cycle. Two current techniques are available for capnography: infrared spectroscopy and mass spectroscopy. Accurate capnography depends on adequate pulmonary blood flow, pulmonary capillary flow, and gas exchange; low dead space; and minimal leakage around the tube. The maximal carbon dioxide tension during exhalation is defined as the end-tidal carbon dioxide. In normal subjects, this differs by approximately 5 mm Hg from the Pa_{CO_2}. End-tidal carbon dioxide monitoring is helpful in multiple conditions, including in the confirmation of tracheal intubation, the evaluation of the respiratory pattern, the determination of dead space ventilation, the evaluation of pulmonary blood flow, and the assessment of cardiac output. A variety of conditions can cause alterations in the end-tidal carbon dioxide: a decrease in the end-tidal carbon dioxide may be a result of decreased pulmonary blood flow, cardiac output, oxygen consumption, or dead space ventilation or of endotracheal tube leakage. An increase in end-tidal carbon dioxide may result from an increase in carbon dioxide production, pulmonary blood flow, or cardiac output. Monitoring of end-tidal carbon dioxide is beneficial in ventilator-dependent patients and can reduce the number of arterial blood gas measurements.

EVALUATION OF RESPIRATORY MECHANICS

One of the most exciting developments in evaluating the respiratory system is the availability of mobile bedside monitoring units capable of evaluating respiratory mechanics. Unlike the cardiovascular system, in which there is a continuous display of the electrical activity of the heart and easy display of heart function through echocardiography, the respiratory system has been largely underevaluated. Formal pulmonary function testing is both cumbersome and of limited availability. Newer devices permit clinicians to display respiratory mechanics continuously, including graphic displays of gas flow, airway pressures, delivered tidal volume, and esophageal pressures. These data allow calculations of compliance, airway resistance, and time constants of the lung, and evaluation of the timing of ventilatory events. The placement of an esophageal balloon allows the evaluation of spontaneous ventilation and the integration of patient-ventilator synchrony. This is especially important in weaning patients with chronic respiratory or cardiorespiratory dysfunction from positive pressure ventilation. In addition, the evaluation of respiratory mechanics can provide information on the effectiveness of each respiratory intervention and on whether side effects of the various respiratory interventions have occurred. The side effects that can be detected by respiratory monitoring include alveolar overdistention, gas trapping, excessive or inadvertent PEEP, peak airway pressures, and patient-ventilator dyssynchrony. Respiratory mechanics should be evaluated in any patient in whom abnormal respiratory convalescence occurs and in patients who require peak airway pressure greater than 30 to 35 cm H_2O, PEEP greater than 6 cm H_2O, or mean airway pressure greater than 10 to 15 cm H_2O.

Invasive Evaluation

BRONCHOSCOPY

Bronchoscopy, either flexible or rigid evaluation, may occasionally be required in the neonatal patient. Flexible bronchoscopy has several advantages over rigid bronchoscopy: its primary advantage is the ability to pass the bronchoscope through the endotracheal tube, which allows maintenance of the airway. A No. 4.5 endotracheal tube is the smallest endotracheal tube through which a flexible bronchoscope with a suction port can pass. Smaller flexible bronchoscopes that allow visualization only are the mainstay of neonatal bronchoscopy. Indications for bronchoscopy include evaluation of stridor, airway compression, and tracheomalacia.

RESPIRATORY SUPPORT FOR SPECIFIC NEONATAL SYNDROMES

One of the primary maxims of medicine is diagnosis before treatment. This approach is critical in the neonate because many newborns may exhibit respiratory symptoms without having respiratory disease. The appearance of respiratory signs in the neonate may focus the physician on lung disease, causing nonpulmonary problems to be overlooked. It is therefore imperative to understand the cardinal signs of respiratory disease in the newborn for an appropriate differential diagnosis, as outlined previously.

The differential diagnosis of common pulmonary and nonpulmonary diseases in the neonate is shown in Figure 54–16. Some of the diagnoses, although appropriate for term infants, rarely occur in premature babies and can be dismissed if the child is born preterm. Meconium aspiration syndrome and primary pulmonary hypertension (persistent fetal circulation), for example, are diseases that are almost always seen in term or post-term infants. In contrast, RDS and pulmonary hemorrhage are primarily problems of the premature infant, with the onset of respiratory signs and symptoms occurring within 4 hours of birth. A child who

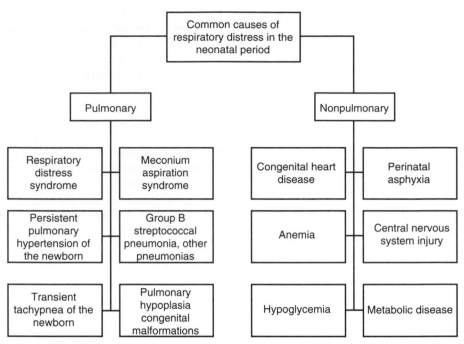

FIGURE 54–16: Common pulmonary and nonpulmonary causes of respiratory distress during the neonatal period.

becomes symptomatic beyond 12 hours of age probably has a different etiology for respiratory distress, such as pneumonia or hypoglycemia. Thus, the differential diagnosis can frequently be narrowed simply by accurately assessing gestational age and by recognizing the timing associated with respiratory signs and symptoms.

In the infant with respiratory disease, several basic studies are valuable in determining the etiology of respiratory signs. In addition, umbilical artery catheters are commonly used in the management of these infants. One helpful test is the hyperoxia test. This test helps to differentiate cyanotic congenital heart disease from pulmonary disease in the critically ill neonate. The test is performed by placing the neonate in a 100% oxygen environment, usually with positive pressure ventilation. The infant with cyanotic heart disease will be unable to generate a Pa_{O_2} of greater than 150 mm Hg because of right-to-left shunting. In contrast, the infant with pulmonary disease can usually achieve an appropriately higher level of oxygenation. When used in a preterm infant, this test should be limited to prevent the potential risk of retinopathy of prematurity.

Initial Care and Stabilization of the Infant With Respiratory Disease

The management of neonatal respiratory disease can be divided into three distinct phases: (1) initial care during the first hours of life, (2) continued acute care, and (3) long-term ventilatory care. Fortunately, few infants enter the long-term ventilatory care phase, which is difficult to manage.

Phase one, initial care during the first hours of life, actually begins prematurely, with the obstetrician and the neonatologist determining the clinical status of the mother and the fetus. Optimal approaches to labor and delivery management are predetermined. Such decisions are fostered by total preparation for any adverse clinical conditions in either the mother or the infant. Appropriately, competent personnel within the delivery room should be experienced in intubation and assisted ventilation of the neonate. These people should be focused on any potential for resuscitation and any other tasks that should be performed to preserve the well-being of infant and mother. Equipment for resuscitation must be totally operational before delivery. Approximately 10% of all deliveries in hospitals require some degree of resuscitation. Most resuscitation is usually as simple as oxygen administration by face mask. Some infants, however, require vigorous resuscitation. These infants are usually at high risk owing to factors of pregnancy. Prompt resuscitation of an infant demonstrating pulmonary signs at the time of birth is strongly advised, rather than waiting for the onset of hypoxemia and acidemia. Once acidemia occurs, surfactant production may decrease, leading to respiratory distress. The acidemic infant is usually more difficult to treat than the infant who is resuscitated early. Therapy can always be reduced or withdrawn as improvement is noted. Anticipation of risk factors requires that someone skilled in endotracheal intubation of the neonate should be present at the delivery. Although most infants needing resuscitation are adequately treated with bag-and-mask ventilation, in some circumstances endotracheal intubation is essential. Selection of the laryngoscope blade is also important. For babies weighing less than 3 kg, a No. 0 Miller blade is adequate. In babies weighing more than 3 kg, a No. 1 blade is necessary to displace the tongue appropriately for easy visualization of the vocal cords. The techniques of intubation and securing the endotracheal tube are critical but often neglected facets of care.

Assurance of an appropriate neutral thermal environment and reduction of cold stress is imperative to resuscitation and subsequent care. Many babies, when exposed to cold stress, will break down brown fat, which is found in abundance in the perispinal and periadrenal regions of the neonate. When this occurs, fatty acids are released and metabolized, and ketosis results. A sudden fall in the core temperature of an infant may therefore result in acidosis, pulmonary vasoconstriction, and respiratory distress with grunting. Once the baby's condition has been stabilized, a number of questions must be answered. First, is the nursery capable of caring for infants with this lung disease? A perinatal center should be capable of caring for babies in the following categories: (1) infants weighing less than 1500 g who have RDS; (2) infants who require early intubation and mechanical ventilation, regardless of their size; (3) asphyxiated infants with pulmonary and neurologic signs; (4) infants who are large for their gestational age and have apparent lung disease; (5) infants with complications related to lung disease, such as pneumothorax, patent ductus arteriosus, intraventricular hemorrhage, infection, and necrotizing enterocolitis; and (6) babies who have neonatal problems unrelated to respiratory distress but who have respiratory difficulties related to diagnoses such as congenital heart disease, severe anemia, seizures, and so forth.

If transport to a perinatal center is necessary, the primary care physician should facilitate transport to minimize delay in ensuring that appropriate infant care requirements are met. Many complications may be encountered during the transport period, including occlusion and dislodgment of the endotracheal tube, tension pneumothorax, fluid and electrolyte disturbances, intraventricular hemorrhage, umbilical catheter–

related complications; infection; and thermal instability. The presence of appropriately trained practitioners during transport can minimize complications to the infant.

Initiation of Ventilatory Assistance in the Symptomatic Neonate With Respiratory Distress (Continuing Care Phase)

Many approaches for the initiation of assisted ventilation have been published. The most common error made in starting ventilatory support is to wait too long before assisting the neonate. In most neonatal lung diseases, some intervention must ensue once an infant has demonstrated pulmonary signs or the baby's condition will progressively deteriorate. The conditions of premature infants can worsen very rapidly.

The symptomatic infant with a birth weight of less than 2 kg and suspected RDS is initially placed on 5 cm H_2O of CPAP, with 40 to 50% oxygen as a clinical reference point. Positive pressure can be applied in a variety of ways. Nasal CPAP and endotracheal CPAP are the most commonly accepted routes of administration. Improvement may occur with increased inspired oxygen and positive airway pressure. A recognized positive response should immediately follow the initiation of CPAP oxygen therapy or assisted ventilation. Such a prompt intervention in the small preterm infant may prevent progressive atelectasis, hypoxemia, and acidemia. In the large infant, however, atelectasis may be indiscernible, and hypoxemia and acidosis from intrapulmonary and intracardiac shunting may lead to an equally poor acid-base balance.

Mechanical Ventilation

The need to initiate mechanical ventilation during the neonatal period is readily recognized. In most instances, progressive deterioration in the infant's blood gas values, acid-base status, and clinical respiratory signs leaves little alternative. A technique using bag-and-mask ventilation with an oxygen source (preferably on an oxygen blender) and a pressure manometer inline to determine appropriate ventilator settings is frequently needed. Such an approach is suggested to reduce the risk of tension pneumothorax from inappropriately adjusted ventilator parameters (Fig. 54–17).

Higher or lower settings for manual inflation may be required, depending on the size of the infant, clinical presentation, and the pulmonary disease. Adjustments can be made promptly to ensure adequate gas exchange. Assessment of clinical indicators and adequate ventilation should be performed. These indicators include chest wall excursion and auscultation of the chest. Breath sounds that mimic faint inspiratory rales are desired. Such sounds indicate the opening of terminal airspaces. If ventilation exceeds this auditory response to breath sounds during the initiation of ventilation, air leakage is often present. In the young infant with decreased connective tissue and reduced cartilaginous support of the airway, the airway distends, and gas flow, which depends on the rigidity of the airway, becomes more turbulent. Turbulent airflow alters the distribution of gas throughout the lung, reduces effective gas exchange, and requires additional increases in ventilatory support to provide adequate patient support. This process leads to progressive airway and lung injury, which is referred to as pulmonary barotrauma. The

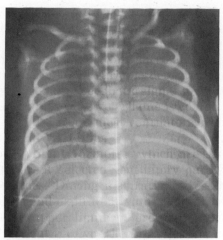

FIGURE 54–17: An infant with classic respiratory distress syndrome. The lung shows diffuse microatelectasis, producing a generalized haziness or "white-out" appearance. Air bronchograms, which reflect the airways surrounded by gasless lung, are also noted. (Courtesy of George Gross, M.D.)

consequences of pulmonary barotrauma are discussed later in this chapter. The goal, therefore, of neonatal mechanical ventilation is to minimize pulmonary barotrauma while achieving optimal gas exchange or to maximize the benefit of ventilation and minimize its complications. Understanding the available ventilatory parameters for neonatal mechanical ventilation greatly assists in meeting this goal. Underventilation of an infant to avoid pulmonary barotrauma, at the expense of adequate gas exchange, should be equally assessed. If an infant is inadequately ventilated and morbidity or mortality ensues, avoidance of barotrauma is of little benefit. Although these points may appear obvious, failure to ventilate adequately because of the presence of pulmonary interstitial emphysema is the most commonly encountered error in mechanical ventilation. If a tension pneumothorax ensues, appropriate emergency treatment should be performed.

Several additional decisions are required with the initiation of mechanical ventilation. First, is the ventilator appropriate for the clinical situation? At present, ventilators with the following three classifications are commonly used for mechanical ventilation of the newborn. These are constant-flow ventilators that may be pressure-cycled ventilators (the ventilator delivers a gas volume up to the point at which a certain preset pressure is reached); volume-cycled ventilators (designed to deliver a consistent volume of gas with each breath, regardless of the pressure required); or high-frequency ventilators (which deliver very small tidal volumes of gas at rates in excess of 150 breaths per minute). High-frequency ventilation has been approved by the US Food and Drug Administration for use in cases of RDS complicated by pulmonary air leakage. In practice, however, these ventilators are used for the rescue treatment of infants with various lung diseases who are unresponsive to conventional mechanical ventilation. Additional discussion of high-frequency ventilation is provided earlier in this text. Most neonatal mechanical ventilation, however, is started with a standard pressure-limited, time-cycled ventilator (Table 54–2).

Pressure-limited ventilators for neonatal lung disease generally offer simplicity of design, compact size, ease of operation, and a decreased capital cost because of the simplicity of ventilator parameters. In contrast, volume-limited ventilators often require a piston and spirometer pneumotach to regulate breath size, thereby necessitating more complex design features and a substantial increase in ventilator cost.

A major design benefit of pressure-limited ventilators is ease of control of peak inflating pressure (PIP). Because PIP is thought to be an important factor in the development of pulmonary air leakage and chronic lung disease (bronchopulmonary dysplasia), the management of PIP levels is important during neonatal mechanical ventilation. With pressure-limited ventilators, the same pressure is delivered to the baby with each ventilator breath. Tidal volume delivery varies in accordance with patient lung compliance and airway resistance. Additionally, the ventilatory pressure-time waveform is also modified by lung forces when fixed inspiratory pressure cycling is utilized.

A pressure-limited ventilator generates adequate tidal volume for appropriate gas exchange when lung compliance and resistance are stable. If an increase in airway resistance or a deterioration in lung compliance occurs, tidal volume and adequate alveolar gas exchange may be reduced. Conversely, immediate changes in airway resistance and compliance in an opposition direction will significantly increase tidal volume. Appropriate airway management, proper patient positioning, and careful assessment of pulmonary parameters ensures consistent alveolar ventilation with pressure-limited ventilators. Currently available graphic analysis of all ventilatory parameters discussed within the text ensures the appropriateness of ventilator adjustments and patient responses.

The volume-cycled ventilator, however, has a role in the management of the chronically ventilator-dependent child, who requires the delivery of a constant tidal volume. In these infants, cyanotic episodes are commonly observed during periods of activity because of the compliance changes occurring within the lung or airway. Progressive hypoxemia may result, as previously discussed, if pressure-limited ventilation is employed.

The application of respiratory support for patients with heart disease is complicated by the need to balance the effects of each respiratory intervention on both the cardiovascular and the respiratory systems. The complex cardiorespiratory interactions that may occur and the diversity of the conditions treated require a patient-tailored approach appropriate for every patient. Respiratory strategies are therefore designed to address the specific pathophysiologic condition present in each patient. This section defines respiratory management strategies that use the principles outlined in the previous sections. Initial ventilator settings are presented, followed by a systematic approach outlined for patient-specific pathophysiologies, respiratory, and cardiovascular conditions.

Goals of Respiratory Support

Varying degrees of ventilatory support may be required, depending on the adequacy of oxygenation and carbon dioxide removal. Despite the wide variety of respiratory support used, all types of support have the following goals: (1) optimizing oxygen delivery by improving the oxygen content of blood (systemic arterial saturation) or by decreasing the oxygen needs of the respiratory muscles through decreasing the work of breathing and (2) improving carbon dioxide elimination. Respiratory interventions are not innocuous and can result in side effects, which were previously outlined. Respiratory support should therefore meet these goals while minimizing the deleterious effects of these interventions on the various organ systems.

Application of Positive Pressure Ventilation

INITIAL VENTILATOR SETTINGS

The initial ventilatory approach for all patients should be one that is simple, meets the needs of the patient, provides the greatest benefit with the lowest risk of complications, and is familiar to the multidisciplinary intensive care team. The criteria for initiating positive pressure ventilation vary according to the intended goals and the pathophysiology present.

Ventilator Management

Once respiratory parameters have been determined and analyzed, the infant should be placed on mechanical ventilation. Arterial blood gas values should be measured every 1 to 2 hours during mechanical ventilation until the infant's condition has stabilized. The frequency of arterial blood gas determination can then be decreased to every 2 to 4 hours. Pa_{O_2} values of 60 to 80 mm Hg and Pa_{CO_2} values of 40 to 50 mm Hg are optimal goals. Some investigators have advocated higher Pa_{CO_2} levels in order to minimize barotrauma. This approach, which is referred to as permissive hypercapnia, must be used cautiously because of the potentially adverse effects of respiratory acidosis on the pulmonary circulation and the central nervous system. Chest excursion and bilateral breath sounds should be routinely assessed (see Fig. 54–17).

Noninvasive monitoring of respiratory function may reduce the necessity for arterial blood gas determinations in the stabilized infant. Such monitoring offers a simple approach to adjustment of mechanical ventilation, as well as weaning from the ventilator. Additional information on the use and techniques of noninvasive monitoring is further detailed within this text. This weaning technique assumes that the primary injury-producing factors in newborn mechanical ventilation are inspired oxygen concentration and PIP. Consequently, these controls are of the first parameter to be decreased as the infant shows signs of improvement.

The time to begin ventilator weaning is often unclear. In many instances, a sudden improvement in arterial blood gas values provides the first clue. An additional marker that may be of value is the observation of the diuretic phase. In most neonates with lung disease, particularly those with RDS, there is a diuretic phase of the disease that precedes improvement in ventilation and oxygenation (Figs. 54–18 and 54–19). Thus, a sudden increase in urinary volume may herald the onset of pulmonary improvement. In addition, bedside computerized pulmonary function assessment is a simple technique for examining compliance and resistance. These techniques effectively monitor ventilatory status as the lung disease becomes less severe. Furthermore, it appears that commercially available ventilator graphics measurements and analysis systems, which have primarily been research tools to date, enable rapid, real-time assessment of neonatal respiratory conditions. These determinations will be valuable in ventilator management and in assessing recovery from many forms of neonatal lung disease.

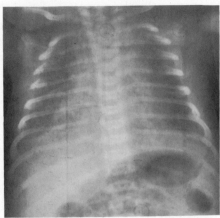

FIGURE 54–18: Transient tachypnea of the newborn. There is an increase in the density of the perihilar markings, reflecting fluid absorption. The right transverse fissure is also seen, which is indicative of fluid in the pleural space. (Courtesy of George Gross, M.D.)

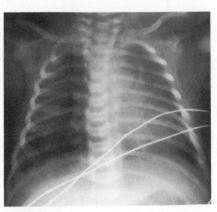

FIGURE 54–19: The same infant seen in Figure 54–18 after a 2-day period. There has been substantial clearing of increased interstitial lung water. (Courtesy of George Gross, M.D.)

Once an infant has achieved low levels of support, a decision must be made with respect to removing the infant from the ventilator. In very low birthweight infants (those weighing less than 1000 g), it is often helpful to continue some ventilation until nutrition is adequate. For these babies, a steady weight gain and an adequate daily caloric intake before extubation are advocated. In the very tiny infant, discontinuation of mechanical ventilatory support may lead to progressive atelectasis because of the inability of the chest wall to act as a strut. The infant often requires reintubation. The use of nasal or nasopharyngeal CPAP after extubation, however, may help to stabilize the chest wall and lung and reduce the need for reintubation.

At the time of extubation, the child should be receiving a CPAP of 2 to 4 cm H_2O and an inspired oxygen concentration of less than 0.4, with a ventilator rate of 4 to 10 breaths per minute. Because of endotracheal tube resistance and the associated increases in the work of breathing, we have found it useful to maintain partial ventilatory support. Several pharmacologic agents have been advocated at the time of extubation. These agents include theophylline, caffeine, corticosteroids, and racemic epinephrine. Evidence for the benefit of all of these drugs is sparse. In general, such agents are omitted as a weaning regimen unless an extubation attempt in the child has already failed and the failure can be attributed to either apnea (in which case theophylline or caffeine may be of benefit) or vocal cord edema (in which case treatment with dexamethasone may be of value). If these agents are used, they should be started 1 to 2 days before the extubation attempt and continued for a minimum of 24 to 48 hours after extubation. Racemic epinephrine is usually administered by inhalation at the time of extubation to reduce laryngeal edema.

THERAPY FOR SPECIFIC PATHOPHYSIOLOGIC CONDITIONS

Pulmonary Artery Hypertension

Therapy for pulmonary artery hypertension is directed at lowering pulmonary artery pressures and improving right ventricular function by optimizing preload and contractility. Patients with elevated pulmonary vascular resistance are sensitive to changes in right ventricular preload. Because of the increased afterload, the right ventricle requires increased right ventricular preload in order to maximize right ventricular stroke volume. Therefore, these patients require an assessment of right-sided filling pressures, which are higher than usual filling pressures (right atrial pressure of 10 to 12 mm Hg). As afterload increases, the end-systolic volume of the right ventricle increases. An increase in right ventricular end-diastolic and end-systolic volume can result in conformational changes in the interventricular septum. Such changes can cause a reduction in left ventricular volume and a reduction in left ventricular stroke volume. Patients with pulmonary hypertension frequently require inotropic agents because of the decreased right ventricular cardiac output demonstrated in the majority of these patients. However, success in using inotropic agents in patients with pulmonary artery hypertension has been very limited. This may be related to the relative insensitivity of the right ventricle to inotropes. Agents such as dopamine, epinephrine, and dobutamine have limited utility in treating patients with pulmonary hypertensive crisis, and these patients are more successfully treated by decreasing the right ventricular afterload. In addition, maintaining right ventricular coronary perfusion pressure through inotropic support may be helpful because right ventricular perfusion occurs primarily during systole.

One of the most successful approaches for reducing pulmonary artery pressures is the manipulation of cardiorespiratory interactions to lower pulmonary vascular resistance. Therapy directed at reducing pulmonary hypertension consists of increasing pH, decreasing Pa_{CO_2}, increasing Pa_{O_2} and PA_{O_2}, and minimizing intrathoracic pressures. Increasing pH has been shown to significantly reduce pulmonary vascular resistance in a variety of studies. Drummond and coworkers showed that by reducing the Pa_{CO_2} to 20 mm Hg and increasing the pH to 7.6, a consistent reduction in pulmonary vascular resistance is obtained in infants with pulmonary hypertension. In addition, maintaining serum bicarbonate levels to achieve a pH between 7.5 and 7.6 while maintaining a Pa_{CO_2} of 40 mm Hg resulted in a similar reduction in pulmonary vascular resistance. Both an increase in pH and a reduction in Pa_{CO_2} could independently result in a reduction in right ventricular afterload. Other studies have shown that increasing both alveolar oxygen (PA_{O_2}) and arterial oxygen (Pa_{O_2}) by increasing the inspired oxygen concentration can also result in a reduction in pulmonary vascular resistance. Increasing the inspired oxygen concentration improved the Pa_{O_2} in patients without a right-to-left shunt and resulted in a reduction in pulmonary artery vascular resistance. Increasing the inspired oxygen concentration in patients with intracardiac shunts resulted in little change in Pa_{O_2}; however, a reduction in pulmonary vascular resistance occurred. This was related to an increase in PA_{O_2} and demonstrates that an increase in both the alveolar and the arterial oxygen content can alter pulmonary vascular resistance. In animal studies, increasing the inspired oxygen concentration has been shown to be a more potent pulmonary vasodilator in neonates than in adults. The use of inspired oxygen to reduce pulmonary vascular resistance has been useful in the intensive care unit and is a frequent mode of interrogating pulmonary vascular responsiveness in the cardiac catheterization laboratory.

Positive pressure ventilation is usually required in patients with pulmonary artery hypertension (Figs. 54–20 and 54–21). The effects of

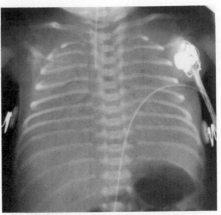

FIGURE 54–20: Group B streptococcal pneumonia in a neonate with lung disease. The chest radiographic findings mimic those seen in the infant with classic respiratory distress syndrome and in fact very probably reflect a combination of respiratory distress syndrome and pneumonia in a critically ill infant. (Courtesy of George Gross, M.D.)

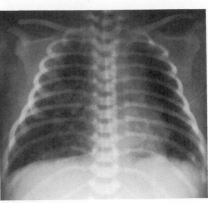

FIGURE 54–21: Meconium aspiration syndrome. There is patchy infiltration of the lung, with relatively clear areas. Some hyperinflation of the lung occurs from gas trapping distal to meconium plugs in the airways. (Courtesy of George Gross, M.D.)

different types of ventilation on pulmonary vascular resistance are not well established. However, a reduction in mean airway pressure has been shown to reduce pulmonary vascular resistance. Patients with pulmonary artery hypertension may benefit from hyperventilation, but because of the detrimental effects of mean airway pressure on pulmonary vascular resistance and right ventricular filling, mean airway pressure should be limited. Therefore, PEEP must be used judiciously in these patients. Low PEEP (2 to 3 mm Hg) may be helpful in preventing alveolar collapse, but high PEEP or high mean airway pressure results in alveolar overdistention and compression of the pulmonary capillaries with a resultant increase in pulmonary vascular resistance. Therefore, an approach to these patients should be directed at reducing right ventricular afterload and improving right ventricular stroke volume by increasing right ventricular preload.

Several differences in lung physiology exist between newborns and infants compared with adults. At the end of normal breathing, many of the smaller infants have reduced functional residual capacity and increased airway collapse. This process results in a ventilation-perfusion mismatch, with segments of lung demonstrating perfusion without ventilation. As these nonventilated lung segments become hypoxic, a secondary hypoxic response can develop, and pulmonary vascular resistance increases. In order to increase lung volumes at the end of inspiration without increasing mean airway pressure, large tidal volumes of 15 to 20 mL/kg are required. Respiratory rates are usually held at 15 to 20 breaths per minute, and respiratory cycles with short inspiratory times and long expiratory phases are used to augment pulmonary blood flow. The short inspiratory times and low rates help to minimize mean airway pressure. In addition, PEEP is held at the minimum required to prevent atelectasis (3 to 5 mm Hg).

Alternative modes of ventilation have been tried for patients with pulmonary hypertension and right ventricular dysfunction because of the detrimental effects of positive pressure ventilation on right ventricular dynamics and the need for hyperventilation. Because HFJV reduces mean airway pressure and pulmonary vascular resistance while maintaining a similar or lower Pa_{CO_2}, it should be ideally suited for patients with right ventricular dysfunction, pulmonary artery hypertension, or both. In selected patients, HFJV decreases mean airway pressure and pulmonary vascular resistance.

COMPLICATIONS OF RESPIRATORY INTERVENTIONS

Oxygen Toxicity

Oxygen therapy is not without risks; therefore, the risk-benefit ratio needs to be continuously evaluated in patients requiring oxygen therapy. Oxygen toxicity can involve multiple organs, including the central nervous system, the retinal structures, the hematopoietic system, the endocrine system, and the respiratory system. The respiratory system is extremely sensitive to oxygen. Although the onset of oxygen toxicity may vary from patient to patient, the contributing events seem to be constant: (1) the degree of oxygen exposure, (2) the length of time over which the exposure occurs, and (3) the pathophysiology of the respiratory system. The universal factor in determining the toxic effects of oxygen is the partial pressure of inspired oxygen: $PI_{O_2} = (Pb - PH_2O) \times FI_{O_2}$, where Pb is the barometric pressure and PH_2O is the partial pressure of water. At sea level, an FI_{O_2} of 1.0 is deleterious to the pulmonary parenchymal structures. The PI_{O_2} is dependent on the atmospheric pressure, and at an increased atmospheric pressure, lower concentrations of oxygen may yield parenchymal injury.

PULMONARY PATHOPHYSIOLOGY

Pulmonary oxygen toxicity is a progressive process. The initial stage involves the development of pulmonary edema, vascular congestion, distention, and capillary endothelial cell damage. This results in increased cellularity of the alveolar septum and interstitial edema. Initially, epithelial cells are spared; however, with prolonged exposure to high concentrations of inspired oxygen, destruction of the oxygen-sensitive type I pneumocytes occurs. Cell injury results in denuation of epithelial cells, which compromises the alveolar basement membrane. The loss of epithelial cells causes the alveolar basement membrane to become exposed and less effective. The progression of oxygen toxicity results in hyperplasia of type II pneumocytes, interstitial fibrosis, and end-stage pulmonary fibrosis.

ABSORPTION ATELECTASIS

Patients with high levels of oxygen may also develop absorption atelectasis. The predominant gas in the alveoli is the inert gas nitrogen. In patients breathing 100% oxygen, a "nitrogen washout" may occur within minutes. Patients with any degree of airway obstruction, as may result from retained secretions, may experience diffusion of oxygen from the alveolus into the pulmonary circulation at a rate greater than that which can be replaced by ventilation. This subsequently promotes a loss of alveolar volume, which finally collapses the aveolar structures. Alveolar nitrogen washout may explain the increase in intrapulmonary right-to-left shunting seen with 100% oxygen ventilation. Patients without pre-existing lung disease or pathology successfully inhibit this response with a natural "sigh" mechanism that periodically recruits atelectatic regions of the lung.

CLINICAL MANIFESTATIONS OF OXYGEN TOXICITY

The initial clinical manifestation of oxygen toxicity is a decrease in tracheobronchial mucus flow and mucus clearance, which may occur after only 3 hours of 100% oxygen exposure. Early signs of oxygen toxicity, which can be demonstrated during the measurement of respiratory mechanics, include a decreased vital capacity, a decreased compliance, a decreased DL_{CO_2}, and an increased $P(A - a)O_2$ gradient. In addition, an increase in the dead space–tidal volume ratio occurs. Surfactant deficiency has also been demonstrated with oxygen toxicity and may be related to the increased permeability of epithelial cells, which results in alveolar edema and a reduction in RLF surfactant.

THERAPY

The primary medical management is directed at limiting the development of oxygen toxicity through limiting the inspired oxygen concentration. Very few data are available to determine the level of oxygen concentration that is "safe" in diseased lungs. In addition, neonates may be less susceptible to the pulmonary effects of oxygen because they may have less superoxide dismustase.

Retinopathy of Prematurity

Retinopathy of prematurity (ROP) occurs predominantly in preterm and low-birthweight infants. The pathophysiology of ROP is dependent on the immaturity of the retina and exposure to ambient or supplemental oxygen. In the preterm infant, the peripheral retina is incompletely vascularized and is therefore susceptible to injury from oxygen. After exposure to oxygen, there is an increase in the gap junction between subjacent cells. This initial injury results in abnormalities of retinal development, with retinal neovascularization and intravitreal fibrovascular proliferation.

ROP has been divided into four separate clinical stages, although the disease process occurs as a continuum. Stage 1 consists of a demarcation line that separates avascular from vascular retina. In stage 2, the line of demarcation assumes a ridge shape. Stage 3 consists of the development of extraretinal fibroblast proliferation. Stage 4 consists of retinal detachment. The clinical progression of ROP is dependent on the patient's condition and on the exposure. The development of stages 1 and 2 does not necessitate progression to higher stages. The end-result of ROP is a spectrum of clinical abnormalities ranging from mild myopia to complete blindness.

The diagnosis and treatment of ROP are intimately linked. Oxygen therapy should be reduced to the minimum in at-risk patients. In addition, screening for ROP at 7 days is recommended for infants who are less than 36 weeks of gestation, those who weigh less than 2 kg, and newborns requiring increased inspired oxygen concentrations. If ROP is present, follow-up screening at regular intervals is required. Success with cryosurgical techniques is encouraging, and cryosurgery should be considered in severe cases.

Barotrauma

Pulmonary complications that occur with the use of positive pressure ventilation and PEEP, referred to as barotrauma, consist of various abnormalities in neonates. Some of the more common ones are noted in the following sections. One of the most common difficulties seen during mechanical ventilation is the acute deterioration of the infant's condition. In such instances, the approach outlined in the previous section should be taken.

PATHOPHYSIOLOGY

Barotrauma has become an all-inclusive term that describes pathologic changes ranging from pulmonary interstitial emphysema to life-threatening events such as tension pneumothorax. The primary offending factor in barotrauma is alveolar overdistention (high peak inflation volume). Barotrauma occurs in infants exposed to a high peak inspiratory pressure. The area of disruption typically occurs at the border of the alveolar base and the bronchovascular sheath. Once in the interstitium, air dissects toward the hilum, enters the mediastinum, and extends into the subcutaneous tissues and the pleural and peritoneal spaces. Barotrauma can present in a variety of forms, including pneumomediastinum, pneumoperitoneum, subcutaneous emphysema, subpleural air cysts, and hyaline membrane formation. (Pulmonary interstitial emphysema manifests as linear air streaking, perivascular blebs, or subpleural air on radiographic examination and may be an early indicator of barotrauma. Pulmonary interstitial emphysema, pneumomediastinum, subcutaneous emphysema, and pneumoperitoneum can lead to patient discomfort but are rarely of major clinical significance.)

PNEUMOTHORAX

Pneumothorax, which develops when a communication between the pleural space and the alveolus or atmosphere occurs, is frequently seen in neonates. Collapse of the lung may be partial or complete. Complete lung collapse occurs when transpulmonary pressure equilibrates with atmospheric pressure. The clinical consequences of pneumothorax are dependent on the pre-existing respiratory status of the patient and the extent of collapse. Symptoms range from the rare asymptomatic presentation to severe respiratory distress or death.

Tension pneumothorax is a life-threatening complication of barotrauma. It occurs when intrapleural pressure exceeds atmospheric pressure. Physiologically, this takes place when air enters the pleural space during inspiration from the atmosphere or alveolus and cannot escape during expiration. The increasing intrapleural pressure causes progressive ipsilateral lung collapse, shift of the mediastinum with contralateral lung compression, and obstruction of venous return to the heart, resulting in compromised pulmonary and cardiac function. The treatment of pneumothorax is the evacuation of pleural air via a closed-chest thoracotomy tube.

FACTORS THAT PREDISPOSE TO BAROTRAUMA

Various conditions increase the risk of barotrauma. They include ventilatory support requiring high peak airway pressures and high levels of PEEP, and pre-existing lung pathology, such as necrotizing pneumonia, acidosis, and RDS.

Bronchopulmonary Dysplasia

Bronchopulmonary dysplasia (BPD) is defined as oxygen dependency at 1 month after birth. BPD was first described by Northway and colleagues in 1967. BPD results from the exposure of the neonatal airway and lung to positive pressure ventilation and prolonged inspired oxygen concentration and is primarily a disease of premature infants. Forty percent of infants with birthweights of less than 1500 g develop BPD. BPD is not limited to low-birthweight infants, however. Term infants with severe lung disease who require prolonged ventilatory support at high pressures may also develop BPD. Other factors that may contribute to BPD include pulmonary air leakage, patent ductus arteriosus, airway injury, free oxygen radicals, nutritional deficiencies, and genetic tendencies, among others.

BPD remains a major management problem in the nursery, despite the advances in treatment outlined in this chapter. In fact, many of these advances may actually cause BPD because they enable these infants to live, whereas they would probably have died in the past. The care of BPD patients is complex. Attention must be paid to improving nutrition because many of these babies are malnourished from their inability to feed. Intravenous nutrition is helpful but does not completely replace enteral nutritional needs. A caloric intake as high as 170 to 200 kcal/kg/day may be needed for growth because caloric expenditure from the increased work of breathing is high in these infants. Acid-base disturbances, primarily respiratory acidosis from the underlying lung disease and metabolic alkalosis as a compensatory response and from diuretic therapy, are commonplace. Cor pulmonale, failure to thrive, and developmental delay are seen in severely affected children who are hospitalized long term.

The management of ventilation in these infants is an important part of their overall care. Once an infant has been diagnosed with BPD, a plan for ventilatory care should be established. A common error in these children occurs when the clinician overestimates the ability of the infant to wean. The child often tolerates a decrease in support initially but tires 24 to 48 hours later and has an acute increase in Pa_{CO_2}. This weaning failure may be due to the increased work of breathing that is present because these infants are exceptionally sensitive to small decreases in support.

Nutrition is essential for recovery in patients with BPD. Growth of the infant often heralds a decrease in lung disease; therefore, optimal caloric intake is essential. Because nutrition in the neonatal period is usually given as infant formula, fluid intake may become excessive for some babies. Diuretic treatment can aid in preventing fluid overload. Furosemide and chlorothiazide are the drugs of choice for these patients. Spironolactone and potassium supplementation should be given as adjuncts to therapy in order to reduce the metabolic alkalosis that occurs with prolonged diuretic use. Bronchodilators are also valuable in some infants with BPD. Pulmonary function testing can aid in defining the optimal drug treatment. The use of multiple bronchodilators should be avoided because this approach may make the airway excessively compliant. This problem can be particularly acute in infants with tracheobronchomalacia.

Dexamethasone reduces acute disease severity in many cases of BPD. The long-term effects, however, are not clearly defined at this time. An initial dose of 0.5 mg/kg/day in two divided doses is given, with a gradual taper over 2 to 3 weeks. Steroids appear to be most effective for the child with exudative disease, which is usually present at 2 to 3 weeks of life. The initiation of steroid therapy during a later stage of BPD is often helpful, although the clinician must be aware of the potential rebound effect that may occur approximately 1 to 2 weeks after discontinuation of the drug.

Tracheobronchomalacia is underdiagnosed in infants with BPD. The introduction of flexible fiberoptic bronchoscopy into the neonatal intensive care nursery has demonstrated that many patients with BPD have some degree of tracheobronchomalacia. It appears that the same factors that produce lung parenchymal disease in these children also damage the airway. Tracheobronchomalacia can be suspected in infants who have frequent cyanotic spells ("BPD spells") that do not respond to bronchodilator therapy. Pulmonary function testing in these infants reveals flow-volume loops that have periods of inspiratory collapse, expiratory collapse, or both. Although it is aesthetically displeasing, the only effective treatment for tracheobronchomalacia is increasing CPAP or PEEP. Often, levels of 10 to 15 cm H_2O are needed to abolish BPD spells. In these infants, recovery may require many months of hospital care. The management of patients with BPD requires appropriate time for tracheostomy and home ventilation. In some cases of chronic ventilator dependency, care can be shifted to the home environment. Many parents find this approach preferable to hospitalization.

WEANING FROM POSITIVE PRESSURE VENTILATION

Noninvasive Monitoring

Weaning from positive pressure ventilation requires the infant to gradually assume the entire work of breathing. Understanding respiratory muscle performance and evaluating this performance in infants are necessary to manage withdrawal (weaning) from positive pressure ventilation. In the past, weaning from mechanical ventilation required arterial blood gas analysis 20 minutes after every ventilator change. For acutely ill babies, this could result in 10 to 15 blood draws per day. Noninvasive monitors of respiratory function have become invaluable in the neonatal intensive care unit in reducing the number of arterial blood gas studies these patients require. Transcutaneous blood gas monitors provide an indirect measure of the partial pressure of oxygen and carbon dioxide from arterialized capillaries in the skin under the electrode. These values are correlated with arterial measurements to establish the basis for continuous trend monitoring. Ventilator changes can then be made and trends observed without the immediate need for blood gas analysis.

Pulse oximeters and capnographs can also be used in the neonatal intensive care unit. Pulse oximetry uses a light absorption technique to measure continuous arterial oxygen saturation and heart rate indirectly. In the presence of normal hemoglobin levels, pulse oximetry values correlate $\pm 2\%$ with direct laboratory measurements. Characteristics of fetal hemoglobin are within the clinical limits of pulse oximeter accuracy and should not affect readings. End-tidal carbon dioxide monitors (capnographs) provide an analysis of exhaled carbon dioxide as a reflection of arterial carbon dioxide. These monitors have recently been redesigned to reduce mechanical dead space and facilitate their use in very low birthweight babies. We have found good correlation with these monitors after the administration of surfactant and resolution of the ventilation-perfusion mismatching seen in RDS. Reliance on noninvasive monitors reduces the need for blood gas sampling and resultant blood transfusion in babies. Stable patients may be effectively weaned with these technologies, thereby reducing the need for direct blood gas measurement to every 4 to 6 hours.

Physiology of Weaning

Successful weaning from positive pressure ventilation depends on various factors, including adequate cardiovascular function, the presence of satisfactory ventilatory reserve, and favorable pulmonary mechanics. During the weaning phase, the patient has a gradual increase in respiratory muscle work, and if the cardiorespiratory system is unable to meet its goals, inadequate gas exchange with resultant hypoxemia and hypercapnea and inadequate oxygen delivery occur.

Criteria for Weaning

Several studies have attempted to define the criteria for weaning in infants. Investigators were unable to find a correlation between maximal negative inspiratory airway pressure and successful removal of positive pressure ventilation in a group of neonates. In a group of older infants receiving postoperative positive pressure ventilation, the combination of a crying vital capacity of greater than 15 mL/kg and a maximal negative inspiratory airway pressure of greater than 45 cm H_2O accurately predicted successful discontinuation of ventilatory support. Failure to meet these criteria was associated with a failure to tolerate the withdrawal of positive pressure ventilation and extubation. In a separate study, Dicarlo demonstrated a reduced mean lung compliance during the acute phase of ventilation in neonates after surgery for congenital heart disease. However, the primary determinant of the inability to extubate was an elevated airway resistance during the weaning phase and postoperative weight gain.

Weaning should be considered when adequate resolution of cardiorespiratory dysfunction has occurred and respiratory mechanics have improved such that the work of breathing is not excessive. Appropriate settings to begin weaning include an FI_{O_2} of 0.50 or less, a PEEP of 5 cm H_2O or less, a peak inspiratory pressure of 30 cm H_2O or less, and a ventilatory frequency of 25 breaths per minute or less.

Ventilator Adjustments

Ventilatory parameters may be progressively reduced as gas exchange stabilizes. Management of sedation and paralysis should also be considered as the patient's condition improves. Ventilatory parameters should be minimized with good gas exchange with the patient sedate. The patient should then be allowed to increase spontaneous efforts through a reduction in paralysis and sedation. Patient-ventilator synchrony is often dependent on sedation during the acute phase of respiratory dysfunction. Ventilator parameters should be readjusted to facilitate patient comfort and minimize the work of breathing as sedation is weaned. A long inspiratory time often contributes to ventilator dyssynchrony during this phase. The longer inspiratory times that facilitated oxygenation in acute lung disease should be reduced to promote patient-ventilator synchrony as the patient increases spontaneous efforts. Patient observation and pulmonary mechanics measurements help to identify the inspiratory time most comfortable for patients.

The most "toxic" ventilator parameter (i.e., the parameter most likely to have a deleterious effect on the patient) should be weaned first. Typically in the neonatal intensive care unit, this is the F_{IO_2}. Care plans should focus on continuous noninvasive monitoring of oxygenation. Transcutaneous PO_2 monitoring or pulse oximetry (Sp_{O_2}) should allow progressive oxygen weaning to maintain a transcutaneous PO_2 of 60 to 80 mm Hg or an Sp_{O_2} of greater than 92%. The F_{IO_2} may be decreased in increments of 3 to 5% to less toxic levels of less than 0.40. PEEP levels should be reduced as F_{IO_2} decreases below 0.40. PEEP level reductions usually occur in 1 cm H_2O increments until a baseline "physiologic" level of 3 to 4 cm H_2O is maintained. Patients are extubated from this PEEP level to preserve the functional residual capacity of the lung. Premature infants often require small increases in F_{IO_2} as activity levels change. F_{IO_2} may be titrated to maintain prescribed Sp_{O_2} levels. The toxic effects of oxygen therapy include retinopathy of prematurity, oxygen toxicity, and bronchopulmonary dysplasia, as previously described.

The next parameter to be assessed for weaning should be the peak inflating pressure (PIP). Delivered tidal volume must be routinely measured at the patient as dynamic compliance improves to avoid overdistention of the lung and reduce barotrauma. PIP should be adjusted to provide a delivered tidal volume of 7 to 10 mL/kg. The adequacy of this parameter can be further assessed by auscultation, noninvasive monitoring, and periodic blood gas sampling. When the adequacy of tidal volume is ensured at a PIP of less than 20 to 25 cm H_2O, the IMV rate can be weaned to reduce ventilatory support further. The rate can be reduced in increments of 2 to 4 breaths per minute to maintain the prescribed Pa_{CO_2} and pH. Transcutaneous PCO_2 and end-tidal carbon dioxide monitors can be used to continuously monitor alveolar ventilation. Pa_{CO_2} levels of 40 to 50 mm Hg are acceptable with a pH of greater than 7.25.

When IMV rates approach fewer than 10 breaths per minute, the F_{IO_2} is less than 0.40, PEEP is 3 to 4 cm H_2O, and PIP is less than 25 cm H_2O, the practitioner should evaluate the patient's readiness for extubation. Other criteria to consider before extubation include the spontaneous respiratory rate, the presence of apnea or periodic breathing, the work of breathing, the amount and consistency of respiratory secretions, the weight gain during the intubation period, vital signs, and chest radiographic findings. Upper airway edema from prolonged intubation should also be assessed. This can be evaluated by measuring the amount of inspiratory pressure required to cause air leakage around the endotracheal tube. If the inspiratory pressure is greater than 25 cm H_2O, a short course of intravenous steroid therapy may be indicated, as well as the use of aerosolized racemic epinephrine after extubation. Neonates with small endotracheal tubes (No. 3.0 or less) are usually extubated from IMV rates of 6 to 10 breaths per minute to minimize the work of breathing associated with the high airway resistance of these small endotracheal tubes. Patients may be extubated to nasal CPAP or the use of an oxy-hood oxygenator, with the F_{IO_2} administered after extubation being initially 5% greater than the F_{IO_2} on the ventilator.

Failure to Wean

Failure to wean from positive pressure ventilation can also result from increased ventilatory requirements that the patient is unable to compensate for. Increased ventilatory requirements may be a result of increased tissue carbon dioxide production, which necessitates increased alveolar ventilation to preserve normocapnea. Intake of excessive carbohydrate calories during enteral and parenteral nutrition can also lead to hypercapnia because of excessive carbon dioxide production. In addition, carbon dioxide production increases with fevers (a 10% increase for each 1°C) and excessive muscle activity (seizures, shivering, and rigor). Conditions that increase the ratio of physiologic dead space to tidal volume, such as low cardiac output, airway obstruction, and excessive positive airway pressure, require an increase in minute ventilation to maintain effective ventilation and normocapnia. Increased ventilatory requirements can also be due to other pathophysiologic conditions. Excessive respiratory drive from psychological stress, neurologic lesions, or pulmonary irritant receptor stimulation may lead to inappropriate hyperventilation and increase respiratory muscle load.

SUMMARY

Respiratory support for neonatal patients requires a thorough understanding of respiratory pathophysiology. Using the principles of respiratory physiology, pathology, and respiratory support, the clinician can develop a management strategy that is matched to the pathophysiology of the patient. This strategy will vary depending on individual variations in the pathophysiology of each patient, and one strategy is not appropriate for all patients. The principles outlined in this chapter allow clinicians the opportunity to maximize neonatal patient care and improve outcome variables. New respiratory care interventions that are forthcoming can be incorporated into the management strategy for these complicated conditions by continuing the pathophysiology-based approach.

Suggested Readings

Adams FH, Fujiwara T, Rowshan G. The nature and origin of the fluid in the fetal lamb lung. J Pediatr 63:881–888, 1963.

Avery ME, Mead J. Surface properties in relation to atelectasis and hyaline membrane disease. Am J Dis Child 97:517–523, 1959.

Bartlett RH, Gazzaniga AB, Jeffries MR, et al. Extracorporeal membrane oxygenation cardiopulmonary support in the newborn. Trans Am Soc Artif Intern Organs 22:80–93, 1976.

Bayliss WM. Surface action. In Principles of General Physiology, 1st ed. London, Longmans, Green, 1915, pp 48–73.

Boros SJ, Mammel MC, Coleman JM, et al. Neonatal high-frequency jet ventilation: Four years' experience. Pediatrics 75:657–663, 1985.

Bose C, Corbet A, Bose G, et al. Improved outcome at 28 days of age for very low birthweight infants treated with a single dose of synthetic surfactant. J Pediatr 117:947–953, 1990.

Carlo WA, Siner B, Chatburn RL, et al. Early randomized intervention with high frequency jet ventilation in respiratory distress syndrome. J Pediatr 117:765–770, 1990.

Carter JM, Gerstmann DR, Clark RH, et al. High frequency oscillatory ventilation and extracorporeal membrane oxygenation for the treatment of acute neonatal respiratory failure. Pediatrics 85:159–164, 1990.

Clements JA, Platzker ACG, Tierney DF, et al. Assessment of the risk of respiratory distress syndrome by a rapid test for surfactant in pulmonary fluid. N Engl J Med 286:1077–1081, 1972.

Collaborative European Group. Surfactant replacement therapy for severe neonatal respiratory distress syndrome: An international randomized clinical trial. Pediatrics 82:683–691, 1988.

Field D, Milner AD, Hopkins IE. Effects of positive end expiratory pressure during ventilation of the preterm infant. Arch Dis Child 60:843–847, 1985.

Fox WW, Spitzer AR, Rozycki HJ. Clinical assessment and management of bronchopulmonary dysplasia. *In* Guthrie R (ed). Neonatal Intensive Care. New York, Churchill Livingstone, 1988, pp 75–90.

Fredberg JT, Glass GM, Boynton BR, Frantz ID. Factors influencing performance of neonatal high frequency ventilators. J Appl Physiol 62:2485–2490, 1987.

Fujiwara T, Chida S, Watobe Y, et al. Artificial surfactant therapy in hyaline membrane disease. Lancet 1:55–58, 1980.

Glass P, Miller M, Short B. Morbidity for survivors of extracorporeal membrane oxygenation: Neurodevelopmental outcome at one year of age. Pediatrics 83:72–78, 1989.

Gluck L, Kulovich MV, Borer RC Jr, et al. Diagnosis of respiratory distress syndrome by amniocentesis. Am J Obstet Gynecol 109:440–445, 1971.

Greenspan JS, Wolfson MR, Rubenstein SD, Shaffer TH. Liquid ventilation of human preterm neonates. J Pediatr 117:106–111, 1990.

Gregory GA, Kitterman JA, Phibbs RH, et al. Treatment of idiopathic respiratory distress syndrome with continuous positive airway pressure. N Engl J Med 284:1333–1340, 1971.

Hall RT, Rhodes PG. Pneumothorax and pneumomediastinum in infants with idiopathic respiratory distress syndrome receiving continuous positive airway pressure. Pediatrics 55:493–499, 1975.

HiFi Study Group. High frequency oscillatory ventilation compared with conventional intermittent mechanical ventilation in the treatment of respiratory failure in preterm infants: Neurodevelopmental follow-up at 16 to 24 months postterm age. J Pediatr 117:939–946, 1990.

HiFi Study Group. High frequency oscillatory ventilation compared with conventional mechanical ventilation in the treatment of respiratory failure in preterm infants. N Engl J Med 320:88–93, 1989.

HiFi Study Group. Pulmonary follow-up of children treated with high frequency oscillatory ventilation compared to conventional mechanical ventilation. J Pediatr 116:933–941, 1990.

Jost JA, Policard A. Contribution experimentale a l'etude du development prenatal du poumon chez le lapin. Arch Anat Microsc 37:323–332, 1948.

Keszler M, Donn SM, Bucciarelli RL, et al. Controlled multicenter trial of high-frequency jet ventilation vs. conventional ventilation in newborns with pulmonary interstitial emphysema. J Pediatr 119:85–93, 1991.

Kwong M, Egan E, Notter RH, et al. Double-blind clinical trial of calf lung surfactant extract for the prevention of hyaline membrane disease in extremely premature infants. Pediatrics 76:585–592, 1985.

Merritt TA, Hallman M, Bloom BT, et al. Prophylactic treatment of very premature infants with human surfactant. N Engl J Med 315:785–790, 1986.

O'Rourke PP, Crone RK, Vacanti JP, et al. Extracorporeal membrane oxygenation and conventional medical therapy in neonates with persistent pulmonary hypertension of the newborn: A prospective randomized study. Pediatrics 84:957–963, 1989.

Pattle RE. Properties, function and origin of the alveolar lining layer. Nature 175:1125–1126, 1955.

Roberts RJ. Employment of pulmonary superoxide dismutase, catalase, and glutathione peroxidase activity as criteria for assessing suitable animal models for studies of bronchopulmonary dysplasia. J Pediatr 95:904–910, 1979.

Spitzer AR, Butler S, Fox WW. Ventilatory response of combined high-frequency jet ventilation and conventional mechanical ventilation for the rescue treatment of severe neonatal lung disease. Pediatr Pulmonol 7:244–249, 1989.

Spitzer AR, Davis J, Clarke WT, et al. Pulmonary hypertension and persistent fetal circulation in the newborn. Clin Perinatol 15:389–414, 1988.

Spitzer AR, Fox WW, Delivoria-Papdopoulos M. Maximum diuresis—A factor in predicting recovery from respiratory distress syndrome and the development of bronchopulmonary dysplasia. J Pediatr 98:476–491, 1981.

Toomasian JM, Snedecor SM, Cornell RG, et al. National experience with extracorporeal membrane oxygenation for newborn respiratory failure: Data from 715 cases. Trans Am Soc Artif Intern Organs 34:140–147, 1988.

Wung JT, James LS, Kilchevsky E, et al. Managements of infants with severe respiratory failure and persistence of the fetal circulation, without hyperventilation. Pediatrics 76:488–494, 1985.

55

Prehospital Respiratory Care*

Jay A. Johannigman, M.D., F.A.C.S.

The clinical presence of cyanosis is most readily detected by examination of the circumoral region, the nail beds, or the base of the tongue.

The efficient and effective management of the airway and respiratory system remains an absolute requisite for successful patient resuscitation. The primacy of the airway is indicated by the tenet "airway, breathing and circulation," which emphasizes the need for effective airway management during resuscitative efforts. Prehospital respiratory management poses the most immediate, and often most complex, challenge to the emergency caregiver. Without the establishment of adequate oxygenation and effective ventilation, all other considerations of care assume secondary importance. The scope of this chapter is threefold:

1. *To identify those patients who require airway assistance*
2. *To describe the many techniques, equipment, and procedures that may be employed to secure the airway and provide oxygenation ventilation*
3. *To describe the tools and techniques that permit the safe transport of the patient who requires airway management*

The most basic tenet of airway management remains the recognition of respiratory distress. In the setting of cardiac arrest and apnea, the need is obvious; however, the diversity of clinical settings and patient conditions often makes accurate assessment a clinical challenge. In the awake, spontaneously breathing patient, the need for airway management may be subtle and easily overlooked, thus mandating a thorough and thoughtful evaluation of each patient based on careful physical examination.

The evaluation of the patient in respiratory distress remains anchored by the physical examination. It must include careful consideration of the patient's appearance, respiratory effort and rate, and auscultatory findings. Anxiety, restlessness, and agitation may be indicative of hypoxia. Diaphoresis, which is a result of increased sympathetic tone, may reflect inadequate organ perfusion or tissue hypoxia, or a combination of both. Cyanosis, a very late sign of hypoxemia, requires at least 5 g of reduced hemoglobin to be clinically detectable. This level of desaturation may not be attained in the trauma patient with acute hemorrhage and resultant anemia. The practitioner must be significantly concerned by the presence of cyanosis but should not attain a false sense of security by its absence.

Assessment of the character and frequency of respiratory effort is a vital part of an accurate patient evaluation. Important physical findings include the patient's ability to speak and the presence of stridor, tracheal deviation, chest wall excursion and the symmetry of excursion, and the use of accessory muscles of respiration. The presence of sternal and supraclavicular retractions, which indicate an attempt to increase ventilation, must alert the practitioner to carefully evaluate the adequacy of ventilation.

---

*The opinions expressed herein are those of the author and do not reflect official policy of the United States Air Force or the United States Government.

Tachypnea is a basic physiologic response elaborated at the brain stem level in response to hypoxia, hypercarbia, and other stressors.

The auscultatory examination, which provides important, complementary information, should be considered an essential component of any evaluation.

The presence of tachypnea should prompt an evaluation of patient status; in most instances tachypnea indicates the need for some form of airway assistance to improve oxygenation or ventilation.

Auscultatory findings provide a simple and convenient means of evaluating the status of the respiratory system. In the noisy and often distracting environment of the prehospital setting, the clinical utility of these findings is often overlooked. A rapid, thorough auscultation of both lung fields may alert the clinician to asymmetry or lack of breath sounds. These findings are of particular importance in the trauma patient in whom a unilateral lack of breath sounds may indicate the presence of a tension pneumothorax requiring immediate intervention.

INDICATIONS FOR AIRWAY MANAGEMENT

A wide variety of indications for airway management based on the patient's physical findings exists. Although some indications appear obvious, others are less apparent. The indications for airway intervention may be divided into three broad categories: *absolute, strong relative,* and *relative* (Table 55–1).

Absolute Indications

Apnea

Apnea accompanying cardiac arrest remains the most common indication for prehospital airway management. Up to 1000 cardiac arrests occur every day in the United States, with the overwhelming majority of these patients requiring airway management.[1] Other causes of apneic arrest include head injuries, spinal cord trauma, blunt traumatic arrest, and overwhelming respiratory failure.

Acute Airway Obstruction

One of the most demanding and urgent indications for airway management is airway obstruction. The most frequent cause of airway obstruction relates to the mechanical obstruction of the upper airway in the unconscious patient in the supine position. Under these circumstances, the tongue relaxes and occludes the airway by obstructing the posterior oropharynx. Once this form of obstruction is recognized by the inability to provide adequate ventilation, it may be readily alleviated by any of a number of maneuvers, such as the chin lift–jaw thrust tech-

TABLE **55–1:** Indications for Airway Management

Absolute Indications
Apnea
Acute airway obstruction
Hypoxia
Penetrating trauma, expanding hematoma of the neck
Strong Relative Indications
Closed head injury
Shock
Thoracic trauma
Relative Indications
The combative or intoxicated patient
Maxillofacial injuries

nique, or through the use of a simple airway (oral or nasal). Other causes of acute airway obstruction in the injured patient may include solid foreign objects, such as dentures, gastric contents, tissue or teeth fragments, or pooled fluids, such as blood or oral secretions. Direct laryngeal trauma such as that which occurs when a driver's throat impacts against the steering wheel may result in life-threatening upper airway obstruction. Depending on the severity of the injury, initial manifestations may include difficulty with phonation, marked anxiety or progressive air hunger, or both, and stridor. This form of airway obstruction, which can often lead to rapid and complete airway obstruction, may mandate the provision of a surgical airway such as a cricothyrostomy or formal tracheostomy.

Hypoxia

Hypoxia may be clinically overt as in the cyanotic patient, or it may be a more subtle finding manifested by restlessness, anxiety, and tachypnea. The absolute determination of hypoxemia requires analysis of arterial blood gases, an adjunct not often available in the prehospital setting. In recent years, the technology to provide reliable, rapid, and portable pulse oximetry has become available. Recent advances in microprocessing, miniaturization, and light-emitting diode technology have made it feasible to measure oxygen saturation portably in the prehospital environment. The use of pulse oximetry allows the rapid and ongoing determination of oxygen saturation, which gives the prehospital provider immediate feedback regarding the effectiveness of therapeutic interventions. In the United States, there are currently more than 20 manufacturers producing various types of pulse oximeters. Many models possess desirable characteristics such as small size, portability, rugged construction, and battery operation, which make them applicable in the prehospital setting. The use of pulse oximetry provides a powerful tool that may supplement the clinical decision-making process in the field.

In most situations, the presence of hypoxia constitutes an absolute indication for airway intervention by providing supplemental oxygen. The one well-recognized exception to this generalization is the patient with chronic obstructive pulmonary disease (COPD). Hypoxemia may be relatively well tolerated in the COPD patient—the so-called blue-bloater; in this type of patient, the addition of supplemental oxygenation may ablate the hypoxemic respiratory drive, thereby resulting in respiratory arrest.

Penetrating Trauma or Expanding Hematoma

Penetrating injuries to the neck, such as those caused by a knife or gunshot wound, are capable of causing vascular injury. A resultant, rapidly expanding hematoma can compromise the upper airway by direct mechanical compression. These same wounding agents may also result in direct mechanical disruption of the upper airway. These injuries may present a sudden and often challenging need for an emergency airway. Lesser degrees of tracheal deviation in penetrating trauma with hematoma should be considered an urgent airway emergency.

Strong Relative Indications

Closed Head Injury

The presence of significant closed head injury may constitute a number of relative indications for airway intervention. The altered sensorium that often accompanies a closed head injury may

---

Oximetry is based on the principle that hemoglobin changes color and light transmission characteristics as its saturation changes. Oxygenated and deoxygenated (reduced) hemoglobin have unique wavelength "signatures," which may be distinguished by their differing light absorbance. Through the introduction of light of two known wavelengths that corresponds to the respective absorbance peaks of oxygenated and reduced hemoglobin, it is possible to calculate the oxygen saturation.

The clinician is often faced with a difficult decision regarding immediate transport with a potentially unstable airway versus a difficult, or even impossible, orotracheal intubation in the field. Unnecessary delay may allow the "golden opportunity" to slip away and necessitate more complex maneuvers under more difficult circumstances.

- Decrease the patient's protective reflexes
- Promote aspiration
- Allow passive obstruction of the upper airway

The use of therapeutic hyperventilation to obtain cerebral vasoconstriction remains one of the cornerstones in early management of increased intracranial pressure in closed head injuries. Finally, the traumatized central nervous system is acutely sensitized to ongoing hypoxemia.

Shock

Shock is defined as a state of inadequate organ perfusion. This definition implies significant tissue hypoxemia. Airway management with enriched oxygen provides a means of maximizing the oxygen content of the circulating blood volume. Patients manifesting evidence of systemic shock should receive enriched oxygen via a source capable of providing an FI_{O_2} of 0.5 or greater. This simple maneuver may significantly ameliorate tissue hypoxia while efforts are directed at reversing the primary cause of circulatory collapse.

Thoracic Trauma

A number of traumatic injuries may disrupt or significantly compromise a patient's ability to maintain effective oxygenation and ventilation. Specific examples of such injuries include flail chest, hemothorax, tension pneumothorax, diaphragmatic disruption, and sucking chest wounds. Airway management may prove necessary to augment ventilation, relieve hypoxemia, and compensate for the loss of functional residual capacity.

Relative Indications

The Combative or Intoxicated Patient

The widespread association of alcohol intoxication, drug use, closed head injury, and trauma has resulted in an increasing number of disoriented, violent, or combative patients who require prehospital airway management. The altered mental status elicited by alcohol, drugs, or injury is accompanied by decreased airway protective responses, so the victim becomes susceptible to gastric aspiration, airway obstruction, and hypoventilation. Such a patient often proves most challenging, since the prehospital care provider must "walk a fine line" in an attempt to determine the adequacy of the patient's ventilatory status. The goal is to accurately distinguish those patients who require assistance (face mask, supplemental oxygen, and so on) from those who require invasive intervention such as endotracheal intubation. In the context of life-threatening injuries, it is sometimes necessary to subdue the violent patient who cannot be adequately restrained. This is especially true during aeromedical evacuation in which a thrashing patient poses danger not only to himself or herself but also to the safety of the aircraft and flight personnel. In this setting, restraint may be attained through the administration of systemic paralytic agents that allow the care provider to achieve and maintain airway control. With the administration of paralytic agents, the prehospital care provider, who is truly taking the patient's life into his or her own hands, must be thoroughly skilled in invasive airway

---

Therapeutic hyperventilation to a Pa_{CO_2} of 25 to 30 mm Hg is most effectively achieved via endotracheal intubation and controlled-assisted ventilation. Efficient administration of enriched oxygen is most reliably attained through endotracheal intubation.

Oxygen delivery is the product of cardiac output and the oxygen content of blood.

Since paralytic agents eliminate the opportunity to perform a neurologic examination, a thorough neurologic examination must be completed and well documented prior to their administration.

Specific caution must be exercised in maintaining cervical spine protection because of the relatively high coincidence of cervical spine trauma in the presence of maxillofacial trauma (12 to 18%).[4]

The chin lift is performed by grasping the midportion of the mandible and lifting anteriorly without extending the neck. The jaw thrust is completed by elevating the angles of the mandible to obtain the same effect.

The oral airway, constructed of rigid plastic, is positioned to prevent the posterior displacement of the tongue. This airway may also serve as a bite block in the unconscious patient, but it is poorly tolerated by the patient with an intact gag reflex. The nasal airway, often more readily tolerated by the semiconscious patient, maintains an adequate upper airway for the spontaneously breathing patient when properly positioned.

management and surgical airway alternatives. The use of paralytic agents in the field by nonphysician providers remains a controversial topic. In a carefully supervised and well-controlled program, the use of paralytic agents by paramedics has been demonstrated to be an effective maneuver.[2, 3] The use of these agents clearly requires a strong commitment to training, ongoing quality assurance, and active supervision.

Maxillofacial Injuries

Despite the increasing availability of supplemental restraint devices, such as seat belts and air bags, significant maxillofacial injuries remain a frequent airway challenge in the prehospital environment. Maxillofacial injuries often occur in patients with concomitant closed head injuries or significant multisystem trauma. In most instances, simple, basic airway maneuvers such as suctioning and careful, protected positioning of the patient, along with supplemental oxygen administration, will provide an adequate airway until arrival at a definitive care facility. When indications for intubation are present in the setting of maxillofacial trauma, it may be necessary to modify the techniques used. Nasotracheal intubation is contraindicated in the patient with midfacial fractures or evidence of a basilar skull fracture ("raccoon's eyes" or cerebrospinal otorrhea). Orotracheal intubation may be difficult or impossible in this setting, so patients with actual or impending airway compromise may require a surgical cricothyrostomy. Readers are referred to excellent descriptions by Phillips[5] or the *Textbook of Advanced Trauma Life Support*[6] for the technique of surgical cricothyrostomy and other surgical airway techniques.

SIMPLE TECHNIQUES FOR AIRWAY MANAGEMENT

Once the clinician determines that airway intervention is required, it is necessary to select the proper technique and equipment to provide an adequate airway. In the spontaneously breathing patient, the provider must strive to achieve two goals:

- Clear and maintain the airway
- Provide a means of supplemental oxygenation

The chin lift and jaw thrust maneuvers are two techniques designed to displace the tongue and mandible anteriorly to relieve passive obstruction of the upper airway by the base of the tongue. These simple maneuvers are often the only intervention required to secure the airway in a spontaneously breathing patient.

Clearing the airway is an obvious but often overlooked prerequisite to more elaborate techniques. Airway compromise due to aspiration of gastric contents or a solid foreign object remains a frequent occurrence that necessitates a thorough evaluation of the upper airway. Visual inspection of the oropharynx with a light and tongue blade, along with the use of a suction device to clear secretions, provides the safest and most effective means of clearing the airway. Digital exploration of the posterior oropharynx, which is less effective, may actually push objects deeper into the oropharynx. The use of the curved McGill forceps provides a means of retrieving objects that are visualized during the inspection. Once the airway has been opened and cleared, the use of an oral or nasal airway may prove necessary to protect the airway from passive reocclusion.

OXYGEN ADMINISTRATION

Oxygen Therapy

For the spontaneously breathing patient, the simplest and most logical way to initiate therapy is through oxygen administration. Oxygen must be regarded as a powerful therapeutic tool that has significant benefits but can also have potentially harmful side effects. Devices that deliver oxygen are commonly grouped into two distinct categories, which assist in the understanding of their capabilities and limitations. Devices that provide only a portion of the total gas volume inspired by the patient are classified as *low-flow or variable performance* devices. As a patient's ventilatory demands or respiratory pattern changes, a variable amount of room air must be incorporated to meet the patient's needs, resulting in a dilution of the final oxygen content.

High-flow or fixed performance equipment supplies all of the patient's inspired flow at a prescribed $F_{I_{O_2}}$. In most instances, the performance of this equipment is not significantly altered by the patient's ventilatory demand or respiratory pattern.

Low-Flow or Variable Performance Devices

The nasal cannula, the simplest and oldest form of oxygen administration, was first described in 1871. It is designed to provide low-flow oxygen via orifices positioned at the nares. The flow provided by the cannula constitutes only a small portion of the patient's total inspiratory flow; therefore, the $F_{I_{O_2}}$ provided at a given flow rate may vary significantly, depending on the patient's respiratory pattern. The ratio of admixture varies with each breath as well as with changes produced by mouth versus nasal breathing patterns. The ability of the nasal cannula to increase the inspired oxygen content plateaus at approximately 6 L/min of flow. Above this level, increases in oxygen flow result in a negligible increase in $F_{I_{O_2}}$. For this reason, as well as patient complaints of nasal dryness at higher flow rates, the maximal delivered flow from a nasal cannula is normally 6 to 8 L/min. Table 55–2 provides an estimate of the range of potential $F_{I_{O_2}}$ obtained with a nasal cannula.

Simple Mask. Commonly employed in the prehospital setting, the simple mask is a disposable, lightweight device designed to cover the nose and mouth. The face seal of the simple mask, which is not form-fitting, readily allows entrainment of room air. The poorer the mask fit, the greater the relative proportion of entrainment occurring with each breath. Even a reasonably well-fitting mask displays a great variability in $F_{I_{O_2}}$ based on the patient's ventilatory pattern. With proper fit, adequate oxygen flow, and a slow and steady inspiratory pattern, $F_{I_{O_2}}$ in the range of 40 to 60% may be achieved. Patients often find these masks hot and uncom-

Examples of low-flow or variable performance devices include the nasal cannula, the simple oxygen mask, the partial rebreathing mask, and the nonrebreathing mask. Examples of high-flow devices include air entrainment masks ("Venturi masks") and aerosol systems.

Note: Studies that quote $F_{I_{O_2}}$ values obtained with the use of a nasal cannula are, at best, rough estimates.

Simple masks must be used with a minimum oxygen flow of 5 L/min to ensure adequate washout of the patient's exhaled carbon dioxide.

TABLE **55–2:** Estimate of the Range of Potential $F_{I_{O_2}}$ with Nasal Cannula

L/Min	$F_{I_{O_2}}$
1	23
2	24–38
3	25–32
4	26–36
5	30–40
6	36–42
10	40–45

fortable as well as irritating to the skin. Some patients, particularly hypoxic ones, complain of feeling claustrophobic with these devices and tolerate them for a short time only. Despite these limitations, the simple mask provides an effective, convenient, and readily available means of administering supplemental oxygenation.

Partial Rebreathing Mask. This mask uses a reservoir to provide oxygen to the patient. During inspiration, oxygen is drawn from the mask, the reservoir bag, and the supply tubing. The mask's reservoir serves as a means of meeting a portion of the inflow demands that occur during peak inspiratory flow. When a patient's peak flow exceeds the reservoir's volume, room air will be entrained, thereby diluting the final $F_{I_{O_2}}$. These devices are called partial rebreathing masks because the first portion of expired gas returns to partially refill the reservoir before the remainder vents to the ambient surroundings. Theoretically, the first portion of exhaled gas is dead space, therefore carbon dioxide does not return to the reservoir. If inflow to the mask is sufficiently high to prevent the reservoir bag from deflating more than one-half its volume during inhalation, no carbon dioxide accumulates during expiration. The partial rebreathing mask provides an $F_{I_{O_2}}$ of approximately 60% if correctly used, with a minimum oxygen inflow of at least 8 L/min.

Nonrebreathing Mask. This mask uses the same basic design as the partial rebreathing mask but incorporates a one-way flap valve between the reservoir bag and the mask and between the mask and the exhalation port. This design prevents any portion of exhaled gas from returning to the reservoir bag. As with the partial rebreathing mask, the patient inspires from the mask, the reservoir, and the supply tubing. If the available oxygen reservoir exceeds the patient's peak inspiratory needs, an $F_{I_{O_2}}$ approaching 100% will be obtained. Practically speaking, this situation occurs only in a patient with a slow, shallow inspiratory pattern. In most patients, a variable amount of room air entrainment occurs during inspiration, thereby diluting the final $F_{I_{O_2}}$. Proper operation of the nonrebreathing mask requires an oxygen flow of at least 10 to 15 L/min to assure flushing of the mask with oxygen and complete filling of the reservoir prior to the next breath. The proper use of the nonrebreathing mask results in an $F_{I_{O_2}}$ of 0.6 to 0.8.

High-Flow or Fixed Performance Devices

High-flow or fixed performance devices are designed to supply a patient's entire inspiratory flow without entrainment of room air and therefore provide a more precise $F_{I_{O_2}}$. There are two commonly used high-flow systems in the prehospital setting:

- Air entrainment masks
- Large-volume aerosols

Air Entrainment Masks. Although often incorrectly referred to as "Venturi" masks, air entrainment masks actually employ the principle of jet drag to achieve their effect. Oxygen under pressure is forced through a narrow orifice at the base of the nozzle (Fig. 55–1). The velocity of the oxygen flow is accelerated at the nozzle because of the change in cross-sectional diameter. This increased velocity creates a *jet drag*, or *shearing* effect, which results in the surrounding room air being "dragged" or entrained into the mask. The resultant $F_{I_{O_2}}$ produced is a function of the proportions of the mixture of oxygen and entrained air.[7] The proportion

With increased patient ventilatory effort, it may be necessary to increase flow to 15 L/min to keep the reservoir bag adequately filled.

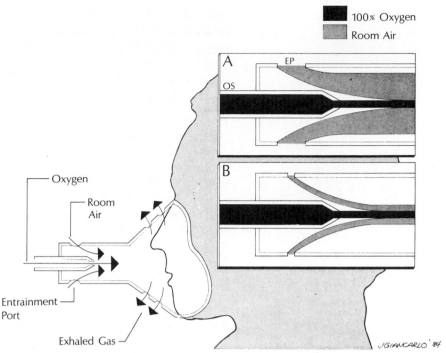

■ 100% Oxygen

▨ Room Air

FIGURE 55–1: Principle of an air entrainment device. Pressurized oxygen is forced through a nozzle (constricted orifice); the increased gas velocity distal to the orifice creates a jet drag or shearing effect that causes room air to be entrained through the entrainment ports. The high flow of gas fills the mask, which has holes, allowing both exhaled and delivered gas to escape. *A* and *B* illustrate that the size of the entrainment ports (EP) determine the amount of room air to be entrained; OS is the oxygen source. *A* illustrates large ports, resulting in relatively higher FI_{O_2}. For any size of entrainment port, the FI_{O_2} is stable; however, the total gas flow will vary with the pressurized oxygen flow. (From Shapiro BA, Harrison RA, Kacmarek RM, et al. Clinical Application of Respiratory Care, 3rd ed. Chicago, Year Book Medical, 1985.)

At FI_{O_2} exceeding 35%, the total flow of the system may fall below a patient's peak inspiratory flow, particularly for patients with COPD or respiratory distress (Tables 55–3 and 55–4). In this situation, dilution of the FI_{O_2} occurs as the patient's demands exceed flow, and room air is entrained.

of mixing is determined by the relationships among the nozzle size, the oxygen velocity, and the size of the entrainment ports. This design allows the creation of a system that provides a relatively high flow at a constant FI_{O_2}. As the desired final FI_{O_2} concentration is increased, the total flow produced by the system decreases (more oxygen, less entrainment).

Air entrainment masks are particularly suited for patients whose hypoxemia cannot be controlled with lower FI_{O_2} devices, such as the nasal cannula. Patients with COPD who tend to hypoventilate at moderate FI_{O_2}s are candidates for an air entrainment mask because it allows more precise, controlled oxygen delivery. Because of its ability to provide relatively high flows, the air entrainment mask is also suited for asthmatics or patients who are hyperventilating.

Aerosol Systems. These systems, which use a variable FI_{O_2} delivery

TABLE **55–3:** Basic Approximation of Inspiratory Flow Rates

Condition of Patient	Minute Ventilation (L/min)	Inspiratory Time (sec)	Peak Inspiratory Flow (L/min)
Normal	7	2	28
COPD	6.5	1.43	39
Respiratory distress	10	0.71	73

COPD, chronic obstructive pulmonary disease.

TABLE **55–4:** Approximate Input Flow and Total Generated Flow by Typical Air Entrainment System

FI_{O_2}	Input Flow	Total Flow
0.24	4	97
0.28	6	68
0.30	6	54
0.35	8	45
0.40	12	50
0.50	12	33

capability via entrainment, incorporate a large-volume aerosol nebulizer to increase the water content of the gas delivered to the patient. These units commonly employ a plastic sleeve at the level of the oxygen orifice. This sleeve may be rotated to vary the entrainment orifice size. The FI_{O_2} may be set at a fixed point or may be variable from 30 to 100%. As with air entrainment masks, as FI_{O_2} increases, total flow decreases. The total flow of the system may fall below the patient's peak demand at or above FI_{O_2}s of 0.4. Large-volume aerosol systems may be interfaced to the patient via many different routes, including the aerosol mask, face tent, tracheostomy collar, and T-piece (Briggs adaptor). Table 55–5 provides a summary of oxygen therapy devices.

THE ASSISTED AIRWAY

When patients cannot sustain their ventilatory needs, the emergency care provider must decide which airway or ventilatory technique best meets those needs. A wide variety of techniques and tools for establishing the airway and maintaining ventilation has been described. The most commonly employed techniques include

- Mouth-to-mouth ventilation
- Mouth-to-mask ventilation
- Bag-valve-mask ventilation
- Positive pressure ventilation through an esophageal obturator airway (EOA), a pharyngotracheal lumen airway, or an endotracheal tube

The multiplicity of devices available for prehospital ventilatory care suggests that no one device or technique is universally applicable or accepted. Agreement has not been obtained regarding which of these techniques is superior. One significant consideration must enter into the decision process—the expertise of the caregiver responsible for initiating resuscitation efforts. Although trained paramedical personnel are increasingly more prevalent in urban areas, they are by no means widely

TABLE **55–5:** Summary of Oxygen Therapy Devices

Device	Flow (L/min)	Approximate FI_{O_2}*
Nasal cannula	1–10	0.23–0.45
Simple mask	5–15	0.40–0.60
Partial rebreathing mask	10–15	0.60
Nonrebreathing mask	10–15	0.60–0.80
Anesthesia bag-valve-mask	15	0.90–1.0
Air entrainment	4–12	0.24–0.50
Aerosol	5–15	0.40–1.0

*FI_{O_2} varies based on inspiratory flow (see text).

available. A substantial number of resuscitation efforts must be initiated by lay persons or basic life support personnel who are not trained in the techniques of invasive airway management. Although most authors agree that the endotracheal tube remains the "gold standard" of airways, the remaining techniques must be thoughtfully evaluated and carefully taught for they continue to represent an important portion of prehospital ventilatory care.

Mouth-to-Mouth Ventilation

Mouth-to-mouth ventilation remains the oldest and simplest resuscitation technique. This easily taught technique is effective in its application but not without its limitations. Mouth-to-mouth resuscitation, which has been criticized for its inability to provide enriched oxygen, may also be associated with significant gastric distention in the setting of altered lung compliance. Studies show that although mouth-to-mouth resuscitation is an effective technique in providing adequate ventilation, it also results in the greatest volume of gastric distention, even when performed by trained personnel.[8] Perhaps the most significant shortcoming of this technique is that most prehospital care givers find direct patient contact unacceptable. In today's era of concern over the transmission of communicable diseases, most notably acquired immunodeficiency syndrome, the question arises whether it is practical to expect that this technique will maintain widespread acceptance.[9] Nevertheless, it remains important because of its simplicity; in addition, trained lay family members can often provide initial bystander cardiopulmonary resuscitation (CPR) for their relatives.

Mouth-to-Mask Ventilation

The technique of mouth-to-mask ventilation offers many advantages for providing ventilation in the prehospital setting. The uncomplicated technique is readily mastered by lay personnel; it also requires simple equipment and avoids direct patient contact. With the use of an oxygen enrichment port attached to the mask, an FI_{O_2} in the 0.6 to 0.9 range can be provided.[10] The use of the mouth-to-mask technique is associated with adequate tidal volume delivery, lower peak airway pressures, and less gastric distention when compared with mouth-to-mouth technique.[8]

Bag-Valve-Mask Ventilation

The bag-valve-mask continues to be the most widely employed initial technique of airway support used by basic life support personnel in the prehospital setting. The widespread use of the bag-valve-mask must be viewed cautiously because of the documented shortcomings of this technique. Multiple investigators[11–12] have demonstrated inherent difficulties with the use of the bag-valve-mask in the one-rescuer situation. The primary problem with this technique is that it often fails to provide the American Heart Association's recommended tidal volume of 800 mL/ breath[14] when employed by a single rescuer.[8, 11] This is particularly true with altered lung compliance, which typically occurs following cardiac arrest.[15] The loss of tidal volume when using the bag-valve-mask at decreased compliance is primarily due to a poor face mask seal. It is a technically difficult feat for one rescuer to adequately maintain head tilt and mask seal with one hand and simultaneously deliver adequate tidal volumes with the second hand. This technique should therefore not be used by a single rescuer as a primary means of resuscitation.

Esophageal Obturator Airway

The EOA has not been proved superior to the basic techniques of mouth-to-mouth or mouth-to-mask ventilation; in fact, it may be markedly inferior to these simple techniques.

Introduced in 1968, EOA[16] subsequently received the endorsement of the American Heart Association. Although a number of studies have suggested that the EOA is capable of providing adequate ventilatory support, an increasingly large body of evidence is accumulating that suggests this airway has serious and significant shortcomings. Multiple studies have demonstrated significant hypercarbia and acidosis associated with the use of the EOA.[17–19] It has also been associated with complications such as pharyngeal lacerations, esophageal perforation, and inadvertent tracheal intubation. Because of these issues, the use of the EOA in the prehospital arena should be re-evaluated.

Pharyngotracheal Lumen Airway

The pharyngotracheal lumen airway, a modification of the EOA concept,[20] includes the option of alternative tracheal or esophageal intubation but also includes a large intraoral cuff to create a pharyngeal seal in the case of esophageal placement of the long tube (Fig. 55–2). This design is proposed to circumvent the problem of obtaining an adequate mask seal, which is often encountered with the use of the EOA. Although experience with this relatively new device is limited, studies have suggested that it offers an advantage over the EOA. Prior to widespread endorsement of this new device, it would be valuable for a prospective, prehospital trial evaluation to demonstrate two key points:

- The pharyngotracheal lumen airway is truly effective in achieving adequate ventilation and oxygenation.
- This device offers a distinct advantage (survival or otherwise) over the simpler basic technique of mouth-to-mask ventilation.

We recently completed a study designed to evaluate the effectiveness of the various techniques used for the noninstrumented airway in the prehospital setting.[8] The study used a resuscitation mannequin adapted to a lung model (Fig. 55–3). A single rescuer provided ventilatory support using one of four techniques: mouth-to-mouth ventilation, mouth-to-mask ventilation, bag-valve-mask ventilation, or a portable ventilator with a mask. The lung, esophagus, and stomach were simulated with a Penrose drain connected through a positive end-expiratory pressure (PEEP) valve to a spirometer. Paramedics were instructed to ventilate the "patient" according to American Heart Association standards (800 mL tidal volume/12 breaths/min) and recording was made of the tidal volume, peak inspiratory pressures, and gastric insufflation volumes. The trials were completed at three levels of lung compliance (0.1 L/cm H_2O, 0.04 L/cm H_2O, and 0.01 L/cm H_2O).

Mouth-to-mouth ventilation produced the largest delivered tidal volume at each level of compliance but was also associated with the greatest proximal airway pressure and largest gastric insufflation volume. Bag-

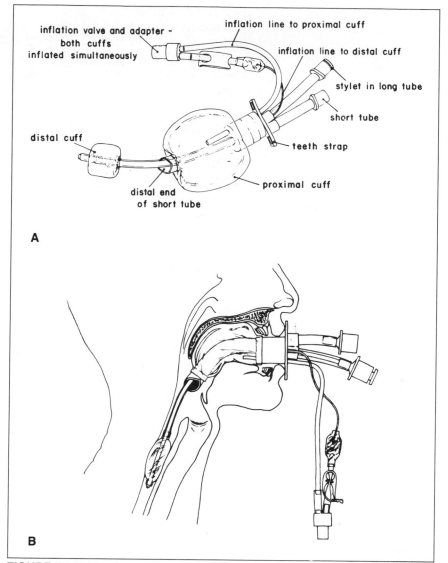

FIGURE 55–2: The pharyngotracheal lumen airway. (From Phillips TF. Airway management. *In* Moore EE, Mattox KL, Feliciano DP [eds]. Trauma. Norwalk, CT, Appleton & Lange, 1991, p 134.)

valve-mask ventilation provided a mean tidal volume of 817 mL at normal compliance but failed to provide adequate volumes at the altered compliance levels. Mouth-to-mask ventilation provided a larger tidal volume than the bag-valve-mask technique and was associated with lower airway pressures and lower gastric insufflation volumes when compared with mouth-to-mouth ventilation (Figs. 55–4 to 55–6).

Two types of portable transport ventilators were evaluated for their ability to provide ventilator-to-mask ventilation. The HARV (Hope automatic resuscitator ventilator; Ohmeda Emergency Care, Orchard Park, NY) has a fixed tidal volume that is determined by the selected ventilatory rate. The Uni-Vent (Impact Medical Corp., West Caldwell, NJ) has a tidal volume control that allows adjustment of delivered volume, as well as a separate rate control. In this study, the Uni-Vent provided a significantly larger tidal volume at all levels of compliance when compared with the HARV (see Fig. 55–4). This observed difference may

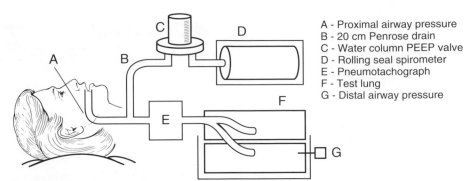

A - Proximal airway pressure
B - 20 cm Penrose drain
C - Water column PEEP valve
D - Rolling seal spirometer
E - Pneumotachograph
F - Test lung
G - Distal airway pressure

FIGURE 55–3: Schematic representation of test device used to evaluate the noninstrumented airway. (From Johannigman JA, Branson RD, Davis KJ, et al. A model to evaluate tidal volume. J Trauma 31[1]:93–98, 1991.)

represent the significance of the rescuer compensating for tidal volume lost to poor mask seal by increasing the delivered tidal volume of the Uni-Vent, a maneuver that is not possible with the fixed tidal volume of the HARV. The overall performance of the technique of ventilator-to-mask ventilation suggested that further study of the use of transport ventilators in the noninstrumented airway should be pursued. The use of a transport ventilator with adjustable tidal volume allows the rescuer to devote full attention and both hands to airway maintenance and the mask seal and also avoid direct patient contact. In addition, these devices generally use a fixed inspiratory time (1.5 seconds) and a controlled flow rate. This combination avoids the high peak flows and pressures that are often generated by rescuers or the bag-valve device. At levels of normal

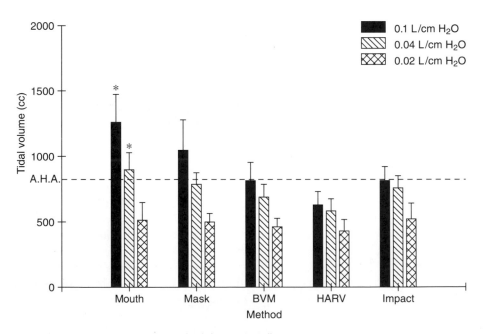

$* = p < 0.05$ vs other methods/same compliance

FIGURE 55–4: Delivered tidal volumes of five methods of ventilation. Error bars represent standard deviation; dashed line represents American Heart Association's recommended tidal volume of 800 cc (mL). (From Johannigman JA, Branson RD, Davis KJ, et al. A model to evaluate tidal volume. J Trauma 31[1]:93–98, 1991.)

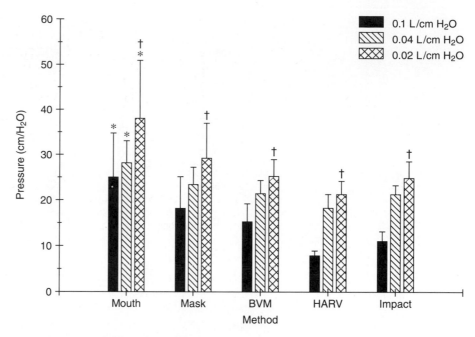

$\dagger$ = p < 0.05 vs other compliances/same method
$*$ = p < 0.05 vs other methods/same compliance

FIGURE 55–5: Proximal airway pressure generated by five methods of ventilation at varying compliance. Error bar represents standard deviation. (From Johannigman JA, Branson RD, Davis KJ, et al. A model to evaluate tidal volume. J Trauma 31[1]:93–98, 1991.)

and one-half normal compliance, the Uni-Vent provided acceptable tidal volumes without gastric insufflation.

Basic life support airway techniques should emphasize the use of mouth-to-mask ventilation for the noninstrumented airway in the prehospital setting. The use of single-rescuer bag-valve-mask ventilation has significant shortcomings that should limit its application. The routine use of the EOA should be discouraged in favor of more effective, simpler techniques. The efficacy of the pharyngotracheal lumen airway must be demonstrated in a controlled prospective study before its implementation can be supported. Finally, the technique of ventilator-to-mask ventilation may provide an extremely effective and acceptable means of ventilation in the prehospital setting. (These devices are described further later in the text.)

ADVANCED AIRWAY TECHNIQUES

Endotracheal Intubation

Endotracheal intubation remains the accepted, preferred method of airway control in the prehospital setting.[21, 22] Endotracheal intubation

- Secures the airway
- Facilitates effective oxygenation and ventilation
- Provides a degree of protection of the bronchopulmonary tree

These advantages have established orotracheal intubation as the mainstay of airway management in cardiopulmonary resuscitation. In trauma, concerns for the degree of cervical hyperextension may accom-

All compliances

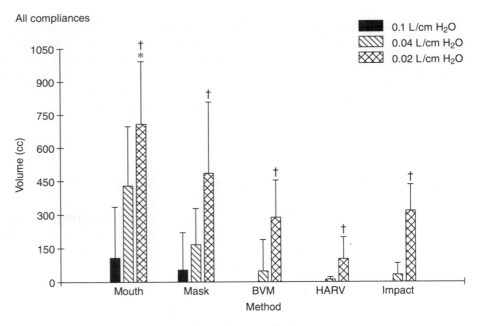

† = p < 0.05 vs other compliances/same method
∗ = p < 0.05 vs BVM, HARV, or impact

FIGURE 55–6: Gastric insufflation volume generated by five methods of ventilation at varying compliance. Error bar represents standard deviation. (From Johannigman JA, Branson RD, Davis KJ, et al. A model to evaluate tidal volume. J Trauma 31[1]:93–98, 1991.)

pany intubation. Some authors maintain that inline cervical traction by an assistant allows safe direct laryngoscopy in the trauma patient.[6] Other authors remain unconvinced that this approach is safe, so they advocate other techniques, such as nasotracheal intubation, percutaneous ventilation, or surgical cricothyroidotomy.[4] Despite the relative divergence of opinion concerning the trauma patient, endotracheal intubation remains the "gold standard" of airway control against which other methods must be compared.

Endotracheal intubation in the prehospital setting has been criticized because of the belief that this technique is too complicated to be mastered by nonphysician personnel. The fallacy of this belief appears in studies demonstrating the proficiency of paramedical personnel.[23] DeLeo[24] was one of the first to demonstrate a paramedical field intubation success rate of 91% which compared favorably with a physician rate of 89%. Jacobs and associates[23] demonstrated a 97% success rate in a study that defined a protocol for endotracheal intubation and limited paramedics to a maximum of three attempts with a time limit of 15 seconds per attempt. In this same study it was noted that the 3% of patients who could not be intubated by paramedics also failed to be intubated by physicians in the emergency room.

When analyzing the data from published reports regarding prehospital endotracheal intubation, it is important to consider the criteria for "successful intubation." Multiple unsuccessful attempts may delay therapy or exacerbate hypoxemia. The documented success rate may reflect a selection bias if paramedics attempt to intubate only the flaccid cardiac arrest patient and not the combative, head-injured patient. Two recent studies of paramedical performance addressed the issue of unnecessary delay resulting from field endotracheal intubation. In these studies,

The benefit-to-risk ratio of prehospital intubation appears to be extremely high when performed routinely in the field by well-trained, supervised paramedical personnel.

paramedics were allowed a maximum of three attempts; each attempt lasted no longer than 15[23] or 45 seconds.[25] All attempts were monitored by direct observation at the scene or via physician telemetry. Both demonstrated success rates greater than 90% and a complication rate less than 5%. The survival advantage imparted by endotracheal intubation is difficult to accurately determine because of the multiple factors involved and the many concomitant advances in advanced life support techniques. Nonetheless, there has been a suggested survival advantage for patients in cardiac arrest who are intubated.[26]

Needle Thoracentesis and Chest Thoracostomy

In the prehospital setting, the development of a tension pneumothorax constitutes a life-threatening emergency. Proper management of this condition requires rapid identification and swift intervention if the patient is to be saved. A tension pneumothorax occurs when air escapes from the lung parenchyma into the pleural space without a means of exit. Subsequent respiratory efforts result in a progressive increase in the intrathoracic pressure of the affected hemithorax. It is important to recognize that the increased intrathoracic pressure results in the life-threatening physiologic alterations. The elevated intrathoracic pressure results in a shift of the mediastinum and impairs central venous return through the inferior and superior vena cava. Hemodynamic and respiratory instability in a thoracic trauma patient should alert the clinician to the possibility of a tension pneumothorax. Other clinical signs associated with the development of this process include absent or diminished breath sounds on the affected side, hyperresonance to percussion, tracheal deviation away from the pneumothorax, and distention of the neck veins. The diagnosis of tension pneumothorax may be overlooked in the prehospital setting because of the application of various extrication-stabilization devices, which may mask the clinical signs (e.g., a cervical collar may obscure tracheal deviation and venous distention). The noisy environment of the trauma scene or the back of an ambulance often precludes effective auscultation. In sum, the clinician must maintain a high index of suspicion to correctly diagnose and intervene in this potentially life-threatening condition.

The patient who presents with thoracic trauma and hemodynamic instability requires immediate intervention. In this situation, it may be difficult to differentiate hypotension resulting from a tension pneumothorax from other life-threatening processes such as cardiac tamponade, massive hemothorax, or hemorrhagic shock. A standard anteroposterior portable chest x-ray film can be invaluable in determining the cause of hypotension in the trauma patient. It is our practice to maintain an x-ray plate on our trauma resuscitation gurney and obtain a chest x-ray film within the first seconds of admission. Often a patient is too unstable in the field to await transport or perform the definitive radiologic studies.

In the hemodynamically unstable patient with thoracic trauma, immediate needle thoracentesis may be necessary to avert hemodynamic collapse. The placement of a needle thoracentesis converts the tension pneumothorax into a simple pneumothorax and permits the restitution of venous return to the heart. If needle thoracentesis is accompanied by a rush of air through the needle, the diagnosis of tension pneumothorax is virtually assured. If there is no return of air or if the patient fails to improve significantly, other clinical conditions such as massive hemotho-

Patients with an acute tension pneumothorax are most affected by hemodynamic insufficiency rather than respiratory embarrassment.

Needle thoracentesis is accomplished by inserting a large-gauge needle (No. 14) into the second intercostal space in the midclavicular line of the affected hemithorax. An alternative site for needle placement is the third or fourth intercostal space in the anterior axillary fold.

rax, cardiac tamponade, or exsanguinating hemorrhage must be considered.

Once needle thoracentesis has been accomplished, the definitive management of a tension pneumothorax includes placement of a chest thoracostomy tube. In most circumstances, a large-bore (No. 32 or No. 36 Fr) chest tube is placed in the fifth intercostal space and connected to a water-sealed, closed-suction drainage system (Figure 55–7). Complete re-expansion of the lung is critical to achieving hemostasis in parenchymal lung injuries. Lung re-expansion is also important for restoring alveolar surface area and improving ventilation and oxygenation.

If a patient with a chest thoracostomy tube in place must subsequently undergo ground transport or aeromedical evacuation, the clinician must be prepared to adapt the drainage system for this purpose. In most instances, the placement of a one-way valve system (e.g., a Heimlich valve) permits safe, efficient transport while eliminating the need for a bulky drainage system. In the prehospital-field setting, the fingertip of a sterile glove may be cut off and placed over the end of the thoracostomy tube to achieve this function.

Incomplete evacuation of blood or air from the pleural space is the primary factor responsible for the development of complications such as empyema and fibrothorax.

THE PHARMACOLOGY OF AIRWAY CONTROL

The use of neuromuscular blockade and paralytic agents to facilitate intubation has been described in the prehospital setting.[2, 3] These agents are most commonly used in the combative multitrauma patient, the closed head injury victim, the drug overdose patient, or the patient with status epilepticus. These situations pose unique airway challenges that require sophisticated and experienced clinical decision-making skills. The most critical primary decision is the determination of the adequacy of the patient's existing airway. Four criteria must be met prior to considering the use of neuromuscular blockade in the prehospital setting:

1. An adequate airway cannot be established or maintained.
2. Transport to a definitive care facility requires significant time.

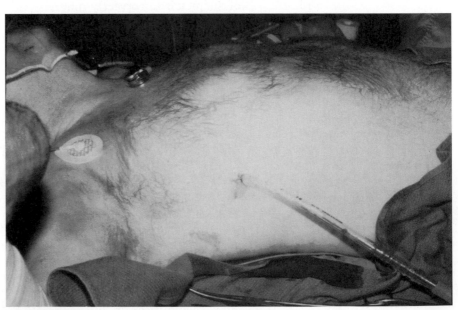

FIGURE 55–7: Placement of a chest thoracostomy tube.

3. Adequate equipment and support material is available.

4. Significant skill and expertise in the techniques of intubation have been acquired through a closely supervised training program.

Neuromuscular blocking agents have long been used by anesthesiologists in the operating room to facilitate intubation. The use of paralytic agents in the emergency room setting has gained increasing acceptance with demonstrated efficacy.[27, 28] An extension of this policy has been the administration of paralytic agents in the prehospital setting by paramedical personnel functioning as members of an aeromedical evacuation service[29] or as part of a strictly controlled prehospital protocol.[2]

It must be emphasized that patients requiring neuromuscular blockade to facilitate intubation are a distinct minority in the prehospital setting. The more skilled and experienced the practitioner, the more likely he or she will be able to provide and maintain an adequate airway without resorting to paralysis for intubation. For a more complete discussion of this topic, the reader is referred to excellent reviews by Storer[30] and Phillips.[5]

CAPNOGRAPHY

Capnography is the recording and analysis of the expired carbon dioxide waveform. The original instrumentation for capnography employed sophisticated infrared spectrophotometers for detecting end-tidal carbon dioxide concentrations. This form of monitoring remains widely used in the operating room environment. Recently, a new disposable device was introduced that is capable of quantitatively detecting end-tidal carbon dioxide concentrations.[31, 32] This device uses a chemically treated indicator strip that colorimetrically determines the concentration of carbon dioxide. The indicator strip dynamically changes color in response to the changing levels of carbon dioxide during a normal ventilatory cycle. With a properly intubated patient, the device cycles from purple as the patient ventilates (0.03 to 0.3% carbon dioxide) to gold as the patient exhales (2 to 5% carbon dioxide), and back to purple with the next ventilatory cycle.

To date, a limited number of studies have evaluated the use of this device as an adjunct to prehospital endotracheal intubation. In an evaluation of the forced expiratory flow end-tidal carbon dioxide detector in the aeromedical setting, the detector identified correct endotracheal tube placement in 31 of 33 patients.[33] In a prospective study of 250 emergency intubations, the use of the carbon dioxide detector displayed an overall sensitivity of 88% and a specificity for tracheal intubation of 92%.[31] The liability of this technique is that it relies on the generation of carbon dioxide as a byproduct of cellular metabolism. In the setting of cardiac arrest, cellular hypoxemia and inadequate pulmonary perfusion may significantly limit carbon dioxide production and elimination. In the non-arrest situation, the use of capnography appears particularly useful and sensitive. In the cardiac arrest patient, particularly the patient with long-standing arrest, the interpretation of a lack of color change requires caution. It may indicate esophageal placement, lack of cellular metabolism, or inadequate perfusion. The use of capnography must be viewed as an adjunct to the basic skills of endotracheal intubation. It is not meant to replace the basic assessment of endotracheal tube position via direct visualization of the vocal cords and auscultation of the lung fields and epigastrium. The ultimate value of this and other adjuncts depends on the training, skill, and clinical acumen of the prehospital care provider. For further discussion of capnography, the reader is referred to an excellent review by Kissinger and colleagues.[34]

TRANSPORT VENTILATION

Once an airway has been established, the prehospital care provider must be concerned with providing efficient and effective ventilation. Traditionally, this has meant the use of a bag-valve device. In the uninstrumented airway, bag-valve-mask ventilation performed by one rescuer usually results in inadequate volume delivery (see earlier discussion). In the intubated patient, the use of a bag-valve device necessitates the total attention of one member of the resuscitation team. In recent years, a number of portable transport ventilators have been developed that may offer distinct advantages for prehospital airway management.

The first generation of transport ventilators was represented by the (in)famous Flynn valve, which was a fixture on most ambulances from the 1950s on. The liability of this device was that it provided extremely high flow and pressures until terminated by the rescuer. The next generation of portable ventilators featured a pressure-cycled design. When used during CPR, simultaneous chest compressions and delivery of a breath often resulted in premature cycling and inadequate tidal volume delivery. This liability led to the widespread abandonment of the concept of prehospital transport ventilation. With recent advances in microprocessor and solenoid technology, the most recent generation of transport ventilators is far removed from its predecessors and is now worthy of consideration. Recent prospective studies have demonstrated that transport ventilators are capable of providing effective oxygenation and ventilation comparable to that provided by a bag-valve device.[35] These studies suggest that in the intubated patient, adequate oxygenation and ventilation are reliably provided by these devices. Although the ventilator is not "better" than manual ventilation, it frees one rescuer to devote attention to other duties, such as drug administration, transport, monitoring, or telemetry communication. Paramedical squads that have used these devices find this to be their major advantage, particularly in today's cost-conscious municipalities in which paramedical crews are often limited to two persons. A disadvantage of the use of a transport ventilator is that it eliminates the rescuers' ability to "feel" patient compliance; this may delay the recognition of airway obstruction or tension pneumothorax. The development of a rugged, inline airway monitor is desirable.

The currently available generation of transport ventilators offers a wide variety of features and capabilities. It is desirable to distinguish between devices that are primarily intended for prehospital applications and devices that are capable of providing more sophisticated (and expensive) needs for intra- and interhospital transport. Aside from the obvious distinctions of size and complexity, prehospital transport ventilators differ from hospital transport ventilators in their configuration. The prehospital ventilator is usually simpler, consisting of only a control module and patient valve. The following represents a brief overview of the desirable features of a prehospital transport ventilator.

Operational Characteristics

The largest application of a prehospital transport ventilator is to provide ventilation for the apneic patient during CPR.[32] As such, the design should be simple and straightforward, emphasizing ease of operation as well as a light and compact design. Ventilators used in prehospital care should be time- or volume-cycled to avoid premature cycling during CPR compressions. The delivered tidal volume should be minimally affected by changes in pulmonary compliance. This characteristic assures adequate tidal volume delivery during cardiac arrest, since studies have suggested a significant decrease in compliance following such arrest.[15] It is preferable that all gas from the cylinder be delivered to the patient and not diverted to pneumatic control of the ventilator. Low-level gas consumption (<5 L/min) for pneumatically controlled ventilators is acceptable, but decreases overall operational time. Portability is essential; generally a weight of less than 4 kg is desirable. If the ventilator is electronically controlled, it should possess a long battery life without needing to be frequently recharged. Lead acid battery systems offer stability of charge and favorable storage capability without excessive weight. Systems that rely on electronic controllers should feature a low-battery warning light to signal when at least 1 hour of useable charge remains. The most important aspect of transport ventilators is their ease of operation. There should be a minimum number of controls, each of which should be clearly labeled as to function and effect. If possible, a diagram of the breathing circuit and its proper assembly should be imprinted on the back panel of the ventilator. Ventilators used for prehospital transport do not require variable $F_{I_{O_2}}$, PEEP, or intermittent mandatory ventilation capability. These ventilators need to provide only reliable, consistent, controlled mechanical ventilation in accordance with American Heart Association standards: 12 breaths/min at 800 mL tidal volume.[14] Ventilators capable of functioning in this fashion will meet the ventilatory needs of the majority of patients, since 95% of patients intubated in the field remain apneic during transport.[32] The placement of an antiasphyxiation valve at the airway allows spontaneous breathing without the added weight, complexity, or gas consumption of a demand circuit.

Tidal volume and rate controls should be independently variable to allow variation in patient size and airway leak and to permit intentional hyperventilation in the setting of closed head injuries. A manual inspiration button is an important, but often overlooked, feature. The addition of this feature allows the rescuer to manually control rate and volume during special situations. This control also allows auscultation of breath sounds to confirm tube placement. The circuit and patient valve should be easily disassembled for decontamination and cleaning. The small size and simplicity of transport ventilators limits their alarm capability and safety features. At a minimum, there should be a high-pressure relief valve that prevents circuit pressure from exceeding a set value—60 or 80 cm H_2O for adults, 30 or 40 cm H_2O for children. Activation of the high-pressure relief valve should be signaled by a visual or audio alarm, or both, to alert the operator of the abnormal condition. The provision of an antiasphyxiation valve at the patient airway allows spontaneous breathing via entrainment of room air in the event of total failure of the ventilator. This valve should allow spontaneous breathing without excessive resistance. Electronically controlled ventilators should signal "low power" when less than 1 hour of usable charge remains. It is also desirable for an alarm to signal when the gas source is exhausted.

The following is a brief list of currently available products that are applicable in the prehospital setting. This list should not be viewed as all-inclusive nor as an endorsement of a particular product, but rather the most widely available units with which I have had experience.

Impact Uni-Vent

The Uni-Vent (Impact Medical Corp., West Caldwell, NJ) (Fig. 55–8) is a pneumatically powered, electronically controlled, time-cycled ventilator designed specifically for prehospital application. The rate is chosen

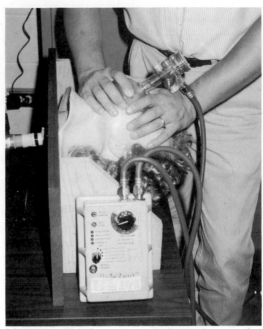

FIGURE 55–8: The Uni-Vent (Impact Medical Corp, West Caldwell, NJ) ventilator.

from one of four settings: adult CPR (12 breaths/min), adult hyperventilation (18 breaths/min), child-infant CPR (14 breaths/min), and child-infant hyperventilation (20 breaths/min). Inspiratory time is fixed at 1.5 seconds for adults and 0.75 seconds for children and infants. Tidal volume is varied by adjusting the flow control. Power is supplied by a lead acid battery that provides up to 10 hours of service when fully charged; a low-battery light signals when 1 hour of power remains. The patient valve contains an exhalation diaphragm, a two-position high-pressure relief valve (60 and 80 cm H_2O), and an antiasphyxiation valve. The Uni-Vent employs a solenoid to regulate gas flow and therefore does not have internal gas consumption. The Uni-Vent, which is simple to operate and durable in construction, has the desirable features of separate rate and adjustable tidal volume controls. I have had extensive experience with this unit following its placement on more than 30 paramedical units in a metropolitan area. The unit proved reliable and rugged and was well received by paramedical personnel. In a prospective evaluation of arterial blood gas results in prehospital resuscitations managed with an endotracheal tube and the Uni-Vent, the results demonstrated no significant difference for patients managed with the Uni-Vent compared with patients manually ventilated with a bag-valve device.[36]

Hamilton MAX

The MAX (Hamilton Medical, Reno, NV) (Fig. 55–9) is a pneumatically powered, electrically operated, time-cycled ventilator. The MAX has controls for rate and tidal volume as well as an aneroid display for airway pressure. A manual inspiratory control is also provided. The unit is powered by four 1.5-V AA rechargeable batteries or by disposable alkaline batteries. A low-battery warning light is positioned on the front panel. An internally mounted demand valve is referenced to ambient pressure and is set to trigger at -2 cm H_2O. Demand flow is provided at

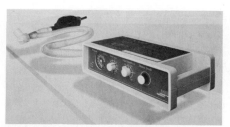

FIGURE 55–9: The MAX (Hamilton Medical, Reno, NV) time-cycled ventilator.

source gas pressure, thus allowing maximal flow for spontaneous breathing. PEEP can be added by using an external PEEP valve, but triggering will not be PEEP-compensated. The solenoid has a fixed inspiratory time of 1 second; expiratory time is adjusted according to respiratory rate. Peak airway pressure is limited by an adjustable pressure regulator from 45 to 90 cm H_2O. Adjustment of the pressure regulator requires removing the ventilator's cover.

Clinical evaluation of the MAX demonstrated it to be a reliable, easy to operate transport ventilator that meets most of the demands of ventilation during transport.[37] Measured delivered tidal volume was altered only at compliances less than 0.04 L/cm H_2O. The lack of PEEP compensation may make triggering more difficult for the patient on elevated levels of PEEP, and therefore it was recommended that the respiratory rate be increased whenever patients were on an assisted mode of ventilation and greater than 8 cm H_2O of PEEP. Peak inspiratory pressure was significantly higher during transport with the MAX ventilator compared with the intensive care unit ventilator. This difference is most probably a reflection of the MAX's fixed 1-second inspiratory time. With careful attention to the limitations described, the MAX can provide adequate ventilation and oxygenation to a majority of patients.

Pneu-Pac 2-R or HARV

The Pneu-Pac 2-R or HARV (Hope automatic resuscitator ventilator) (Ohmeda Emergency Care, Orchard Park, NY) (Fig. 55–10) is a flow or pressure controller that is time-triggered, flow- or pressure-limited, and time-cycled. It is pneumatically powered and controlled with an optional patient valve that allows delivery of an FI_{O_2} of 1.0 or 0.45. The Pneu-Pac or HARV has a single control that simultaneously adjusts rate and tidal volume. As rate is increased, the delivered tidal volume and inspiratory time decreases with inspiratory flow fixed at 40 L/min (Table 55–6). Peak pressure can be limited with nonadjustable, replaceable valves provided by the manufacturer (40, 60, and 80 cm H_2O). The relative simplicity of the Pneu-Pac makes it suitable for use in the prehospital arena, but its effectiveness may be limited by the inability to control tidal volume. In a study of the noninstrumented airway, the Pneu-Pac failed to provide the American Heart Association's recommended tidal volumes during mouth-to-mask ventilation.[8] This finding was particularly pronounced at levels of decreased compliance, which may reflect the inability of the rescuer to increase the delivered tidal volume of the unit to compensate for volume lost due to a poor mask seal. A second important consideration is that if a PEEP valve is attached to the expiratory port, spontaneous breathing is prohibited.

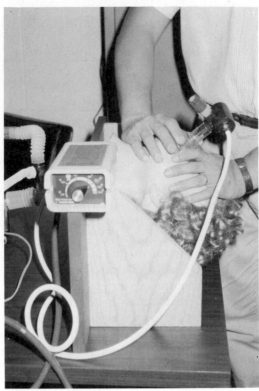

FIGURE 55–10: The Pneu-Pac (Ohmeda Emergency Care, Orchard Park, NY) ventilator.

Auto Vent 2000 and 3000

The Auto Vent ventilators (Life Support Products, Irvine, CA) are pneumatically powered, pneumatically controlled, time-cycled ventilators designed for prehospital care. Both the 2000 and 3000 units employ a spool-valve mechanism to control gas flow. The Auto Vent 2000 has separate rate and volume controls with a fixed inspiratory time of 1.5 seconds. The Auto Vent 3000 offers the additional feature of a two-position inspiratory time switch (1.5 or 0.75 second), which therefore provides a wider range of tidal volumes. The Auto Vent units have a demand valve that connects to the patient airway to provide the delivery of 100% oxygen during spontaneous respiration. The demand circuit has a fixed flow of 48 L/min; if patient demand exceeds this level, it results in entrainment of room air through a side port. The high-pressure alarm

TABLE **55–6:** Respiratory Rate and Tidal Volume Provided by the Pneu-Pac 2-R or HARV Ventilator

Rate (breaths/min)	Volume (mL)
11	1450
12	1100
13	900
14	700
16	500
19	400
21	340

is fixed at 45 cm H_2O with activation resulting in an audible alarm. The Auto Vent devices are easy to operate while fulfilling most of the criteria for prehospital ventilation. The relatively low value for the nonadjustable pressure relief valve (45 cm H_2O) may result in inadequate ventilation in the patient with decreased compliance or in cardiac arrest. The use of the demand valve circuit creates weight at the airway, which may result in inadvertent kinking or accidental extubation.

Stein Gates Omni Vent

The Omni Vent (Stein Gates, Atchison, KS) is a pneumatically powered, pneumatically controlled, time-cycled ventilator that provides controlled mechanical ventilation only. Rate and volume are adjusted by two uncalibrated controls (inspiratory time-volume and expiratory time), whereas airway pressure is continuously monitored. The uncalibrated controls may potentially make this a difficult product to accurately employ; no alarm functions are provided.

Transport ventilation in the prehospital setting has proved to be an efficient and effective means of providing ventilatory support. In a controlled, prospective trial, it was shown to be as effective as manual ventilation with a bag-valve device, and it freed one rescuer to devote attention to other aspects of the resuscitation.[32] The use of a transport ventilator in conjunction with an endotracheal tube represents the "gold standard" of prehospital ventilatory support. The application of a transport ventilator can provide a steady state of adequate ventilation and oxygenation, even during difficult situations such as transport down stairs, prolonged vehicular extrication, or overland transport. The selection of a transport ventilator should be tailored to its application. It must be remembered that the majority of patients who require prehospital ventilatory support will be in apneic respiratory arrest. Perhaps the most common mistake is purchasing a ventilator that is more sophisticated than necessary, rendering the unit more difficult to understand, operate, and maintain. For the prehospital setting, a simple control mode ventilator with an air entrainment valve meets most needs. It is desirable for the ventilator to have separate, calibrated controls for rate and tidal volume. Simple alarm functions, including high peak inspiratory pressure and loss of power and gas source, are desirable. Rather than being sophisticated, these ventilators must be rugged and reliable if they are to survive in the prehospital environment. Prior to their purchase, these units should be placed in an extended field trial to ensure that they meet the demands of the service. I have participated in a trial program in which 15 paramedical services in a metropolitan area were equipped with a transport ventilator. The ventilators proved to be dependable and efficient and were readily accepted by paramedical personnel, who quickly became adept in their application.

SUMMARY

The provision of adequate oxygenation and ventilation remains a vital challenge to the prehospital care provider. The clinician must combine expertise with a well-founded understanding of the technical aspects of the tools of the trade. The most sophisticated prehospital ventilatory device will surely fail in the hands of the ill-prepared practitioner.

Conversely, ventilation may be efficiently performed by the skilled therapist who uses the simple basic tools of airway control.

References

1. Textbook of Advanced Cardiac Life Support. Dallas, TX, American Heart Association, 1987, p 3.
2. Hedges JR, Dronen SC, Feero S, et al. Succinylcholine assisted intubations in prehospital care. Ann Emerg Med 17(5):469–472, 1988.
3. Berve MO. Easing intubation with succinylcholine. Journal of Emergency Medical Services 15(11):60–67, 1990.
4. Jorden RC, Rosen P. Airway management in the acutely injured. *In* Moore EE, Eiseman B, Van Way CW III (eds). Critical Decisions in Trauma. St. Louis, CV Mosby, 1984.
5. Phillips TF. Airway management. *In* Moore EE, Mattox KL, Feliciano DP (eds). Trauma. Norwalk, CT, Appleton & Lange, 1991.
6. American College of Surgeons Committee on Trauma: Advanced Trauma Life Support Course for Physicians. Chicago, 1989.
7. Spearman CB. Effects of changing jet flows on O_2 concentrations in adjustable air entrainment masks. Respir Care 25:1266, 1980.
8. Johannigman JA, Branson RD, Davis KJ, et al. Techniques of emergency ventilation: A model to evaluate tidal volume, airway pressure, and gastric insufflation. J Trauma 31(1):93–98, 1991.
9. Fluck RR, Sorbello JG. Mouth-to-mouth resuscitation by lay rescuers—should they or shouldn't they? Respir Care 35(8):831, 1990.
10. Johannigman JA, Branson RD. Levels of oxygen enrichment during mouth-to-mask breathing. Respir Care 36:99–103, 1991.
11. Hess D, Baran C. Ventilatory volumes using mouth-to-mouth, mouth-to-mask and bag-valve-mask techniques. Am J Emerg Med 3:292–296, 1985.
12. Elling R, Politis J. An evaluation of emergency medical technicians' ability to use manual ventilation devices. Ann Emerg Med 12:765–768, 1983.
13. Harrison RR, Maull KI, Keenan RL, et al. Mouth-to-mask ventilation: A superior method of rescue breathing. Ann Emerg Med 11:74–76, 1982.
14. Healthcare Provider's Manual For Basic Cardiac Life Support. Dallas, TX, American Heart Association, 1988.
15. Ornato JP, Bryson BL, Donovan PJ, et al. Measurement of ventilation during cardiopulmonary resuscitation. Crit Care Med 11(2):79–82, 1983.
16. Don Michael TA, Lambert EH, Mehran A. Mouth-to-lung airway for cardiac resuscitation. Lancet 2:1329, 1968.
17. Auerbach PS, Geehr EC. Inadequate oxygenation and ventilation using the esophageal gastric tube airway in the prehospital setting. JAMA 250:3067–3071, 1983.
18. Smith JP, Bodai BI, Aubourg R, et al. A field evaluation of the esophageal airway. J Trauma 23:317–321, 1983.
19. Smith JP, Bodai BI, Seifkin A, et al. The esophageal obturator airway: A review. JAMA 250:1081–1084, 1983.
20. Niemann JT, Rosborough JP, Myers R. The pharyngotracheal lumen airway: Preliminary investigation of a new adjunct. Ann Emerg Med 13:591, 1984.
21. McCabe CJ, Browne BJ. Esophageal obturator airway, ET tube and pharyngeal-tracheal lumen airway. Am J Emerg Med 4:64–71, 1986.
22. Pepe PE, Copass MK, Joyce TH. Prehospital endotracheal intubation. Rationale for training emergency medical personnel. Ann Emerg Med 14:1085–1092, 1985.
23. Jacobs LM, Berrizbeitia LD, Bennett B, et al. Endotracheal intubation in the prehospital phase of emergency medical care. JAMA 250:2175–2177, 1983.
24. DeLeo BC. Endotracheal intubation by rescue squad personnel. Heart Lung 6:851–854, 1977.
25. Stewart RD, Paris PM, Winter PM, et al. Field endotracheal intubation by paramedical personnel—Success rates and complications. Chest 85:341–345, 1984.
26. Geehr EC, Bogetz MS, Auerbach PS. Prehospital tracheal intubation versus esophageal gastric tube airway use: A prospective study. Am J Emerg Med 3:381–385, 1985.
27. Thompson JD, Fish S, Ruiz E. Succinylcholine for endotracheal intubation. Ann Emerg Med 11:526–529, 1982.
28. Roberts DJ, Clinton JE, Ruiz E. Neuromuscular blockade for critical patients in the emergency department. Ann Emerg Med 15:152–156, 1986.
29. Syverud SA, Borron SW, Storer DL, et al. Prehospital use of neuromuscular blocking agents in a helicopter ambulance program. Ann Emerg Med 17(3):236–242, 1988.
30. Storer DL. The pharmacology of airway control. Emerg Care 7(2):64–77, 1991.
31. MacLeod BA, Heller MB, Gerard J, et al. Verification of endotracheal tube placement with colorimetric end-tidal CO_2 detection. Ann Emerg Med 20(3):267–269, 1991.
32. Anton WR, Gordon RW, Jordan TM, et al. A disposable end-tidal CO_2 detector to verify endotracheal intubation. Ann Emerg Med 20(3):271–275, 1991.

33. Campbell RC, Boyd CR, Shields RO, et al. Evaluation of an end-tidal carbon dioxide detector in the aeromedical setting. J Air Med Trans 9:13–15, 1990.
34. Kissinger DP, Hamilton IN, Rozycki GS. The current practice of pulse oximetry and capnometry/capnography in the prehospital setting. Emerg Care 7(2):44–50, 1991.
35. Hurst JM, Davis K, Branson RD, et al. Ventilatory support in the field: A prospective study. Crit Care Med 17:527, 1989.
36. Johannigman JA. Unpublished data.
37. Johannigman JA, Branson RD, Campbell RS, et al. Laboratory and clinical evaluation of the MAX transport ventilator. Respir Care 35:952–959, 1990.

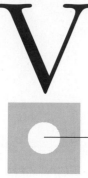

Respiratory Therapy Department Management

56

Managing Organizational Change

Delorese Ambrose, Ed.D.

Key Terms

Culture
Lifestyle Integration
Total Quality Management

If you have ever gone white water rafting, you have a good sense of what it is like to run an organization in the 1990s: before you can catch your breath after one maneuver, another challenge comes around the bend. As you begin to navigate the new challenge, an even more awesome one surfaces up ahead. There is little time to plan, yet planning is what you need. There is not enough time to gather your wits, yet wit and creativity will keep you securely anchored to your raft. Your resources are limited to little more than a life jacket, yet you need all the resources you can get to remain afloat.

This metaphor for today's work climate, made popular by management expert Peter Vaill who calls it "permanent white water," can be aptly applied to the health care industry. Workers in health-related fields discuss the "white water" phenomenon daily. They talk about the "constant changes" and make comments about "having to do more with less" in a climate of uncertainty, mergers, and down-sized organizations. They reflect on the challenges of regulatory issues and their concerns that technology and information are advancing at a faster rate than they can adapt to.

Fortunately in white water rafting, as in organizational life, humans are remarkably resilient. Their survival instincts enable them to make it back to shore aided by the skill of a white water guide. This guide is analogous to an effective organization manager: someone who repeatedly scopes out the environment and develops sound strategies for maneuvering through threatening conditions. Such a guide understands the importance of flexibility and adaptability—a willingness and ability to change the course of action to ensure survival.

If our health care organizations are to survive and flourish, administrators, professionals, and other employees must have the vision and skill required to successfully negotiate the rapids of change. We need to constantly monitor the external and internal environment, anticipate change, and effectively manage the process of change. We must motivate and enable all employees, suppliers, and customers to participate in the process.

This chapter explores the human and organizational dynamics of change and provides techniques for managing such change. This chapter

- Outlines some external and internal driving forces for change in the health care industry
- Defines the concept of "organizational change"
- Identifies both systemic and human barriers to change
- Offers tactics for reducing resistance and building commitment to change

EXTERNAL DRIVING FORCES FOR CHANGE

Technology

Innovations in health care technology require all employees to engage in continuous learning and retooling. In some areas, automation replaces manual labor with technology, redefining the method and meaning of patient care. In just about every area, computerization and elaborate information systems allow instant access to data and more efficient collaboration across disciplines. Yet although these advances provide positive benefits in terms of the precision and timeliness of patient care, they also produce new stresses and challenges for managerial and technical professionals, and even in some cases for the patient.

Competition and Marketplace Trends

Rising health care costs, more demanding health care consumers, a movement toward home health care, shortages of certain health professionals, and the emergence of health care conglomerates are a few of the trends that have combined to fuel massive changes in our health care environment. They have led to an increased focus on marketing and health care consumer–driven approaches to service.

As the sameness of the industrial era gives way to customization, health care facilities have been challenged to provide service in ways that bring into greater focus the unique needs of individual care recipients. "Patient-focused" approaches are now viewed as key to innovation and quality service. As a result, many health care organizations have adopted industrial models of "total quality" management to ensure continuous process improvement aimed at providing the best care possible.

Legal and Regulatory Pressures

Legal and regulatory challenges require suppliers of health care to be more innovative as they strive to provide the most cost-effective and high-quality care. Mergers, acquisitions, and the disappearance of small, less competitive hospitals are examples of new patterns driven by the rapids of change.

These conditions have created a "ripple effect" in the health care environment. Administrators and other employees find that they must adjust how they manage profits, structure, tasks, technology, and employees to achieve organizational goals in the face of external threats and opportunities.

INTERNAL DRIVING FORCES FOR CHANGE

Rising Costs and Decreasing Profits

Declining admissions, decreasing corporate dollars through benefits plans, and decreased reimbursement for indigent care seriously threaten the financial viability of some hospitals. At the same time, hospital management must remain committed to quality care and to the education and development of professionals—all of which are costly. The changes that are driven by these internal issues include the development of programs and strategies to provide new sources of income while maintaining a successful operation.

Reorganization for Greater Efficiency and Effectiveness

Glaring inefficiencies exist in most health care facilities. Booz Allen, a leading management consulting firm, estimates that 84% of the value-added activities performed by hospital personnel include scheduling, record keeping, supervising, and attending meetings, rather than direct care.

Increasingly, health care providers are becoming concerned about the impact of cumbersome practices and approaches on their ability to provide the best service for patients. The growing focus on total quality management with its emphasis on the health care consumer's need has been one outgrowth of this concern. Hospitals and other care facilities are moving to more "matrixed" arrangements to improve how human and technologic resources are deployed. The cross-functional team approach that is used by a respiratory care team (composed of a physician leader, nurses, a respiratory therapist, a physical therapist, social workers, a psychologist, and a dietitian) requires both technical and interpersonal skills. In fact, in all sectors there is a movement from the staid bureaucracies of the past to flexible, responsive interorganizational units in which professionals from various disciplines collaborate to meet consumer needs.

Employee Activism

Internal change is often driven by employee pressure, whether through formal unionized efforts or more informally. As hospitals trim operating budgets, they create more anxieties as workers face an uncertain future in which they are being asked to "do more with less." Working parents bring pressure to bear on management to change internal policies concerning child care, parental leave, job-sharing, work at home, and so forth. Many employers experience what they perceive as a shift from the traditional corporate loyalty to self-interest and "lifestyle integration." To avoid employee dissatisfaction, organizational leaders wrestle with ways to promote a more "employee-centered" climate.

Demographic Trends

Finally, the makeup of the work force provides a growing catalyst for change. The health care industry, like other industries, is experiencing an influx of immigrants, whereas women and minorities are making advances in professional areas. Estimates suggest that foreign-educated physicians currently compose 20% of licensed practitioners in the United States. In addition, many laboratory and technical workers, as well as unskilled or semiskilled hospital workers, are immigrants. The potential for interpersonal conflict in this increasingly diverse workplace has created a need for changes aimed at managing differences. Many hospitals, such as Mount Sinai in New York and Magee-Women's Hospital in Pittsburgh, now add training in dealing with diversity as part of their supervisory training. Baxter Healthcare Corporation is becoming recognized for its global program that focuses on preparing employees to work across cultures nationally and internationally.

Clearly, health care employees must become adept at both embracing and managing change. As health care organizations restructure their delivery systems to improve patient care, employees at all levels will be affected. Developing competence, versatility, and confidence in working through the challenges of uncertainty and transition will play a major role in improving quality and ensuring organizational survival. This requires an understanding of the nature and dynamics of change as well as basic skills in managing change.

WHAT IS "ORGANIZATIONAL CHANGE"?

The external and internal driving forces cited earlier are just a few of the reasons that today's health care administrators and employees are preoccupied with the notion of "organizational change." This type of change falls into at least two broad categories: developmental and transformational.

Developmental Change

During the routine performance of work, we constantly make developmental changes—minor modifications designed to fine-tune existing procedures or practices. A supervisor who changes the layout of the reception room furniture to make it more "user friendly" is initiating a developmental change that may have important ramifications for guest relations. An administrator who takes a course in conducting effective meetings may return with new ideas on how to make meetings more efficient. As the administrator implements these ideas, staff members may be required to modify their behaviors.

These developmental changes are necessary to ensure continuous improvement of service by facilitating the process of day-to-day management aimed at efficiency and effectiveness.

Transformational Change

In contrast to the day-to-day developmental changes, transformational change encompasses larger scale transitions. When strategic decisions are made to alter the way an organization is run, far-reaching changes are usually necessary. For example, when new technology is introduced into a department, employees must learn new skills, reorganize themselves both physically and emotionally, and develop new working relationships. The degree and nature of their interaction with the consumer may change as well. Typically, such changes cause both the agents of the change and the "changees" (those required to change) to feel disoriented and challenged. As a result, transformational changes tend to be met with much more resistance than day-to-day developmental changes. The discussion that follows elaborates on why this is so and how to manage such resistance.

SYSTEMIC BARRIERS TO CHANGE

Barriers to organizational change are either systemic (embedded in the culture) or human (in an individual's emotional or rational responses). To execute any change successfully, the change agents must be able to manage both the systemic and human resistance. They must be able to "diagnose" the culture and identify the culture-related barriers to change. They must then engage everyone in the process of reshaping the culture to facilitate the change. To do this, they must first understand what organizational culture means.

An organization's culture is the set of underlying assumptions that drive behaviors within the organization. Over time, as the organization successfully resolves its challenges, it develops practices that work. These approaches and the values and beliefs surrounding them become embedded in the organization's psyche so that its members begin to internalize these practices as part of a belief system that dictates "the way things get done around here."

For example, a facility headed by an autocratic, task-oriented administrator who believes that individuals are basically lazy and must be monitored closely will, over time, create a culture whose values reflect a lack of trust and concern for task over concern for individuals' needs. Such a culture may not value input from employees and may be experienced as rigid and bureaucratic. The reward systems may further reinforce this culture because only persons who are themselves autocratic and inflexible get promoted to influential positions. The culture thereby propagates itself. To unfreeze this culture and move it in the direction of participatory management that supports and involves employees requires great skill in transformational change management.

To change an organization's culture, we must understand how culture works. Culture exists on three levels.

- At the superficial, more readily observed, level are the *artifacts* of culture: the language that is used, the way individuals are treated, the physical layout of a facility, how individuals interact in meetings, and what behaviors get rewarded or punished.
- At the less visible level are the *values* that inform the culture and dictate the choices of the artifacts. These values include beliefs about what is important. They reflect convictions about how to deal with individuals, broad judgments about what is good or bad for the organization, the philosophies that get expressed in slogans such as "the customer is first" or "excellence in all we do" or employee gems of wisdom like "it is who you know around here that counts."
- Finally, at the invisible level of culture are the deeply embedded, out of awareness, *assumptions* that truly drive the organization. They include underlying beliefs about human nature (individuals are lazy or work is natural), the nature of "truth" (the facts speak for themselves or truth is relative), and the reason for the organization's existence (to make a profit or to do good).

These assumptions pose the greatest barriers partly because they are out of conscious awareness and partly because they are so deeply held as the basis for the organization's survival. Organization members are initially unable to perceive how enslaved they are to the prevailing cultural mindset. It is not unusual, for example, to find managers who ask employees to take risks in order to innovate, yet punish them if they fail, or managers who solicit candid feedback only to "shoot the messenger" if they do not like what they hear. Such managers are verbalizing one set of new "cultural values," whereas their behaviors are still being shaped by the prevailing deeply embedded cultural assumptions. This sort of contradiction, in the face of efforts to lead organizational change, only leads to employee morale problems and poor service to the consumer.

One way to foster cultural change is to challenge old assumptions, bring them into conscious awareness, and replace them with new ones. In this way a conscious change can affect the choices we make at the level of artifacts and values. As new approaches at the visible levels are tried with success, changes in visible behaviors, policies, and rewards will reinforce these successes.

In this process, remember that, as Figure 56–1 shows, hidden assumptions shape and are shaped by organizational values. Values, in turn, shape and are shaped by artifacts. These artifacts, the visible manifestations of culture, both symbolize and reinforce that culture.

All of this suggests that transformational change must be driven by a philosophy (assumptions and values) that sets the direction and supported by the establishment of a structure and the deployment of resources (artifacts) to move the organization in that direction.

The Philosophy Behind the Change

Strategic decisions to change are typically linked to a set of values, beliefs, and norms that inform the change agents' vision of the direction the organization ought to take and how it ought to get there. At Chicago's Mercy Hospital, for example, initiatives are under way to change the culture so that (1) employees' ideas are sought and valued as a way of improving service and (2) service delivery is patient-focused. As in many other hospitals embarking on achieving similar goals, change agents must find ways to gain commitment and support from both medical and hospital staff. At the same time, they must make sure that the vision and direction take into account the consumer's (patient's) needs and perspectives. One approach used at Mercy was to schedule a staff retreat that included medical and hospital staff as well as former inpatients. Together they shared ideas and recommended strategies for achieving their goals.

As health care organizations pursue quality care, many are changing

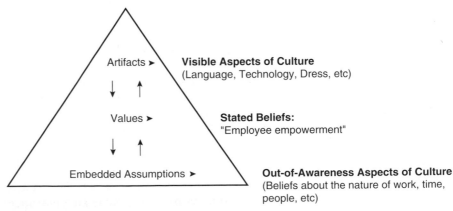

FIGURE 56–1: Three aspects of culture.

their values or philosophy. They are moving from an autocratic, "top-down" style to a more participative culture. In his book *Thriving on Chaos*, Tom Peters suggests that this approach is necessary for organizational renewal. He urges deference to the front line as a means of ensuring that employees "closest to the action" bring their first-hand experience to bear on solving organizational problems. In the spirit of this philosophy, many organizations are moving from monocultural perspectives based on blind conformity, to multicultural perspectives that embrace and value the diversity of their employees and customers.

In a well-managed change effort, then, the philosophy sets the direction, and the structure and resources are the pathways to getting there.

The Structure and Resources that Support the Change

Some organizations are driven by a highly mechanistic functional structure. In such organizations, complexity, formalization, and rigid hierarchic relationships are assumed to assure stability and effectiveness. In a climate of rapid change and constant challenges, the opposite may be required. Instead, the bureaucratic processing systems may become so unwieldy that the bulk of the employees' time and energy is spent on data gathering and processing, relaying information via complex formalized communication channels, and working the chain of command in ways that compromise productivity and eventually quality.

The consumer-driven or patient-focused facility is structured in more "organic" ways. It is organized to be less complex, less formalized, and more adaptable. It allows cross-functional teams to operate collaboratively by removing bureaucratic constraints.

Related to structure are the resources for change, which include skills, technology, time, personnel support, money, well-laid plans, and resourcefulness—the creativity and risk taking needed to get to the desired end state. Without adequate resources change will not occur. Even if the philosophy and structure are sound, individuals will become frustrated if the tools, time, and support needed to effect the change are unavailable.

Three aspects of culture

- Artifacts
- Values
- Assumptions

In effecting transformational change, all three aspects of culture must be managed. For the sponsors and agents of change, this translates into having a philosophy or vision of the change and the ability to provide the structure and resources to effect the change. None of this will work, however, if the individuals are not motivated to participate in the process.

HUMAN BARRIERS TO CHANGE

Individuals resist change. It is human nature to do so. A primary reason is that every change involves loss. Individuals see change as giving something up. When confronted with change, they instinctively ask "What is in it for me?" If the incentives to change are not perceived, and if rewards are not clearly linked to the change, individuals resist. The perceived losses take many forms:

- *Loss of security or control.* Perhaps we seek the comfort of the status quo as part of a basic survival mechanism that enables us to manage our lives with some degree of certainty. Why, for example, do individuals return to the same seat at staff meetings time after time? Why do we follow the same sequence when getting dressed in the mornings? Often the answer is simply "because we have always done it that way."

We do it the way we have always done it because it enhances our sense of safety and control over our environment. We hold on to organizational policies and practices long after they have outlived their original intent because they are familiar ways of defining "how things work around here."

Yet, paradoxically, individuals also understand and value the importance of change. Most employees I talk to in the course of my consulting practice want to change for the better. They are anxious to give feedback to managers, suppliers, and customers on ways to improve processes, products, or services. They want to move on to better jobs, create more jobs (or less, depending on who is talking), take on more rewarding or stimulating positions, cut back on "red tape," improve communications, find ways to work more efficiently, and even (for some) "return to the good old days!" In each case, they express an interest in change—moving away from the status quo.

The resistance to change is nothing more than a predictable psychological discomfort with letting go of what is familiar about the old situation. In other words, the fact that individuals resist change initially does not necessarily mean they do not want it or that they do not see the value in it. It could also be simply because of the anxiety that comes from disengagement from the security of what is familiar.

- *Loss of Identity*. This is tied to the employee's sense of role clarity and organizational self-worth. A technician who has worked a long time to develop expertise in a given procedure has invested a lot of himself or herself in the process. This person may be identified as an expert, therefore deriving a sense of comfort and esteem from this fact. When new technology is introduced, this technician loses competence, if only temporarily, and is no longer "the expert." In some cases, the entire job may be eliminated, eradicating that person's sense of "professional self" as well. Although he or she may agree with or may even have initiated the change, there remains a part of the unconscious that resists it.

- *Loss of Competence*. Related to the loss of identity is the loss of competence that accompanies change. Sometimes this loss is simply a justifiable concern about the change agent's and the changee's lack of skills in the new ways. At other times, it has to do with the change agent's or the changee's perception that the proposed change is really a bad idea. There is always the possibility that a proposed change is not in the organization's best interest. Therefore, management should not dismiss employee complaints as "mere human resistance to change." If "red flags are raised," the issues should be examined carefully. The change agent should weigh the cost of maintaining the status quo against the cost of changing and apply appropriate risk management tactics if he or she decides to proceed with the change.

REDUCING RESISTANCE TO CHANGE

The following tactics are useful in overcoming systemic and human resistance to change. If managed well, they also serve to build commitment to change.

- *Clearly communicate* rationale, overall direction, and specific goals for the proposed change. Use every medium of communication available: face-to-face discussions, written memorandums or proposals, group meetings, and bulletin boards. Do this continually until everyone hears and understands the message. This is critical because without sufficient information and clear communication of the vision, organization members create their own version of the proposed changes. They may even imagine the worst and circulate these fears among the workers, resulting in further resistance and morale problems.

- *Provide intensive training.* As suggested earlier, a major source of resistance to change is the loss of competence individuals experience when asked to change directions or procedures. Stories abound with examples of employees refusing to use new technology because of lack of proper orientation and skill building.

- *Involve everyone* in planning and implementing goals. Individuals are more likely to commit to changes they help to shape. This is an important step in addressing the loss of security or control that accompanies change. When everyone is actively involved, the organization benefits by having a wider array of ideas and experiences to draw from. When leading change, the wise manager gets to know everyone's unique talents and needs. He or she then focuses on helping them find ways to get their needs met as they further the organization's goals.

- *Look for ways to build consensus and support.* The autocratic manager of change may successfully gain short-term compliance. This means that he or she may get individuals to do something by using the power of his or her position to influence them. The more effective manager of change understands the importance of being consultative—asking individuals for input and ideas and encouraging them to suggest solutions and "own" the process as well as the outcomes. If the change is a long-term transformational effort, it is particularly important to take the time necessary to test assumptions and gain consensus before forging ahead. Without a reasonable consensus, or if conflicting assumptions exist, change efforts will unravel in the long run.

- *Leave room for changees to exercise creativity* as they influence outcomes. The most effective change agents create a climate in which individuals can try out new ideas, take risks, and learn from their mistakes. Although the decision to change and the overall direction of the change might be non-negotiable, they recognize that there is much room in the implementation of change for those affected by it to help shape the outcomes in positive ways. The payoffs associated with this approach include increased motivation and satisfaction and better quality results.

- *Model the way.* To maintain credibility and trust, change agents must act with integrity. They must consistently demonstrate commitment and good faith. They must do what they say they are going to, and they must do it in a manner that is congruent with the stated philosophies or assumptions underlying the change effort. I am reminded of a general manager, allegedly a major sponsor of a total quality effort, who in addressing a group of supervisors told them "all this customer involvement stuff is okay, but it is profits that really count!" This general manager later approached our consulting firm perplexed by his employees' lack of ownership and teamwork.

- *Provide the resources that engender success.* It is short-sighted to ask individuals to change without providing the time, tools, coaching, support, and structure that enable them to successfully execute the plan.

Without resources, both change agent and changee will become frustrated and ineffective.

• *Set manageable goals and a clear action plan.* Here, again, involvement in the process by everyone affected by the change is crucial. The goals should be realistic for the time and resources available. The plan should be straightforward, "doable," and broken down into manageable steps. Activities within this plan should also be prioritized, and participants should be encouraged to look for areas in which they can have the most meaningful organizational impact in both the short and long term. This brings us to the final strategy:

• *Look for opportunities to celebrate successes.* Individuals need ongoing positive reinforcement in the face of change. By breaking the action plans into manageable steps, participants can celebrate the accomplishment of each step as a milestone along the way. Exemplary change agents focus on gains, not losses. They observe individuals doing something well and reward them. They view mistakes as developmental opportunities so that rather than focusing on, "Who's to blame?" they ask, "What went wrong, and what did it teach us?"

The preceding discussion identified the systemic or cultural barriers to change as well as the pattern of human resistance to change. At the systemic level, I suggested that the existing philosophy, structure, and resources will impede change unless the change agent is skilled at diagnosing and reshaping organizational culture. At the human level, I suggested that predictable "losses" are associated with change. These losses may also block change unless the change agent can find ways to minimize them and build commitment to the process.

MANAGING PLANNED ORGANIZATIONAL CHANGE

To successfully manage planned change, the manager may be guided by the following questions:

• What are the driving forces for change in our organization?
• What are the restraining forces (systemic and human)?
• Is there a perceived need or opportunity that calls for change?

If a decision is made to change based on the first three questions:

• Do we have a clear vision of where we are headed?
• Do we have sufficient support and other resources to create the future we envision?
• Do we have the skills to go there?
• Do we have clear action plans that specify the steps to take, whom to involve, how to achieve the goal and by when?
• Have we developed a process for monitoring and feedback?

As these questions imply, a well-executed effort to change must be supported by strategic, planned steps. As Figure 56–2 shows, change is undertaken in response to a driving force—an event or series of events that "upsets, or could upset, the apple cart." The awareness that this force creates may be experienced by organization members as a threat (pain) or an opportunity. Once a decision has been made to act, a process of planning must begin. This requires careful data gathering and analysis, which provides the data necessary to develop the right goals and objectives. This leads to action—the deployment of resources to effect the

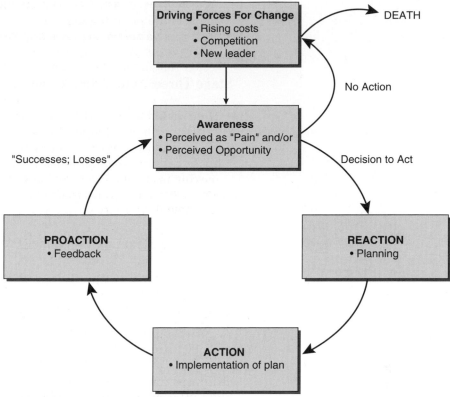

FIGURE 56–2: The process of change.

change. The results of the chosen action or actions provide additional feedback, which becomes an internal catalyst for developmental changes or midcourse corrections. At each stage in this cyclic process, the change agent must manage the systemic and human barriers to change. The following are useful questions and tactics that will facilitate the management of each phase.

Stage One: Awareness

Be continually aware of your external and internal environments. Frequently ask the following questions:

- What are the driving forces for change in our organization?
- What are the barriers to change (systemic and human)?
- Is there a condition (threat or opportunity) that calls for change?

Stage Two: Proaction (Planning)

Key questions at this stage include:

- What is the present state?
- How well positioned are we internally to ward off threats and capitalize on opportunities?
- What data do we need to gather to answer these questions?
- What actions do we need to take?

- Who will be affected by the change, and how? How can we involve them in the planning process?
- How can we turn resistance and barriers into driving forces?

Stage Three: Action (Implementation)

- How should we deploy our resources to effect the change?
- What training and other forms of support do we need to implement?
- How should we structure ourselves to carry out the changes?
- What reward systems must we implement to support individuals in moving in the direction of change?
- How can we integrate their wisdom and input in the process?

Stage Four: Reaction (Feedback)

- What new information do we now have (successes, failures, resistance, and so forth)?
- What needs to happen now? (Return to stage one.)

As the preceding model suggests, the process of planned change is cyclical. To effectively lead a change effort, the agents must conceptualize change as a spiral continuum. With each iteration, the organization's readiness for change is strengthened, especially if successes are documented, celebrated, and reinforced by the reward structure.

SUMMARY

Change management theorists generally agree that the process of effecting organizational change must be approached in the same way that one would deal with any transition or personal loss. First, individuals must come to terms with the need for, or the inevitability of, the change. The change agent must "upset the apple cart" and in so doing challenge the status quo. Next, the change agent must move individuals in the direction of the change by providing support and direction. Finally, the change agent must restabilize the organization in the "new state" until external and internal driving forces call for new changes.

This is usually as depicted in the following three stages. In each case, I have listed tactical choices as a guide.

Unfreezing

- Explain the rationale for change.
- Analyze the payoffs and costs and emphasize the cost of not changing.
- Be specific about what is and is not changing.

Transitioning

- Communicate, communicate, communicate!
- Allow individuals to vent their frustrations and allow their resistance to surface.

- Involve changees as partners.
- Model the way—"walk the talk."
- Be positive—no one follows a pessimist.
- Be forward-looking—visionary.
- Plan small wins and celebrate each step.
- Provide resources: training, budget technology, time, individuals, and other resources.

Refreezing

- Acknowledge and reward individuals for their contributions.
- Continue to model commitment.
- Evaluate what works well and what needs to be improved and communicate both progress and challenges.

Above all else, in this age of the "quick fix," contemporary managers must remember that to transform our organizations, we must first transform our own thinking and our willingness to entertain change in ourselves. We must develop the insight and the patience to acknowledge that real, lasting change is usually fraught with false starts and frustration and that it requires the ability to consistently stay the course.

Suggested Reading

Beckhard R, Harris RT. Organizational Transitions: Managing Complex Change. Reading, MA, Addison-Wesley, 1987.

Kanter RM. The Change Masters. New York, Simon and Schuster, 1983.

Peters, T. Thriving on Chaos. New York, Alfred A. Knopf, 1987.

Schein EH. Organizational Culture and Leadership. San Francisco, Jossey-Bass, 1985.

Vaill P. Managing as a Performing Art. San Francisco, Jossey-Bass, 1989.

57

Managing Quality in Health Care*

Thomas H. Breedlove, Ann Parks Linn,
and Philip Crosby Associates, Inc.

Key Terms

Culture
Management
Organization
Process
Quality

THE NEED FOR QUALITY MANAGEMENT

Providers of health care have always been concerned about quality. After all, consumers of health care services want, expect, and *deserve* nothing less than quality services from their practitioners, their hospitals, nursing homes, health maintenance organizations, clinics, health insurers, clinical laboratories, urgent care and drop-in centers, and therapists. In the tough marketplace of the 1990s, however, managing quality is not just desirable but is the price of survival. Consumers are getting smarter and becoming more active in judging quality. Individuals and organizations willing to consume health care services on blind faith are disappearing rapidly. Competition has arrived on the health care scene, as it has in just about every other industry. Governments, employers, direct consumers, and physicians themselves are demanding more, better, smarter, smoother, and cost-effective services.

In the past, definitions of technical and functional quality were left to health care professionals. This is not so any longer. It seems as if lawyers and jurors are defining standards of medical practice more than doctors are. Functional quality, or *how* the service is provided, is getting more attention in today's market-oriented environment. Health care organizations often have to show that their care is as good or better than their competitors'—in both the technical and clinical sense and also from the viewpoint of the consumer. For the health care industry, quality of care may indeed become the major marketing issue of this decade.

The decade of the 1990s looms as a critical crossroads at which a litany of problems and challenges bombard the health care field. Health care providers must face not only rising costs and competition in their markets but also shortages of trained professionals, a need to improve working relationships, a larger aging population, an increasing incidence of viral diseases, and an escalating need for long-term care. At the same time, the debate grows, Who is going to pay for all this?

Add to that burden a dramatic increase in regulatory requirements. The federal government, the Joint Commission on the Accreditation of Healthcare Organizations, employer groups, and insurance carriers are among those trying to address skyrocketing health costs and patient dissatisfaction. They are designing and imposing various criteria for performing clinical procedures. The sanctions and nonpayment associated with failing to meet these criteria can send a damaging blow to a health care provider's balance sheet.

There are also technologic changes. Health care executives and professionals have to keep up with the dizzying pace of technology and how it affects health care delivery. They have to balance critical demands

---

*Copyright © 1995, Philip Crosby Associates, Inc.

such as the need for costly new diagnostic tools and the availability of an ever-widening range of alternative therapies against the reality of shrinking capital resources.

Despite the growing shortage of nurses, studies still show that as much as 40% of a nurse's time is spent on administrative tasks. Other studies show that up to 20% of that time could be saved if technology at a nursing station and the bedside were linked to centralized hospital information systems.

There is also the matter of malpractice, which begs a crucial question, "Why didn't you do it right the first time?"

Health care organizations are caught in a tight squeeze. They face enormous pressures to reduce costs while at the same time maintain quality services. In the midst of all this, individuals within the health care industry are still arguing over definitions of quality. There is no need to do that. Health care providers have traditionally looked at quality in terms of quality assurance. With the focus on clinical outcomes, quality was either "good" or "bad" and something for the practitioners or the clinicians to worry about. Patient outcome statistics, however, are only one measure of quality performance and, although important, are not adequate in today's highly competitive business environment. A new "technology" in quality is called for.

PROGRESS REPORT*

Administration: Fresh Look at Systems Reduces Overtime $50,000/Month; Receivables Down by 10 Days

Historically, health care administrators have looked at "bottom line" results, that is, outcome results, and have not been systems-motivated. As the chief executive officer (CEO) of one of the top 100 community hospitals in the United States said, "We have not looked at processes and I think the reason for that is, like water, we all flow to the easy path. Hospital systems are very complex and we have found, through the quality initiative, that the systems are more complex than the employees or even the management understands. That is why the quality process is so important. Management may arbitrarily change a system to achieve one goal and 'downstream' affect four or five other departments negatively. From that perspective, this has helped us change the way we think to flow analysis or systems analysis. In order to make decisions now, management needs to get the input of the individuals who are going to be affected. This is quite an opportunity in health care."

By going back and looking at their systems, this hospital was able to produce some real quality-improvement success stories. By taking a hard look at the patient registration process, they were able to change the way they registered patients and cut overtime by $50,000 a month. They have also been able to reduce the amount of time it takes to receive payment by 10 days.

According to the CEO, "We went to the employees. We sat them in this room and said 'What are we not doing?' We found out that the work flow was never explained to the employees. We found out that we were

---

*The progress reports presented in this chapter are based on actual case histories of Philip Crosby Associates, Inc. (PCA) health care clients who have implemented the quality improvement process. Client names are not used in these reports, however, because it is PCA's policy to protect the confidential nature of client relationships.

not educated about the new version of the software. The employees came up with more than 200 suggestions on how to improve the process. We have implemented probably 120 of these suggestions and 50 or 60 are computer fixes that we are working on with IBM to implement. As a result, our receivables are going down and greatly improving compared with other facilities our size. I didn't do that. The director of finance didn't do that. The employees did it."

PROGRESS REPORT

Purchasing: Communication Buys Pacemaker Savings

It is not unusual for a physician to state a preference for a particular manufacturer or model—especially when it comes to something like pacemakers. However, many of these decisions are very personal and not necessarily cost-effective for the health care facility buying the equipment.

When one hospital found they were purchasing pacemakers from four different manufacturers—with prices from "the basement to the attic"—they decided to use the Crosby Quality Improvement Process to bring in the physicians who used pacemakers and open communication on the subject. An awareness of the price variations and a discussion of differences helped to break down prejudices. As a result, the hospital was able to "buy smarter" and save about $50,000 a year.

WHAT IS QUALITY?

Additional standards of quality can and should be applied to the health care structure and process as well as patient outcomes. To do that in this modern, competitive arena, quality must have a universal meaning that understood by everyone and a definition that works. That definition can be stated in a simple, direct sentence: "Quality is conformance to requirements." It means every individual doing what he or she is supposed to do every time.

To attend to quality, everyone has to know what the requirements are. The organization must view quality as meeting specific expectations. This definition has nothing to do with "goodness," except as meeting standards is good. Quality starts with setting requirements for everyone. Its measurement entails the degree to which those requirements are met. Requirements have to be defined in a straightforward manner—whether it is how to conduct business, how to treat a patient, how to deliver care, or how to diagnose a disease. Once the requirements are defined, a process can be put into place that causes them to happen. Starting at the beginning, rather than looking retroactively at what went wrong, can help ensure a positive outcome.

Quality can be looked at as expectations and how they have been met. If you want individuals to do things right the first time, you have to tell them exactly what it is you expect. Performance can then be measured against clearly understood expectations. It is the job of top management to establish this culture that encourages attention to quality and rewards conformance to requirements. Any health care institution that hopes to be around in the 21st century must manage quality in this way.

As in every industry, quality in health care is not a finished product but a process of continuous improvement. This is true not only in direct clinical situations but also in preventive care, holistic care, hospice care, substance abuse treatment, and so on. It is also true among the insurance and benefits organizations that help pay for this care.

PROGRESS REPORT

Respiratory Therapy: Eliminating Outdated Procedures Saves Dollars, Improves Care

The respiratory services area of a large hospital used quality management to look at the processes the staff members performed every day to see if efficiency could be improved. They learned that just because they had "always done it that way" did not necessarily mean that they were doing it the best way *now*.

Historically, the respiratory care services department had been one of the hospital's revenue generators, but things had changed. With diagnostic related groups (DRGs) and prospective payment systems now in place, the department was forced to turn from the role of revenue generator to one of revenue saver.

Because a hospital gets paid a certain amount of money for a patient with a disease, it really does not matter if the patient's stay is 2 days, 4 days, or 20 days, so it has become imperative to release patients as quickly as possible while giving them the best quality care. It is just as important to make sure they are well when they leave because if they come back, the hospital does not receive reimbursements for readmittance.

Through a systematic approach of looking at their processes, this respiratory care department aggressively set out to assess therapies. Many of the systems had been in place for a long time; it was always thought that they were indicated. In the end, they found they could perform therapy at a lower cost and even eliminate some therapies that were not really beneficial to the patient. For example, an apparatus that is used every day in many hospitals is a simple bubble bottle, a piece of equipment that bubbles oxygen before it gets to patients who are receiving low-flow oxygen supplementation. The respiratory care department conducted a survey of patients and therapeutic outcomes and mapped out a process flow. They found that the bubble bottle did not improve patient comfort and did not provide any real benefit to the patient, especially at low flows of oxygen. By eliminating the use of bubble bottles in patients receiving low-flow oxygen, the department saved the hospital $11,000—a savings that will occur every year from now on.

All the employees in the respiratory care department were involved in this effort to make the processes they use every day work more smoothly and efficiently. Management learned to listen, teams worked together to improve systems and procedures, and communication opened up with other areas of the hospital. By installing a system for getting orders to the respiratory care department from the nursing unit (there had never been one before!), 320 missed treatments every quarter were eliminated.

Quality management also helped the department establish appropriate therapeutic guidelines for arterial blood gas measurements. They were able to modify Blue Cross Blue Shield guidelines to meet both College of American Pathologists and Joint Commission on the Accreditation of Healthcare Organizations–mandated regulations. A system is in place for evaluating every blood gas measurement in the hospital and establishing that it is indeed needed. If, in contrast, it is not needed, the physician is contacted for clarification of the order, and it is all carried out with no additional time or expense.

According to the respiratory care department supervisor, the department has been able to improve existing therapy and patient care, eliminate unnecessary therapy, and terminate respiratory therapy in the shortest amount of time; employee morale has also skyrocketed.

"They are the individuals who do the work. They needed to be involved. They understand the processes better than we do," he said. "Prior to the initiation of our quality management system, the department meetings were pretty much a one-way street. Our department head would talk and the staff would listen. Since the quality initiative, the department meetings have become animated. We have an awful lot of give-and-take between the respiratory therapy staff and the department head and the supervisors. They can actually voice their opinions and have them acted on within a short time. When therapists can see that what they are saying is being acted on within the week, they can actually say, 'Hey, this is worth working for.'"

TOTAL COMMITMENT TO QUALITY

Today's health care providers must take managing quality to a new level—beyond what has been done or thought in the past. This change in thinking can be summed up in a few statements:

- Quality management can provide an important competitive edge and improve bottom line performance.
- Effective quality management demonstrates an organization's high regard for its consumers and can be the best differentiator between competitors.
- As competition increases, those who *do not* understand quality management run a big risk of failure.
- Quality is a matter of *policy*.
- Senior management needs to be involved.

For the rest of this decade and into the next century, management's major weapon in facing its challenges is nothing short of a total commitment to quality and quality management. Quality management must transcend the entire organization and energize all its members—whether they work in housekeeping, management, billing, dietary, or maintenance departments or in the laboratory, pharmacy, or nursing units, or are physicians.

This *total* quality management means a complete culture change for the entire organization—a concern for the interrelationships among all associates with one another and with their "customers" in a very basic service delivery sense.

In the tight marketplace of the 1990s, health care providers are competing for capital, human resources, and customers (health care consumers). Although it is of utmost importance that costs be contained, it makes little sense to contain costs if the staff does not work harmoniously together or if customers are lost.

A hospital can have the best doctors, the best nurses, and the most up-to-date technology, but to thrive in the marketplace of the 1990s, more than the finest medical product is needed. That fine medical product has to be wrapped in an overall delivery system in which employees are consumer-oriented and care about meeting the requirements of the customer 100% of the time.

PROGRESS REPORT

Pharmacy: Brainstorming Sessions Result in Reduction in Medication Errors

A hospital's pharmacy staff used the quality process to "brainstorm" ways to improve its drug distribution process. A major reduction in incident reports was the result.

The pharmacy's director started out by asking the staff pharmacists to review when they had problems with nursing and then invite nurses in to talk about it. He called the nursing managers and had them pick two staff duty nurses to participate in a brainstorming session with two staff pharmacists.

"I put them in our pharmacy library for 45 minutes with a preamble that they were to do no finger-pointing, no blaming; just simply sit and discuss their processes on 'each side of the fence' and ways to overcome problems that occur. After all, nursing is our principal customer in this department," the Director of Pharmacy said and added, "I will not come back into the room unless I hear screams or reports of blood-letting."

The meetings between staff pharmacists and staff nurses were productive and out of them came a multitude of ideas for the pharmacy to consider how to improve its own process. Using these ideas, brainstorming sessions were held for the pharmacy staff. So many ideas came forth that a work group of three staff pharmacists and four pharmacy technicians was formed to consider, revise, and review the process of drug distributions throughout the institution. The work group met routinely with the rest of the staff and as they progressed, more individuals were asked for their input. The group found several ways to reduce the potential for medication errors and to increase the work flow and efficiency in the department.

According to a staff pharmacist who participated in the work group, "Because of the quality initiative, there is a lot more cooperation between the nursing and pharmacy departments now, and it has made a big difference in the department itself. Everyone throughout the department has a better attitude and is looking for ways to solve problems on a daily basis—because of that, it is a better place to work."

The group found that interruptions were a big part of the problem. Phones would ring and they would have to stop filling the order, answer the phone, go get the pharmacist, and come back. Also, their location near the service window did not help. Individuals were constantly coming to the window for medications while the technicians were trying to do their work. This resulted in a number of errors because the technicians would forget what they were doing or would forget to put something in the drawer. Corrective action involved locating the technicians away from the phones and away from the service window where they did not have interruptions. It was just that easy, and errors decreased significantly.

WHAT ARE THE CUSTOMERS' REQUIREMENTS?

The quality of service actually delivered to external customers often will make the difference between keeping them as customers or losing them.

Customer satisfaction must be a key goal of any quality effort. It's a matter of attitude. How conscientiously a service provider focuses on its customers can make or break its future. Today—in finance, transportation, health care, entertainment, government, or any other service industry you can identify—quality service is more than a smile for the customer. Behind the scenes of every service organization, for example, there is an infrastructure of support, information systems, technology, supplier relations, communications, training, and so on. That infrastructure can be working smoothly to deliver competitive quality support or it can be outmoded, cumbersome, and more a part of an organization's business problems than part of the solution to those problems.

The term *external customers* describes those individuals who pay us for what we do. There also are *internal* customers, however, who are vital to success. These are the individuals in an organization—the managers and employees—who depend on quality work from their coworkers. That includes just about everyone. Nowhere is this more important than in clinical health care. The relationships among physician, nurse, pharmacist, laboratory technician, radiologist, and so on are crucial. Each must receive quality output from coworkers if he or she is to deliver quality health care services. Each person is not only a customer but also a *supplier* in a work process (Fig. 57–1). To service customers effectively, everyone in the organization must know the requirements of his or her job and meet them.

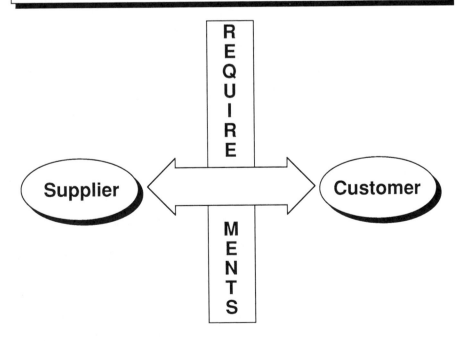

FIGURE 57–1: The customer–supplier relationship comprises both external customers (those who pay for a service) and internal customers (one's coworkers).

PROGRESS REPORT

Seniors Served Required Diets on Time and "Right the First Time"

An off-site program for seniors, primarily Alzheimer's victims, had difficulty receiving meal trays from the dietary office on time and right. Each client was supposed to get a different, personalized meal according to his or her physician's recommendation, which was not always easy. Meals were irregular. They came in late, cold sometimes and at times incomplete, for example; utensils and condiments were missing. Often the number of meals delivered differed from the number of meals ordered. Sometimes if they were supposed to be low in sodium, they came with regular amounts of sodium, if they were for diabetic clients, there were cookies on the tray. To compound the problem, the meal tickets were placed on the tray in such a manner that they got wet; when the staff removed the ticket from the tray, the ticket broke in half and the staff had no way of knowing what tray belonged to which person.

The situation caused tremendous hassle and added work for the staff. They had to leave and go to the main facility for the correct meals or microwave other food themselves to fulfill the clients' dietary needs.

The program director tried for 2 years to clear up this problem with the food service department. However, it was not until the two departments were able to clearly define the problem using the quality process that "customer-supplier" requirements were agreed on and the problem was resolved. After just 6 weeks, the meal trays were error-free.

The problem was defined as the dietary office not meeting the requirements stated by the off-site facility staff in terms of ordering and receiving the lunches. A root cause was determined to be communication between the dietary office and the food line. A measurement system helped to pinpoint when requirements were not met, and a daily measurement chart that is monitored by both the dietary office and the off-site facility is now a permanent part of corrective action for the meal tray problem. Daily phone contact and regularly scheduled meetings provide an opportunity for the two department directors to discuss any nonconformance.

According to the Director of Food Services, "This problem with the auxiliary site was as an opportunity for us to show that we could be a good supplier and we could meet our customers' needs every time."

"The greatest benefit has been to the clients," said the off-site program director. "They now receive their *proper* lunches—on time, and warm."

PROGRESS REPORT

Emergency Room: Diversion Hours Drop from 350 to Zero in 1 Year

One cold January day, the president and CEO of a large medical center set out to regenerate his organization—to take a fresh look at the staff and their relationships with the community they served. He saw the medical center's customers as its patients, physicians, visitors, and all fellow employees.

The CEO began his process by going to school along with 200 of the medical center's managers to learn management techniques of the quality improvement process—ones that would replace negative hours of repeated work with positive time devoted to customer requirements.

A month later, he put the quality process to work on a long-standing and emotionally charged problem. Patients requiring emergency admission often spent more than 8 hours in the emergency room or found themselves being sent to another hospital. The CEO asked a team of nurses and administrators to use the quality process to study the situation. They found that patients awaiting emergency admission were diverted to other hospitals 50% of the time at a cost of 350 hours a month. When they investigated the root causes of the problem, they saw that employee communication was inconsistent and unclear, certain critical care beds were being occupied by patients who could be moved to "step down" units for less acute care, and beds on nursing units were often unused because of a shortage of nurses.

The procedures for emergency admissions were quickly clarified, and one administrator became responsible for the movement of patients from the emergency room to nursing units. All employees involved began to perform in accordance with clearly stated requirements. Within 2 months, the monthly diversion hours dropped from 350 to 150 hours.

Later that same year, three additional critical care beds were made available, and in December diversion hours dropped to 6 hours for the month. When a new critical care evaluation system was started in January of the next year, monthly diversion hours dropped to zero and have been at zero ever since.

THE ROAD TO WELLNESS

Everyone has to work together on quality. Managing quality in health care must be a corporate mission, those "at the top" must be committed to it and communicate about it effectively throughout the organization. Today's health care professionals are discovering that quality management translates into "business wellness," just as properly administered clinical procedures apply to personal wellness. The road to wellness is one of understanding the work processes involved in providing health care and managing them for success. It is a systematic approach. Wellness occurs in health care organizations when there is a focus on the processes of providing health care and not just on the outcomes of clinical procedures.

In order to produce desired symptoms of wellness, health care providers have to change their processes. The businesses of health care providers, and all other organizations, are made up of work processes that have been put in place to produce a desired result. When the outcome of the process produces waste, patient dissatisfaction, and frustration for those participating in the process, the process is saying, "I need help." (To better understand the condition of your organization take the test provided in Figure 57–2.)

There is a solution—a way to move through the healing process. It is not easy, but it is feasible. Help comes from focusing the providers of health care on the *processes* in which they are involved, not on each other. Problems happen by design, not by accident. The solution—focusing on the process—seems clear, but doing so is more complex. Health care organizations, by their very nature, are complicated enterprises with a large number of departments that often operate independently.

ETERNALLY SUCCESSFUL ORGANIZATION GRID

Read through the grid below and check the boxes that most closely correspond to your organization at the present time. This exercise will help focus improvement actions.

	COMATOSE	INTENSIVE CARE	PROGRESSIVE CARE	HEALING	WELLNESS
QUALITY	Nobody does anything right around here. ☐	We finally have a list of customer complaints. ☐	We are beginning a formal Quality Improvement Process. ☐	Customer complaints are practically gone. ☐	People do things right the first time routinely. ☐
GROWTH	Nothing ever changes. ☐	We bought a turkey. ☐	The new product isn't too bad. ☐	The new group is growing well. ☐	Growth is profitable and steady. ☐
CUSTOMERS	Nobody ever orders twice. ☐	Customers don't know what they want. ☐	We are working with customers. ☐	We are making many defect-free deliveries. ☐	Customer needs are anticipated. ☐
CHANGE	Nothing ever changes. ☐	Nobody tells anyone anything. ☐	We need to know what is happening. ☐	There is no reason for anyone to be surprised. ☐	Change is planned and managed. ☐
EMPLOYEES	This place is a little better than not working. ☐	Human Resources has been told to help employees ☐	Error Cause Removal programs have been started. ☐	Career path evaluations are implemented now. ☐	People are proud to work there. ☐

FIGURE 57–2: This chart can be used to evaluate the condition of one's business.

Needless to say, there are many interdepartmental requirements. Often these requirements are not necessarily communicated from one department to another. That can repeatedly result in hassle and having to do things over; for example, an order is filled out incorrectly; the wrong room number is recorded and the patient has moved to a different room. Everything is processed with the old number, and the laboratory comes up to the wrong room—the errors just multiply with a mushrooming effect.

Quality management helps break down communication barriers among individuals at all levels and in all functional areas of the hospital. That can go a long way toward helping them work together to improve the efficiency and effectiveness of the hospital's systems.

To have the organization members working on processes, rather than on each other, two factors are required: a common focus and common knowledge.

PROGRESS REPORT

Short-Stay Surgery: Updating Charging Procedure Results in Six-Figure Savings

During a quality education class, a billing department manager identified a problem her department had with producing error-free work because of inputs received from other departments in the hospital—especially the pharmacy. In fact, she pointed out, every bill created for a short-stay surgery patient had to be recreated, redone, or reworked. On the surface, it looked like the hospital's change to a new computer system was to blame. As a result of the change, the pharmacy department was no longer able to clearly identify short-stay surgery patients, for whom there was a different charging structure. It seemed like a fairly simple process to fix at the time, but the more the hospital looked into the problem, the more extensive it became.

Through the process of analyzing how they were charging for pharmacy services in relation to short-stay surgery, the hospital found that there were other areas that were not being handled properly. As a result, they realized that by correcting this one area, they could receive in excess of $100,000 in additional revenue.

"Without the quality process, it may have been 2 years before we were able to identify the problem," said the Senior Vice President of Operations. "Using the work process flow sheets, we were able to really tie down all the various inputs and outputs and clearly identify the total extent of the problem. Going through the quality process itself forces a certain discipline on the organization and on the employees within the organization to really make certain that all parts of an issue are examined. I think in the past we would have fixed the problem without totally solving it and that, herein, is where the real difference is in the quality process."

A corrective action task force made up of personnel from the operating room, pharmacy, supply, accounting, and billing departments worked together to tackle the short-stay surgery problem.

"These individuals thoroughly enjoyed working with each other and obtaining a thorough understanding of how the entire organization works," said the Senior Vice President of Operations. "A lot of folks did not understand how what they did in their own area affected what happened later on down the line. Therefore, it was a great learning experience for the individuals involved, and I suspect that they not only solved the problem we had identified but also many other problems along the way."

Basically the task force found that the services the hospital was providing were based on a set charging mechanism that had been used for a number of years but no longer reflected either the true cost in providing the service or all the inputs that were going into that service. Actually, the hospital was not even sure how much it cost them to perform each specific type of outpatient surgery. Because the hospital was not properly costing out their services, it was not properly charging for those services.

According to the Senior Vice President of Operations, "These things are not always easy to spot. Traditionally, a manager such as myself may look at it and feel that the system is working properly. When you have a large organization such as a hospital there are so many various inputs and outputs that you are often not totally aware of all of the details that are going into the system. Individuals learn to accept something less than 'error-free,' and because they learn to live with these problems, they do not always surface and do not always become known to management. We found there was a significant amount of hassle that management certainly did not realize existed and that the employees helped to identify for us. There was a lot of excess paperwork that was totally unnecessary. The problem was so significant that after we corrected it and implemented the solution, we saw a dramatic improvement in the bottom line of the entire hospital."

A COMMON FOCUS

The common focus consists of the work processes needed to provide health care. It includes all clinical and administrative procedures. All work can be viewed as a process—a series of actions that produces a result (Fig. 57–3). The flow of a piece of paper or information through the organization involves a process, perhaps many, and processes can be defined, planned, measured, and improved. Take, for example, the admitting process at a hospital. It involves getting specific information from a patient; that information directs much of the hospital activity. In essence it is the order-entry point. Getting admissions information right is crucial to providing a smooth way for the patient. Correct information about insurance helps ensure that bills are paid promptly. A patient's history of allergies influences the choice of medication the doctor prescribes.

All the different jobs in a process have to work together if quality is to be attained. The most talented and wonderful brain surgeon would get nowhere without a whole team of individuals, each meeting his or her own requirements. The brain surgeon has to understand that his or her work is related to the work of others in a process by which quality is attained because everyone has conformed to the requirements of their jobs. Everyone in the process depends on others in the process.

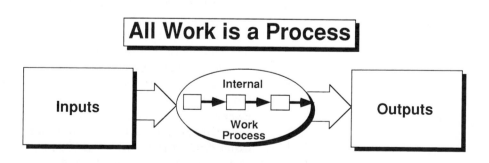

FIGURE 57–3: A process can be defined as a series of actions that produces a result, and all aspects of an organization's function are composed of processes.

The members of a well-run organization know how the process is doing. Is it producing quality results? Is the focus on process prevention, not just process outcome? Are all the required steps being performed right all the time or just most of the time? How much does all of it cost?

PROGRESS REPORT

Radiology: Measurement Helps Film Library and Staff Shine

Using the tools learned in the quality education process, a radiology department identified a problem it was having with its film library. Measurement showed that at the end of the day there were as many as 300 to 400 cases that had not been processed, which meant that those films could not be read by the radiologists and that the reports were not available for the referring physicians. Through corrective action that involved changes in procedures, staffing, and assignments, the number of cases that were not processed at the end of the work day dropped to an average of 30 and as low as zero on some shifts.

According to the Associate Director of Radiology and Diagnostic Energy, "We found that a large part of the problem was that we needed more space, which we were able to obtain on the lower levels of our hospital. We could therefore keep more films in the hospital facility rather than our outside facility for film storage. We also established a procedure for scheduling so that we now have a centralized scheduling system; we can now get adequate information prior to the patient coming into the radiology department. This means that when they are here for their study, their previous films are available for comparison. Also, by processing the films more expeditiously, we have reduced turnaround time. We now supply the report on the floor for the referring physicians much faster then we did before.

"We were having a problem getting films to the operating room so that they had them when they did the surgeries. By working with the operating room through the quality process and using process models, we were able to come up with new procedures. The operating room is now giving us more complete information. We are able to get the films pulled and get them there and we are able to supply the service needed by the physicians. There were as many as 10 cases a day that involved 30 additional phone calls to get the films to the operating room. Now we are down to maybe one or two a day with one or two phone calls, so we have made a lot of progress."

That progress did not come easy, however. "There was a lot of apprehension when we first started doing the measurement," the Associate Director said, "especially when we were behind 300 or 400 cases a day. Everyone felt very threatened by it, but as we progressed and as they saw some of the new procedures take hold and work, they became really excited when they only had 100 cases left at the end of the day, or 50, or none. That was great! They became very accountable and were very proud of what they were accomplishing. I remember arriving at 8:30 one morning and walking through the file room to see how things were going. There was a big 0 written by the employee that had just finished the midnight shift—outlined in yellow, very bright, with a big star beside it. Everyone was very excited and happy because obviously the first shift was starting with no films to catch up on from the night before, so it was a great accomplishment for everyone. That is a morale booster. Especially when you can see the progress—it definitely is a morale booster."

COMMON KNOWLEDGE

To competently focus on this, or any work process, the second ingredient, common knowledge, is required (at Philip Crosby Associates, Inc., this knowledge is referred to as the four *Absolutes of Quality Management*) (Fig. 57–4). This knowledge helps individuals understand that quality is performing the job agreed to in order to accomplish the work process requirements. It also helps individuals apply prevention to work processes and to measure how much mistakes cost.

QUALITY MANAGEMENT STRATEGY

Knowing what to do is important; knowing how to make it happen is also critical.

Common knowledge means having the ability to incorporate quality management into the business strategy and planning of the organization. It all starts with top management's commitment to making quality management part of the organization's policy and practices and then requiring it to be incorporated into the culture and activities of the organization.

There are four critical elements for bringing everything (and everyone) together when it comes to quality:

- A clear policy statement and top management commitment to it
- Top to bottom involvement
- A management communications process that focuses on customer, client, or patient requirements and the support to fulfill those requirements
- A management-backed process that gives every individual the tools and education that will permit them to practice prevention in every job task

These are the elements that make the quality management process

ABSOLUTES OF QUALITY MANAGEMENT™

- **Quality has to be defined as conformance to requirements, not as goodness.**

- **The system for causing quality is prevention, not appraisal.**

- **The performance standard must be error-free, not "that's close enough."**

- **The measurement of quality is the Price of Nonconformance, not indexes.**

FIGURE 57–4: Common knowledge is essential when focusing on a work process.

successful. Despite the best intentions, the best measurement programs, and the best technologies, quality improvement *programs* are likely to fail if they lack even one of these elements.

The word *program* does not just apply when quality is involved. Program denotes something that comes to an end. There is no end to the quality process; it is a way of life. There is no finish line.

COMMITMENT OF TOP MANAGEMENT

Although many executives might truly believe in total quality for their organizations, their behavior does not *demonstrate* their long-term commitment. We are talking about leadership:

- Setting clear quality strategy, policy, goals, and objectives and insisting on appropriate action plans
- Changing processes and technologies so that they will enhance the quality of services and control long-term costs in doing so
- Sharpening the organization's focus on the customer
- Making quality management an integral part of the strategic and financial plans
- Helping suppliers meet the standard of "error-free"
- Promoting the involvement of all employees in achieving quality improvement and giving them the tools they need
- Recognizing and rewarding quality accomplishments
- Becoming a personal example

Quality means doing every task right the first time.

Many CEOs put the blame for poor quality on the work force, not on themselves. When executives look only to the work force, only to those who discover the errors, they are ignoring the fact that the real problem most likely rests somewhere back up the line—perhaps too close to senior management for comfort. Quality is a management issue. The management team has the responsibility for quality. It does not belong to the quality department. Paying "lip service" to quality without direct senior management commitment will not achieve conformance to requirements. Quality improvement starts with a commitment at the top of the organization to see that a sharp quality focus is ingrained into the *established thinking* and culture of the organization. That is the job of senior management—ensuring that the quality policy, the quality focus of the organization, is in place and working. An appropriate policy is "We will deliver error-free services to our customers, internal and external, on time, every time" (Fig. 57–5). Nothing else is acceptable. In other words, there is *much* that the senior management of an organization can do, and must do, to ensure prevention of errors—to ensure that things are done right the first time.

PROGRESS REPORT

CEO's Office: Show 'Em! Responsibility Starts at the Top

When employees first hear about the total quality management process, they often try to dismiss it as just another fad—another one of *those* "programs." It is up to the management staff to *show them* that things are going to be different, not just today but forever.

"This is a CEO-driven process," said the CEO of a large medical

Quality Policy

Monmouth Medical Center*
is committed to quality in everything
it does.

Quality demands that
each of us understand the
requirements of
our job.

Quality is
an ongoing process
of defining the requirements
of those we serve
and meeting those requirements
every time.

Management will support
all employees
by eliminating barriers
to quality.

*Reprinted with permission of Monmouth Medical Center, Long Branch, New Jersey.

FIGURE 57–5: Monmouth Medical Center's policy on quality.

center. "Frankly, I have become a 'quality fanatic.' Everything I do involves the quality process and I must tell you it has changed my personal life. I was one of those guys who was never on time for meetings. Now I am on time for every meeting. I was one of those guys who used to keep people in a meeting room for an inordinate time droning on and on and on. I don't do that any longer. We have an agenda and 'quality' is the first item on it; we start when we are supposed to start and we end when we are supposed to end."

This CEO shows his personal commitment "out in the trenches" every day by making *quality rounds,* visiting "nose to nose" with employees, helping them with measurements, and talking with them about the requirements of their jobs. "It is important to give the employees the accolades that they rightfully deserve," he said. "There are a lot of people in this organization who are working very, very hard and are committed to this process. We have to be supportive of that."

This CEO is so committed to *using* the quality process that he keeps a framed copy of the five-step problem elimination process on his desk and on his coffee table. No matter where he is conducting business in his office, when someone comes in to see him and talks about a problem they are experiencing, he immediately goes to the framed five steps and says, "Let's talk about that. Have you analyzed the problem and defined your problem? What's the fix?" He goes through the steps with the employee.

"I want to get their thinking process moving in that direction," he said. "The first couple of times that we did it, it was very, very amusing because I took them by surprise. Now they come in prepared and they know what the boss is going to ask them. I have also gone to the extent of giving my senior managers a framed copy that they, in turn, keep on their desks, again trying to demonstrate to this organization the commitment of this senior management team to the overall quality improvement process."

EDUCATION

Management must create an environment that communicates the need for work processes that result in quality and the necessary systems to support that desire.

Since all employees are involved in the work processes of the organization, and each one contributes to its success or failure, each needs to know what is expected of him or her. Success comes when everyone in an organization knows that his or her main job is meeting requirements precisely—the importance of doing things right the first time.

Everyone needs quality improvement tools, techniques, and skills, such as how to analyze a work process to see if it is producing the desired results, to make quality happen. With these skills they can measure processes, identify and correct problems, and work together as teams to reduce cost. Preventing errors and eliminating repeated work should be part of every corporate culture because doing things right the first time saves money and improves customer satisfaction.

HOW MUCH DOES IT COST TO DO THINGS WRONG?

The cost of doing things wrong (the price of nonconformance [PONC]) even a small percentage of the time can make an organization noncompetitive. It costs a lot to do things wrong. After working with hundreds of service providers in many industries, Philip Crosby Associates, Inc. has found that almost without exception, 40% of operating costs in service businesses "go down the drain" in waste and inefficiency.

The price of nonconformance (Fig. 57–6) can be reduced dramatically when the culture of the organization changes to one of doing things right the first time—prevention. Problems in an organization are caused, and just about anything that is caused can be prevented. A tool called a process model can be used to identify the root causes of why things go wrong (Fig. 57–7). No business organization can afford to implement problems or lurking "time-bombs" that can become problems. It is essential to strive for *anticipatory* problem solving. Preventive action is second only to executive commitment in the quality process. Prevention can be encouraged. Remember parents repeatedly telling their children the old adages that an ounce of prevention is worth a pound of cure and that a stitch in time saves nine. Individuals generally get more personal satisfaction when they anticipate problems and design them out of their products and services than they do in fixing problems.

Effective quality management means reduced hassle for staff and

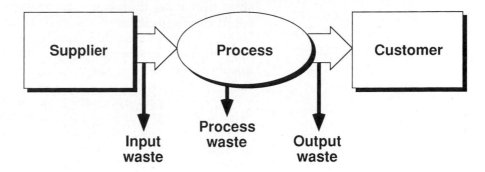

FIGURE 57–6: The price of nonconformance, which results from inefficiency and waste, hurts the competitiveness of an organization.

patients—symptoms of a healthy organization; however, it takes the participation of everyone and a continuous effort.

PROGRESS REPORT

Cardiology Clinic: Identifying PONC Brings Attention to Patient No-Show Problem

A cardiologist who had been in practice for 15 years clearly admits that he used to have the idea that everything he had done for that 15 years was the way he ought to continue to do it. After quality management education, he learned to look at the *process* of delivering patient

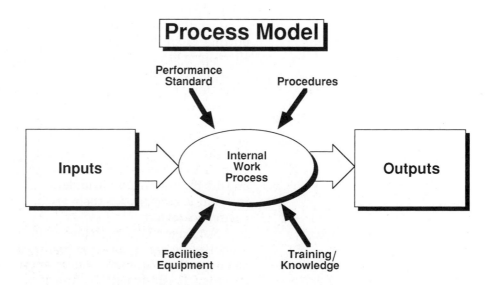

FIGURE 57–7: A process model can be used when evaluating the causes of inefficiency and waste.

care from the standpoint of looking at all the little "nooks and crannies" to find ways to make things just a little bit better. To start, he sat down with his secretarial staff and asked them what problems *they* saw in the department. One of the problems identified was patients who did not show up for appointments—particularly new patients. Using measurement, the physician and his staff looked at a 6-week period and found eight patients in that time frame who did not come for their scheduled appointments. In frustration, the staff realized that patients were given appointments so far in the future that they probably went to some other facility.

The physician approached the administration about the problem. "That's interesting information" came the reply, and nothing happened. The physician then returned to his staff secretaries and asked them to calculate the price of nonconformance related to these patient "no-shows." They computed not only the cost of lost revenue from these unkept appointments but also the amount of laboratory data, x-rays studies, and electrocardiograms that were *not obtained or performed* because those patients did not show up. The figure was about $5000 for that 6-week period, which amounted to about $45,000 annually.

The physician now had the "ammunition" he needed. He took that number back to the administration and the next day had a solution for the problem. By calling new patients on the phone 1 week before the scheduled appointment to make sure that they were coming and that they knew how to get there has reduced the number of "no-shows" to virtually zero. As an added bonus, the secretaries and receptionists on the physician's staff were especially pleased to have participated in this problem-solving effort and, at their level, are eagerly looking into other processes for improvement.

SUMMARY

Quality management consists of the policy, education, witness, and action that are necessary to prevent errors in an organization and make things happen as planned.

Quality cannot be achieved by "lip service." It cannot be achieved by putting catchy slogans on the wall. It cannot be achieved by one-time, short-term efforts. There are no magic pills. It is not a program. It can be achieved only by hard work and continuous effort that saturates everything we do—from the courteous way we answer our phones to the way we integrate technology into our operations.

Senior management has a special responsibility to keep "pushing ahead." They must encourage all of the individuals in their organizations to define what quality means to them in their work and then provide them with the tools to achieve improvement. They must insist that everyone in the organization understand who depends on whom—who the internal customers for their work are and precisely what the external customers expect.

No longer is it possible to speak of "acceptable quality." Today's marketplace *demands* error-free work, new levels of organizational efficiency, and an intimate understanding of customer requirements. Quality must be designed into every service provided and every business operation.

Quality is achievable. An organization is successful when quality improvement is woven into its fabric and culture. The health care providers featured in the progress reports presented in this chapter have made a definite commitment to "wellness." They have determined that they want to do things right routinely, manage change properly, grow purposefully, cause employees to be proud to work there, and most importantly, understand and meet their customers' needs (Figs. 57–8 and 57–9).

Health care operations are unique in that they have a great many disciplines and interests wrapped up into one organizational package. Often there is the opportunity for inefficiency and waste in the interface of these disciplines. However, when everyone has a common language of quality, when everyone knows what the requirements are, and when everyone knows that management is serious about conforming to those requirements, there is less hassle and everyone works as a team. Cooperation solves almost everything.

Prevention of illness is built into the concept of the science of health care. Prevention of problems and waste in the management and operation of health care institutions is just as important. There is no need to careen from problem to solution and back again. Individuals can learn to eliminate old problems and prevent new ones. Quality management is nothing less than a win-win situation for health care providers and patients. Everyone works together to improve processes and systems. Patient care improves, whereas time and money are saved.

No more cold meal trays left uneaten on 7E. No more unexpected changes to the operating room schedule. No more angry early morning phone calls. No more medication errors. No more late laboratory reports. No more short staffing. No more test results missing from the chart. No more failed audits. No more red on the bottom line. No more hassle. No more patients going someplace else.

PROGRESS REPORT

Hospital-wide Employee Recognition Puts on a Happy Smile

Recognition is a vital part of the quality improvement process. In fact, it is a thread woven throughout the entire process that allows an

Characteristics of an Eternally Successful Organization

Quality –	**People do things right the first time routinely**
Growth –	**Growth is profitable and steady**
Customers –	**Customer needs are anticipated**
Change –	**Change is planned and managed**
Employees–	**People are proud to work there**

©1988 Philip B. Crosby. All Rights Reserved.

FIGURE 57–8: To be successful, an enterprise must practice quality management, manage growth and change, and provide a workplace that employees are proud of.

A Personal Commitment

- **Understand requirements**

- **Work together to meet them**

- **Recognize nonconformance**

- **Prevent problems**

- **Do It Right The First Time**

FIGURE 57–9: Each individual must personally commit to providing quality health care.

organization to recognize individual as well as team achievements. An organization that does not take the time to recognize that it is making progress misses a large part of what the quality improvement process is all about—feeling good about what each individual does to make his or her workday life and that of the patients better.

When setting up their recognition program, the staff of a satellite health care facility determined first that there were certain tenets that were important to them:

- Recognition had to be meaningful.
- It had to be close to the event.
- It had to have value for the organization as a whole.
- It should be appreciated by the people who received it.
- It had to be simple to implement.

The process they came up with allowed them to accomplish all of these things. It allows for any member of the organization to identify what they believe is a success story. A success story is defined as one that involves an improvement in the process of providing quality within the organization that will result in direct improved patient care and may result in a cost savings to the organization. The employee writes up the success story and then gives it to his or her supervisor who validates the information and submits the story to the organization's Quality Improvement Team for consideration. It is again evaluated and then passed on to the steering committee for the recognition process. At that point, a member of senior management goes out to the recipient on the job and presents him or her with a "Quality Achiever" ribbon. An article about the recipient is then printed in the organization's internal publication and a photograph goes up on a special bulletin board dedicated solely to the quality improvement process.

"I think it works very well," said a Quality Improvement Team member. "Any time you see a smiling face on a person walking around with a ribbon on their name badge, you know they have had a good day!"

58

Ethics and Patient Care

Joseph E. Vincent and Stephen E. Lammers

This chapter introduces the respiratory therapist to the major concepts in medical ethics, the way in which those concepts are relevant to the everyday practice of respiratory care, and discussions of the major ethical issues that respiratory care practitioners face. It should not be viewed as a substitute for a full treatment of ethical issues in medicine. Our aim is not only to make the respiratory care practitioner aware of current issues in medical ethids but also to prepare the respiratory care practitioner for the future. It is our hope that as new matters are raised, the practitioner will know what questions to ask and what difficulties to avoid. In this chapter, the term *ethics* describes the critical study of what makes actions right or wrong, good or bad.

There is one misunderstanding about ethics that should be discussed—ethics is simply a matter of opinion and thus it does not really matter how you act, because any person's opinion on an action is as good as any other person's. Certainly, many different points of view are expressed in our society today. However, it is not the case that within health care it is simply a matter of opinion how one acts toward patients. This chapter shows how health care professionals and society have developed norms for the behavior of health care professionals. These professionals must understand these norms and use them to guide their actions. Respiratory care practitioners should learn to reflect on the sources of these professional and societal norms, because then they will have learned how to use ethical reasoning in the context of health care.

ETHICAL THEORIES

Teleological Theories and Utilitarianism

Outside of a religious context, ethics in western culture is thought about in two major ways. The first way, called *teleological*, looks at the ends or purposes of an action. In ethics, this means that an action is justifiable if it brings about good results, as opposed to evil results.

Teleological thinking can take many forms, the most popular form being *utilitarianism*, which itself takes two forms. The first form, known as *act utilitarianism*, claims that it is generally possible to calculate the amount of good or evil produced by an action. Those actions that produce the most good or the least harm are the actions that persons ought to perform. Thus, deceiving a patient should be evaluated by examining the consequences of the deception. If these consequences are good, deception is permitted. If they are bad, it is forbidden. This form of utilitarianism has been subjected to a number of criticisms. Many persons question whether one is readily able to calculate the utility of every action performed; it is not only time-consuming but individual biases enter into the calculations so that the calculations may be unreliable.

The second form of utilitarianism, *rule utilitarianism*, argues that

1153

instead of focusing on acts, we should focus on justifying moral rules that are an amalgam of human experience reflected on over time. Rule utilitarians propose that if individuals follow the rules, they will, over the long run, maximize the good they do and minimize the harm. The rule is justified by the calculus of good and bad results, not the particular action. Thus, there is a rule against deceiving patients. One utilitarian-based reason for this rule is that health care personnel have learned that patients will not trust them if the patients believe that they may be deceived by the health care personnel. Patient mistrust is a bad result; therefore, deception is ordinarily forbidden.

Utilitarianism is not the only form of teleological thinking, although it is the most popular one. Another form of teleological thinking that is important for professional persons examines an action and judges whether the action leads to an increase or decrease in the virtues necessary to be a good professional. This is known as *virtue ethics*. This philosophy starts with a list of virtues necessary to be, for example, a good physician, and then looks at daily actions and reflects on whether these actions lead to an increase or decrease in virtue. Actions that lead to an increase in virtue are good and those that lead to a decrease in virtue are bad. For example, in this point of view, deceiving a patient is wrong, not only because of the impact it has on the patient but also because it does not help the professional develop the virtue of truthfulness necessary to be a good professional. Only professionals who have developed the virtue of truthfulness will be able to sustain the trust of patients and their fellow professionals. Virtue ethics is an important philosophy to consider for persons developing professional lives.

Deontological Theories

A second way in which persons think about ethics is by asking whether proposed actions are right independent of their consequences. This is called *deontological reasoning*, which takes various forms.

Some philosophers argue that certain actions are wrong because they violate divine commands. Thus stealing is wrong because it is a violation of the commandment, "Thou shalt not steal." Other thinkers argue that actions can be wrong based on a hypothetical social contract. Defenders of the social contract perspective argue, for example, that the killing of the innocent is wrong because all of us have agreed not to kill unless in self-defense. Still other thinkers say that actions are to be judged on whether they respect or violate a person's rights. For example, all human beings have a right to the truth; persons who deceive us violate our rights. Deception is itself enough cause to call an action wrong, no matter how good the results.

Whatever basis they use—divine commands, social contract, or human rights—most deontological theorists focus on moral rules to guide our behavior. An action that breaks one of the rules is wrong. Deontologists are clear about the distinction between harms and wrongs. An action may be wrong even if no harms result from it. Thus, even if a patient is "successfully" deceived for whatever reason, that act of deception is wrong because it violates a moral rule.

Both teleological and deontological theories have been defended and criticized. These criticisms are part of a large literature in philosophical ethics. For our purposes, it is not important whether one thinks that any particular form of teleological or deontological reasoning is the most appropriate way to reason in ethics. Here we focus on four moral principles that can and have been justified according to both teleological and deontological reasoning. Once the four principles have been discussed, we turn to the application of those principles in the context of health care.

ETHICAL PRINCIPLES

Respect for Persons—Autonomy

Autonomy, perhaps the most important principle in modern medical ethics, is sometimes called *respect for autonomy* or simply *autonomy*. This means that the medical relationship should begin with the awareness of the patient as a moral agent. As such, a patient is entitled to govern himself or herself, freed as much as possible from internal or external constraints. When individuals achieve a certain minimum of self-governance such that they are judged to have the capacity to make decisions, these decisions ought to be respected.

It is often difficult to tell whether or not a person is autonomous. It involves making decisions about persons in their totality. It is preferable to focus on autonomous choices. These are choices that are intentional, made with appropriate understanding, and free of outside influences. There is one possible misunderstanding. An action can be autonomous and at the same time be part of the belief system of a particular community. As long as the patient freely accepts the belief system as his or her own, and acts according to that belief system, the action cannot be ruled as nonautonomous because it flows from his or her belief. Thus, a Jehovah's Witness' refusal of blood can be an autonomous action for a patient who freely accepts the life of a Witness.

Respect for persons gives rise to positive and negative duties. The negative duty is that health care personnel are to avoid deception and coercion of patients; in brief, there is a duty not to deceive or coerce. However, there is a positive obligation as well. Health caregivers must disclose information necessary for decision-making and maintain an atmosphere in which autonomous decision-making is supported. The most important practice in health care that is a sign of its commitment to respect for autonomy is the practice of asking patients for their consent. (Informed consent is discussed in detail further on.)

> Respecting a decision is not the same as agreeing with a decision; it involves not interfering with a decision that is made autonomously.

Nonmaleficence

One of the most important duties that all persons owe others is the duty not to harm them. In medicine, this is captured by the maxim, "First, do no harm." According to Beauchamp and Childress,[1] nonmaleficence is often mixed up with beneficence. We think that it should be separated, because health care provides a context in which there can be conflicts between these two obligations.

This does not mean that distinguishing these two principles is easy. Beauchamp and Childress do it in the following way:

- Nonmaleficence
- One ought not to inflict evil or harm.
- Beneficence

- One ought to prevent evil or harm.
- One ought to remove evil or harm.
- One ought to do or promote good.

The importance of the principle of nonmaleficence is that it reminds us that all harms must be justified by a greater good.

However these principles are ultimately distinguished, nonmaleficence demands that all persons forego causing harm. This is a prima facie rule, one that all must obey unless a stronger rule overrides it. Thus, in medicine, the physician causes harm by cutting a patient to remove an infected appendix. In this case, the expected good for the patient gives reason to proceed with the surgery. Medical personnel make decisions like this every day. The danger is that they become so used to these decisions that they do not realize they cause harm as they go about doing good.

The usual discussions of nonmaleficence focus on preventing grave harms, such as death or debilitating injury. Further, such discussions usually focus on the responsibilities of the health caregivers. In fact, the duty of nonmaleficence extends beyond health caregivers and becomes very important when persons are making decisions for others.

Harms can be caused by other than deliberate action. For example, harm can occur because of negligence on the part of the respiratory care practitioner. This means that there is an ethical as well as legal obligation to exercise due care in fulfilling one's professional responsibilities.

When nonmaleficence is being considered, it is important to take into account what the patient considers to be harm. A particular patient may think that he or she will be harmed by the use of medical technology that others find acceptable. This leads to the second conclusion about nonmaleficence. Not only must health caregivers balance harms and benefits to patients but also they must bring patients into the process of determining what counts as a harm and what counts as a benefit.

Beneficence

The third ethical principle of great importance is the principle of beneficence. Some argue that at one time, this was the central ethical principle in medicine. In ordinary language, beneficence suggests charity or kindness toward another. In fact, beneficence is an obligation and is used to describe all those actions that aim to benefit other persons.

Even the simplest action can be seen to be an act of beneficence, such as helping a child cross the street where there is heavy traffic.

In medicine, beneficence takes on special importance. It is simply assumed that one of the ends of medicine is patient benefit. Indeed, this assumption has often led to misunderstandings that because health care personnel intend to benefit patients, patients should accept their ministrations. Thus beneficence can sometimes cause tension when the intention to benefit conflicts with the patient's desire not to be treated. However, just because a patient may refuse an action that is beneficent in intention does not mean that health caregivers are excused from the obligation of beneficence. Indeed, it is important for health caregivers to establish that patient wishes are actually autonomously expressed; otherwise, patient wishes may be overridden. This view is called weak paternalism. Strong paternalism would justify overriding patient wishes even when the patient is fully autonomous.

Finally, not only is it important to provide benefit and remove harm but it is also often necessary to weigh the benefits being sought against the harms that may or will be done. One must first weigh the proposed benefit against the risk of harm and then weigh the harms that are a known outcome of the procedure against the proposed benefits, for example, an amputation in which one first weighs the risks of surgery against the proposed outcome of survival and then examines the known harm of amputation (the loss of a limb) and weighs that harm against the proposed benefit (life). Thus beneficence is not simply the obligation to benefit another but also an obligation to balance harms and benefits when both occur. This is called cost-benefit or risk-benefit analysis.

Justice

The fourth ethical principle, justice, is related to three distinct ideas in our society—fairness, entitlement, and desert. By trying to incorporate all three of these ideas into our discussion of justice, we intend to develop a discussion relevant for health care.

Fairness demands that, insofar as we can, we treat persons equally. Two respiratory care practitioners who received the same numerical test scores deserve the same letter grade for that test.

Entitlement reminds health caregivers that they often deal with what is owed to patients. Recipients of health care are owed that care as theirs, not as something that is the charity of the rest of society.

Finally, desert reminds us that to deny certain benefits to individuals under certain conditions is to treat them unjustly. For example, a respiratory care practitioner who has successfully completed a course of study deserves the recognition associated with that accomplishment, such as a diploma or a certificate.

There are three major types of theories of justice, each having its own distinctive conceptions of fairness, entitlement, and desert. According to Beauchamp and Childress, these are egalitarian theories, which emphasize the importance of equal access to all important goods; libertarian theories, which insist on rights; and utilitarian theories, which focus on the outcomes so that the public good is enhanced.

Most commentators think that, up until now, much of the health care in the United States has been developed under the influence of utilitarian theory.

Utilitarian theories of justice follow the type of thinking already identified in the discussion of utilitarian theory. In brief, one seeks the policy or policies that most enhance health in the aggregate; if one needs both public and private funding in order to accomplish this, so be it.

Defenders of the libertarian theory, in the absence of a societal agreement about how to distribute the benefits and burdens of health care, argue for a market-based system, in which health care is distributed based on one's ability to pay for it.

Libertarian theories focus not on outcomes but on fair procedures. Libertarians leave it up to the marketplace to determine how health care is to be distributed. Even organ exchanges should be handled under this market model, rather than the current system of organ donation. Libertarians argue that if we leave such decisions open to other types of decision-making, such as government, inevitably we find that private property is expropriated through one kind of taxation or other. Governments will take private monies in order to finance the government-developed health care plan instead of allowing individuals to purchase whatever health care they desire with their own monies. For libertarians, the individualist model of free choice is central to questions of justice in health care. Systems that are imposed and not freely chosen are unjust.

What is important for egalitarians is that no one would be without a basic minimum of health care.

The major alternative to a libertarian perspective is some form of egalitarianism. Egalitarians insist that some goods and services must be distributed equally, independent of a person's ability to pay. Different egalitarian theorists develop the implications of this claim in slightly different ways, but the general picture is consistent. Everyone should be provided with a decent minimum of health care so that differences among members of society with respect to health would be eliminated, at least for primary health care. Most theorists think that the United States is wealthy enough that the decent minimum would be adequate for the health care of most of the members of society. Maximal health care, beyond the level of the decent minimum, would be available to those who could pay for it.

As should be obvious by now, issues of justice in health care most often focus on distributive justice. What discussions of distributive justice presuppose is that health care is a scarce good, that not all of us can have all the health care we desire, and that some way must be found to constrain or limit our access to health care. The difficulties begin, of course, when theorists propose how we should make those difficult decisions. (We briefly discuss the most important alternatives for helping us make those decisions further on.)

PROFESSIONAL AND PATIENT ISSUES

Medical Uncertainty, Including Risk-Benefit Assessments

Any discussion of professional and patient issues in medicine proceeds under the presumption of medical uncertainty. Although many tools and tasks can reduce the margin of uncertainty in medicine, they do not eliminate it. This uncertainty exists at many different levels, including diagnosis. This is one of the prime functions of a physician, and diagnostic judgments are inexact and fallible. The consequence is that patients sometimes are treated for a disease they do not have or are not tested for the disease they do have.

Uncertainty can sometimes lead to extensive testing in order to attempt to eliminate uncertainty. Unfortunately, this testing can be performed when it is not appropriate, and it also can be performed in order to avoid making a decision. This can put patients at risk, cause discomfort and pain, and increase the cost of their health care.

Beyond diagnosis, physicians notoriously have difficulty in making prognostic judgments, especially judgments about the life span of persons with terminal illness. Physicians have been frequently surprised by patient outcomes, making them wary about prognostic judgments. In reaction to this uncertainty, they may be tentative or reluctant in making predictions about outcomes.

Uncertainty does not end with diagnosis and prognosis. It extends to therapeutics and research as well. Physicians can know the risks and benefits of a particular therapy for the population at large but not know what is going to happen in a particular case.[2]

Risk and benefits of the same treatment might be, and often are, markedly different for different patients.

The uncertainty becomes even more complex when different studies report different results about the same therapeutic intervention. For example, there is much discussion about the effectiveness of cardiopulmonary resuscitation (CPR) for the elderly. One study reports decreased effectiveness for persons older than 69 years of age.[3] Another study reports no statistically significant difference for different age groups.[4] Inappropriate conclusions may be drawn from either study.

Uncertainty gives rise to a number of ethical questions for the respiratory care practitioner. The practitioner will be asked questions by patients and family members, who will themselves be uncertain about matters (uncertain in the sense that they do not have information). Practitioners must be cautious in responding to these queries for information. They should be clear about what is certain and what is unknown at any given point. If they are not, patients and families will suffer much distress that could have been avoided with careful communication.

Uncertainty has a number of other important effects on the discussion of ethical issues in medicine. First, medical personnel should work to eliminate uncertainty when possible. The medical care team seeks to help the patient and avoid doing harm. Second, medical personnel should avoid irreversible life and death ethical decisions in situations of great medical uncertainty. Again, this is mandated in order to avoid harm.

Truthfulness

Truthfulness is one of the practical implications of "respect for persons" that is often overlooked in everyday medical activity. Most often it is overlooked not because persons wish to be deceitful but because the imperative, "Tell the truth"" is in competition with other realities in medicine, including the realities of human relationships.

Consider, for example, the following question from a spouse, "How is my husband doing?" The natural inclination on the part of many members of the health care team is to give an answer that is sometimes no more than their own opinion. Since another member of the health care team can be asked the same question and have another opinion, there is the possibility of confusion on the part of the spouse. In response to this potential problem, health care team members often answer with a guarded response. "What did the physician say?" "What did the nurse tell you?" What has happened here is that members of the health care team rightly want consistent information conveyed to the patient or surrogate, or both. This is important so that patients and families are not confused. Yet, in the desire to maintain consistency, there is the possibility that the professional judgments of the members of the health care team will not be communicated clearly.

It should be clear by now that truthfulness is more than the correspondence of our statements with the facts. Obviously, factual accuracy is essential. This means that health care personnel are obligated to tell, insofar as it is possible to know, what the facts are. In addition, attempts to deceive the patient are not permitted. The only exception to this is the therapeutic privilege. In that case, one has to be convinced that knowing the factual truth of the situation will harm the patient's health. Invoking this privilege should be an extremely rare event; all presumptions should be that members of the medical team should relay the factual truth to the patient or surrogate, or both. The respiratory care practitioner cannot invoke the therapeutic privilege. That is the responsibility of the attending physician alone.

The factual truth should include an assessment of what is not known as well as that which is known. As we have already pointed out, there is much uncertainty in medicine, and when that uncertainty might be important for patient decisions, the uncertainty should be shared with patients and their families. Factual accuracy is only part of truthfulness. It is not simply that the patient and surrogate are owed the factual truth. They are owed this as theirs, as something they do not have to discover for themselves. The truth is not the health professional's, with the patient having the obligation to find it out.

There is a third element of telling the truth that is important. That element is empathy, which is part of the professional responsibility of health care professionals. What medical professionals tend to forget is that a part of what patients want to know is whether they will continue to be cared for. For them, the truth of the case is not simply the factual information that is known, along with all that is unknown, but also the promise of competent care and that the ill person will not be abandoned. When the patient or surrogate understands that competent, caring treatment will be provided no matter how bleak the diagnosis and prognosis, he or she is free to take charge of his or her life and to cooperate, insofar as possible, with the health care team.

Informed Consent

Informed consent is a necessary condition of autonomy. Although it is sometimes considered the legal arm of autonomy, it is an integral part of the decision-making process within health care. Some persons confuse the process of informed consent with the written consent form. Obtaining the signature of a patient on a consent form does not assure informed consent. In addition, autonomy encompasses both decisions to consent and to refuse treatment, and the process for either consenting to or refusing treatment is encompassed in the usual usage of informed consent.

Four components of informed consent-refusal must be fulfilled if autonomous decisions are to be achieved:

- Adequate information
- Comprehension of the information
- Voluntariness
- Competency or capacity of the patient

These assume mutual participation and respect between the patient and the provider and demand genuine communication and agreement about the course of action.

Accurate information may be judged by two standards. The first is based on the information commonly provided by competent practitioners in the community or specialty. The second is the reasonable person concept, in which adequate information allows reasonable persons to make prudent choices on their own behalf. In any case, the person must have enough information concerning the diagnosis and prognosis, as well as the benefits, burdens, and alternatives of a treatment plan, to make an autonomous decision consistent with his or her value system. If the amount of information is overwhelming or is presented in a biased, insensitive, or inappropriate manner, even if the facts are correct and complete, the information may not be "adequate."

The information must be given in an understandable way. This seems self-evident. The most obvious example of this is being certain that the patient understands the language used to impart the information. If not, a translator should be obtained to provide the necessary translation. The patient's level of education also determines the kind of language that will be comprehensible in this process. Minimizing medical jargon and technical terms is essential for many patients, whereas for others it would be demeaning or insulting. The art of medicine is needed to help assess the needs of the individual patient or family under the circumstances of illness and anxiety.

The standard of voluntariness may have both external and internal components. This means that there should be no coercion from within or without. Hints of abandonment or ignoring suffering if the proposal is refused by the patient may not allow the individual to make an autonomous decision and act on that decision. This type of coercion may also come from other outside forces, such as the family and friends. Within the patient, feelings of guilt, remorse, anxiety, depression, and hostility, among other emotions, may prevent autonomous thought and action and

Informed consent is central to both the ethical and legal relationship between the patient and the provider of health care.

The entire process of achieving informed consent-refusal requires time, patience and understanding on the part of the caregiver.

The health care provider should neither subtly nor blatantly threaten the patient to urge acceptance of a procedure or treatment plan.

Physicians and other health professionals should also remember that they are influenced by their own personal values and unconscious motivations, which they bring to their role as providers.

Religious beliefs may appear irrational to the nonbeliever, but if it is an established system of values such as those of Jehovah's Witnesses, holding these beliefs does not indicate incapacity or loss of autonomous decision-making ability. Choosing and acting on these beliefs should not pose a threat to others.

provide a coercive internal environment that may be difficult to recognize and even more difficult to overcome. This standard has many nuances and, like the next standard, capacity or competency, presents a continuing challenge to the patient-provider relationship in the context of informed consent. It may be impossible to eliminate an element of coercion when the patient is weak, helpless, and at the mercy of others.

Informed consent requires the patient's capacity to understand and integrate the information into his or her value system for living. It must be put into the context of a real person who had a full life preceding the decision. Health professionals are advised to use the term *capacity*, since competency is a legal term and is determined only by the courts. However, in everyday parlance, the two terms are frequently used interchangeably, devoid of the legal finality. At the bedside or in the office, decisions must be made, and the evaluation of the patient's capacity to make and carry out autonomous choices may be made by assumption or intention. Competency does not necessarily mean rationality. Patients may hold unusual beliefs that appear irrational to others but are important parts of the patient's value system. In general, the ethical principle of autonomy requires that these beliefs be respected even though they appear mistaken to others. For the health professional for whom beneficence and, in the recent past, paternalism has had a powerful ethical influence, it is difficult to stand by and watch a patient make a choice that seems so personally detrimental and injurious. However, it is the patient's life and the patient's choice as long as it is consistent with who he or she is and does not injure third parties. Saying this does not relieve the professional of the responsibility of providing ongoing information and an alternative perspective on the patient's choice if the professional thinks the patient is choosing unwisely.

Emergency care, when there is no valid way of knowing the patient's wishes or value system, precludes the need for capacity determination or informed consent. A comatose or unresponsive patient does not present a dilemma about capacity; he or she has none. Most other patients who seek out or are brought to the health professional fall at the other end of the capacity spectrum. They are alert, oriented, and capable of understanding and processing information for decision-making. However, there is a group of patients who fall into an indeterminate area in which their capacity is questioned and it is suspected they are unable to make autonomous decisions and therefore cannot give informed consent or refusal.

Over the years, it has become evident that capacity (competency) is not an all-or-nothing phenomenon.[5] Some persons have the capacity to make some decisions but not others, depending on the complexity and probabilities associated with the decision. Some illnesses allow a person to have adequate capacity intermittently but not at all times. Sometimes a treatment such as hemodialysis will restore capacity so that the patient can have self-determination. The level of capacity needed for autonomous decision-making varies with the gravity of the decision to be made. The greater the risk of danger, regardless of the decision, the higher the standard of competence needed for making that decision. A high benefit-burden ratio allows a lower level of understanding, comprehension, and reasoning than when the outcomes of treatment are less certain and the potential side effects more severe. The degree of suffering and pain that diagnostic and treatment procedures will cause must be weighed by the patient against the potential benefit or benefits. This can be exemplified by contrasting treating a pneumococcal pneumonia with penicillin and

Having a completed values history would be helpful to health care providers and families in determining the authenticity and constancy of patient's decisions.

treating an incurable cancer with a toxic chemotherapeutic agent. The capacity needed to process the benefits and burdens and arrive at a deliberate decision is greater in the latter scenario than in the treatment of a common pneumonia.

The authenticity and constancy of the decision with the patient's previous life history are important. Refusal of a treatment that seems rational to most persons may be consistent for the patient who has lived a life of stark independence, rejecting authority to his or her detriment throughout life. The choice may be totally "in character" for this person and consistent with and authentic to his or her previous decisions and actions.

The problem of depression complicates the determinations of capacity for autonomous decision-making in some patients. How much depression is "normal" and "acceptable" under the circumstances of a particular person's life and illness? When is the patient internally coerced by the depression to such a degree that the capacity for decision-making is impaired, preventing autonomous thinking? These are difficult questions and even with psychiatric aid and evaluation, the answers sometimes are not clear.

The entire process of informed consent requires mutual respect, extensive ongoing dialogue, and patience and persistence in the patient-provider relationship. In modern medicine, it often benefits from a team approach in providing information to and promoting understanding by the patient as well as in evaluating the patient's capacity for giving informed consent-refusal.

Surrogacy

A surrogate is an individual or institution who speaks for another person when that person is incapable of making autonomous decisions.

Surrogates have an ethical obligation to speak for the patient within certain principles of conduct. Surrogates should not act on the basis of what they would want for themselves if they were in a similar situation. Rather, they should make decisions for the patient using the principle of "substituted judgment" or "best interest."

The surrogate tries to mimic what the patient would say if he or she could make autonomous decisions.

When the previously competent patient is no longer able to make competent decisions, the extension of autonomy may be provided by a surrogate. This person may be a court-appointed guardian. In some jurisdictions, a family member who has a bonded and loving relationship with the person who is ill becomes the surrogate in practice. There may or may not be a legally established order for determining who speaks for the patient. In some states, practice has established a hierarchy similar to the order of authority for giving autopsy permission after death. The law in most states requires a court order granting guardianship even to family members before they can consent to or refuse medical care on behalf of an adult family member.

Substituted judgment requires the surrogate to know the patient's value system and his or her wishes concerning treatment during illness and the attitude toward suffering, disability, and death. This presumes discussions of preferences with the patient when he or she is competent and experience with the person's actions and reactions during living prior to the illness and the onset of incompetence. The surrogate attempts to place himself or herself into the patient's heart and mind and make decisions consistent with the patient's wishes, desires, and convictions.

If the surrogate has no way of knowing the patient's preferences because they had never been expressed or clarified, the principle of "best interest" should be used for decision-making. This principle involves weighing the benefits and burdens and determining what course of action would serve the patient best using some more objective, socially shared values. What would most reasonable persons in the same situation decide? This stretches the concept of autonomy and falls more appropriately under the principle of beneficence. In some jurisdictions, as exemplified by the Cruzan decision in Missouri (discussed further on), best interest standards are not enough and even substituted judgment standards are set very high in order to withdraw or withhold life-sustaining therapy. What the court in Missouri required was "clear and convincing evidence" of the patient's wishes. Some have argued that this demands direct instructions or documentation of the patient's preferences and wishes prior to the onset of incompetency (e.g., written living wills or durable powers of attorney).

Advance Directives

A person can extend his or her autonomous wishes and decisions regarding medical care into the portion or portions of his or her life when he or she will become incompetent by providing documented information while still competent. Informally, this is carried out by expressions to family members, friends, or professional persons indicating attitudes and convictions about life and death and medical care. This "hit or miss" approach is often never fully developed or clarified, and a great deal of doubt or uncertainty arises when the decisions must be made. However, the usual surrogate decision-making process depends heavily on this communication. Using an advance directive that is written and witnessed is a more formal expression of a person's wishes.

Another legally formalized way of extending one's wishes is through the "durable power of attorney for health care." The patient, while competent, designates a willing person to make health care decisions if and when the patient becomes incompetent. The power does not become effective until incompetency is declared. Unlike a usual power of attorney, which becomes null and void when the person no longer has capacity for autonomous decision-making, the "durable" power starts when the patient becomes incompetent and lasts through incompetency. This presumes that the patient informs the surrogate of his or her wishes and attitudes toward health care while competent. The surrogate with durable power of attorney then uses substituted judgment to make decisions for the patient, especially concerning medical treatment. The presence of a person with whom the health care team can communicate allows an ongoing exchange between competent persons in the decision-making process; it is more of a "living document" than the customary living will or written advance directive.

For many persons, the term *living will* is synonymous with the advance directive, which is broader and more generic in meaning. Living wills historically have been rejectionist documents stating, often in vague and confusing terms, the medical care that is not wanted if the patient is in a certain condition, such as terminal illness. Often they do not include conditions that are not terminal or the problems that surround the "hopelessly" ill. In 35 states, the law requires medical certification of a terminal condition before the document can be executed.

Living wills can be helpful to health caregivers and families. However, living wills often fail to capture the complexity of the conditions of modern medical care. For example, there are living wills that use vague phrases such as "no reasonable expectation of recovery from extreme physical and mental disability." Phrases like these compound the problematic decision-making for these patients. There is the possibility of

In most states in the United States there is "living will" legislation making these documents legally binding but also, in some instances, restricting the contents of these directives (Fig. 58–1).

Artificial means, heroic measures, life-sustaining procedures, extraordinary, and *treatments that only prolong the process of dying* are terms and phrases that have too many conflicting meanings to be useful and helpful.

To My Family, My Physician, My Lawyer
And All Others Whom It May Concern

Death is as much a reality as birth, growth, and aging—it is the one certainty of life. In anticipation of decisions that may have to be made about my own dying and as an expression of my right to refuse treatment, I _____ being of sound mind, make this statement of my wishes and instructions concerning treatment. (print name)

By means of this document, which I intend to be legally binding, I direct my physician and other care providers, my family, and any surrogate designated by me or appointed by a court, to carry out my wishes. If I become unable, by reason of physical or mental incapacity, to make decisions about my medical care, let this document provide the guidance and authority needed to make any and all such decisions.

If I am permanently unconscious or there is no reasonable expectation of my recovery from a seriously incapacitating or lethal illness or condition, I do not wish to be kept alive by artificial means. I request that I be given all care necessary to keep me comfortable and free of pain, even if pain-relieving medications may hasten my death, and I direct that no life-sustaining treatment be provided except as I or my surrogate specifically authorize.

This request may appear to place a heavy responsibility upon you, but by making this decision according to my strong convictions, I intend to ease that burden. I am acting after careful consideration and with understanding of the consequences of your carrying out my wishes. *List optional specific provisions in the space below. (See other side)*

_____ **Durable Power of Attorney for Health Care Decisions** (Cross out if you do not wish to use this section) _____

To effect my wishes, I designate _____,
residing at _____ (Phone #) _____ ,
(or if he or she shall for any reason fail to act, _____ (Phone #) _____ ,
residing at _____) as my health care surrogate—
that is, my attorney-in-fact regarding any and all health care decisions to be made for me, including the decision to refuse life-sustaining treatment—if I am unable to make such decisions myself. This power shall remain effective during and not be affected by my subsequent illness, disability or incapacity. My surrogate shall have authority to interpret my Living Will, and shall make decisions about my health care as specified in my instructions or, when my wishes are not clear, as the surrogate believes to be in my best interests. I release and agree to hold harmless my health care surrogate from any and all claims whatsoever arising from decisions made in good faith in the exercise of this power.

I sign this document knowingly, voluntarily, and after careful deliberation, this _____ day of _____, 19 _____.

_____
(signature)

Address _____

_____

I do hereby certify that the within document was executed and acknowledged before me by the principal this_____ day of _____, 19 _____.

_____
Notary Public

Witness_____

Printed Name _____

Address _____

_____

Witness_____

Printed Name _____

Address _____

Copies of this document have been given to:

(Optional) My Living Will is registered with Concern for Dying (No. _____)
Distributed by Concern for Dying, 250 West 57th Street, New York, NY 10107 (212) 246-6962

FIGURE 58–1: An example of a living will. (Reprinted by permission of Concern for Dying, 250 W. 57th Street, New York, NY, 10107.)

added confusion if the living will uses imprecise terms delineating the types of medical interventions that may be used or terminated.

Emanuel has suggested a more comprehensive and detailed document which they prefer to call an advance care document.[6] In this document, various scenarios of illness for an incompetent patient are presented and the person, while competent, can make choices about different kinds of interventions they would want, reject, or like to try under the described circumstances. The response can also be "I don't know." This type of document, in conjunction with the durable power of attorney for health care, can provide a more complete picture of the incompetent patient's wishes and a better chance of extending the autonomous decisions of the person who is ill.

All advance directives can suffer from the same deficiencies as informed consent-refusal of the competent patient. The documents should be completed using the same principles as informed consent-refusal: adequate information, comprehension, voluntariness, and competency.

In states that do not have living will legislation, the ethical force of these expressions of autonomous decisions should be honored and incorporated into the health providers' care of the patient. Federal legislation has been passed requiring that patients be asked whether they have a living will when entering a health care program such as a hospital, nursing home, hospice, and so forth. Coupled with this legislation is a plan for widespread societal education about advance directives. As societal conversation is promoted concerning these issues of life and death decisions, competent patients should be better prepared to make their preferences known in a meaningful and effective way, which would allow their wishes to be followed more accurately if and when they become incompetent.

Confidentiality

Remember that confidentiality belongs to the patient.

Confidentiality is one of the most taken for granted and, at the same time, one of the most ignored realities in medicine. It is not surprising that it is ignored. First, unlike earlier times in the practice of medicine, many persons see the medical record. This includes persons who are not part of the medical care team, for example, persons who work for insurance companies. Second, not only do many persons see the record but confidentiality can be ignored without the abuses appearing to be malicious. Part of the lore of medicine is the odd or unusual case. In the process of giving the details of the interesting case, medical personnel often violate the confidentiality of the patient. This does not refer to the exchange of information among members of the medical team but to telling persons who come into contact with team members. The patient may indeed have given permission for caregivers to exchange information; this does not mean that the patient gave permission to tell luncheon partners who work in a different critical care unit about the patient's problems. Yet this kind of conversation occurs frequently.

Within the limits of law and reality, the patients are the persons who can choose what should be concealed and what may be revealed about them. Confidentiality is not the right of the hospital, or the physician, or the medical care team. Recognizing this may save some time when there are discussions about the limits of confidentiality. This does not mean that there are not limits on patient confidentiality. There are legal requirements, such as the obligation of a physician to report a gunshot wound. There are moral limits, such as the case of the child-molesting father who wants his molestations to remain a secret. This means that there are times when medical personnel are obligated to tell. There are also situations about which there are legitimate differences of opinion. For example, there is a variety of opinion about whether physicians have an obligation to inform sexual partners of human immunodeficiency virus (HIV)-positive patients about the partner's HIV status if the HIV-positive patient refuses to do so.

Given that there will be a time when disclosure is mandated, and that there will be a time when it is forbidden, how do medical personnel decide what to do? There are no absolute rules to guide us. Conversation with trusted peers can be a source of ethical insight. Medical personnel cannot go back to a time when confidentiality could be taken for granted. What respiratory care practitioners can do is keep in front of themselves the obligation to keep confidences, recognize that there are legal as well as moral limits on this obligation, and strive to be discreet in their discussions of matters about patients.

Belief Systems

As our society becomes more pluralistic, there is no doubt that health care workers will come into contact with persons who have beliefs that differ from theirs. Historically, health care workers have had difficulty dealing with persons who held religious beliefs that were radically at odds with the beliefs of the majority of persons in our society. The issue of religious identity often comes up when persons wish to refuse or limit health care; those treatment refusals or limitations appear irrational. In the United States, this issue has arisen most often with Jehovah's Witnesses.

Jehovah's Witnesses believe that they are forbidden to take blood or blood products. Thus they refuse to consent to blood transfusions for themselves or their children. This is a case in which respect for persons is in tension with beneficence. In the case of a competent adult Jehovah's Witness, the principle of respect for persons is thought to be the more important principle, and thus the wishes of the Jehovah's Witness not to be transfused should be honored. However, it is different in the case of children. Children are not competent adults. In their case, others can act beneficently on their behalf. Following this principle, hospitals routinely go to court to have a guardian appointed who will consent to transfusions for the child.

The medical treatment of Jehovah's Witnesses must be handled with special sensitivity on the part of all members of the health care team, not simply because persons owe respect to every person but because there are differences of belief among Jehovah's Witnesses themselves. This makes the treatment of an individual Jehovah's Witness something that has to be carefully managed. Some Witnesses believe that they will be condemned to punishment if they consent to receive blood or blood products, but that if they do not consent and blood or blood products are given, they are relieved of any responsibility before their God. Other Witnesses believe that they will be condemned if they have a blood transfusion whether or not they consented.

This means that members of the health care team must listen carefully to what they are being told by Witnesses. Generally, they will discover that the Witnesses do desire medical care and will be cooperative with members of the health care team. However, their refusal of blood and blood products is part of who they are, and it is at that point that they put a limitation on the health care team, a limitation that must be respected as other treatment limitations of competent adults are respected.

Professional Roles and Team Membership

Because the diagnostic and therapeutic aspects of medicine have become so complex and sophisticated, there has been a need for persons to specialize their intellect and energies to apply this knowledge. This specialization has had far-reaching effects in the delivery of medical care to patients, for good and for ill.

Specialization allows a practitioner to become expert in a more manageable body of knowledge and techniques, providing in-depth application of these to the patient. It brings current and "cutting edge" theories and practices within a specialty to the patient-practitioner encounter. At the same time it has necessitated involvement of multiple persons in the care of a single patient in order for various aspects of the patient's needs to be provided expertly. This may lead to fragmentation of care and uncoordinated efforts. Conversely, this type of care has the potential for producing a whole that is greater than the sum of the parts if the individual efforts of the specialists are integrated and applied in a unified way. Here the concept of the team arises, in which many talents are focused to accomplish a known common objective. The full potential of each individual member is encouraged within the framework of the team's objectives and, ideally, the contributions of all the members of the team are melded into a seamless whole. This usually requires the leadership and authority of someone to "coach," "conduct," or "edit" the efforts on behalf of the patient. When that integration does not occur, the patient might perceive fragmentation, confusion, and isolation. Without appropriate application, the process lacks warmth, compassion, and patient-centered interest and instead becomes mechanical and uninvolved.

The roles of the individual practitioners in the care of the patient require definition and clarification. In the United States, even the roles of physicians, who have an oath tradition, have become unsure and ill-defined. One accepts certain personal risks and responsibilities when one enters the health professions; these should be made apparent and real to each practitioner during the educational and developmental process. The issues of truth telling, confidentiality, trustworthiness, and nonabandonment are a part of this identity. The meaning of caring, compassion, and service in the delivery of competent care should be understood and incorporated into the practice of each professional.

The role of the respiratory care practitioner is evolving, but there is little doubt that he or she plays a significant and important part in the collective effort of health care providers. The ethical tenets and processes that are considered in this chapter are relevant and applicable to the respiratory care practitioner. What is sometimes not so clear is how the therapist carries them out within the framework of the "team" and how the efforts of the practitioner are integrated into the patient-centered objectives. This can probably best be accomplished by having well-informed, dedicated practitioners who communicate and interact freely with the other members of the health care team. There are many issues that need to be resolved among the various members of the team. Authority, expertise, responsibility, and accountability within the health care arena are some of the important and ongoing issues that must be dealt with, seeking resolutions that provide the best care or cure, or both, to the patient as a human being who has a unique value system and a life experience outside the health care practitioner–patient relationship. Respiratory care practitioners can and should play an important role in resolving these issues.

Patient Advocacy

One term that has come into vogue in health care is *patient advocacy*. Various members of the health care community have claimed the role of patient advocate. Teams in medicine should have the patient as their focus of attention, and this focus on the patient is everyone's responsibility. However, this focus does not constitute patient advocacy. Patient advocacy involves doing only what patients want. Health care providers have additional responsibilities, however, which may preclude fulfilling the advocacy role. At the same time, the term *patient advocacy* reminds us that the patient is the focus of our efforts.

SELECTED TOPICS

Brain Death

The respiratory care practitioner often participates in the care of patients who are suspected of being or have been declared "brain dead." Brain death, a modern medical designation of death, has become a legal designation of death in most of the United States. Through the Uniform Determination of Death Act, consistent state laws have been passed in most states that equate brain death with clinical and legal death. This new definition of death historically grew out of the Harvard Committee Criteria for Brain Death published in the *Journal of the American Medical Association* in 1968.[7] Confusingly, as pointed out by Cranford,[8] they used the term *irreversible coma*, a concept that includes conditions that are different from brain death. Prior to the Brain Death Act, death was declared only when the person stopped breathing and the heart stopped beating.

Certainty of diagnosis is a requirement for the determination of death. No false-positive results can be tolerated; the patient's lack of neurologic function must be irreversible. No one meeting these criteria has ever improved and a person who is brain dead seldom can have cardiac function maintained beyond a few weeks or, rarely, months, and by definition has no ventilatory drive. There is no ethical question of withholding or withdrawing treatment or care from a person with brain death. Brain death is death that requires only those duties due a corpse.

The declaration of brain death requires a knowledgeable physical examination, specifically a designated neurologic evaluation. Although laboratory testing is sometimes warranted and used, brain death can be diagnosed with a physical examination performed by a physician who is capable of carrying out a thorough and accurate neurologic examination. There should be a known cause for the completely unresponsive state. Certain conditions, such as hypothermia and drug intoxication (especially barbiturates), must be ruled out. The patient has no reaction to deep pain and exhibits no movement (although some spinal reflexes may be present). Seizures or posturing (decorticate, decerebrate) preclude the diagnosis of brain death.

By definition, any patient being evaluated for brain death is on ventilatory support. A person who is brain dead has no function of the brain stem and consequently will have no ventilatory drive or function subserved by the cranial nerves. The pupillary, corneal, and oculovestibular reflexes are absent. There are no oculocephalic reflexes (doll's eyes). Heartbeat, as well as other vegetative functions related to internal homeostasis, can continue, since these functions are semiautonomous.

Two bedside tests should be part of every examination for brain death. The first test is caloric stimulation of the vestibular nerve. This is performed by placing ice water in the ear canals and observing for appro-

---

The Brain Death Act defines death as follows: "An individual who has sustained either

• Irreversible cessation of circulatory and respiratory functions
• Irreversible cessation of all functions of the entire brain, including the brain stem, is dead."

Any person who can swallow, gag, or cough is not brain dead.

Semiautonomous—not completely dependent on the integrity of the brain stem.

priate ocular responses (nystagmus). The brain dead patient has no oculovestibular reflexes bilaterally.

The second bedside test involves the respiratory care practitioner's participation. The ventilated patient must be tested for apnea—complete lack of respiratory drive even in the face of hypercapnia. At the same time, the patient must be protected from hypoxemia during the test to avoid any additional hypoxic damage to the central nervous system. Each respiratory care department should have an approved protocol for this procedure. The goal is to allow the P_{CO_2} to rise to at least 60 mm Hg and observe for any signs of ventilatory effort on the part of the patient. The hypercapnia assures maximal ventilatory stimulus. Prior to disconnecting the patient from the ventilator, he or she is hyperoxygenated with 100% oxygen; an oxygen catheter delivering supplemental oxygen is then inserted into the endotracheal or tracheostomy tube. The pretest arterial blood gas determination will indicate the state of ventilation and how much the P_{CO_2} will have to rise to meet the test goal.

Carbon dioxide tension will rise at 3 to 4 mm Hg/min, and the length of time needed to reach a P_{CO_2} of 60 mm Hg can be calculated. The patient is observed closely during this time off the ventilator. If there is no sign of ventilation initiated by the patient's brain stem, an arterial blood gas determination should be performed and the patient placed back on the ventilator. If the arterial blood analysis shows the desired hypercapnia, the patient can be declared apneic with maximal ventilatory stimulation, which is supportive of the diagnosis of brain death.

In some cases, the physician will want an electroencephalogram (EEG) to determine the lack of electrical activity in the brain (a flat EEG), although this is not always required. Other tests such as a brain scan, cerebral arteriogram, or computed tomographic scan of the brain may be indicated in certain clinical settings.

When brain death is declared, there are no longer any ethical issues regarding withholding or withdrawing therapy. The patient may be removed from the ventilator, along with any other diagnostic or therapeutic apparatus. In some cases, the viability of the internal organs may need to be maintained for a time until they can be removed for transplantation to a living recipient. For this purpose, the body is ventilated and oxygenated while the circulatory status is supported. Although the body may appear alive with electromechanical heart function maintained, the person is dead, clinically and legally.

Occasionally, ventilation and other supportive physiologic maneuvers will be maintained until the family is prepared emotionally for the death. However, a family or surrogate should not be given the option to maintain a corpse in this situation. It may require kind and compassionate explanations from the health care providers, since the loved one does not appear dead in the traditional sense. Sensitivity to the family's emotional needs is needed, along with other services that provide psychological and social support.

A flat EEG is not synonymous with brain death, since some patients with persistent vegetative state (PVS) have flat EEGs as well.

Persistent Vegetative State

The persistent vegetative state (PVS) presents an ethically and clinically more difficult patient condition than brain death. The definition and diagnosis are more imprecise; therefore a greater margin for error exists.

PVS should be distinguished from coma, which is a sleep-like (eyes closed) unarousable state resulting from extensive damage to the reticular activating systems of the brain stem. Coma patients usually do not have long-term survival, even with maximal medical-nursing care because they often have impaired cough, gag, and swallowing reflexes, which makes them prone to aspiration and infection.

In PVS, the brain stem and ascending reticular activating system are relatively intact. Cerebral hemispheres are the part of the central nervous system that is destroyed, often secondary to ischemia or hypoxia, or both. A high metabolic rate of the cerebral cortex makes it particularly vulnerable to deprivation of blood flow and oxygen, whereas the brain stem is relatively resistant to ischemia and hypoxia. Loss of oxygen or blood flow, or both; for 4 to 6 minutes is known to cause extensive destruction of the cerebral cortex. This neocortical death has also been referred to as cognitive death. The initial phase may be manifested as coma, but later the condition becomes "eyes-opened" unconsciousness. There are wake-sleep cycles, and the eyes wander without sustained visual pursuit. This patient is unconscious, unaware of self or surrounding environment. The pupils react to light, and the protective gag, cough, and swallowing reflexes are usually normal. This is a major reason that these patients can live for long periods (longest recorded is 38 years) with appropriate care. Some will smile meaninglessly or may chronically chew or clamp their teeth, and most have impaired motor functions with varying degrees of weakness, spasticity, posturing, and contractures of the limbs. They are incontinent of urine and stool.

Positron emission tomography in patients with PVS shows severely depressed energy metabolism uniformly distributed throughout the cortical and immediate subcortical areas of the cerebral hemispheres. This is equivalent to what is found during deep general anesthesia in normal persons. Although these patients often require mechanical ventilation after the initial insult, they usually can be weaned from the ventilator and have adequate respiratory drive and control on their own. In addition, the retention of the protective reflexes of cough and gagging makes these patients less prone to aspiration, secretion retention, and pneumonia.

Armstrong and Colen[9] describe the state: "These are not patients with diminished capacity. They are unable to give or, what is far more important, perceive love on even the most primitive of levels. Rather, they are nonmentative organ systems, artificially sustained—like valued cell lines in cancer laboratories."

The prognosis for return of any awareness varies with age and the cause of the initial insult. After cardiac arrest, few PVS patients regain awareness after 1 month and essentially none regain cognition after 3 months in the vegetative state. Even for young persons who have a better prognosis for some recovery, a conservative criterion for no recovery of consciousness after head trauma would consist of observed unawareness for at least 12 months. Brain trauma and subarachnoid hemorrhage have a better prognosis for improvement than does asphyxia.

Do patients with PVS feel pain or have the capacity to suffer? Physiologic evidence indicates that persons without cortical function cannot "feel" pain and therefore cannot experience pain and suffering. However, subcortical reactions to stimuli can produce facial movements and other signs that we associate with conscious human suffering. These patients cannot experience dyspnea, thirst, hunger, or pain.

At present, PVS is not equivalent to death medically, ethically, or legally. There is general agreement that the usual characteristics of

The degree of certainty of the diagnosis and prognosis of PVS is less absolute than that of brain death. The EEG varies in PVS from flat (silent) to normal, with less than 5% in the normal range.

personhood are lacking, since there is permanent and irreversible lost of conscious interaction between the patient and the environment. The patient is a body bereft of its cognitive functions and personality.

Judgments of Futility and Hopeless Illness

Often the respiratory care practitioner hears about a case described as "hopeless" or "futile." For our purposes, these terms are equivalent. Sometimes their meaning is unclear. A person might be "hopeless" because he or she will never be able to live independently; another person might be "hopeless" because he or she is at the end stages of terminal illness and is expected to die shortly. What becomes clear is that there is no agreement on a definition of a "hopeless" or "futile" case; in that situation, language must be used carefully.

If futility is defined in terms of goals that incorporate the wishes and values of the patient, an end-point for comparison exists, and decisions can be measured against these goals. For example, if an unweanable, terminally ill, yet alert patient on a ventilator has a goal of living until a favorite grandchild graduates from college next month, it would not be futile to continue ventilator support and treatment. Once the goal has been met, the ventilator may be futile therapy if the patient considers it too burdensome and does not want to prolong dying. At that point, the patient may consider the continuation of care futile because medically there is no hope of being successfully weaned from the ventilator. Conversely, if the grandchild is not due to graduate for another 2 years, the goal of this patient may be unrealistic and therefore unattainable. In that situation, the continuation of therapy may be considered "hopeless" or "futile."

Ideally, the medical care team and the patient should set the treatment goals together; however, this is not always possible. What is important is to involve the patient in this process when it is possible so that the medical care team is not judging a situation hopeless when the patient finds it satisfactory. The more difficult problem arises when families insist that "everything must be done." Often this leads to a situation in which medical care personnel have conflicting feelings. On the one hand, they would like to follow the wishes of the family. On the other hand, in their best medical judgment the goals of the family are unrealistic and would subject the patient to treatments that would not be effective. Yet the family insists.

What might be done? Medical care personnel should remember the following points. First, their primary responsibility is to the patient and not to the patient's family. Second, if in the judgment of the medical care team, the given therapy is not going to assist a treatment goal, team members are not obliged to begin or continue treatment. This does not mean that they should do nothing for the patient; treatment goals can change from life-preserving to palliative care. What is important to remember is that judgments of futility relate to treatment goals and that physicians and patients should be involved in the discussion of the goals.

Withholding and Withdrawing Medical Therapy

Ethically, legally, and clinically, autonomy or self-determination has become the key principle in the United States for delivering medical

Incompetent—does not have the necessary capacity to make the decision.

services to and interacting with individual patients. Judge Cordozza's ruling in 1914 that "Every human being of adult years and sound mind has the right to determine what shall be done to his (her) own body," has been used to substantiate case law while generally being accepted by ethicists, including deontologists and teleologists. The process of withholding and withdrawing treatment depends on informed consent-refusal, which is integral to autonomous action. Therefore, adequate information given in a noncoercive and understandable way to a person who has the capacity to make the decision is vital to making a decision for withholding and withdrawing medical treatments. If the person is incompetent, autonomy is extended by and through a surrogate, usually a close family member who is bonded to the patient. A surrogate may also be someone who has a durable power of attorney for health care for the patient. Sometimes a court-appointed guardian will be necessary.

For many years, physicians and other health care providers believed and acted as though withdrawing a therapy was ethically and legally different from withholding a therapy. Withdrawing therapy was equated with "active euthanasia," directly causing death, whereas withholding treatment was thought to be "passive euthanasia" or letting death happen. It was a distinction between commission and omission, which neither ethically nor legally has a reasoned basis. Death may occur as surely in the patient who needs ventilator assistance but refuses it as in the patient who has the ventilator withdrawn following its initiation. The cause of death in both instances is the disease process, whatever has caused the respiratory system to become damaged to the point that it cannot supply the patient's physiologic needs. The intent is not "to kill" but to allow the disease to run its course because the patient or his or her surrogate, in conjunction with medical caregivers' information and advice, finds it too burdensome or undesirable to endure. The therapy need not be futile for all treatment goals for this decision to be made. In fact, true futility requires withholding or withdrawing whatever the futile treatment is, since the treatment cannot meet the goals of the health care team and the patient.

"Do Not Resuscitate" Orders

"Do not resuscitate" (DNR) orders were among the first issues regarding withholding therapy. For years physicians were fearful and many refused to write a DNR order, thinking they would be legally or ethically vulnerable. As the principle of autonomy replaces the paternal beneficence of yesteryear, the patient, in consultation with the physician, must decide for himself or herself whether CPR is appropriate to his or her life values and wishes. Once the decision is made, with informed consent-refusal principles being satisfied, the order must be written and followed.

Careful definition of CPR is needed to avoid confusion. Generally CPR refers to the response of a person or team to evidence of sudden death (loss of pulse or respirations, or both) in a person. This response consists of the ABCs of resuscitation: ensuring a patent Airway, providing Breathing (ventilation), and substituting for or restoring spontaneous Circulation (closed-chest cardiac massage or electrical therapy). The term *resuscitation*, often used more broadly to include fluid resuscitation or giving vasoactive drugs without artificial ventilation or closed-chest cardiac massage, must be distinguished from basic CPR. However,

Some institutions have devised a DNR order sheet that incorporates other forms of therapy that may be withheld or withdrawn. This provides a clear communication link to everyone involved in the care of these patients. Ideally, it provides a better chance of truly following the patient's wishes.

some patients may want to preclude the use of several treatment modalities, so there needs to be a mechanism for allowing this but not confusing it with a simpler, more limited, DNR order.

A DNR order does not mean abandonment or "no care," nor does it preclude aggressive therapy or intensive care. Unless modified by other requests, it simply means that if the patient stops breathing or becomes pulseless, mechanical respiration, closed-chest cardiac massage, and electrical defibrillation will not be provided to attempt to interrupt the patient's dying. If the withholding or withdrawing of medical care is intended to go beyond the DNR order, specific orders should be written to accommodate and clarify such requests. It is preferable that the patient considered and decided his or her wishes prior to acute illness so that the decision might be integrated into the value system of the patient. Mechanisms for promoting conversation about death and dying and medical therapies under various conditions should be initiated while persons are well and thinking clearly. Studies show that contrary to the medical providers' impressions in the past, patients do want to discuss their wishes concerning DNR orders and withholding and withdrawing medical treatments.

Withholding and Withdrawing Ventilator Therapy

The management of withholding or withdrawing ventilator care within the ethical-legal framework of our society can be looked at as a prototype of medical therapy to be accepted or refused by a patient.

Ventilator therapy, which is involved with an essential of life—breathing, is performed with equipment that is often considered "high technology", "artificial," or "extraordinary," which are words with confusing connotations. Unlike the beliefs of many health care providers in the recent past, it is no longer necessary or proper to think that once a therapy such as ventilatory support is initiated it cannot be withdrawn. This approach assumed that not starting the therapy, for example, a ventilator, was different ethically and legally from withdrawing the therapy; this is a throwback to the notion that withholding therapy is passive euthanasia and acceptable, whereas withdrawing the ventilator would constitute active killing or active euthanasia, which is unacceptable. The same process, which involves informed consent to assist autonomous decision-making by the patient, is required to withhold ventilator care when medically indicated as is required to withdraw ventilator care that has been started.

The ethical principles and professional roles of the health care providers must be integrated into the decision-making process. Physicians and other providers must be certain that the diagnosis, prognosis, benefits, burdens, and alternatives are presented and clearly understood by the patient.

The first level of decision-making concerns the futility of a given modality. If a treatment is medically futile, it should not be offered or begun. The physician is not required to offer futile therapy. Actually, it may be unethical to provide futile therapy in the first place. Unfortunately, the nature of medical decision-making, which depends on weighing probabilities, makes futility a difficult fact to establish in many situations. The various ways of defining futility complicates matters. Notwithstanding these problems, futile treatment need not and, indeed, should not be given.

A competent patient has the right to decide what should be done. After the conditions of informed consent have been satisfied, the patient may choose or reject the ventilator both prospectively and retrospectively after having begun ventilator therapy. As with all difficult decisions,

The President's Commission[10] advocated the development of "objective societally shared criteria for benefit and burden evaluation to determine best interest." In our pluralistic society there is no social consensus regarding best interest; convictions vary from sustaining life at any cost in any condition to ending life when the patient can no longer respond to affection or interact in a caring and loving relationship.

thorough communication, which is time-consuming and emotionally demanding, is required.

When the patient does not have the capacity to make a decision about withholding or withdrawing therapy, in most states a close family member will act as the surrogate. This person requires the same information as the patient to make a decision about accepting or rejecting ventilator therapy. As pointed out earlier; the surrogate does not do what he or she would do for himself or herself but uses one of two principles for decision-making, substituted judgment or best interest. When the surrogate knows the patient well and bonds in some significant way, the surrogate tries to make the same decision he or she believes the incapacitated patient would make. This presumes that the patient has expressed and clarified his or her wishes while competent and has expressed his or her values regarding health care through word and deed over many years. If the surrogate does not know what the patient would choose under the circumstances, the alternative principle for decision-making is called "best interest." Under this principle, the benefits and burdens of the therapy are evaluated in light of the prognosis; the decision that most reasonable persons would choose for themselves is then adopted.

Once the decision to withdraw the ventilator is made and accepted, the mechanism for discontinuation becomes paramount. The comfort of the patient should be maintained, which may require therapy with analgesics or sedation, or both. This might contribute to an earlier death. This is similar to the situation in which large doses of narcotics are required to relieve the pain of terminal cancer, with the treatment of the pain perhaps hastening the person's death. This exemplifies the concept of "double effect." The doctrine of double effect justifies an action or omission if certain criteria are satisfied:

- One does not will the evil outcome, for example, the narcotic-sedation is given to relieve the dyspnea and pain, not to kill the patient.
- The act itself is not evil, for example, there is nothing in itself morally wrong in refusing a treatment or using a narcotic to control pain or discomfort.
- The good does not follow directly from the evil, for example, it would be wrong to kill a person in order to relieve their dyspnea; the evil of killing results in the relief of their suffering.
- There is a proportional good involved, for example, the dyspnea or feeling of suffocation is severe and causes great pain, suffering, and anxiety, which is relieved by the narcotic-sedative.

Withholding and Withdrawing Artificial Nutrition and Hydration

The issue of withholding and withdrawing medical therapies becomes more controversial when it involves the administration of fluid and nutrition. The emotional and societal connotations that surround eating and drinking, feeding, nourishing, and supporting often set them apart from other forms of medical treatments. It is considered a comfort care or human caring modality by many, and so should never be withdrawn. For many others, it is a form of medical treatment that may be withheld or withdrawn using the same principles discussed concerning ventilator care—futility, autonomy, substituted judgment, and best interest. It is complicated by the advent of new technologic ways of providing fluid and nourishment. The problem is not whether to refuse food and water to a person who can eat and drink normally but whether a tube in the stomach or a tube in the superior vena cava should be maintained to allow the delivery of nourishment to the patient by mechanical means.

Over the history of humankind, the "old fashioned" mode of dying for large numbers of patients has been from malnutrition. The disease processes prevented the person from eating and drinking adequately, and gradually starvation either caused or contributed significantly to the death. The technology was not available to intervene. In our view, this is comparable to the availability of oxygen and ventilation until the discovery of oxygen and the development of mechanical ventilation. Disease processes prevented life by causing hypoxia or respiratory acidosis, or both; nothing was available medically to interrupt the process. It would seem consistent to hold that the withholding or withdrawing of mechanically or artificially delivered food and water is similar to the withholding or withdrawing of another essential process of life, breathing. In our society, the ethical and legal consensus does not seem to have evolved to clarify this issue at this time. What the respiratory care practitioner should remember is that the central issue is whether artificial nutrition and hydration is a medical therapy, like other therapies, or ordinary care.

Resource Allocation

One of the most hotly contested topics in medical ethics today is the allocation of resources. Health care resources are scarce and they are likely to become more scarce; therefore, important decisions will have to be made about allocating the available resources. The health care system in the United States is a mixed system, that is, it has utilitarian, libertarian, and egalitarian elements. Thus there is no one principle that has been used by our society up until now.

The central question of justice remains given that not everyone can have all the health care resources they desire. How should society's resources be distributed? Should this be done on the basis of need, or some notion of desert, or the ability to pay, or should all persons be treated according to some version of equality? We could give everyone the same amount of health care dollars to spend or we could say that we will use "first come, first served" as a way of allocating medical care. In any case, some persons will benefit and others will be burdened. This is an area in which no one should be under the illusion that they will be able to satisfy the health care demands of everyone.

What are some of the ways in which health care rationing questions arise in respiratory care? There are at least two concerns. First, there is the allocation of a hardware resource, such as an intensive care bed. If a number of patients would benefit from intensive care, and there are more patients than beds, someone has to decide who to admit and who to deny admission to the unit. Some would argue that the person with the greatest need should be admitted first, others for the person who would probably obtain the greatest medical benefit, and still others would argue for a first come, first served method. We will not be making an argument here for what system of allocation should be used. What we wish to do is indicate what we think are impermissible grounds for allocation of scarce health care resources.

Ethical decisions about the use of feeding tubes, gastrostomy tubes, vena cava catheters, and so on for the delivery of nutrients and fluids should be similar to the decisions surrounding the uses of mechanical ventilation.

Medical need is more important than ability to pay when it comes to therapeutic interventions.

Any allocation based on race, religion, or creed is not justifiable morally or legally. In addition, judgments of social worth or lifestyle are also morally problematic. Further, judgments based on age need to be carefully scrutinized. Finally, we think that allocation of resources based on ability to pay bears a heavy burden of proof, a burden likely to be met only for experimental therapies, not for regular therapeutic interventions.

One mistake is to think that only medical hardware is in scarce supply and so it must be allocated. Often, medical personnel are scarcer than hardware. Some of the most difficult decisions concern the assignment of scarce personnel to patients, all of whom might benefit from more personal attention. Again, many different forms of rationing have been suggested.

Euthanasia

The Dutch legal system no longer prosecutes physicians for carrying out euthanasia.

Some ethicists propose that the distinction between active and passive euthanasia is artificial or forced and contend that voluntary active euthanasia is as legitimate and necessary as withholding and withdrawing therapy.

In our culture, the word *euthanasia*, which is derived from roots meaning "good death," connotes intentionally causing a patient's death, usually to relieve suffering in accordance with the patient's wishes. In the United States and in most countries of the world, euthanasia is illegal and a felony. Despite this, ethical and legal debate rages about the definition and justification or repudiation of euthanasia. In the Netherlands, there exists a process for providing euthanasia to patients who desire it. Patients who desire euthanasia must meet certain criteria.

Historically, euthanasia was divided into categories, usually active and passive. Active euthanasia usually meant "killing intentionally," similar to the meaning of euthanasia in our culture today. Passive euthanasia, which was permissible and was considered "letting death happen," encompassed the issues of withholding and withdrawing medical therapies; the disease process was allowed to take its course. Euthanasia requires an agent other than the patient to carry out the final act. Unlike the therapies to relieve suffering, which may have a "double effect," the intent of the agent of euthanasia is to cause the death of the person. Examples of these kinds of actions include injection of lethal doses of potassium chloride to stop the heart or anesthetizing the patient with a short-acting barbiturate and then injecting a paralyzing agent to stop ventilation. These actions have no therapeutic purpose, so the intent is to kill the patient.

Besides the ethical and theologic controversy surrounding this issue, there is a debate about who would or should be the agent. Many argue that if physicians assume this role, a conflict will exist between the basic role and principles of physicians and the therapeutic trust between the patient and physician.

The arguments against euthanasia are compelling, both as a general practice and as a practice involving physicians. There is not space here to develop all of the arguments on this issue. Suffice it to say that the introduction of euthanasia has the potential for changing the relationship between physicians and patients and of opening up the possibility of subtle and not so subtle pressures placed on dying persons so that they "ask" to be killed.

In "assisted suicide," the physician provides the "means" for the self-inflicted death and refrains from any attempts at resuscitation.

Assisted suicide can be defined as a situation in which someone, usually a physician, provides the lethal agent or agents and information for a patient to end his or her own life. This is usually in the context of terminal illness accompanied by serious distress and suffering. It is usually presumed that all other attempts to relieve the suffering have failed; the patient perceives the condition to be intolerable. Often, in anticipation of this, patients seek assistance in preparing to bring about their death when they choose. Unlike euthanasia, the agent of the death is the patient rather than the physician. Like euthanasia, the purpose is to cause death directly. The whole issue of assisted suicide is complex and problematic. There are differences of opinion about the morality of assisted suicide. In 1989, a panel of medical experts endorsed the morality of assisted suicide but the endorsement was not unanimous; two physicians could not consider assisted suicide a moral alternative for patients or physicians.[11, 12]

Experimentation on Human Beings

Occasionally, a respiratory care practitioner may be asked to participate in an experiment. Modern medicine has progressed in part because of experimentation, so respiratory care practitioners should be willing to participate with other members of the health care team in developing new knowledge. At the same time, some caveats are in order because experiments open up serious ethical questions.

One of the safeguards established by the federal government to protect patients is the requirement that all experimentation that carries some risk has to be approved by an institutional review board (IRB). Usually, each hospital or medical center will have its own IRB, whose task it is to decide the acceptability of the research. Respiratory care practitioners might be asked to join an IRB as members. The IRB examines whether or not patients are protected in experiments. In the first place, patients have to be protected by being asked to give consent for an experiment in which they will participate. Everything said about informed consent applies here. Second, the IRB attempts to ascertain whether there is a real need to do the experiment, since it is not just to put persons at risk unless there is good reason to do so. For example, a well-established experiment should not be repeated unless there is something controversial about its results.

Federal regulations about experimentation change from time to time, so it is important to be abreast of the latest rules. Someone in the hospital should have responsibility for keeping abreast of these matters and informing the members of the IRB and investigators of the changing requirements. In this way, everyone will know his or her responsibilities to patients and to the medical community.

However, the most important moral claim surrounding experimentation is that the patient must be informed. This means that, among other things, the patient must understand that this is an experiment and not therapy; the patient must be told that they do not have to enroll; and the participants should be assured that they can drop out at any time without prejudice. Although often the only part of an experiment a member of an IRB sees is a description of the scientific information sought and the informed consent form, the IRB member must remember that a vulnerable human being will be reading this document. Among other things, that means it will be someone who will often misunderstand the point of the experiment and will instead assume that what they are being asked to do is part of a therapeutic regimen. When this misunderstanding occurs, it is everyone's responsibility to see that it is corrected as soon as possible. Patients should not be deceived, even inadvertently.

SIGNIFICANT COURT CASES

Quinlan

The landmark case of Karen Ann Quinlan in New Jersey in 1976 marks a significant change in the day-to-day approach to medical ethical issues in the care of patients in our society. The New Jersey Supreme Court reversed a lower court refusal to appoint Karen Ann Quinlan's father as guardian. He had asked for the power to authorize the "discontinuance of all extraordinary procedures" that sustained his daughter's "vital processes." The New Jersey Supreme Court based the right for termination of treatment on the constitutional right of privacy, this was the first decision to enunciate this right as a basis for withholding or withdrawing life support from a terminal patient. It left the decision-making to the guardian, family, and physician. It also promoted review by a hospital "ethics committee," which in New Jersey was better known as a "prognosis committee." The court discouraged the necessity of using the judicial system to confirm or approve such decisions. It also emphasized the need to center the decision-making within the patient-doctor-family relationship.

Interestingly, the condition of Karen Ann Quinlan was miscalculated, since she was expected to die when the ventilator was removed. For 9 years following the withdrawal of the ventilator, Karen Ann lived with artificial tube feedings, which her father decided should not be discontinued. She was not terminally ill as assumed by the court decision.

Following the Quinlan decision, there was a flurry of activity to develop "living will legislation" in most states and to establish ethics committees in most hospitals. The lay press as well as professional journals presented and continued to emphasize medical ethical questions, dilemmas, processes, and procedures written from many points of view.

The 1980s may well be called the growth decade for medical ethical issues and ideas becoming integrated into the fabric of North American society. The mature phase of that growth can be expected in the 1990s.

Bartling

The Bartling vs. Superior Court case that took place in California in 1984 is an instructive and important court case for providers of care to patients with respiratory disease, especially those patients receiving ventilatory support. Seventy-year-old William Bartling, who had emphysema, arteriosclerosis, and an abdominal aortic aneurysm, experienced a pneumothorax as a result of a needle biopsy of a lung cancer. The resultant respiratory failure required mechanical ventilation; he was unable to be weaned from ventilatory support successfully. He tried to disconnect himself from the ventilator and remove the endotracheal tube on several occasions and had to be restrained physically to prevent this.

Mr. Bartling requested that the ventilator be removed even though he might die without it. He executed a nonstatutory living will document designating his wife as his proxy through a durable power of attorney for health care decisions. He and his family also signed documents releasing the hospital and doctors from liability for compliance. The trial court in California said that Mr. Bartling could not be removed from the ventilator because he was not comatose or terminally ill. The court did agree that he was legally competent.

The case was heard by the court of appeals, which reversed the decision of the trial court, holding that the right to disconnect life support equipment was not limited to comatose or terminally ill persons. The court agreed that Mr. Bartling was legally competent and had the right to refuse treatment; therefore, the ventilator could be removed even if he might die after the therapy was discontinued. The court also stated that the patient's periodic wavering did not justify the hospital's or physicians' conclusions that his decision-making capacity was impaired.

The right to refuse treatment according to the appeals court is based on the constitutional right of privacy, which "guarantees to the individual the freedom to choose or to reject, or refuse to consent to, intrusions of his bodily integrity. The right of a competent adult to refuse medical treatment is a constitutionally guaranteed right which must not be abridged." The court also stated that there could be no civil or criminal liability for carrying out Bartling's instructions and that no advance court approval would be necessary.

Mr. Bartling died 5 months after his original application to a court and the day before the court of appeals heard the case.

Satz vs. Perlmutter

Abe Perlmutter was 70 years old and ventilator-dependent because of amyotrophic lateral sclerosis (Lou Gehrig's disease). He was conscious and competent but had some difficulty communicating. He decided, and his family concurred knowing that he would die, that the ventilator should be removed. He indicated that his suffering was intense. He tried several times to disconnect himself from the ventilator but was reattached when the alarm alerted his caregivers.

The state attorney general argued that anyone who disconnected the ventilator, as the patient requested, would be guilty of assisted suicide. The petition to the Broward County Circuit Court to disconnect the ventilator was appealed to the district court of appeals. This court declared that the patient's right to privacy and self-determination provided the basis for Mr. Perlmutter to have the mechanical respirator removed despite the inevitability of death; it rejected the contention of "self-murder," because Mr. Perlmutter's illness was not self-inflicted. This is consistent with the notion that withholding or withdrawing life-sustaining therapies is not the cause of death in these patients; it is the underlying disease process that causes death. It follows that the person who does not start or who disconnects the ventilator (or any legitimate therapy) under these circumstances is not the agent of the death.

Mr. Perlmutter died 40 hours after the ventilator was removed with his family at his bedside. Fifteen months after his death, the Florida Supreme Court unanimously affirmed the appeals court opinion.

Cruzan

Nancy Cruzan was a young woman who suffered severe central nervous system injuries in an automobile accident in 1983, which left her in PVS maintained by tube feedings and supportive care.

In 1987, her parents requested that the food and fluid administrations be stopped because they felt that their daughter would not want to be sustained in this noncognitive condition. The parents and several of Nancy's friends had heard her state while well and competent that she would not want to be maintained in a helpless and hopeless state if she were unaware of her surroundings. The caregivers and the hospital agreed as did the local court. However, the State of Missouri contended that food and fluid could not be withdrawn because there was no "clear and convincing" evidence that this would be the wish of the patient.

Eventually, the case was heard by the United States Supreme Court, which upheld the state's right to demand "clear and convincing" evidence, which was not present in this case. The written opinions, however, assumed a patient's right to privacy and self-determination and also assumed that food and fluid under these circumstances were medical therapies that could be withheld or withdrawn like other medical therapies if the other conditions of autonomy and informed refusal were satisfied. Nevertheless, the court supported the right of the State of Missouri to decide on the conditions that should be met, in this case, "clear and convincing evidence" of wishes, which would require an advance directive in writing specifically refusing artificial feeding.

After this US Supreme Court decision, the State of Missouri later reversed its decision to oppose the parents' request; the feeding tube and administered feedings were stopped, allowing Nancy Cruzan to die 12 days later.

SUMMARY

This chapter has provided an introduction to the major concepts in medical ethics, some examples of how those concepts are helpful to the practice of respiratory therapy, a discussion of the major ethical issues in respiratory care, and a summary of some of the critical court cases. The chapter is not meant to substitute for a more intensive course in ethics but has provided therapists with the tools to begin reflection on issues which arise in the care of patients. That reflection is best continued with other respiratory therapists, other members of the patient care team, the patient, and if appropriate, members of the patient's family.

Therapists should know that ethics is a field which has seen change in the past and it is safe to say that there will be change in the future. For that reason, continuing education in medical ethics should be part of the ongoing education of respiratory therapists.

References

1. Beauchamp TL, Childress JF. Principles of Biomedical Ethics, 3rd ed. New York, Oxford University Press, 1989.
2. Murphy DJ, Matchar DB. Life-sustaining therapy—A model for appropriate use. JAMA 264:2103, 1990.
3. Murphy DJ, Murray AM, Robinson BE, et al. Outcomes of cardiopulmonary resuscitation in the elderly. Ann Intern Med 111:201, 1989.
4. Linn BS, Yurt RW. Cardiac arrest among geriatric patients. Br Med J 2:25, 1970.
5. Drane J. Competency to give an informed consent. JAMA 254:925, 1984.
6. Emanuel E. A review of the ethical and legal aspects of terminating medical care. Am J Med 84:291, 1988.
7. Ad Hoc Committee of Harvard Medical School to Examine the Definition of Brain Death. A Definition of Irreversible Coma: Report of the Ad Hoc Committee of the Harvard Medical School to Examine the Definition of Brain Death. JAMA 205:337, 1968.
8. Cranford RE. The persistent vegetative state: The medical reality (getting the facts straight). Hastings Cen Rep 18:27, 1988.
9. Armstrong PW, Colen BD. From Quinlan to Jobes: The courts and the PVS patient. Hastings Cen Rep 18:37, 1988.
10. President's Commission for the Study of Ethical Problems in Medicine and Biomedical and Behavioral Research: Deciding to Forego Life-sustaining Treatment: Ethical, Medical, and Legal Issues in Treatment Decisions. Washington, DC, Superintendent of Documents, 1983.
11. Wanzer SH, Adelstein SJ, Cranford RE, et al. The physician's responsibility toward hopelessly ill patients. N Engl J Med 310:955, 1984.
12. Wanzer SH, Federman DD, Adelstein SJ, et al. The physician's responsibility toward hopelessly ill patients—A second look. N Engl J Med 320:844, 1989.

Suggested Reading

Barker DJP. Time trends in cancer mortality in England and Wales. Br Med J 288:1325, 1984.

Bedell SE, Delbanco TL, Cook EF, et al. Survival after cardiopulmonary resusitation in the hospital. N Engl J Med 309:569, 1983.

Bone RC, Rackow EC, Weg JG, et al. Ethical and moral guidelines for the initiation, continuation, and withdrawal of intensive care, an ACCP/SCCM consensus panel. Chest 97:949, 1990.

Council on Ethical and Judicial Affairs. Guidelines for the appropriate use of do-not-resuscitate orders. JAMA 265:1868, 1991.

Council on Scientific Affairs and Council on Ethical and Judicial Affairs. Persistent vegetative state and the decision to withdraw or withhold life support. JAMA 263:426, 1990.

Dagi TF. Role responsibilities in clinical bioethics: The dialectic of consultation: Comments on the case presented by Barbara Springer Edwards. J Clin Ethics 1:79, 1990.

Dresser RS, Boisaubin EV Jr. Ethics, law and nutritional support. Arch Intern Med 145:122, 1985.

Emanuel LL. Advance directives for medical care—A case for greater use. N Engl J Med 324:889, 1991.

Guidelines for the determination of death: Report of the medical consultants on the diagnosis of death to the President's Commission for the Study of Ethical Problems in Medicine and Biomedical and Behavioral Research. JAMA 246:2184, 1981.

Hanson GC. Cardiopulmonary resuscitation: Chances of success. Br Med J 288:1324, 1984.

Jonsen AR, Siegler M, Winslade WJ. Clinical Ethics, 2nd ed. New York, Macmillan, 1986.

Lambert P, Gibson JM, Nathanson P. The values history: An innovation in surrogate medical decision-making. Law Med Health Care 18:202, 1990.

LaPuma J, Schiedermayer DL. Outpatient clinical ethics. J Gen Intern Med 4:413, 1989.

Lee WR. Medicine in the workplace. Br Med J 288:1326, 1984.

Marsden C. Ethics of the "doctor-nurse game." Heart Lung 19:422, 1990.

McCrary SV, Botkin JR. Hospital policy on advance directives. JAMA 262:2411, 1989.

Moss AH. Informing the patient about cardiopulmonary resuscitation. J Gen Intern Med 4:349, 1989.

President's Commission for the Study of Ethical Problems in Medicine and Biomedical and Behavioral Research: Defining death: a report on the medical, legal and ethical issues in the determination of death. Washington, DC, Superintendent of Documents, 1981.

Schneiderman LJ, Jecker NS, Jonsen AR. Medical futility: Its meaning and ethical implications. Ann Intern Med 112:949, 1990.

Schneiderman LJ, Spragg RG. Sounding board, ethical decisions in discontinuing mechanical ventilation. N Engl J Med 18:984, 1988.

Singer PA, Siegler M. Sounding board, euthanasia—A critique. N Engl J Med 322:1881, 1990.

Smedira NG, Evans BH, Grais LS, et al. Withholding and withdrawal of life support from the critically ill. N Engl J Med 322:309, 1990.

Sprung CL. Changing attitudes and practices in foregoing life-sustaining treatments. JAMA 263:2211, 1990.

Task Force on Ethics of the Society of Critical Care Medicine. Consensus report on the ethics of foregoing life-sustaining treatments in the critically ill. Crit Care Med 18:1435, 1990.

Vincent R, Martin B, Williams G, et al. A community training scheme in cardiopulmonary resuscitation. Br Med J 288:617, 1984.

59

Legal Aspects of Clinical Care

Vincent F. Maher, Esq.

Doctors (sic) are the same as lawyers; the only difference is that lawyers merely rob you, whereas doctors rob you and kill you, too.

ANTON CHEKOV

HISTORY

The quotation ascribed to Chekov unfortunately but accurately describes not only the perceptions of and relationships between and among the professions but also among individuals in general. Such relationships are not unique to modern times. Hammurabi, some 2000 years before the Christian era, codified existing laws, one of which said in part that if a physician injured a slave, restitution in kind had to be made for the slave; if, however, the physician injured a free man, the physician would lose his hand.

In the 14th century, the first English medical malpractice case records a plaintiff suing a surgeon for the negligent treatment of a wound. Although the surgeon won the case on a technicality, the court said that had the physician, J. Mort, been shown to have used less than due and reasonable care, the plaintiff would have won. The phrase "due and reasonable care" is language that has subsequently been passed into our common law or case law legal tradition, which is based on a principle known as *stare decisis*, or precedent. In 1794, in the first medical malpractice case in colonial America, a husband successfully sued a surgeon for the negligent treatment and wrongful death of his wife following a mastectomy. The identical "due and reasonable" criterion was applied to determine liability.

The wave of tort activism sweeping the United States has resulted in dramatic changes for allied health care providers. Prior to examining these issues, let us refresh our collective memories regarding our system of government in the United States, because this system has everything to do with the current discussion.

GOVERNMENTAL STRUCTURE

The United States of America is a federated republic within a democratic framework. This simply means that

- There is a central government to which the states voluntarily belong and cede some degree of sovereignty in order to advance their own good and that of the greater number of individuals and states.
- Citizens are democratically elected by their peers to hold public office through an elective process outlined by statutes.

The three branches of government, each of which serves as a check and balance to the others, include the executive branch (central federal government headed by the President and Vice President), the legislative branch (a bicameral Congress consisting of the Senate and the House of Representatives), and an independent judiciary, the judges of which are appointed for a specific term of years or for life. Within the states, there are complementary systems headed by governors and then local mayoralties, town supervisors and so on; state and local legislatures; and a state and local judiciary. In order to prevent problems with the political pecking order, there is deference to the 11th amendment of the US Constitution, a.k.a. the supremacy clause, which simply states that when there.is a conflict within or among the states and the federal government, the rulings of the federal government shall take precedence. When the federal government yields jurisdiction, is silent on, or refuses to address an issue, the states retain sovereignty. This, as you can easily surmise, can lead to disparities in interpretation and implementation of essential or appropriate government services and also sets the stage for legal battles, such as the celebrated Cruzan, Quinlan, Bouvier, and Conroy cases, the right of a state such as Oregon to legislatively ration access to health care, or the ability to contain or control people such as Jack Kevorkian.

PROFESSIONAL ACCOUNTABILITY

The case that began the demystification of the medical community of the "modern era" is *Darling v. Charleston Community Memorial Hospital* (33 Ill. 2d N.E. U.S. 326, 211 NE2d 253 [1965]), *cert denied*, 383 US 946 (1966), which held that the hospital negligently reviewed the credentials of its medical staff. The court added that the medical and nursing staff failed to render proper and acceptable care to a 16-year-old football player whose leg ultimately required amputation because of the negligent medical care and treatment of a fracture. As a result of this case, the charitable immunity previously enjoyed by hospitals and their employees was eliminated. Simply put, no longer did the physician stand alone, accountable to the patient for his or her acts and those of others as "captain of the ship." Increasingly, once relatively immune allied health care providers found themselves the targets of litigation. This shift in professional occupational liability exposure has prompted, changed, or modified relationships among patients, institutions, and providers.

LEGAL FRAMEWORK FOR PRACTICE

The respiratory therapist (RT) is subject to legal theories arising from a number of sources. These include local, state, and federal statutes that govern RT practice, national and local standards of care established by national RTs, peer review, and hospital accreditation organizations, institutional policies, the professional literature, and case law, also known as common law.

CONTRACT LAW

Contract law establishes the foundation of RT and patient or RT and institution relations. Contracts signify a meeting of competent adult minds for legal purposes, in mutual understanding of rights, duties, and obligations of the parties for consideration (money, goods, or a promise to perform a service). Contracts may be express (written or oral), or implied in fact.

When an RT accepts a position with a provider organization, there is an agreement derived in accordance with common and accepted health care practices. The contract generally requires the RT to provide services according to standard and accepted practices and procedures for a fee or salary; the institution provides the RT with patients, facilities, properly functioning equipment, adequate and trained staff, a safe work environment, and a compensation package.

The contract described may be an express contract between the named RT and the facility, it may be a more general employment agreement used for all employment categories, or it may be a handshake. Regardless of contract format, good faith is presumed and duties and obligations are created between the parties, the breach of which is actionable at law. Proof of the existence of a handshake or oral agreement is a difficult matter, which formerly left the employee at the "short end of the stick." However, in the case *Hatson v. Idaho Falls Consolidated Hospitals, Inc.* (V. III Idaho 44, 720 P. 2d 632 [Idaho 1986]), the court ordered a hospital to pay damages to a nurse's aide based on representations made to employees in the employee handbook. The employee was required to sign the handbook as a receipt of acceptance.

Similarly, RTs and patients enter into contractual agreements, which may be formal, as commonly seen in home care settings. Alternatively, these agreements may be implied when RT services are provided to an inpatient or when health care is provided to a patient who is temporarily or permanently incompetent or incapacitated. These contracts create a professional fiduciary duty between the RT and the patient. Specifically, the RT will provide proper, acceptable, and reasonable RT services and the patient, when able, will cooperate with the treatment modalities and provide direct or indirect (insurance) financial reimbursement for these services. This contractual relationship ultimately sets the stage for potential actions in negligence. This occurs when the professional does not know or ignores the limits of his or her professional knowledge (and practice)—*Sermchief v. Gonzales* (60 S.W. 2d 683 [Mo 1983]) (en banc).

Finally, contracts may create exclusive relationships between providers or provider groups and facilities. This simply means that group A enters into an exclusive relationship with General Hospital. General Hospital yields hiring control and frequently billing matters to the group. If an individual seeks employment at the facility, he or she must be referred to the group. Exclusive contracts in this scenario have been held to be constitutional, for example, *Hyde v. Jefferson Parish Hospital District* (104 U.S. S. CT. RPTR. 5051 [1984]). Should a facility move to a product line management or faculty practice approach to provider services, one must inquire about the nature of the contractual relationship and the term of years. This is relevant as follows. Group A enters into an exclusive contract with General Hospital for a term of 10 years. In the ninth year, provider bids are invited. Group X wins the contract. Does group X have an obligation to retain the employees, including RTs, when they assume the exclusive relationship with General Hospital? The answer is no, although this is unusual, particularly with "ancillary staff." If there have been problems within the department, however, there should be no expectation of continued employment.

NEGLIGENCE

Negligence is a subdivision of the law of torts, which holds individuals accountable for their foreseeable acts or omissions that result in injuries to third parties. When professionals are involved as the wrongdoers, simple negligence becomes professional negligence or malpractice. The act or omission that constitutes the malpractice is delimited against specific and reasonable professional standards (Joint Commission on the Accreditation of Healthcare Organizations, national respiratory care standards, institutional policies and procedures, the professional literature and so on) and is situationally defined by an expert witness who is a peer or, in the case of respiratory therapy, a physician who is a pulmonologist or anesthesiologist.

Once a duty of care has been established between the hospital or RT and the patient, the provider must render reasonable and proper care in accordance with national standards promulgated by statute, specialty, peer review, and accreditation bodies. Failure to do so, either by an act or by omission, results in a breach of that duty for which the patient may sue for damages.

Breach of duty—proximate cause of the injury either as the cause in fact or as conduct so closely connected with the result and of sufficient significance to legally justify imposition of liability.

The breach of duty provides a basis for an action only if there is an injury to the patient with resulting damages either of a monetary or psychological nature, the latter commonly referred to as pain and suffering. Unless the patient (now a plaintiff) through his or her attorney proves all four elements of negligence: duty, breach of duty, injury, and damages, there is no actionable claim under a negligence theory (Prosser, 1971). A case from the Indiana Court of Appeals in 1982 illustrates the point. In this case, the court found nurses and an "inhalation therapist" liable for their failure to apprise a supervisor that an endotracheal tube had been in place longer than the dictates of a hospital protocol. The patient suffered permanent tracheal injury and successfully sued for damages, *Sisters of St. Francis v. Catron* (435 N.E. 2d 305 [Ind. 1982]). Suppose, in contrast, that a patient's ventilator humidifier runs dry because the RT forgot to check it on rounds; the RT only refills it a half hour later when summoned to ascertain the cause of the ventilator alarm. Because, in this example, no harm occurred to the patient, there is no actionable claim even though in fact the RT was negligent when he or she failed to fill the humidifier, resulting in the patient receiving unhumidified inspiratory gases.

An exception to the patient's burden of proof is a legal evidentiary inference referred to as *res ipsa loquitur*: "the thing speaks for itself." For example, the misassembly of a ventilator results in a patient's demise or severe brain damage. Proper practice requires the examination, check out, and documentation thereof of the equipment prior to its use on a patient.

In a negligence suit, most RTs are usually protected from liability for negligent acts by their employing institution under a doctrine of *respondeat superior*, literally translated as the superior responds or answers. A loose translation captures more of the colloquial and legal reality, that is, "I only work here, she (or he) is in charge." When an RT fully complies with appropriately and commonly established practice protocols, this principle usually protects the facility-employed RT from individual, personal liability.

An exception to this immunity, most commonly presents itself when the RT exceeds the scope of practice established by the hospital or institution, for example, intubates or draws blood for arterial blood gas determinations by stick when prohibited from doing so, or if the RT practices, formally or informally, outside of the facility environment, for example, by giving advice to a neighbor regarding a "croupy" child, which the neighbor relies on and something goes wrong because the neighbor did or did not do something to or for the child based on the RT's advice.

Although state and national certification and even licensure standards exist to protect the public, they may permit a depth and breadth of activities performed by the RT; however, a hospital or institution retains the privilege of circumscribing or restricting that practice, even on an individual basis, that is, privileges. Conversely, the hospital or institution may not expand the level of practice beyond that created by statute. For example, RTs are commonly taught principles and techniques of endotracheal intubation, but many find that their employer insists that such functions be carried out only by physicians or anesthesia personnel. In this example, potential personal liability is avoided when the RT does not perform endotracheal intubation. Conversely, a hospital may not use RTs in practice areas for which they are not formally educated or trained, for example, electrocardiographic monitoring in an intensive care unit.

Should an RT not perform a protocol in accordance with a hospital policy and procedure manual, the hospital has the right to countersue an RT under a theory of indemnification. In this way, the institution seeks to hold itself harmless by recovering any monies paid to a plaintiff by the institution on behalf of the negligent acts of their RT. In the past such an event would never have occurred for many reasons, not the least of which is public relations in a tight market; however, recent conversations I have had with various hospital risk managers have resulted in the discovery that when an employee exceeds or fails to comply with institutional policies and procedures, not only does the institution refuse to pay a patient for the negligent acts of the employee but it also refuses to defend the negligent RT in a lawsuit. Once again, this refusal applies only to an employee who exceeds or ignores the scope of institutional practice or who engages in other illegal acts, for example, drug misappropriation, sexual abuse of a patient, and so on.

Caveat:
If you "moonlight" in another facility, make sure that you are familiar with the policy and procedure manual of that facility because what is permissible in one facility, for example, performing an arterial blood gas determination, may not be in another facility even in the same city or county.

ASSAULT AND BATTERY

The quickest way for a health care provider to find himself or herself on the wrong end of a lawsuit is to ignore the patient's wishes or directives. If modern case law has done anything, it has gone to great lengths to eliminate paternalism by recognizing that patients are autonomous, competent, and capable of making their own decisions, even if those decisions are other than what the provider's would be. This issue was particularly and eloquently stated as follows by the eminent Justice Cardozo in 1914: "Every human being of adult years and sound mind has the right to determine what shall be done with his (her) own body," *Schloendorff v. Society of New York Hospital* (211 N.Y. 125 [1914], 105 N.E. 92 [1914]). Similar sentiments were expressed by the court in *Natanson v. Kline* (350 P2d 1093, 1104 [Kan 1960]). "Anglo-American law starts with the premise of thorough-going self-determination. It follows that each (person) is considered to be the master of his own body, and he may, if of sound mind, expressly prohibit the performance of life-saving surgery, or other medical therapy."

Battery is simply an unconsented touch of the person or of an object that is continuous with the patient, for example, a cane. Providers may be held liable for battery when a procedure is performed on a patient without the patient's consent. In the case *Kohointek v. Hafner* (366 N.W.2d 633 [Minn. App. 1985]) review granted (July 11, 1985), the court held that the administration of oxytocin to a conscious, cooperative patient in labor without her consent constituted a battery.

Assault is the act of placing another in severe apprehension for their well-being. Touch is not required. This happens when we threaten our patients, for example, "Mr. Jones, if you go near that tube again, I'm going to tie your hands and you into the chair."

INFORMED CONSENT

Although much anxiety centers on the issue of informed consent, it merely requires the provider of a procedure to discuss the reasonable or common risks, benefits, goals and alternatives, if any, of the proposed treatment to the patient, who then determines whether or not the procedure will be carried out.

DURABLE POWER OF ATTORNEY–HEALTH CARE PROXY

Note: A durable power of attorney is a formal undertaking that requires a writing and witnesses and can even supersede the decisions of a spouse or offspring.

In the event that a patient is unable to answer for himself or herself, the next of kin or the patient's power of attorney or health care proxy must be consulted for consent. A durable power of attorney or a health care proxy is a legal construction permitting patients, while competent and able, to designate a decision maker. The decision maker will act in their stead and in accord with their wishes when they are unable to do so for themselves. The decision maker may be any competent adult, not necessarily a spouse or adult child, whose decisions supersede even those of legal next of kin.

STAFFING

Various courts in the United States, for example, *Leavitt v. St. Tanmany Parish Hospital* (396 So.2d 406 [La. App. 1981]) and *Czinbinsky v. Doctors Hospital* (188 Cal. RPTR. 685 [App. 1983]) have held facilities liable for failing to provide adequate staff to render patient care in accordance with standard and accepted procedures. This in and of itself does not relieve the RT of the obligation to perform a job in a proper fashion, but it does extend the base of potential liability to an institution that insists on acutely or chronically functioning in a short-staffed manner.

DEFAMATION

Another area in which RTs may find themselves at legal risk is that of defamation by slander or libel. Defamation is a character attack of one person made by another through word (slander) or writing (libel). The critical element is that the defamation is made to another person, that is, it is publicized to a third party. Depending on the circumstances, the plaintiff may be required to prove malice on the part of the defendant.

An RT may find himself or herself liable as follows: While caring for a ventilated patient, the RT says to nursing staff, "Dr. Jones is a real idiot. I wouldn't let her take care of my gerbil." The RT then writes in the patient record, "This patient would not have sustained a need for such prolonged mechanical ventilation if Dr. Jones weren't so inept and would follow my recommendations." Dr. Jones may sue the RT for damages based on slander in the former example or libel in the latter example.

The only defense to such an action based in defamation is the truth. Suppose for the sake of argument that the RT can muster sufficient support to give credence to the statements, resulting in a dismissal of the defamation action. Is the case closed? Not necessarily. The physician may choose to sue the RT individually. Note that the hospital does not represent the RT in this situation, that is, for intentionally interfering with the physician-patient relationship (tortious interference with a contract). The legally appropriate thing to do in this type of a situation is to document only facts and objective clinical findings, keep your thoughts to yourself or, if the physician, nurse, or other RT is truly (i.e., objectively v. subjectively) dangerous or incompetent, or both, make a protected statement to the medical director, RT Supervisor nursing administration, hospital risk manager, or general counsel.

PRIVACY

Invasion of privacy is an intentional tort in which one deliberately seeks out and violates the privacy of another in situations in which reasonable expectations of privacy exist. An RT would violate another's privacy by reading the chart of a patient to whom the RT is not rendering care or by making inquiry of other staff members about specifics of a patient's condition when there is no professional provider-patient relationship. Typically this situation presents itself when the RT reads the chart of a well-known inpatient—for example, politician, movie star, community leader, cleric, or school teacher—or the chart of a neighbor or a neighbor's friend (to report to the neighbor on the friend's condition). When this occurs, the RT violates the expectations of patient privacy that exist. The RT may be liable in damages for this tort should the patient become aware of the act and suffer injury and damages such as embarrassment or ostracism as a result.

Violations of confidentiality are actionable when an RT discusses patient matters with others who have no professional relationship with the patient. Not uncommonly, a patient's conditions and idiosyncrasies are bantered about in elevators, cafeterias, employee lounges, public transportation, and even in local taverns and coffee klatches. Such bantering clearly violates not only norms of common decency but also the patient-provider relationship. Discussions of a patient's condition are properly held only with immediate caregivers or with others for whom the privilege of confidentiality has been waived by the patient, for example, minister, family, insurance company, and so on.

ACQUIRED IMMUNODEFICIENCY SYNDROME

Acquired immunodeficiency syndrome (AIDS), an area of contemporary practice, presents a most difficult legal and ethical dilemma to providers. It is a commonly held precept that if you are a health care provider, a professional, you may not, by virtue of your licensure, refuse to care for a patient entrusted to your care and expertise. Indeed, health care lore is replete with tales and legends of selfless providers who, at great threat to personal safety, cared for victims of plague and pestilence. Many of these individuals acquired the illnesses and died themselves. Today, to formally refuse to care for a person with AIDS could subject the provider to charges of discrimination based on handicap or abandonment by the patient or to insubordination or other disciplinary action by hospital administration, or both. The latter could, in turn, also find itself the object of a discrimination lawsuit.

Because AIDS, currently a fatal disease, is an admittedly political "hot potato," it has given pause to this previously unquestioned professional duty by all sectors of the health services industry. Staffing in many hospitals and cities with large human immunodeficiency virus–positive populations is becoming more and more of a problem. Compounding this issue is the unfortunate manner in which some seropositive providers have been treated (terminated, ostracized, slandered) by their employing institutions, even when they were exposed and underwent seroconversion secondary to patient care and contact, for example, *Ayoun v. Johns Hopkins Medical Center*, among others.

A number of cases in the United States have mandated that employers may not discriminate against providers with AIDS, particularly when the providers are in minimal patient care contact areas, for example, pharmacists—*Smith v. Westchester Co Medical Center, NY*. Similarly, providers have been ordered to retain seropositive staff in patient care areas until or unless such staff are unable to function in their designated professional capacity, *Doe v. New York Hospital*, GA-00035041487-DN, City of New York, Human Rights Commission. Although not specifically on point as an AIDS case, the matter *Arline v. School Board of Nassau County*, 772 F. 2d 759 (Fla., 1985), which mandated the retention of a teacher with tuberculosis because the risk to the students was negligible, has been analogized to AIDS.

It certainly bears watching to see whether seropositive providers will be restricted in their practices by state or federal action. Based on mid-1990s reports, a dentist in Florida and a surgeon in Baltimore allegedly infected some of their patients. Restrictions of this sort will likely result in further secretiveness among a seropositive provider population or in flat-out refusal to provide treatment to seropositive patients or high-risk populations. Of interest is the increasing amount of legal random serum testing of house staff by institutions.

The dilemma faced by all concerned is real because there is a commonly acknowledged duty to warn others of a condition that may imperil them or expose them to an unreasonable increase in personal risk, for example, *Tarasoff v. Regents of University of California* (17 Cal.3d 425, 551 P. 2d 334, 131 Cal. RPTR. 14 [1976]). Once the physician reasonably determines that a patient poses a serious danger, ". . . the physician must take action to protect the foreseeable victim of that danger" *Lipari v. Sears, Roebuck and Co.* 497 F. Supp. 185 (1980) and *Gill v. Hartford Accident and Indemnity Company* (337 So.2d 420 [Fla. 1976]).

Of further interest is a 1993 jury verdict from California that awarded damages to a health care provider (surgical technician) who was unknowingly exposed to an HIV-positive patient and who subsequently underwent seroconversion. The jury held that the patient had a duty to warn the health care providers of his HIV status.

SUMMARY

This chapter discussed relevant legal principles that are regularly involved in RT practice. The legal principles discussed should be understood solely as an introduction to the issue and as an attempt to facilitate provider-patient relations rather than to polarize them. When medical and legal expectations are understood by all involved, the risk of professional liability on an individual and corporate level diminishes. Further, political issues surrounding a national health care agenda may prompt tort reform.

Should a respiratory care practitioner find himself in a legal situation that requires specific advice, the opinion of qualified legal counsel should always be sought. This can be done by referral from a friend who has satisfactorily used competent legal services or by contacting one's professional association or the county bar association for a referral.

Suggested Reading

American College of Legal Medicine. Legal Medicine: Legal Dynamics of Medical Encounters. St. Louis, CV Mosby, 1991.

Bouvia v Superior Court 225 Cal. RPTR. 297 (1986).

Carroll P, Maher V. RTs beware! You too could be sued. Adv Respir Ther December 19, 1988.

Carroll P, Maher V. RTs must heed certification rules. Adv Respir Ther November 27, 1989.

Carroll P, Maher V. Court case tests employee health issue. Adv Respir Ther August, 1989.

Carroll P, Maher V. RT and the law: Competence. Adv Respir Ther March 20, 1989.

Carroll P, Maher V. Legal aspects of contagious infectious diseases. Adv Clin Care July/August, 1989.

Fiesta J. The Law and Liability: A Guide for Nurses, 2nd ed. New York, John Wiley & Sons, 1988.

Fiscina S, Boumil M, Sharpe D, Head M. Medical Liability. St. Paul, West Publishing, 1991.

Hall M, Ellman IM. Health Care Law and Ethics. St. Paul, West Publishing, 1990.

Quinlan 70 N.J. 10, 355 A. 2d 647 N. J. 1976).

Conroy 486 A. 2d 1209 (N. J. 1985).

In the Matter of Claire Conroy, A-108 (1985).

Mackauf S (ed). Hospital Liability. New York, Practicing Law Institute, 1986.

Maher V. Legal aspects of ethical decision making. JNYSNA December, 1989.

Maher V. Legal savvy: The nurse and the law. Nursing November, 1989.

Maher V, Badin R. A Rehnquistean bed. JNYSNA December, 1990.

Maher V. Legal issues and update on AIDS. Adv Clin Care January, 1991.

Northrup C, Kelly M. Legal Issues in Nursing. St. Louis, CV Mosby, 1987.

Pozgar GD. Legal Aspects of Health Care Administration, 5th ed. Rockville, MD, Aspen Publishers, 1993.

Prosser W. Law of Torts, 4th ed. 1971 sec 30 note 1 at 236–237.

Rhodes AM, Miller RD. Nursing and the Law, 4th ed. Rockville, MD, Aspen Publishers, 1984.

Vocational Rehabilitation Act of 1973. 29 USC sec 504 and 794.

60

◨

Key Terms

Affective Domain

Attitude

Cognitive Domain

Psychomotor Domain

Patient, Community, and Staff Education

David D. Rice, Ph.D., R.R.T.

WHY EDUCATION IS AN ESSENTIAL PROFESSIONAL SKILL

The ability to promote learning is as essential to professional practice as are the more traditionally identified clinical skills of observation, assessment, communication, treatment planning, evaluation, and adjustment. Education is a recognized specialty within respiratory care and other medical professions. More importantly, respiratory care practitioners outside the education specialty frequently support the learning process. This participation in the ongoing enterprise of learning is essential for the survival of the profession. The facilitation of patient learning is essential for effective clinical practice. The ability and willingness of patients to comply with treatment protocols is a prerequisite for successful clinical outcomes. Even within hospital settings, patients frequently share the responsibility for basic therapy. This may result in significant savings and satisfactory clinical outcomes if appropriate patient instruction and monitoring are provided. With declining personnel resources for patient instruction and monitoring, respiratory care practitioners must be proficient in these critical roles to serve the best interests of their patients and their profession. Most respiratory care personnel work within large, complex organizations. Part of the professional transition from solo practice to an organizational setting is acceptance of the responsibility for supporting and nurturing organizational life. Traditionally, this may be viewed as the responsibility of administrative and supervisory personnel, with the workers participating as directed. In more participatory models, particularly with professional staff (employees) the responsibility is more widely shared. Some may question whether respiratory care, particularly as it exists within large teaching hospitals, is truly a profession. Perhaps as Houle suggests in a broader context, this is the wrong question. It may be more productive to ask how respiratory care practitioners might establish respiratory care as a profession and themselves as professionals.[1]

Education Is an Essential Component of Professional Life

One of the traditional characteristics of a profession is the acceptance of responsibility for education and regulation of current and future members of the profession. Members of the respiratory care profession should be educated by other members of the profession. Respiratory therapy technicians and therapists fill the key faculty leadership roles in preprofessional education. Like other professional programs, individuals from related disciplines and professions support the full-time professional faculty. A physician medical director and subject area specialists from arts and science disciplines are critical. A substantially larger group of clinical instructors and preceptors typically supports the care faculty. These individuals provide the direct supervision of clinical learning.

1191

With few exceptions (e.g., specialty rotations in which members of other health care professions may provide appropriate supervision), these individuals are respiratory care professionals. They serve in a variety of role definitions and employment models but share the common thread of commitment to advancing their profession through preparation of future practitioners. This role is the most frequent entry point for participation in formal professional education. Members of the profession have a similar responsibility for education beyond initial professional entry. In addition to fulfilling a professional obligation, participation provides significant personal benefit. Jason observed "A well accepted, but surprisingly ignored principle is that one of the most effective ways to pursue one's own learning is to engage in the instruction of others."[2]

Education Is an Essential Component of Clinical Practice

Patient education is essential in clinical practice. From the earliest days of clinical education, it should be evident that the correct installation of a nasal cannula, following valid written orders, and supported by blood gas analysis, holds little value if the patient removes the device as soon as the therapist leaves the room. Jason has identified the following as essential goals of patient education: information, understanding, modified lifestyle, and compliance with the treatment plan.[2] Providing information about medical devices and therapy is relatively comfortable territory. Attempts to modify lifestyle or promote compliance involve influencing patient attitudes and motivation (particularly as reflected in unsupervised and unmonitored behavior). Occasionally, even seasoned educators retreat from this type of outcome involving the affective domain to the more familiar and predictable territory of knowledge and intellectual capabilities. The affective domain borders on mysticism. In contrast, clinicians are not offered this escape. The judgment of clinical outcomes does not accept the conclusion that "the treatment would have been successful if the patient had been willing to breathe deeply." The practitioner is expected to make a concerted effort to modify patient behavior and attitudes.

Drug administration with a metered dose inhaler also involves training patients to perform a physical task (the psychomotor domain). Accurate dosage requires correct positioning and coordination of manual manipulation with inhalation. Customary professional standards for medication delivery include responsibility for the end result of timely delivery of the correct dosage to the patient. Even when this task is shared with the patient, professional behavior must go beyond the unsupported assumption that the patient can use the device correctly. Evaluation and feedback are also essential. Perhaps the frequently repeated clinical instructor's admonition that "no task is completed until the paperwork is done," should be modified to state that "no clinical task is complete until the teaching is done and patient learning has been demonstrated." To do less would be to retreat from a significant opportunity to behave professionally.

Education Is a Central Component of Organizational Life

Since most respiratory care practitioners work within organizations, they may be required to assume the additional responsibility of supporting the training needs of the organization. Respiratory care practitioners frequently play an active role in clinical training beyond their own department. Respiratory care frequently plays an active role in cardiopulmonary resuscitation training. In institutions in which interdisciplinary models are encouraged, training initiatives for clinical units may involve teachers from several professions. Even under more traditional models, respiratory therapists may be asked to share their expertise in mechanical ventilation, cardiopulmonary diagnostics, and bronchodilator therapy with other professional groups. If respiratory care practitioners can respond with high-quality learning activities, their professional image improves, and the individual practitioner's professional standing is reinforced.

Education Is an Essential Component of Personal Development

In addition to the responsibility for supporting the educational needs of other professionals, patients, and organizational colleagues, professionals have a responsibility for maintaining their own personal well-being and growth. Wedemeyer suggests that Carl Sandburg's advice, although originally directed to a youth coming of age, is also relevant to learners of any age who he describes as nontraditional or "back door" learners.[3]

> Tell him to be alone often and get at himself and above all tell himself no lies about himself whatever the white lies and protective fronts he may use amongst other people. Tell him solitude is creative if he is strong and the final decisions are made in silent rooms. Tell him to be different from other people if it comes natural and easy being different. Let him have lazy days seeking his deeper motives. Let him seek deep for where he is a born natural. Then he may understand Shakespeare and the Wright Brothers, Pasteur, Pavlov, Michael Faraday and free imaginations bringing changes into a world resenting change. He will be lonely enough to have time for the work he knows as his own.[4]

Adults cannot assume that someone else will assume responsibility for personal learning goals. Traditional formal education depends heavily on goals, methods, activities, and assessments that are selected and implemented by someone other than the learner. This environment offers little opportunity to develop the skills necessary for self-directed learning. Students should recognize their own self-interest in developing independent learning skills. Some of these skills may be borrowed from the study of the teaching-learning process.

Conclusion—Education Should Not Be Left to the Specialists

The ability to facilitate learning is an essential capability for all respiratory care professionals. Like other specialty areas, success as an educator requires specific knowledge, skills, intellectual strategies, and the willingness and discipline to put these competencies into practice. The recognition of education as an important specialty is reflected in most respiratory care department organizational charts and in the specialty section designations of the American Association for Respiratory Care. Other professions grant similar recognition to education. Chemistry, medicine and nursing have their own education specialty journals.

Some have gone so far as to suggest that education should be considered the exclusive domain of specialists. Human resource development professionals argue for a centralized educational program run by education professionals outside the operating departments.[5] The control of hospital inservice programs by adult education specialists rather than subject specialists has also been advocated.[6] Some respiratory care professionals have called for formal training and credentialing for respiratory care educators. The notion that education should be left to the educators is quite common. It is not uncommon for individuals (including some educators) to suggest that since education is the exclusive domain of a specialty, there is no reason for educational skills to be included in initial professional preparation. Somehow, when the identical logic is applied to other specialties such as pulmonary function or neonatal respiratory care, it is immediately rejected, and the need for comprehensive preparation is reaffirmed. Since educational competencies are related to success in professional life, clinical practice, and organizational life, as well as in personal development, inclusion of basic fundamentals during initial professional preparation is justified. If we choose to behave as professionals, the systematic facilitation of learning must be promoted as a universal responsibility.

HOW LEARNING OCCURS

Change of Behavior

Learning is most universally defined as a change in behavior. This definition is commonly limited to purposeful or intentional changes. Some authors further limit the definition of learning by specifying the types of outcomes. Herman limits the outcome to more effective behavior and in particular the development of survival behaviors.[7] The following three recurring elements of the definition can provide a useful framework for teachers:

- Learning involves change in behavior.
- Learning can be influenced by purposeful activity.
- Learning should be focused toward desirable changes.

Simple behavioral models rarely represent a complete picture of reality. Teachers must remember that they do not control all the conditions of the learning environment. Teacher-directed learning activities represent only a portion of the total environment; the student, groups of students, parents, television, and random events also influence behavior. Therefore, it should be no surprise that the outcomes are not entirely predictable, standardized, or even desirable. The model still provides a useful focus for directing the influences that can be made by teachers and formal learning systems.

Stimulus-Response and Chaining

Classic conditioning, which provides a theoretical starting point for the examination of learning can be demonstrated in the laboratory. This technique, which provides the basis for some animal training, requires carefully controlled conditions to ensure that other influences are not determining behavioral change. Application of classic conditioning to the modification of complex human behaviors is of limited value. It does merit consideration as an illustration of the essential elements and conditions that occur in other more complex learning-teaching models. Figure 60–1 summarizes the three stages of classic conditioning, as reflected in Pavlov's classic experiment. Behavioral models usually include a stimulus, a response, and reinforcement. In this classic example, physiologic reinforcement or reward is built into the unconditioned stimulus, the smell of food. Classic conditioning requires careful sequencing or concurrence of events, repetition, and control of extraneous conditions.

During classic conditioning, the conditioned and unconditioned stimuli must occur at the same time, that is, they must be concurrent. Thorndike and Skinner examined the effects of conditions that exist after a particular behavior occurs. The consequences of three contingencies were described:[7]

1. Behavior that is followed by desirable or favorable consequences (positive reinforcement) is more likely to be repeated.

2. Behavior that is followed by no particular associated consequences (nonreinforcement) is less likely to recur (extinction).

3. Behavior that is followed by undesirable consequences (negative reinforcement or punishment) is likely to be modified or hidden to avoid the negative consequences.

This variation of classic conditioning, known as operant or instrumental conditioning, is an underlying principle that can be applied in most attempts to purposefully modify animal or human behavior. Understanding and applying this principle is essential for effective teaching (and management).

Most evidence suggests that rewarding desirable behavior (positive reinforcement) is more effective than punishment (negative reinforcement) following undesirable behavior. Positive reinforcement includes several operational advantages:

• It is generally easier to administer.
• It has fewer side effects.
• It is effective even when repeated frequently.

STAGE ONE		UNCONDITIONED ⟶	UNCONDITIONED
		STIMULUS	RESPONSE
Before			
Conditioning		*Smell of Food*	*Salivation*

STAGE TWO	UNCONDITIONED +	CONDITIONED ⟶	UNCONDITIONED
	STIMULUS	STIMULUS	RESPONSE
During			
Conditioning	*Smell of Food*	*Ringing of Bell*	*Salivation*

STAGE THREE		CONDITIONED ⟶	CONDITIONED
		STIMULUS	RESPONSE
After			
Conditioning		*Ringing of Bell*	*Salivation*

FIGURE 60–1: Classic conditioning.

Positive reinforcement can usually be delivered with little delay following demonstration of the desirable behavior that is being reinforced. As a result it is clearly linked to the particular behavior that is being reinforced. In contrast, punishment is seldom administered immediately. Most settings require punishment to be administered only after the requirements of "due process" have been satisfied. During the delay associated with the judicial process, supervisory review, academic hearing, or the return of a second parent, many other behaviors are likely to occur. Even when the punishment is verbally linked to a particular behavior, the linkage with a specific behavior is often clouded; a mixture of positive and negative behaviors may be associated with the consequence. It should not be surprising that students receiving frequent negative reinforcement (punishment) for poor performance in a class learn to dislike and avoid the subject or the teacher, or both.

Some punishments (especially those involving violence) require teacher behaviors that are not considered desirable. The modeling of negative behavior by the teacher may inadvertently provide a stimulus or reinforcement for inappropriate behavior in students. The administration of positive reinforcement is more likely to model positive student behaviors. Careful review of the outcomes associated with each of the three contingencies outlined earlier, is a reminder that negative reinforcement is unlikely to result in extinction or elimination of the undesirable behavior. Negative reinforcement frequently leads to behavior that is modified or concealed to avoid the particular negative consequence. Consequently, the careful balancing of positive reinforcement with the systematic and predictable withholding of rewards (nonreinforcement) is the most universally applicable model for changing behavior. If nothing else is retained from this chapter, this principle will provide a valuable tool for teaching and supervision.

Individual stimulus-response associations can be linked together to form more complex behavior. This process is called *chaining*. When the chaining involves the association of names and specific objects, it can be classified as a verbal association. Verbal associations can be linked together or chained to provide the basis for learning of verbal information. These essential prerequisite abilities are included in Gagné's hierarchy of learning outcomes.[8] Since they are usually well established in early childhood, they are not often identified in most descriptions of school learning.[9]

Behavioral Theory

Behavioral theory is built on the assertion that behavior is determined by predictable (and therefore potentially controllable) relationships among specific stimuli, responses, and reinforcers. Skinner, the best known proponent of this theory, contends that human behavior is essentially determined by external forces.[10] This view is not shared by all psychologists. Cognitive psychologists emphasize conscious thought and Freudians emphasize unconscious processes in determining individual human behavior.[7] Social psychologists deal with additional factors in studying group behavior. The view of external factors determining human behavior also conflicts with commonly held views of personal freedom and self-determination.

Recognition that behavioral theory shares the limitations in scope and permanance associated with all scientific knowledge does not diminish its usefulness. Behavioral theory is the central foundation for promoting purposeful changes in behavior. Several critical elements have been well established. Effective learning is promoted by precise definition of intended outcomes. Behavior is not random; appropriate stimuli are needed if specific behaviors are to be demonstrated. Control of the environment is a prerequisite for control of behavior. In particular, careful provision of timely and appropriate (preferably positive) reinforcement is an essential component of any effective learning model. Even if we question the completeness of a behavioral model, these critical elements have been well documented as useful tools in promoting effective learning, regardless of the target population, desired outcomes, or model employed.

Systems Theory

The application of systems theory has played a major role in the development of modern educational theory and practice. Unlike behavioral theory, with its clear origins in psychology, systems theory is drawn from work in several different fields, including operations analysis, physical science, engineering, computer science, and management. Consequently there is less standardization of terminology, symbols, and patterns of application. Elements of the systems approach have been repackaged in a variety of educational models, including programmed instruction, individualized instruction, Mastery Learning,[11] Performance Based Instructional Design,[12] Teach-Practice-Apply, and the Personalized System of Instruction.[13] Each of these approaches or models is an extension of the key elements and processes of systems theory.

In its most general sense, the systems approach is a structured thought process that is particularly suited to problem solving and design applications. Most definitions of a system include a set of defined elements, defined goals or outcomes, and operations that typically involve interaction among the elements.[14]

Systems approaches are almost always associated with visual representations. In the customary visual representation of systems, the elements are shown as boxes. This reflects the notion of defined boundaries dividing the components or variables that are considered within a particular system and those that are excluded from consideration. This is a critical step in designing new systems and using old ones. Failure to consider the boundaries of a particular system can lead to unpredictable results when systems are applied to new elements or in new environments.

In some situations, the process elements may be identified as a "black box," suggesting that the processes contained in the box may not be well understood or even fully controlled (Fig. 60–2). In educational

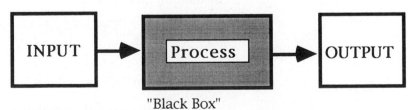

"Black Box"

FIGURE 60–2: Basic visual representation of a systems model.

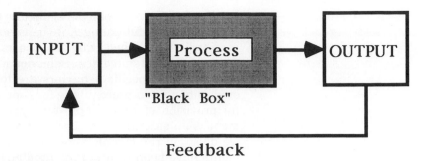

FIGURE 60-3: A feedback loop.

systems, behavioral theory is a major component of the process box. Since the conditions in most learning situations are not totally defined or controlled, the notion of a "black box" may be appropriate.

Most systems include a feedback loop (Fig. 60–3). This is typically illustrated by an arrow from the output box back to the input box. Another presentation in familiar flowcharting symbols adds additional meaning to the notion of feedback (Fig. 60–4). This representation suggests the involvement of predefined criteria (goals), measurement or evaluation of the outputs, a comparison, and corrective action. In addition to changing the inputs to the system as suggested earlier, the corrective action could involve modification of the process, the evaluation procedures, or even reconsideration and reassessment of the original goals or criteria. This could be illustrated with additional arrows returning to the appropriate boxes. The flowcharting representation also suggests the possible, and in fact typical, linkage to other subsystems of a larger (or macro) system. Once a particular learning activity has been successfully completed, the student should be directed to the next appropriate activity.

Systems approaches are equally applicable to the design of complex programs or curricula and to the design of individual units of instruction. Since the formal study of curriculum and instruction are often considered as distinct fields of inquiry, some authors focus almost exclusively on one level of application. It should be recalled that micro- and macrosystems operate concurrently. Individual microinstructional systems (or units) may involve cycles measured in hours; macrosystems (curricula or programs) typically involve cycles measured in months and years. Ideally, micro- and macroelements of a system are linked in the process of curriculum review and revision. As Romiszowski suggests, the systems approach is a scientific methodology including the following stages:[14]

• Definition of the problem in systems terms
• Analysis to identify alternatives
• Selection of an optimal solution
• Implementation under controlled conditions
• Evaluation and revision

In essence, it is a structured thought process using systems terminology and methodology.

Communication Theory

Both teachers and learners spend considerable time communicating information. Examination of the communication process may provide

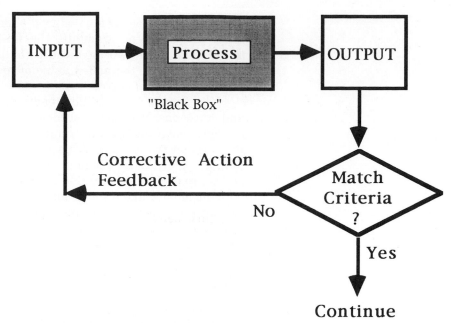

FIGURE 60–4: Another, more complex representation of a feedback loop.

valuable insights. Communication models are described in almost every introductory management text but are noticeably lacking in similar education materials. The basic steps included in Figure 60–5 are relabeled and rearranged in a variety of patterns.

Unfortunately, many formal educational settings place most of the emphasis on the sender and the message. The professor or guest speaker has the special status of expert; therefore he or she is the unquestioned source of the message. The channel is assumed to be a lecture (supplemented with a few slides if they are readily available). The receivers can be easily forgotten once the lights are lowered. Feedback, which is postponed until the next major examination, may or may not relate to the message that was actually transmitted. There is little opportunity for necessary correction.

Closer examination reveals that the expert's knowledge of the subject covers most but not all of the applicable information. Most of this information is also found in the assigned text, although some of the information is contradictory. The lecturer's notes include a selected portion of his or her total information base. Ideally, this narrowing is based on a rational selection process, with careful consideration of the course goals and objectives. Reality may involve a form of intellectual recycling. Common sources include the lecturer's own student notes for the same course, lecture notes for a recent lecture on a similar topic to a more or less similar audience, or a not so recent clinical or research presentation

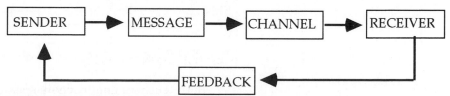

FIGURE 60–5: The basic elements of a communications model.

(with the added advantage of good slides). If the lecturer is a good note taker and a recent graduate, the first source may be reasonably on target. The other two have the potential of offering some useful information and have the added value of reinforcing (or destroying) the "expert" status of the speaker.

The lecture notes will be read with only a few major content errors and omissions. Most of the students will have reasonable attention levels (at least early in the hour) and will attempt to accurately record the information transmitted. This involves tradeoffs: record half the information legibly or try for more with the hope of later translation. If the slides are copied, substantial chunks of spoken text will be missed. The student must make a quick judgment about whether the slide was prepared to emphasize key elements of the lecture or was used only because of ready availability. Whatever choices were made, the result is significantly less comprehensive and accurate than the instructor's original. Since there is little opportunity to process the information for several hours or days, transfer to long-term memory is unlikely. When the notes are "reviewed" weeks later for the examination, the net effect is scarcely different from first exposure to a new information source, and one of questionable accuracy. The process has not facilitated learning. Furthermore, it has not even provided an accurate information base for later individual learning during the final preparation for the examination. The communication model does not represent all of the conditions for learning—it is not a sufficient guide for effective teaching. It does represent the conditions necessary for effective information transfer. Careful attention to each component of the model can avoid many common breakdowns in the teaching-learning process. Whether the information being transmitted represents the instructions for learning activities, the critical verbal information of a subject, or the response of a student, accurate and timely completion of communication cycles is essential.

Since learning is more directly associated with student actions than with instructor actions, particular attention should be placed on the feedback segment of the cycle. As Figure 60–6 suggests, the first four elements of the communication model are involved in the transmission and interpretation of feedback. Feedback from students should not always be taken at face value. A "yes" response to the question, "Do you understand the procedures I just explained?" may have a variety of meanings. The affirmative response could mean any of the following:

1. Yes, I understand the steps you followed but have no idea why the procedure was used.

2. Yes, I understand why you performed the procedure but have no idea how the steps are actually performed.

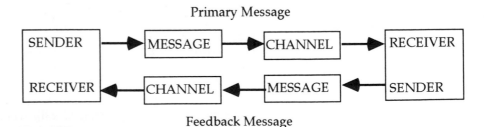

FIGURE 60–6: Another view of the feedback message.

3. Yes, I think my notes are complete, so I can learn it before the test.

4. Yes, I understand what you are looking for, and although I did not understand anything you said, I am confident that the text will explain it better than you can.

5. Yes, I am showing proper respect for your presentation and your status as a professor; in my culture it would be impolite to criticize the performance of an elder and unthinkable to attribute my lack of comprehension to the poor quality of their presentation.

6. Yes, I want you (and my peers) to believe that I understand the procedure.

7. Yes, I have learned to avoid the verbal abuse associated with admitting a lack of understanding.

8. Yes, I would like to move on to the next topic.

Skillful teachers learn to decode these messages and, when necessary, select alternative communication channels that involve actual performance of the desired behavior. Recitation, skill checks, or quizzes may be more meaningful than interrogation.

Adult Learning Theory

Although adult education is established as a field of educational inquiry, its boundaries with other areas of study are not always precise. Of the several definitions that have been stated, the following reflects the traditional focus of academic discipline:

> Adult education is the process by which men and women (alone, in groups or in institutional settings) seek to improve themselves or their society by increasing their skills, knowledge, or sensitiveness; or it is any process by which individuals, groups or institutions try to help men and women improve in these ways.[15]

Studies in vocational education, continuing education, inservice training, human resource development, and nontraditional education overlap with the traditional boundaries of adult education. This overview examines the areas of lifelong learning and lifespan learning. When the overlapping domains of these specialty areas are surveyed, a substantial body of literature can be found dealing with the unique characteristics of adult learners, the range of needs that can be addressed by adult education, and the methods and techniques that are unique and distinct from those of elementary, secondary and, unfortunately to a substantial degree, postsecondary or higher education.

Lifelong Learning

It was once common practice for vocational skills to be passed from one generation to the next with little need for modification. Now the formal education and training of each new generation includes substantial new information and techniques. Furthermore, individuals in technical professions are faced with the prospect of obsolete knowledge and skills long before retirement. The concept of "half-life" has been applied to the knowledge component of professional curricula.[16] In most professions, lifelong learning is achieved through independent learning or through individual selection of educational programs offered by colleges and professional associations. A realistic approach to continuing education for health professions is based on a medical problem-solving strategy that includes the following steps:[17]

- Recognize difficulty.
- Analyze and diagnose.
- Prescribe therapy.
- Implement therapy.
- Assess outcomes.

Since colleges and professional associations are not likely to support the type of individual analysis required to implement the model, employers must assume at least a portion of the responsibility for maintaining the professional skills of their employees.[18]

Several factors have led to increasing acceptance of the need for lifelong learning. Each year the rapid expansion of technical information and skills leads to a significant knowledge gap. Over time, the normal process of forgetting results in a retention gap. As shown in Figure 60–7, these knowledge gaps combine and become technical obsolescence. Unless progressive obsolescence is stemmed by appropriate continuing education, quality and productivity will decline rapidly. In respiratory care, obsolescence decreases the potential level and scope of practice. Without continuous or periodic updating, practitioners who could be offering the benefit of extended clinical experience must be relegated to routine roles to avoid compromising patient safety. Even if obsolescence is confined to a few individuals, the resentment of therapists who are "rewarded" for their own professionalism by carrying the additional load can result in an entire department becoming dysfunctional.

Lifelong education could promote equality because access would not be restricted by the barriers of traditional education.[16] Unfortunately, individuals who were unsuccessful with traditional education may lack essential skills and motivation to seek out learning opportunities involving even greater individual initiative later in life. Learning can be more closely matched with rapidly changing job requirements. Greater (or at least more easily recognizable) economic returns have been claimed by adult learning programs. The ability to transfer responsibility for costs from the government to individuals and their employers may be an even stronger political advantage. A combination of social and economic factors have led to more frequent employment changes and new demands

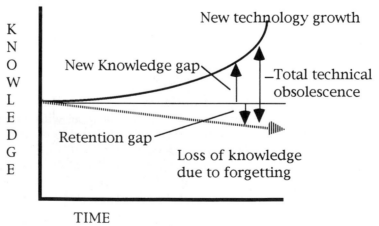

FIGURE 60–7: Time-dependent knowledge gaps for technically educated people. (Developed by John P. Klus.)[19]

for flexible work schedules. When these factors are combined with the growing frustration surrounding the failure of traditional educational systems to achieve universal literacy and employability, it becomes clear that lifelong education is no longer a luxury.

Lifespan Learning

As individuals progress through the stages of human development, both the goals and methods of learning undergo substantial changes. Wedemeyer has described three types of lifespan learning.[3] Newborns are confronted with a new, physiologically hostile environment. Their most immediate learning needs focus on survival. Being without the tools of language or structured learning experiences, their response is largely instinctive. Their primary focus can be described as *survival learning.* As the child interacts with the parents and other elements of the environment, external factors exert increasing control over learning. The child must attend to expectations and learning activities that are determined by others; they must make the transition to *surrogate learning.* When the child enters school, surrogate learning becomes the predominant mode because most of the activities, methods, and expectations are determined by others. Other types of learning continue, particularly outside of school. As the child matures, basic learning processes are established and an independent self-concept is formed; some of the goals, content, and methods of learning will be internally controlled by the individual. This type of *independent learning* is primarily focused on self-actualization or identity and is achieved through individually determined activities. Figure 60–8 depicts an estimate of the relative intensity or importance of each type of learning during different stages of development.

The Methodology—Pedagogy, "Androgogy," and "Appropriogogy"

Many factors influence learning. Studies in elementary and secondary schools have identified a long list of factors that influence learning. Important student characteristics include intelligence, self-esteem, val-

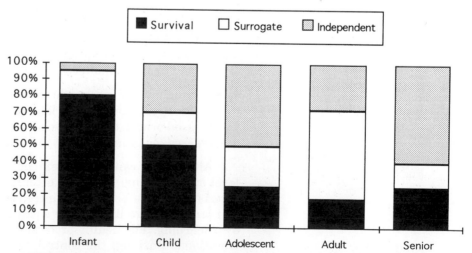

FIGURE 60–8: An estimate of the relative intensity of three kinds of life span learning at different times in life. (Based on data from Robert Clasen.)

ues, and attitudes. Institutional characteristics are influenced by public policy and the choices of individual teachers. Important instructional variables include goals, strategies, time on task, teacher-pupil relations, methods, and quality of instruction. Environmental characteristics of the home, school, and peers may present conflicting influences. Most of these factors also influence learning by adult students. Additional factors have been identified that are of particular importance with adult students:[20]

- Personal goals
- Organizational policies
- Expectations of the future
- Lifestyles
- Feelings and emotions

Of the three lifespan learning types, independent learning is most closely matched with popular definitions of adult learning. It is not a precise match because individually initiated, participatory group learning is not specifically addressed in the lifespan model. Jason has suggested two sets of skills that are necessary for success in independent learning. Individuals must be able to identify learning deficiencies; this requires the capability and inclination to critically and accurately assess individual skills and performance. Once the deficiencies have been identified, individuals must be able to select or create appropriate independent learning activities to correct the deficiencies. Most formal education for the health professions does little to encourage the development of either skill. The rigorous evaluation systems and the highly competitive nature of many programs may actually discourage the openness that is essential for valid self-assessment. Most educational programs could be characterized as highly structured, other-directed, group-paced and didactically focused; these patterns do little to develop the capacity for independent learning.[2] Few employers do much better. Employees are rarely rewarded for open disclosure of skill deficiencies or faulty performance. Most inservice education, which is directed at institutional or group needs, is delivered in traditional settings. It should be no surprise that health professionals often prefer traditionally structured group learning activities when continuing education is sought.

Knowles has popularized the terms *androgogy* and *pedagogy* as a way of distinguishing between the methods of adult and child learning. Both deal with the art and science of learning. "Pedagogy" deals with the teaching of children. "Androgogy" deals with helping adults learn.[21] As the wording implies, the distinction goes beyond the difference in the age level of the target population. The distinctions are based on four assumptions about changes that occur as a learner becomes more mature:[22]

- Increased level of independence and self-direction
- Increased reservoir of experience as a basis for learning
- Increased orientation to developmental tasks and societal roles
- Increased focus on solutions to current practical problems

Although it cannot be assumed that all adults will have the same level of educational maturity, attention to these four adult learner characteristics in the design can increase the likelihood of success. Mature learners are more likely to be successful if they are "in control" of their own learning. For health professionals who have been successful with traditional learning, the control over selection of learning experiences may be sufficient. Experienced allied health and nursing personnel are likely to seek opportunities for more independent and self-directed professional practice. There is particular interest in programs that prepare practitioners for new roles in supervision, leadership, specialty practice roles, and education. Learning experiences should be related to the accumulated experience of the learners. In adult groups, particularly groups of professionals, the combined knowledge and experience base of the students is likely to exceed the knowledge of an individual instructor in many important areas of inquiry. The effective adult educator is forced to abandon the familiar role of subject expert for the less familiar and potentially vulnerable role of facilitator. The adult educator must be prepared to continue learning.

Since adult learners are balancing a number of different social roles and developmental tasks at the same time, successful learning experiences must provide sufficient flexibility to allow students to adjust their activities when conflicting roles emerge as critical. Adult learners may also be professionals, employees, parents, spouses, and neighbors. Adult learners are less likely to put the rest of their lives on hold to complete educational tasks, particularly if they seem unrelated to their own current development needs. If education is truly a lifelong endeavor, the traditional expectation of putting other life activities and goals on hold becomes rather farcical. Traditional-aged college students also balance a variety of activities and obligations, but campus life is artificially structured around the weekly and term schedule. College students are also expected to temporarily suspend normal housekeeping and maintenance functions. Family obligations can usually be packaged during their breaks. Working adult students do not have a dining commons or breaks from their work obligations. Their learning activities must accommodate continuation of a reasonably normal life.

The focus on practical solutions for current problems is of particular importance. Adult students are generally more interested in concrete, current, practical applications. They would rather be problem-focused than discipline-focused. The only limitation to this as a distinguishing characteristic of adult learners is the serious doubt as to whether younger students actually prefer or benefit from a focus on academic disciplines, accumulated knowledge, and hypothetical abstractions. Even if it should be shared with the young, the focus on the solution of real problems is a major element of effective learning.

The ultimate goal is to match learning methods with the needs of individuals and not to implement a particular model of adult learning. Considering the difficulty many traditional students have in making the transition to independent learning, the time may have come to go beyond "pedagogy" and "androgogy" to the new realm of "appropriogogy."

CLASSIFYING LEARNING OUTCOMES

More complex learning outcomes associated with school learning have been classified in various ways to assist in the study of learning processes and instructional strategies. Bloom's taxonomy,[23] which is probably the most widely used classification, divides learning outcomes into cognitive, affective, and psychomotor domains. Romiszowski suggests that interpersonal or interactive skills are sufficiently important and unique to constitute a fourth domain.[14] Gagné divides the same universe of educational outcomes into five categories: intellectual skills, cognitive strategies, verbal information, attitudes, and motor skills.[9] The similarity of affective and psychomotor domains to attitudes and motor skills is quite evident. Intellectual skills and cognitive strategies generally correspond to the cognitive domain. Closer examination of the subdivisions of the Bloom and Gagné classifications reveals similar hierarchic approaches but significantly different divisions of possible outcomes. Guilford has proposed a nonhierarchic model that could be represented as a three-dimensional matrix with three independent divisions of operation, content, and product.[23] Romiszowski suggests another three-dimensional model that combines several existing approaches; objectives are classified by immediacy (short, medium, or long term), performance type (domain), and source (e.g., job requirement, individual-felt need, or societal aim).[14] Foshay describes six domains of learning: intellectual, emotional, social, physical, aesthetic, and spiritual.[24] Most students and teachers have at some time questioned the classification of a particular objective. This is hardly surprising when the crazy quilt created by combining the "road maps" of individual theorists is examined. No individual classification scheme should be expected to unambiguously classify all possible educational outcomes into discrete pockets.

The Cognitive or Intellectual Skills Domain

The lack of uniformity becomes even more apparent when the variety of approaches to subdivision of the cognitive domain are examined. The subdivision of Bloom's three domains is well developed. Figure 60–9 lists the major subdivisions of the cognitive domain.

Gagné divides intellectual skills into seven hierarchic levels:[9]

```
1.00   KNOWLEDGE
       1.10    Knowledge of specifics
               1.11      Knowledge of terminology
               1.12      Knowledge of specific facts
       1.20    Knowledge of ways and means of dealing with specifics
               1.21      Knowledge of conventions
               1.22      Knowledge of trends and sequences
               1.23      Knowledge of classifications and categories
               1.24      Knowledge of criteria
               1.25      Knowledge of methodology
       1.30    Knowledge of the Universals and Abstractions in a field
               1.31      Knowledge of principles and generalizations
               1.32      Knowledge of theories and structures

2.00   COMPREHENSION
       2.10    Translation
       2.20    Interpretation
       2.30    Extrapolation

3.00   APPLICATION

4.00   ANALYSIS
       4.10    Analysis of elements
       4.20    Analysis of relationships
       4.30    analysis of organizational principles

5.00   SYNTHESIS
       5.10    Production of a unique communication
       5.20    Production of a plan, or proposed set of operations
       5.30    Derivation of a set of abstract relations

6.00   EVALUATION
       6.10    Judgements in terms of internal evidence
       6.20    Judgements in terms of external criteria
```

FIGURE 60–9: Condensed outline of Bloom's Cognitive Domain Taxonomy. (From Bloom BS. Taxonomy of Educational Objectives I: Cognitive Domain. New York, David McKay, 1956.)

- Stimulus-response
- Chaining
- Verbal associations
- Discriminations
- Concepts
- Principles and rules
- Problem solving

In his classification, cognitive strategies and verbal information are treated as separate domains. Gagné's use of verbal information is not the same as knowledge (Fig. 60–10). Bloom's subdivisions of knowledge resemble the hierarchic divisions of intellectual skills (Fig. 60–10), but these divisions also resemble the comprehension, application, and analysis sequence.[22] Attempts to correlate the various subdivisions are not very successful.

As imperfect as they are, taxonomies are useful in designing curricula to ensure an appropriate distribution in the levels or complexity of learning objectives. They are also useful in designing instruction. It is generally recognized that learning is most effective when there is a logical progression from less complex (lower order) objectives to more complex (higher order) objectives. Gagné's classification of learning outcomes is particularly suited to analysis of the hierarchic nature of related learning outcomes.[9]

The Psychomotor Domain

The psychomotor domain includes the development of physical skills and capabilities. The distinction from cognitive or intellectual skills is relatively straightforward. In fact, there is relatively little attention to this domain in the general literature on instructional design and methodology. Romiszowski characterized it as the neglected domain and sug-

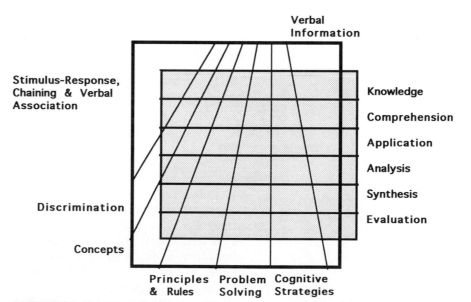

FIGURE 60–10: The "crazy quilt" of learning outcomes. (Data from Bloom BS. Taxonomy of Educational Objectives, Handbook I: Cognitive Domain. New York, David McKay, 1956; Gagné RM, Briggs LJ. Principles of Instructional Design, 2nd ed. New York, Holt, Rinehart and Winston, 1979.)

gested that this neglect was the result of educational researchers' assessment of this domain as unworthy of serious research.[25] The traditional separation of academic disciplines, the organization of university departments, and the library classification systems may have been equally responsible for this assessment. It is not unusual for physical education and vocational-technical education departments to be independent from other academic units doing research on instructional design research. Since there are few shared courses or research projects, the limited awareness of these areas should be no surprise. It is not unusual for items that we consider to be of closely related content to be classified under different major subject headings within the common library classification systems. Books dealing with "respiratory care" can be found in several different places in most library collections. Many researchers had specific discipline-based interests. Gagné's interest in mathematics education, rather than a disdain for the physical, led to an emphasis on intellectual skills. The material is there but may require some additional effort to locate. The psychomotor domain is a major focus in physical education, vocational-technical education, and business education. The development of physical or psychomotor skills is of obvious importance in a field like respiratory care. Knowledge of procedures like drawing blood gases or suctioning or simply connecting tubing is no substitute for the actual performance of essential physical skills.

Bloom and associates have developed a taxonomy for classifying psychomotor objectives. As in the other domains, there are several alternative classifications. The hierarchic structure of physical skills is of particular importance in designing learning systems. Basic mobility and manipulation capabilities, strength and endurance, and the correct use of tools are essential prerequisites for many clinical skills. Some classifications also reflect stages of skill development. The following sequence is a workable classification for objectives as well as a framework for designing instructional systems for psychomotor skills:[25]

- Knowledge of what is to be done
- Step-by-step performance
- Performance with reduced visual control
- Automatization to reduce conscious control of each step
- Generalization of the skill to new applications

The developmental stages should not be carried to the absolute extremes for most clinical skills. Drawing blood gases with eyes closed or making ventilator checks without conscious control does not reflect the intent of the model. Skilled practitioners should develop greater ability to use nonvisual cues. Most complex procedures must be somewhat automatic for efficiency; other skills such as cardiopulmonary resuscitation must be automatic for clinical effectiveness. Few clinicians will be using identical equipment and procedures 5 years after graduation.

Although clearly identifiable as a unique domain, the development of psychomotor skills is clearly related to the other domains. Physical skills frequently involve a knowledge component. The mastery of complex physical skills usually begins with the cognitive learning of a sequence of steps. Popular sports and games involve combinations of physical and cognitive components. The acquisition and application of cognitive skills frequently involves the application of psychomotor tools such as writing, typing, drawing, and turning pages. Physical activity may also have a significant impact on the individual's physiologic readiness for cognitive activity as well as in the formation of attitudes.

The Affective Domain

From a behavioral perspective, we would expect that once the required intellectual and psychomotor capabilities had been acquired, the presence of a particular stimulus would result in a predictable response. Everyday experience tells us that human behavior is not always this predictable. Students, colleagues, and patients who have previously demonstrated the requisite capabilities do not always demonstrate desired behaviors. Assuming that the capabilities are actually present, an examination of Figure 60–11 suggests three possible explanations for this phenomenon. First the stimulus may lack essential characteristics associated with the learned behavior. Performance with a specific category of patients may not automatically transfer to performance with all patients. Such differentiation may have been deliberately or inadvertantly reinforced during the learning process. In this event, the underlying cognitive learning process may need to be modified. A second possibility is that the environmental conditions discouraged or interfered with performance of the desired behavior. Missing essential materials, equipment, or tools may make it impossible to perform the task. If so, the external conditions must be modified to allow successful performance. It is also possible that the environment contains other more powerful stimuli, so behaviors conflict.

If these explanations are eliminated, it is likely that individual predispositions or attitudes are influencing the actual performance. Perhaps the individual has chosen not to carry out a particular action for some combination of internal conditions. The individual may have acted appropriately out of respect for the patient's expressed wishes or inappropriately because of prejudice toward an individual's gender, age, race, ethnicity, or disease state. The examination of attitudes is the historical domain of social psychology—a region of ambiguity that creates discom-

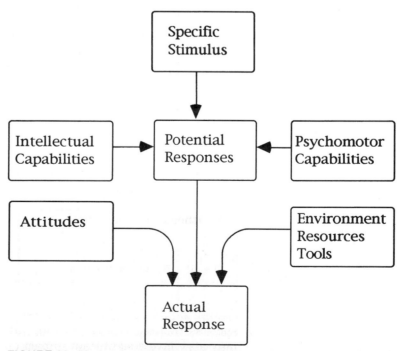

FIGURE 60–11: A systems model for the stimulus-response relationship.

fort for many strict behaviorists. It is also an area of imprecise and often conflicting terminology.

Martin and Briggs summarize several different approaches to classification of affective outcomes.[20] The most widely used taxonomy by Krathwohl and colleagues[26] describes five progressive levels and 13 sublevels, ranging from "awareness" to "characterization." The full range of the hierarchy does not apply to all affective outcomes. For example, objectives dealing with interest realistically begin with awareness and may extend as far as acceptance or preference for a value; higher levels of the taxonomy are more meaningful for more complex outcomes, including attitudes, values, and adjustment. Figure 60–12 illustrates the rela-

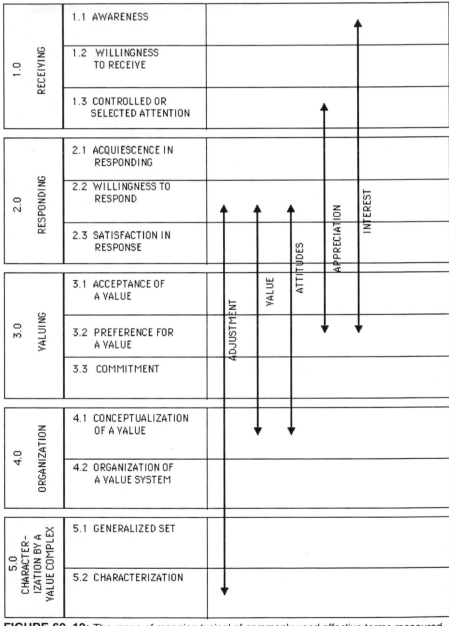

FIGURE 60–12: The range of meaning typical of commonly used affective terms measured against the taxonomy continuum. (From Krathwohl DR, Bloom BS, Bertram B, Masia BB. Taxonomy of Educational Objectives—Handbook II: Affective Domain. New York, David McKay, 1964 [reprinted 1971].)

An attitude is a mental and neural state of readiness, organized through experience, exerting a directive or dynamic influence upon the individual's response to all objects and situations with which it is related.

tionship of common affective terms to the major levels represented in the taxonomy.

Gagné describes attitudes as internal states that influence individual choices and action.[8] Alternate terminology, such as "response tendencies" and "readiness to respond," reflect the notion that attitudes change the probability of an action rather than determine a particular outcome. Allport's definition of attitude has survived the test of time.[27]

The frequent practice of labeling everything that is not cognitive or psychomotor as the "affective domain" is not completely accurate. Martin and Briggs have recognized that the division between cognitive and affective domains is not consistent with learning theory or effective instructional practice.[20] The teaching of affective domain objectives typically involves cognitive and verbal information components. Conversely, cognitive learning is strongly influenced by attitude, values, and affective elements that are seldom formally recognized.[8]

Attitudes have been described as including cognitive, affective, and behavioral components.[8] The cognitive component includes conscious thought processes and elements that have been formalized or defined as beliefs. The affective component includes feelings and preferences. Of particular significance in describing this component are the dimensions of seeking-avoiding and liking-disliking. The behavioral component is reflected in the common definitions of attitudes as predisposition, disposition, readiness, or willingness to perform particular actions, behaviors, or tasks. Several studies have shown that behavior does not always match particular indicators or measures of attitudes, beliefs, and values.

The lack of agreement on the wording (as well as the underlying intent) of attitudinal objectives will be problematic to most educators. The discomfort may account for the frequent denial and tokenism in addressing this domain of learning. Fortunately, attention to the affective domain is increasing. Professional schools are including objectives dealing with attitudes, human relations, values, and ethics in their formal curricula. Accrediting agencies such as the Joint Review Committee for Respiratory Therapy Education are supporting this practice in respiratory care programs.

HOW TEACHERS INFLUENCE LEARNING

Common Elements of Significant Models

There are more educational models than could be listed on this page. They represent a variety of conceptual approaches, discipline foundations, and intended applications. Some deal with the design of large instructional systems or curricula. Others deal with individual learning events. Some focus on the activities of the teacher, whereas others examine the individual learner. Some are simple linear listings, whereas others involve multiple nested cycles, overlapping circles of activity, or the recurrent iterations of a helix. Newcomers understandably find it difficult to make sense of the maze. Experienced educators select a model they find useful (usually the one they learned in graduate school) or adjust to the blurred theoretical background and adopt a more intuitive approach to the art of teaching. Educational experts avoid the problem altogether by ignoring everything that does not match their favorite model (usually the one they wrote).

This attempt to find a useful core of common understanding will not be totally immune to the pitfalls identified earlier. The models of Briggs and Gagné have the unfair advantage of author influence during graduate studies at The Florida State University. To maintain neutrality, a starting point that predates the education of the author (or any reader of this chapter) has been selected.

Johann Friedrich Herbart (1776 to 1841) wrote an essay entitled *The Science of Education.*[27a] His followers have suggested five steps as the basis for effective instruction:[28]

- Preparation
- Presentation
- Association
- Generalization
- Application

Even a brief introduction to systems theory should be enough to realize that the lack of a feedback loop is an obvious deficiency. Allen adds testing, a possible mechanism for feedback, and reduces the list to four essential teaching operations:[29]

- Preparation
- Presentation
- Application
- Testing

These approaches provide some shared common ground but do not offer specific or useful guidance for the new teacher. Herman offers some additional details as seen in Table 60–1.[30] The additional detail is helpful, but there may be some holes. Although application could be included in the analysis of the learning task (as reflected in various taxonomies of educational outcomes), it is also an important learning activity to support retention.

Performance-based instructional design provides a useful, highly structured (systems approach) guide for the development of larger instructional systems (curricula); it also offers some useful suggestions about the development of lesson flow:[31]

- Objective
- Rationale
- Need-to-know information
- Demonstration
- Guided practice
- Evaluation
- Feedback

The teach-practice-apply paradigm[32] rearranges similar elements in a way that recognizes that the instructional world is not entirely linear. The three major events teach, practice, and apply are presented as re-

TABLE **60–1:** Herman's Guideline for Effective Teaching

Preparation	Specify behavioral goals
	Analyze the learning task
	Assess entry behavior
Presentation	Provide cues
	Feedback
	Reinforcement
	Self-pacing
Application	No parallel
Testing	Evaluate, record, and adjust

lated and possibly overlapping events that should be practiced in recurring cycles as new topics and levels of complexity are added (Table 60–2).

Finally, returning the author's initial bias, Gagné and Briggs provide a listing of instructional events that incorporates most of the items already suggested.[9]

- Gaining attention
- Informing the learner of the objective
- Stimulating recall of prerequisite learning
- Presenting the stimulus material
- Providing "learning guidance"
- Eliciting the performance
- Providing feedback about performance correctness
- Assessing the performance
- Enhancing retention and transfer

The list reflects a systems approach and terminology that is consistent with important behavioral concepts. For those who wish to expand their investigation of the instructional process, specific variations of the instructional events to achieve particular types of learning outcomes are also well developed.[8] An added advantage is the availability of a carefully matched model for the design of instructional systems.[8] Some stages of the instructional design model could be viewed as belonging to the preparation stage of an instructional model. This includes defining course objectives and sequencing them to reflect the need for prerequisite information-skills and the category or level of educational outcome expected.

If the actions and events described in these models are compiled, we obtain a "laundry list." The wording is awkward, some items overlap, and a clear sequence is no longer evident. The composite is not a good model (Table 60–3).

With some editing and the addition of critical questions that must be addressed in designing instructional activities, it is possible to compile a checklist that may be useful to practitioners who are preparing for instructional assignments.

Recommendations for Establishing the Conditions for Learning

Learning is more related to what students do than what teachers do. In planning learning activities, place first priority on defining what the students will do both in and out of class. The teacher's activities should be determined by asking what needs to be done to ensure that students will have the necessary resources, stimulus materials, feedback, and reinforcement to carry out their own learning activities. This does not

TABLE **60–2:** The Teach-Practice-Apply Paradigm

Teach	Establish set (attention, recall, motivation, and focus)
	Deliver instruction (lecture, demonstrate, and dialogue)
Practice	Strengthen concepts
	Monitor student work
	Reinforce students
	Provide feedback
Apply	Assign independent work
	Provide extension activities
	Lend skills to new areas

TABLE **60–3:** Composite List of Learning Applications

Preparation	Implementation	Evaluation
Specify behavioral goals	Gain attention	Testing
Analyze learning tasks	Communicate objectives	Feedback
Objectives	Recall of prerequisites	Record
Rationale	Provide cues	Adjust
Need-to-know information	Present stimulus materials	
Assess entry behavior	Presentation	
	Demonstration	
	Learning guidance	
	Elicit performance	
	Guided practice	
	Provide feedback	
	Reinforcement	
	Self-pacing	
	Retention and transfer	
	Association	
	Generalization	
	Application	

imply individual instruction. In fact, many learning outcomes related to the workplace require coordinated group actions; it is unrealistic to think that individual learning will always provide the necessary conditions for learning. In the same way that effective supervisors must delegate responsibility for performance to their staff, effective teachers must focus on bringing together the necessary resources and delegating responsibility to the learners. An effective teacher is manager of the conditions of learning.

Like other management activities, this can be approached from a systems perspective involving recurring cycles of planning, implementation, evaluation, and correction. Preparation for learning activities involves determining in advance how an instructor will *attempt* to structure and influence a particular learning event. Preparation can occur at the program, course, week, lesson, or single objective level. It can involve a formal group process extending over several months or can occur as a practitioner is walking to a patient's room. Planning examines the entire cycle, including the items listed under implementation and evaluation. The complexity of the process is less important than the systematic and insightful answering of several critical questions presented in Table 60–4.

Once the entire checklist has been completed on paper (or in the teacher's head), the instructional activities can be put into action. The answers that were included in the plan may need to be modified if the planning assumptions do not match reality. By using the planning questions and answers as the teaching plan, the instructor (like any good manager) can determine when revisions are necessary. During the evaluation steps, similar adjustments may be required. Although the plan should be viewed as a flexible guide, changes must be made in response to specific needs, with each change recorded so that an accurate summative evaluation of the learning process can be made. Outcomes should be assessed against what actually occurred rather than what was initially planned if accurate decisions are to be made about which activities, approaches, and techniques should be retained or modified.

SUMMARY

As professionals, respiratory care practitioners must assume responsibility for their own learning as well as facilitate learning for patients,

TABLE **60–4:** Recommendations for Establishing the Conditions of Learning

	Preparation
Goals	What should the learner be able to *do* at the end of this learning event? How will the teacher and the learner know that the goal has been accomplished?
Rationale	Why is this goal really important? Who says it's important? Will the learner recognize its importance? If not, how can the teacher help them discover its importance?
Objectives	What smaller steps (or objectives) need to be accomplished before the goal can be achieved? How will the teacher and learner know that the individual steps have been satisfactorily accomplished? What does the learner need to *do* first before the new behavior can be realistically attempted?
Information	What information needs to be available to achieve the goal? What portion of the information needs to be stored in the learner's brain, and what portion will be just as useful obtained from an available reference source?
Analysis	What type (domain, level, complexity) of learning is involved in each step? How should the steps be sequenced from simple to complex?
Learner Readiness	What abilities, skills, information, attitudes is the teacher assuming that the learner will already have? How will the accuracy of these assumptions be evaluated?

	Implementation
Teaching Plan	How will each of the essential conditions of learning be established?
Attention	How will the learner's attention and interest be focused on the learning activity?
Communicate	How will the learner be informed about the objectives? How will the learner be informed about the planned learning activities? How will teacher and learner expectations be defined?
Promote Recall	How will the learner be assisted in recalling (or if necessary refreshing) essential prerequisite skills and knowledge? (This could lead to its own planning cycle.)
Stimulus	What cues will be given to the learner to initiate attempts to demonstrate the desired behavior? What conditions, resources, materials, tools, and events (real or simulated) are necessary for appropriate performance? (For example when learning cardiopulmonary resuscitation, chest compressions, even if perfectly performed, should *not* be demonstrated on another student or in response to stimuli other than the lack of a pulse.)
Demonstration	How will the correct performance of the goal or desired behavior be described, specified, demonstrated, or modeled for the learner? (Occasionally this step is skipped and the learner is led through a series of steps to discover the desired solution. If skillfully accomplished, reinforcement and potential for transfer are built into the process from the beginning. If time is limited and specific behaviors are intended, demonstration is the most efficient and effective approach.)
Guidance	What assistance or guidance will be provided to encourage, focus, and direct the learner's initial attempts?
Performance	Once the preliminary steps have been mastered, how will the learner be given the opportunity (and an appropriate stimulus) to demonstrate the desired behavior (expected outcome or goal)?
Feedback	How will the learner or the teacher, or both, assess the correctness of initial performance and provide necessary confirming and corrective feedback?

Table continued on following page

TABLE **60–4:** Recommendations for Establishing the Conditions of Learning *Continued*

	Implementation
Guided Practice	How will the learner practice the behavior or skill with increasing levels of independence and complexity as correct behavior is documented?
	How will the learner unlearn and relearn if specific errors or deficiencies are detected?
Reinforcement	How will correct performance (or approaches to correct performance) be *positively* reinforced?
Retention	How will long-term retention of the capability be promoted through repetition, connections with similar capabilities, and recurrent performance and assessment cycles? (This may involve its own planning and implementation cycle.)
Association	How will connections with other knowledge, skills, proficiencies, and interests be encouraged?
Generalization	How can this behavior be established as part of a broader set of skills, knowledge, and capability?
Application	How can this behavior be applied in a variety of situations and problems?
Transfer	How will this capability be extended to other related situations, tasks, and approaches?

	Evaluation
Summative Evaluation	How will the success of the learning cycle be assessed?
Testing	How will mastery of the behavior specified in the original goal be formally evaluated or tested?
Record	How will the results of this evaluation be documented in program records and individual learner records?
Feedback	How will the results of this evaluation be communicated to the learner?
	How will the results of this evaluation be summarized and communicated to those responsible for the larger learning system (e.g., the program)?
Adjustment	How will the results of the evaluation be used to influence the learner's progress in the larger learning system (repeat this cycle, return to an earlier cycle, progress to the next step or skip ahead to something more challenging)?
	How will the cumulative results of the evaluation be used to modify or adjust the larger learning system? (For less formal planning systems this could be restated as "How could I do it better next time?" Increased complexity is not necessarily better planning!)

professional colleagues, organizational associates, and the next generation of respiratory care practitioners. Skills must be developed to effectively manage the variety of learning conditions that match the full range of learning outcomes and meet the complex needs of individual learners. Essential clinical proficiency cannot be neglected.

References

1. Houle CO. The comparative study of continuing professional education. Convergence 3(4):7–9, 1970.
2. Jason H. The health-care practitioner as instructor. *In* Fostering the Growing Need to Learn. Monographs and Annotated Bibliography on Continuing Education and Health Manpower. Rockville, MD, US Department of Health Education and Welfare, Public Health Service, Health Resource Administration, 1974.

3. Wedemeyer CA. Learning at the Back Door, Reflections on Non-Traditional Learning in the Lifespan. Madison, The University of Wisconsin Press, 1981.
4. Sandburg C. The People, Yes. New York, Harcourt Brace, 1936, pp 18–19.
5. Dickinson G, Coolie V. The provision of inservice education for health manpower. *In* Fostering the Growing Need to Learn. Monographs and Annotated Bibliography on Continuing Education and Health Manpower. Rockville, MD, US Department of Health Education and Welfare, Public Health Service, Health Resource Administration, 1974.
6. Campbell AB. The adult educator in the hospital setting. Adult Leadership 10:331–332, 335, 1991.
7. Herman TM. Creating Learning Environments: The Behavioral Approach to Education. Boston, Allyn and Bacon, 1977.
8. Gagné RM. The Conditions of Learning and Theory of Instruction, 4th ed. New York, Holt, Rinehart and Winston, 1985, pp 36–40.
9. Gagné RM, Briggs LJ. Principles of Instructional Design, 2nd ed. New York, Holt, Rinehart and Winston, 1979.
10. Skinner BF. Science and Human Behavior. New York, Macmillan, 1953.
11. Carrol JB. A Model of School Learning. Teachers College Record 64(8):723–733, 1963.
12. Pucel DJ. Performance-Based Instructional Design. New York, McGraw-Hill, 1989.
13. Keller FS, Sherman JG. PSI, The Keller Plan Handbook. Menlo Park, CA, Benjamin, 1974.
14. Romiszowski AJ. Designing Instructional Systems, Decision Making in Course Planning and Curriculum Design. New York, Nichols Publishing, 1981.
15. Houle CO. The Design of Education. San Francisco, Jossey-Bass, 1972, p 32.
16. Copley AJ. Lifelong Education; A Psychological Analysis. New York, Pergamon Press, 1977.
17. Charters AN, Blakely RJ. The Management of Continuing Learning; A Model of Continuing Education as a Problem-Solving Strategy for Health Manpower. *In* Fostering the Growing Need to Learn. Monographs and Annotated Bibliography on Continuing Education and Health Manpower. Rockville, MD, US Department of Health Education and Welfare, Public Service, Health Resource Administration, 1974, p 3.
18. Dickinson G, Verner C. The provision of inservice education for health manpower. *In* Fostering the Growing Need to Learn. Monographs and Annotated Bibliography on Continuing Education and Health Manpower. Rockville, MD, US Department of Health Education and Welfare, Public Health Service, Health Resource Administration, 1974, p 177.
19. Hutchison DJ. The process of planning programs of continuing education for health manpower. *In* Fostering the Growing Need to Learn. Monographs and Annotated Bibliography on Continuing Education and Health Manpower. Rockville, MD, US Department of Health Education and Welfare, Public Health Service, Health Resource Administration, 1974. (Based on Klus JP. Time Dependent Knowledge Gaps for Technically Educated People [Need for Updating and Broadening]. Madison, University of Wisconsin Extension.)
20. Martin BL, Briggs LJ. The Affective and Cognitive Domains: Integration for Instruction and Research. Englewood Cliffs, NJ, Educational Technology Publications, 1986.
21. Hutchison DJ. The process of planning programs of continuing education for health manpower. *In* Fostering the Growing Need to Learn. Monographs and annotated bibliography on Continuing Education and Health Manpower. Rockville, MD, US Department of Health Education and Welfare, Public Health Service, Health Resource Administration, 1974. (Based on Knowles M. The Modern Practice of Adult Education. New York, Association Press, 1978.)
22. Bloom BS. Taxonomy of Educational Objectives, Handbook I: Cognitive Domain. New York, David McKay, 1956.
23. Guilford JP. The Nature of Human Intelligence. New York, McGraw-Hill, 1967.
24. Foshay WR. An alternative for task analysis in the affective domain. J Instruct Dev 1(2):24, 1978.
25. Romiszowski AJ. Producing Instructional Systems, Lesson Planning for Individualized and Group Learning Activities. New York, Nichols Publishing, 1984, p 37.
26. Krathwohl DR, Bloom BS, Bertram B, Masia BB. Taxonomy of Educational Objectives—Handbook II: Affective Domain. New York, David McKay, 1964 (reprinted 1971).
27. Allport GW. Attitudes. *In* Murchison C (ed). Handbook of Social Psychology. Worcester, MA, Clark University Press, 1935, p 819.
27a. Herbart JF. The Science of Education, Its General Principles Deduced from its Aim and the Aesthetic Revelation of the World. Translated from the German with a biographical introduction by Felkin HM and Felkin E. London, Swan Sonnenschein & Co., Ltd., 1904.
28. Gwynn JM. Curriculum Principles and Social Trends. New York, Macmillian, 1960.
29. Allen CR. The Instructor: The Man and The Job. Philadelphia, JB Lippincott, 1991, p 129.
30. Herman TM. Creating Learning Environments, The Behavioral Approach to Education. Boston, Allyn and Bacon, 1977, pp 126–130.
31. Pucel D. Performance-Based Instructional Design. New York, McGraw-Hill, 1989.
32. Reinhartz J, Reinhartz D. Teach-Practice-Apply: The TPA Instructional Model. Washington, DC, National Education Association, 1988, pp 7–12.

61

▣

Key Terms

Case Mix Management

Cost Shifting

Full-Time Equivalent (FTE)

Motivation

Payer Mix

Productivity

Prospective

Relationship-Oriented

Retrospective

Task-Oriented

The per capita cost (the cost per individual) of America's health care will effectively double from 1990 ($2551) to the year 2000 ($5551). The total cost of health care will follow a similar pattern as the 1990 cost of $647.3 billion will more than double to $1.53 trillion by the year 2000. Add to this equation the fact that there are now more than 33 million uninsured US citizens and it becomes increasingly clear that problems are substantial.

Management Principles

Eric D. Bakow, M.A., R.R.T.

The goal of this chapter is to provide the reader with information vital to managing health care in the 1990s. Although space does not permit a detailed description of every relevant topic, this chapter addresses issues that form an important foundation for understanding the direction of health care into the next century. This requires an understanding of financial concerns because this single topic largely controls the future of health care; economic survival must first occur for a health care organization to fulfill its mission. Managing an organization that produces computer chips or one that specializes in organ transplantation presents similar concerns when it comes to topics such as sources of revenues and expenses, productivity, and budgeting. The goal here is to provide insight into each as it relates to effective management of a hospital service. The chapter ends with a discussion of leadership, since all health care managers require this skill to provide the necessary direction in these difficult times.

HEALTH CARE IN THE 1990s

First a few words about the health care environment. This discussion begins with this important perspective because forces from outside of health care significantly affect the actions of those providing the service. As certain environments are known to have a direct impact on organ function (i.e., occupational lung disease), so the political, economic, technical, and social spheres have a similar influence on health care.

If all the goods, services, and products marketed by the United States were lumped together, the end sum would be the gross national product. It is estimated that by the year 2000, the health care industry will account for a full 15% of the gross national product; up from 12% in 1990 and about a third higher than 1986.[1] This increase indicates that a large share of the goods and services produced by the United States is in the form of health care, and its rate of increase is substantial. Health care has priced itself out of the reach of most individuals, with the exception of the well-to-do. The old thinking that health care is a "right of citizenship" is now a matter for the ethicists to resolve. Add the notion that technology is burgeoning throughout the medical field and one adds another cost mechanism to exceed our wildest projections. Lastly, the disintegration of the US social structure has become an increasingly popular topic because it has ramifications for all industries. The social fabric is a link that ties values, aggression, compassion, and the like to a functional structure that weathers the stressors of life. Without this structure the society falls apart. The purchase of health care without any mechanism for payment happens all the time, only now it is called indigent care or charity.

Another important element of the health care environment concerns demographic trends of the US population. The so-called "graying" of

The agenda for health care of the future is clear: There will be a shift toward the care of the elderly with a concomitant increase in chronic health problems as a focus of this care. Therefore, long-term care facilities, elder care, home care, and the like will become major players in this complicated field.

America, a single trend worthy of attention, has universal ramifications. The total number of persons aged 65 years and older has shown a steady increase over the past 50 years; in 1940 only 6.8% of the population fell into this age group, but by the year 2030, about 20% of the population will be 65 years of age or older.[2] This represents a projected 65 million persons. This group of individuals is more likely to be female than male, to live alone, and to be in a pattern of declining income. Additionally, this same population has a high incidence of chronic disease and as such become likely candidates for inpatient admissions and recipients of federal and state health care benefits. Because chronic health problems increase with advanced age, these patients become somewhat overrepresented in hospital admissions. For example, individuals 65 years or older accounted for only 11.6% of the population in 1986 but were responsible for 19.6% of all physician contacts, 27.2% of all hospital discharges, and 35.3% of hospital days of care.[3]

Health care in the 1990s and beyond will be very different from that of a decade ago. Taken collectively, the issues previously described form the economic and social realities for those who provide care. There is much more to the story than space allows here—health maintenance organizations, preferred provider organizations (PPOs), ethical considerations of rationed care, national health care insurance, and so on. However, these realities can also be opportunities for real change and with it real improvements in the health care system. These are the challenges of health care managers.

HEALTH CARE FINANCES

Retrospective costs, that is, actual costs for providing care, were calculated after the care was rendered and might include the actual costs of service, other operating costs, educational costs, and so on.

Financial issues are, perhaps, the single most important factor affecting health care in the 1990s. Reimbursement of hospitals in the past was comparatively straightforward, with federal and state health care reimbursement (Medicare and Medicaid) and private insurance (Blue Cross, commercial insurers) providing payment for a hospital's operating costs. Added to the cost of the hospital admission (e.g., for a cholecystectomy) were costs imbedded in the bill for building an operating room or to finance expansions of staff to provide new services. This "cost plus" system was responsible for an increase of $42 billion in Medicare Part A payments in the period 1967 to 1984. In this period, hospital room rates increased 450%.[3] This huge growth in the health care industry had both a positive and a negative impact on the future. Because of the reimbursement system, a quantum leap in health care technology was able to occur. Obviously, a large part of today's innovations were made possible by the financial opportunities of the past. However, it was not long before Congress recognized the need to change its spending habits and passed PL 97-248, the Tax Equity and Fiscal Responsibility Act, in 1982 and PL 98-21, the Social Security Amendments of 1983. Thus, financial restraints imposed by federal reimbursement policies would reshape the health care industry into a more productive and efficient system.[4] This system was unlike its predecessor because payment was no longer retrospective. Prospective payment, as was contained in this legislation, established a fixed payment for service prior to care being rendered for Medicare beneficiaries. The Health Care Financing Administration, the federal agency responsible for administrating the Medicare program, classified 467 diagnoses into groups of similar medical problems called

The difference between the PPS payment and the total costs expended in the care of the patient is termed the *contribution margin*.

The process of shifting huge increases in costs to commercial insurers in the form of inflated charges, known as *cost shifting*, is a recognized method of net revenue generation by many health care organizations. However, it is only a matter of time until a prospective payment is incorporated into the commercial insurer's realm. Again, the process is more complicated than presented here. Commercial insurers negotiate pricing with hospitals. They may receive a volume discount for their patients and may only pay a certain percentage of the hospital charge.

"For profit" hospitals will use excess revenue as a return to investors in the organization (i.e., those who may own stock). "Not for profit" facilities will use this excess to reinvest in the organization in the form of capital projects, structural improvements, or funding research.

Depending on the hospital mission, charitable or indigent care is also a source of expense. This form of expense can assume 2 to 5% of the hospital's payor mix and therefore represents a significant expense.

diagnosis-related groups (DRGs). DRGs are now the cornerstone for the prospective payment system for Medicare reimbursement.

As an example, consider a patient with chronic obstructive pulmonary disease, which is DRG 88. Under a prospective payment system (PPS), the hospital knows it will be reimbursed $3120 for the care of this patient. (Actually the calculated payment is a product of a complex equation, which has been greatly simplified for this illustration.) The hospital must provide the service at a cost less than $3120 for revenue to exceed expenses. If the hospital's costs are in excess of $3120 for this care, it is "in the red." The goal of management is to maintain this margin in a positive state (i.e., PPS payment exceeds costs). The reimbursement picture is more complicated than this. "Outlier" payments exist for patients who receive a different level of care than would be considered average, and the hospital can change the DRG to add in complications (arising after admission) or comorbidities (present at admission) to increase the payment rate. The idea is that the presence of complications consumes more resources and therefore the provider should be eligible for an increase in compensation. Clearly, there is a limit to the number of services the hospital can offer at a loss if it intends to survive the 1990s and remain a viable health care provider. To do so, hospitals must reduce the cost for a DRG by:[5]

- Reducing the prices paid for resources (i.e., personnel, equipment)
- Reducing the patient's length of stay (this increases the volume of patients the institution can serve, which should reduce the daily cost per patient)
- Reducing the intensity of the service (more complicated conditions require more resources)
- Improving production efficiency (increase the number of patients the service can see without increasing the input of resources to the service)

There are some exceptions to a PPS—commercial insurance carriers for instance. Have you ever wondered how a hospital can charge $5 for an adhesive bandage (Band-aid) or $8 for an aspirin? Commercial insurers actually pay hospital charges for services. This is different from costs of a service, as will be explained later in this chapter.

Like all businesses, the hospital must be a financially viable organization to offer the services described in its mission statement. To do this, there must be revenues in excess of operating costs for the institution. Regardless of the type of hospital, its sources of revenues and expenses will be similar and are worthy of explanation.

Sources of revenues for hospitals can be either patient- or nonpatient-generated. Few patients today assume full financial responsibility for their health care bill; when they do they are termed *self-pay* patients. These patients account for a small percentage (usually 5 to 8%) of the total mix of payment to the hospital called *payor mix*. The remainder of patient-related reimbursement is from third-party payers, who can be the federal (Medicare) or state (Medicaid) governments, self-insured employers, or commercial insurance. Nonpatient sources of revenues include investments, grants, private contributions, foundations, tax support, and miscellaneous sources such as gift shops and cafeterias.

Hospital expenses are distributed among several broad categories but differ in scope, depending on the status of the hospital (profit vs nonprofit vs government) and the type of institution (university vs community). Regardless of the nature of the institution, the single largest source of operating expense is that of personnel, namely, salary and wage expenses. This one expense category can consume 60 to 75% of a given hospital operating budget. Other expense categories include employee benefits (which can add up to 25% above the salary of the employee), supplies (disposable equipment, small equipment, drugs, gases, office equipment, and so on), purchased services (such as purchased maintenance contracts, per diem assistance or equipment rentals), depreciation (the use of capital equipment, such as ventilators or computed tomography scanners, in generating revenues over time), and overhead (electricity, sewer, and water costs and insurance premiums for both employee and hospital).

Expenses can be further categorized to identify their *origin* within the organization and to provide a framework for thinking about their relationship to the volume of hospital procedures. For the purpose of this discussion, the terms *cost* and *expense* will be used interchangeably. Costs can be categorized as either direct or indirect based on their original cost objective or the allocation for dollars.[5] For example, salaries and supplies are direct costs because their original cost objective is well defined (i.e., to provide for salaries and equipment), whereas depreciation, plant support (electricity, air conditioning, heat) and employee benefits could be classified as indirect costs. In the latter example, the cost objective is not readily identifiable without some arbitrary method of accounting.

Costs can also be placed in the larger context of volume of hospital procedures (output of the organization, department, or nursing unit). Costs can be fixed, variable, semifixed, or semivariable. Fixed costs are independent of hospital output and are a function of time only. These expenses are constant over time, with examples being depreciation costs, mortgage, some personnel costs, and so on. The mortgage of the facility must be paid, regardless of whether one or 1000 patients are receiving care. Semifixed costs change over time and are "output-sensitive." For example, seasonal adjustments to staffing for clinical departments show an incremental increase over a fixed base of expenses. Trauma units, most notably, may need additional staffing to handle the summer surge of patients using this service. Variable costs are those that move in direct relationship to output; as patient volume increases by 15%, supply costs will increase by a similar amount. Semivariable costs have elements of both fixed and variable costs,[5] that is, there is a fixed basic requirement per month, and as volume of use increases, so does the cost. Utility costs are good examples because they have a basic, fixed monthly behavior but respond to variations in the weather. In general, the more heat or air conditioning one uses, the higher the utility expense.

Let us now attempt to synthesize the preceding information into a concrete example. Suppose City General Hospital is considering expanding its respiratory care service to its sister hospital, Suburban General Hospital, which was recently acquired in a merger. Suburban General Hospital was a 200-bed, underused extended care facility without a respiratory care services, but as part of a new strategy, it will be marketing its services to a broader base of patients, so a respiratory care service is now necessary. Tables 61–1 and 61–2 represent a basic feasibility study for the respiratory care service. A few assumptions were made: There will be a 5% increase in wages, revenues, patient volume, and operating costs in years 2 through 5. Indirect expenses were calculated as a flat 18% of the total operating costs. The personnel costs include FICA (federal income tax) and 8% benefits (that is pretty lean). The department was initially designed for a total of 20 individuals—one director, 15 staff

TABLE **61–1:** Feasibility Summary for the Respiratory Care Services—SGH

Revenues and Expenses	Fiscal Year				
	1992	*1993*	*1994*	*1995*	*1996*
Net patient service revenue	$970,806	$1,121,281	$1,295,079	$1,495,817	$1,727,668
Operating expenses					
Salaries and fringes	$672,500	$706,125	$857,747	$900,634	$1,061,029
Indirect expenses	$150,516	$158,175	$187,271	$196,923	$227,866
Department director	$49,150	$51,608	$54,188	$56,898	$59,743
RC staff	$527,507	$553,882	$697,891	$732,786	$854,917
Billing	$22,118	$23,224	$24,385	$25,604	$26,884
RC assistants	$73,726	$77,412	$81,282	$85,347	$119,485
Drugs and gases	$12,000	$13,800	$15,870	$18,251	$20,988
Medical and surgical supplies	$144,000	$151,200	$158,760	$166,698	$175,033
Purchased services	$5000	$5250	$5513	$5788	$6078
Small equipment	$2000	$2100	$2205	$2315	$2431
Instruments	$450	$0	$0	$0	$0
Uniforms	$250	$275	$303	$333	$366
Total operating expenses	$986,716	$1,036,925	$1,227,668	$1,290,942	$1,493,790
Excess (loss) of revenues over expenses	($15,910)	$84,356	$67,412	$204,875	$233,878

Procedure	Charges	Costs
Drug aerosol	$45.00	$10.00
Oxygen	$25.00	$5.00
Ventilators	$250.00	$100.00
IS	$25.00	$5.00
CPT	$75.00	$10.00
BIPAP	$100.00	$25.00
ABGs	$35.00	$5.00
PFTs	$50.00	$10.00

Payer Mix		Reimbursement	
MA/MC	36%	MA/MC	DRG (see text)
BC	40%	BC	60% of charges
Other	24%	Other	Charges

members (therapists and technicians), one billing clerk, and three aides. The department will grow over the 5-year interval to 26 full-time equivalents (FTEs), with an increase in clinical staffing to 20 individuals and aides to four individuals.

Note that the total operating expense for Tables 61–1 and 61–2 are composed mainly of personnel costs (approximately 67%). A large variable in this financial analysis involves the kinds of payers the hospital will have. In Table 61–1, Medicare and Medicaid represent 36% of the total; Blue Cross represents 40%; and "other" (commercial insurers) represents 24%. This is the "payer mix" for the hospital. Under this assumption, the department actually has a positive excess of revenues over expenses. Now, in reality, payer mix is quite complicated and may be composed of 15 to 20 different organizations that all differ in the amount of reimbursement they provide to the hospital. Federal and state insurance programs usually reimburse costs plus a small percentage (our example assumed Medicare and Medicaid reimbursed for costs only). Others might reimburse a percentage of charges, such as in our example of Blue Cross providing 60% of the charges. Only commercial insurers and "self-pay" individuals currently reimburse full charges, as did the "other" category in the example. In Table 61–2, the payer mix was changed to Medical Assistance, Medicare, and Medicaid representing 60%; Blue Cross representing 30%; and "other" representing 10%. This is probably more realistic, as the first payer mix was quite lucrative.

TABLE **61–2:** Feasibility Summary for the Respiratory Care Services—SGH

Revenues and Expenses	Fiscal Year				
	1992	*1993*	*1994*	*1995*	*1996*
Net patient service revenue	$723,025	$835,094	$964,533	$1,114,036	$1,286,712
Operating expenses					
Indirect expenses	$152,556	$160,215	$189,311	$198,963	$228,286
Department director	$49,150	$51,608	$54,188	$56,898	$59,743
RC staff	$527,507	$553,882	$697,891	$732,786	$854,917
Billing	$22,118	$23,224	$24,385	$25,604	$26,884
RC assistants	$73,726	$77,412	$81,282	$85,347	$119,485
Drugs and gases	$12,000	$13,800	$15,870	$18,251	$20,988
Medical and surgical supplies	$144,000	$151,200	$158,760	$166,698	$175,033
Purchased services	$5000	$5250	$5513	$5788	$6078
Small equipment	$2000	$2100	$2205	$2315	$2431
Instruments	$450	$0	$0	$0	$0
Uniforms	$250	$275	$303	$333	$366
Total operating expenses	$988,756	$1,038,965	$1,229,708	$1,292,982	$1,494,210
Excess (loss) of revenues over expenses	($265,731)	($203,871)	($265,174)	($178,946)	($207,499)

Procedure	Charges	Costs
Drug aerosol	$45.00	$10.00
Oxygen	$25.00	$5.00
Ventilators	$250.00	$100.00
IS	$25.00	$5.00
CPT	$75.00	$10.00
BIPAP	$100.00	$25.00
ABGs	$35.00	$5.00
PFTs	$50.00	$10.00

Payer Mix		Reimbursement	
MA/MC	60%	MA/MC	DRG (see text)
BC	30%	BC	60% of charges
Other	10%	Other	Charges

The overall process of manipulating payer mix to optimize the return of gross revenue is known as *case mix management*. This is a difficult and complex process, as the payer mix changes significantly from unit to unit within the hospital.

With this adjustment it can be noted that the department now becomes a significant liability to the organization, with losses exceeding $200,000 per year for 4 years of the 5-year period.

The difference in the two models is that Table 61–1 represents a 56% net of gross revenues, whereas Table 61–2 nets only 42% of gross revenues. In other words, the department was originally recovering $0.56 for every $1 of charges, and this was reduced to $0.42 for each dollar. This represents a 25% loss in revenues in the face of increasing operating costs for each of the years of the model. Obviously, the payer mix is an element that management needs to control, which can be accomplished, for example, through negotiated rate setting for services to industries that might purchase the hospital services. Some patient care units may receive only 3 to 5% of gross revenues (e.g., those with an inordinately high mix of elderly patients), whereas others may appreciate a 50 to 60% return. One can readily see a future in which commercial insurers no longer reimburse 100% of charges but develop a fixed prospective payment schedule instead. This will only further stress an already marginal financial environment for health care organizations.

Productivity

As already mentioned, the principal expense for the health care organization is in the form of personnel costs, that is, wages and benefits.

Mathematically, productivity can be expressed as

Productivity = Q^O/Q^I

It is important therefore to determine the effective use of this resource in pursuing the mission of the organization.

Productivity monitoring has its traditions in the late 1800s and early 1900s in a process known as *scientific management.*[6] A popular study of 1924, the Hawthorne study (from which the often used *Hawthorne effect* originated) was designed to identify the effect of the level of plant lighting on the production level of employees. The classic definition of productivity is the relationship between qualities of outputs (Q^O) from a given system and quality of inputs (Q^I) in that same system.[7]

Outputs for the organization vary according to the level used as a reference; outputs for the hospital versus the division versus the department. Outputs could then range from mortality-morbidity to diagnostic tests to patient days. Alternatively, it might take the form of treatments or total service output (procedures) for a given department. Examples of inputs are total operating expenses, worked or paid hours per FTE. Some prefer to eliminate the idea of a treatment per se and instead substitute a raw measure of output, termed the relative value unit. This is a unitless number that identifies all output processes, such as treatments, equipment repair, or travel time to yield a measure that might take the form of relative value units per worked hour as a productivity measure.

Managers of a clinical service are often required to address changes in service (the addition or deletion of services) in terms of their effect on manpower needs. To this end, a productivity analysis can be useful in this decision-making process. One method of arriving at such an endpoint is through the development of time standards that tie together service volume (in terms of numbers of procedures performed) and staff time to provide the service. A time standard represents an average amount of time needed to perform a given task. Several different tasks would require a time standard for each given task. The fact that this number is an average represents a major problem: Tasks that have a high degree of time variability are less accurately represented by this technique. In other words, if a given treatment can realistically take 5 to 25 minutes per treatment, depending on prevailing patient conditions, a standard of 12.5 minutes could significantly underestimate true labor needs. In cases such as this, it may be necessary to break down the procedure into its most frequently used forms, such as an initial treatment versus a daily treatment or an emergency versus a routine procedure. This further discrimination of the task can lead to a more homogeneous allotment of time needed to perform the procedure and improve the accuracy of the standard.

Time standards can be purchased externally (the American Hospital Association's Monitrend or the American Association of Respiratory Care [AARC] Uniform Reporting Manual) or they can be internally determined. This latter method can be a difficult process. Perhaps the best approach is to formulate a comprehensive plan of action that describes the utility and the source of the data to be collected. Some starting point for the analysis might include the following questions: How accurate do the data need to be? How many data points need to be collected to achieve a truly representative sample? How will the information be used? How will the data be collected?

There are several techniques to answer the question regarding how the data are collected. Decisions of this sort should be addressed by others in the organization that might have a vested interest in the ultimate use of the data. For example, if the information is to serve as a primary vehicle for staffing requests, it would be prudent to solicit the input of a management engineering department or its equivalent from within the organization. The bottom line to such an endeavor is the ultimate utility of the data, and to that end credibility is key. Rejection of one's conclusions by the vice president of the division is less likely if he or she believes the data are accurate and unbiased.

Collection of the data can take the form of rigorous questioning of the staff regarding the perceived time needed for a given task (the Delphi technique), having staff maintain a diary of time per procedure, or by actual time motion studies. These studies measure time in performing the task along with "down time," such as travel time to the patient, charting, discussions with family and physicians, and so on. Time motion studies requires a rather large investment by the organization to achieve this degree of accuracy and are the preferred method if the data are to play an important role in the decisions for staffing needs. Indexing the total time for a given service by some element of input then completes the equation used earlier.

Let us suppose that a respiratory care department wishes to develop such standards for a productivity system to offer a new metered dose inhaler service to outpatients. A time motion study is performed, determining that a complete treatment requires 9.75 minutes per treatment. Because of the homogeneity of the patient population, there is little variation in the time measurements, and they are considered to be reliable (i.e., reproducible). A projected volume for this service is 10 patients per day, 5 days per week, or 2600 patients per year. You could then arrive at a staffing need by the following calculation:

$$\text{needed FTEs} = \frac{(2600 \text{ patients/year}) (0.16 \text{ hour/patient})^*}{1920 \text{ worked hours/FTE} \dagger}$$

The needed staff for this change in service is 0.22 FTE.

This calculation has been simplified to illustrate a point. In reality, however, it is more complicated; services in the hospital are usually offered 24 hours per day, and treatments are often not performed one at a time. Additionally, process variables such as performing therapy in three different wings of the hospital or all on one unit must be considered. Some might also add a productivity "target" to the preceding equation that further defines the expectations of the staff needed. Service demands are also not consistent; just the opposite is true and staffing for peaks and valleys in service can be quite challenging. Finally, the revenue side of the equation must be considered to balance the expenses incurred for providing the service, although managed care models increasingly minimize the role of revenue analysis for such decisions.

Budgeting

The list of operating expenses in Tables 61–1 and 61–2 represents a simplified approach to all the expenses that a department must plan and control. The largest expense category is personnel costs and to a large degree an operating budget must plan, identify, and justify its budget around this single issue. The budgeting process has been known to be a

---

*9.75 min/60 min/hr

†Worked hours incorporates 2 weeks of vacation (80 hr/yr) and 40 hr/yr for each: sick time and holiday time; all subtracted from 2080 hr/FTE/year. (One then monitors the performance of this therapy with a productivity profile such as treatments per worked hour to identify trends in the service.)

Fiscal year—a 12-month period that is named by the year in which the period ends

An FTE is an individual or groups of individuals that work 2080 hours per year. These are *paid* hours that incorporate holiday, vacation, and sick time into the 2080 hours. Two employees may each work 1040 hours per year in a permanent, part-time job, and each would be 0.5 FTE.

Careful monitoring of productivity trends can be helpful in understanding the appropriateness of staffing levels.

A different technique for projecting future trends in a given data point would be to use a regression equation such as the least squares method.[9] This involves the mathematical manipulation of at least 5 years of data to determine a probable trend for some future interval.

source of confusion and fear for management neophytes, but viewed in the most basic terms, the budget represents an operational plan.[8] This plan, which usually covers a period of 1 year, describes the expense categories that are necessary to achieve organizational objectives and the financial resources that will be used to accomplish this task.

The operational budgeting process usually begins 6 months prior to the beginning of the next fiscal year. For example, many fiscal years start July 1, 199a and end June 30, 199b; the budget for this interval would be called fiscal year 199b. Many methods for developing a budget exist, but only two, historical base and zero base budgets, are described here.

By far, the more common budgetary process is the historical process. This procedure begins with some underlying assumptions concerning the next fiscal year. This is a necessary component because the proverbial crystal ball still does not exist, so the next best approach is to make assumptions regarding important operational issues. Topics that may be included in these assumptions are projected patient volume, the implementation of new programs, changes to existing clinical programs, or the emergence of new external forces such as regulatory mandates or reimbursement changes. This is a difficult process because the answers to many of the issues are not readily known.

The next step in the process is to review historical data in light of the assumptions. These data provide a mechanism to formulate the baseline budget for the next fiscal year. Of primary concern is the wage and salary budget, since it represents the major portion of the budgeted dollars. The standard unit for personnel is the FTE. The determination of how many FTEs the department or work unit will need for the next fiscal year will largely be driven on the basis of the assumptions that define the environment for the next year. Will new services begin during this time, will jobs be redesigned, or will the service be decentralized? These are only a few of the possibilities for directions in a clinical service that will have a major impact on the personnel needs of the department.

Another consideration in deriving a personnel budget is productivity. Increasing the scope of a clinical service may not require the need for additional personnel if a strategy of improving productivity of the existing staff allows for the provision of new service demands. All available information should be used in the derivation of the personnel budget because this is the single most important aspect of preparing an operating budget. Recall that in Table 61–1 the wage and salary component of the theoretical department was about 67% of total operating expenses.

Historical data for the supplies for the current fiscal year are also reviewed to determine the baseline for the next fiscal year. For example, the medical-surgical equipment expense category (disposable equipment, adapters, tubing, water, and so on) is reviewed for the past 6 months to determine an average value for each month. This figure is then annualized to project a dollar amount that represents a 12-month or annual interval. Let us assume the department spent $6350 per month (an average figure based on actual spending) on medical-surgical supplies for the period June through December. This figure would annualize to $76,200 for a 12-month interval ($6350 × 12—An alternative method calculates the dollars on a daily basis. Suppose the actual spending for the same 6-month interval, 181 days, was $38,100. This equals $210.50/day × 365 = $76,832).

Table 61–3 lists expense line items that more accurately depict the magnitude of a complete operating budget. By reviewing historical data

TABLE **61–3:** Typical Budgeted Expenses for an Ancillary Department

Wage and Salary Expense
Therapists
Technicians
Assistants
Supervisors
Director
Medical director and other physician consulting salaries
Biomedical technician
Supplies
Medical-surgical
Medical gases
Drugs
Small equipment
Office supplies
Postage
Slides
Book and journals
Printing
Repair maintenance supplies
Purchased Services
Purchased repair-maintenance contracts
Purchased services (per diem)
Other Expenses
Travel and meetings
Uniforms
Utilities
Telephone

in light of operating assumptions for each of the categories, one can derive a new baseline budget.

A second method of budget preparation is known as zero-based budgeting. This process involves the total justification of a given expense for it to be included in the next year's budget. In other words, the baseline budget is zero, and the expense category is justified as though it were a completely new program or expense. Typically, most budgets incorporate some line items as zero-based, thus forcing the author to provide a detailed explanation for the need of this resource allocation.

After thorough review by the department director, medical director, and administrator, the budget is usually passed on to the finance department. Their charge is to assure that the budget is in compliance with the spending guidelines for the organization (perhaps a 4% overall reduction in spending was designated as a "target" for each cost center) and to review the document for accuracy. This department, in association with the chief financial officer, compiles the budgets from all cost centers to construct a global picture of the institution's spending for presentation to the executive staff. The budget must then receive approval from the board of directors before it can be implemented.

Managed Care

Much of this section has focused on the impact of prospective payment systems on the financial status of health care providers. It is clear that this system has radically changed the way hospitals do business in the 1990s. However, this system is destined to evolve a step further and place a significant increase in financial risk on the doorstep of most hospitals in this country. The national emphasis on health care reform brings managed care products to the marketplace of many American cities. These systems rely on preventive health care, utilization review, primary care "gatekeepers," and a host of other strategies to manage the care of patients enrolled in this type of coverage plan. The concept goes well beyond the scope of this chapter, but many have an understanding of how health maintenance organizations operate from the flurry of media coverage.

However, one of many payment possibilities for physicians and hospitals is much different from those described previously and warrants a brief description here. Consider how most of us purchase health care coverage today. A common practice is to purchase some form of health care insurance that may be jointly purchased with an employer and may have some out-of-pocket expenses (in the form of "copayments" or deductibles) associated with it. Usually, these expenses are for medications or a flat portion of a hospitalization, say $250, that is the insured's responsibility for payment.

Let's say that a typical family pays $75 per month for health care insurance; the employer picks up the rest of the monthly tab. Let's also imagine that one member of this family of four has a minor surgical procedure (tonsillectomy), one member makes several office visits (the oldest son has asthma), and unfortunately, a parent is hospitalized for a discectomy that same year. Now, let's add up the dollars and see how this works. The total cost for this fictional family this year was $900 in monthly premiums, a $250 deductible for the discectomy, and $100 for copayments for asthma medications, bringing the total bill to $1250. But what were the actual costs of this family's medical care for the year? Let's assume that this care was provided in Efficient Hospital Systems, Inc., a for-profit chain that is as efficient as it gets in health care, and that the total bill for the care described here was $9760 for the discectomy, $2150 for the tonsillectomy, and $425 for the office visits. These charges totaled $12,335 but were discounted to the insurance company for a new total of $11,101. The family's bill was $1250, and the total cost was $11,101; who made up the difference in these two figures? Obviously, the insurance company assumed the burden of this hypothetical scenario because it was paid on a capitated basis. That is, it received prospective monthly payments from the insured family that did not change, even though the family required much more care than the sum total of their premiums and out-of-pocket expenses.

Now, what has this to do with hospital reimbursement? Many managed care plans feature a capitated payment schedule to both physicians and hospitals; it is a prospective monthly payment (usually stated as per member per month) that is a flat fee to these providers, who now assume the financial risk of providing health care, as did the insurance company in the previous paragraph. The costs of providing care for illness that exceed the capitated payment represent a financial loss for the provider. The strategies to achieve financial viability in the capitated environment are to reduce inpatient admissions per enrollee and to reduce the cost per inpatient admission. There is very little margin for the bottom line to absorb until it becomes red and the system must quickly contract to avoid disaster.

LEADERSHIP

Earlier, this chapter presented a number of trends that will shape health care over the next decade and the resulting challenges to managers to survive these changes. Clearly, there needs to be strong leadership at all levels of an organization to seize the opportunities that present themselves in the process of change. Effective leadership makes the difference in determining who will prosper and who will fail during these times.

Classically, management is the process of planning, leading, organizing, and controlling an organization. However, some now separate leading from the traditional view of management. Both managers and leaders are charged with three basic tasks:

- Determine what is to be accomplished.
- Establish an environment conducive to the process.
- Assure the job is performed.

Kotter describes a model that clarifies distinct differences in the manner that managers and leaders reach these end-points.[10] Table 61–4 identifies Kotter's differences between managing and leading. These distinctions are subtle yet offer practical insights to leadership. Every manager must cope with the complexity of the organization—the politics, the paperwork and the administrative channels for accomplishing the goals of the organization. This is not leadership, however. *Change* is the only consistent attribute of the 1990s, and it is the leader who adopts this additional focus in moving the organization to a new position. As Kotter notes, "More change always demands more leadership,"[10] and so it is the leader who will provide an environment that facilitates this process.

Kotter also describes other attributes of effective leaders. The most imaginative vision is destined to failure if the leadership cannot articulate its specifics to the work unit. Imbedded in this concept is the ability to effectively communicate the vision. This implies more than simply being able to talk to large groups of individuals. Implicit is the need to stress the values of the audience one is addressing to make the concept important to these individuals.[10] Kotter also identifies the need for credibility in this process. This involves the track record of the individual delivering the message, the content of the message, the leader's reputation for integrity and trustworthiness, and the consistency between words and deeds.[9]

At the heart of leadership is the notion of motivation or the ability of the leader to change the behavior of the individuals in the work unit, not by pushing them in the right direction but by attending to basic human needs for achievement—a sense of belonging, recognition, self-esteem, a feeling of control over one's life, and the ability to live up to

TABLE **61–4:** Differences Between Managing and Leading

Management (Coping with Complexity)	Leadership (Coping with Change)
Planning and Budgeting Involves goal setting with detailed actions and resources committed to achieving goals; is deductive in nature	*Setting a Direction* Involves developing a vision and strategies needed to achieve the change; is inductive in nature
Organizing and Staffing Involves job formation to accomplish goals, providing qualified staff in jobs, and monitoring for success	*Aligning Individuals* Involves communicating the vision to create "coalitions" to staff who are committed to the new direction
Controlling and Problem-solving Involves monitoring, identifying problems and their solutions to meet organizational goals	*Motivating and Inspiring* Involves keeping the process on track and recognizing the importance of human needs, values, and emotions

one's ideals.[10] There are several motivational theories that are relevant, but they are beyond the scope of this chapter. However, I will include a few practical points regarding motivation.

Before discussing motivation, a few general comments are in order. It is difficult to generalize motivational theory and information to larger groups of diverse individuals, as tempting a thought as that might be. Rakich and colleagues clarify three important ground rules that help one approach the individuals in a specific work group.[6]

1. *No one is an average person.* This may sound trite at first but it is one of those universal truths (well, almost). Individuals differ in every conceivable manner, so taking one, simple approach to dealing with the needs of a group of individuals is destined to failure.

2. *Individuals work to satisfy their own needs.* The items listed further on are a potpourri of concerns that many individuals share, but the relative importance of each to any one individual varies significantly. Therefore, motivating a group of individuals is difficult if one assumes all needs are the same.

3. *Individuals respond to leadership,* that is, effective leaders can help those around them meet their needs and at the same time achieve organizational goals.

Herzberg and associates developed a two-dimensional theory of motivation that identified a "maintenance" dimension that, when lacking, tends to dissatisfy employees and when present, usually tends to be a weak motivator. The second dimension of this theory involves a "motivational" dimension that, when present, can serve as a strong motivator[10] (Table 61–5). Interestingly enough, salary is not listed as a motivational factor. In fact, the notion of pay as a motivator is thought to be important only when the following circumstances exist:[11]

- It is linked to individual job performance.
- This linkage occurs in such a way that the employee can control the aspects under evaluation.
- The pay increases are sufficiently large to be meaningful.

Often all three of these criteria are difficult to fulfill and as such, pay as a motivational tool cannot be used reliably.

Again, Herzberg's factors differ in priority for each individual, so a generalized ranking of factors will not be applicable to different popula-

TABLE **61–5:** Herzberg's Two-Dimensional Motivational Theory

Maintenance Dimension
Organizational policy and administration
Technical supervision
Interpersonal relations with supervisor
Interpersonal relations with peers
Interpersonal relations with subordinates
Salary
Job security
Personal life
Work conditions
Status
Motivational Dimension
Achievement
Recognition
Advancement
The work itself
The possibility of growth
Responsibility

tions of employees. However, it is important to note that factors appearing in the "motivational" dimension are often variables for which many managers have some element of control. Pritchett and Pound refer to many of these factors in their description of "team reconstruction."[12] They speak of spending "soft currency" in the form of "psychological paychecks." They recommend everything from a simple pat on the back to empathy and understanding to bigger titles and special assignments to soliciting suggestions and opinions.

The only limit is imagination and a willingness to satisfy the emotional needs of the staff in the workplace. As Pritchett and Pound put it:

> Most managers don't realize the importance that their acceptance and approval carry with subordinates. As a result, they waste this most precious resource through sheer neglect—like a bank account they never touch, money they never spend, that could be freely used to motivate and improve employees' quality of work life . . . When it comes to handing out psychological paychecks, you should spend extravagantly.[12]

MANAGEMENT STYLE

Much has been written concerning management style, as in theories X, Y, or Z. The first two theories were advanced by McGregor in delineating a spectrum of management style that occupies two ends of a continuum.[13] At one end, theory X maintains that the average worker has an inherent dislike for work and therefore needs direct control to assure the achievement of organizational objectives. Additionally, this theory assumes the worker prefers this direct supervision because he or she has little ambition. At the other end of the continuum is a completely different concept of the employee and his or her view of the workplace. Work may actually be a source of satisfaction, and individuals may be capable of self-control in the context of their work environment. Importantly, theory Y contends that lack of ambition, avoidance of responsibility, and emphasis on security (as found in theory X) are not inherent human characteristics.

In contrast to the preceding models, Ouchi developed theory Z as an opposing paradigm that recognizes that workers exhibit both theory X and theory Y characteristics.[14] The strategy for managers, therefore, is to maximize the desirable characteristics while controlling and modifying those attributes that are counterproductive to organizational goals. Ouchi stressed the need to involve the workers in operational issues as a means to improve productivity and quality for the organization.

In keeping with Kotter's overriding theme that management and leadership are different skills, we will now focus on describing leadership styles.

Although several personality traits are common to effective leaders, the role of the environment must be considered in any analysis that describes how these leaders make decisions. To this end, Fiedler developed a contingency model of leadership.[15] This model integrates an analysis of leadership styles into three situational (environmental) factors:

1. Leader-member relations—this quantifies the relationship of the leader and work group members and is the most important variable in the three situations.

2. Task structure—the degree to which the tasks of the work group are defined.

Task-oriented style describes the leader's actions that define leader-follower relationships, establish definite standards of performance, specify standard operating procedures, and determine who does what.

Relationship-oriented style describes the leader's attitude toward followers, the warmth of the leader-follower relationships, the leader's willingness to listen, and the degree of mutual trust between the leader and the follower.[11]

3. Leader position power—the scope of the leader's legitimate power base.

Each of the three situations is divided into positive and negative possibilities that result in a grid of combinations. Each combination of the preceding situations is assigned a numeral from 1 to 8 that expresses a range of situations from most favorable (1) (i.e., when a leader is likely to have a *large* influence on the function of a work group) to least favorable situations (8) (i.e., when a leader is likely to have *minimal* influence on the function of a work group). The leadership styles used in this model are task-oriented and relationship-oriented.

Fiedler maintains that these two styles are at opposing ends of a continuum of behavior and that they represent an underlying need structure of the leader that motivates the use of each style in various situations. Fiedler also argues that leadership style is a function of one's personality and therefore cannot be readily changed.[16] Fiedler does suggest, however, that instead of changing the leader one should focus on changing the leader's environment.[16] For example, the leader's power position can be changed by assigning him or her sole authority for a project. Perhaps the task structure could be changed by assigning a situation in only the most abstract terms if that better matches the individual's style. Lastly, one could change the leader-member relations by controlling the make-up of the work group to better pair style and members.

Task-oriented leaders perform better at the ends of the continuum when good leader-member relations are coupled with structured tasks or when poor leader-member relations are combined with unstructured tasks. In other words, the task-oriented leadership style seems to be most effective in having a task accomplished by a group effort when the situations are very favorable or very unfavorable. The nondirective, relationship-oriented style is most effective in situations that are intermediate in difficulty.[16]

It could be argued that more "situations" exist than have been factored into Fiedler's analysis or that it may be difficult to characterize one individual as either task-oriented or relationship-oriented; probably, traits of both exist in the same manager. The contingency model is still worthy of attention, however, as it places the style of the leader into the larger context of the immediate environment.

A second leadership style, proposed by Tannenbaum and Schmidt is termed *participative leadership.*[17] This model is a continuum of leadership behavior, from "boss centered" to "subordinate centered."

Several strong arguments favor the use of a more subordinate-centered leadership style. Providing constructive input for the direction of the organization is an important motivational strategy because it offers a sense of control for the staff in this process. Direction that tends to be "bottom-up," as opposed to "top-down," also tends to be accepted more readily because the work group may perceive "ownership" of the change process. Involving employees in decision-making brings many perspectives and differing experiences to the project. This process can provide a wider range of options along with an enriched experience for those who participate.

A leader can use a wide range of behaviors. It would be misleading to think that only one arm of this paradigm would be used by any individual. Clearly there are times when a more autocratic style is preferred. Consider the example of a disaster: Panic and chaos could result if the manager called a participative discussion regarding assignments to the disaster drill. Quick change that precludes participative involvement demands the use of more authority by the manager. It is the effective leader who understands the appropriate urgency of the environment and adjusts his or her style as needed. Effective leaders will then "slide" across the continuum, invoking the style that best fits the situation at hand. Even Fiedler agrees that effective leadership involves a change in behavior from a directive to a more permissive style when the environment indicates the need to do so.[16]

True power is that which can be given to others, but this is a difficult task for those who may feel a bit out of control in the process.

Not all aspects of participative leadership can be construed positively. Many managers who engage in this style of leadership may find the process threatening. Clearly, the leader of the group needs to have a clear sense of self so that power can be delegated to those at the table. Some managers may also feel that the participative style is a form of relinquishing responsibility by the very nature of the process. This notion was addressed by Tannenbaum and Schmidt in a recent retrospective commentary on their original work.[17] They point out that the leader in the group process must be willing to be held accountable for the quality of the decisions made and that he or she must also be willing to assume the necessary risks that accompany this process. Again, the limiting factor for many in engaging in this process may well be their ability to cope with ambiguity and a perceived loss of control.

Involving a group to work through problems or to flesh out a new direction for an organization can create its own stumbling blocks. For example, the scope of the task must be manageable by the group and within the boundaries of the expertise of the participants. It may not be appropriate for a group of technically oriented individuals to work out the details of a complicated budget unless the leadership is willing to invest the energy to provide the necessary background information. Instead, this group might be better equipped to provide some feedback on upcoming capital purchases of technical equipment. Time becomes an increasingly scarce commodity. Since this process is not efficient, it is imperative that sufficient time be provided for the process to be successful. Good group dynamics are needed to keep the members on target. In fact substantial direction may be necessary to start the process. Pritchett and Pound refer to "pointing your team toward magnetic north" as a means of setting the stage for the vision or the process that confronts the team.[12] Groups being as they are, it is more than likely that not all will want to participate. Some staff members may feel that "that is management's job" and elect to be on the periphery. Mandatory attendance for all workers is a possibility, but this must be weighed against the possible disruptive potential of this strategy. Finally, this process must be entered with an atmosphere of sincerity and commitment by all. Failure by the leaders to follow through with the process only undermines respect and future credibility. The long-term consequences of a half-hearted attempt are grim, indeed.

The issue now becomes how to decide which leadership style to use. Tannenbaum and Schmidt describe three basic forces the manager should consider to make this decision: forces in the manager, forces in the subordinates, and forces in the situation.[17]

- Forces in the manager include the manager's value system, his or her confidence in subordinates, his or her own leadership inclinations, and feelings of security in an uncertain situation. Delegation of responsibility leads to increased uncertainty, and this may be unsettling for many who must assume responsibility for the end product.
- Forces in the subordinates: Do they have high needs for independence, a readiness to assume more responsibility, the necessary understanding and experience to manage the problem?

- Forces in the situation: the type of organization (i.e., its values, traditions, the size of the work groups), group effectiveness (i.e., the experience of the members, cohesiveness, mutual acceptance, and so on), the problem itself, the pressure of time.

Cerebral face—operating with words and numbers of rationality. Insightful face—rooted in the feel and images of the manager's integrity.

Obviously, this difficult decision-making process requires a balance of fact and judgment—what Mintzberg terms the *cerebral face versus the insightful face.*[18] Leadership is not a science that can be reduced to a mathematical expression; therefore, one must rely on more intuitive, common sense approaches to determine exactly how to lead in a given situation. The glaring omission of a strict definition of leadership in this chapter was purposeful to avoid having the reader walk away with a "pat" definition of leadership. Leadership is many things; therefore, the situation, the individuals, and the leader must all be known to provide any meaningful answer to this dialectic.

Finally, our discussion of leadership would not be complete without an *almost* universal truth: not everyone can be the leader. What, then, of the other intelligent, well-motivated individuals who demonstrate a positive potential for the organization? Kelley answers this question with the notion that followers play an important and necessary role in the organization.[19] Followers should be groomed, trained, and used to the advantage of both worker and organization. Followers become the informal leaders of the organization, who act as a stabilizing force when the going gets a bit rocky. Followers also become role models that effective leaders can reward with "soft currency," which in time pays major dividends. An effective followership also becomes a core of self-managed individuals who can assume new responsibilities and enhance their quality of work life. It is clear that an effective organization of the 1990s will need to balance each side of the equation with both dynamic leadership and followership.

SUMMARY

A major goal of this chapter was to stress the business aspect of the health care arena and to draw parallels to perhaps better-known industries. The reason for this emphasis is clear: the next few years are likely to harbor radical changes in the very fabric of this industry. Major players in the field, such as academic medical centers, are especially vulnerable. This uncertainty and prospect for change require all who choose health care as a profession to understand clearly the business of health care. It is hoped that the need for other portions of this chapter is also self-evident. The nuts and bolts of management were presented as an impetus to further reading. Details on expenses, budgeting, and productivity were offered as insight into how the business is run. The last section focused on leadership as an intentional strategy to demonstrate that effective leaders are not born but are products of a motivation to understand their task and develop the skills that promote leadership. It is after all leadership, and a healthy dose of followership, that will be required to navigate through the difficult and challenging times ahead. That which seems impossible is often a perceptual problem, and this chapter was intended as a start to seeing things differently, so that someday the impossible may be realized.

References

1. Vincenzino GB. Statistical Bulletin. Metropolitan Life Insurance Company, January/March, 1991, pp 2–11.
2. Rice GP. Health and long term care for the aged. AEA Papers and Proceedings 179(2):343–348, 1989.
3. Valinsky W, Starkman JL. The impact of DRGs on the health care industry. Health Care Management Rev 12(3):61–74, 1987.
4. Fray WM, Metwalli AM. Tax Equity and Fiscal Responsibility Act of 1982: An incentive to improve productivity in health care. Health Care Management Rev 12(2):31–35, 1987.
5. Cleverley WO. Essentials of Health Care Finance, 2nd ed. Rockville, MD, Aspen Publishers, 1986.
6. Rakich JS, Longest BD, Darr K. Managing Health Services Organization, 2nd ed. Philadelphia, WB Saunders, 1985, p 265.
7. Fink DS. Productivity Management: Planning, Measurement and Evaluation Control and Improvement. New York, John Wiley & Sons, 1985, p 43.
8. Herkimer AG. Understanding Health Care Budgeting. Rockville, MD, Aspen Publishers, 1988.
9. Kotter JP. What liters really do. Harvard Business Rev May-June, 1990.
10. Herzberg F, Mausner B, Snyderman B. The Motivation to Work, 2nd ed. New York, John Wiley & Sons, 1959.
11. Pringle CD, Jennings DF, Longenecker JG. Managing Organizations, Functions and Behaviors. Columbus, OH, Merrill Publishing, 1988.
12. Pritchett T, Pound R. Key Reconstruction: Building a High Performance Work Group During Change. Dallas, Pritchett Publishing, 1992.
13. McGregor D. The Human Side of Enterprise. New York, McGraw-Hill, 1960, pp 33–34.
14. Ouchi WG. Theory Z: How American Businesses Can Meet the Japanese Challenge. Redding, MA, Addison-Wesley, 1981.
15. Fiedler FE, Chemers MN. Leadership and Effective Management. Glenview, IL, Scott, Foresman, 1974.
16. Fiedler FE. Engineer the job of manager. Harvard Business Rev, September-October:115–122, 1965.
17. Tannenbaum R, Schmidt WH. How to choose a leadership pattern. Harvard Business Rev, May-June:162–180, 1973.
18. Mintzberg H. Manager job: Folklore and fact. Harvard Business Rev, March-April:170, 1990.
19. Kelley RE. In praise of followers. Harvard Business Rev, November-December:142–148, 1988.

62

Research and Statistics for the Clinician

Robert L. Chatburn, R.R.T.,
and Dean Hess, M.Ed., R.R.T.

The scientific method is a systematic, objective, ordered approach to gathering and solving problems.

What is clinical research and how does it relate to respiratory care? The parallels and relationships between clinical respiratory care and clinical research may be closer than most therapists realize. Research provides the scientific basis for respiratory care practice. *Clinical research* is actually an approach to clinical practice that can be used in everyday patient care.

SCIENCE AND THE SCIENTIFIC METHOD

Research is an objective approach to finding answers to questions based on the *scientific method*. Science is simply organized curiosity. Science is based on data. Unlike anecdotal evidence (e.g., clinical experience), science can be replicated and validated. Science and research are meant to be unbiased—good research *determines whether* rather than *proves that* and seeks not to *prove* but rather to *improve*.

The scientific method can be described as a series of steps that lead from a question to answer (and usually to questions). Figure 62–1 illustrates these steps by way of analogy.

Step 1: *Formulate a concise problem statement*. It is helpful to think in terms of (1) what you see happening and (2) why it is important. In the example, the problem is to identify an unknown coin. The statement might be "I need to identify this coin so that I can spend it."

Step 2: *Generate a hypothesis*. It is difficult to describe how this is done because it is an act of creativity. One can best prepare by thoroughly studying all aspects of the problem so that the mind becomes fertile ground for appropriate hypotheses to reveal themselves. In the example, the hypothesis is that the coin is a penny.

Step 3: *Define rejection criteria*. The hypothesis will be judged on the basis of some objective, measurable criteria that must be defined before conducting the experiment. For the coin example, objective and measurable criteria include color and size.

Step 4: *Make a prediction*, that is, state the study hypothesis in terms of the rejection criteria. For example, if the coin is a penny minted in the United States, it will have a copper color and a diameter of 1.9 cm.

Step 5: *Design and carry out the experiment*. The rejection criteria define the type of measurements required in the experiment. A sample of the coin in question must be obtained and observations made regarding color and size.

1236

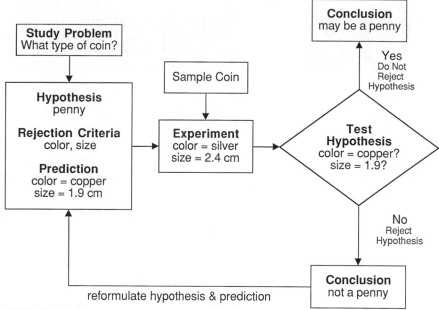

FIGURE 62–1: The scientific method in the form of an algorithm. In this example, the scientific method is used to determine the identity of a coin.

Step 6: *Test the hypothesis.* Note that it is the hypothesis, not the experimental unit (e.g., the coin) that is being tested. The hypothesis is tested by comparing the prediction with the data from the experiment. If the data contradict the prediction, the hypothesis is rejected. A new hypothesis must then be generated along with another prediction based on the rejection criteria. If, however, the data are consistent with the prediction, the hypothesis is not rejected. Strictly speaking, the hypothesis is not accepted either but rather is held as a temporary explanation of reality until other data are available that would suggest a more useful hypothesis. The life span of hypothesis is inversely proportional to the amount of scientific study devoted to it. In our example, we conclude that the coin may be a penny. We do not blindly accept that it *is* a penny because other reasonable hypotheses have not been tested (e.g., that the coin is of a foreign denomination with the same physical characteristics as a US penny.)

It is important to be thoroughly familiar with this process since it is the basis of all scientific research. Of course, not all research is designed to test a hypothesis. Some of the steps may be eliminated, for example, for descriptive studies (e.g., new product evaluations).

WHY CLINICIANS NEED TO KNOW ABOUT RESEARCH METHODOLOGY

Only a disappointingly few clinicians actually conduct formal research projects. Nonetheless, all clinicians should have a basic working knowledge of research methodology for the following reasons:

1. Everyday clinical practice requires answers to questions. Similar to the research process, answering practical questions should be system-

atic and objective. One can accomplish this by developing an inquiring approach to clinical respiratory care—in other words, asking questions when things do not seem right and acting on data rather than on experience alone. A scientific approach to clinical practice will base clinical decisions on data as much as possible. This means, for example, administering oxygen to a patient with chronic obstructive pulmonary disease to treat documented hypoxemia, not because "that's the way we always do it." A trial of positive end-expiratory pressure is a good example of application of the scientific method to clinical practice. The clinical question is "What level of positive end-expiratory pressure produces the best oxygen delivery for a hypoxic patient?" Optimum oxygen delivery may be defined in terms of a specific range of cardiac output and oxygen content of arterial blood. Data (e.g., Pa_{O_2}, cardiac output, and so on) are then collected at several levels of positive end-expiratory pressure to objectively answer the question.

2. The results of research studies are published in the scientific literature. It is important that clinicians be able to critically assess the methodology of these studies. The conclusions of a published research study should never be accepted on faith without a critical evaluation of the methods and results on which the conclusions are based. An understanding of research methodology causes the scientific literature to "come to life" and have meaning.

3. Quality control and quality assurance programs (such as those mandated by the Joint Commission on Accreditation of Healthcare Organizations and the Clinical Laboratory Improvement Act '88) require systematic data collection and analysis. An example of this is the Levey-Jennings plot used in the blood gas laboratory. This plot is generated from quality control data. It requires statistical analysis (e.g., calculation of means and standard deviations) as well as a thoughtful interpretation of results (e.g., Is the analyzer in or out of control?).

4. A basic knowledge of research methodology is needed if one wishes to design and conduct formal research projects for publication. Such studies are necessary to establish the scientific basis for respiratory care. Ideally, these studies should be designed and conducted by respiratory care practitioners and physicians interested in respiratory care practice.

RESEARCH METHODOLOGY: COMPONENTS OF CLINICAL RESEARCH

For formal research projects, the novice can get started by helping others with their projects. Research requires teamwork, and a good place to get some hands-on experience with clinical research is to join a team doing research. The components of clinical research follow.

Generate an Idea

Many legitimate ideas for research projects result from irritations or frustrations that occur during routine clinical activities.

The research process begins with an idea, which, in turn, comes from clinical experience. Ideas for research projects can be fostered by developing an inquiring attitude, seeking answers to clinical questions from colleagues and the literature, and from searching for improvements in patient care.

TABLE **62–1:** Examples of Study Questions

Good study questions:
- What is the relationship between the dependency level of chronic ventilator patients and their length of hospitalization?
- Are day-to-day peak flow variations predictive of the need for hospitalization in asthmatics?
- Is there a relationship between the frequency of turning and the development of atelectasis in comatose patients?
- Does the use of pulse oximetry decrease the incidence of retinopathy of prematurity in preterm infants?

Poor study questions:
- Do respiratory therapists know their legal liabilities?
- Is intravenous magnesium sulfate useful in the treatment of asthma? ·
- Are positive expiratory pressure masks useful in cystic fibrosis?
- Do transcutaneous P_{CO_2} monitors work in adults?

Develop the Study Question

Good research is the result of a good study question. A practical study question has five attributes: it is focused, clear, brief, "doable," and has a measurable outcome. Many projects fail because the study question is too broad in scope, too vague, cannot be answered with the available resources, or has no tangible outcome. Table 62–1 provides some examples of good and poor study questions.

State the Null Hypothesis

The null hypothesis is usually a statement of no difference between or among treatments of experimental conditions (Table 62–2). The null hypothesis is a statistical concept based on the desire to minimize the possibility of concluding that there is a difference among data groups when in fact no difference exists. It can usually be generated by rewording the study question. A null hypothesis is usually not necessary for descriptive studies in which there is only one group of data.

Search the Literature

An early and important step in the research process is a thorough search of the literature. The search provides an orientation to what is known related to the research question and provides ideas for the methods to be used when designing the study. The literature search helps to determine whether the question is worthy of further investigation (i.e., the question may already have been answered by others). Also, what aspects of the question are likely to be of interest to your peers? When conducting a search, check as many related studies as possible. Look for

TABLE **62–2:** Examples of Statements of the Null Hypothesis

- There is no difference in the length of hospitalization between chronic ventilator patients with a high dependency level and those with a low dependency level.
- There is no difference in the number of hospital admissions per year for asthmatics with high day-to-day peak flow variations and those with stable day-to-day peak flows.
- There is no difference in the frequency of atelectasis in comatose patients who are turned side-to-side every 2 hours and those who are turned once per shift.
- There is no difference in the incidence of retinopathy of prematurity in preterm infants who are monitored with pulse oximetry and those in whom pulse oximetry is not used.

Note: the journal *Respiratory Care* is found in CINAHL but not in Medline.

current review articles and examine the reference sections for leads. Computerized search facilities such as Medline and CINAHL (Cumulative Index to Nursing and Allied Health Literature) are particularly useful. Rely on primary references (i.e., the original medical journal articles) rather than secondary references (i.e., interpretations of articles found in books).

Consult An Expert

Before the research protocol is written, it is a good idea to get some input from others about the project. This may include colleagues who have performed similar research as well as someone familiar with statistics. Expert advice at this point in the process can help to refine the study question, assess the experimental methodology, and develop an implementation plan. A statistician can be particularly helpful in determining the sample size for study.

Design the Experiment

There are a number of issues that should be considered when designing the experiment.

Study Type. There are three basic study designs: the case study, the device or method evaluation, and the original clinical study. The case study is a description of a case with exceptional teaching value. There is usually no need for statistical analysis and no hypothesis testing involved in a case study, so this form is particularly good for the novice researcher. A device or method evaluation focuses on a description of methodology and usually requires at least descriptive statistical analyses such as means, standard deviations, linear regression, and error intervals. An original study is the most advanced study design and usually involves hypothesis testing by more sophisticated statistical procedures such as *t*-tests and analysis of variance.

Designs that are prospective but less scientifically rigorous (e.g., ones with no random assignment of groups) are called *quasiexperimental.*

A *retrospective study* is one in which the study is designed after the data are recorded (Fig. 62–2). An example might be a quality assurance project in which the medical records of patients who have been mechanically ventilated for the past year are reviewed to determine the incidence of accidental disconnection. This project illustrates some of the problems with retrospective studies: There may have been disconnections that were not recorded and the consequences of the disconnects that were recorded may be unknown. A special type of retrospective study is the *case control study.* With this design, the study group (cases) with the trait of interest is retrospectively compared with a matched control group. An example might be a study that retrospectively compares a group of mechanically ventilated patients who experienced barotrauma (cases) to a matched group (in terms of age, diagnosis, and so on) of mechanically ventilated patients who did not experience barotrauma (controls). A *prospective study* is one in which the study is designed before the data are collected (Fig. 62–3). A major advantage of the prospective design is that the researcher has control over the quality of all aspects of the study. Generally, prospective designs are favored over retrospective designs. A *controlled clinical trial* is a special type of prospective study (Fig. 62–4). With this design, subjects are prospectively

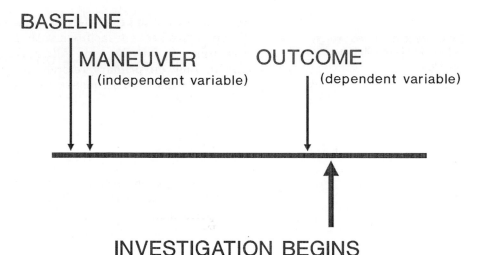

FIGURE 62–2: The retrospective study design. The horizontal line indicates the progression of time.

and randomly assigned to an experimental (treatment) group or control (placebo) group.

Types of Variables. A *variable* is a characteristic or entity that can take on different values. A *qualitative variable* is one that is descriptive in a categoric rather than a numeric sense (e.g., gender is a qualitative variable). A *quantitative variable* is measurable using a meaningful scale of numbers (e.g., temperature). A *discrete variable* is a quantitative variable with gaps or interruptions in the values it may assume (e.g., bed size of a hospital or the number of children in a family; the variables are expressed as integers because fractions have no meaning). A *continuous variable* can take on any value, including fractional ones, in a given range of values (e.g., temperature and pH). The *independent variable* is manipulated by the researcher. The *dependent variable* changes in response to manipulations of the independent variable. When a clinician administers oxygen to a patient and measures the change in Pa_{O_2}, the FI_{O_2} is the independent variable and the Pa_{O_2} is the dependent variable. A *confounding variable* is anything other than the independent variable

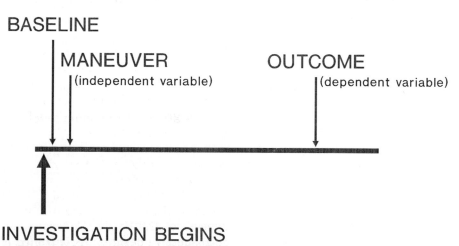

FIGURE 62–3: The prospective study design.

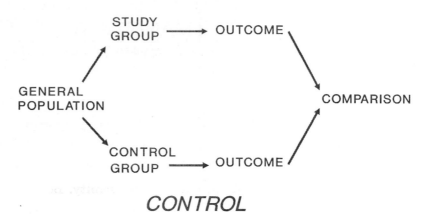

FIGURE 62–4: The design for a controlled clinical trial.

that affects the dependent variable. In the previous example, changes in the patient's secretions would be a confounding variable affecting the relationship between FI_{O_2} and Pa_{O_2}. It is important for the researcher to recognize potential confounding variables and control for their effects; otherwise, the confounding variable will bias (i.e., add error to) the results of the study.

Experimental Unit. The researcher must decide whether to use human subjects, an animal model, a bench model, or a mathematical model. Although human subjects or an animal model often may be desirable, it may be more feasible to use bench or mathematical models because of ethical and regulatory issues. If human subjects or animal models are used, the researcher must be careful to follow all institutional and regulatory guidelines.

Assignment to Treatments. Ideally, groups of experimental units should be *randomly* assigned to different treatments so that each subject has an equal likelihood of being assigned to the experimental or control group. Random assignment can be produced by a table of random numbers (available in statistics books) or, more commonly, by computer software (e.g., a spreadsheet). A pocket calculator can be used to generate a random number sequence by the following procedure:

1. Select a seed number between 0 and 1 and add it to the value of π (i.e., pi).
2. Raise the result to the fifth power.
3. Take the fraction portion (i.e., the numbers to the right of the decimal place) as the random number.
4. Use the fraction portion as the new seed number and repeat the procedure for more random numbers.

Blinding means that either the subject or the researcher does not know to which group the subject has been assigned; *double blind* means that neither the subject nor the researcher knows the assignment (the strongest design to prevent bias). A *crossover* design is one in which the subject is included in both the treatment and control groups with the order usually randomly assigned.

Assessment of Outcome. It is important to choose an appropriate measure of outcome. It may be inappropriate, for example, to use pulse oximetry to assess changes in arterial oxygenation during suctioning if the arterial P_{O_2} is high (i.e., large changes in Pa_{O_2} may not be detected by changes in oxygen saturation if the changes occur on the flat portion of the oxyhemoglobin curve). It is also important that all measurement systems be calibrated to assure accurate data. Care must be taken to minimize the effect of measurement itself on the outcome variable. For example, if an indirect calorimeter is used to measure changes in oxygen consumption with different modes of ventilation, it is important that the placement of the calorimeter in the patient circuit not increase the work of breathing (which would increase oxygen consumption and bias the results). Another concern is that of variability among observers when the outcome involves a subjective measure such as breath sounds.

Assessment of Practicality. Because of the personal commitment involved, the process of identifying and defining a research project can be very nearsighted. After all the effort put into developing a study, it may become difficult for an investigator to see that others might not be interested in supporting the project or that feasibility problems make the study's implementation questionable. Thus, before beginning the study, it is necessary to step back mentally and evaluate the overall practicality of the project in a larger context. The major considerations are

- Significance or potential benefits of the study results
- Measurability of research variables
- Duration and timing of the study
- Availability of research subjects
- Availability of equipment and funds
- Knowledge and experience of investigators

Most research projects can be implemented without extra funds or with equipment donated by vendors. It is better to consider funding to be the result of a good research effort than to expect funding before the initiation of a project.

Write the Protocol

A brief yet detailed research protocol should be written to serve as a set of instructions for investigators and a means to communicate your plans to others (e.g., the hospital's investigation review board). The study proposal should be clear and convincing to anyone who reads it. The protocol should include the following

- *Title*: The project should be given a title that clearly identifies the research topic.
- *Rationale and review of literature*: The justification for the study should be clearly stated. A theoretical basis or framework should be established if possible. A brief review of the literature should be provided to establish the rationale for the study and justify the choice of the particular research design that will be used.
- *Inclusion-exclusion and assignment criteria*: The specific criteria for inclusion and exclusion of subjects should be stated. Further, the methods used to assign subjects to the experimental and the control groups should be described (e.g., randomization, convenience sample and so forth).
- *Length of study*: The researcher should estimate the length of time

required to complete the study and the number of subjects to be included in the study.

- *Techniques for data capture*: This information will often be in the form of a data collection sheet, which needs to be developed by the researcher to capture all the data generated by the project. The data sheet should be easy to use and designed in a manner to facilitate analysis of the results. Some researchers prefer to record all data in a laboratory notebook. A notebook has the added advantage of providing a place to record notes, illustrations of experimental setups, and miscellaneous information that will most assuredly be forgotten by the time the paper is written.

- *The specific methods that will be used*: The specific methodology that will be used in the project should be outlined. Enough detail should be provided to serve as a guide for conducting the research project. The methods that will be used should also provide enough detail so that anyone can replicate the study.

Obtain Permission

Criminal law, civil law, and the ethics of society do not allow the potential risk of harm to a human subject for research purposes without consent.

Perhaps the most important aspect of research ethics is the design of a valid and legitimate research protocol; it is unethical to expose human subjects to potential harm in a research project of dubious value. It is also unethical to breach the confidentiality of patient information for research purposes.

It is important to gain the necessary permission to conduct the research. Permission should be gained from your immediate supervisor as well as any others that the study will affect (physicians, nursing staff, laboratory personnel, and so on). If the study involves the potential for risk to human subjects, the research protocol will likely need approval by the hospital's institutional review committee (sometimes called committee for protection of human subjects). Any research project that has the potential for risk to the subject requires his or her informed consent. Informed consent from the subject (or the subject's legal guardian) is usually obtained with a signature on a form that describes the study along with the potential benefits and risks in layman's terms. The decision to participate in a research project must be voluntary, and the subject must be allowed to withdraw from participation at any time. It is important to follow the specific institutional rules related to research projects involving human subjects or animals.

Collect the Data

Data collection will go much more smoothly if the appropriate attention is directed toward the initial preparatory steps. Too frequently, the novice researcher progresses too quickly to this step without the necessary planning. Many times, data collection requires a long-term commitment to the project. Most studies take longer for data collection than originally anticipated. The research team must find ways to maintain enthusiasm for the project during the lengthy, and often tedious, data collection period. The researcher must also expect unanticipated problems during the implementation of the project and be willing to modify the protocol as necessary.

Reject or Concede the Hypothesis

Based on the data analysis, a decision is made to reject or not reject (i.e., concede) the null hypothesis. To reject the null hypothesis is to say that there *is* a difference between the groups, and to concede the difference is to say that there is *no* difference between the groups. Analysis of the data is based on statistical principles. There is a tendency to confuse research with statistics. Statistical procedures are simply one standardized way to test hypotheses. Fortunately, one does not need to be a statistician to conduct research. Although a basic understanding of statistical principles is an asset to the researcher, the statistical calculations and manipulations can be performed by a computer and the appropriate statistical software. It is more important for the clinician-researcher to know what test to use than to understand the theoretical basis of the calculations involved.

The first step in data analysis is aggregation of the data. This is commonly performed by entering the data into a computer spreadsheet or database. From here, the data can be exported to statistical, graphic, and word processing software. The statistical basis for hypothesis testing is discussed later in this chapter. However, it is important to recognize the difference between *statistically significant* and *clinically important*. With a very large sample size, statistical significance might be demonstrated for a very small and thus clinically unimportant difference between groups. Conversely, a clinically important difference may not be statistically significant if the sample size is too small. The choice of an appropriate sample size will be discussed later.

Write the Paper or Abstract

Research findings that are not shared through publication are of limited value. The research is not over until the results are published. The results may also be presented in abstract form at a regional, national, or international meeting. The format of the paper or abstract is dictated by the specific medical journal in which you intend to publish your results. Every journal has a section that gives instructions to authors about how to prepare the manuscript, including length of abstract, how to handle figures, and the style to use for references. There are many different styles used in medical journals, so one must check what is required before beginning to write. The journal *Respiratory Care* accepts three basic types of research manuscripts: case studies, device-method evaluations, and original studies. The case study should be written to contain the following sections:

- Statement of problem or question
- Presentation of evidence
- Validity of evidence
- Implications of evidence
- Conflicting or supporting evidence from the literature
- Case summary

The device-method evaluation should include the following sections:

- Description of device or method
- Evaluation methodology
- Results (measured data, including tables and graphs)
- Descriptive statistics
- Relevant clinical experience
- Conclusion

The original study should contain:

- Abstract: a synopsis of the important findings
- Introduction: describes study problem, relevant references, and specific hypotheses
- Methods: complete description of experimental setup, including statistical procedures used to analyze data
- Results: data obtained from measurements in experiment, including tables and graphs as appropriate, and results of statistical analyses
- Discussion: explains the meaning of the results and relationship of findings to other published reports if available
- Conclusion: gives the "take-home" message
- References: a list of related published studies

The following presents some mistakes that novice researchers often make when writing manuscripts. They should be avoided.

- Failure to state explicit hypothesis (when one does not know which harbor they are making for, no wind is the right wind)
- Using the wrong evaluation procedure (study what other researchers have done)
- Using the wrong statistics (do not use inferential statistics when descriptive statistics will suffice; use analysis of variance instead of multiple t tests; use limits of agreement rather than correlation to show accuracy of devices)
- Expected data not included (the hypothesis dictates the experimental design)
- Data do not address study question ("off on a tangent")
- Unsupported claims ("the emperor has no clothes")
- Failure to follow publishers instructions to authors ("look before you leap")
- Failure to write from an outline (lazy person's mistake)

The summary of this chapter contains more information about writing manuscripts.

Incorporate the Findings into Practice

Clinical research should be viewed as part of clinical practice, not separate from it. What is learned from the research findings should be incorporated into clinical situations. This is particularly appropriate for studies that pass the rigors of peer review and are confirmed by other published studies.

Perform Another Study

The results of a research project may answer some questions, but usually more questions are raised. This often results in one developing a series of research projects in a specific area of interest.

BASIC STATISTICS FOR DATA ANALYSIS

A complete review of statistical concepts is beyond the scope of this chapter. However, this chapter covers some of the basic descriptive procedures commonly used for device-method evaluation studies.

Descriptive Statistics

Levels of Measurement

Measurements result in data (singular: datum). However, not all data may be treated the same way mathematically, depending on their information content, which is classified according to three levels or scales (Table 62–3). A *nominal* scale, the most primitive, refers to qualitative variables whose values are generally categories (e.g., male, female). Numbers, which are used here to name or distinguish categories, are purely arbitrary. An *ordinal* scale applies when the values of the numbers indicate relative high and low values of the variable (e.g., pain measured on a scale of none = 0, mild = 1, severe = 2). For an *interval* scale, it is assumed that equal, uniform intervals between numbers represent equal intervals in the variable being measured (e.g., the Celsius temperature scale). The mathematically strongest level is the *ratio* scale, in which numbers represent equal intervals and start with an absolute zero. This allows ratio statements, such as "4 is twice the value of 2." Some examples include the Kelvin temperature scale, height, and weight. Although higher levels of measurement can be reduced to lower levels (e.g., from ratio to ordinal), the reverse is generally not true. The lower, or more primitive, the level of the measurement, the more restricted and less mathematically sophisticated is the statistical analysis.

Frequency Distributions

When a data set is obtained, it should be organized for inspection through a frequency distribution, which can represent the data numerically (i.e., in a table) or graphically. Regardless of how sophisticated the data analysis will be, looking at it in tabular or graphic form is a most useful procedure. This simple form suggests further analyses and may prevent inappropriate analyses.

In representing data, a frequency distribution is distinguished from a grouped frequency distribution. In a *frequency distribution*, the data are ordered from the minimum to the maximum value, and the frequency of occurrence is given for each value of the variable. With a *grouped frequency distribution*, values of the variable are grouped into classes. For example, if values range from 1 to 100, it is not practical or helpful to use a frequency distribution that is an ordered list of 100 different values. Rather, the data should be grouped into, say, values from 1 to 10, 11 to 20, and so forth. Usually, grouping the data into 10 to 20 classes is recommended.

Table 62–4 illustrates both an ungrouped and a grouped frequency distribution. In constructing a frequency distribution, the minimum and the maximum values of the variable are found first, the values are listed in order, the number of occurrences for each value in the ordered list is tallied and the percentage and cumulative percentages are calculated

---

TABLE **62–3:** Examples of Nominal, Ordinal, and Continuous Measurements

Nominal Measurements	**Continuous Measurements**
• Mortality (dead or alive)	• Arterial Po_2
• Sex (male or female)	• Urine output
• Breath sounds (present or absent)	• Body temperature
	• Birth weight
Ordinal Measurement	
• Body size (small, medium, large)	
• Pulse amplitude (strong, weak, normal)	

TABLE **62–4:**   Frequency Distributions, Ungrouped and Grouped

Data Set 6, 5, 3, 7, 3, 2, 4, 6, 5, 4, 6, 4, 3, 2, 8, 7, 4, 5, 5, 5

Variable Values	Tally		Frequency	Percentage	Cum Percentage
2	11		2	10	10
3	111		3	15	25
4	1111		4	20	45
5	1111		5	25	70
6	111		3	15	85
7	11		2	10	95
8	1		1	5	100
		Total:	20	100%	

Grouped Frequency Distribution:

Interval		Frequency	Percentage	Cum Percentage
2–3		5	25	25
4–5		9	45	70
6–7		5	25	95
8–9		1	5	100
	Total:	20	100%	

From Rau JR. Data analysis. *In* Chatburn RL, Craig KC (eds). Fundamentals of Respiratory Care Research. East Norwalk, CT, Appleton & Lange, 1988, pp 191–248.

(computer software is available to do this). The percentage is obtained from the frequency divided by the total number of values. The cumulative percentage accumulates the percentage of each value. For example, the value of 3 occurs three times, or 15%, (3/20) × 100. After we include the value of 3, we have accumulated 25% of the total observations in the distribution.

In the ungrouped frequency distribution, the class interval is actually one. Every value between the minimum and maximum is included. If the range of values is extremely large, it is preferable to group values into classes and represent the frequency of each class, as shown in Table 62–4. The ability to "see" information in the numbers is lost with more than 20 intervals, and many prefer 10 to 12 intervals.

The goal of constructing a frequency distribution is to allow inspection of the data by summarizing, organizing, and simplifying the data without misrepresenting it. In Table 62–4, the values of the variable tend to occur most frequently in the middle range and to be relatively infrequent at extreme values (the "tails" of the distribution as viewed in graphic form). This is visually apparent in the tally marks and confirmed in the percentage column, which shows the largest percentages for the middle values of 4 and 5. Also, the cumulative percentage grows most rapidly in the middle range. When the value of 4 is added, the cumulative percentage jumps from 25% to 45%, and adding 5 brings it to 70%. Almost three fourths of the values are included at that point. A researcher would want to know how values are distributed since this may be of significance for interpreting results. For example, a survey of patterns of practice in respiratory care revealed the data shown in Table 62–5. From the table we can conclude that most institutions surveyed have a policy requiring a ventilator circuit change every 48 hours. We can say that the "standard of care" seems to be to change the circuit at least every 48 hours because the cumulative frequency shows that this statement applies to the majority (i.e., 89%) of respondents.

If one wishes to see literally how the data are distributed, a graphic

A frequency distribution makes it possible to observe how the numbers are distributed, to see patterns or trends, and to begin extracting information from the mass of numbers.

TABLE **62–5:** The Variance, Standard Deviation, and Coefficient of Variation With a Set of Sample Values

Data Set 2, 3, 5, 6

Variance

$$\text{Variance, } S^2 = \frac{\sum\limits_{i=1}^{n} (X_i - \overline{X})^2}{n - 1}$$

Calculation:

$$\overline{X} = \Sigma X_i / n = 16/4 = 4$$

Value of X	$(X - \overline{X})$	$(X - \overline{X})^2$
2	-2	4
3	-1	1
5	1	1
6	2	4
	$\Sigma = 0$	$\Sigma = 10$

Sample variance, $S^2 = 10/(4 - 1) = 3.33$

Standard Deviation

$$\text{Standard deviation, } S = \sqrt{\frac{\sum\limits_{i=1}^{n} (X_i - \overline{X})^2}{n - 1}} = \sqrt{S^2}$$

Sample standard deviation, $S = \sqrt{3.33} = 1.83$

Coefficient of Variation

Coefficient of variation, $CV = (S/\overline{X}) \times 100$

$CV = (1.83/4) \times 100 = 45.6\%$

From Rau JR. Data analysis. *In* Chatburn RL, Craig KC (eds). Fundamentals of Respiratory Care Research. East Norwalk, CT, Appleton & Lange, 1988, pp 191–248.

presentation of the frequency distribution is desirable. Figure 62–5 shows a histogram of fictitious Po_2 values from a patient in an intensive care unit. Figure 62–6 shows the same data in the form of a percentiles plot, showing the cumulative percentages.

Measures of Central Tendency

There are three statistics used to represent the typical value in a distribution. Each statistic is a single number or an index that characterizes the center, or average value, of the whole set of data. These are the mean, the median, and the mode.

Summation Notation. Summation is a mathematical operation common in statistical calculations. The summation notation is denoted by the capital Greek letter sigma (Σ) and simply indicates addition over the values of a variable. The general representation of the operator is:

$$\sum_{i=1}^{n} X_i$$

which is read "the summation of X_i for i equal 1 to n." This means that all the values of X_i are added together:

$$\sum_{i=1}^{n} X_i = X_1 + X_2 + \cdots + X_n$$

The subscripted variable, X_i, which is read "X sub i," is used to denote

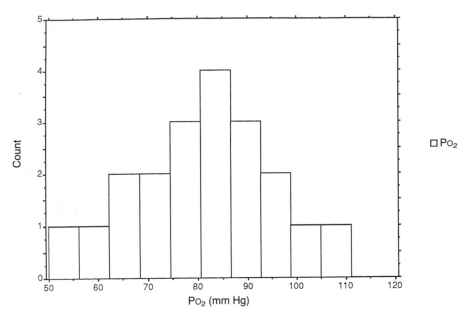

FIGURE 62–5: A histogram or bar graph.

specific values of the variable. For instance, X_1 is one value of X_i, X_2 another, and so on. An example should make the use of the summation operator clear. Let the variable X have three values, each of which is given by a subscripted variable $X_1 = 3$, $X_2 = 4$, and $X_3 = 2$. Then

$$\sum_{i=1}^{3} X_i = X_1 + X_2 + X_3 = 3 + 4 + 2 = 9$$

The Mean. The mean is the sum of all the observations divided by the number of observations. The symbol for the mean is $\overline{X}$ for a sample mean or μ for a population mean. The equation is

$$\overline{X} = \frac{\sum_{i=1}^{n} X_i}{n}$$

where X is the variable and there are n values. For example, let us use the preceding values of X (3, 4, and 2), so n = 3. The mean is then (3 + 4 + 2)/3 = 3.

The Median. The median is the 50th percentile of a distribution or the point that divides the distribution into equal halves. The median is the value below which 50% of the observations occur. For grouped observations, an equation is used to find the exact value of the median. It is conceptually clearer to use the following rules. For an *odd* number of observations, the median is the value that is equal to (n + 1)/2, where n is the number of observations. For example, if we have 1, 3, 5, 6, and 7 as our data, n is 5. The median is (5 + 1)/2 = third value = 5. Notice that this equation gives the number of the observation, not its value.

With an *even* number of observations, the median is equal to the sum of the middle values divided by 2. For example, if we have 1, 3, 5, 6, 7, and 9 as data, the median is (5 + 6)/2 = 5.5. This equation gives the

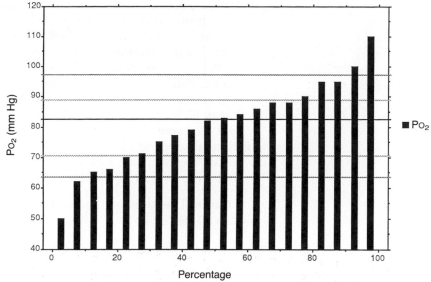

FIGURE 62–6: The same data as in Figure 62–5 but graphed as a percentile plot showing cumulative percentages. The horizontal lines indicate the 10th, 25th, 50th, 75th, and 90th percentiles. Such a plot allows us to conclude that in this example, 75% of the blood gas values were below 90 mm Hg or that 90% were above 60 mm Hg.

value of the observation that divides the data set (even if it does not actually exist in the original data).

The Mode. The mode is the most frequently occurring observation in the distribution. The mode is found by inspection, or counting. In Table 62–4, the mode is the value 5, which occurs five times. In a histogram, the mode is represented by the highest bar.

Interpretation and Application. The mean is the most sophisticated measure of central tendency, is influenced by every value in the distribution, and assumes at least an interval level of measurement. The mean is inappropriate for a qualitative variable with a nominal or ordinal level of measurement. What sense is there in calculating the mean of political affiliations, which have been coded with the values 1, 2, and 3 for Republican, Democrat, and other? Of course we could calculate a number, but it is inappropriate for the variable. The mean is termed an *interval* statistic.

The median, which is considered an *ordinal* statistic, is less sophisticated than the mean. The median requires only ranking of numbers, not equal intervals. If a single value skews the distribution and hence displaces the value of the mean, the median may give a more typical representation of the data than does the mean. For instance, if all the salaries in a data set range from $10,000 to $14,000 except for one person who earns $25,000, the mean will be increased, whereas the median will probably better represent the average salary.

The mode is a *nominal* statistic, since it requires only a nominal level of measurement. The qualitative variable, political affiliation, is a good example for using the mode to typify the observations. With a nominal level of measurement, we cannot appropriately calculate a median or mode.

Measures of Dispersion

Most research studies provide at least two descriptive statistics: one measure of central tendency and one measure of dispersion. Measures of dispersion indicate the variability or how spread out the data are. These measurements include the range, variance, standard deviation, and coefficient of variation. The need for a measure of central tendency and dispersion to characterize a distribution more fully is seen in Figure 62–7. We have two different distributions of pH values, both with the same mean. Although both center on the same value, they do not "distribute" the same. The range and variability are different. If we had only the mean (7.4) to characterize the data, we would conclude the distributions are the same. However, although they are the same with regard to their central tendency, they are quite different in their dispersion. Note that pH is a continuous variable and measurable at a ratio level (there is a true zero as well as equal intervals).

Range. The range is the distance between the smallest and largest values of the variable:

$$\text{Range} = X_{max} - X_{min}$$

where X_{max} and X_{min} are the maximum and minimum values in the distribution. The range is the simplest measure of dispersion and is very informative to a researcher. Although the range is the actual distance between the smallest and largest values, it is more informative to provide the actual minimum and maximum values themselves.

Variance and Standard Deviation. The variance is the average squared deviation of the values from the mean. The standard deviation is the square root of the variance. Equations and an example of the variance and standard deviation are given in Table 62–5. There is a difference in the equation for the variance, depending on whether a sample with n observations is used to estimate the population variance or whether a population itself with the total collection of N observations is used. For a *sample,* the variance, S^2, used to estimate the variance of a population is

$$S^2 = \frac{\sum\limits_{i=1}^{n} (X_i - \overline{X})^2}{n - 1}$$

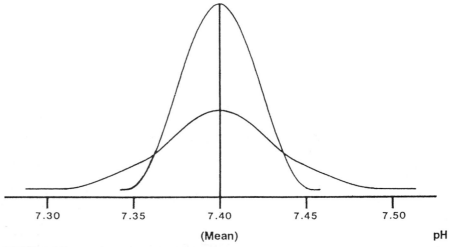

FIGURE 62–7: Two distributions of pH values with the same mean but different amounts of dispersion.

If the data collected actually make up the entire population, the variance is calculated as

$$\sigma^2 = \frac{\displaystyle\sum_{i=1}^{N}(X_i - \overline{\mu})^2}{N}$$

We use Roman letter S^2 and $\overline{X}$ for the variance and mean of a *sample,* but Greek letters σ^2 and $\overline{\mu}$ to indicate the *population* variance and mean. The square root of the variance, S or σ, is called the *standard deviation.* The standard deviation is often abbreviated SD.

One common way of viewing data using both the mean and standard deviation is the Levey-Jennings plot used in quality control systems (Fig. 62–8).

Coefficient of Variation. The coefficient of variation expresses the standard deviation as a percentage of the mean. The equation for the coefficient of variation (CV) is simply

$$CV = \frac{S}{X} \times 100$$

The coefficient of variation is not useful as a single value but is applicable when comparing the dispersion of observations, for example, with two different instruments or methods intended to measure the same variable.

Correlation Coefficient

A coefficient of correlation is a descriptive measure of the degree of relationship between two variables. This is the first statistic that involves *two* variables. The concept of a correlation implies that two varia-

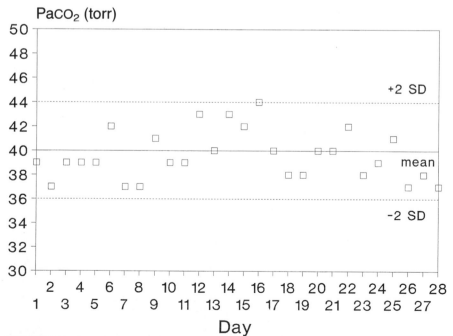

FIGURE 62–8: An example of a Levey-Jennings plot for the quality control of P_{CO_2} measurements in the blood gas laboratory.

Table 62–6 gives an example of the calculation of a Pearson r correlation coefficient using the formula

$$r = \frac{\Sigma xy}{\sqrt{\Sigma x^2 \Sigma y^2}}$$

where $x = X - \bar{X}$ and $y = Y - \bar{Y}$, which are the deviation scores. The term xy is the crossproduct of the deviation scores for X and Y.

bles covary, that is, a change in variable X is associated with a change in variable Y. The most common correlation coefficient with a continuous variable measurable on an interval level is the Pearson product-moment correlation coefficient (the Pearson r). Another basic assumption of the Pearson r is linearity. The relation of the two variables is such that a visual inspection of a scattergram (i.e., a plot of the data points on an X-Y coordinate system) shows the data to be grouped around a straight (versus curved) line.

The Pearson r statistic, which ranges in value from -1 to $+1$, indicates two aspects of a correlation, the *magnitude* and *direction*. Figure 62–9 illustrates some possible values for a Pearson r statistic and their meaning. A negative r value indicates an inverse relation: X increases and Y decreases (Fig. 62–9*B*). A positive value indicates a positive or direct relation (Fig. 62–9*A* and *C*). The closer the absolute value is to unity, the stronger and more perfect the relation, whereas a value approaching zero indicates a lack of linear relationship (Fig. 62–9*D*). However, there may be a strong curvilinear relationship.

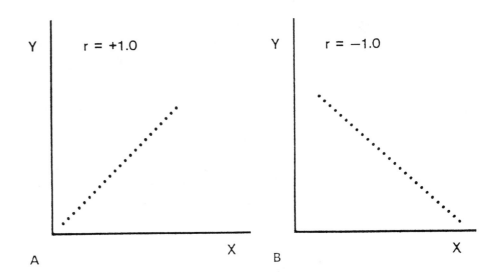

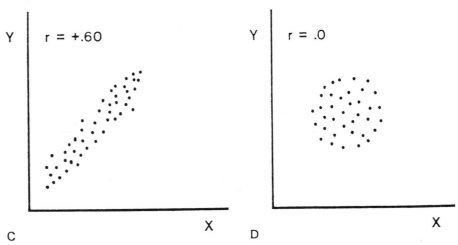

FIGURE 62–9: Illustration of four Pearson r values, indicating varying aspects of the linear relation between variables X and Y.

TABLE **62–6:** Calculation of the Pearson Product-Moment Correlation
Coefficient

$$r = \frac{\Sigma xy}{\sqrt{\Sigma x^2 \, \Sigma y^2}} \quad , \quad \begin{matrix} x = X - \overline{X} \\ y = Y - \overline{Y} \end{matrix}$$

X	Y	$(X - \overline{X})$	$(Y - \overline{Y})$	x^2	y^2	xy
1	2	−3	−2.2	9	4.84	6.6
3	3	−1	−1.2	1	1.44	1.2
2	4	−2	−.2	4	.04	.4
6	5	2	.8	4	.64	1.6
8	7	4	2.8	16	7.84	11.2

$\overline{X} = 4 \quad \overline{Y} = 4.2$ $\qquad\qquad\qquad\qquad\qquad\qquad \Sigma x^2 = 34 \quad \Sigma y^2 = 14.8 \quad \Sigma xy = 21$

$$r = \frac{21}{\sqrt{34 \times 14.8}} = 0.936$$

From Rau JR. Data analysis. *In* Chatburn RL, Craig KC (eds). Fundamental of Respiratory Care
Research. East Norwalk, CT, Appleton & Lange, 1988, pp 191–248.

Regression

When there is a linear relationship between two variables, we often
wish to use the value of one variable to predict the value of the other
variable (avoiding the necessity of measuring the second variable). Of
course, both variables have to be measured initially to establish the
presence of a correlation. This is possible using least squares analysis
and simple regression. When we measure X and predict Y, Y is said to
be *regressed* on X. The term *simple* indicates that Y is predicted from
only one variable and not several simultaneously, which would involve
multiple linear regression. The regression line is referred to as being fit
to the data by a *least squares* criterion because it is the line that minimizes the squared error (i.e., distance or deviation) between points on
the line and the actual points on the graph. Figure 62–10 illustrates this
line for the correlation data in Table 62–4. Such a line can be described
with a linear equation of the form

$$\hat{Y} = a + bX$$

where $\hat{Y}$ is the predicted value of Y for the given value of X in the
equation and a and b are the Y intercept and slope of the line, respectively. Values of a and b are obtained from the equations shown in Figure
62–10. In practice, the equation of the line is first obtained by solving for
a and b; the line can then be drawn by establishing two points. The value
of a gives us the Y intercept, which is the value of Y when X equals zero.
If we calculate $\hat{Y}$ for one other value of X, we can fit the line on the
graph. In effect, the line gives us the predicted value of Y for every value
of X.

Measures of correlation exist for the lower levels of measurement.
The Spearman rank coefficient can be used with ordinal levels of data,
and the phi coefficient with nominal levels. Explanations of these statistics can be found in standard statistical textbooks.

Inferential Statistics

Probability and the Normal Distribution

The basic idea of inferential statistics is to use measurements from
a sample to make *inferences* about the population from which the sample
came. Such inferences are only guesses however; the basic concepts of

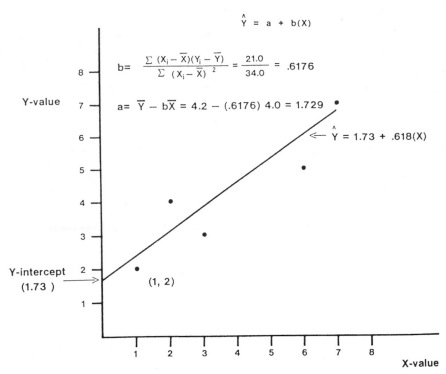

FIGURE 62–10: An example of simple linear regression, giving the line of best fit for data in Table 62–4.

probability must be understood to ensure that the guesses are reasonably accurate.

The probability of an event (e.g., a mistake) can be defined as the relative frequency, or proportion of occurrence of that event out of some total number of events. Since probability is a proportion, it always has values between 0 and 1 inclusively. For example, the probability of obtaining an ace from a deck of well-shuffled cards is 4 in 52, or .77. There are four aces (the event of interest) in a total of 52 cards (or alternative events). A frequency distribution may be drawn so that it shows the relative frequency of a variable rather than the raw count. Such a distribution is called a *probability distribution.*

The concept of a probability distribution is essential to inferential statistics, and the key to making probability statements about events is to have the appropriate probability distribution. Many biologic variables such as height, weight, and pH can be adequately described by what is known as a "normal" distribution. This is a particular distribution described with certain mathematical function (the Gaussian function). Probabilities can be obtained whenever one is willing to assume that a variable follows this distribution.

On a graph of a probability distribution, the curve represents the probability of particular values along the horizontal axis. If the line is drawn perpendicular from any two points on the horizontal axis up to the curve, the enclosed area represents the probability of observing values of the variable on the horizontal axis between and including these two points. Figure 62–11 illustrates the areas under the normal curve. In a normally distributed variable, the mean is at the center of the distribution and is therefore also the median and the mode. The curve in Figure 62–11 is called a standard curve because the areas are indicated

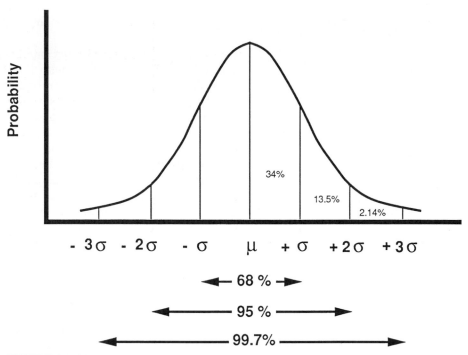

FIGURE 62–11: Areas under a standard normal curve.

for standard deviation units from the mean (rather than the original measurement units of the variable on the horizontal axis such as inches, mm Hg, and so on). Thus, the mean itself, regardless of its value from actual data, is zero standard deviations away from itself.

In a standard normal curve, approximately 68% of the data values are included if an area around the mean of ± 1 standard deviation is taken. If the area extends ± 2 standard deviations from the mean, approximately 95% of the values are included in the distribution, and 99.7% of all the values at ± 3 standard deviations. Probabilities for various multiples of the standard deviation can be found in statistical tables. However, tables are usually created in terms of "Z scores" where

$$Z = \frac{\text{observed value} - \text{mean value}}{\text{standard deviation}}$$

For example, a Z score of $+1.5$ would indicate that the observed value of X is one and one-half standard deviations above the mean. Using a table of Z scores, we could find the probability of observing a data value that was this far from the mean.

Sampling Distributions

A statistic such as the mean, $\overline{X}$, will have different values for different samples even though the samples all come from the same population. In fact, it can be shown that the possible values of $\overline{X}$ make up a probability distribution, known as a sampling distribution, which is the distribution of all values of a statistic when it is computed from random samples of the same size from a given population.

For a sampling distribution of mean values, the mean of the sample, $\overline{X}$, is the best estimate of the mean value of the distribution. An estimate of the distribution's standard deviation, often called the *standard error of the mean* ($\sigma_{\overline{x}}$), is estimated as:

$$\sigma_{\bar{x}} \approx \frac{S}{\sqrt{n}}$$

where S is the standard deviation of the sample and n is the sample size. The standard error of the mean is simply the standard deviation of all possible values of $\bar{X}$ in the sampling distribution.

There are many types of sampling distributions described in statistical textbooks. For most purposes, however, only two types are important: the normal distribution and the t distribution (which looks like a normal distribution but is more spread out). Also, we are usually only concerned with testing hypotheses about mean values, which further simplifies the statistical procedures one needs to be familiar with. Generally, when the sample size is greater than about 30, statistical procedures based on the normal distribution are used, otherwise the t distribution is used. We can go one step further and simply always use the t distribution because when the sample size gets large enough, the t distribution is equivalent to the normal distribution.

Confidence Intervals

A mean value, $\bar{X}$, calculated from a single sample is called a *point estimate* of the population mean. As an estimate, we accept the fact that it may be in error, that is, it may be different from the true population mean, μ. We want to estimate how far away μ might be from $\bar{X}$ and how much confidence we should place in this estimate. We will assume that $\bar{X}$ has approximately a t distribution (because we do not know the standard error of the distribution and the sample size may be small). Probability values (i.e., areas under the distribution curve) associated with different distances away from the distribution mean can be obtained from a statistical table. These distances are expressed in standardized form, exactly like Z scores. In other words, the t values in the table are

$$t_{\alpha/2, n-1} = \frac{\bar{X} - \mu}{S/\sqrt{n}}$$

where the subscripts on t indicate the specific confidence level and "degree of freedom," which are determined by the sample size and affect the shape of the t distribution. The Greek symbol α indicates the amount of error that can be tolerated. The acceptable error in medical research is usually 5%, expressed in decimal form (0.05) in statistical tables. An error of 5% results in a 95% confidence level. The sample size, n, is used to calculate the sample mean ($\bar{X}$) and sample standard deviation (S). The degrees of freedom, n − 1, determine the spread of the t distribution. For example, the value of the t statistic at the 95% confidence level for a sample size of 11 (i.e., 10 degrees of freedom) is 2.228. Figure 62–12 illustrates this for a 95% confidence level. Multiplying this value for t by the standard error of the sample data, we get the distance of the observed value of $\bar{X}$ from μ in the original units (i.e., the units used to measure the sample data such as mm Hg).

We now have the background for calculating a *confidence interval,* which is the interval of possible values for the mean at the desired confidence level. The expression for the confidence interval (CT) for the true population mean is

$$CI = X \pm t_{\alpha/2, n-1} \times \frac{S}{\sqrt{n}}$$

The general procedure is to

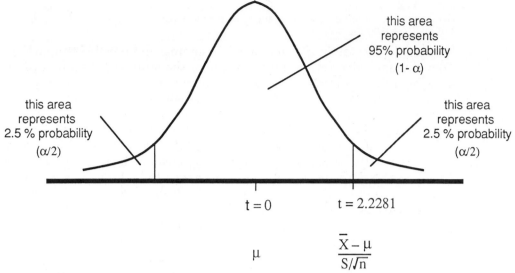

this area
represents
95% probability
(1- α)

this area
represents
2.5 % probability
(α/2)

this area
represents
2.5 % probability
(α/2)

t = 0

t = 2.2281

μ

$\dfrac{\bar{X} - \mu}{S/\sqrt{n}}$

FIGURE 62–12: Areas under a *t* distribution for a sample size of 11. The *t* value (from a table) represents the distance between an observed value of a sample mean and the true population mean in units of sample standard deviations. The *t* value will change for different sample sizes or confidence levels. Notice that the ends of the distribution (i.e., the "tails") each contain exactly half of the acceptable error, so the *t* value is known as a "two-tailed" *t* value.

1. Calculate the sample mean and standard deviation.
2. Determine the desired confidence level for the interval (the higher the confidence level, the wider the interval will be).
3. Look up the required *t* value in a statistical table.
4. Substitute these values into the preceding equation.

For convenience, Table 62–7 lists values for $t\sqrt{n}$ for different sample sizes. One simply multiplies the appropriate value from Table 62–7 (depending on the desired confidence level and sample size) by the sample standard deviation and then adds and subtracts the result from the sample mean to construct the confidence interval.

For example, suppose we performed an experiment that produced a set of 20 Pa_{O_2} measurements with a mean value of 83 mm Hg and a standard deviation of 5 mm Hg. We wish to construct a 95% confidence interval that contains the true mean value of the population of Pa_{O_2} values from which the sample was taken. From Table 62–7, starting at n = 20 and reading over to the column for a 95% confidence level, we obtain the factor 0.468 (which represents the two-tailed *t* value with 19 degrees of freedom at the α = 0.025 level). The confidence interval (CI) is then

$$CI = \bar{X} \pm \left(\frac{t_{\alpha/2, n-1}}{\sqrt{n}} \right) \times S$$

$$CI = 83 \pm 0.468 \times 5$$

$$CI = 83 \pm 2.3$$

$$CI = (80.7,\ 85.3)$$

It is tempting to conclude that the true average Pa_{O_2} for the population is between 80.7 mm Hg and 85.3 mm Hg. However, this is not strictly true. Rather, the confidence interval is interpreted as follows: If the

TABLE **62–7:** Factors for Determining (a) Confidence Intervals for the Mean, (b) Confidence Intervals for the Standard Deviation, (c) Error Intervals for Individual Values (n = sample size)

(a)

	Confidence Level	
	95%	**99%**
n	$\dfrac{t_{\alpha/2}}{\sqrt{n}}$	$\dfrac{t_{\alpha/2}}{\sqrt{n}}$
6	1.05	1.65
8	0.838	1.24
10	0.715	1.03
12	0.635	0.898
15	0.555	0.700
20	0.468	0.640
25	0.412	0.560
30	0.374	0.504
40	0.320	0.429
50	0.284	0.379

(b)

	95% Confidence Level	
n	k_L	k_U
6	0.59	2.25
7	0.61	2.05
8	0.63	1.92
9	0.65	1.82
11	0.68	1.69
16	0.72	1.51
21	0.75	1.42
26	0.77	1.36
31	0.79	1.32
36	0.80	1.29
40	0.81	1.27
51	0.83	1.23
61	0.84	1.21
71	0.85	1.19
81	0.86	1.18
91	0.87	1.17
101	0.88	1.16

(c)

	Confidence Level	
	95%	**99%**
n	k_I	k_I
2	37.67	188.49
4	6.73	11.15
6	4.41	6.35
8	3.73	4.94
10	3.38	4.27
12	3.16	3.87
14	3.01	3.61
16	2.90	3.42
18	2.82	3.28
20	2.75	3.17
25	2.63	2.97
30	2.55	2.84
35	2.49	2.75
40	2.45	2.68
45	2.41	2.62
50	2.38	2.58
100	2.23	2.36
1000	2.04	2.07
∞	1.96	1.96

Data from Walpole RE, Myers RH. Probability and Statistics for Engineers and Scientists. New York, MacMillan, 1989; and Weisbrot IM. Statistics for the Clinical Laboratory. Philadelphia, JB Lippincott, 1985.

experiment was repeated 100 times and 100 confidence intervals were calculated, 95 of those intervals would contain the true (but still unknown) population mean.

A confidence interval for the standard deviation can also be constructed. However, it is based on the chi-squared distribution, which is not symmetric like the t distribution. This means that the form of the confidence interval cannot be expressed by adding or subtracting the same factor as can the confidence interval for the mean. Rather, the confidence interval (CI) for the true population standard deviation is

$$CI = S \times k_L, S \times k_U$$

where k_L is the factor for the lower limit of the confidence interval and k_U is the factor for the upper limit from Table 62–7. For example, if the standard deviations of eight measurements is 12.7, the 95% confidence interval for the true population standard deviation is

$$CI = (12.7 \times 0.63, 12.7 \times 1.92) = (8, 24.4)$$

Error Intervals

Many studies involve the assessment of new devices or methods compared with existing standards. Also, there are many statistical concepts involved.[1] We will simplify and discuss only three cases. For example, when a new batch of blood gas analyzer control solutions is purchased, it is necessary to verify the manufacturer's specifications for the expected lower and upper limits of the measured value for the analyte. In addition, the performance of a new blood gas analyzer might be evaluated by examining measurements of control solutions with known P_{O_2} values. Another example might be comparison of P_{O_2} data from a new model of blood gas analyzer with measurements from a currently used blood gas analyzer. These are actually three different problems. In the first case, it is necessary to determine a range of values within which any given individual measurement should fall when measuring a known value, known as a *tolerance interval*. In the second case, we wish to determine the range of values for the difference between the known (assumed true) value and the actual measured values to assess the *inaccuracy* of the measurement system. In the third case, the true value is not known, so we can only assess the range of values for the difference between one measurement system and another to assess *agreement* (Fig. 62–13). In each case data on measurement error are used to construct *error intervals*.

In assessing where *individual measurements* might fall, we are interested in determining the range of values, which should include the true value with a specified degree of confidence. If the true mean and standard deviation of an infinite number of repeated measurements were known, a 2σ (i.e., a two standard deviation) tolerance interval (TI) could be expressed as:

$$TI = \mu \pm 1.96\sigma$$

This interval includes exactly 95% of the observed measurements and thus it can be said with 95% confidence that the true value lies within this range of values. In this special case, the confidence level coincides with the proportion of measurements encompassed by the tolerance interval. However, μ and σ are unknowable. Therefore, we must substitute the appropriate point estimates $\overline{X}$ and S. Because of the random error involved with estimating the population mean and standard deviation,

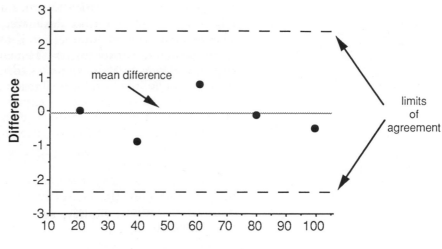

Mean Value of Pair (agreement study)
or True Value (accuracy study)

FIGURE 62–13: A plot of sample data pairs. The data pairs are either from an accuracy study (in which measured values are compared with known values) or from an agreement study (in which values from two different measurement systems are compared). For an accuracy study, the known (true) values are plotted along the horizontal axis. For an agreement study, the true values are unknown, so the mean value of each data pair is calculated as an estimate of the true value and these values are plotted along the horizontal axis.

the proportion of the population of measured values covered by the tolerance interval is not exact. As a result, the confidence level must be calculated based on the uncertainty of the point estimates of the population parameters. The *tolerance interval* (TI) is expressed as[2, 3]

$$TI = \overline{X} \pm k_1 S$$

where $\overline{X}$ is the sample mean value and S is the sample standard deviation of repeated measurements of the known quantity. The factor k_1 is determined so that one can assert with the desired confidence that the true value lies within the specified tolerance limits. The value of k_1 is selected from Table 62–7 by determining the desired confidence level and the number of observations in the data set, n. Values for k_1 are calculated to include 95% of the population of observations in the error interval.

Because of the use of point estimates for the population mean and standard deviation, the tolerance interval given by the aforementioned equation is associated with a double probability. There is one probability *that a given measurement will lie within the specified interval* for a given set of measurements (determined by the proportion of observations specified for the interval) and there is one probability (i.e., the confidence level) *that we will be correct* in assuming that a given measurement falls within the tolerance interval. In general, the smaller the sample size and the more confidence we want to have in the error estimate, the larger the interval will be.

If a measurement system was perfectly accurate (i.e., no errors), the measurement values would exactly equal the true values. In real life, of course, there are differences due to measurement errors. There are two basic types of measurement errors. One is called systemic error or bias. The other type is random error or impression. To assess the inaccuracy of a measurement system, we need estimates of these two types of errors

Bias represents a constant difference between two measurements and can be caused, for example, by improper calibration.

Random error causes differences that change unpredictably and may be due to a wide variety of environmental factors (e.g., temperature and electromagnetic variations).

from experiments in which known quantities are repeatedly measured. Bias error is estimated as the mean difference between measured and assumed true values. Imprecision is estimated as the standard deviation of the repeated measurements. Thus, inaccuracy can be expressed as the sum of the bias and impression. An *inaccuracy interval* (II) is made in a fashion similar to the tolerance interval:

$$II = \bar{d} + k_1 S$$

where $\bar{d}$ is the mean difference between measured and true values, S is the standard deviation of the differences, and k_1 is selected as described for tolerance intervals.

Assessing agreement between two measurement systems is similar to assessing accuracy, except that instead of repeatedly measuring one level of a known quantity, several levels of the known quantity are selected, and split samples are measured by both systems. For example, in assessing the agreement between old and new models of blood gas analyzers, several samples of patient blood would be split in half and analyzed through each device. The difference between the measured values from the two machines is used along with the standard deviation of the differences to make a statement about agreement. Bland and Altman[5] have suggested a statistic called the *limits of agreement,* which is the mean difference plus or minus two standard deviations. Although this is easy to calculate, it is only a point estimate. Alternatively, an *agreement interval* (AI) similar to the tolerance interval and the accuracy interval can be expressed as

$$AI = \bar{d} \pm k_1 S$$

where $\bar{d}$ is the mean difference between measured values from the two devices and S is the standard deviation of the differences. k_1 is selected as described for tolerance intervals.

Hypothesis Testing

Hypothesis testing takes many forms, but most often entails testing hypotheses about mean values from samples. The study hypothesis can be that

- A given sample comes from a population with a known mean.
- One sample mean (e.g., from a treatment group) is different from another sample mean (e.g., from a control group).
- Three or more sample means do not all come from the same population.

The first two types of hypotheses involve fairly simple *t* tests, which are reviewed further on. The third is most appropriately handled with a procedure called analysis of variance, which is beyond the scope of this chapter but can be found in most statistical textbooks.

In hypothesis testing, there are actually two hypotheses: the null hypothesis, symbolized H_0 (which states that there is no difference between mean values) and the alternate hypothesis, symbolized H_a (which states that there is a difference). The alternate hypothesis can be stated as either $\mu_1 > \mu_2$ (implying a "one-tailed test" where α is all in either the upper or lower tail of the distribution) or $\mu_1 \neq \mu_2$ (for a "two-tailed test" where α is equally divided between both tails of the distribution as seen in Figure 62–12). There are also two decisions that can be made as a result of the test: reject or not reject the null hypothesis. It follows logically that there are four possible combinations of the decision and reality, as illustrated in Figure 62–14. To simplify the discussion, let us suppose that the actual population mean is either 100 or 103. This implies that if the null hypothesis is true, distribution of values center on 100, whereas if the alternative hypothesis is true the distribution centers on 103 as shown in Figure 62–14. The decision matrix in Figure 62–14 indicates two states of reality (i.e., the null hypothesis is true or it is false) and two types of possible decisions (accept or reject the null hypothesis). There are two ways to be wrong and two ways to be right. Rejecting a true hypothesis is called a *type I error,* and the probability of this error is symbolized by the Greek letter α. Accepting a false null hypothesis is called a *type II error* and is symbolized by the Greek letter β. The probabilities of the two correct decisions are calculated from α and β as shown in Figure 62–14.

In performing a statistical test, we specify a predetermined value of α, which sets the significance level. Naturally, we would like to keep α low, but Figure 62–14 shows that as we decrease α, we increase β. One way to keep α low and also to lower β is to decrease the variability, or spread, of the two distributions. There are sampling distributions, or distributions of the statistic $\overline{X}$. The standard deviation of the $\overline{X}$ values is

Actual Case

	H_0 true ($\mu = 100$)	H_0 false ($\mu = 103$)
accept H_0	correct prob = $1 - \alpha$	Type II error prob = β
reject H_0	Type I error prob = α	correct prob = $1 - \beta$

Decision

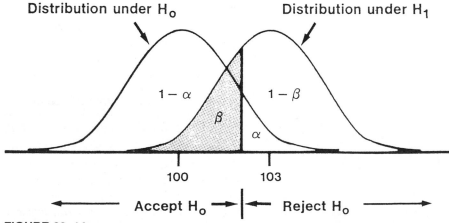

FIGURE 62–14: Illustration of the probabilities for type I and type II errors and their relationship to each other.

given by the standard error of the mean. The smaller the standard error, the less variability or spread in the distributions. Recall that the standard error is the population standard deviation divided by the square root of the sample size. Thus to decrease the standard error, decrease the spread of the distributions, and decrease the chances of making an erroneous decision during hypothesis testing, we need only increase the sample size.

Which type of error is more serious is relative to the research question. If a new drug is investigated, a definite effect, that is, a large difference, would be wanted to conclude the drug is effective. A small value for α would be desirable because we would rather accept a false null hypothesis (type II error) than reject a true null hypothesis (type I error). In other words, it is preferable to throw out a drug as ineffective when it really is effective than to foist a truly ineffective drug on the public thinking it is significant. Alpha is made small, although β increases. Alternatively, when testing for accuracy of a monitor, only a very small difference is needed before we say the difference is significant. A large α is desired so that the difference is more likely to be called significant. In this case, it is preferable to reject a true null hypothesis (type I error) than to accept a false null hypothesis (type II error). It is preferable to reject the conclusion of accuracy even though the monitor is accurate (because we already have accurate, though perhaps older, monitors) than to accept that the monitor is accurate when it is not.

With this information as background, we can now describe three basic hypothesis tests, the single-sample test and two types of two-sample tests for the difference between means. In each case, a t value will be calculated based on the statistic of interest (e.g., mean value of measurements or mean difference between pairs of measured values).

The t value will have the general form:

$$t = \frac{\text{(value of sample statistic)} - \text{(hypothesized value of population statistic)}}{\text{standard deviation of statistic}}$$

Given the t value calculated from the sample data, the associated probability or p $value$ (i.e., the probability of the sample statistic being as great as or greater than the one observed) is then obtained from a statistical table of values for the t distribution. If the p value obtained from the table is greater then the preset α level (usually set at 0.05), the null hypothesis is rejected.

A way to simplify the test and make the table easier to read is to list only the values of t (called *critical values*) that are associated with specific probabilities at common significance levels (e.g., 0.05 and 0.01). If the absolute value of the calculated t value is *larger* than the critical t value, the p value is *less* than the preselected significance level, and the null hypothesis is rejected. Table 62–8 lists critical t values.

Test with a Single Sample Mean. This test involves comparing a mean value from a single sample (e.g., the mean weight of premature babies in your hospital's nursery) with a value that represents the true (or assumed true) mean of a given population (i.e., the mean weight of all premature babies in all nurseries across the United States). The null hypothesis is that the sample was taken from the population with the given mean value (i.e., all premature babies). The alternate hypothesis is that the sample came from some other population with some other (unknown) mean value. The t value is calculated as:

$$t = \frac{\overline{X} - \mu}{S_{\overline{X}}}$$

where

$\overline{X}$ = sample mean
μ = assumed population mean if H_0 is true
$S_{\overline{X}}$ = standard deviation of the mean = $S/\sqrt{n}$
n = number of observations in sample

The *absolute value* of the calculated t value is then compared with the critical t value at the specified significance level (Table 62–8) with n − 1 degree of freedom. If the calculated value for t is larger than the critical t value in the table, the null hypothesis is rejected (the sample came from some other population); otherwise it is not rejected (the sample may have come from the specified population).

Example: Suppose you weighed a random sample of 10 premature infants in your hospital's nursery and calculated a mean weight of 1.1 kg with a standard deviation of 0.4 kg. A medical journal article has stated that the national average weight for a premature infant is 1.6 kg. Does your hospital's nursery have babies whose weight is significantly different from those in other nurseries nationwide? The null hypothesis is that your sample came from a population of babies who weigh, on average, 1.6 kg. The alternate hypothesis is that your sample mean was far enough away from 1.6 kg to indicate that it came from a different population. You accept the conventional significance level of 0.05. The calculated t value from your sample statistics is

$$t = \frac{1.1 - 1.6}{0.4/\sqrt{10}} = -3.95$$

The absolute value of −3.95 is 3.95. There are n − 1 = 9 degrees of freedom. In Table 62–8, we first look at the degrees of freedom = 9. We then look across to the critical value of t under the column for significance level = 0.05. The critical t value is 2.262. Because the calculated t value is *larger* than the critical value, you reject the null hypothesis and

TABLE **62–8:**   Critical Values for Two-Tailed t Statistic

df	Significance Level 0.05	0.01	df	Significance Level 0.05	0.01
1	12.706	63.657	18	2.101	2.878
2	4.303	9.925	19	2.093	2.861
3	3.182	5.841	20	2.086	2.845
4	2.776	4.604	21	2.080	2.831
5	2.571	4.032	22	2.074	2.819
6	2.447	3.707	23	2.069	2.807
7	2.365	3.499	24	2.064	2.797
8	2.306	2.896	25	2.060	2.787
9	2.262	3.250	26	2.056	2.779
10	2.228	3.169	27	2.052	2.771
11	2.201	3.106	28	2.048	2.763
12	2.179	3.055	29	2.045	2.756
13	2.160	3.012	30	2.042	2.750
14	2.145	2.977	40	2.021	2.704
15	2.131	2.947	60	2.000	2.660
16	2.120	2.921	120	1.980	2.617
17	2.110	2.898	∞	1.960	2.576

df, degrees of freedom.

conclude that the babies in your hospital's nursery are no different from those in other nurseries.

Test with Two Independent Sample Means. In this case, you have two *independent* samples and you wish to determine if they both come from the same population. Independent means that the specific values (or experimental subjects) in one sample have no obvious connection to those in the other sample. The null hypothesis is that both samples came from the same population. The alternate hypothesis is that the samples came from different populations. The study is designed so that the only obvious difference is the way they were treated in the experiment. Thus if the result of the test is that the samples came from different populations, you would assume that the treatment caused the difference. For example, suppose you wanted to see if the mode of ventilation has any effect on the length of stay in the intensive care unit for postoperative cardiac patients. A group of patients is selected who have the same age, diagnosis, and so on to assume they come from the same population with respect to intensive care unit stay. They would be randomly assigned to either continuous mandatory ventilation (CMV) or synchronized intermittent mandatory ventilation (SIMV). Their mean lengths of stay would be compared to see if they were different enough to warrant the conclusion that the mode of ventilation caused them to be in two different populations (i.e., that ventilatory pattern affects mean length of stay). The t value is calculated as

$$ t = \frac{\overline{X}_1 - \overline{X}_2}{S_{\overline{X}_1 - \overline{X}_2}} $$

where

$$ \overline{X}_1 = \text{mean of sample 1} $$
$$ \overline{X}_2 = \text{mean of sample 2} $$
$$ S_{\overline{X}_1 - \overline{X}_2} = \text{the estimated standard deviation of the statistic } \overline{X}_1 - \overline{X}_2 $$

$$ S_{\overline{X}_1 - \overline{X}_2} = \sqrt{\frac{(n_1 - 1)S_1^2 + (n_2 - 1)S_2^2}{n_1 + n_2 - 2}\left(\frac{1}{n_1} + \frac{1}{n_2}\right)} $$

in which

$$ n_1 = \text{number of observations in sample 1} $$
$$ n_2 = \text{number of observations in sample 2} $$
$$ S_1^2 = \text{variance of sample 1} $$
$$ S_2^2 = \text{variance of sample 2} $$

The *absolute value* of the calculated t value is then compared with the critical t value at the specified significance level (Table 62–8) with $n_1 + n_2 - 2$ degrees of freedom. If the calculated value for t is larger than the critical t value in the table, the null hypothesis is rejected (the two samples come from different populations with different means), otherwise it is not rejected (the two samples may have come from the same population).

Example: The next 24 patients who are admitted to the intensive care unit are randomly assigned to either CMV or to SIMV. The mean ($\pm$S) length of stay for the 11 CMV patients is 39.3 $\pm$ 5 hours, and for the SIMV group (13 patients) it is 31.5 $\pm$ 3 hours. It appears that the CMV group had a longer stay. Was it really different? To find out, the calculated t value is

$$t = \frac{39.3 - 31.5}{\sqrt{\dfrac{(11-1)5^2 + (13-1)3^2}{11+13-2}\left(\dfrac{1}{11}+\dfrac{1}{13}\right)}} = 4.69$$

The absolute value of 4.69 is 4.69. There are $11 + 13 - 2 = 22$ degrees of freedom. In Table 62–8, we first look at the degrees of freedom = 22. We then look across to the critical value of t under the column for significance level = 0.05. The critical t value is 2.074. Because the calculated t value is *larger* than the critical value, you reject the null hypothesis and conclude that the mode of ventilation did affect length of stay.

Test with Two Dependent Sample Means. In this case, you have two *dependent* samples and you wish to determine if they both come from the sample population. Dependent means that the specific values (or experimental subjects) in one sample are obviously connected to those in the other sample. This is the case, for example, when each experimental subject is given two different treatments and thus each acts as their own control. The null hypothesis is that both samples came from the same population. The alternate hypothesis is that the samples came from different populations. The study is designed so that the only obvious difference is the way subjects were treated in the experiment. Thus if the result of the test is that the samples came from different populations, you would assume that the treatment caused the difference. For example, suppose you wanted to see if body position has any effect on oxygen saturation for patients with chronic obstructive pulmonary disease. A group of patients is selected with the same age, diagnosis, and so forth so that it can be assumed they come from the same population with respect to oxygen saturation. They are randomly assigned to either a sitting or prone position and their saturation is measured in each position by pulse oximeter. The mean saturation for the sitting position is compared with the mean saturation for the prone position to see if they were different enough to warrant the conclusion that the body position caused saturations to be in two different populations (i.e., that position affects mean saturation). The t value is calculated as

$$t = \frac{\bar{d}}{S_{\bar{d}}}$$

where

d = the difference between pairs of observations (i.e., one from each group)
$\bar{d}$ = mean difference
$S_{\bar{d}}$ = standard deviation of the mean difference = $S_d/\sqrt{n}$
n = number of paired observations
S_d = standard deviation of the differences

The *absolute value* of the calculated t value is then compared with the critical t value at the specified significance level (Table 62–8) with $n_1 - 1$ degrees of freedom. If the calculated value for t is larger than the critical t value in the table, the null hypothesis is rejected (the two samples come from different populations with different means); otherwise it is not rejected (the two samples may have come from the same population).

Example: Fifteen patients with chronic obstructive pulmonary disease are selected for the study. Each patient's saturation is measured once while sitting and then once while prone, with the order varied randomly. There are 30 measurements in all. The difference between the sitting and the prone measurements for each patient is calculated, resulting in 15 differences. The mean of these 15 numbers is 4 and the standard deviation is 8. The *t* value is

$$t = \frac{4}{8/\sqrt{15}} = 1.94$$

The absolute value of 1.94 is 1.94. There are $15 - 1 = 14$ degrees of freedom. In Table 62–8, we first look at the degrees of freedom $= 14$. We then look across to the critical value of *t* under the column for significance level $= 0.05$. The critical *t* value is 2.145. Because the calculated *t* value is *smaller* than the critical value, you accept the null hypothesis and conclude that the position did not affect saturation.

Determining Sample Size and Power

For each hypothesis test, care was taken to keep α, the probability of a type I error, low. As discussed earlier, the lower α becomes, the higher β becomes. Typically, novice researchers pay no attention to β so when the results of a test suggest not to reject the null hypothesis, the conclusion of no difference is blindly accepted even though the probability of making a type II error is quite high. Therefore, it is desirable to keep β low along with α. In other words, if the results of the test are "negative," we want to be reasonably sure that if the null hypothesis is really false we would have rejected it. From Figure 62–14, it can be seen that the probability of correctly rejecting the null hypothesis is one minus β, which is called the *power* of the test.

The power of the test, at any given significance level, is directly proportional to both the sample size and the treatment effect (i.e., the difference between two mean values). An intuitive understanding of this is gained by looking at Table 62–8. For a given treatment effect (i.e., the difference between two mean values), the smaller the sample size the larger the critical value of *t* becomes. This means that one is more likely to conclude no difference for small versus large sample sizes. In fact, a given treatment effect that results in a conclusion of no difference can be changed to a conclusion of a significant difference just by increasing the sample size.

The power of a test can be determined after the experiment is concluded, but it will be unfortunate if it turns out that the results are negative and the test has little power because the sample size was picked arbitrarily and was too small. The experimental results then have little value or can even be misleading. For instance, in the preceding example in which it was concluded that body position had no effect on saturation, the power is less than 0.2. Thus, if there was a difference in saturation, there would have been less than a 20% chance to detect it with a sample size of only 15. Clearly, it is much better to determine beforehand how large the sample size should be to obtain the desired power at the desired significance level. The nomogram in Figure 62–15 is designed to facilitate this choice. To estimate the required sample size, the size of the treatment effect must first be postulated by deciding how large a difference in the measured variable would be clinically significant. There must also be some estimate of the variability (i.e., standard deviation) of the measured

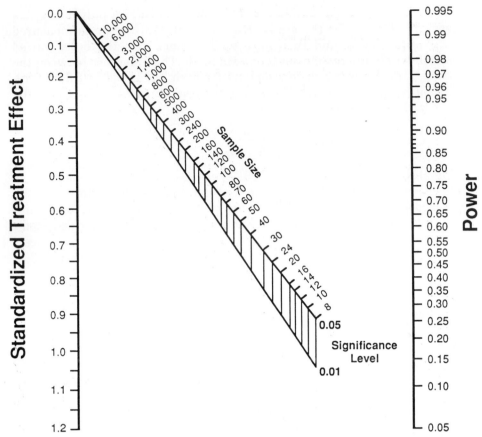

FIGURE 62–15: Nomogram showing relations among standardized effect size, sample size, and statistical power. Treatment effect size is standardized by dividing the postulated difference due to treatment by the estimated population standard deviation. (Adapted from Altmand DG. Statistics and ethics in medical research. III. How large a sample? Br J Med 281:1336–1338, 1980.)

outcome variable. To avoid the problem of different measurement units, the effect size is standardized as follows:

$$\text{standardized effect size} = \frac{\text{postulated difference}}{\text{estimated sample standard deviation}}$$

On the nomogram, a straight line connecting the standardized effect size with the desired power will run through the sample size required at the desired significance level. For example, suppose we wish to evaluate the effect of a new type of chest physiotherapy on the amount of sputum produced during a treatment. From previous experience (e.g., a small pilot study) with patients with cystic fibrosis, we expect that the weight of sputum produced during routine chest physiotherapy will be about 20 ± 7 g. We decide that an average difference (either increase or decrease) of about 5 g would indicate a significant treatment effect. The standardized effect size is 5/7 = 0.7. From Figure 62–15 we see that to get a power of 0.8, we will need to include about 65 patients in our study. Notice that if we settle for a lower power or expect a larger effect size, we can use a smaller sample.

SUMMARY: COMMUNICATING THE RESEARCH RESULTS

Any research project that is important enough to require careful thought in design and sustained effort in data gathering, merits a writ-

TABLE **62–9:**   Review Questions for a Research Manuscript

I. Introduction
   A. Is the topic clearly identified?
   B. Is the reason for performing the study given?
   C. Is the research question clearly stated?
   D. Are the background information and references adequate to introduce the study question?
   E. Is the study hypothesis stated? (This does not apply to a descriptive study.)
   F. Is the writing clear?
II. Methods
   A. Are the study design and execution described in enough detail so that a reader could duplicate the study?
   B. If applicable, were theoretical assumptions reasonable?
   C. Was the study design appropriate for answering the study question-hypothesis?
   D. If appropriate, is there information regarding calibration of measurement systems?
   E. Were appropriate statistical tests chosen and identified in this section?
   F. If illustrations are appropriate, are they provided and are they adequate?
III. Results
   A. Does this section provide both a general description of the results and specific representative data?
   B. Are all the findings you would expect from the study question and design presented here?
   C. Are results of statistical analysis presented?
   D. Are the data meaningful?
   E. Do the findings answer the study question?
   F. Are appropriate tables or figures, or both, presented?
   G. The results should not repeat any of the description of the method section. Has the author followed this rule?
IV. Discussion
   A. Does the discussion present the principles, relationships, and generalizations shown by the results?
   B. If appropriate, does this section point out any exceptions to the findings or any unsettled points?
   C. If appropriate, does this section discuss any limitations of the study?
   D. If appropriate, does this section show how the study findings agree or contrast with previously published reports?
   E. If appropriate, does this section discuss the theoretical implications of the findings?
   F. Are references cited thoroughly and properly?
   G. Is all of the discussion relevant?
V. Miscellaneous
   A. Are the mathematical calculations in this paper correct?
   B. Are the figure legends adequate?
   C. Are the table titles adequate?
   D. Are references accurate (e.g., dates and page numbers)?
   E. Is medical terminology used correctly?
   F. Does the paper's title accurately reflect its content?
   G. Is the abstract informative—briefly outlining the *methods* and giving *specific results* and *conclusions*?

Someone once said that to become familiar with a subject, one should teach it; to understand a subject, one should write about it; but to master a subject, one must read what one has written.

ten report at its conclusion. Such a report serves at least two purposes. First, it forces the researcher to review the entire thought process involved, from the initial recognition of a clinical problem through the formation of a conceptual model relating the pertinent variables to the comparison of this model with reality using actual measurements. Any flaws or ambiguities in this train of thought becomes evident once the events are recreated in a written report. A research report is a teaching instrument in the sense that it provides a concise view of the background and current perspective on a specific topic. A second, more obvious function of a research report is to expand the scientific community's knowledge base. If the report is published, it will become an immortal piece of the ever-changing puzzle we call scientific knowledge.

Publication of an article in a scientific journal can also result in personal benefits for the author. It is a measure of professional success, which may contribute to tenure, status, lecture tours, and consulting jobs.

There are two major types of written reports—abstracts and papers. Both types have the same general format: title, introduction, methods, results, and discussion. However, the abstract, which is much more condensed, is usually limited to one double-spaced page. Abstracts in most medical journals are often not reviewed by peers, whereas papers are usually sent to at least two expert reviewers. Each medical journal has its own requirements regarding the format of submitted material. The requirements of the journal *Respiratory Care* for both abstracts and papers follow:

When submitting material for possible publication in a medical journal, there are several things to keep in mind. First, the written material will be subjected to critical review, which may be a new experience for you. Make sure that you follow the instructions to authors found in the journal in which you intend to submit the article. Be familiar with the style of writing in that journal and make sure that your paper will be of interest to the people who read that journal. *Always* make an outline *before* you begin to write and be prepared to change both the outline and the paper as it progresses. Any good paper, or even an abstract, is usually rewritten at least three, and as many as a dozen, times before it is ready. Always try to get someone with experience to be your mentor. Research requires on-the-job training.

Try not to let your ego get in the way of learning when you read the reviewer's comments. If you are lucky, the comments will help you rewrite some sections of the paper or collect more pertinent data. Occasionally, reviewers' comments are unsupported, misguided, and even malicious. It is the responsibility of the journal editor to help "smooth the waters" in these situations.

Finally, make sure that you critically review the manuscript yourself, as if you were a reviewer, to maximize your chance of acceptance. Table 62–9 shows a list of items that reviewers for *Respiratory Care* consider when reviewing your manuscript. Remember, unless your manuscript is rejected as being totally without merit (a rare occurrence), make any sensible revisions suggested by the reviewers and resubmit it. Most individuals get discouraged and will not "go the extra mile," but it is worth it a hundred times over when you see your name in print.

References

1. Chatburn RL. Fundamentals of Metrology: Evaluation of instrument error and method agreement. Respir Care 35:520–545, 1990.
2. Hofmann D. Measurement errors, probability and information theory. *In* Sydenham PH (Ed). Handbook of Measurement Science, vol 1. Theoretical Fundamentals. New York, John Wiley & Sons, 1982, pp 241–275.
3. Walpole RE, Myers RH. Probability and Statistics for Engineers and Scientists. New York, Macmillan, 1989, pp 264–266, 242–244, 638–639.
4. Weisbrot IM. Statistics for the Clinical Laboratory. Philadelphia, JB Lippincott, 1985, p 179.
5. Bland JM, Altman DG. Statistical methods for assessing agreement between two methods of clinical measurement. Lancet 1:307–310, 1986.
6. Altmand DG. Statistics and ethics in medical research. III. How large a sample? Br J Med 281:1336–1338, 1980.

Suggested Reading

Beveridge WIB. The Art of Scientific Investigation. New York, Vantage, 1953.
Bland M. An Introduction to Medical Statistics. New York, Oxford University Press, 1987.

Chatburn RL, Craig KC. Fundamentals of Respiratory Care Research. Norwalk, Appleton & Lange, 1988. (Out of print from original publisher but available from Daedalus Enterprises, PO Box 29686, Dallas, TX, 75229-9998.)

Cleveland WS. The Elements of Graphing Data. Monterey, CA, Wadsworth Advanced Books and Software, 1985.

Kanare HM. Writing the Laboratory Notebook. Washington, DC, American Chemical Society, 1985.

Katz MJ. Elements of the Scientific Paper. A Step by Step Guide for Students and Professionals. New Haven, Yale University Press, 1985.

Lanham RA. Revising Prose, 2nd ed. New York, Macmillan, 1987.

Marks RG. Analyzing Research Data. Belmont, CA, Lifetime Learning Publications, 1982.

Marks RG. Designing a Research Project. Belmont, CA, Lifetime Learning Publications, 1982.

Rubin SA. The Principles of Biomedical Instrumentation. A Beginner's Guide. Chicago, Mosby-Year Book, 1987.

Webster JG. Medical Instrumentation. Application and Design, 2nd ed. Boston, Houghton Mifflin, 1992.

Wilson, EB Jr. An Introduction to Scientific Research. New York, Dover, 1990.

Index

Note: Page numbers in *italics* refer to illustrations; page numbers followed by t refer to tables.

A

A line, 364
A waves, on cardiac inspection, 184
Abdomen, distention of, 747–750
 ascites and, 749–750
 causes of, 747–748
 intestinal, 748–749
 in abnormal breathing patterns, 43, *45*
 injured, delayed surgical closure of, 646
  diagnostic imaging in, 637–638, *638*
  early management of, 646
 muscles of, in ventilatory control system, 35–36, 124, 178
 surgery of, 646, 675
Abdominal pain, acute, 743–745, 756
 causes of, 744t
 cholecystitis and, 756
 extra-abdominal conditions simulating, 744t
 laboratory diagnostic data on, 745t
 pancreatitis and, 758
 peptic ulcer and, 755
Accelerated idioventricular rhythm, 307
Accelerated junctional rhythm, 309
Acetaminophen, overdose with, 779
Acetazolamide, for sleep apnea, 817
Acetylcholine, antimuscarinic agents and, 979–981
 in myasthenic syndrome, 889
 receptors for, in myasthenia gravis, 888
 release of, 16
Acetylcysteine, action and uses of, 991–992
Acid(s), acute renal failure and, 619
 in gastric contents, adult respiratory distress syndrome and, 835, 836
  aspiration pneumonia and, 660, 835, 837
 volatile and fixed, 70
Acid phosphatase, 352
Acid-base balance, alignment nomogram for, 378, *379*
 disorders of, compensatory responses to, 72, 73t
 types of, 72
 in vitro analyzers for, 369t
 physiology of, 70–72
Acidosis, definition of, 72
 dyspnea and, 57

Acidosis *(Continued)*
 hyperchloremic, 76–77
 in hypokalemia, 87t
 lactic, 74–75
 metabolic, 73–77
  anion gap, 74–76, 347
   normal (hyperchloremic), 76–77
  classification of, 74, 74t
  definition of, 73
  in cardiopulmonary resuscitation, 413
   sodium bicarbonate for, 416–417
  ischemic or hypoxic origin of, 416
  mechanisms of, 73, 771t
  near-drowning and, 843
  peripheral chemoreceptor responses to, 122
  methanol or ethylene glycol poisoning and, 70
  pulmonary vasoconstriction and, 870–871
  renal tubular, proximal and distal, 76–77
 respiratory, causes of, 79t, 79–81
  chronic obstructive pulmonary disease and, 508
  respiratory pattern changes and, 177
  salicylate overdose and, 75
  uremic, causes and management of, 75
Acinus, 12
Acquired immunodeficiency syndrome (AIDS), 340. See also *Human immunodeficiency virus (HIV)*.
 glucocorticoids for, 985–986
 legal aspects of, 1188–1189
 opportunistic infections with, 340–341
 pneumonia with, 830–831
 trimethoprim-sulfamethoxazole for, 998
 zidovudine for, 999
Acrocyanosis, tissue perfusion and, 214
Actinomycosis, pleural effusion and, 918–919
Action potential, of cardiac muscle cell, 278, *278–279*, 280
Activated partial thromboplastin time, 344
Acute chest syndrome, 801
Acute renal failure. See *Renal failure, acute.*
Acute tubular necrosis, intrinsic renal failure and, 616

Acute tubular necrosis *(Continued)*
 recovery from, 627
Adenosine, blood flow regulation and, 160
Adenosine triphosphate, evolutionary development of, 3
 hydrolysis of, formula for, 158
 metabolism of, anaerobic, 158
  magnesium and, 92
  tissue oxygenation and, 170
 muscle contractility and, 37
 oxidative phosphorylation and, 157–158
Adenovirus, pneumonia due to, 820, 822
Adenylate kinase, cerebrospinal fluid, 268
Adrenergic agonists other than epinephrine, in cardiopulmonary resuscitation, 417
Adrenergic nerves, blood flow and, 160
Adult respiratory distress syndrome, 731–733
 barotrauma and, 194, 666–667
 conditions associated with, 732t
 diagnosis of, 731–732, 732t
 gastric acid aspiration and, 835, 836
 hyaline membrane formation in, 664–666, 667
 incidence of, 731
 pathophysiology of, 731
 PEEP and, 22, *23*, 667–669
 pulmonary edema and, 194
 signs of, 194
 treatment of, 669, 732–733
Adults, learning by, characteristics of, 1204
 methods of, 1203–1205
 types of, 1201–1203
Advance care document, 1164
Advance directories, 1163–1165
Advanced life support, 632
Adventitial sounds, 181, *183*
Aerobic capacity, in exercise stress test, 933, *933*
Aerobic metabolism, oxygen supply and oxygen transport levels in, 164–166
Aeromedical transport, 632–633
Aerosol delivery, of oxygen therapy, 513–514, 1097–1098
Aerosol therapy, 539–560
 antibiotic, 485, 995, 996t

ISBN 0-7216-2844-3

9 780721 628448